MELLONI'S
ILLUSTRATED

MEDICAL
DICTIONARY

Ida Dox

Technical Lexicographer
Medical Communicator
Georgetown University Schools
of Medicine and Dentistry

Biagio John Melloni, Ph.D. (candidate)

Professorial Lecturer in Anatomy
Chairman, Department of Medical-Dental Communication
Georgetown University Schools
of Medicine and Dentistry
Medical Art Editor
American Family Physician

Gilbert M. Eisner, M.D., F.A.C.P.

Adjunct Associate Professor of
Physiology and Biophysics
Georgetown University School
of Medicine

Clinical Associate Professor of Medicine
Georgetown University Hospital

Senior Attending Physician
Washington Hospital Center

MELLONI'S
ILLUSTRATED
MEDICAL
DICTIONARY

THE WILLIAMS & WILKINS COMPANY
Baltimore

Made in the United States of America

Library of Congress Cataloging in Publication Data

Dox, Ida.
   Melloni's illustrated medical dictionary.

   1. Medicine—Dictionaries. I. Melloni, Biagio John, joint author. II. Eisner, Gilbert M., joint author. III. Title.
R121.D76   1978   610'.3   77-2952
ISBN 0-683-02642-9

Composed and printed at the
Waverly Press, Inc.
Mt. Royal and Guilford Aves.
Baltimore, Md. 21202, U.S.A.

PREFACE

The rapid expansion and accumulation of knowledge required in the health sciences, coupled with a decrease in the time available to acquire this knowledge, has created the need for a new dictionary of health-science terminology that helps the reader to quickly and easily assimilate this terminology. The current choice of dictionaries is between the comprehensive volumes that require an in-depth professional and scientific background, or abridged versions of such volumes, and the glossary type that are limited in scope to a particular discipline. *Melloni's Illustrated Medical Dictionary* provides another choice.

This new dictionary is a compilation of approximately 25,000 terms that comprise the common core of information for all of the health sciences, as well as a large number of terms most frequently used in the distinctive language of particular subspecialties, and was developed especially for students of the health sciences. It is anticipated that it will also be useful as a reference book for the general public interested in a brief and "to the point" explanation of medical terms.

A number of departures from the formats of other dictionaries have been utilized to present a wide range of information in a concise manner. In one particular aspect it is unique: it is the first dictionary of its size and scope to incorporate approximately 2,500 illustrations as visual components of the textual definitions of its terms.

The illustrations were expressly designed to be simple and specific for enhanced initial visual impact, with enhanced understanding of the meaning of the definitions and improved retention of their content. Each illustration is integrated with a specific term and its definition for the dual purpose of further elucidating the term while at the same time precluding the need for a lengthier definition by visually "completing" it. This integration of illustration and text is intensified by judicious use of color to identify, highlight, and correlate each illustration with the respective term and its definition.

To facilitate location of a desired term the first and last terms of those alphabetized on a page are printed in color at the outside of the bottom margin of each page. Each term on the page is printed in a type that is larger and bolder than that used for its definition. When a term has more than one definition, each is clearly distinguished by a number.

Main entry and subentry formating of major anatomic terminology groupings, such as arteries, bones, muscles, nerves, and veins, has been replaced by illustrated tables alphabetized within the text. Terms comprising certain arbitrary groupings, such as diseases, syndromes, signs, symptoms, acids, etc., have been individually alphabetized as main entries. Tables of measurements, conversions, dosages, etc. are graphically presented on the pages where the subject terms of the respective calculations are located.

The most important and commonly used chemical compounds and drugs have been included as defined entries. Some of the more widely used brand names are cited at the end of the definitions, but are not included as defined entries.

Synonyms of defined terms are cited in the definitions and are also included as cross reference entries to the defined terms. The more frequently used synonym is located at the beginning of a definition; others are located at the end of a definition.

The terms included in this dictionary were selected with the intended audience in mind. Arbitrary inclusions and exclusions were avoided through an extensive review of the current professional literature and by constant consultation with health science specialists. To reflect contemporary developments, terms that were only recently introduced but are gaining wide acceptance have been included. A limited number of obsolete terms were retained for historical perspective. A substantial number of colloquialisms were also included, and by liberal use of cross references are closely interrelated with their professional equivalents.

Special attention has been given to the vocabulary used in the definitions. The definitions are simply, clearly, and concisely worded and usually do not begin with a broad conceptual statement. Whenever possible, the use of words that would require additional reference has been avoided. When the understanding of one entry is complemented by that of another, appropriate cross references provide the necessary correlation.

If this dictionary enables the reader to grasp clearly the meaning of terms of the health-science vocabulary in the least possible time, through words and pictures, it will have realized its purpose.

ACKNOWLEDGEMENTS

Although dozens of our colleagues at various institutions have generously contributed of their time and expertise in helping to shape the definitions in this dictionary, we are particularly indebted to Dr. Rona Eisner, Dr. Joseph Bellanti, Dr. Melvin Blecher, Dr. Mortimer Lorber, and Dr. Jacques Quen.

A book of this nature could not have been brought to completion without the more than usual cooperation of the publisher. We are especially grateful to Mr. Dick M. Hoover for his encouragement and support from the earliest planning stages of the book, and to Mr. William R. Hensyl, Dictionary Managing Editor, for his editing of the manuscript. We are also grateful to Mr. Robert C. Och, Mr. Wayne J. Hubbel, Mrs. Joanne Janowiak, Mr. Norman W. Och, and Ms. Anne G. Stewart. For their respective editorial and production expertise, we thank them.

HOW TO USE THIS DICTIONARY

Each illustration is integrated with a specific term and its definition on that page. Brown correlates the respective illustration (or any of its parts) with the appropriate entry in the text below

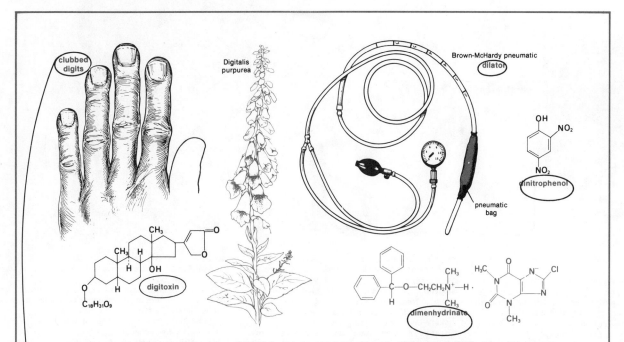

clubbed digits

Digitalis purpurea

Brown-McHardy pneumatic dilator

pneumatic bag

digitoxin

$C_{18}H_{31}O_9$

dinitrophenol

dimenhydrinate

magnetic waves); e.g., the tendency of light rays to bend in the direction of an obstacle.

diffuse'. 1. Spread out; not circumscribed, localized, or limited. **2.** To move by diffusion.

diffu'sion. 1. The process of uniformly spreading out or scattering; the passage of the molecules of one substance between the molecules of another to form a mixture of the two substances. **2.** Dialysis.

digas'tric. Having two bellies, as the digastric muscle.

Dige'nea. A subclass of flatworms or flukes (class Trematoda); parasitic in man and other mammals.

diGeorge's syndrome. Congenital thymic aplasia; see under aplasia.

digest'. 1. To break up food into simpler, assimilable compounds by the muscular and chemical action of the digestive tract. **2.** To absorb mentally.

diges'tant. An agent that aids the process of digestion.

diges'tion. The process taking place in the alimentary canal whereby the nutritive components of food are converted into substances that can be absorbed by the intestine; the decomposition of materials into simpler compounds.

diges'tive. Relating to digestion.

dig'it. A finger or toe.

    clubbed d.'s, a bulbous enlargement of the fingertips, seen in some cases of heart disease and certain pulmonary disorders; also called drumstick or clubbed fingers.

dig'ital. 1. Pertaining to, performed by, or resembling a digit or digits, especially a finger. **2.** Possessing digits.

digital'is. 1. Foxglove, a plant of the genus *Digitalis.* **2.** Digitalis (USP), a drug obtained from the dried leaves of *Digitalis purpurea,* used in the treatment of heart disease, especially for congestive heart failure and some supraventricular tachyarrhythmias.

digitaliza'tion. The treatment of an individual with digitalis or a related cardiac glycoside, to achieve a desired therapeutic effect.

dig'itate. Having fingerlike processes.

digita'tion. A finger-like process.

digitox'in. A glycoside obtained from *Digitalis purpurea;* used in the treatment of congestive heart failure.

dig'itus, *pl.* **dig'iti.** Latin for finger.

digox'in. A glycoside obtained from the leaves of *Digitalis lanata;* used in the treatment of congestive heart failure.

DiGuglielmo's syndrome. Erythremic myelosis; see under myelosis.

dihy'drate. A compound having two molecules of water.

dihydro-. Combining form denoting the addition of two hydrogen atoms.

dihydroergot'amine (D.H.E. 45). A crystalline compound produced by the hydrogenation of ergotamine; used in the treatment of migraine headache.

dihydrostreptomy'cin. Compound made by the hydrogenation of streptomycin and having antibiotic properties.

dihydrotachys'terol (AT 10). A synthetic sterol that produces effects similar to those of vitamin D.

diiodoty'rosine (T₂, DIT). A precursor of the thyroid hormone thyroxin; also called iodogorgoic acid.

dil. Abbreviation for dilute or diluted.

dilata'tion. 1. The condition of being enlarged, occurring normally, artificially, or as a result of disease; said of a tubular structure, a cavity, or an opening. **2.** Dilation (1).

    gastric d., acute distention of the stomach with fluid and air; commonly seen following surgery or trauma.

dila'tion. 1. The act of stretching or dilating. **2.** Dilatation (1).

di'lator. Instrument for enlarging a passage or cavity.

dil'do, dil'doe. An object having the approximate size and shape of an erect penis; used to produce sexual pleasure by vaginal insertion.

dil'uent. A substance which reduces the concentration of a solution.

dilu'tion. 1. The process of reducing the concentration of a solution or substance. **2.** A weakened solution or substance; an attenuated mixture.

dimenhy'drinate. Drug used in preventing and treating motion sickness; Dramamine®.

dimen'sion. Any measurable distance.

    vertical d., in prosthodontics, the distance between two points on the face, one above and one below the mouth, usually in the midline; it may be measured when the opposing occlusal surfaces are in maximum contact (occlusal vertical dimension) or in rest position, when the jaws are not in contact (rest vertical dimension).

di'mer. A chemical compound composed of molecules that consist of two identical simpler molecules.

dimercap'rol. (BAL). A compound used as an antidote for lewisite and other arsenic poisoning; also called British antilewisite.

dimeth'yl sulfox'ide (DMSO). An industrial solvent occasionally used in medicine as a skin penetrant to facilitate absorption of medications from the skin; also called methyl sulfoxide.

dimor'phism. The property of occurring in two forms.

dinitrophe'nol (DNP). A drug which causes an increase in rate of metabolism by interruption of the coupling of oxidation and phosphorylation; not used clinically because of its toxicity.

dinu'cleotide. One of the compounds into which nucleic acid splits on hydrolysis; it may split into two mononucleotides.

diop'ter. The unit used to designate the refractive power of a lens or an optical system.

dioptom'eter. An instrument for measuring refraction and accommodation of the eye; also called dioptrometer.

diop'tric. 1. Relating to the unit of refractive power of lenses. **2.** Refractive.

diop'trics. The science of the refraction of light.

dioptrom'eter. See dioptometer.

diot'ic. In audiology, denoting an arrangement in which each ear receives the same signal.

diox'ide. An oxide containing two atoms of oxygen per molecule.

dipep'tidase. One of the protein-splitting enzymes that causes the breakdown of a dipeptide into its two constituent amino acids.

dipep'tide. Two amino acids linked by a peptide bond.

diphenhy'dramine hydrochlo'ride. An antihistamine used in the prevention and treatment of motion sickness, postoperative nausea, nausea and vomiting of pregnancy, and some allergies; Benadryl®.

diphenylhydan'toin. An anticonvulsant agent, used primarily to treat epilepsy; Dilantin®.

diphos'phonates. Synthetic substances similar to the pyrophosphates in structure but not biologically hydrolyzed; in vitro they prevent hydroxyapatite crystal formation; it has been suggested that they coat the bone surface and prevent bone resorption.

diphosphopyr'idine nu'cleotide (DPN). Old term for nicotinamide adenine dinucleotide (NAD).

diphthe'ria. An acute contagious disease caused by a bacillus, *Corynebacterium diphtheriae;* marked by inflammation of the upper respiratory tract, fibrin formation (false membrane) of the mucous membranes, and elaboration of soluble exotoxin which acts on the heart and cranial or peripheral nerve cells.

diph'theroid. 1. Resembling diphtheria. **2.** A bacterium resembling the organism that causes diphtheria.

diphyllobothri'asis. Infestation with *Diphyllobothrium latum* (broadfish tapeworm), caused by ingestion of inadequately cooked, infected fish.

Diphylloboth'rium. A genus of tapeworms (family Diphyllobothriidae); formerly called *Dibothriocephalus.*

129

synonym of defined term

synonym cross reference to defined term

boldface numbers distinguish multiple definitions

diffuse | Diphyllobothrium

abbreviation or symbol for defined term

first and last entry on the page to facilitate location of the desired term

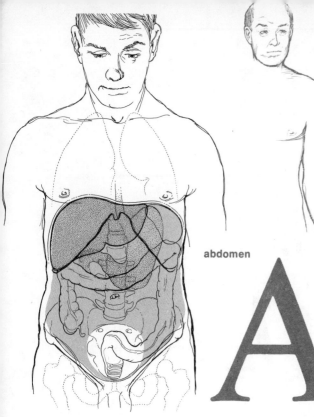

abduction

abdomen

abortion
(threatened)

Aa

α. Alpha. For terms beginning with α, see under specific term.

A. Symbol for (a) mass number; (b) type of human blood; (c) Argon.

a. Abbreviation for (a) accommodation; (b) anode; (c) area; (d) artery; (e) type of human blood.

Å. Symbol for Angstrom unit.

°A. Symbol for degree absolute.

a-, an-. Prefix denoting without, lacking, or away from.

ab-. Prefix denoting from, off, away from.

Ab. Abbreviation for antibody.

abaissemen't. French for a lowering or depression.

abarogno'sis. Loss of sense of weight estimation.

abarthro'sis. See diarthrosis.

abartic'ular. Not affecting, or far from, a joint.

abarticula'tion. 1. Dislocation. **2.** Diarthrosis.

aba'sia. Inability to walk due to impaired motor coordination.

aba'sic. Related to or afflicted with abasia.

abax'ial, abax'ile. Not located on the axis of the body or any structure.

ab'domen. Area of the body between the thorax and pelvis containing the viscera; belly (1).

  acute a., an incapacitating condition characterized by intense abdominal pain, which may or may not be associated with fever, nausea, vomiting, and shock.

abdom'inal. Pertaining to the abdomen.

abdominal'gia. Pain in the abdomen.

  periodic a., familial Mediterranean fever (1); benign paroxysmal peritonitis; disorder of unknown cause, marked by abdominal pain recurring at regular intervals and accompanied by fever, inflamed peritoneum, and sometimes purpura.

abdom'ino-. A combining form denoting association with the abdomen in any way.

abdominocente'sis. Puncturing of the abdominal wall for drainage purposes.

abdominoposte'rior. Denoting position of the fetus in the uterus in which its abdomen is turned toward the mother's back.

abdominos'copy. Examination of the abdomen, especially visual examination of the abdominal organs.

abdominothoracic. Relating to the abdomen and thorax.

abdominovag'inal. Relating to the abdomen and the vagina.

abdominoves'ical. Relating to the abdomen and urinary bladder.

abdu'cens. 1. Denoting the sixth cranial nerve. **2.** Term used with the names of muscles or

nerves that abduct a part.

abdu'cent. Denoting structures that serve to abduct a part.

abduct'. To draw away from the median line of the body or from an adjacent part or limb.

abduc'tion. Movement of a part away from the middle line; act of turning outward.

abduc'tor. A structure, such as a muscle, that draws a part away from an axis of the body; opposite of adductor.

abembryon'ic. Located away from the embryo.

aber'rant. Deviating from the normal or expected course, as a duct taking an unusual direction.

aberra'tion. 1. A deviation from the normal. **2.** Unequal refraction of light rays passing through a lens, resulting in the formation of an imperfect image.

ab'ient. Having the tendency to avoid, or move away from, a stimulus.

abiogen'esis. The origin of living matter from nonliving matter; a theory of spontaneous generation.

abiogenet'ic. Of or relating to spontaneous generation.

abiol'ogy. The study of nonliving or inorganic things.

abio'sis. Lifelessness.

abiot'rophy. General term denoting degenerative changes of tissues due to genetic causes.

abir'ritant. 1. Relieving irritation. **2.** A substance having this property.

ablate'. To remove.

abla'tio. 1. Detachment. **2.** Removal.

  a. placentae, abruptio placentae; see under abruptio.

abla'tion. 1. Detachment. **2.** Surgical removal or amputation.

alepha'ria, ableph'aron. Congenital absence of the eyelids, partial or total.

ableph'arous. Without eyelids.

ablep'sia, ablep'sy. Blindness.

ab'luent. A substance that has cleansing properties.

ablu'tion. The act of cleansing.

ablutoma'nia. Abnormal concern with cleanliness.

abneu'ral. Away from the central nervous system or from the dorsal aspect.

abnor'mal. Not normal; departing from the usual position, structure, or condition.

abnormal'ity. The condition or state of being abnormal.

ABO blood group. ABO factors; the international (Landsteiner) classification of human blood types according to their compatibility in transfusion;

typed as A, B, AB, or O.

ab'oclusion. Absence of contact between two or more opposing teeth.

abo'ral. Distant from or opposite to the mouth.

abort'. 1. To terminate pregnancy before the fetus is viable. **2.** To arrest the usual course of a disease. **3.** To cease growth or development; to cause to remain rudimentary.

abor'tient. 1. Aborting. **2.** An abortifacient; a drug that produces abortion.

abortifa'cient. Anything that produces abortion.

abortigen'ic. Abortifacient.

abor'tion. 1. Interruption of pregnancy before the fetus has attained a stage of viability, usually before 28 weeks of gestation; characteristic symptoms are vaginal bleeding and expulsive uterine contractions. **2.** The arrest of a disease or natural process before completion.

  accidental a., abortion due to an injury.

  complete a., elimination of the entire contents of the uterus (fetus, placenta, and membranes).

  elective a., induced abortion without specific medical indication.

  habitual a., see recurrent abortion.

  incomplete a., expulsion of the fetus while all or part of the placenta remains in the uterus.

  induced a., intentionally caused abortion.

  inevitable a., condition characterized by severe vaginal bleeding and uterine contractions, accompanied by cervical dilatation that has advanced beyond any hope of preventing the expulsion of the uterine contents.

  missed a., one in which the fetus dies and is retained in utero for two months or longer.

  recurrent a., loss of three or more successive pregnancies; also called habitual abortion.

  septic a., abortion in which the embryo and maternal genital tract are infected.

  spontaneous a., the termination of a previable conception without apparent cause.

  therapeutic a., instrumental termination of a pregnancy for medical or psychiatric reasons.

  threatened a., slight vaginal bleeding with or without feeble uterine contractions, in the absence of cervical dilatation.

abor'tive. 1. Causing abortion. **2.** Cutting short, arresting; said of a disease. **3.** Failing to reach completion; partially developed.

abou'lia. See abulia.

abra'chia. Absence of arms.

abrade'. To rub or wear away the external layer by friction, as to scrape away the epidermis from a part; to excoriate.

abra'sion. 1. A superficial injury, in which the skin or mucous membrane is scraped away. **2.** The

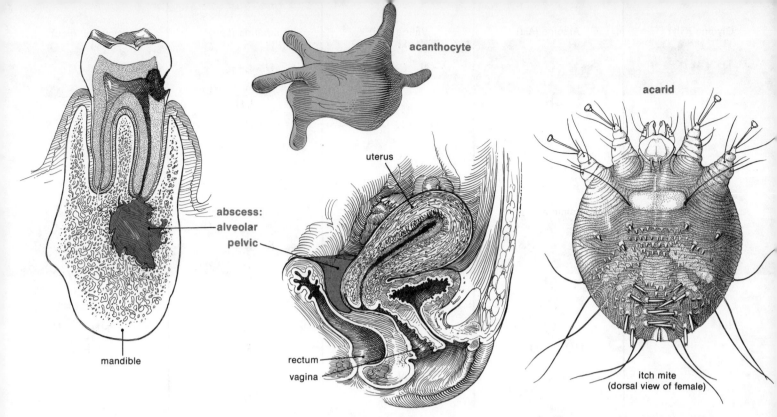

acanthocyte

abscess:
alveolar
pelvic

mandible

uterus

rectum

vagina

acarid

itch mite
(dorsal view of female)

process of wearing down of a tooth by friction; usually applied to excessive wear such as that caused by the use of an abrasive dentifrice.

abra'sive. 1. Producing abrasion. **2.** A material used in dentistry for grinding or polishing.

abreac'tion. A form of psychotherapy, called catharsis by Freud, in which emotional release is attained by recalling a forgotten (repressed), painful experience.

abrup'tio. A tearing off.

 a. placentae, premature separation of the normally implanted placenta from its uterine attachment after the twentieth week of gestation; also called placental abruption and ablatio placentae.

abruption, placental. Abruptio placentae; see under abruptio.

ab'scess. Localized accumulation of pus.

 acute a., one of short duration, producing a throbbing pain and fever; also called hot abscess.

 alveolar a., a collection of pus in the tooth socket, resulting from dental caries; it causes a constant, severe, throbbing pain and swelling.

 appendicular a., one in the area of the vermiform appendix.

 chronic a., a long-standing collection of pus without inflammation; also called cold abscess.

 cold a., see chronic abscess.

 extradural a., one situated between the skull and the outer covering of the brain (dura mater); it is usually an extension of infection of the middle ear or frontal sinus.

 gingival a., a localized, painful, inflammatory lesion of the gingiva, usually arising from a periodontal pocket.

 hot a., see acute abscess.

 mammary a., an abscess in the breast, generally seen during the lactation period or on weaning.

 orbital a., an abscess within the ocular orbit, frequently an extension of purulent sinusitis.

 palmar a., a collection of pus in the palm of the hand, resulting from a puncture injury.

 pelvic a., an abscess located in the pelvic cavity, usually in the rectouterine pouch.

 periapical a., an abscess occurring in the alveolus near the apex of a tooth root, usually due to death of the tooth pulp.

 periodontal a., a localized, purulent inflammation in the gingiva corium, infrabony pockets, or periodontal membrane; it may be acute or chronic.

 periurethral a., one involving the tissues around the urethra, causing strained, painful urination.

 subdiaphragmatic a., one between the diaphragm and the liver or between the diaphragm and the spleen and stomach; also called subphrenic abscess.

 subphrenic a., see subdiaphragmatic abscess.

abscis'sa. The horizontal coordinate which, together with a vertical one (ordinate), forms a frame of reference for the plotting of data.

ab'solute. Complete; unrestricted; unadulterated.

absorb'. 1. To take in as through pores or interstices. **2.** To incorporate or take up gases, liquid, light rays, or heat. **3.** To neutralize an acid.

absor'bable. Capable of being absorbed.

absor'bent. Anything that can incorporate a substance into itself.

absorptiom'eter. 1. An instrument used to measure the solubility of gas in a liquid. **2.** An instrument for measuring the layer of liquid between two glass plates; used as a hematoscope in the analysis of blood.

absorp'tion. 1. The taking up of substances by the skin or other tissues. **2.** The taking up of part or all of the energy of incident radiation by the medium through which radiation passes, resulting in reduction of radiation intensity.

abster'gent. 1. Cleansing or purgative. **2.** An agent having such properties.

ab'stinence. A refraining from the indulgence of something, as sexual intercourse or stimulants, by one's own choice; also called self-denial.

ab'stract. 1. A preparation containing the soluble elements of a drug mixed with lactose. **2.** A summary of a book or literary article.

abu'lia. Pronounced diminution of the will power; inability to make decisions; also written aboulia.

abuse'. Improper use, particularly excessive use of anything; maltreatment.

 child a., physical maltreatment of a child, usually by parents.

 drug a., the excessive use, generally self-administered, of any drug, most commonly an agent that acts on the central nervous system, without regard for accepted medical practice.

 self a., masturbation.

abut'ment. A supporting structure; in dentistry, a natural tooth or root used to anchor and support a partial denture appliance.

 intermediate a., a natural tooth, without other natural teeth in proximal contact, which is used as an abutment, in addition to the primary or terminal abutments.

a.c. Abbreviation for Latin *ante cibum*, before meals.

Ac. Chemical symbol for the element actinium.

aca'cia. The dried gummy exudate from a tropical tree of the genus *Acacia*; used in the preparation of medicinal drugs; also called gum arabic.

acalcero'sis. Calcium deficiency in the body.

acalcu'lia. A form of aphasia characterized by inability to do simple arithmetic.

acan'tha. 1. The spine. **2.** The spinous process of a vertebra.

acanthesthe'sia. Condition in which there is a sensation of pressure with a sharp point.

Acan'thia lectula'ria. A species of flat blood-sucking insects with a disagreeable odor; also called bedbug and *Cimex lectularius*.

acan'thion. A projection on the anterior nasal spine.

acan'tho-. A combining form denoting thorns or spines.

acanthoadenocarcino'ma. Adenoacanthoma.

Acanthoceph'ala. A phylum of parasitic worms having a proboscis with hooked spines for attachment to the host.

acanthocephali'asis. Infestation with acanthocephalids.

acanthoceph'alid. Any worm of the order Acanthocephala.

Acanthocheilone'ma. A genus of parasitic worms, commonly called filaria; the adults live mainly in the body cavities or the subcutaneous tissues, while the larvae exist in the peripheral blood.

acanthocheilomeni'asis. Infestation with *Acanthocheilonema perstans.*

acan'thocyte. An abnormal red blood cell having several protoplasmic projections that give it a thorny appearance; seen in the disorder acanthocytosis and in some forms of liver disease.

acanthocyto'sis. A familial condition marked by the presence in the blood of large numbers of acanthocytes and a marked decrease in serum β-lipoproteins; may be associated with steatorrhea and progressive neurologic disease.

acan'thoid. Having the shape of a spine; spinous.

acanthokeratoder'mia. See hyperkeratosis.

acanthol'ysis. Disintegration of the layers of the skin.

acantho'ma. Carcinoma of the epidermis.

acantho'sis. Thickening of the prickle-cell layer of the skin.

acap'nia. See hypocapnia.

ac'ari. Plural of acarus.

acari'asis. 1. Any disease caused by mites, especially of the genus *Acarus*. **2.** Infestation with mites.

 sarcoptic a., see scabies.

acar'icide. Any agent that destroys mites.

ac'arid. A mite or tick; any member of the order Acarina.

Acar'idae. A family of small mites (order Acarina) some of which cause skin eruptions in humans.

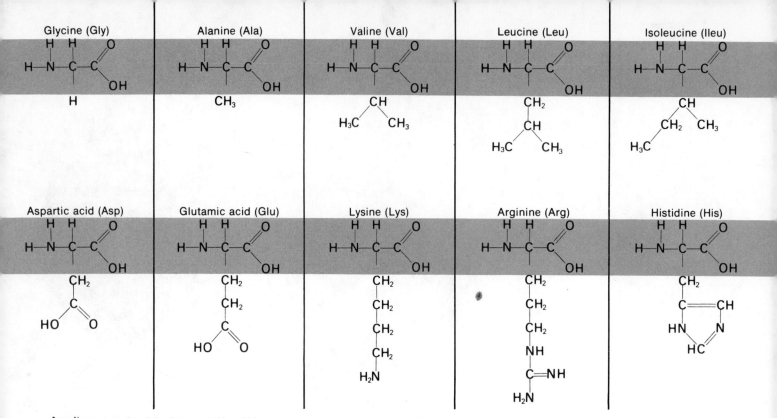

Glycine (Gly) · **Alanine (Ala)** · **Valine (Val)** · **Leucine (Leu)** · **Isoleucine (Ileu)**

Aspartic acid (Asp) · **Glutamic acid (Glu)** · **Lysine (Lys)** · **Arginine (Arg)** · **Histidine (His)**

Acari'na. An order of the class Arachnida, which includes mites and ticks.

acarino'sis. Acariasis.

acarodermati'tis. A skin rash caused by mites (acari).

ac'aroid. Resembling a mite.

acarol'ogy. The science that deals with the study of mites and ticks.

acaropho'bia. Abnormal fear of mites (acari), or of small particles.

ac'arus, *pl.* **ac'ari.** A mite or tick.

acar'yote. See akaryocyte.

acatalep'sia, acat'alepsy. 1. Lack of comprehension, as in mental deficiency. **2.** Impossibility of arriving at certain or definite knowledge.

acatapha'sia. Loss of the power to formulate one's thoughts correctly.

acata'posis. Difficulty in swallowing, or inability to swallow.

acathamathe'sia. Loss of the power of understanding.

acau'dal, acau'date. Without a tail.

acau'line. A term applied to a group of stemless fungi.

accel'erant. Accelerator.

accelera'tion. Increased speed of action, as of pulse or respiration.

accel'erator. Anything (drug, device, nerve, or muscle) that increases speed of action or function.

accel'erin. Accelerator globulin; see under globulin.

accentua'tion. Intensification.

accent'uator. A substance that increases the action of a tissue stain.

accep'tor. A substance that unites with a chemical group or ion of another substance (the donor), thus allowing a chemical reaction to proceed.

accesso'rius. Accessory; said of certain glands, nerves, etc.

acces'sory. Supplementary; having a subordinate function to a similar but more important structure.

acces'sory sign. Any sign that usually, but not always, accompanies a disease.

ac'cident. An unexpected, unintentional, undesirable event, or an unforseen complication in the course of a disease.

   cerebrovascular a., cerebral vascular a., occlusion or rupture of an artery in the brain; also called stroke and apoplexy.

acclima'tion. Acclimatization.

acclimatiza'tion. The adaptation or adjustment of an individual or plant to a new environment.

accolé form. See under form.

accommoda'tion. Alteration in the convexity of the lens of the eye to attain maximal sharpness of a retinal image of an object, distant or near.

accom'modative. Relating to accommodation.

accouchement'. French for childbirth or labor.

accrementi'tion. 1. Reproduction by budding. **2.** Growth by gradual external addition.

accre'tio cor'dis. Adhesion of the pericardium to adjacent structures, such as the chest wall, pleura, or diaphragm.

accre'tion. Slow accumulation of deposits, as on the surface of a tooth.

acel'lular. Having no cells.

acenesthe'sia. Loss of the normal sense of physical existence.

acen'tric. 1. Not centrally located. **2.** Denoting a chromosome fragment lacking a centromere.

aceph'alocyst. A cyst filled with liquid; one of the stages in the development of a sterile tapeworm; it does not give origin to daughter cysts which contain tapeworm heads (scoleces).

acer'vuline. Occurring in cluster forms.

acervulo'ma. Intracranial tumor or meningioma containing acervulus.

acer'vulus. Brain sand; a sandlike matter occurring in the pineal body and near the choroid plexus; composed chiefly of calcium carbonate.

aces'cence. 1. Slight acidity. **2.** The process of becoming sour.

acetab'ular. Of or relating to the acetabulum.

Acetabula'ria. A genus (phylum Chlorophyta) of single-celled alga which may grow as tall as 10 centimeters and which possesses a distinctive cap; used in the study of molecular biology.

acetabulec'tomy. Surgical removal of the acetabulum.

acetab'uloplasty. Surgical restoration of the hip socket or acetabulum.

acetab'ulum. The cup-shaped cavity in the lateral surface of the hipbone in which the head of the femur fits.

acetal'dehyde. A colorless liquid, CH_3CHO, with a pungent odor; an intermediate in yeast fermentation of carbohydrate and in alcohol metabolism in man; also called acetic aldehyde.

acetam'ide. A colorless crystalline substance, CH_3CONH_2; an amine of acetic acid, used as a solvent.

acetamin'ophen. *N*-Acetyl-*p*-aminophenol; a white, crystalline powder, used to reduce pain and fever.

acetan'ilide. A white crystalline substance, obtained from the action of acetic acid upon aniline; formerly used to relieve pain and fever.

ac'etate. Any acetic acid salt.

acetazol'amide. A diuretic that inhibits the action of carbonic anhydrase in the kidney, promoting the loss of bicarbonate and sodium; the effect is to produce a mild acidosis and to alkalize the urine; Diamox®.

ace'tic. Relating to, or containing, vinegar.

   a. acid, a colorless, organic acid with a pungent odor.

   glacial a. acid, a caustic liquid containing 99.5 per cent acetic acid; used to remove corns and warts.

acet'ify. To convert to vinegar or acetic acid.

acetoace'tic acid. A colorless, syrupy acid, $CH_3COCH_2 \cdot COOH$; one of the ketone bodies, occurring in excessive quantities in the urine of diabetics.

Acetobac'ter. A genus of bacteria (family Pseudomonadaceae) having elongated or rod-shaped forms, sometimes flagellated; important in the production of vinegar.

acetol'ysis. The splitting of an organic compound by the introduction of the elements of acetic acid.

acetomor'phine. Heroin.

acetonaph'thone. Naphthylmethyl ketone, $C_{10}H_7COCH_3$; a derivative of naphthalene, occurring in the shape of needles.

ac'etone. A colorless, volatile, extremely flammable liquid with an ethereal odor, CH_3COCH_3; generally used as an organic solvent.

acetone'mia. The presence of relatively large amounts of acetone or acetone bodies in the blood, as occurs when there is incomplete oxidation of large amounts of fat, as in diabetic acidosis or starvation.

acetone'mic. Characterized by acetonemia.

acetonu'ria. The presence of acetone in the urine; it occurs in poorly controlled diabetes mellitus and in starvation from incomplete oxidation of fats.

acetophenet'idin. See phenacetin.

ace'tum, *pl.* **ace'ta. 1.** Vinegar. **2.** A solution of a drug made with acetic acid.

acetyl. A radical or combining form of acetic acid, CH_3CO.

acetyla'tion. The introduction of a radical group of acetic acid (acetyl) into an organic compound.

acetylcho'line (ACh). The acetic acid ester of choline, $CH_3 \cdot CO - OCH_2CH_2 - N(CH_3)_3OH$; the chemical transmitter of the nerve impulse across a synapse; also released by the endings of parasympathetic nerves (cholinergic nerves) upon stimulation; produces cardiac slowing, vasodilation, increased gastrointestinal activity, and other parasympathetic effects; it is hydrolyzed and inactivated by the enzyme cholinesterase; available as acetylcholine bromide and acetylcholine chloride.

acetylcholines'terase. See cholinesterase.

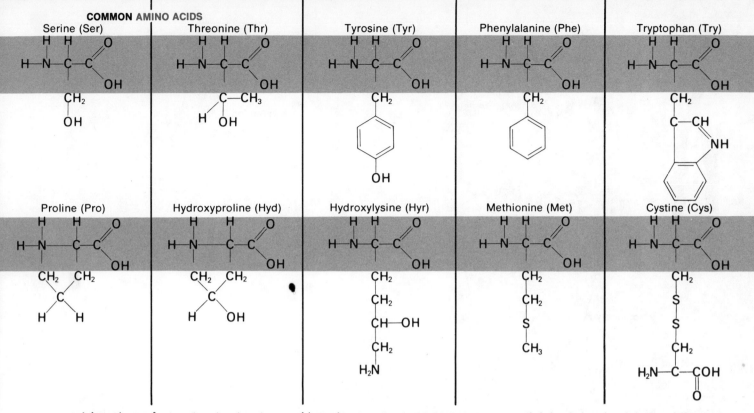

COMMON AMINO ACIDS

Serine (Ser) · Threonine (Thr) · Tyrosine (Tyr) · Phenylalanine (Phe) · Tryptophan (Try)

Proline (Pro) · Hydroxyproline (Hyd) · Hydroxylysine (Hyr) · Methionine (Met) · Cystine (Cys)

acetylcoen′zyme A. A product of condensation of coenzyme A and acetic acid.

acetylcys′teine. An agent used in the treatment of some bronchopulmonary disorders to reduce the viscosity of mucus; Mucomyst®.

acet′ylene. A colorless, flammable, explosive gas, C_2H_2, with a disagreeable garlic odor; made by the action of water on calcium carbide; formerly used as an anesthetic.

acetylphos′phate. A high-energy phosphate that takes part in the metabolism of bacteria.

acetylsalicyl′ic acid. Aspirin; an antipyretic, analgesic agent of value in the treatment of arthritis and other inflammatory conditions.

acetylstrophan′thidin. A synthetic cardiac glycoside with the most rapid onset of action of all the digitalis preparations.

ACh. Abbreviation for acetylcholine.

achala′sia. Failure to relax; referring especially to sphincter muscles of the esophagus.

ache. A dull pain.

Achil′les. A mythical Greek hero who was invulnerable except in the heel.

   A. bursa, see bursa of calcaneal tendon.

   A. tendon, see tendon, calcaneal.

achillodyn′ia. Pain in or about the calcaneal tendon (Achilles tendon); also called achillobursitis.

achillor′rhapy. Repair of a torn calcaneal tendon (Achilles tendon).

achillotenot′omy. Achillotomy.

achillot′omy. Surgical division of the calcaneal tendon (Achilles tendon).

   plastic a., elongation of the calcaneal tendon by plastic surgery.

achlorhy′dria. Absence of hydrochloric acid in the stomach; also called gastric anacidity.

achlorop′sia. A form of color blindness restricted to green.

achlupho′bia. A morbid fear of darkness.

acho′lia. Deficiency of bile.

acholu′ria. Absence of bile pigments from the urine.

achondroplas′ia, achon′droplasty. Congenital abnormality in the process of ossification in cartilage, resulting in dwarfism and deformity; also called chondrodystrophia and chondrodystrophy.

achor′date, achor′dal. Without a notochord; denoting animal forms classified below the chordates.

achore′sis. Reduction of the capacity of a hollow organ, as of the bladder, caused by permanent contraction.

achroma′sia. 1. Absence of normal pigmentation of the skin. **2.** Lack of staining reaction in a cell. **3.** Achromatopsia.

ach′romate. A totally color blind individual who sees colors as different shades of gray.

Achromatia′ceae. A family (order Beggiatoales) of colorless, motile bacteria that have spherical, ovoid, or rod shapes, contain globules of sulfur or crystals of calcium carbonate, and exist in both fresh and marine water.

achromat′ic. 1. Colorless. **2.** Refracting light without separating it into its component colors. **3.** Staining poorly. **4.** Characterized by color blindness.

achro′matin. The part of the cell nucleus that is only faintly stained by dyes.

achromatophil′ia. The condition of being resistant to the action of stains.

achromatop′sia. Total color blindness; also called achromasia (3) and achromatopia.

achromato′sis. Lack of natural pigmentation, as in the iris or the skin.

achro′matous. Colorless.

achro′mia. See leukoderma.

Achromobac′ter. A genus (family Achromobacteraceae) of nonpigment-forming, rod-shaped bacteria found in fresh water and soil.

achro′mocyte. Phantom corpuscle; see under corpuscle.

achromotrich′ia. Lack or loss of color in the hair.

achy′lia. A rare condition marked by the absence of gastric juices.

achy′lous. 1. Without gastric juice or other digestive secretion. **2.** Without chyle.

aci′cular. Needle-shaped; said of some crystals or leaves.

acid. A compound capable of donating a hydrogen ion (proton) to a base; any substance that turns litmus indicators red and combines with a base to form a salt. For individual acids, see specific names.

   amino a., any organic acid containing one or more amino groups (NH_2) and a carboxyl group (CO_2H); forming the essential components of proteins.

   chenic a., chenodeoxycholic a., a natural bile acid in man; it reduces the stone-forming tendency of bile and dissolves cholesterol gallstones by decreasing the hepatic secretion of cholesterol.

   dibasic a., an acid containing molecules with two displaceable hydrogen ions.

   essential fatty a., a polyunsaturated fatty acid indispensable for nutrition; its absence causes a specific deficiency disorder and it cannot be fabricated by the body (must be obtained from the diet); e.g., linoleic acid and linolenic acid; originally called vitamin F.

   fatty a., any of a large group of organic acids made up of molecules containing a carboxyl group at the end of a long hydrocarbon chain; the carbon content may vary from C_2 to C_{34}.

   inorganic a., an acid composed of molecules that do not contain carbon atoms; e.g., hydrochloric acid, boric acid, etc.

   monobasic a., an acid containing molecules with one displaceable hydrogen ion.

   nonessential fatty a., the main form of circulating lipid.

   nonesterified fatty a. (NEFA), the main form of circulating fatty acid used for energy.

   organic a., an acid composed of molecules containing carbon atoms; e.g., ascorbic acid, amino acid, etc.

   polybasic a., an acid containing molecules with three or more displaceable hydrogen ions.

   polyunsaturated fatty a., any unsaturated fatty acid with two or more double bonds; e.g., linoleic acid (two double bonds) and arachidonic acid (four double bonds).

   resin a.'s, a class of organic compounds derived from certain plant resins; e.g., abietic acid and pimaric acid; also called rosin acids.

   saturated fatty a., a fatty acid in which the carbon chain is connected by single bonds, and is incapable of accepting any more hydrogen, i.e., all the available valence bonds of the carbon chain are filled with hydrogen atoms; e.g., stearic acid and palmitic acid.

   unsaturated fatty a., a fatty acid in which the carbon chain has at least one double bond, and is capable of accepting additional hydrogen atoms; e.g., oleic acid.

acide′mia. An increase in the hydrogen ion concentration of the blood; a fall below normal in pH (in man, a fall below pH 7.4). Cf acidosis.

acid-fast. Denoting bacteria that, once stained with acids such as basic fuchsin, are not decolorized by acid-alcohol.

acidifi′able. Capable of being made acid.

acid′ify. 1. To make acid. **2.** To become acid.

acid′ity. 1. The quality or state of being acid. **2.** The acid content of a fluid.

acid′ophil. Eosinophilic leukocyte; see under leukocyte.

acido′sis. A process tending to produce an increase in hydrogen ion concentration in body fluids; if uncompensated it produces a lowering of pH; commonly used synonymously with acidemia.

   metabolic a., acidosis caused by excessive production or ingestion of acid other than carbonic acid or loss of base.

   renal a., acidosis caused by defective elimination of acid or excessive loss of bicarbonate by the kidneys.

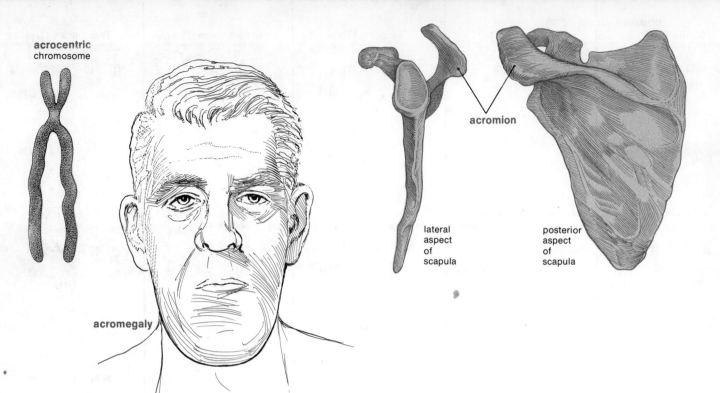

acrocentric
chromosome

acromegaly

acromion

lateral
aspect
of
scapula

posterior
aspect
of
scapula

respiratory a., defective elimination of carbon dioxide (CO_2) by the lungs, leading to excessive accumulation of carbonic acid (H_2CO_3).

acidos'teophyte. A sharp-pointed outgrowth of bone.

acidot'ic. Relating to, or suffering from, acidosis.

acid'ulous. Slightly sour or acid.

acidu'ria. Acid in the urine.

acidu'ric. Capable of living under acid conditions; said of some bacteria.

ac'idyl. A term used to denote any acid radical.

ac'inar. Of or relating to an acinus.

ac'ini. Plural of acinus.

acini'tis. Inflammation of an acinus.

ac'inous. Resembling a bunch of grapes or made up of minute sacs (acini).

ac'inus, pl. **ac'ini. 1.** A minute saclike dilatation. **2.** The smallest division of a gland.

ac'lasis. Continuity of structure provided by pathologic tissue which arises from, and is continuous with, normal tissue.

acleistocar'dia. Condition in which the foramen ovale of the heart fails to close.

acmesthe'sia. Sensation of a pinprick in the skin.

ac'ne. An eruption caused by inflammation of the sebaceous glands.

a. ciliaris, acne on the free edges of the eyelids.

a. rosacea, see rosacea.

a. vulgaris, chronic acne, occurring commonly on the face, chest, and back of adolescents and young adults.

ac'neform, acne'iform. Resembling acne.

acocan'thera. A poisonous substance extracted from the leaves and stems of *Acocanthera venenata,* used by some natives of Africa as an arrow poison.

acogno'sia, acog'nosy. The study or knowledge of remedies.

acol'ogy. Therapeutics.

aco'lous. Without limbs.

aco'mia. Baldness.

acon'ative. Without volition.

cis-**aconitic acid.** A product of dehydration of citric acid; an intermediate in the tricarboxylic acid cycle.

acopro'sis. Absence or extreme diminution of fecal matter in the intestines.

acore'a. Congenital absence of the pupil of the eye.

aco'ria. Lack of a feeling of satisfaction after eating.

acous'ma. The sensation of hearing imaginary sounds; also called acouasm.

acousmatagno'sia. Failure to recognize sounds; also called mind deafness.

acousmatamne'sia. Inability to recall sounds.

acous'tic. Of or relating to sound or to the sense of hearing.

acousticopho'bia. Abnormal fear of sounds.

acous'tics. The branch of science concerned with the study of sound, its generation, propagation, and perception.

acquired. Developed after birth, in contrast to congenital or hereditary.

ac'ral. Relating to the extremities or peripheral parts of the body.

acra'nia. Congenital absence of the skull, or a portion of it.

ac'rid. 1. Pungent, caustic, or sharp to the taste or smell. **2.** Causing an irritation.

ac'ridine. Dibenzopyridine; a coal tar derivative, $C_{13}H_9N$, occurring in colorless crystals and having a strong, irritating odor.

acris'ia. Uncertain course of a disease.

acrit'ical. Without a crisis.

acro-. Combining form denoting extremity, end, tip, or summit.

acroagno'sis. Absence of sensory recognition of a limb.

acroanesthe'sia. Lack of sensation in the extremities.

acroatax'ia. Lack of muscular coordination of the fingers and toes.

acrocen'tric. Denoting a chromosome whose centromere is situated close to one end.

acrocephal'ic. Relating to or affected with acrocephaly.

acrocephalosyndac'tyly, acrocephalo-syndac'tylism. Congenital malformation consisting of a high-domed skull and complete or partial webbing of the digits; also called Apert's syndrome.

acroceph'aly. Congenital malformation marked by a high-domed skull.

acrochor'don. A small, soft, pedunculated growth, occurring usually on the neck or eyelids.

acrocyano'sis. A chronic circulatory disorder characterized by cold, cyanotic, sweaty hands and feet; the skin is a mottled blue and red; the condition is intensified by cold and emotion.

acrodermati'tis. Inflammation of the skin of the hands or feet.

a. chronica atrophicans, dermatitis of the extremities accompanied by atrophy of the skin.

a. vesiculosa tropica, dermatitis of the fingers, occurring in hot climates, in which the skin becomes glossy with numerous small vesicles.

acrodolichome'lia. Abnormal largeness of hands and feet.

acrodyn'ia. A disorder affecting infants and young children, marked by irritability, stomatitis, loss of teeth, insomnia, and redness of fingers, toes,

cheeks, nose, and buttocks; also called pink disease and erythredema.

acroesthe'sia. 1. Abnormally increased sensitivity. **2.** Pain in the extremities.

acroge'ria. Premature aging of the skin of the hands and feet.

acrogno'sis. Sensory perception of the limbs and their parts in relation to one another.

acrohyperhidro'sis. Abnormally increased sweating of the hands and feet.

acrokerato'sis verruciform'is. Condition marked by warty growths on the hands and feet.

acromegal'ic. Relating to or afflicted with acromegaly.

acromeg'aly. A disease marked by progressive enlargement of the head, face, hands, feet, and internal organs due to a disorder of the pituitary gland, with overproduction of growth hormone after the normal growth period has ended; also called Marie's disease.

acromelal'gia. A disease affecting the extremities, especially the feet, and marked by dilation of the blood vessels, headache, vomiting, and redness, pain, and swelling of the toes and fingers.

acrometagen'esis. Congenital deformity of the extremities.

acro'mial. Of or relating to the acromion.

acromic'ria. Abnormal smallness of bones of the head, hands, and feet; the converse of acromegaly.

acromioclavic'ular. Of or relating to the acromion and clavicle.

acromiocor'acoid. Of or relating to the acromion and the coracoid process.

acromiohu'meral. Of or relating to the acromion and humerus.

acro'mion. The flattened process extending laterally from the spine of the scapula and forming the most prominent point of the shoulder; also called acromial process.

acromioscap'ular. Pertaining to the acromion and the body of the scapula.

acromiothora'cic. Relating to the acromion of the scapula (shoulder blade) and the thorax; also called thoracicoacromial.

acrom'phalus. Abnormal protuberance of the navel.

acromyco'sis. Any disease of the limbs caused by a fungus.

acromyoto'nia. Rigidity of the hands or feet, resulting in spasmodic deformity.

ac'ropachy. Thickening (clubbing) of the tips of fingers and toes with proliferation of bone tissue and swelling; also called pachyacria.

acroparesthe'sia. A vasomotor-trophic disorder marked by attacks of numbness and prickly or tin-

acidosteophyte | **acroparesthesia**

6

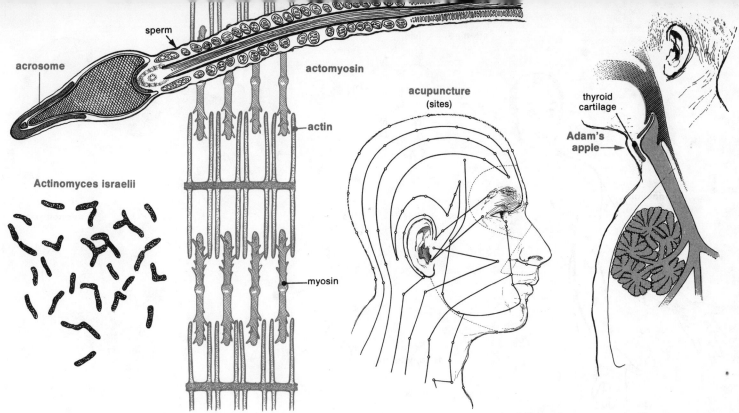

sperm
acrosome
actomyosin
actin
acupuncture
(sites)
thyroid cartilage
Adam's apple →
Actinomyces israelii
myosin

gling sensations in the extremities, chiefly the tips of the fingers and toes.

acropho′bia. Morbid fear of high places.

acroposthi′tis. Inflammation of the prepuce.

acroscleroder′ma. Hardening of the skin of the fingers and toes; also called sclerodactyly.

acrosclero′sis. Thickening of the skin and subcutaneous tissue of the hands and feet due to swelling and thickening of fibrous tissue; scleroderma of the hands and feet.

ac′rosome. The dense structure covering the anterior half of the head of a spermatozoon; it contains the enzyme hyaluronidase which aids the penetration of the egg by the sperm during fertilization.

acrot′ic. 1. Of, affecting, or located on the surface of the body. **2.** Pulseless.

acrotrophodyn′ia. Neuritis of the extremities as a result of exposure to prolonged cold and moisture.

acryl′ic. Denoting any derivative of acrylic acid, used in the construction of dental and medical prostheses. See also resin.

ACTH. Abbreviation for adrenocorticotrophic hormone.

ac′tin. A muscle protein which, together with myosin, is responsible for muscular contraction.

ac′tinism. The property of radiation that produces chemical changes or activity.

actin′ium. A radioactive element, symbol Ac, atomic number 89, atomic weight 227; found in uranium ores and possessing no stable isotopes.

actino-. A combining form denoting (a) radiation or radioactivity; (b) radial or ray form.

Actinobacil′lus. A genus of small, gram-negative, aerobic bacteria (family Brucellaceae) that cause disease in cattle and hogs; some species attack humans.

  A. mallei, see *Pseudomonas mallei.*

  A. pseudomallei, see *Pseudomonas pseudomallei.*

actinodermati′tis. Inflammation of the skin caused by radiation.

actin′ogen. A radioactive element.

actinogen′esis. See radiogenesis.

actin′olite. Any substance that undergoes marked changes in the presence of light.

actinom′eter. Any of several instruments for measuring the intensity and chemical effects of actinic rays.

Actinomy′ces. A genus of nonmotile, nonacid-fast bacteria (family Actinomycetaceae), occurring in groups of radiating club-shaped rods superficially resembling fungi; some varieties are used in the production of antibodies; also called ray fungus.

  A. bovis, a species that causes actinomycosis or lumpy jaw in cattle.

  A. griseus, *Streptomyces griseus.*

A. israelii, the causal agent of human actinomycosis.

Actinomyceta′ceae. A family of bacteria (order Actinomycetales) having filamentous shapes with a tendency to branch and resembling both bacteria and fungi; some varieties are pathogenic.

actinomy′cin. An antibacterial substance found in some soil bacteria.

actinomyco′sis. Disease of cattle and hogs, sometimes occurring in man, caused by *Actinomyces bovis* and marked by the formation of slow-growing granulomas from which pus-discharging abscesses develop; the infection affects mostly the jaws and neck, sometimes spreading to the lungs and alimentary tract; also called lumpy jaw.

actinoneuri′tis. Neuritis caused by prolonged exposure to any radioactive substance.

actin′ophage. Any virus that destroys actinomycetes.

ac′tion. 1. The performance of an act, movement, or function. **2.** The transmission of energy.

  ball valve a., the periodic or intermittent blockage of a tubular structure by a foreign body.

  cumulative a., suddenly increased intensity, as the effect of a drug that had been previously administered with moderate or negligible effect.

  sparing a., the lowering of the requirement for an essential food factor in the diet caused by the presence of another food factor which, by itself, is not essential.

  specific dynamic a., the increase in heat production during digestion; from 4 to 6 per cent for carbohydrates to 30 per cent for proteins.

activa′tion. 1. Stimulation. **2.** The act of making radioactive.

ac′tivator. 1. A substance that stimulates the action of another. **2.** An agent that accelerates a reaction.

  allosteric a., one that enhances enzyme activity when bound to a site other than the active site of the enzyme molecule.

ac′tive. Capable of functioning or changing; requiring energy, as contrasted to passive.

active transport. See transport, active.

activ′ity. 1. The condition of being active. **2.** The intensity of a radioactive element. **3.** The release of electrical energy by nerve tissue.

actomy′osin. A unique contractile protein with a linear molecular shape, formed by the union of actin and myosin; it is responsible for the contraction of muscle fibers.

acu′ity. Acuteness, distinctness.

  visual a., clearness of vision; dependent on the size and sharpness of the image on the retina, the sensitivity of the nerves, and the interpretative abil-

ity of the brain.

acu′leate. Thorny; covered with sharp points.

ac′upressure. Compression of a blood vessel by inserting needles in surrounding tissues.

acupunc′ture. A modality developed in China for certain types of anesthesia and treatment of various disorders; fine stainless steel needles are inserted into specific areas of the body; it is thought to work through the body's autonomic nervous system; also called neuronyxis.

acu′sis. Normal hearing.

acute. Denoting a disease or symptoms of abrupt onset or lasting a relatively short period of time; opposite of chronic.

acute brain syndrome. Sudden, often reversible, impairment of brain function, secondary to other conditions, such as drug ingestion or systemic metabolic disorders; manifested by faulty perception and interpretation, usually associated with delirium.

acyanoblep′sia. Inability to see the color blue; also called blue blindness.

acyanot′ic. Not marked by cyanosis.

acye′sis. 1. Sterility in the female. **2.** A non-pregnant state.

acyl. Any radical derived from an organic acid by the removal of the hydroxyl group.

acyla′tion. The introduction of an acyl radical into a compound.

acys′tia. Congenital absence of the urinary bladder.

Acystosporid′ia. An order of parasitic sporozoa that includes the genus *Plasmodium*, the malarial parasite.

A.D. Abbreviation for Latin *auris dextra.*

ad. A Latin preposition denoting to; used in writing prescriptions.

ad-. Prefix meaning increase, motion toward, proximity, dependence, and intensified action.

-ad. Suffix denoting direction toward.

adac′tyly. Congenital absence of fingers or toes.

adamantino′ma. See ameloblastoma.

Adam's apple. Laryngeal prominence; the thyroid cartilage of the larynx which forms a subcutaneous projection in the midline of the neck.

Adams-Stokes syndrome. A syndrome characterized by fainting and sometimes convulsions due to prolonged asystole; seen usually when there is a failure of effective contraction in the course of complete heart block or when heart block supervenes on a sinus rhythm; sometimes Cheynes-Stokes respiration may occur; also called Stokes-Adams or Morgagni-Adams-Stokes syndrome.

adapta′tion. 1. The adjustment of the pupil of the eye to variations in the intensity of light. **2.** Altera-

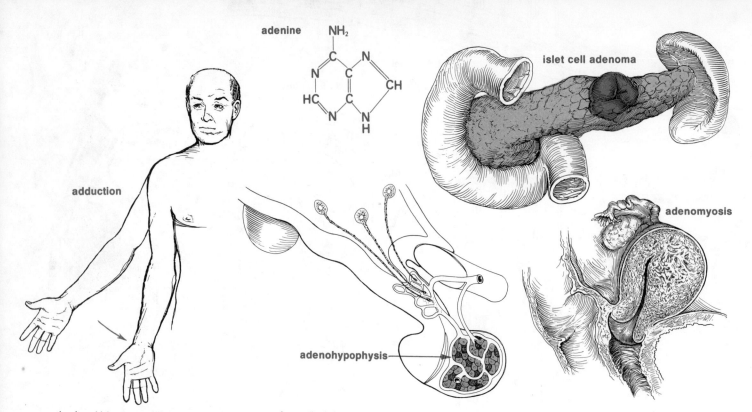

adenine

islet cell adenoma

adduction

adenomyosis

adenohypophysis

tion by which an organism becomes fit for a new environment. **3.** The decreased response of a sense organ to repeated stimuli.

dark a., eye adjustment to reduced illumination (sensitivity to light is greatly increased).

light a., eye adjustment to increased illumination (sensitivity to light is reduced).

ad'der. European viper; see under viper.

ad'dict. One who has a strong dependence upon some practice which has progressed beyond voluntary control.

drug a., an individual with a psychologic and physiologic dependency on drugs.

addic'tion. Strong habituation to some practice, beyond voluntary control.

drug a., compulsive use of a habit-forming drug, the deprivation of which gives rise to symptoms of distress, or withdrawal symptoms, and compulsion to take the drug again; also called pharmacopsychosis.

addiso'nian. 1. Characterized by features of Addison's disease. **2.** Someone suffering from Addison's disease.

Addison's anemia. See anemia, pernicious.

Addison's disease. Primary adrenocortical insufficiency; adrenocortical insufficiency caused by destruction of the adrenal cortex, a disease characterized by chronic deficiency of hormones concerned with mineral metabolism and glycostasis; findings include striking skin pigmentation, anemia, hypotension with small heart, severe dental caries, and stiffness of the cartilages of the ear; hyponatremia is present and, later, there may be azotemia and hyperkalemia; also called addisonism.

addition. In pharmacology, the quality of two drugs (e.g., epinephrine and norepinephrine) that act on the same receptors whereby doses of one drug can substitute for those of the other, in proportion to their relative potency.

ad'ditive. Any substance that is added to another material to fulfill a specific purpose, i.e., to improve it, strengthen it, etc.

addu'cent. Bringing toward or together; performing adduction; denoting some adductor muscles, as the adducens oculi.

adduct'. To pull or draw toward the median line of the body.

adduc'tion. Movement of a part toward or beyond the median line; act of turning inward.

adduc'tor. A structure, such as a muscle, that draws a part toward an axis of the body; opposite of abductor.

ad'enase. An enzyme that converts adenine into hypoxanthine; present in the liver, pancreas, and spleen.

adenasthe'nia. Abnormal reduction in the activity of a gland.

adendrit'ic. Denoting a nerve cell without dendrites, such as certain cells in the spinal ganglia.

adenec'tomy. Surgical removal of a gland.

adenecto'pia. The presence of a gland somewhere other than its normal position.

ad'enine. A white, crystalline purine derivative, $C_5H_5N_5$; one of the constituents of ribonucleic acid (RNA) and deoxyribonucleic acid (DNA).

a. arabinoside (Ara-A), a substance that acts intracellularly to inhibit viral replication; used in the treatment of some viral infections such as those caused by cytomegalovirus.

a. nucleotide, see adenylic acid.

adeni'tis. Inflammation of a lymph node or gland.

adeno-. Combining form denoting gland or glands.

adenoacantho'ma. A malignant tumor made up of a glandular tissue.

ad'enoblast. Embryonic cell from which glandular tissue develops.

adenocarcino'ma. A malignant tumor with cells arranged in a glandlike pattern.

ad'enocele. A benign, cystlike tumor derived from glandular tissue.

adenocysto'ma. A benign, epithelial, glandlike tumor associated with cysts.

adenodias'tasis. The presence of glands or glandular tissue in other than their normal sites.

adenoepithelio'ma. Tumor made up of glandular and epithelial tissues.

adenofibro'ma. A benign tumor made up of connective tissue with some glandular elements.

adenofibro'sis. The formation of a fibrous tissue in a gland.

adenohypophys'eal, adenohypophys'ial. Of or relating to the anterior portion of the pituitary gland.

ad'enohypoph'ysis. The anterior or glandular portion of the pituitary gland (hypophysis).

ad'enoid. 1. Resembling a gland. **2.** Pharyngeal tonsil.

adenoidec'tomy. Surgical removal of the adenoids.

adenoidi'tis. Inflammation of the pharyngeal tonsil.

ad'enoids. Enlargement of the pharyngeal tonsil.

adenolipo'ma. Benign tumor of fat tissue containing some glandular elements.

adenolipomato'sis. Condition marked by the presence of several subcutaneous adenolipomas, especially in the neck, axilla, and groin.

adenolym'phocele. Cystic enlargement of a lymph node.

adenolympho'ma. Papillary cystadenoma lym-

phomatosum; see under cystadenoma.

adeno'ma. Benign tumor of epithelial tissue with a glandlike structure.

acidophilic a., adenoma of the anterior portion of the pituitary gland; made up of acidophil cells and causing acromegaly and giantism.

a. psammosum, one occurring especially in the anterior lobe of the pituitary gland, containing a great number of calcifications.

a. sebaceum, a tumor of the face made up of sebaceous glands; appears as a collection of reddish and yellowish papules and is associated with mental deficiency.

basophilic a., tumor of the anterior lobe of the pituitary gland; composed of basophil cells and associated with Cushing's syndrome.

chromophil a., an acidophilic or a basophilic adenoma.

chromophobe a., a tumor composed of chromophobe cells in the anterior pituitary gland, associated with hypopituitarism.

eosinophilic a., tumor of the eosinophilic cells of the anterior pituitary gland, causing giantism and acromegaly.

islet cell a., a tumor of the pancreas, made up of tissue similar in structure to that of the islets of Langerhans.

malignant a., adenocarcinoma.

oxyphil, oxyphilic a., acidophilic adenoma.

oxyphil granular a., a tumor of the parotid gland made up of oxyphilic granular cells.

adeno'matoid. Resembling an adenoma.

adenomato'sis. Condition marked by the formation of multiple glandular tumors.

familial polyendocrine a., the presence of tumors in several endocrine glands.

pulmonary a., the presence in the alveoli and distal bronchi of abundant mucus and mucus-secreting columnar epithelial cells of neoplastic origin; characterized by the production of very large amounts of sputum.

adenom'atous. Relating to adenoma or glandular overgrowth.

adenomyo'ma. A benign tumor composed of muscle tissue, found in the uterus and uterine ligaments.

adenomyo'sis. The presence of adenomatous growths in smooth muscle, as the invasion of the uterine musculature by endometrium.

adenomyxo'ma. A benign tumor made up of glandular and mucous tissue.

adenop'athy. Disease of glands, especially of the lymphatic glands.

adenosarco'ma. A malignant tumor containing glandular tissue.

adder | adenosarcoma

8

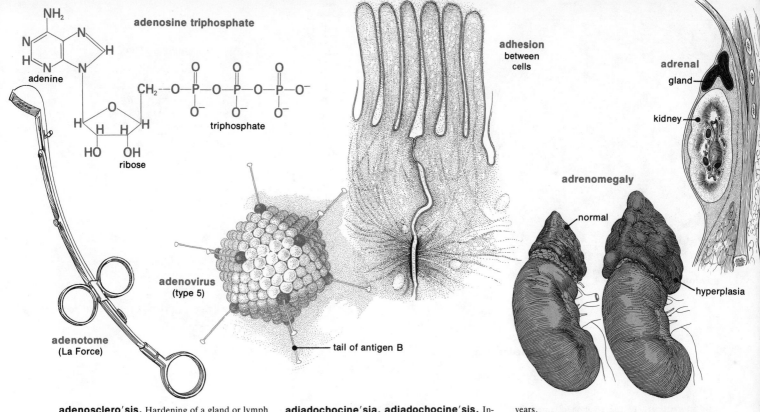

adenosine triphosphate

adenine

triphosphate

ribose

adenovirus
(type 5)

adenotome
(La Force)

tail of antigen B

adhesion
between
cells

adrenal
gland

kidney

adrenomegaly

normal

hyperplasia

adenosclero'sis. Hardening of a gland or lymph node.

ad'enose. Relating to a gland.

aden'osine. An organic compound, $C_{10}H_{13}N_5O_4$, derived from nucleic acids; composed of adenine and a pentose sugar.

  a. diphos'phate (ADP), a product of the hydrolysis, and the substrate for the biosynthesis, of adenosine triphosphate (ATP).

  a. monophos'phate (AMP), see adenylic acid.

  a. triphos'phatase (ATPase), an enzyme, present in muscle tissue, that promotes the splitting off of a phosphate group from adenosine triphosphate.

  a. triphos'phate (ATP), organic compound present in all cells; upon hydrolysis, it yields the energy required by a multitude of biologic processes.

adeno'sis. Any disease of the glands, especially one affecting the lymph nodes.

ad'enotome. A surgical instrument for the removal of adenoids.

adenotonsillec'tomy. Surgical removal of adenoids and tonsils.

ad'enovi'ruses. A group of DNA viruses that multiply in the nuclei of cells; some members cause infections of the respiratory tract and occasionally the eye; others have been extensively used in experimental studies of cancer.

ad'enyl. A radical, $C_5H_4N_4$; a constituent of adenine.

  a. cyclase, an enzyme that catalyzes production of cyclic AMP from ATP; also written adenylcyclase.

adenyl'ic acid. One of the hydrolysis products of all nucleic acids, occurring in all tissues and participating in high-energy phosphate transfer; also called adenosine monophosphate (AMP) and adenine nucleotide.

adenylosuccin'ic acid. An intermediate in biosynthesis of adenylic acid.

ADH. Abbreviation for (a) antidiuretic hormone; (b) alcohol dehydrogenase.

adhe'sio interthalam'ica. A band of gray matter, frequently absent, connecting the two halves of the thalamus across the third ventricle of the brain; also called massa intermedia.

adhe'sion. 1. The union of two surfaces. 2. A fibrous band that abnormally unites two parts.

  fibrinous a., adhesion composed of fine strands of fibrin.

  fibrous a., one composed of a group of fibrinous adhesions.

  primary a., the adhesion or healing of a wound without suppuration or the formation of granulations; also called healing by first intention.

adhesiot'omy. Surgical division of adhesions.

adiadochocine'sia, adiadochocine'sis. Inability to perform rapid alternating movements (e.g., pronation and supination).

adiaphore'sis. Deficiency of persipiration.

adiaphoret'ic. Characterized by or causing adiaphoresis.

adip-, adipo-. Combining form meaning fat.

adipec'tomy. See lipectomy.

adip'ic acid. Acid formed by the oxidation of fats.

ad'ipocele. See lipocele.

ad'ipocere. A waxy substance formed on decomposing dead bodies under humid conditions.

adipogen'ic. See lipogenic.

adipoki'nin. A hormone of the anterior pituitary gland important in the metabolism of lipids.

adiponecro'sis. Necrosis of fat.

ad'ipose. Of or related to fat; fatty.

adipo'sis. Excessive accumulation of fat in the body, either local or general.

adipos'ity. A bodily state in which the proportion of the body weight composed of fat is excessive; the body weight may not exceed normal (feature that distinguishes it from obesity).

ad'itus. A general anatomic term denoting approach or entrance to an organ.

ad'juvant. That which aids or assists, as a substance which enhances the response to an antigen.

  Freund's complete a., a mixture of mineral oil, plant waxes, and killed tubercle bacilli; used with antigen to increase antibody production.

  Freund's incomplete a., Freund's complete adjuvant minus the tubercle bacilli.

ad lib. Abbreviation for Latin *ad libitum,* as much as desired.

adner'val. Near or in the direction of a nerve.

adnex'a. Appendages; parts accessory to the main organ.

adoles'cence. The stage in human growth from the onset of puberty to the attainment of full physical development.

adoles'cent. 1. Of or relating to adolescence. 2. A person during the period of adolescence.

ado'ral. Toward or near the mouth.

ADP. Abbreviation for adenosine diphosphate.

adre'nal. 1. Located near the kidney. 2. The adrenal gland.

adrenalec'tomize. To remove the adrenal glands.

adrenalec'tomy. Surgical removal of the adrenal glands.

adren'aline. See epinephrine.

ad'renarch. 1. Puberty induced by hyperactivity of the adrenal cortex. 2. A physiologic change in which the function of the adrenal cortex is increased, occurring at approximately the age of nine years.

adrener'gic. Term applied to nerve fibers of the sympathetic nervous system that, upon stimulation, release the chemical transmitter norepinephrine (and possibly small amounts of epinephrine) at their post-ganglionic endings.

adrenocor'tical. Relating to the adrenal cortex.

adrenocorticomimet'ic. Having a function similar to that of the adrenal cortex.

adrenocorticotroph'ic, adrenocorticotrop'ic. Stimulating the function or growth of the cortex of the adrenal gland.

adrenocorticotro'phin, adrenocorticotro'pin. Adrenocorticotropic hormone; see under hormone.

adrenogen'ic. Produced or originating in the adrenal glands.

adrenogenital syndrome. Metabolic disorder caused by hyperfunction of the adrenal cortex, usually associated with premature virilization and, in the female, with pseudohermaphroditism and sexual infantilism; caused by a congenital deficiency in the ability to form cortisol with a compensatory increase in ACTH serving to cause hypersecretion of other adrenal steroids.

adren'ogram. X-ray picture of an adrenal gland.

adrenolyt'ic. 1. Inhibiting the action of sympathetic (adrenergic) nerves. 2. Having an inhibitory influence on the action of or response to epinephrine (adrenaline).

adrenomeg'aly. Enlargement of the adrenal glands.

adrenopri'val. Absence of adrenal function.

adrenos'terone. A male sex hormone (androgen), $C_{19}H_{24}O_3$, present in the adrenal cortex.

adrenotox'in. Any substance toxic to the adrenal glands.

adrenotroph'in, adrenotrop'in. Adrenocorticotrophic hormone; see under hormone.

adrenot'ropism. The predominance of adrenal influence in endocrine function.

adsorb'. To attach one substance to the surface of another.

adsor'bate. A substance adhered to the surface of another by adsorption.

adsor'bent. A substance that attracts and holds on its surface another substance.

adsorp'tion. The process by which gas molecules or small particles in solution are attracted by, and attached to, the surface of another substance.

adult'. A fully grown individual.

adul'terant. 1. Anything added to a substance which makes it impure or inferior. 2. Any of various materials added to a hallucinogenic drug in the hope of enhancing its potency.

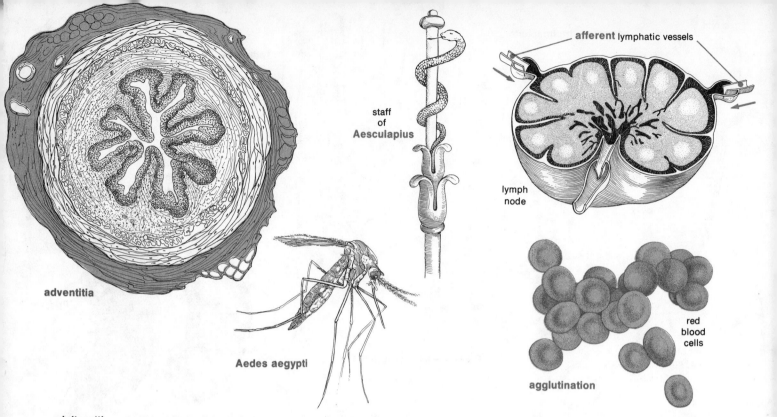

adventitia

staff of Aesculapius

Aedes aegypti

afferent lymphatic vessels

lymph node

red blood cells

agglutination

adultera′tion. 1. The addition of foreign substances to a product. **2.** Alteration of a substance by the addition of material of cheaper and inferior qualities.

advance′ment. Surgical procedure in which the tendon of a muscle is detached and reattached at an advanced point; used to correct strabismus.

adventi′tia. The outer, loose connective tissue covering of a structure such as a blood vessel, thoracic duct, or ureter; also called extima.

adventi′tial. Relating to the outer layer of a blood vessel.

adynam′ia. Weakness; asthenia.

Ae′des aegyp′ti. An important species of mosquito, the carrier of yellow fever and dengue; it may also transmit filariasis and encephalitis; it generally breeds near houses; also called tiger mosquito.

a′erated. Containing air, carbon dioxide, or oxygen.

aera′tion. 1. The act of airing. **2.** The saturation of a fluid with a gas. **3.** The oxygenation of blood in the lungs.

a′erobe. Any organism capable of growing in the presence of air.

aero′bic. Growing only in the presence of air; also called aerobiotic.

aerobio′sis. Life in an oxygen-containing environment.

aerobiot′ic. See aerobic.

a′erocele. Distention of a small body cavity with gas.

a′erogen. A gas-producing microorganism.

aerogen′esis. Production of gas.

aerogen′ic. Gas producing, such as certain bacteria.

aeropha′gia. The swallowing of air, usually accompanying emotional disorders; also called aerophagy.

aero′phagy. See aerophagia.

a′erophil, aerophil′ic. Air loving; an organism that requires air for proper growth.

aeropho′bia. Abnormal fear of drafts or of fresh air.

aerosinusi′tis. Inflammatory condition of paranasal sinuses caused by difference between pressures within the sinuses and that of the atmosphere; also called barosinusitis.

a′erosol. Relatively stable suspension of liquids or solids in air, oxygen, or inert gases which is dispersed in the form of a fine mist, usually for therapeutic purposes.

aeroti′tis me′dia. Inflammation of the middle ear caused by a sudden increase in atmospheric pressure, as on descent in an aircraft from a high altitude, when obstruction of the auditory tube does

not permit equalization of pressures within and without the middle ear; also called aviator's ear.

Aescula′pian. Of or relating to the healing art; medical.

Aesculap′ius. The Roman god of healing.

staff of A., a rod encircled by a single snake; symbol of the medical profession and emblem of the American Medical Association, the Royal Army Medical Corps, and the Royal Canadian Army Medical Corps.

aes′tival. See estival.

afeb′rile. Without fever.

af′ferent. Conveying a fluid or a nerve impulse toward an organ or area.

afferent loop syndrome. Chronic partial obstruction of the duodenum and jejunum following gastrojejunostomy, resulting in distention and pain after eating.

affin′ity. In chemistry, the attractive force of two substances for each other.

afibrinogene′mia. Marked deficiency of fibrinogen in the blood.

AFIP. Abbreviation for Armed Forces Institute of Pathology.

af′terbirth. The placenta and fetal membranes expelled from the uterus after childbirth.

afterdis′charge. The discharge of impulses from a reflex center after stimulation has ceased.

af′terimage. The continued visual sensation or image perceived after the physical stimulus has been removed.

af′terload. In cardiac muscle, the force against which the ventricle ejects once contraction of the muscle fibers begins; for the left ventricle this is equivalent to aortic diastolic pressure.

af′terpains. Cramps due to uterine contractions after delivery.

afterpoten′tial. The small upward deflection following the sharp main deflection (spike) in an oscillograph record of the electrical potential of a stimulated nerve.

aftersensa′tion. Sensation persisting after the stimulus that caused it has been removed.

Ag. 1. Abbreviation for antigen. **2.** Symbol for silver.

agalac′tia. Condition in which milk in the breasts is absent after childbirth.

agalorrhe′a. Absence or arrest of milk flow.

agammaglobuline′mia. Condition marked by virtual absence of γ-globulin in the blood, inability to form antibody, and frequent attacks of infectious diseases.

agamogen′esis. Asexual reproduction, as by budding, cell division, etc.

ag′amous. Reproducing by agamogenesis.

aganglio′no′sis. Congenital absence of ganglia.

a′gar. A gelatinous material prepared from seaweed; used as a culture medium for bacteria because it is not affected by most bacterial enzymes, and as a laxative because its bulk increases greatly upon absorption of water.

blood a., bouillon solidified with 1 per cent agar and mixed with blood.

chocolate a., agar mixed with fresh blood and then heated, which gives it a chocolate brown color; used as a culture medium for *Neisseria*.

Sabouraud's a., bouillon solidified with 1 per cent agar, mixed with 1 per cent Chassaing's peptone and 4 per cent maltose or mannite; used for growth of fungi; also called French proof agar.

age. The period of time during which a person has lived.

biologic a., the age measuring the degree of physical maturity of an individual; for children, usually determined by a roentgenogram of the bones (bone age).

bone a., see biologic age.

chronologic a., the time from the date of birth; calendar age.

mental a., the age level of intellectual ability as measured by standardized tests.

agen′esis, agene′sia. Absence or abnormal development of a part.

agen′italism. Symptoms occurring in the absence of secretions of the ovaries or testes.

agenoso′mia. Congenital absence or defective development of the genitals and protrusion of the abdominal organs through an incomplete abdominal wall.

a′gent. Anything capable of producing an effect upon an organism.

blocking a., a drug that blocks the transmission of a nerve impulse at a synapse.

chelating a., a compound that combines with metals to form a complex (chelate); used in medicine to render poisonous metal compounds nonpoisonous.

Eaton a., *Mycoplasma pneumoniae*; one of the main causes of primary atypical pneumonia.

sclerosing a., any compound used in the treatment of varicose veins.

ageu′sia. Absence of the sense of taste.

agglutina′tion. 1. the clumping of cells or microorganisms when exposed to a specific immune serum. **2.** The process of joining together in the healing of a wound.

group a., the clumping together of several related varieties of bacteria in the presence of serum specific for one of that group.

agglu′tinin. An antibody that causes particulate

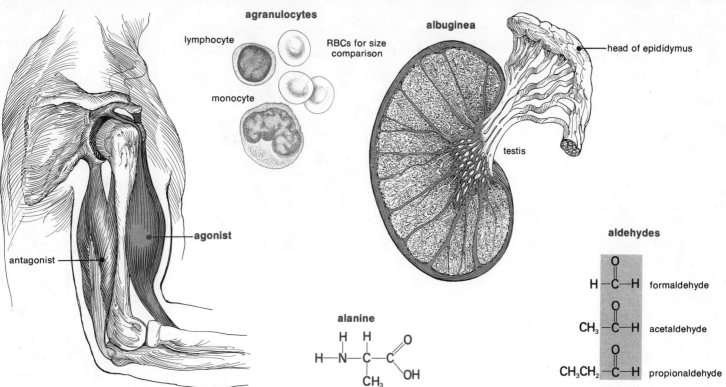

agranulocytes

lymphocyte

monocyte

RBCs for size comparison

albuginea

head of epididymis

testis

alanine

$$H_2N-C(H)(CH_3)-C(=O)-OH$$

aldehydes

$$H-\overset{O}{\underset{}{C}}-H \quad \text{formaldehyde}$$

$$CH_3-\overset{O}{\underset{}{C}}-H \quad \text{acetaldehyde}$$

$$CH_3CH_2-\overset{O}{\underset{}{C}}-H \quad \text{propionaldehyde}$$

agonist

antagonist

---

antigens, such as bacteria or other cells, to adhere to one another, forming clumps.

cold a., agglutinin that causes clumping of human group O red blood cells at temperatures from zero to 5°C.

agglutin′ogen. An antigenic substance that stimulates the formation of a particular antibody (agglutinin) that causes clumping of cells containing the antigen.

agglutinogen′ic. Causing the production of an agglutinin.

agglu′tinoid. An agglutinin that has lost its ability to produce clumping but can still combine with its corresponding agglutinogen.

ag′gregate. 1. To crowd together. **2.** The mass or cluster thus formed.

agit. Abbreviation for *agita,* Latin for shake, stir; used in prescription writing.

aglaucop′sia. Inability to distinguish green; also called green blindness.

aglomer′ular. Having no glomeruli.

agly′cone, aglu′cone. The noncarbohydrate group of a glycoside.

agnogen′ic. Of unknown cause; idiopathic.

agno′sia. Loss of ability to comprehend the meaning of sensory stimulation, such as auditory, visual, olfactory, tactile, and gustatory sensations.

ag′onist. 1. A muscle in a state of contraction opposing the action of another muscle, its antagonist, which at the same time relaxes. **2.** A drug that can interact with receptors (specific sites in certain cells) and initiate a drug response; e.g., acetylcholine.

agorapho′bia. Abnormal fear of open spaces.

agranulocytope′nia. See agranulocytosis.

agran′ulocytes. Agranular leukocytes; a group of so-called nongranular white blood cells that contain nonspecific (azurophilic) granules; it includes the lymphocyte and the monocyte; normally it constitutes from 37 to 42 per cent of the total white blood cell population.

agranulocyto′sis. A state marked by a great reduction of granular white blood cells (polymorphonuclear leukocytes); often used to describe a syndrome including the hematologic change plus constitutional symptoms and the development of infected ulcers in the mouth (agranulocytic angina), throat, intestinal tract, and sometimes the skin; the acute form is most frequently drug induced but may be seen in acute leukemia; the chronic form is of unknown etiology and is seen more frequently in women; also called agranulocytopenia.

agraph′ia. Loss of the power to communicate ideas in writing, due to a cerebral lesion.

AHF. Abbreviation for antihemophilic factor.

AHG. Abbreviation for antihemophilic globulin.

AID. Abbreviation for (a) autoimmune disease; (b) artificial insemination donor.

air. The mixture of gases that make up the earth's atmosphere, composed of approximately 78 per cent nitrogen, 21 per cent oxygen, and lesser amounts of carbon dioxide, argon, ammonia, neon, helium, and organic matter.

alveolar a., air remaining in the lungs after a normal expiration in which the O_2 and CO_2 tensions are in equilibrium with those of the arterial blood.

residual a., former name for residual volume; see under volume.

tidal a., air that enters and leaves the lungs during normal respiration; also called tidal volume.

A.K. Abbreviation for above the knee, referring to site of amputation.

akar′yocyte. Any cell without a nucleus, such as a mature red blood cell; also called acaryote.

akine′sia. Loss or impairment of voluntary muscular action.

akiyami. See hasamiyami.

a′la, *pl.* **a′lae. 1.** Any winglike structure. **2.** Axilla.

al′anine. An amino acid of the pyruvic acid family; found widely in proteins.

alanine aminotransferase. An enzyme that transfers amino groups from an α-amino acid to (usually) a 2-keto acid; also called glutamic pryruvic transaminase (GPT).

a′lar. Of or relating to any winged structure or to the armpit.

alas′trim. A contagious eruptive disease resembling a mild form of smallpox.

al′ba. White; term used to describe certain anatomic structures which appear whitish, such as the linea alba.

Albers-Schönberg disease. See osteopetrosis.

al′binism. Absence of pigment in the skin, hair, and irises; it may be partial or complete; also called congenital leukoderma.

albi′no. A person marked by albinism.

Albright's syndrome. A polyostotic fibrous dysplasia of bone marked by dense overgrowth of bone and cystic transformation, most commonly involving several areas of the skeleton; accompanied by pigment spots on the skin and sexual precocity (principally in females).

albugin′ea. A thick connective tissue capsule surrounding the testis.

albu′min, albu′men. A protein in many animal and vegetable tissues, including human plasma, soluble in water and coagulable by heat; a principal constituent of egg white.

radioiodinated serum a. (RISA), **iodinated** [131]I

serum a., human serum albumin iodinated with ^{131}I which emits beta and gamma radiation; used for determining blood and plasma volumes and cardiac output, and for detection of brain tumors.

albuminif′erous. Producing albumin.

albuminocytologic dissociation. See dissociation, albuminocytologic.

albu′minoid. 1. Resembling albumin. **2.** A scleroprotein.

albuminu′ria. Urinary excretion of albumin in excess of the normal daily amount; see also proteinuria.

al′cohol. 1. A colorless, flammable fluid, C_2H_5OH; obtained from fermented sugars and starches; used as a solvent, antiseptic, preservative of specimens, and in the preparation of drugs and intoxicating beverages. **2.** CH_3H_2OH; the alcohol of wine, whiskey, etc.; produced by several microorganisms fermenting different substrates; also called ethanol and ethyl or grain alcohol.

absolute a., alcohol containing not more than 1 per cent of water (by weight).

acid a., 70 per cent ethyl alcohol containing 1 per cent hydrochloric acid.

a. dehydrogenase, (ADH), an enzyme present in the liver which promotes the dehydrogenation of ethyl alcohol to acetaldehyde.

denatured a., alcohol that has been rendered unfit to drink by the addition of other chemicals.

methyl a., CH_3OH; a colorless, flammable liquid, soluble in water or ether; used as an industrial solvent and in the manufacture of formaldehyde; also called methanol, wood alcohol, and pyroxylic spirit.

rubbing a., a mixture of about 70 per cent of absolute alcohol and varying quantitites of water, denaturants, and perfumed oils; used as a rubefacient.

wood a., see methyl alcohol.

alcohol′ic. 1. Relating to or containing alcohol. **2.** A person addicted to alcohol.

al′coholism. A pathologic condition, mainly of the nervous and gastroenteric systems, caused by excessive consumption of alcohol.

acute a., condition caused by excessive drinking of alcoholic beverages; also called drunkenness and intoxication.

chronic a., addiction to alcohol, often accompanied by damage to the health of the individual.

al′dehyde. 1. Any of a group of organic compounds obtained from oxidation of the primary alcohols and containing the group CHO. **2.** Acetaldehyde.

a. dehydrogenase, an enzyme, important in the metabolism of ethyl alcohol, which promotes the

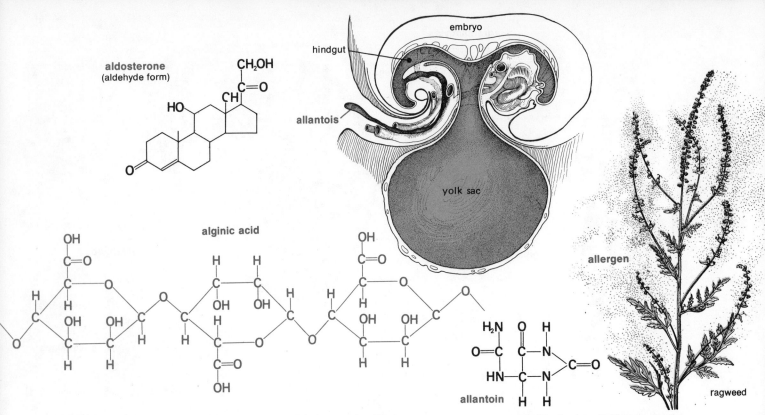

aldosterone
(aldehyde form)

alginic acid

allantois

hindgut

embryo

yolk sac

allergen

allantoin

ragweed

oxidation of acetaldehyde to acetic acid.

al′dolase. An enzyme in muscle extract that catalyzes the reversible cleavage of fructose 1,6-diphosphate to yield dihydroxyacetone phosphate and glyceraldehyde.

aldopen′tose. A sugar containing five carbon atoms and the aldehyde group—CHO.

aldos′terone. A potent electrolyte-regulating hormone secreted by the zona glomerulosa of the adrenal gland which causes retention of sodium in the body by enhancing sodium reabsorption by the cells of the distal tubule of the kidney, in addition to the cells of the gastrointestinal tract, and the sweat and salivary glands; the reabsorption of sodium is usually accompanied by an increased secretion of potassium ions.

aldoster′onism. Excessive secretion of aldosterone by the adrenal cortex; also called hyperaldosteronism.

  primary a., a syndrome in which (1) a tumor in the cortex of the adrenal gland (Conn's syndrome), or (2) hyperplasia of the adrenal gland without obvious cause, is responsible for excessive aldosterone secretion; the syndrome is characterized by hypertension, hypokalemic alkalosis, and weakness.

  secondary a., aldosteronism caused by excessive stimulation of the adrenal gland, frequently associated with fluid-retaining states.

Aldrich syndrome. See Wiskott-Aldrich syndrome.

aleuke′mia. Deficiency of white corpuscles in the blood; denoting leukemic diseases in which the white blood cell count in peripheral blood is normal or deficient; also called aleukemic leukemia.

aleuke′mic. Relating to or characterized by aleukemia.

alex′ia. A form of aphasia in which brain damage causes inability to grasp the meaning of written or printed words; also called visual aphasia and word blindness.

alex′in. See complement.

ALG. Abbreviation for antilymphocyte globulin.

alge′sia. Increased sensitivity to pain.

algesiom′eter. See odynometer.

algesthe′sia. Perception of pain.

al′ginate. An irreversible hydrocolloid salt of alginic acid which is extracted from marine kemp; used primarily for making dental impressions, particularly for partial dentures.

al′ginic acid. A colloidal polysaccharide obtained from marine kemp; used in the making of alginate, a widely used dental impression material.

algopho′bia. A morbid fear of pain.

algorith′m. Any procedure (either mechanical or through step-by-step instructions) designed to solve a particular type of problem.

align′ment. In dentistry, the line along which the teeth, natural or artificial, are arranged.

al′iment. Food.

alimen′tary. Of or relating to food or nutrition.

alimenta′tion. The process of providing nourishment; also called feeding.

aliphat′ic. Relating to, or denoting, the fatty series of hydrocarbon compounds in which the carbon atoms are arranged in open chains rather than closed rings; also called fatty and oily.

alkale′mia. A decrease in the hydrogen ion concentration of the blood; an increase beyond normal of pH (in man, a pH greater than 7.43). Cf alkalosis.

alkales′cent. Becoming alkaline.

al′kali. Any of a group of basic compounds capable of combining with fatty acids to form soaps.

alkalim′etry. The measurement of the degree of alkalinity in a substance.

al′kaline. Relating to, containing, or having the reaction of an alkali (base).

alkalin′ity. The state of being alkaline.

al′kalize, al′kalinize. To make alkaline.

al′kaloid. A class of compounds present in certain plants that strongly affect human physiology; e.g., morphine (opium poppy), quinine (cinchona bark), reserpine (snake root), caffeine (tea leaves and coffee beans), cocaine (coca leaves), LSD (ergot fungus), nicotine (tobacco leaves), etc.

alkalo′sis. A process tending to produce a decrease in hydrogen ion concentration in the body fluids; if uncompensated, it leads to a rise in pH; commonly used synonymously with alkalemia.

  hypokalemic a., alkalosis characterized by a low serum potassium concentration; characteristic of the most commonly seen form of metabolic alkalosis.

  metabolic a., the state resulting from excessive retention of alkali or excessive loss of acid; common causes include prolonged vomiting or gastric drainage, diuretic therapy, and excessive adrenal corticosteroid secretion or administration; characterized by an elevation of the plasma bicarbonate concentration and a tendency to an alkaline arterial pH; when the arterial pH is actually more alkaline than normal, the condition should, strictly speaking, be called alkalemia.

  respiratory a., the state resulting from hyperventilation and reduction of pCO₂ in body fluids.

al′kalot′ic. Relating to, or marked by, alkalosis.

alkap′ton. See homogentisic acid.

alkaptonu′ria. A hereditary condition in which homogentisic acid (alkapton) is not broken down to simpler compounds in the body but is excreted in the urine, which gives it a dark brown color when exposed to air; also called homogentisuria.

allanti′asis. Poisoning caused by the ingestion of sausage containing the toxins of *Clostridium botulinum.*

allan′toin. A nitrogenous crystalline substance, C₄H₆N₄O₃; present in allantoic fluid, fetal urine, and some plants.

allan′tois. A diverticulum that extends from the hindgut of the embryo, appearing at about the 16th day of development; it forms part of the umbilical cord and the placenta.

al′lele. One of a series of two or more contrasting genes that occupy the same position in homologous chromosomes and determine the heredity of a particular trait; the term is shortened from allelomorph.

alle′lic. Relating to two or more different genes that occupy the same position in homologous chromosomes.

al′lelism. The existence of two or more contrasting genes that occupy the same position in homologous chromosomes.

alle′lomorph. See allele.

al′lergen. A substance that stimulates an allergic reaction in the body.

allergen′ic. Capable of stimulating an allergic reaction.

aller′gic disease. A disease resulting from allergy or any response stimulated by an allergen; the gamut includes superficial lesions, as urticaria, to deep-seated lesions, as polyarteritis nodosa.

al′lergoids. Chemically weakened substances (allergens) that can cause an allergic reaction.

al′lergy. Hypersensitivity (1); the altered reactivity to a substance, which can result in pathologic reactions upon subsequent exposure to that particular substance.

  bronchial a., asthma.

  contact a., cutaneous reaction caused by direct contact with a substance to which the person is hypersensitive.

  drug a., unusual sensitivity to a drug or chemical.

allo-. Combining form meaning other, or denoting a condition differing from the normal or usual.

alloan′tibody. An antibody from one individual which reacts with an antigen present in another individual of the same species.

alloan′tigen. Homologous antigen; an antigen produced by one individual which incites the formation of antibodies in another individual of the same species; also called isoantigen.

alloarth′roplasty. The surgical construction of an artificial joint.

alloche′tia, alloche′zia. The passage of feces through an abnormal opening.

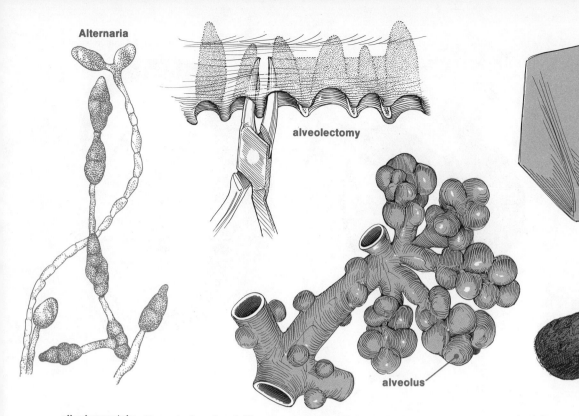

Alternaria

alveolectomy

amalgamator

alveolus

Amanita phalloides

allochroma'sia. Change in the color of skin or hair.

allocor'tex. The primitive part of the cerebral cortex, such as the olfactory cortex, which is not laminated.

allog'amy. Cross-fertilization; fertilization by the union of the ovum from one organism with the spermatozoon from another.

allogen'eic, allogen'ic. Relating to genetically dissimilar individuals of a single species.

 a. disease, either an acute or a chronic disease resulting primarily from a reaction to a graft.

al'lograft. A graft derived from a genetically dissimilar individual of the same species; also called allogeneic graft and homograft.

alloimmune'. The condition of being immune to an allogeneic antigen.

allom'erism. The state of having different chemical composition but the same crystalline form.

allomor'phism. A change in the shape of cells caused by mechanical factors.

allopla'sia. See heteroplasia.

al'loplast. An inert foreign body implant.

al'loploid. An organism arising from the combination of two or more sets of chromosomes from different ancestral species; also called allopolyploid and hybrid.

al'losome. A chromosome that differs from the ordinary chromosome (autosome); a sex chromosome.

allos'terism. The alteration of an enzyme's activity by regulatory molecules that are noncompetitively bound to sites other than the active or catalytic site of the enzyme molecule.

allotransplanta'tion. The transplantation of tissue from one individual to another of the same species but without the identical genetic makeup.

allox'an. A reddish, crystalline substance, $C_4H_2N_2O$; a product of oxidation of uric acid; capable of destroying the islets of Langerhans and, hence, inducing experimental diabetes.

alloy'. A mixture of two or more metals.

alo'chia. Absence of vaginal discharges (lochia) after childbirth.

al'oes. A purgative, brownish-yellow powder derived from plants of the genus *Aloe*.

al'oform. A wing-shaped structure, as the pterygoid bone of the skull.

alope'cia. Baldness.

 a. areata, a. circumscripta, complete loss of hair in patches chiefly on the scalp.

 a. capitis totalis, complete hair loss from the scalp.

 a. congenitalis, absence of hair at birth.

 a. furfuracea, loss of hair associated with dandruff; also called alopecia pityrodes.

 a. hereditaria, premature loss of hair, an inherited trait; also called alopecia simplex.

 a. senilis, loss of hair normally occurring in old age; also called senile alopecia.

 a. totalis, a. universalis, total loss of hair from all parts of the body.

al'pha. 1. The first letter of the Greek alphabet, α; used to denote the first in order of importance. **2.** In chemistry, denotes a location immediately adjacent to the functional group of atoms in a molecule. For terms beginning with alpha see under specific term.

alpha particle. See particle, alpha.

Alport's syndrome. Hereditary nephritis associated with deafness.

ALS. Abbreviation for (a) antilymphocyte serum; (b) amyotrophic lateral sclerosis.

al'ter. To castrate a male animal.

alter'nans. Alternating.

Alterna'ria. A genus of soil molds having dark-colored conidia; prevalent in air and usually considered to be a common laboratory contaminant; a common allergen in bronchial asthma.

al'um. Any double sulfate of a trivalent metal (aluminum, iron, etc.) and a univalent metal (sodium, potassium, etc.); used medicinally as an astringent and a styptic.

alu'minum. A silvery-white, metallic element of extremely light weight; symbol Al, atomic number 13, atomic weight 26.97; its compounds are used therapeutically as antacids and astringents.

 a. chloride, a white or yellowish-white powder, $AlCl_3 \cdot 6H_2O$; used in 10 to 25 per cent solution as an antiperspirant, deodorant, or astringent.

 a. hydroxide, a. hydrate, a white tasteless powder, $Al(OH)_3$; used externally as a drying powder because it takes up water, and internally as an antacid; also called hydrated alumina.

 a. hydroxide gel, a preparation containing from 3.6 to 4.4 per cent of aluminum oxide (AlO_3) in the form of aluminum hydroxide; used to reduce stomach acidity; also prepared in tablet form, which is the dried aluminum hydroxide gel.

alveolal'gia. Dry socket; see under socket.

alve'olar. Of or relating to an alveolus.

alveolec'tomy. Surgical removal of diseased tissue from the alveolar process, following the removal of teeth, in preparation for the fitting of a dental prosthesis.

alve'oli. Plural of alveolus.

alveolin'gual. Relating to the surface of the alveolar process adjacent to the tongue.

alveoli'tis. Inflammation of alveoli.

alveolot'omy. The surgical opening of a tooth socket for drainage and treatment purposes.

alve'olus. 1. See tooth socket. **2.** An air sac of the lungs. **3.** One of the honeycomb pits in the mucous membrane of the stomach.

al'veus. 1. A canal. **2.** The layer of white fibers in the brain which covers the area of the hippocampus adjacent to the lateral ventricle.

Alzheimer's disease. A progressive brain disease occurring in persons 40 to 60 years of age, marked by generalized atrophy of the brain; chief symptoms include disorientation, difficulty in walking, and speech disorders; also called presenile dementia.

amal'gam. An alloy of mercury and other metals, as the mixture of silver, tin, and mercury, used in dentistry for filling cavities in the teeth.

amal'gamate. To make an amalgam by dissolving a metal in mercury.

amalgama'tion. The process of dissolving a metal in mercury to form an alloy.

amal'gamator. In dentistry, a device for mixing amalgam mechanically.

Amani'ta. A genus of fungi.

 A. phalloides, poisonous mushroom which, upon ingestion, causes severe gastrointestinal symptoms, followed by damage to the kidneys, liver, and central nervous system; also called death cup and death angel.

aman'tadine hydrochlo'ride. An antiviral agent used in preventing illness in individuals exposed to respiratory infection from Asian (A_2) strain of influenza virus; also used in treating Parkinson's disease; Symmetrel ®.

amaril'la. International term for yellow fever.

amauro'sis. Complete loss of vision.

 a. centralis, blindness caused by disease of the central nervous system.

 a. fugax, temporary blindness lasting a few minutes.

 toxic a., blindness due to inflammation of the optic nerve caused by the presence in the system of a poisonous agent such as alcohol, tobacco, lead, etc.

amaurot'ic. Relating to, or suffering from, blindness.

ambeno'nium chlo'ride. A chemical compound that inhibits the production of the enzyme cholinesterase; used in the treatment of chronic progressive muscular weakness (myasthenia gravis); Mytelase Chloride®.

ambidex'trous. Being equally skillful with both hands.

ambisex'ual. Of, relating to, or affecting both sexes.

ambisexual'ity. Having characteristics of both sexes.

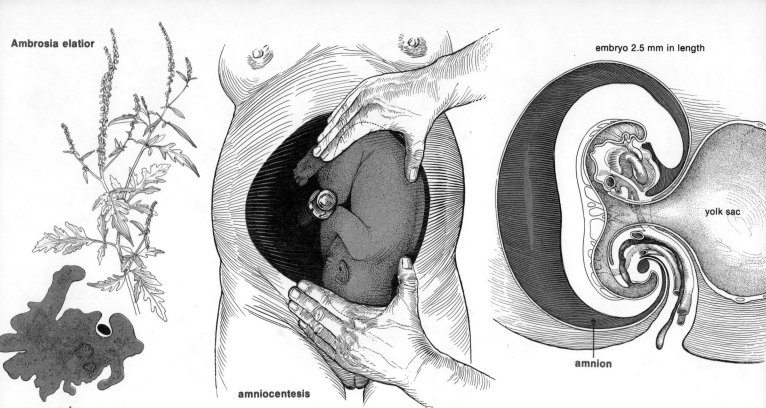

Ambrosia elatior

embryo 2.5 mm in length

yolk sac

amnion

amniocentesis

ameba

ambiv′alence. The existence of contrasting emotional feelings, such as love and hate, about a person or object.

amblyacou′sia. A slight degree of hearing impairment.

amblyo′pia. Dimness of vision without a detectable lesion or disease of the eye.

am′blyoscope. A device consisting primarily of two angled tubes which can be made to swivel to different degrees of convergence or divergence; used for training an amblyopic eye to share equally with the other eye in binocular vision.

ambocep′tor. Archaic term denoting rabbit antisheep red cell antibody; presently called hemolysin.

Ambro′sia ela′tior. Common ragweed that produces highly allergenic pollen capable of causing hay fever and asthma in some individuals; pollination period is from August through October.

am′bulatory, am′bulant. Capable of walking about; said of a patient who is not confined to bed.

ame′ba. Any protozoan of the genus *Amoeba*.

amebi′asis. The condition of being infected with *Amoeba histolytica*.

ame′bic. Pertaining to, resembling, or caused by amebas.

ame′bicide. Anything that destroys amebas.

ame′boid. Resembling an ameba.

amebo′ma. A tumor-like mass sometimes formed in the wall of the colon due to chronic infestation with amebas.

ameio′sis. A type of cell division in which gametes are formed without reduction in chromosome number.

amelanot′ic. Denoting certain types of unpigmented skin growths.

amel′ia. Congenital absence of a limb or limbs.

amelifica′tion. The development of tooth enamel.

ameliora′tion. Improvement; lessening of the severity of symptoms.

amel′oblast. The epithelial cell in the developing tooth that produces layers of matrix which become calcified to form rods of tooth enamel; when it completes its function of enamel formation, the ameloblast becomes part of the enamel cuticle (Nasmyth's membrane); also called adamantoblast and emailloblast.

ameloblastofibro′ma. A benign tumor composed of epithelial cells of a developing tooth (ameloblasts) and dense connective tissue.

ameloblasto′ma. A tumor derived from epithelial tissue characteristic of the enamel organ, occurring mainly in the molar region of the mandible; also called adamantinoma.

ameloblastosarco′ma. A malignant neoplasm derived from odontogenic tissue and containing a large number of ameloblasts.

amelogen′esis. Enamel formation.

amenorrhe′a. Absence of menstruation.

amenorrhe′al, amenorrhe′ic. Relating to, or accompanied by, absence of menstruation.

ametro′pia. A refractive disorder of the eye in which parallel rays of light do not focus on the retina, but either in front or it (myopia) or behind it (hyperopia).

axial a., one caused by the lengthening of the eyeball on the optic axis.

am′ide. An organic compound derived from ammonia by the substitution of an acyl radical for hydrogen.

amido-. A prefix denoting the presence in a compound of the radical NH_2 along with the CO radical.

amina′tion. The formation of an amine.

am′ine. Any of a group of organic compounds derived from ammonia by replacement of one or more hydrogen atoms by hydrocarbon radicals.

amino-. Combining form denoting the presence of the radical NH_2 in a compound.

aminoace′tic acid. See glycine.

ami′no acid. See under acid.

aminoacide′mia. The presence of amino acids in the blood as a result of congenital metabolic disease.

aminoacidu′ria. The presence of excessive amounts of amino acids in the urine, or the presence of amino acids not usually found in the urine.

p-aminobenzo′ic acid (PABA). Para-aminobenzoic acid; a factor of the vitamin B complex; it is an essential growth factor for bacteria, therefore, it nullifies the bacteriostatic effects of the sulfonamide drugs used in the treatment of some collagen diseases.

γ-aminobutyric acid (GABA). Gamma-aminobutyric acid; a substance in the brain, especially in the basal ganglia and neocortex, that plays a role in cortical transmission.

p-aminohippu′ric acid (PAH). Para-aminohippuric acid; a substance used in clearance studies to determine the total amount of plasma flowing through the kidneys; it is almost entirely removed from the plasma in a single passage through the kidney; also called *p*-aminobenzoylglycine.

δ-aminolevulin′ic acid (ALA). Delta-aminolevulinic acid; $NH_2CH_2COCH_2CH_2COOH$; an important intermediate in the biosynthesis of porphyrin; excessive levels are found in the urine in acute intermittent porphyria.

aminoph′ylline. A xanthine derivative containing 85 per cent anhydrous theophylline and 15 per cent ethylenediamine; it increases cardiac output and coronary blood flow and exerts a mild diuretic action; when administered by slow intravenous injection, it often relieves acute bronchospasm, acute pulmonary edema, and paroxysmal nocturnal dyspnea.

aminopy′rine. An odorless, white, crystalline compound, $C_{13}H_{17}N_3O$; used to reduce fever and pain in rheumatism, neuritis, and pulmonary tuberculosis; also called amidopyrine and pyramidon.

p-aminosalicyl′ic acid (PAS, PASA). Para-aminosalicylic acid; a crystalline compound which retards the growth of bacteria; used as an adjunct in the treatment of tuberculosis.

amito′sis. Direct division of a cell simply by elongation and division of the nucleus and cytoplasm into two new cells, unlike the ordinary process of cell reproduction (mitosis).

ammo′nia. A colorless, volatile, pungent, alkaline gas, NH_3, soluble in water, forming ammonia water; formed in the body as a product of protein metabolism; usually converted to urea by the liver or excreted by the kidney to facilitate H^+ excretion.

ammoni′acal. Of or relating to ammonia.

ammo′niated. Combined with or containing ammonia.

ammo′nium. A chemical ion (NH_4).

a. chloride, a white crystalline compound, NH_4Cl; used as an expectorant and as an acidifying agent; also called sal ammoniac.

amne′sia. Impairment of memory.

anterograde a., inability to recall events after injury or disease.

retrograde a., amnesia for events preceding injury or disease.

amne′siac. An individual suffering from loss of memory.

amnes′tic. Causing amnesia.

amniocente′sis. Withdrawal of amniotic fluid, usually performed through the abdominal wall using a needle.

amniog′raphy. Roentgenography of the pregnant uterus after injection of an opaque solution into the amniotic fluid.

am′nion. The thin, tough, innermost layer of the membranous sac that surrounds the fetus; also called the "bag of waters."

amnioni′tis. Inflammation of the amnion.

amniorrhe′a. The premature escape of amniotic fluid (liquor amnii).

amniot′omy. Surgical rupture of the fetal membranes for the purpose of inducing labor.

Amoe′ba, *pl.* **Amoe′bae.** A genus of one-celled protozoans existing in water, soil, or as parasites, having a changeable shape, and moving by means of pseudopodia; some species cause disease in man.

ambivalence | Amoeba

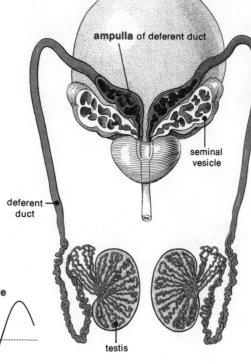

amphiarthrosis

vertebrae

amphitrichous

amplitude

ampulla of deferent duct

deferent duct

seminal vesicle

testis

coronal section of brain

amygdala

optic chiasma

amor'phia, amor'phism. The state or condition of being without a definite form.

amor'phous. Lacking a definite shape or structure.

AMP. Abbreviation for adenosine monophosphate; see adenylic acid.

am'pere. The unit of electric current strength, equal to the current yielded by one volt of electromotive force against one ohm of resistance.

amphet'amine. Any of a group of synthetic chemicals that stimulate the central nervous system; pharmacologically classified as sympathomimetic amines; slang names: speed, uppers, and bennies.

amphiarthro'sis. A joint or articulation that allows only slight motion, e.g., between the bodies of the vertebrae; also called amphiarthrodial joint.

amphibol'ic. 1. Uncertain. **2.** In an energy-generating system, the functional overlap between metabolic intermediates and adenylate compounds.

amphipath'ic. Relating to molecules possessing groups with characteristically different properties, e.g., molecules that are hydrophobic at one end and hydrophilic at the other end.

amphit'richous, amphit'richate. Having flagella or a flagellum at both ends, as in certain microorganisms.

amphixeno'sis. A transmissible disease of vertebrates caused by a microorganism, such as *Trypanosoma cruzi*, which can inhabit either man or animal as its maintenance host. Cf anthropozoonosis and zooanthroponosis.

ampho-. Prefix meaning two or double.

am'phophil. Denoting certain cells that stain readily with either acid or basic dyes.

amphor'ic. The quality of a sound sometimes heard in auscultation, described as that produced by blowing over the mouth of a bottle.

am'plitude. One of three measurements of the vibration of a sound wave (others are frequency and wavelength); the vertical vibrations that reflect the intensity of sound.

am'pule, am'poule, am'pul. A small glass container sealed to preserve the sterile condition of its contents, which are used primarily for subcutaneous, intramuscular, or intravenous injections.

ampul'la. A saclike dilation of a canal, as seen in the semicircular canals of the inner ear.

a. of deferent duct, a. of vas deferens; the dilation of the duct just before it is joined by the duct of the seminal vesicle.

a. of Vater, the short dilated tube formed by the union of the pancreatic and common bile ducts just before they empty into the duodenum; also called greater papilla.

phrenic a., the normal expansion of the lower end

of the esophagus.

ampulli'tis. Inflammation of an ampulla, especially of the dilated end of the deferent duct of the testis.

amputa'tion. The removal of a limb or any appendage of the body.

root a., the surgical removal of the apical portion of the root of a tooth.

amputee'. A person with one or more amputated limbs.

double a., a person with two amputated limbs.

amyg'dala, *pl.* **amyg'dalae. 1.** Any almond-shaped anatomic structure, such as a tonsil. **2.** One of two ovoid masses of gray matter, located in the front part of the temporal lobe of the brain, in the roof of the terminal portion of the inferior horn of the lateral ventricle; also called amygdaloid nuclear complex.

amyg'dalase. A glucoside-splitting enzyme.

amyg'daloid. Almond-shaped.

am'yl. A univalent organic radical (C_5H_{11}).

a. nitrate, a flammable and volatile yellow liquid, $C_5H_{11}NO_2$; used as a motor depressant, and inhaled to relieve pain in angina pectoris.

am'ylase. An enzyme that promotes the splitting of starches.

pancreatic a., one present in pancreatic juice; also called amylopsin.

salivary a., one present in saliva; also called ptyalin.

α-amylase. See α-1,4-glucan-4-glucanohydrolase.

β-amylase. See α-1,4-glucan maltohydrolase.

am'ylin. The insoluble constituent or cellulose of starch.

amylogen'esis. Starch formation.

am'yloid. 1. Resembling starch. **2.** An abnormal protein-polysaccharide complex deposited in various organs or tissues.

amyloido'sis. Accumulation of an abnormal protein, amyloid, in various tissues of the body.

primary a., amyloidosis which is not caused by another disease, usually involving the tongue, intestinal tract, lungs, skin, and skeletal and heart muscles.

secondary a., amyloidosis resulting from a chronic disease, such as tuberculosis, rheumatoid arthritis, osteomyelitis, etc.; usually affecting the liver, kidneys, and spleen.

amylopec'tin. A polysaccharide found in the insoluble component of starch.

amylopha'gia. Abnormal craving for starch; also called starch eating.

amylop'sin. Pancreatic amylase; see under amylase.

amylos'e. The relatively soluble component of

starch.

amyoto'nia. Lack of muscular tone.

a. congenita, amyotonia occurring in infants, affecting only the musculature innervated by spinal nerves; also called Oppenheim's syndrome.

amyotro'phic. Relating to muscular degeneration or atrophy.

amyot'rophy. Wasting or degeneration of muscles.

ANA. Abbreviation for American Nurses' Association.

anab'asis. The progression or increase in severity of a disease.

anabol'ic. Promoting or exhibiting anabolism.

anab'olism. The process by which living tissues build complex compounds from substances of a simple constitution; an energy-consuming constructive metabolic process; the reverse of catabolism.

anabolis'tic. Having constructive metabolic properties, such as the ability to build complex molecules out of simple ones.

anacid'ity. Lack of acidity; especially, lack of hydrochloric acid in the gastric juice.

anaclit'ic. Having a psychologic dependence on others, as the normal dependence of an infant on its mother or mother substitute.

a. depression, see under depression.

anacrot'ic. Having an abnormal pulse, evidenced in a pulse tracing in which the ascending line of the curve has a small additional wave or shoulder, as in aortic stenosis; also called anadicrotic.

anadicrot'ic. See anacrotic.

ana'erobe. An organism that does not grow when freely exposed to air.

facultative a., a microorganism that can grow in either the presence or absence of free oxygen.

anaero'bic. Growing in the absence of oxygen.

anaerogen'ic. Producing no gas.

anagen'esis. Regeneration of tissue or structure.

a'nal. Relating to or near the anus.

analep'tic. A central nervous system stimulant; a restorative medication.

analge'sia. Absence of sensibility to pain; during labor, analgesia may be induced by intermittent administration of certain inhalation anesthetics in concentrations lower than those required for surgical anesthesia.

analge'sic. 1. Relieving pain. **2.** A medication that relieves pain without affecting consciousness; the most commonly used analgesic is aspirin (acetylsalicylic acid).

anal'gia. The condition of being without pain.

anal'ogous. Similar in function or appearance, but not in origin or development.

an'alogue. 1. An organ or part similar in function

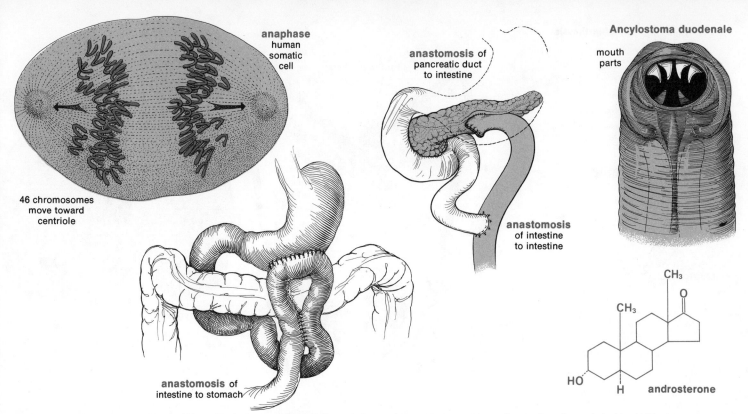

anaphase
human
somatic
cell

46 chromosomes
move toward
centriole

anastomosis of
pancreatic duct
to intestine

anastomosis
of intestine
to intestine

anastomosis of
intestine to stomach

Ancylostoma duodenale

mouth
parts

androsterone

to one in another organism of a different species but different in structure or development. **2.** A chemical compound similar in structure to another but dissimilar in composition.

anal′ysand. A patient who is being treated with psychoanalysis.

anal′ysis, *pl.* **anal′yses. 1.** The separation of a substance into its simple constituents. **2.** Psychoanalysis.

adsorption a., see chromatography.

chromatographic a., see chromatography.

dermatoglyphic a., the analysis of the variety of pattern configurations of epidermal ridges for abnormal characteristics.

gastric a., aspiration and study of the stomach contents after the ingestion of a test meal.

gravimetric a., determination by weight of the exact proportions of the components of a substance.

qualitative a., determination of the nature of the constituents of a substance.

quantitative a., determination of the quantity, as well as the nature, of the components of a substance.

spectrum a., determination of the components of a gas by means of a spectroscope.

volumetric a., quantitative analysis by weight.

an′alyst. See psychoanalyst.

analy′zer, analy′zor. 1. A polarizing filter used to determine the direction of polarization of a beam of light. **2.** One of two filters in an instrument used for the study of a polarized beam of light (polariscope).

wave a., an apparatus by means of which complex wave forms are separated into their component frequencies.

anamne′sis. 1. The act of recalling to memory. **2.** The history of a patient's illness.

an′aphase. The third stage of cell division by mitosis, during which the two chromatids of each chromosome separate and migrate along the spindle fibers toward opposite poles.

anaphore′sis. 1. The motion of electrically charged particles in solution toward a positive pole or anode. **2.** Reduction of sweat secretion.

anaphylac′tic. Characterized by a markedly abnormal or extreme sensitivity to a biologically foreign protein.

anaphylactogen′ic. 1. A substance that produces an exaggerated or severe reaction to the presence of a foreign protein. **2.** Anything that reduces immunity.

anaphylac′toid. Resembling anaphylaxis.

anaphylax′is. An immediate, severe hypersensitivity reaction, sometimes fatal, induced by a second injection of an antigen.

slow-reacting substance of a., a potent contractor of smooth muscle in the bronchi released from the lungs of allergic humans on challenge with specific pollens.

anapla′sia. 1. The loss of normal differentiation of cells, as in tumor cells. **2.** A reversion of cells to an embryonic state in which reproductive activity is very pronounced.

anaplas′tic. Of or relating to plastic surgery.

anar′thria. Loss of ability to articulate properly.

anasar′ca. Generalized massive edema in subcutaneous tissue; may be due to cardiac, renal, or hepatic disease, and to starvation.

anas′tole. Retraction of the margins of a wound.

anas′tomose. 1. To open one into the other; said of blood vessels. **2.** To create by surgery a channel between tubular structures, as intestines or blood vessels.

anastomo′sis. 1. A connection between tubular structures. **2.** The surgical or pathologic formation of a channel between tubular structures, as blood vessels or intestines.

anastomot′ic. Relating to an anastomosis.

anatom′ic, anatom′ical. 1. Relating to anatomy. **2.** Relating to structure as opposed to function.

anatomic snuffbox. A more or less triangular depression formed on the radial aspect of the wrist when the thumb is extended and abducted.

anat′omist. A specialist in anatomy.

anat′omy. The science of the body structure of an organism and its parts.

comparative a., the study of the bodies of different animals in relation to one another.

dental a., the branch of anatomy that deals with the external and internal structure of teeth and the surrounding tissues.

developmental a., see embryology.

gross a., study of structures as seen without the aid of a microscope.

microscopic a., see histology.

pathologic a., the study of diseased or injured tissues.

topographic a., the study of the location of the various organs and parts of the body and their relations to one another and to the surface of the body.

an′chorage. 1. The surgical fixation of a prolapsed organ. **2.** In dentistry, a tooth or part of a tooth to which a bridge, crown, filling, etc. is attached; in orthodontics, the teeth used as support for an appliance.

an′cillary. Subordinate; auxiliary.

anconi′tis. Inflammation of the elbow joint.

Ancylos′toma. A genus of nematode parasites which attach themselves to the mucosa of the duo-

denum where they suck the blood of the host, causing anemia; they enter the body of man in the larval stage, usually through the skin of the feet and ankles.

A. duodenale, a variety of hookworm characterized by the presence of two pairs of teeth; species predominate in southern Europe, coastal North Africa, northern India, and Japan; also called "Old World" hookworm and *Uncinaria duodenalis.*

ancylostomi′asis. Hookworm disease; infestation with the parasite *Ancylostoma duodenale* or *Necator americanus,* causing anemia by the destruction of red blood cells; in children the infection may result in mental and physical retardation; also called miner's, brickmaker's, or mountain anemia and uncinariasis.

cutaneous a., the appearance of small itchy vesicles at the site of entrance of the *Ancylostoma* larvae, usually on the feet, prior to the manifestation of intestinal symptoms; also called ancylostomiasis dermatitis and ground itch.

andro-. Combining form denoting the male sex.

an′drogen. A substance (usually a hormone) that stimulates the development of male sex characteristics.

androgen′ic. Relating to an androgen or producing male characteristics.

androg′ynous. Relating to female pseudohermaphroditism (a true female with masculine characteristics).

an′droid. Manlike.

androp′athy. Any disease peculiar to the male sex.

andros′terone. An androgen (male sex hormone) derived from testosterone metabolism.

anecho′ic. Denoting absence of echoes in an area studied with sonography.

ane′mia. Any condition in which the concentration of hemoglobin in the blood is below the normal for the age and sex of the patient; usually there is also a reduction in the number of red blood cells per mm^3 and in the volume of packed red blood cells per 100 ml of blood.

Addison's a., see pernicious anemia.

aplastic a., anemia characterized by bone marrow insufficiency or failure to produce a normal number of cells for discharge into the blood stream; usually, but not always, associated with a hypocellular bone marrow and frequently with reduction of all the formed elements of the blood (pancytopenia).

congenital hypoplastic a., chronic pure red blood cell aplasia; a form occurring in young infants and marked primarily by depletion of erythroid tissue in the bone marrow, resulting in pallor, listlessness, and poor appetite; minor associated congeni-

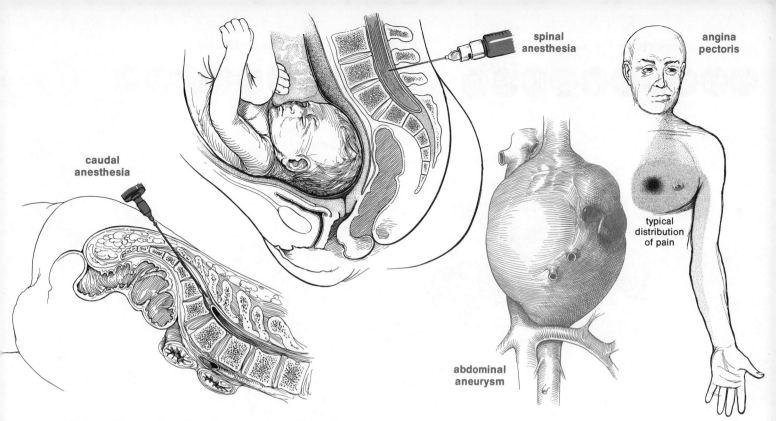

caudal anesthesia

spinal anesthesia

angina pectoris

typical distribution of pain

abdominal aneurysm

tal abnormalities are often observed; also called erythroid hypoplasia.

congenital spherocytic a., see spherocytosis.

Cooley's a., Mediterranean a., see thalassemia.

hemolytic a., anemia resulting from abnormal destruction of red blood cells in the body.

hypochromic a., anemia characterized by a decrease in the hemoglobin content of the red blood cells, i.e., reduced mean corpuscular hemoglobin concentration (MCHC).

hypochromic microcytic a., anemia characterized by a decrease in the hemoglobin concentration of red blood cells and by smaller than normal cells, i.e, decreased mean corpuscular volume (MCV); usually caused by iron deficiency.

iron deficiency a., hypochromic microcytic anemia.

macrocytic a., any anemia in which the average size of circulating red blood cells is greater than normal, i.e., the mean corpuscular volume (MCV) is increased. See also megaloblastic anemia.

Marchiafava-Micheli a., paroxysmal nocturnal hemoglobinuria; see under hemoglobinuria.

megaloblastic a., any anemia usually caused by deficiency of vitamin B₁₂ or folic acid; characterized by macrocytic erythrocytes and an increased number of megaloblasts in the bone marrow; includes pernicious anemia and the anemias caused by folic acid deficiency, such as sprue, "blind loop" syndrome, and megaloblastic anemia of pregnancy.

myelophthisic a., myelopathic a., anemia resulting from the destruction of blood cell-forming (hemopoietic) tissues by space-occupying lesions.

normochromic a., anemia in which the hemoglobin concentration in the red blood cells is within the normal range, i.e., the mean corpuscular hemoglobin concentration (MCHC) is from 32 to 36 per cent.

nutritional a., anemia resulting from lack of some essential materials in the diet, as iron or vitamins.

pernicious a., Addison's a., a chronic progressive, megaloblastic anemia, occurring mostly in individuals in the fifth decade or older; caused by a lack of secretion of the intrinsic factor (enzyme-like) present in normal gastric juice, which is necessary for adequate absorption of vitamin B₁₂; it is frequently associated with neurologic damage.

primary refractory a., any of several persistent, frequently advanced anemias, that is not the result of any other primary disease (e.g., chronic disease of the liver or kidneys) and that does not respond to any treatment except blood transfusions; also called aregenatory or hypoplastic anemia, and progressive hypocythemia.

refractory a., aplastic anemia.

sickle cell a., a hereditary chronic anemia, peculiar to Negroes, in which a large portion of the red blood cells have a crescent or sickle shape, due to the presence of an abnormal hemoglobin (hemoglobin S); also called drepanocytosis.

ane′mic. Of or pertaining to anemia.

anenceph′aly. A congenital developmental defect consisting of absence of the vault of the skull, with an exposed, poorly developed, degenerated brain, resulting from the neural tube's failure to close in the cephalic area; the affected infant usually dies within a few days after birth.

aner′gic. 1. Relating to a diminished or absent response to specific antigens. **2.** Marked by abnormal lack of energy.

an′ergy. 1. Lack of response to the injection of an antigen. **2.** Inability to react; sluggishness.

an′eroid. Not using or containing fluid.

anesthe′sia. Partial or total loss of sensation, with or without loss of consciousness, due to injury or disease, or induced by the administration of a drug.

caudal a., anesthesia produced by the injection of an anesthetic solution into the caudal part of the spinal canal.

crossed a., anesthesia on one side of the body caused by a lesion on the opposite side of the brain.

epidural a., anesthesia produced by the injection of an anesthetic agent into the extradural space.

field block a., anesthesia produced by injecting the anesthetic solution in such a way as to create a wall around the operative field.

general a., a state of unconsciousness and complete loss of sensation produced by the administration of an anesthetic, either by inhalation, intravenously, or intramuscularly; also called surgical anesthesia.

intraneural a., local anesthesia produced by injecting the anesthetic solution into a nerve trunk.

local a., anesthesia of a limited area of the body.

nerve block a., anesthesia produced by injecting the anesthetic solution around and near a nerve.

rectal a., general anesthesia produced by introducing the anesthetic solution into the rectum.

saddle block a., anesthesia of the area of the buttocks, perineum, and inner thighs produced by injection of the anesthetic agent low in the dural sac.

spinal a., (1) anesthesia of the lower part of the body produced by injecting an anesthetic agent in the subarachnoid space around the spinal cord; (2) anesthesia due to injury or disease of the spinal cord.

anesthesiol′ogist. A physician who specializes in anesthesiology.

anesthesiol′ogy. The branch of science concerned with the study and administration of anesthesia.

anesthet′ic. A drug that produces anesthesia.

anes′thetist. A person trained to administer anesthetics.

anes′thetize. To render insensible with anesthesia.

anes′trus. The interval of sexual quiescence between two estrous cycles in mammals or prolonged failure of estrus in a mature animal.

an′euploid. An organism having an abnormal number of chromosomes.

aneuploi′dy. The state of having an abnormal number of chromosomes.

an′eurysm. A circumscribed sac-like bulging of a blood vessel, usually an artery.

abdominal a., aneurysm of the abdominal aorta.

dissecting a., one in which blood forces its way between the layers of an arterial wall, causing them to separate; the blood may enter through an intimal tear or by interstitial hemorrhage.

exogenous a., traumatic a., one due to trauma to the affected vessel.

false a., a blood clot within the wall of an artery.

fusiform a., a spindle-shaped dilatation of an artery.

mycotic a., one caused by growth of microorganisms within the vessel wall.

ventricular a., dilatation of the ventricular wall of the heart.

aneurys′mal. Of or relating to an aneurysm; also called aneurysmatic.

aneurysmec′tomy. Excision of an aneurysm.

ANF. Abbreviation of antinuclear factor.

angiecta′sia, angiecta′sis. Dilatation of a blood vessel or a lymphatic.

angii′tis, angi′tis. Inflammation of a blood or lymph vessel.

hypersensitivity a., inflammation of a blood vessel as a manifestation of an allergic reaction to a specific substance.

an′gina. A severe strangling pain.

abdominal a., pain occurring in the abdominal area as a result of ischemia of the intestine.

a. decubitus, attack of angina pectoris precipitated by the recumbent position, usually occurring at night.

a. pectoris, constricting pain in the chest due to insufficient blood supply to the heart muscle, usually precipitated by effort and relieved rapidly by rest or nitrites; the pain is usually retrosternal and frequently radiates to the precordium, the left shoulder and arm, or the neck.

Ludwig's a., painful inflammation and pus formation in the area of the submaxillary gland, usually

angiotensin I (decapeptide)

Asp—Arg—Val—Tyr—Tle—His—Pro—Pre—His—Leu → **angiotensin II (octapeptide)** Asp—Arg—Val—Tyr—Ile—His—Pro—Pre + His Leu

hydrolyzing enzyme

cornea

venous sinus of sclera

anterior chamber angle

iris

superior angle of scapula

Inferior angle of scapula

sternal angle

body of sternum

anisocoria

resulting from a tooth infection.

Vincent's a., fusospirochetal pharyngitis; see pharyngitis, fusospirochetal.

an'ginal. Relating to, or of the nature, of angina.

an'gioblast. 1. Embryonic tissue from which blood cells and blood vessels are formed. **2.** A vessel-forming cell.

angioblasto'ma. See hemangioblastoma.

angiocardiog'raphy. X-ray examination of the heart and great vessels following the intravenous injection of radiopaque material.

angiocardiop'athy. Any disease of the heart and blood vessels.

angioede'ma. Angioneurotic edema; giant hives, an allergic reaction in the skin or underlying tissue.

angiogen'esis. The formation of blood vessels.

an'giogram. A roentgenogram of a vessel obtained by outlining the structure with a radiopaque material.

angiog'raphy. 1. Description of vessels. **2.** X-ray examination of blood vessels after injection of a radiopaque material.

selective a., the injection of radiopaque solution through a catheter into the vessels of the specific area of the body to be studied.

an'gioid. Resembling a blood vessel.

angiokerato'ma. A skin disorder consisting of a varying number of multiple violaceous (violet or purple discoloration) lesions; also called telangiectatic wart.

angiokerato'sis. The occurrence of angiokeratoma.

angiol'ogy. The study of blood and lymph vessels of the body.

angio'ma. A tumor composed of dilated blood vessels (hemangioma) or lymph vessels (lymphangioma).

cavernous a., cavernous hemangioma; see under hemangioma.

angiomato'sis. A condition marked by the presence of multiple angiomas.

retinocerebral a., see von Hippel-Lindau disease.

angio'matous. Resembling a tumor made up of dilated vessels (angioma).

angioneuro'sis. Paralysis or spasm of blood vessels caused by disease or injury to the vasomotor nervous system.

angiop'athy. Disease of blood vessels or lymphatics.

angioplas'ty. Surgical reconstruction of a blood vessel.

angiopoiet'ic. Causing the formation of blood vessels.

an'giospasm. Vasospasm; spasmodic contraction of a blood vessel.

angiosteno'sis. Constriction or narrowing of one or more blood vessels.

angioten'sin. A peptide present in the blood and formed by the action of the enzyme renin on a globulin in the blood plasma; renin splits off from its substrate a decapeptide known as angiotensin I, which is then changed by a converting enzyme to the octapeptide angiotensin II, a potent vasoconstrictor and stimulator of aldosterone synthesis and release; formerly known as hypertensin.

angiotensin'ogen. An α_2-globulin, also known as renin substrate; it has no pressor activity in the intact form but is acted upon by the enzyme renin which splits off a decapeptide unit, angiotensin I; formerly known as hypertensinogen.

an'giotome. A segment of the vascular system of the embryo.

angiot'onin. See angiotensin.

an'giotroph'ic. Relating to nutrition of blood and lymphatic vessels; also called vasotrophic.

angle. The figure formed by two lines or planes diverging from a common point; the space between two lines or planes diverging from a common point.

acromial a., the palpable point where the lateral border of the acromion joins, and becomes continuous with, the spine of the scapula.

a. of convergence, the angle between the line of vision and the median line.

a. of the jaw, the angle formed by the lower edge of the body of the mandible and the posterior edge of the ramus.

a. of Louis, see sternal angle.

anterior chamber a., angle formed at the junction of the iris and cornea; also called iridocorneal or filtration angle, and angle of the iris.

carrying a., the angle made by the axes of the arm and forearm when the forearm is extended.

cerebellopontine a., space at the junction of the cerebellum and pons.

critical a., the angle of incidence (angle made with the perpendicular by a light ray passing from one medium to another) which results in a refracted ray; if the angle of incidence is greater than 90°, the ray is reflected.

filtration a., anterior chamber angle.

inferior a. of scapula, the angle formed by the junction of the lateral and medial borders of the scapula.

line a., the angle formed by the junction of any two surfaces of a tooth.

point a., the meeting of three tooth surfaces at a point, forming a corner.

pontine a., cerebellopontine angle.

sternal a., the angle or ridge on the anterior surface of the sternum (breastbone) at the junction of its body and manubrium; also called angle of Louis.

superior a. of scapula, angle formed by the junction of the superior and medial borders of the scapula; formerly called medial angle.

ang'strom, Ang'ström (Å, A). A unit of length equal to a ten-thousandth of a micron; 10^{-7} mm; used especially to measure the length of light waves or other electromagnetic radiation and cytologic ultrastructures.

Anguil'lula. *Strongyloides.*

anhidro'sis. Marked deficiency of sweat.

anhidrot'ic, anidrot'ic. Anything that diminishes the secretion of sweat.

anhy'drase. An enzyme that promotes the removal of water from a compound.

anhy'dride. A compound (oxide) derived from an acid by the abstraction of water.

anhy'drous. Without water.

an'iline. An oily, colorless or brown compound derived from benzene; used in the preparation of dyes.

an'ion. A negatively charged ion that is characteristically attracted to the positively charged anode; indicated as a minus sign, e.g., Cl⁻.

anion'ic. Relating to or containing a negatively charged ion; attracted to the anode or positively charged pole when a current is passed through a solution.

anirid'ria. Complete or partial absence of the iris; also called irideremia.

aniseiko'nia. A defect of vision in which the image of an object seen by one eye is of a different size than the one seen by the other eye.

anisochroma'sia. Condition in which only the periphery of the red blood cells is colored while the central portion is almost colorless, as in certain types of anemias caused by iron deficiency.

anisochromat'ic. Not of the same color.

anisocor'ia. A condition in which the pupils of the two eyes differ in size.

anisocyto'sis. Abnormal variation in size of the red blood cells.

anisometro'pia. Difference in the refractive power of the two eyes.

anitrog'enous. Non-nitrogenous.

ankle. The joint between the foot and the leg formed by the articulation of the tibia and fibula above with the talus below.

ankylobleph'aron. Adhesion of the upper and lower eyelids.

an'kylogloss'ia. Tongue-tie.

an'kylosed. Denoting an abnormally immobilized joint.

angina | ankylosed

18

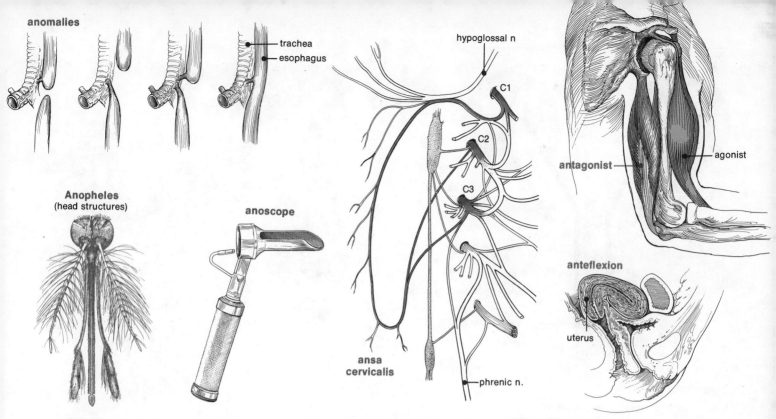

anomalies
- trachea
- esophagus

Anopheles
(head structures)

anoscope

hypoglossal n

C1

C2

C3

ansa
cervicalis

phrenic n.

antagonist

agonist

anteflexion

uterus

ankylo′sis. Abnormal immobility and fixation of a joint.

　artificial a., see arthrodesis.

　bony a., abnormal fusion of the bones forming a joint; also called true ankylosis.

　dental a., fixation of a tooth to its socket as a result of ossification of the surrounding membranes.

　fibrous a., one caused by the presence of fibrous bands between the bones forming the joint.

　true a., see bony ankylosis.

ankylot′ic. Marked by or relating to ankylosis.

an′lage. Primordium (2); the embryonic structure from which the adult organ is developed.

anneal′. To soften a metal by controlled heating and cooling; the process makes a metal more easily adapted and bent.

anneal′ing. In dentistry, the heating of gold leaf for the purpose of removing contaminants prior to its insertion into a cavity.

an′nular. Circular or ring-shaped.

an′nulus. Anulus.

an′ode. The positive pole of a galvanic battery; also called positive electrode.

anodon′tia. The congenital absence of a tooth or teeth.

an′odyne. An agent that has pain-relieving qualities.

anogen′ital. Relating to the anus and genitalia.

anomalo′pia. Partial color blindness in which perception of red or green is less than normal.

anom′aly. Anything marked by considerable deviation from the normal.

　Ebstein′s a., distortion and downward displacement of the tricuspid valve, resulting in impaired function of the right ventricle.

　Pelger-Huét nuclear a., inherited anomaly of neutrophilic leukocytes characterized by nonlobulation of their nuclei.

ano′mia. Inability to name, or to recall the names of objects; also called optic aphasia.

Anoph′eles. A genus of mosquitoes of the family Culicidae, some members of which transmit the malaria parasite to man.

anophthal′mos. Congenital absence of a true eyeball.

anop′sia. 1. Failure to use one eye, as in strabismus. **2.** Hypertropia.

anor′chidism, an′orchism. Congenital absence of the testis, unilaterally or bilaterally.

anoret′ic. 1. Having no appetite. **2.** An agent that tends to depress appetite.

anorex′ia. Loss of appetite.

　a. nervosa, condition marked by great loss of appetite leading to emaciation and metabolic derangement, attended by serious neurotic symptoms;

occurs predominantly in white, middle class, adolescent females with a tendency toward mild obesity.

anorex′iant. Anything that results in appetite loss (anorexia).

a′noscope. An instrument for inspecting the anus and lower rectum.

anosigmoidos′copy. Visual examination of the anus, rectum, and sigmoid colon with the aid of an instrument.

anos′mia. Absence of the sense of smell.

anosogno′sia. Unawareness, real or assumed, of a physical illness or defect.

anov′ular, anov′ulatory. Denoting a menstrual period not accompanied by ovulation.

anoxe′mia. Hypoxemia; deficiency of oxygen in the arterial blood.

anox′ia. Abnormal reduction of oxygen in body tissues; also called oxygen deficiency and hypoxia.

an′sa, pl. **an′sae.** Any looplike structure.

　a. cervicalis, a nerve loop in the cervical plexus consisting of fibers from the first three cervical nerves, some of which accompany the hypoglossal nerve for a short distance.

　a. hypoglossi, ansa cervicalis.

　Henle′s a., nephronic loop; see under loop.

ant. An insect of the family Formicidae.

　fire a., an aggressive South American ant (genus *Solenopsis*), now commonly seen in the southern United States, whose sting can cause severe allergic reactions, including difficulty in breathing, sweating, nausea, itching, and periods of unconsciousness; it is the only insect in the United States whose sting produces a pustule (a pus-containing eruption).

antac′id. An agent that reduces the acidity of the gastric juice or other secretions; the most commonly used agents include aluminum hydroxide, magnesium hydroxide, and calcium carbonate.

antag′onism. Mutual resistance or opposition as between muscles, drugs, bacteria, etc.

antag′onist. Acting in opposition or tending to nullify the action of another; said of muscles, drugs, etc.

　competitive a., see antimetabolite.

antebra′chial. Of or relating to the forearm.

antecar′dium. See precordium.

an′te ci′bum (a.c.). Latin for before meals.

antecub′ital. Located in front of the elbow.

anteflex′ion. A type of displacement characterized by an abnormal bending forward of the upper part of an organ.

anteloca′tion. Denoting the forward displacement of an organ, e.g., the uterus, as a whole.

antemet′ic. Tending to control nausea and vomiting.

antemor′tem. Before death.

antena′tal. Occurring before birth; also called prenatal.

antepar′tum. Before childbirth.

ante′rior. In front; ventral.

anterior tibial compartment syndrome. Ischemic myositis and necrosis of the muscles of the anterior compartment of the leg resulting from vascular insufficiency secondary to specific vessel disease or injury, or to segmental spasm of the anterior tibial artery; seen in some young people following unaccustomed strenous activity.

antero-. Prefix meaning before.

anteroinfe′rior. Located in front and below.

anterolat′eral. In front and to one side.

anterome′dial. In front and toward the middle.

anteroposte′rior. 1. Relating to both front and back. **2.** Directed from the the front to the back.

anterosupe′rior. In front and above.

antever′sion. The leaning forward of an organ, such as the uterus, as a whole, without bending.

antevert′ed. Tilted forward.

anthe′lix. See antihelix.

anthelmin′thic, anthelmin′tic, antihelmin′thic. Able to destroy or expel intestinal worms.

anthrace′mia. The presence of *Bacillus anthracis* in the blood.

anthraconecro′sis. Degeneration and transformation of tissue into a dry black mass; also called black gangrene.

anthracosilico′sis. Fibrous hardening of the lungs due to continuous inhalation of coal and stove dust.

anthraco′sis. Disease caused by accumulation of carbon in the lungs.

anthracot′ic. Marked by anthracosis.

anthrax′. An acute infectious disease of wild and domesticated animals which may be transmitted to man either directly or by contact with hides or hair infected with the anthrax bacillus; the characteristic lesion in man resembles a carbuncle.

　cutaneous a., (1) a skin disease appearing on the exposed areas of the face, neck, hands, or arms; it begins as a papule that becomes vesicular, then necrotic with a purple to black crust surrounded by extensive edema; also called malignant pustule and anthrax boil. (2) a localized disease of cattle and horses marked by swellings due to infection of skin abrasions and wounds with the anthrax bacillus; also called carbuncular fever.

　gastroenteric a., see intestinal anthrax.

　intestinal a., a form of internal anthrax marked by headache, fever, vomiting, bloody diarrhea, prostration, and frequently hemorrhage from mu-

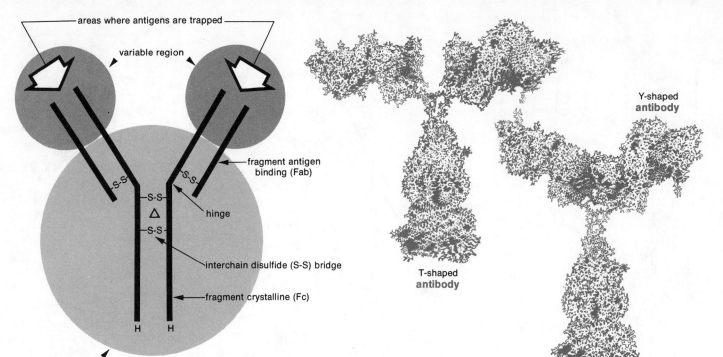

areas where antigens are trapped

variable region

fragment antigen binding (Fab)

hinge

interchain disulfide (S-S) bridge

fragment crystalline (Fc)

constant region

structure of an **antibody**

Y-shaped **antibody**

T-shaped **antibody**

cous membranes; death usually occurs; also called gastroenteric anthrax.

 pulmonary a., internal anthrax caused by inhalation of dust containing the anthrax bacillus; marked by chills, fever, rapid respiration, cough, pain in the back and legs, and extreme prostration; also called wool-sorters' disease.

an'throne. A substance used as a reagent to detect the presence of carbohydrates.

anthropo-. Combining form meaning man or human.

anthropog'eny, anthropogen'esis. The scientific study of man's origin and development, both individual and racial.

anthropol'ogy. The branch of science concerned with the origin, development, and behavior of man.

anthropom'etry. The study of comparative measurements of the human body for use in anthropologic classification.

anthropomor'phism. The attribution of human qualities to inanimate objects, animals, or natural phenomena.

anthropopho'bia. Abnormal aversion to human companionship.

anthropozoono'sis. Disease of man acquired from lower vertebrates that harbor the pathogenic organisms, e.g., trichinosis, rabies, etc.; cf. zooanthroponosis and amphixenosis.

anti-. Prefix meaning against or counteraction.

antialler'gic. Denoting anything that prevents, or alleviates, an allergic reaction.

anti-angiogen'esis. The prevention of new vessel sprouts from penetrating into an early tumor implant; a technique, currently experimental, for prevention of cancer growth.

antibacte'rial. Destructive to or preventing the growth of bacteria, e.g., spermine, the principle self-sterilizing factor in semen.

antibio'sis. The association of two organisms whereby one is affected detrimentally.

antibiot'ic. Any substance, as penicillin or streptomycin, derived from fungi or bacteria, that destroys or inhibits the growth of microorganisms.

 broad-spectrum a., an antibiotic which is effective against a variety of microorganisms, particularly against both gram-negative and gram-positive bacteria.

an'tibody. A three-lobed globulin containing two short and two long chains of protein, found in the blood and other body fluids, that can be incited by the presence of antigen (microorganisms, foreign proteins, etc.); it has a destructive influence on the antigen that stimulated its formation, thus producing immunity; the structure has considerable flexibility and is "hinged," so that it can pivot from a

taut T-shape to a forked Y-shape.

 natural a.'s, antibodies which occur naturally in the body without known antigen stimulation.

antichol'agogue. An agent that reduces the secretion of bile.

anticholiner'gic. Inhibiting the action of a parasympathetic nerve.

anticholines'terase. An agent that inhibits the action of cholinesterase.

anticoag'ulant. Any substance that prevents coagulation of blood.

antico'don. The three-base sequence of transfer RNA which pairs with a codon in messenger RNA.

anticom'plement. A substance that neutralizes the action of complement (material in normal serum that helps to destroy pathogens).

anticomplemen'tary. Having the ability to neutralize the action of complement.

anticonvul'sive. Any substance that serves to prevent or arrest convulsions.

antidepres'sant. 1. Counteracting depression. **2.** Any agent used in treating pathologic depressive states; also called psychic energizer and thymoleptic.

antidiarrhe'al, antidiarrhet'ic. An agent that alleviates diarrhea.

antidiure'sis. Reduction of urinary excretion.

antidiuret'ic. An agent that causes reduction of urine formation.

an'tidotal. Relating to an antidote.

an'tidote. An agent that counteracts the effects of an ingested poison, either by inactivating it or by opposing its action following absorption.

antidrom'ic. Conducting an impulse in a reverse direction of the normal.

antiemet'ic. 1. Preventing or arresting nausea. **2.** A drug that prevents or relieves nausea and vomiting by exerting its effects on the vestibular apparatus of the ear, the chemoreceptor trigger zone, the cerebral cortex, or the vomiting center of the brain.

antien'zyme. A substance that neutralizes the action of an enzyme.

antiepilep'tic. An agent that tends to prevent an epileptic convulsion.

antifibrinol'ysin. A substance that retards the disintegration of fibrin in blood clots.

antifun'gal. Destructive to fungus.

an'tigen. A foreign substance which stimulates an immune response; the immune response may be in the form of antibody formation and/or cell-mediated immunity.

 Australia a., hepatitis-associated antigen.

 endogenous a., any antigen found within an individual.

 exogenous a., any antigen originating from the

individual's environment, e.g., pollen.

 hepatitis-associated a. (HAA), antigen found in the sera of patients afflicted with hepatitis, believed to be associated with the type B virus; originally found in the serum of an Australian aborigine; also called hepatitis B or Australia antigen.

 hepatitis B a. (HBAg), hepatitis-associated antigen.

 heterologous a., an antigen common to more than one species; also called heterogenetic antigen.

 homologous a., an antigen produced by one individual which incites the formation of antibodies in another individual of the same species; more specifically, a genetically controlled antigenic determinant that distinguishes one individual of a given species from another; also called isoantigen and alloantigen.

 T a., antigen present in nuclei of cells infected by certain tumor viruses; thought to be an early virus-specific protein.

antigen'ic. Pertaining to or having the properties of an antigen, especially that of inciting the formation of antibody.

antigenic'ity. The property of being antigenic.

an'tigenize. The administration of an antigenic substance to an individual or animal.

antihe'lix. The curved prominence on the external ear parallel to and in front of the helix; also called anthelix.

antihemagglu'tinin. A substance that checks the action of hemagglutinin.

antihemol'ysin. An agent that inhibits the action of a hemolysin.

antihidrot'ic. See antisudorific.

antihis'tamine. Any of several drugs used to counteract the action of histamine in the treatment of allergic symptoms.

antihistamin'ic. Tending to neutralize the action of histamine; said of an agent having such an effect and used to relieve the symptoms of allergy.

antihyperten'sive. Anything that reduces the blood pressure.

anti-inflam'matory. Relieving inflammation.

antimala'rial. Denoting an agent that prevents or cures malaria.

antimetab'olite. In general, a substance that is chemically similar to an essential metabolite but interferes with, or prevents, its effective utilization; also called competitive antagonist.

antimitot'ic. Anything that arrests mitosis.

antimon'ic. Relating to or containing antimony.

antimo'nium. Antimony.

an'timony. A toxic, irritating, grayish, metallic element; symbol Sb, atomic number 51, atomic weight 121.77.

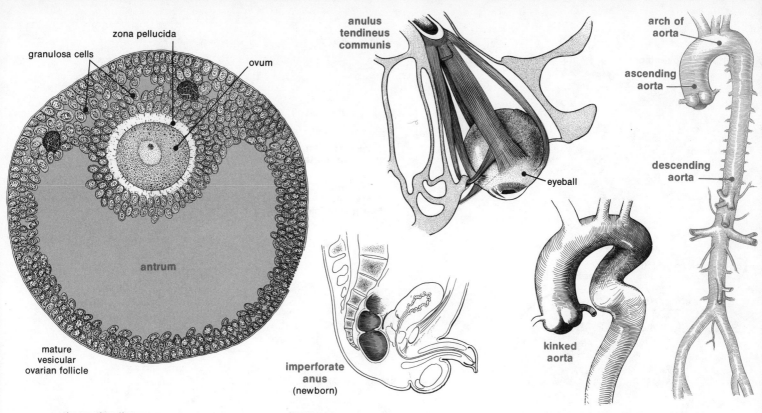

granulosa cells

zona pellucida

ovum

antrum

mature
vesicular
ovarian follicle

anulus
tendineus
communis

eyeball

imperforate
anus
(newborn)

arch of
aorta

ascending
aorta

descending
aorta

kinked
aorta

antimyasthen′ic. Tending to relieve the symptoms of myasthenia (muscular weakness).

antimycot′ic. Fungicide.

antinaus′eant. 1. Preventing nausea. **2.** An agent having such properties.

antiox′idant. A substance that prevents oxidation.

antiperistal′sis. Reverse peristaltic action of the intestines by which their contents are forced upwards.

antiper′spirant. An agent that inhibits the secretion of sweat.

antiphagocyt′ic. Inhibiting ingestion and digestion by cells (phagocytosis).

antiprothrom′bin. A substance that inhibits the conversion of prothrombin into thrombin, thus preventing coagulation of blood.

antiprurit′ic. Relieving itching.

antipyret′ic. 1. Reducing or tending to relieve fever. **2.** A medicine that reduces or relieves fever.

antipy′rine. A colorless, slightly bitter substance derived from coal tar; used to relieve pain and fever.

antirachit′ic. Tending to cure rickets.

antirheumat′ic. Tending to prevent or cure rheumatism.

antiscorbu′tic. Curing or preventing scurvy.

antisecre′tory. Inhibitiing secretions.

antisep′tic. A germicide or, under special conditions, a bacteriostat; generally used on living tissue.

an′tiserum. A human or animal serum containing specific antibodies.

antispasmod′ic. An agent that prevents or relieves involuntary muscular contractions.

antisudorif′ic. Antihidrotic; arresting the secretion of sweat.

antithrom′bin. A substance that counteracts the action of thrombin, thus preventing coagulation of blood.

antitox′in. Antibody produced in the blood and other body fluids in response to the poison of a microorganism, usually bacterial exotoxins.

antitra′gus. A projection on the external ear opposite the tragus and behind the opening of the external auditory canal.

antitrepone′mal. Destructive to treponemes (bacteria of the genus *Treponema*).

antivi′tamin. Any substance that prevents the biologic functioning of a vitamin.

antivivisec′tion. Opposition to experimentation on living animals.

antivivisec′tionist. One who is opposed to experimentation on living animals.

an′tral. Relating to an antrum (body cavity).

antrec′tomy. Surgical removal of the walls of an antrum, especially the mastoid antrum.

an′troscope. An instrument for examining an antrum or hollow space, especially the maxillary antrum.

antros′tomy. The formation of an opening or stoma, sometimes permanent, into any antrum for draining purposes.

antrot′omy. Incision into an antrum.

an′trum. A bodily chamber or cavity.

follicular a., the fluid-filled cavity within the developing ovarian follicle.

pyloric a., the dilated pyloric end of the stomach; it marks the beginning of the pyloric canal.

tympanic a., a cavity in the mastoid part of the temporal bone extending from the middle ear chamber and communicating with the mastoid air cells.

an′ulus. A ring-shaped structure.

a. inguinalis profundus, the orifice in the transversalis fascia forming the internal opening of the inguinal canal; also called deep or abdominal inguinal ring.

a. inguinalis superficialis, the orifice in the aponeurosis of the external oblique muscle forming the external opening of the inguinal canal; also called superficial, subcutaneous, or external inguinal ring.

a. tendineus communis, a fibrous ring in the ocular orbit that surrounds the optic foramen and part of the superior orbital fissure; it serves as the origin of four eye muscles; also called ligament of Zinn.

anure′sis. Total retention of urine in the bladder; failure to urinate.

anuret′ic. Relating to anuresis.

anu′ria. Complete suppression of urine; in clinical use, denoting less than 100 ml urine daily for an adult of average size.

anu′ric. Relating to anuria.

a′nus. The lower opening of the digestive tract.

imperforate a., congenital absence of anal orifice.

an′vil. See incus.

anxi′ety. A state of apprehension, uneasiness, and fear out of proportion to the real threat; the chief characteristic of the neuroses, commonly accompanied by somatic symptoms.

a. syndrome, rapid heart beat, difficulty in breathing, and profuse sweating accompanied by panic.

castration a., fear of loss of genital organs or genital function, as punishment for forbidden sexual or aggressive feelings; also called castration complex.

separation a., a feeling of danger, apprehension, and distress upon separation from a needed person.

aor′ta. The largest blood vessel in the body; the main trunk of the systemic arterial circulation, arising from the upper part of the left ventricle from which it receives blood for delivery to all tissues except the lungs.

abdominal a., the terminal part of the aorta, extending from the diaphragm to the pelvis where it divides into the common iliac arteries.

arch of the a., the curvature by which the aorta changes its course from cephalad to caudad and from which arise the brachiocephalic trunk, left common carotid, and left subclavian arteries.

ascending a., the first part of the aorta between its origin from the heart and the arch; it is about 3 cm in diameter.

descending a., the part of the aorta between the arch and the bifurcation.

kinked a., pseudocoarctation.

aor′tic. Relating to the aorta.

aortic arch syndrome. Condition seen in any of a group of disorders marked by narrowing and occlusion of one or more of the large arterial vessels originating from the aortic arch (brachiocephalic trunk, left subclavian, and left common carotid arteries); such narrowing and occlusion lead to diminished or absent pulse in the neck and arms; caused by inflammatory and/or atheromatous changes with secondary thrombosis. See also pulseless disease.

aorti′tis. Inflammation of one or more of the layers of the wall of the aorta.

rheumatoid a., aortitis associated with rheumatoid arthritis.

aort′ogram. X-ray picture of the aorta, utilizing contrast material.

aortog′raphy. Roentgenography of the aorta after the injection of a radiopaque medium.

retrograde a., aortography after forcing the radiopaque material through one of the aortic branches, in a direction opposite the bloodstream.

translumbar a., roentgenography after injection of the radiopaque material into the abdominal aorta.

aortoiliac occlusive disease. Gradual obstruction of the terminal portion of the aorta by atherosclerosis; associated clinical features include intermittent claudication of the lower back, buttocks, thighs, or calves, and atrophy of the limbs; there may also be trophic changes and impotence; also called Leriche's syndrome.

aortop′athy. Disease of the aorta.

aortot′omy. Incision into the aorta.

ap′athy. Indifference; lack of emotion.

ap′atite. A calcium fluoride phosphate, $Ca_5F(PO_4)_3$.

APC. Abbreviation for (a) a mixture containing aspirin, phenacetin, and caffeine; (b) atrial premature contraction.

aperiod′ic. Occurring irregularly.

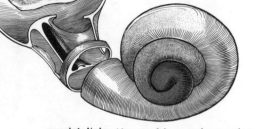

aperture of sphenoid sinus

aperture of maxillary sinus

apex (cochlea)

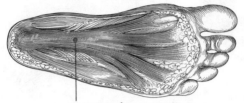

median aperture of fourth ventricle

lateral aperture of fourth ventricle

after Brödel

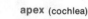

aponeurosis (plantar)

aponeurosis (pharyngeal)

---

aperistal'sis. Absence of the normal contractions of the intestines.

apertogna'thia. Open bite; see under bite.

ap'erture. 1. An opening, hole, or gap. **2.** An opening, usually adjustable, in an optical instrument that limits the amount of light passing through the lens.

   a. of maxillary sinus, a large, irregular aperture through which the maxillary sinus communicates with the nasal cavity.

   a. of sphenoid sinus, an orifice in the anterior wall of the sphenoid sinus through which the sinus opens into the nasal cavity.

   lateral a. of fourth ventricle, foramen of Luschka, one of two lateral openings on the roof of the fourth ventricle of the brain, communicating with the subarachnoid cavity.

   median a. of fourth ventricle, foramen of Magendi, an opening in the midline of the roof of the fourth ventricle of the brain, communicating with the subarachnoid cavity.

a'pex, *pl.* **ap'ices.** The tip or pointed end of a conical structure, as the heart or lung.

   orbital a., the back part of the orbit.

   root a., the tip of the root of a tooth.

apex beat. See beat, apex.

apexcar'diogram. A graphic record of the chest wall movements produced by the apex beat of the heart.

Apgar score. See score, Apgar.

apha'gia. See dysphagia.

apha'kia. Absence of the lens of the eye.

aphalan'gia. Absence of toes and fingers.

apha'sia. A general term for language disorders (reading, writing, speaking, or comprehension of written or spoken words) due to brain dysfunction, not a result of disease of the vocal organs or intellectual deficiency.

   amnesic a., inability to remember words.

   ataxic a., motor aphasia.

   auditory a., word deafness; the individual distinguishes words from other sounds but does not understand them.

   central a., aphasia caused by a lesion of the cerebral cortex.

   global a., complete loss of the power to communicate verbally.

   mixed a., a mixture of sensory and motor aphasia.

   motor a., loss of the ability to communicate by writing, speaking, or signs.

   optic a., anomia; inability to name an object recognized by sight.

   receptive a., sensory aphasia.

   sensory a., inability to understand spoken or written words, gestures, or signs.

visual a., alexia; inability to comprehend written words; also called word blindness.

apha'sic, apha'siac. Relating to or afflicted with aphasia.

apho'nia. Loss of the voice.

   hysteric a., inability to speak due to hysteria.

aphon'ic. Relating to aphonia.

aphrodis'ia. Sexual desire.

aphrodis'iac. Any agent that intensifies sexual desire.

aph'tha, *pl.* **aph'thae.** A small white patch on a mucous membrane, commonly seen in the mouth.

aph'thous. Relating to or having aphthae.

ap'ical. Relating to the apex of a structure, as the tip of the root of a tooth, the top of a lung, or the cardiac apex.

apicoect'omy. Surgical removal of the apical portion of a tooth root; also called apicectomy.

apicos'tomy. The surgical formation of an opening through the alveolar bone to the tip of a tooth root.

apitu'itarism. State in which the pituitary body has ceased to function.

APL. Abbreviation for anterior pituitary-like hormone.

aplana'sia. Absence of spherical or monochromatic aberration; also called aplanatism.

aplanat'ic. Denoting an optical system or lens free from spherical or monochromatic aberration.

apla'sia. Complete or partial failure of a tissue or an organ to develop.

   congenital thymic a., a syndrome characterized by numerous clinical features, all related to some failure in development of the third and fourth pharyngeal pouches; the parathyroid glands are either underdeveloped or absent, often leading to tetany due to parathyroid insufficiency; the thymus is similarly underdeveloped or absent, leading to an increased vulnerability to those infections usually resisted by the cell-mediated portion of the immune response; also called DiGeorge's syndrome and thymic alymphoplasia.

aplas'tic. 1. Pertaining to defective development. **2.** Relating to defective regenerative processes.

apne'a. Cessation of respiration.

apneumati'ic. Denoting a collapsed lung.

apneumato'sis. Congenital airless state of the lungs (atelectasis).

ap'ocrine. Relating to a gland in which some of the apical portion of the gland is discharged along with the secretory product; seen in axillary sweat glands.

apod'ia. Congenital absence of feet.

apoen'zyme. A protein that requires a coenzyme to function as an enzyme; the protein portion of an enzyme.

apofer'ritin. A protein of the small intestine; it combines with iron to form ferritin, which is thought to regulate the absorption of iron in the intestinal tract.

apo'lar. Without poles or processes, as certain nerve cells.

apomor'phine hydrochlo'ride. A white crystalline derivative of morphine; used as an emetic, expectorant, and hypnotic.

aponeuror'rhaphy. See fasciorrhaphy.

aponeuro'sis. A pearly white, iridescent, fibrous sheet, composed of closely packed, mostly parallel collagenous bundles; serves as a connection between a muscle and its attachment.

   epicranial a., the aponeurosis of the scalp; it covers the upper part of the skull, connecting the frontal and occipital bellies of the occipitofrontal muscle; also called galea aponeurotica.

aponeurot'ic. Relating to an aponeurosis.

ap'oplexy. Rupture of a vessel into an organ, usually referring to a cerebral vascular accident with sudden loss of consciousness; also called apoplectic stroke.

appara'tus. 1. A group of instruments or devices used together or in succession to perform a specific task. **2.** A group of organs or structures that collectively perform a common function.

   Benedict-Roth a., One used in the estimation of basal metabolic rate by measuring the amount of oxygen used during quiet breathing; also called Benedict-Roth calorimeter.

   central a., the centrosome and centrosphere.

   Golgi a., a ubiquitous heterogeneous organelle in a cell consisting of a bowl-shaped, reticular network of saccules, vesicles, and vacuoles; in most cells it is located around or in the vicinity of the nucleus, but in some cells (e.g., spinal ganglion cells) it is fragmented and distributed throughout the cytoplasm; it temporarily stores and packages secretory products; also called Golgi body and Golgi complex.

   juxtaglomerular a., the juxtaglomerular body (granular epitheloid cells in the terminal part of the afferent arteriole of the kidney) together with the macula densa (the thickened epithelial cells in the wall of the distal convoluted tubule where it contacts the afferent arteriole).

   lacrimal a., the tear-forming and tear-conducting system, consisting of the lacrimal gland and ducts and associated structures.

   Tiselius a., a device used to separate proteins from solution and to determine the molecular weight and the isoelectric point.

   Van Slyke a., apparatus used to measure the amount of respiratory gases in blood.

   Warburg's a., apparatus used to measure the oxy-

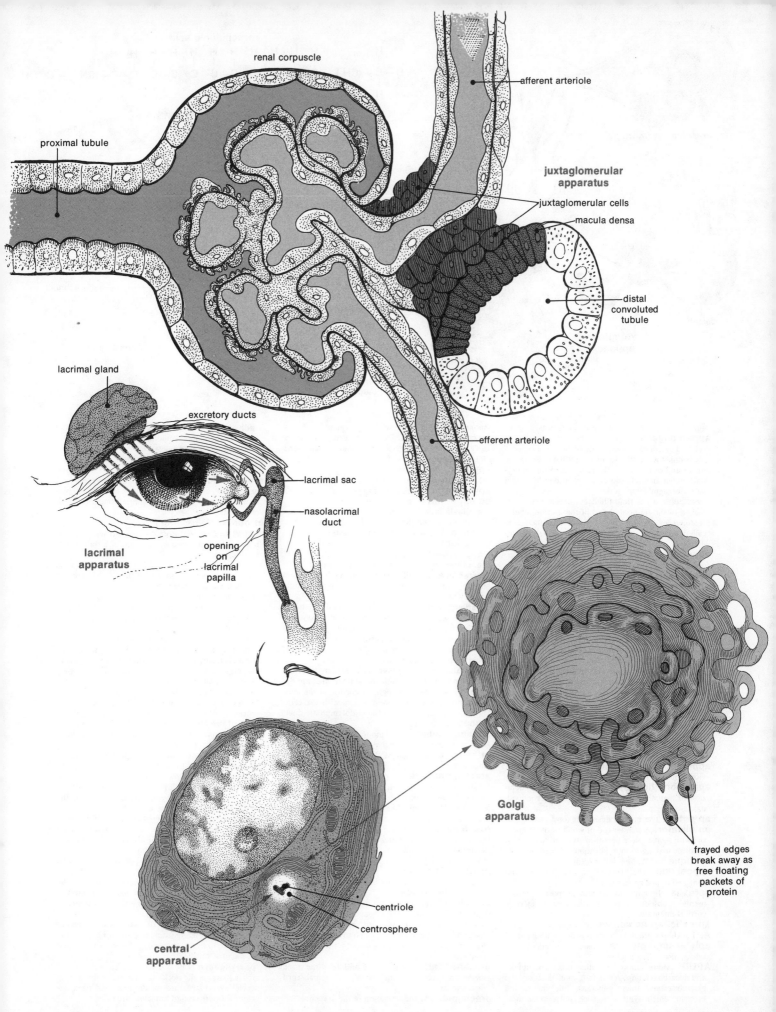

renal corpuscle

proximal tubule

afferent arteriole

juxtaglomerular apparatus

juxtaglomerular cells

macula densa

distal convoluted tubule

efferent arteriole

lacrimal gland

excretory ducts

lacrimal sac

nasolacrimal duct

lacrimal apparatus

opening on lacrimal papilla

Golgi apparatus

frayed edges break away as free floating packets of protein

centriole

centrosphere

central apparatus

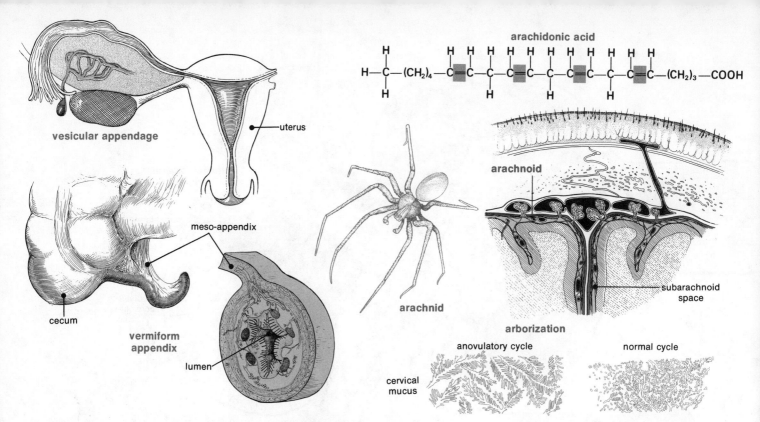

vesicular appendage

uterus

meso-appendix

cecum

vermiform appendix

lumen

arachidonic acid

$$H-C-(CH_2)_4-C=C-C=C-C=C-C=C-C-(CH_2)_3-COOH$$

arachnoid

arachnid

subarachnoid space

arborization

anovulatory cycle | normal cycle

cervical mucus

---

gen consumption of incubated tissue slices.

appen′dage. Any part in close but subordinate relation to a main structure; also called appendix.

  testicular a., a minute, oval, cystlike body on the upper end of the testis, the remnant of the embryonic mullerian duct; also called hydatid of Morgagni and Morgagni's appendix.

  vesicular a., a fluid-filled cystlike structure attached to the fimbriated end of the uterine tube, a remnant of the embryonic mullerian duct; also called hydatid of Morgagni and Morgagni's appendix.

appendec′tomy. Surgical removal of an appendix, especially the vermiform appendix.

appendiceal. Of or relating to an appendix.

appendici′tis. Inflammation of the vermiform appendix.

appendicolithi′asis. The presence of stones in the vermiform appendix.

appendic′ular. Relating to the appendix.

appen′dix, *pl.* **appen′dices.** An appendage, especially the vermiform appendix.

  a. ceci, vermiform appendix.

  epiploic a., one of several small peritoneal sacs extending from the serous coat of the large intestine, except the rectum; also called appendix epiploica and epiploic appendage.

  Morgagni's a., (1) testicular appendage; (2) vesicular appendage; see under appendage.

  vermiform a., the slender, worm-shaped tubular structure extending from the blind end of the cecum; also called appendix vermiformis.

appercep′tion. Comprehension based on previous knowledge or memories of past experiences.

appersona′tion, appersonifica′tion. A delusion of assuming the character of another individual.

ap′petite. The natural desire for food.

ap′plicator. A slender rod of wood or other material with a small piece of cotton attached to one end; used for making local applications of medicine.

appliqué form. See under form.

apposi′tion. The placing in contact of two adjacent and opposing surfaces.

aprax′ia. Inability to execute purposeful movements in absence of paralysis, due to a defect in cortical integration.

aprax′ic, aprac′tic. Relating to apraxia.

APT. Abbreviation for alum-precipitated toxoid.

apty′alism, aptya′lia. Absence or deficiency of saliva; also called asialism.

APUD. Abbreviation for amine precursor uptake and decarboxylation; refers to epithelial cells of the gastrointestinal tract, pancreas, bile ducts, and bronchi which synthesize such polypeptide hor-mones as gastrin, secretin, and glucagon.

apyknomor′phous. Denoting a cell whose stainable elements are not closely placed, which therefore does not stain deeply.

apyret′ic. Without fever.

apyrex′ia. Absence of fever.

apyrex′ial. Of or relating to apyrexia.

aq′ua, *pl.* **aq′uae.** Latin for water.

  a. pluvialis, rain water.

  a. regia, a. regalis, nitrohydrochloric acid.

aquat′ic. Relating to or living in water.

a′queduct. A canal.

  a. of Sylvius, see cerebral aqueduct.

  a. of the cochlea, perilymphatic aqueduct.

  cerebral a., a small canal connecting the third and fourth ventricles of the brain; also called aqueduct of Sylvius.

  perilymphatic a., a fine bony canal extending from the scala tympani (near the round window) of the internal ear to the subarachnoid space of the meninges, permitting the perilymph of the internal ear to be in direct contact with the cerebrospinal fluid; also called aqueduct of the cochlea.

  vestibular a., a thin bony canal leading from the medial wall of the vestibule of the internal ear to the posterior surface of the petrous portion of the temporal bone, where it communicates with the cerebrospinal space; it houses the endolymphatic duct.

a′queous. Watery.

aqueous humor. See humor, aqueous.

Ar. Chemical symbol for the element argon.

ar′abinose. A sugar, $C_5H_{10}O_5$, used in culture media.

arachido′nic acid. A polyunsaturated fatty acid, $C_{20}H_{32}O_2$, essential in nutrition; used in the treatment of infant eczema.

arach′nid. Any member of the class of arthropods, Arachnida.

Arach′nida. A class of arthropods (subphylum Chelicerata) that includes such forms as spiders, scorpions, mites, and ticks, characteristically having four pairs of legs.

arach′nidism. Systemic poisoning following the bite of a spider, especially of the black widow and brown recluse spiders.

arach′noid. 1. Having the appearance of a cobweb. 2. The middle of the three membranes covering the brain and spinal cord, between the dura mater and the pia mater; attached to the dura mater but separated from the pia mater by the subarachnoid space.

arachnoi′dal. Relating to the middle of the three membranes covering the brain and spinal cord (arachnoid).

arachnoidi′tis. Inflammation of the arachnoid.

adhesive a., inflammation of the arachnoid and adjacent pia mater, sometimes causing obliteration of the subarachnoid space.

arachnopho′bia. An inordinate fear of spiders.

arbores′cent. Treelike; branching.

arboriza′tion. Denoting (a) the branching of nerve fibers and capillaries; (b) the tree-shaped pattern sometimes formed by the dried smear of cervical mucus.

ar′borize. To ramify or branch.

arbovi′ruses. Arthropod-borne viruses that multiply in the arthropod's tissues and are transmitted by bite to vertebrates.

arc. 1. Anything shaped like an arch or a bow. **2.** The luminous line formed by the electric current crossing a gap between two electrodes.

  mercury a., an electric discharge through mercury vapor in a vacuum tube, producing ultraviolet rays.

  reflex a., the path followed by a nerve impulse in the production of a reflex act.

arch. Any of several curved structures of the body.

  aortic a.'s of the embryo, a series of six arterial channels encircling the embryonic pharynx (gut) in the mesenchyme of the pharyngeal arches; they never exist all at the same time.

  a. of the aorta, the curved portion of the aorta between the ascending and descending parts of the thoracic aorta; also called aortic arch.

  a.'s of the foot, the two sets of arches (longitudinal and transverse) formed by the bones of the foot.

  branchial a., pharyngeal arch.

  cortical a.'s of kidney, the portion of kidney substance (cortex) located between the bases of the pyramids and the renal capsule.

  costal a., an arch formed by the borders of the inferior aperture of the thorax, comprised of the costal cartilages of ribs seven to ten.

  dental a., (1) the composite structure of the natural teeth and the alveolar ridge; (2) the curved contour of the remains of the alveolar ridge after the loss of some or all of the natural teeth.

  glossopalatine a., anterior pillars of the fauces; see under pillar.

  longitudinal a., the anteroposterior arch of the foot, formed by the seven tarsal and five metatarsal bones and the ligaments binding them together.

  neural a., see vertebral arch.

  palatoglossal a., one of two folds of mucous membrane extending from the posterior edge of the soft palate to the lateral wall of the pharynx, behind the palatine tonsil.

  pharyngeal a., one of a series of five mesodermal arches (bars) in the neck region of the embryo from which several structures of the head and neck develop; formerly called branchial arch.

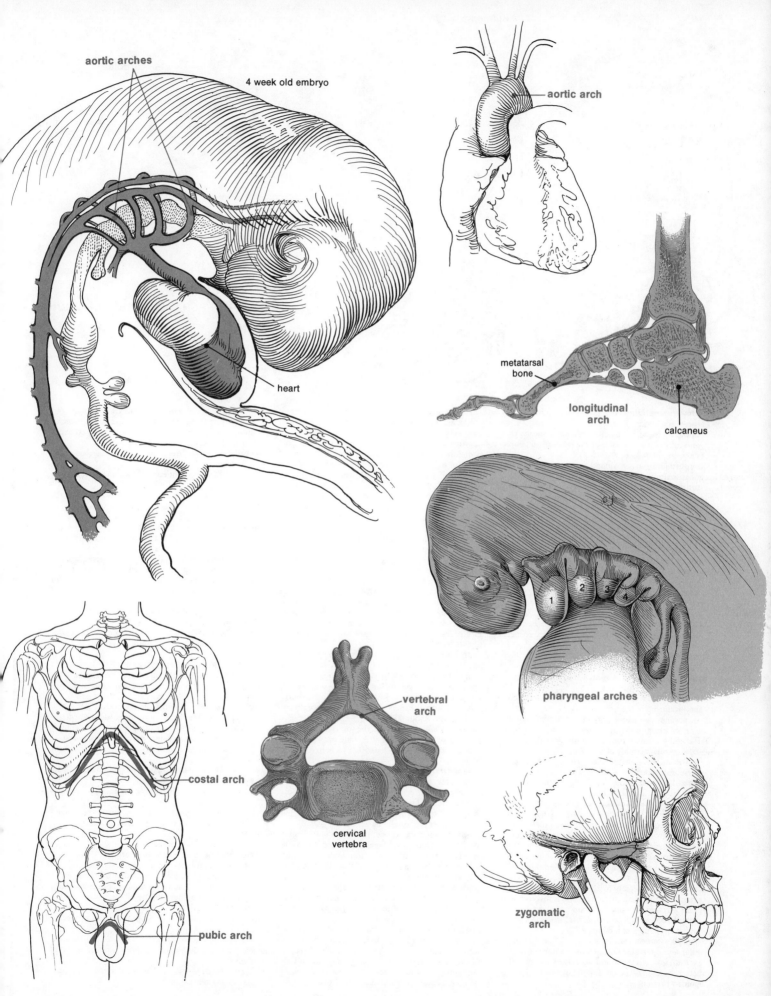

aortic arches

4 week old embryo

aortic arch

heart

metatarsal
bone

longitudinal
arch

calcaneus

pharyngeal arches

costal arch

vertebral
arch

cervical
vertebra

pubic arch

zygomatic
arch

25

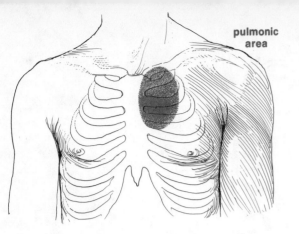

pulmonic area

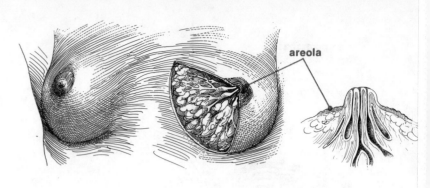

areola

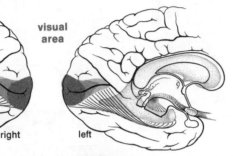

visual area

arginine

$$H_2N-\underset{\underset{NH}{|}}{C}-NH-CH_2-CH_2-CH_2-\underset{\underset{H}{|}}{C}-COOH \qquad \underset{NH_2}{}$$

right   left

pharyngopalatine a., posterior pillars of the fauces; see under pillar.

pubic a., arch on the pelvis formed by the convergence of the inferior rami of the ischium and pubic bones on either side.

supercilliary a., an arched prominence above the upper margin of the orbit.

tendinous a. of pelvis, a condensation of parietal pelvic fascia which arches from the posterior surface of the pubis to the spine of the ischium.

transverse a., the arch of the foot formed by the proximal parts of the metatarsal bones anteriorly and the distal row of the tarsal bones posteriorly.

vertebral a., neural a., the arch on the dorsal side of a vertebra which, with the vertebral body, forms the foramen in which the spinal cord is lodged.

zygomatic a., the arch formed by the zygomatic process of the temporal bone and the temporal process of the zygomatic bone.

archen'teron. The primitive digestive cavity of the embryo at the gastrula stage; also called primary gut.

arcta'tion. Stricture; narrowing.

ar'cuate. Arched.

ar'cus, *pl.* **ar'cus.** Any arch-shaped structure; an arch.

a. juvenilis, a grayish-white ring around the cornea, occurring in the young.

a. senilis, an opaque grayish ring around the cornea, occurring in the aged; also called gerontoxon.

ARD. Abbreviation for acute respiratory disease.

a'rea. A distinct part of a surface or space.

aortic a., area on the chest over the cartilage of the second right rib.

apical a., area about (a) the tip of the root of a tooth; (b) the apex of a lung.

a. of cardiac dullness, normally a small triangular area on the lower left side of the sternum which, on percussion of the chest, produces a dull sound; it corresponds to the portion of the heart not covered by lung tissue.

a. cribrosa, area of the renal papilla containing 20 or more pores through which the urine oozes into the minor calyces.

auditory a., region of the cerebral cortex concerned with hearing, occupying the transverse temporal gyri and the superior temporal gyrus.

basal seat a., the portion of oral structures that is available to support a denture.

Broca's speech a., area comprised of the triangular and opercular portions of the inferior frontal gyrus; it governs the motor aspects of speech and is better developed in the left hemisphere of right-handed persons.

Brodmann's a.'s, the 47 areas of the cerebral cortex mapped out according to the arrangement of their cellular components.

controlled a., in radiography, the space in a room containing the radiation source.

frontal a., portion of the cerebral cortex in front of the central sulcus (fissure of Rolando).

Little's a., a highly vascular area of the anterior portion of the nasal septum; frequent site of nosebleed.

macular a., the part of the retina that contains a yellow pigment, is used for central vision, and appears to be free of vessels when viewed with an ophthalmoscope.

mirror a., the reflecting surface of the lens of the eye and the cornea when illuminated with the slit lamp.

motor a., precentral cortex a., portion of the cerebral cortex comprised of the anterior wall of the central sulcus (fissure of Rolando) and adjacent portions of the precentral gyrus; its stimulation with electrodes causes contraction of voluntary muscles; also called primary motor area.

non-controlled a., in radiography, the office space, corridors, and other offices or rooms adjacent to the area containing a radiation source.

postcentral a., postrolandic a., the sensory area of the cerebral cortex, just posterior to the central sulcus (fissure of Rolando); it receives sensory stimuli from the whole body.

posterior palatal seal a., the soft tissue along the junction of the soft and hard palate on which pressure can be applied by a denture to help its retention.

precentral cortex a., see motor area.

premotor a., area immediately in front of the motor area, concerned with integrated movements.

pulmonic a., area of the chest at the second left intercostal space where flow sounds across the pulmonic valves are usually heard best.

subcallosal a., an area of the cortex in the medial aspect of each cerebral hemisphere, located immediately in front of the lamina terminalis and caudoventral to the subcallosal gyrus; also called parolfactory area of Broca.

tricuspid a., the area of the chest over the lower part of the body of the sternum (breastbone), where the heart sounds produced at the right atrioventricular valve are heard most distinctly.

visual a., area of the occipital lobe of the cerebral cortex concerned with vision; it consists of (a) sensory or striate part, occupying the walls of the calcarine sulcus (occasionally extending around the occipital pole onto the lateral surface of the hemisphere); concerned with recognition of size, form,

motion, color, illumination, and transparency; (b) psychic or parastriate part, surrounding the sensory portion; associates visual impressions and past experiences for recognition and identification.

area'tus, area'ta. Denoting circumscribed areas or patches.

areflex'ia. A condition in which the reflexes are absent.

are'ola. 1. One of the minute spaces in a tissue. **2.** A ringlike pigmented area around a central point, as the pigmented area around the nipple on the breast.

are'olar. Relating to an areola.

argent'affin, argent'affine. Denoting cells that have an affinity for silver salts.

argentaffino'ma. A tumor of the gastrointestinal mucosa, believed to arise from the Kulchitsky glands; found most often in the appendix but also in the small intestine, stomach, and rectum; also called carcinoid.

argenta'tion. Staining with a silver salt such as silver nitrate.

argen'tous. Relating to or containing silver; denoting a compound containing silver in its lower valency.

argen'tum. Latin for silver.

ar'ginase. A liver enzyme that promotes the splitting of the amino acid arginine into urea and ornithine.

ar'ginine. An essential amino acid, $C_6H_{14}N_4O_2$, derived from the digestion or hydrolysis of protein.

ar'gon. A colorless, odorless, gaseous element, constituting about one per cent of the earth's atmosphere; symbol A, atomic number 18, atomic weight 39.6.

Argyll-Robertson pupil, Argyll-Robertson symptom. See under pupil.

argyr'ia. Chronic silver poisoning causing a permanent grayish discoloration of the skin, conjunctiva, cornea, and internal organs due to the prolonged use of preparations containing silver compounds.

argyro'sis. Argyria.

arhyth'mia. Arrhythmia.

ariboflavino'sis. See hyporiboflavinosis.

arith'metic mean. In statistics, the sum of numerical data divided by the number of items.

arm. The upper limb of the human body, especially between the shoulder and the elbow.

arm'pit. See axilla.

arrest'. To prevent or stop function, progress, growth, or motion.

cardiac a., acute failure of the heart to provide adequate circulation to the brain and other vital organs.

cardiopulmonary a., failure of circulation and pulmonary ventilation.

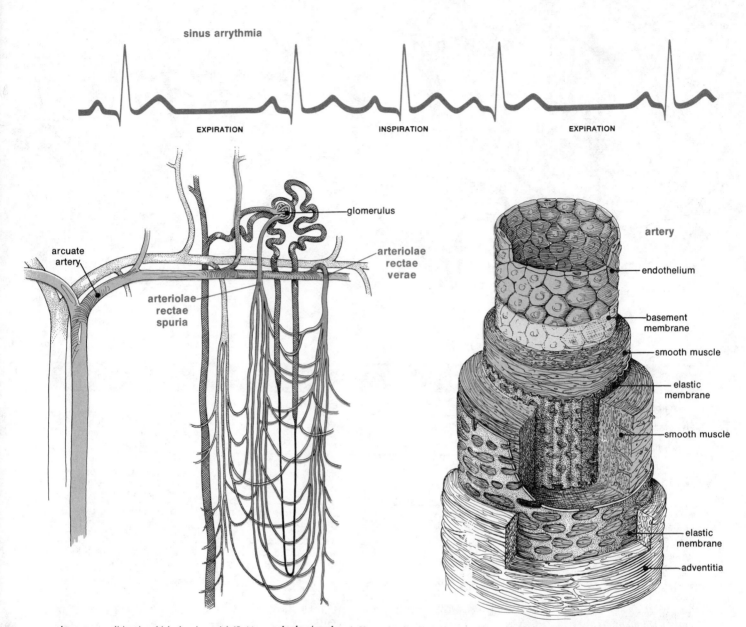

sinus arrythmia

EXPIRATION INSPIRATION EXPIRATION

glomerulus

arteriolae rectae verae

arcuate artery

arteriolae rectae spuria

artery

endothelium

basement membrane

smooth muscle

elastic membrane

smooth muscle

elastic membrane

adventitia

sinus a., condition in which the sinoatrial (S-A) node of the heart fails to send impulses to the atria, resulting in a temporary cessation of cardiac contraction.

arrhenoblasto´ma. An extremely rare tumor of the ovary that causes masculinization.

arrhyth´mia. Irregularity, especially of the heart beat.

sinus a., a variation in the rhythm of the heart beat usually related to breathing (slower during expiration, more rapid during inspiration); also called juvenile arrythmia because it is commonly found in children.

arrhyth´mic. Without rhythm.

ar´senic. A highly poisonous metallic element; symbol As, atomic number 33, atomic weight 74.9; some of its compounds are used in medicine.

ar´senous. Relating to or containing arsenic; denoting a compound of arsenic in a low valency.

arsphen´amine. An organic compound of the arseno-type; its discovery by Ehrlich in 1907 represented a major advance in the treatment of syphilis; also called Salvarsan® and diarsenol.

arte´ria, *pl.* **arte´riae.** Latin for artery.

arte´rial. Relating to the arteries.

arteriecta´sia. Dilation of the arteries.

arteriec´tomy. Surgical removal of a segment of an artery.

arte´riogram. X-ray picture of an artery into which a radiopaque material has been introduced.

arteriog´raphy. 1. X-ray visualization of an artery or arteries after injection of a radiopaque substance. **2.** A treatise on, or description of, the arteries. **3.** Sphygmography.

arte´riola, *pl.* **arte´riolae.** Arteriole.

arteriolae rectae spuriae, the straight vessels which arise from the juxtaglomerular efferent arterioles of the kidney and parallel the nephronic (Henle's) loop; also called vasa recta spuria.

arteriolae rectae verae, the true vasa recta; the straight vessels which arise directly from the arcuate arteries of the kidney and parallel the nephronic (Henle's) loop.

arterio´lar. Relating to an arteriole or arterioles.

arte´riole. The smallest subdivision of the arterial tree preceding the capillary; it possesses muscular walls which, by contracting and relaxing, can alter the flow of blood into the body tissues.

arterioli´tis. Inflammation of the arterioles.

arteriolonecro´sis. Degeneration or destruction of arterioles, as in malignant hypertension.

arteriomo´tor. Causing contraction or dilation of arteries.

arterionecro´sis. Death of arterial tissues.

arterioplas´ty. Replacement of a segment of an artery.

arterior´rhaphy. Suture of an artery.

arteriosclero´sis. Arterial sclerosis; disease of the arteries resulting in the thickening and loss of elasticity of the arterial walls; commonly known as hardening of the arteries.

a. obliterans, the arteriosclerotic narrowing of the lumen of the arteries supplying the extremities.

Mönckeberg's a., a form of arteriosclerosis marked by the formation of ringlike calcifications in the middle layer of arterial walls, especially of small arteries; also called medial calcific sclerosis and medial calcinosis.

arteriosclerot´ic. Relating to or marked by arteriosclerosis.

arteriosteno´sis. Constriction of an artery or arteries.

arteriot´omy. Incision into the lumen of an artery.

arteriove´nous. Relating to both arteries and veins.

a. oxygen difference, the difference in the content of oxygen between arterial and venous blood.

arteri´tis. Inflammation of an artery.

a. deformans, chronic inflammation of the inner layer of an artery (intima).

a. obliterans, inflammation of the inner layer of an artery causing the closure of the artery's lumen.

temporal a., cranial a., disease of older persons involving the temporal arteries, and frequently leading to blindness by involvement of the ophthalmic and retinal arteries.

ar´tery. A vessel that transports blood away from the heart to different parts of the body; in the normal state after birth, all arteries conduct oxygenated blood except the pulmonary arteries which transport unoxygenated blood from the heart to the lungs.

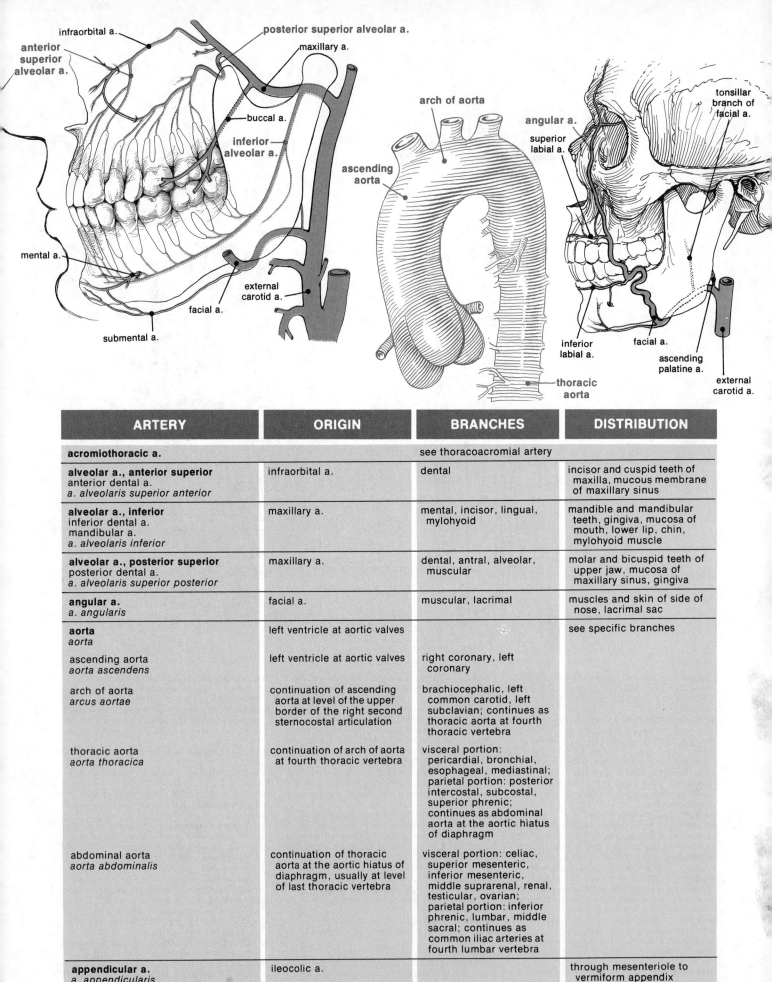

Labels (top illustrations):

infraorbital a.
posterior superior alveolar a.
anterior superior alveolar a.
maxillary a.
buccal a.
inferior alveolar a.
mental a.
external carotid a.
facial a.
submental a.
arch of aorta
ascending aorta
tonsillar branch of facial a.
angular a.
superior labial a.
inferior labial a.
thoracic aorta
facial a.
ascending palatine a.
external carotid a.

ARTERY	ORIGIN	BRANCHES	DISTRIBUTION
acromiothoracic a.		see thoracoacromial artery	
alveolar a., anterior superior anterior dental a. *a. alveolaris superior anterior*	infraorbital a.	dental	incisor and cuspid teeth of maxilla, mucous membrane of maxillary sinus
alveolar a., inferior inferior dental a. mandibular a. *a. alveolaris inferior*	maxillary a.	mental, incisor, lingual, mylohyoid	mandible and mandibular teeth, gingiva, mucosa of mouth, lower lip, chin, mylohyoid muscle
alveolar a., posterior superior posterior dental a. *a. alveolaris superior posterior*	maxillary a.	dental, antral, alveolar, muscular	molar and bicuspid teeth of upper jaw, mucosa of maxillary sinus, gingiva
angular a. *a. angularis*	facial a.	muscular, lacrimal	muscles and skin of side of nose, lacrimal sac
aorta *aorta*	left ventricle at aortic valves		see specific branches
ascending aorta *aorta ascendens*	left ventricle at aortic valves	right coronary, left coronary	
arch of aorta *arcus aortae*	continuation of ascending aorta at level of the upper border of the right second sternocostal articulation	brachiocephalic, left common carotid, left subclavian; continues as thoracic aorta at fourth thoracic vertebra	
thoracic aorta *aorta thoracica*	continuation of arch of aorta at fourth thoracic vertebra	visceral portion: pericardial, bronchial, esophageal, mediastinal; parietal portion: posterior intercostal, subcostal, superior phrenic; continues as abdominal aorta at the aortic hiatus of diaphragm	
abdominal aorta *aorta abdominalis*	continuation of thoracic aorta at the aortic hiatus of diaphragm, usually at level of last thoracic vertebra	visceral portion: celiac, superior mesenteric, inferior mesenteric, middle suprarenal, renal, testicular, ovarian; parietal portion: inferior phrenic, lumbar, middle sacral; continues as common iliac arteries at fourth lumbar vertebra	
appendicular a. *a. appendicularis*	ileocolic a.		through mesenteriole to vermiform appendix

artery | artery

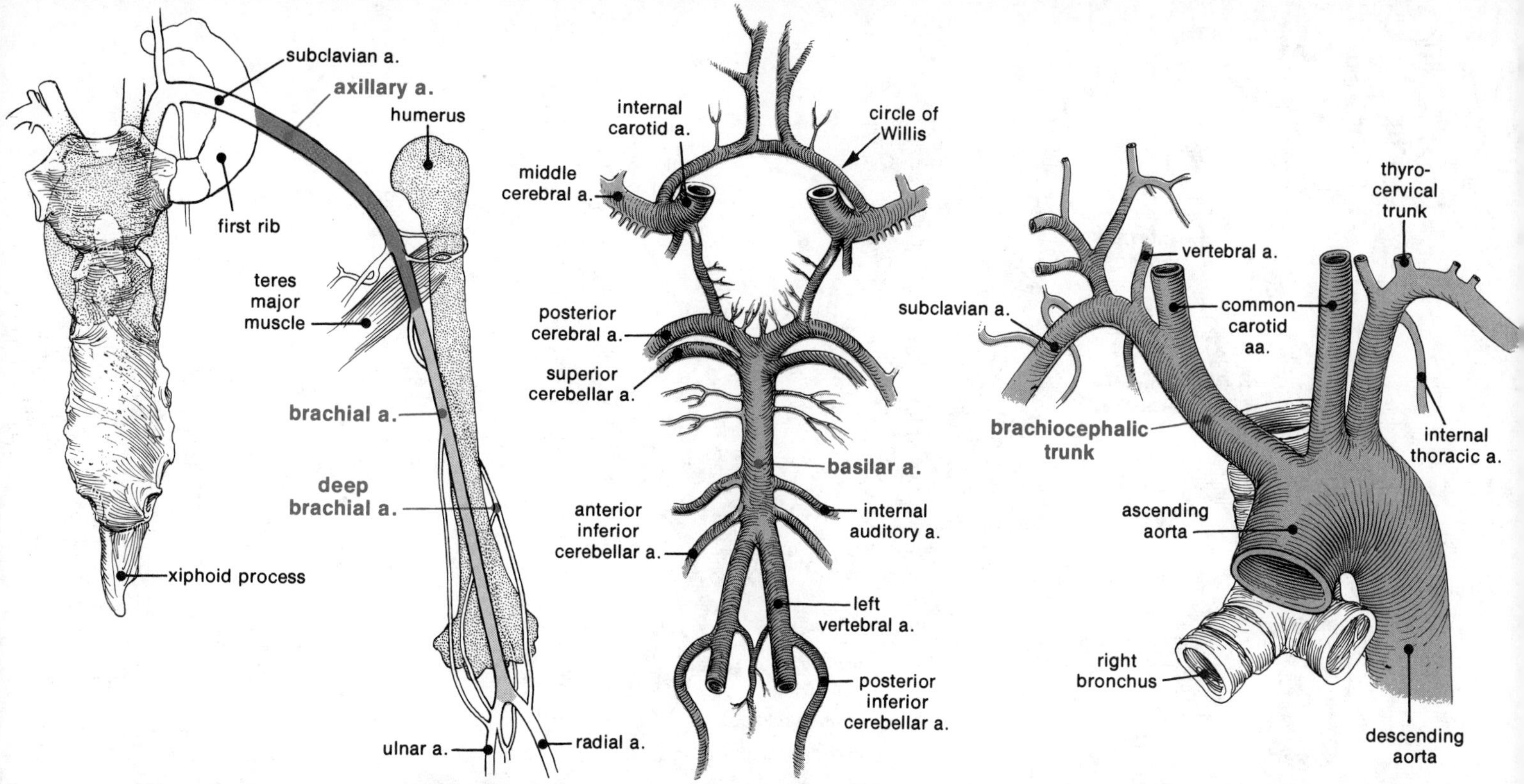

subclavian a.

axillary a.

humerus

first rib

teres major muscle

brachial a.

deep brachial a.

xiphoid process

ulnar a.

radial a.

internal carotid a.

middle cerebral a.

circle of Willis

posterior cerebral a.

superior cerebellar a.

anterior inferior cerebellar a.

basilar a.

internal auditory a.

left vertebral a.

posterior inferior cerebellar a.

vertebral a.

subclavian a.

thyro-cervical trunk

common carotid aa.

brachiocephalic trunk

internal thoracic a.

ascending aorta

right bronchus

descending aorta

ARTERY	ORIGIN	BRANCHES	DISTRIBUTION
arch, deep palmar	see palmar arch, deep		
arch, plantar	see plantar arch		
arch, superficial palmar	see palmar arch, superficial		
arcuate a. of foot metatarsal a. *a. arcuata pedis*	dorsal a. of foot	second, third, and fourth metatarsal arteries	instep of foot
arcuate a.'s of kidney *aa. arcuatae renis*	interlobar a.	interlobular, afferent, arteriole	parenchyma of kidney
auditory a., internal	see labyrinthine artery		
auricular a., deep *a. auricularis profounda*	maxillary a.	temporomandibular	cuticular lining of external acoustic meatus, outer surface of tympanic membrane, temporomandibular joint
auricular a., posterior *a. auricularis posterior*	external carotid a.	stylomastoid, auricular, occipital, parotid	middle ear, mastoid cells, auricle, parotid gland, digastric, stapedius, and neck muscles
axillary a. *a. axillaris*	continuation of subclavian a. in axilla, becoming brachial a. in arm	first part: highest thoracic; second part: thoracoacromial, lateral thoracic; third part: subscapular, posterior humeral circumflex, anterior humeral circumflex	pectoral muscles, muscles of shoulder and upper arm
basilar a. *a. basilaris*	from junction of two vertebral arteries	pontine, labyrinthine, anterior inferior cerebellar, superior cerebellar, posterior cerebral	pons, internal ear, cerebellum, pineal body, ventricles, posterior part of cerebrum
brachial a. *a. brachialis*	continuation of axillary a. at distal margin of tendon of teres major muscle	deep brachial, nutrient of humerus, superior ulnar collateral, inferior ulnar collateral, muscular	muscles of shoulder, arm, forearm, and hand; elbow joint
brachial a., deep superior profunda a. *a. profunda brachii*	brachial a.	ascending, radial collateral, middle collateral, muscular, nutrient	humerus, elbow joint, muscles of upper arm including triceps and deltoid
brachiocephalic trunk innominate a. *truncus brachiocephalicus*	beginning of arch of aorta	right common carotid, right subclavian, thyroidea ima, thymic	right side of head, neck and upper arm, thyroid and thymus glands

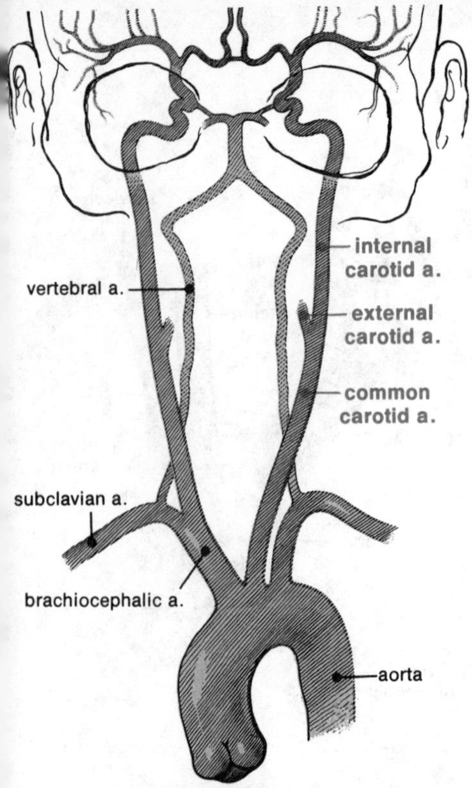

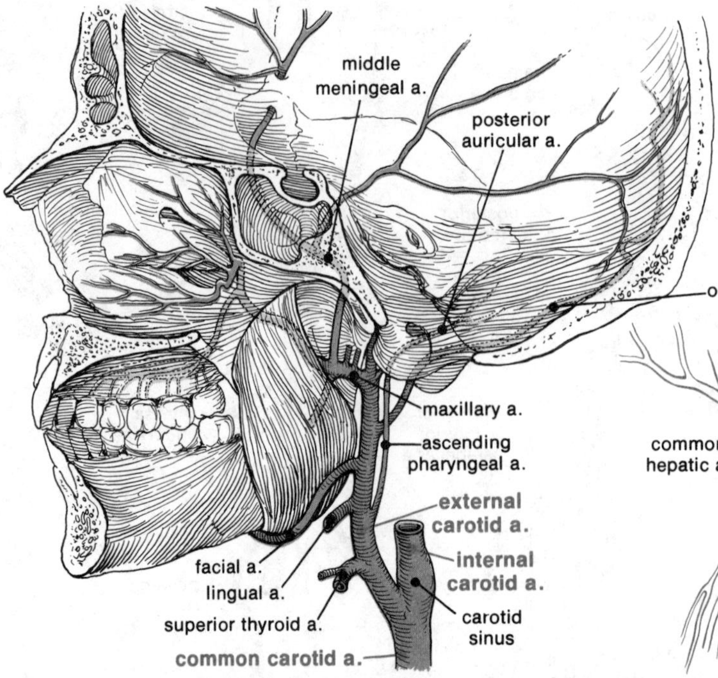

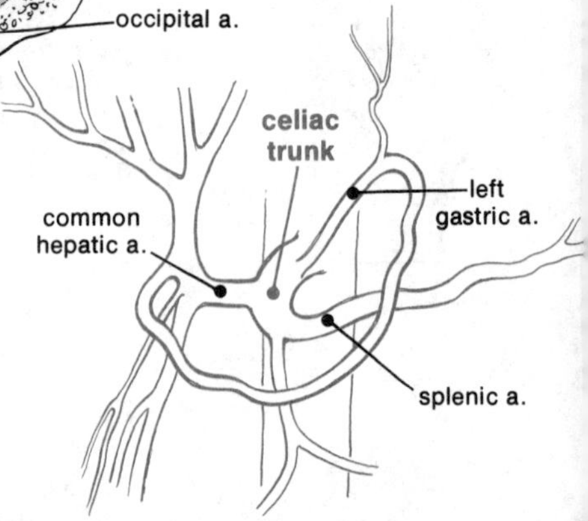

ARTERY	ORIGIN	BRANCHES	DISTRIBUTION
bronchial a.'s *aa. bronchiales*	right side: first aortic intercostal; left side: thoracic aorta		bronchial tubes, alveolar tissue of lungs, bronchial lymph nodes, esophagus
buccal a. buccinator a. *a. buccis* *a. buccalis*	maxillary a.	muscular	buccinator muscle, mucosa of maxillary gums, mucosa and skin of cheeks
a. of bulb of penis *a. bulbi penis*	internal pudendal	bulbourethral	bulb of penis, posterior part of corpus spongiosum, bulbourethral gland
a. of bulb of vaginal vestibule *a. bulbi vestibuli vaginae*	internal pudendal a.		bulbus vestibuli, erectile tissue of vagina
calcaneal a.'s, medial internal calcaneal a.'s *rami calcanei mediales*	posterior tibial a.		skin and fat in back of calcaneal tendon and heel; muscles on tibial side of sole
capsular a.'s, middle	see suprarenal arteries, middle		
carotid a., common *a. carotis communis*	right side: bifurcation of the brachiocephalic trunk; left side: highest part of arch of aorta	external carotid, internal carotid	head
carotid a., external *a. carotis externa*	carotid a.	superior thyroid, ascending pharyngeal, lingual, facial, occipital, posterior auricular, superficial temporal, maxillary	anterior aspect of face and neck, side of head, skull, dura mater, posterior part of scalp
carotid a., internal *a. carotis interna*	common carotid a.	cervical portion: none; petrous portion: caroticotympanic, artery of the pterygoid canal, cavernous, hypophyseal; cavernous portion: ganglionic, anterior meningeal, ophthalmic, anterior cerebral, middle cerebral; cerebral portion: posterior communicating, anterior choroidal	middle ear, brain, hypophysis, trigeminal ganglion, meninges, orbit
celiac trunk celiac artery *truncus celiacus*	abdominal aorta, just caudal to aortic hiatus of diaphragm	left gastric, common hepatic, splenic	esophagus, stomach, duodenum, spleen, pancreas, liver, gallbladder, greater omentum

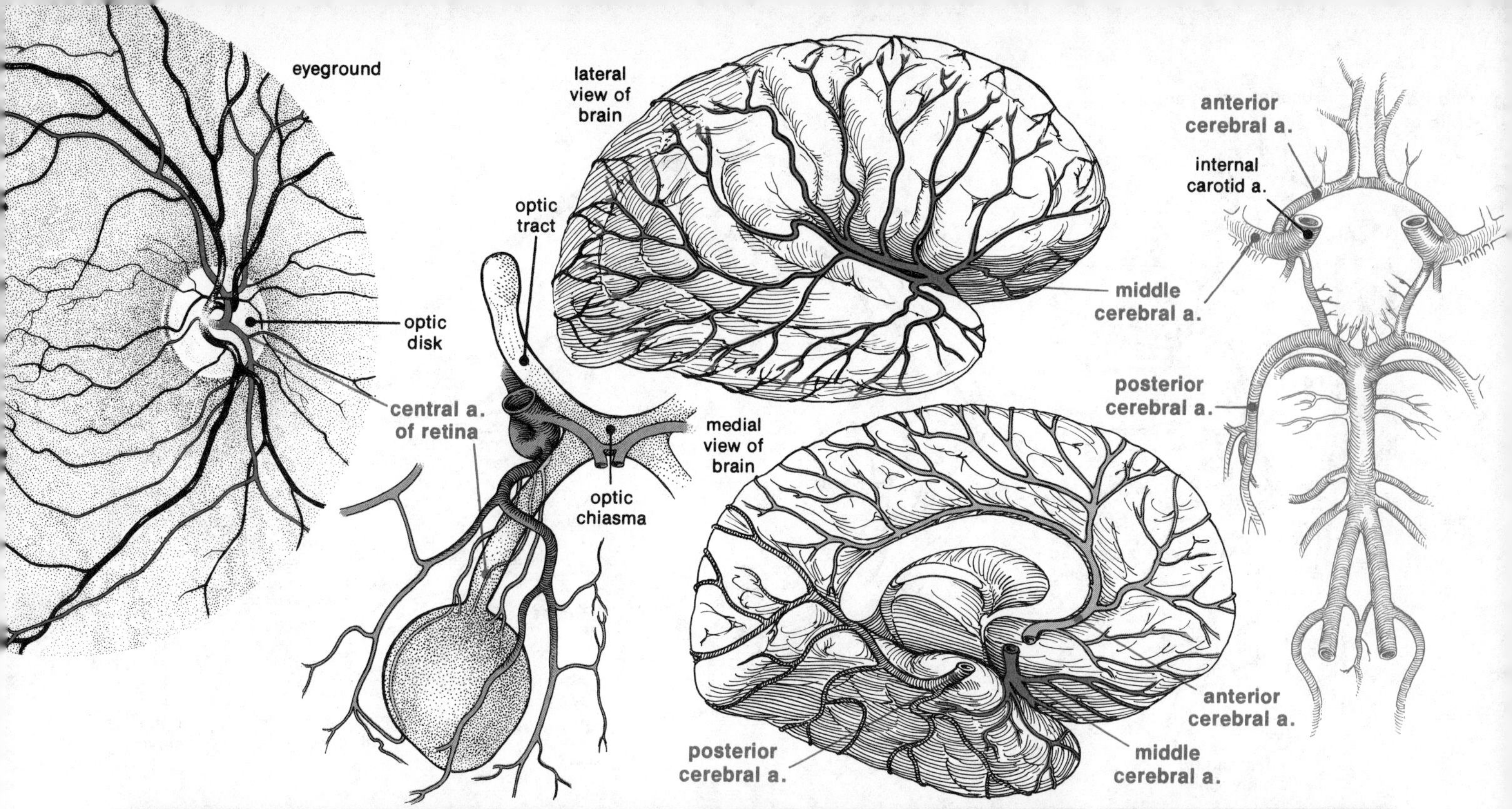

eyeground

optic disk

central a. of retina

optic tract

optic chiasma

lateral view of brain

medial view of brain

optic disk

posterior cerebral a.

middle cerebral a.

anterior cerebral a.

internal carotid a.

middle cerebral a.

posterior cerebral a.

anterior cerebral a.

ARTERY	ORIGIN	BRANCHES	DISTRIBUTION
central a. of retina *a. centralis retinae*	ophthalmic a. or lacrimal a.	nasal, temporal	retina
cerebellar a., anterior inferior *a. cerebelli inferior anterior*	basilar a.	labyrinthine a.	anterior part of inferior surface of cerebellum
cerebellar a., posterior inferior *a. cerebelli inferior posterior*	vertebral (largest branch)	medial, lateral	inferior surface of cerebellum, medulla oblongata, choroid plexus of fourth ventricle
cerebellar a., superior *a. cerebelli superior*	basilar a. near its termination	medial, lateral	superior surface of cerebellum, vermis of cerebellum, pineal body, pia mater, anterior medullary velum, choroid plexus of third ventricle
cerebral a., anterior *a. cerebri anterior*	internal carotid at the medial extremity of the lateral cerebral sulcus	medial striate, orbital (inferior), prefrontal (anterior), middle posterior; the anterior communicating artery connects the two anterior cerebral arteries across the longitudinal fissure	orbital, frontal, and parietal cortex, caudate nucleus, putamen, globus pallidus, internal capsule, corpus callosum, olfactory lobe
cerebral a., middle *a. cerebri media*	internal carotid	central portion: lateral striate; cortical portion: inferior lateral frontal, ascending frontal, ascending parietal, parietotemporal, temporal	lateral surface of cerebral hemisphere; basal nuclei, putamen, caudate nucleus, globus pallidus, internal capsule
cerebral a., posterior *a. cerebri posterior*	terminal bifurcation of basilar a.	central, choroidal, cortical	medial and posterior surface of thalamus, walls of third ventricle tela choroidea and choroid plexus of third ventricle uncus, fusiform gyrus, inferior temporal gyrus; cuneus, lingual gyrus, occipital lobe; precuneus
cervical a., ascending *a. cervicalis ascendens*	inferior thyroid a.	spinal	muscles of neck, vertebral canal, vertebrae
cervical a., deep *a. cervicalis profunda*	costocervical trunk (occasionally from the subclavian a.)	spinal, muscular	spinal cord, deep neck muscles
cervical a., superficial *a. cervicalis superficialis*	thyrocervical trunk	ascending, descending	trapezius and neighboring muscles

31

artery | artery

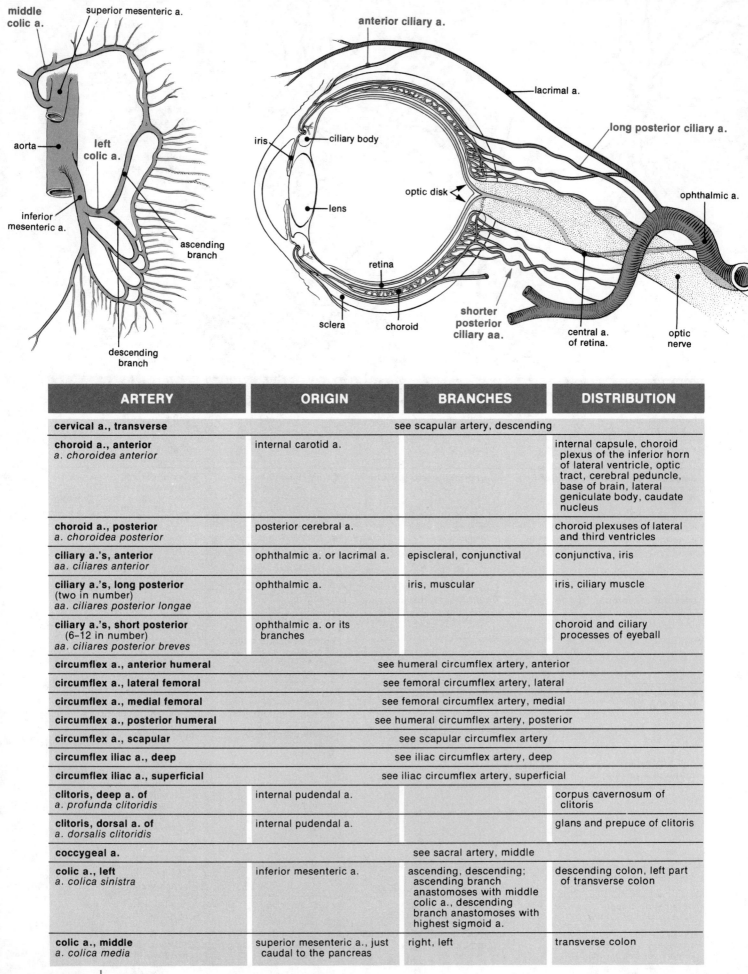

Labels for top-left diagram:
- middle colic a.
- superior mesenteric a.
- aorta
- left colic a.
- inferior mesenteric a.
- ascending branch
- descending branch

Labels for eye diagram:
- anterior ciliary a.
- lacrimal a.
- long posterior ciliary a.
- iris
- ciliary body
- optic disk
- ophthalmic a.
- lens
- retina
- shorter posterior ciliary aa.
- central a. of retina.
- optic nerve
- sclera
- choroid

ARTERY	ORIGIN	BRANCHES	DISTRIBUTION
cervical a., transverse	see scapular artery, descending		
choroid a., anterior *a. choroidea anterior*	internal carotid a.		internal capsule, choroid plexus of the inferior horn of lateral ventricle, optic tract, cerebral peduncle, base of brain, lateral geniculate body, caudate nucleus
choroid a., posterior *a. choroidea posterior*	posterior cerebral a.		choroid plexuses of lateral and third ventricles
ciliary a.'s, anterior *aa. ciliares anterior*	ophthalmic a. or lacrimal a.	episcleral, conjunctival	conjunctiva, iris
ciliary a.'s, long posterior (two in number) *aa. ciliares posterior longae*	ophthalmic a.	iris, muscular	iris, ciliary muscle
ciliary a.'s, short posterior (6–12 in number) *aa. ciliares posterior breves*	ophthalmic a. or its branches		choroid and ciliary processes of eyeball
circumflex a., anterior humeral	see humeral circumflex artery, anterior		
circumflex a., lateral femoral	see femoral circumflex artery, lateral		
circumflex a., medial femoral	see femoral circumflex artery, medial		
circumflex a., posterior humeral	see humeral circumflex artery, posterior		
circumflex a., scapular	see scapular circumflex artery		
circumflex iliac a., deep	see iliac circumflex artery, deep		
circumflex iliac a., superficial	see iliac circumflex artery, superficial		
clitoris, deep a. of *a. profunda clitoridis*	internal pudendal a.		corpus cavernosum of clitoris
clitoris, dorsal a. of *a. dorsalis clitoridis*	internal pudendal a.		glans and prepuce of clitoris
coccygeal a.	see sacral artery, middle		
colic a., left *a. colica sinistra*	inferior mesenteric a.	ascending, descending; ascending branch anastomoses with middle colic a., descending branch anastomoses with highest sigmoid a.	descending colon, left part of transverse colon
colic a., middle *a. colica media*	superior mesenteric a., just caudal to the pancreas	right, left	transverse colon

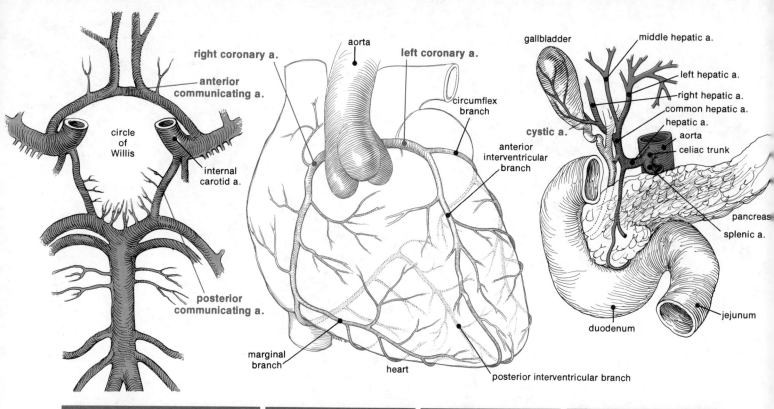

circle of Willis

right coronary a.

anterior communicating a.

internal carotid a.

posterior communicating a.

aorta

left coronary a.

circumflex branch

anterior interventricular branch

marginal branch

heart

posterior interventricular branch

gallbladder

middle hepatic a.

left hepatic a.

right hepatic a.

common hepatic a.

hepatic a.

aorta

celiac trunk

cystic a.

pancreas

splenic a.

duodenum

jejunum

ARTERY	ORIGIN	BRANCHES	DISTRIBUTION
colic a., right *a. colica dextra*	superior mesenteric a. or iliocolic a.	descending, ascending	ascending colon
collateral a., inferior ulnar anastomotica magna a. *a. collateralis ulnaris inferior*	brachial a., about 5 cm proximal to elbow	posterior, anterior, anastomotic	triceps, elbow joint, round pronator muscle
collateral a., middle *a. collateralis media*	deep brachial a.	muscular anastomotic	elbow joint, triceps muscle
collateral a., radial *a. collateralis radialis*	deep brachial a.	muscular, anastomotic	triceps, elbow joint, brachioradial and brachial muscles
collateral a., superior ulnar inferior profunda a. *a. collateralis ulnaris superior*	brachial a., distal to middle of arm	muscular, articular, anastomotic	elbow joint, triceps muscle of arm
communicating a., anterior *a. communicans anterior cerebri*	anterior cerebral a. (connects the two anterior cerebral arteries across the longitudinal fissure of the brain)	anteromedial	anterior perforated substance of the brain
communicating a., posterior *a. communicans posterior cerebri*	internal carotid a.	posterior communicating artery branches; anastomoses with the posterior cerebral artery	base of brain between infundibulum and optic tract; internal capsule, anterior third of thalamus; third ventricle
conjunctival a.'s, anterior *aa. conjunctivales anterior*	anterior ciliary a.'s		conjunctiva
conjunctival a.'s, posterior *aa. conjunctivales posterior*	medial palpebral a.		conjunctiva
coronary a., left *a. coronaria sinistra*	aorta at left adjacent or left posterior aortic sinus (of Valsalva)	anterior descending, circumflex, left atrial	left atrium, left and right ventricle, septum
coronary a., right *a. coronaria dextra*	aorta at left adjacent or right anterior aortic sinus (of Valsalva)	right atrial, posterior descending, preventricular, transverse	right atrium, anterior part of right ventricle, septum
costocervical trunk superior intercostal a. *truncus costocervicalis*	subclavian a.	deep cervical; continues as the highest intercostal a.	deep neck muscles, first and second intercostal spaces, spinal cord
cremasteric a. external spermatic a. *a. cremasterica*	inferior epigastric a.		cremaster muscle, coverings of spermatic cord
cystic a. *a. cystica*	right hepatic a.	superficial, deep	gallbladder

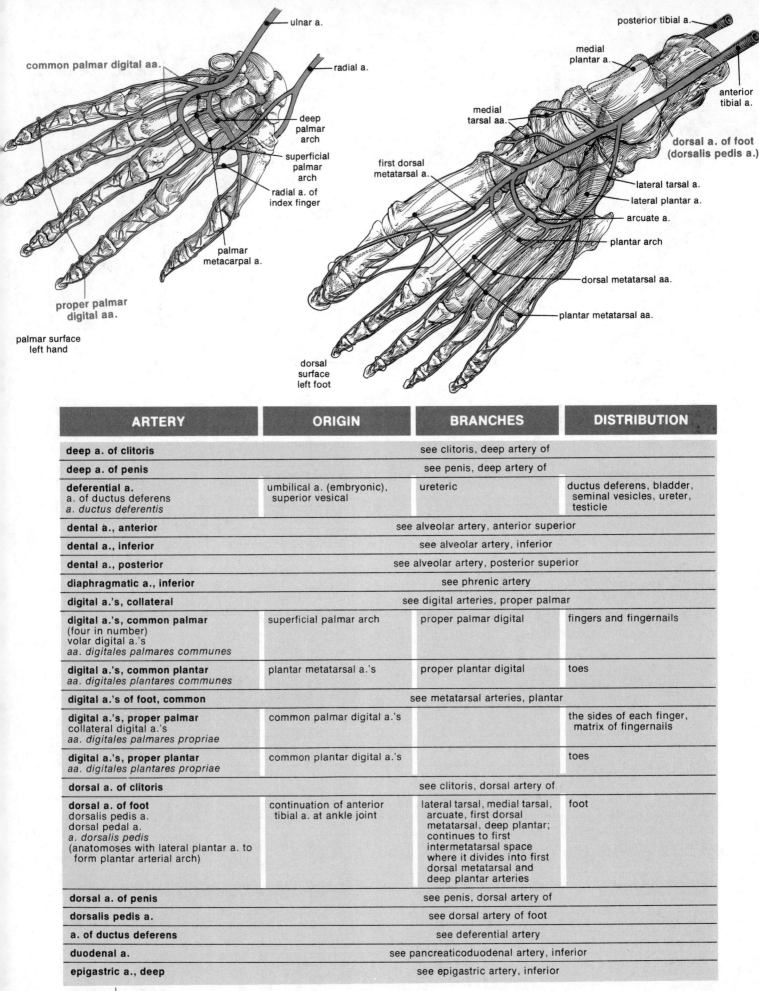

common palmar digital aa.

ulnar a.

radial a.

deep palmar arch

superficial palmar arch

radial a. of index finger

palmar metacarpal a.

proper palmar digital aa.

palmar surface left hand

posterior tibial a.

medial plantar a.

anterior tibial a.

medial tarsal aa.

first dorsal metatarsal a.

dorsal a. of foot (dorsalis pedis a.)

lateral tarsal a.

lateral plantar a.

arcuate a.

plantar arch

dorsal metatarsal aa.

plantar metatarsal aa.

dorsal surface left foot

ARTERY	ORIGIN	BRANCHES	DISTRIBUTION
deep a. of clitoris	see clitoris, deep artery of		
deep a. of penis	see penis, deep artery of		
deferential a. a. of ductus deferens *a. ductus deferentis*	umbilical a. (embryonic), superior vesical	ureteric	ductus deferens, bladder, seminal vesicles, ureter, testicle
dental a., anterior	see alveolar artery, anterior superior		
dental a., inferior	see alveolar artery, inferior		
dental a., posterior	see alveolar artery, posterior superior		
diaphragmatic a., inferior	see phrenic artery		
digital a.'s, collateral	see digital arteries, proper palmar		
digital a.'s, common palmar (four in number) volar digital a.'s *aa. digitales palmares communes*	superficial palmar arch	proper palmar digital	fingers and fingernails
digital a.'s, common plantar *aa. digitales plantares communes*	plantar metatarsal a.'s	proper plantar digital	toes
digital a.'s of foot, common	see metatarsal arteries, plantar		
digital a.'s, proper palmar collateral digital a.'s *aa. digitales palmares propriae*	common palmar digital a.'s		the sides of each finger, matrix of fingernails
digital a.'s, proper plantar *aa. digitales plantares propriae*	common plantar digital a.'s		toes
dorsal a. of clitoris	see clitoris, dorsal artery of		
dorsal a. of foot dorsalis pedis a. dorsal pedal a. *a. dorsalis pedis* (anatomoses with lateral plantar a. to form plantar arterial arch)	continuation of anterior tibial a. at ankle joint	lateral tarsal, medial tarsal, arcuate, first dorsal metatarsal, deep plantar; continues to first intermetatarsal space where it divides into first dorsal metatarsal and deep plantar arteries	foot
dorsal a. of penis	see penis, dorsal artery of		
dorsalis pedis a.	see dorsal artery of foot		
a. of ductus deferens	see deferential artery		
duodenal a.	see pancreaticoduodenal artery, inferior		
epigastric a., deep	see epigastric artery, inferior		

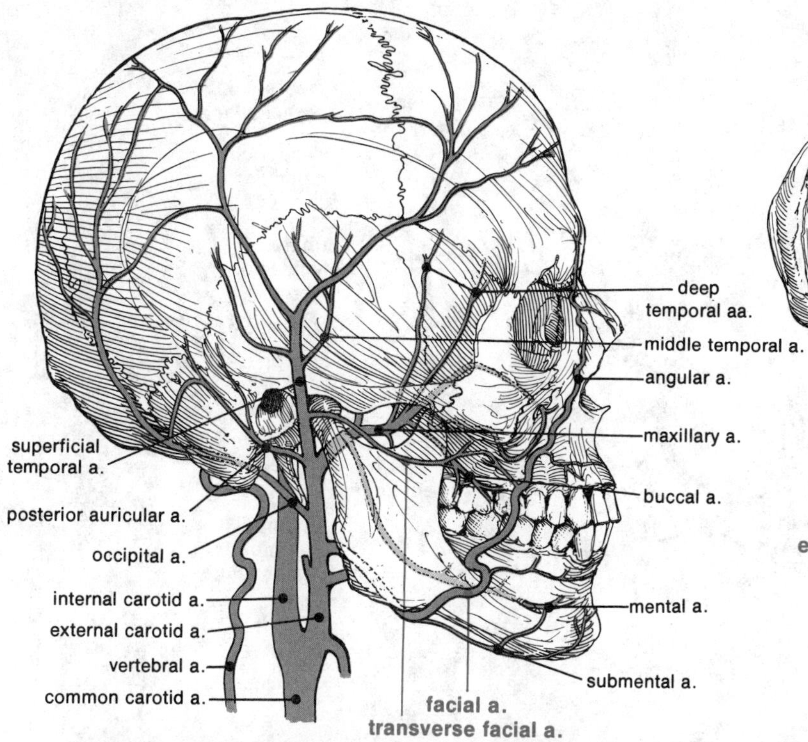

deep temporal aa.
middle temporal a.
angular a.
maxillary a.
buccal a.
superficial temporal a.
posterior auricular a.
occipital a.
internal carotid a.
external carotid a.
vertebral a.
common carotid a.
mental a.
submental a.
facial a.
transverse facial a.

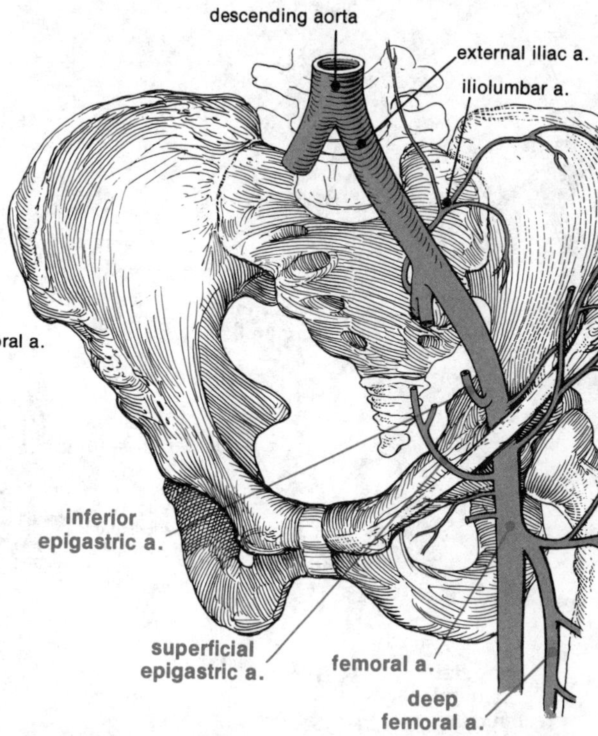

descending aorta
external iliac a.
iliolumbar a.
inferior epigastric a.
superficial epigastric a.
femoral a.
deep femoral a.

ARTERY	ORIGIN	BRANCHES	DISTRIBUTION
epigastric a., inferior deep epigastric a. *a. epigastrica inferior*	external iliac, immediately above inguinal ligament	cremasteric, pubic, muscular	cremaster and abdominal muscles, peritoneum
epigastric a., superficial *a. epigastrica superficialis*	femoral a. about 1 cm below inguinal ligament		lower part of abdominal wall, superficial subinguinal lymph nodes
epigastric a., superior *a. epigastrica superior*	internal thoracic a.	cutaneous, muscular, peritoneal, phrenic, hepatic	skin, muscles, and fascia of upper part of abdominal wall; diaphragm, peritoneum, faliciform ligament of liver
episcleral a. *a. episcleralis*	anterior ciliary a.		iris, ciliary body
esophageal a.'s (four to five in number) *aa. esophagei*	thoracic aorta		esophagus
ethmoidal a., anterior *a. ethmoidalis anterior*	ophthalmic a.	meningeal, nasal	anterior and middle ethmoid air cells, frontal sinus, dura mater, nasal cavity
ethmoidal a., posterior *a. ethmoidalis posterior*	ophthalmic a.	meningeal, nasal	posterior ethmoid air cells, dura mater, nasal cavity
facial a. external maxillary a. *a. facialis*	external carotid a.	neck portion: ascending palatine, tonsillar, glandular, submental; facial portion: inferior labial, superior labial, lateral nasal, angular, muscular	face, tonsil, palate, labial glands and muscles of lips, submandibular gland, ala and dorsum of nose, muscles of expression
facial a., deep		see maxillary artery	
facial a., transverse *a. transverse faciei*	superficial temporal a. while still in parotid gland	glandular, muscular, cutaneous	parotid gland and duct, masseter muscle, skin of face
femoral a. *a. femoralis*	continuation of external iliac a. immediately distal to inguinal ligament	superficial epigastric, superficial iliac circumflex, superficial external pudendal, deep external pudendal, muscular, descending genicular, deep femoral	integument of abdominal wall, groin, and perineum; muscles of thigh, external genitals, inguinal lymph nodes
femoral a., deep profunda femoris a. *a. profunda femoris*	femoral a.	medial femoral circumflex, lateral femoral circumflex, perforating, muscular	muscles of thigh, hip joint, head and shaft of femur, gluteal muscles

artery | artery

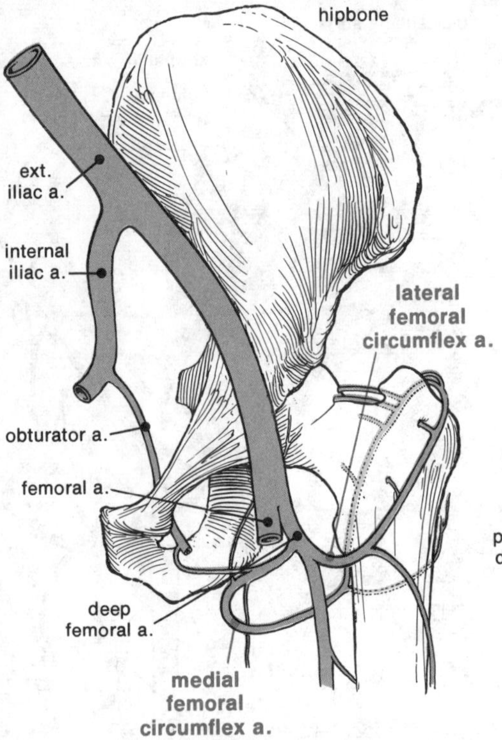

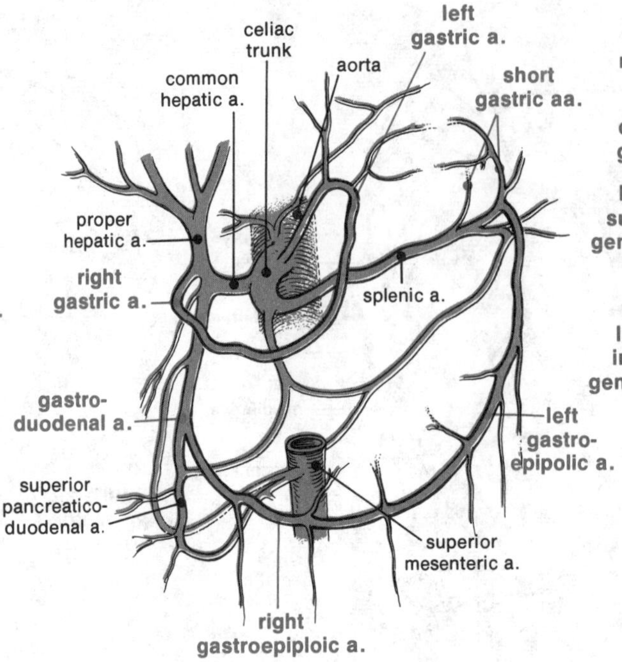

hipbone

ext. iliac a.

internal iliac a.

obturator a.

femoral a.

deep femoral a.

medial femoral circumflex a.

lateral femoral circumflex a.

celiac trunk

left gastric a.

aorta

common hepatic a.

short gastric aa.

proper hepatic a.

right gastric a.

splenic a.

gastro-duodenal a.

superior pancreatico-duodenal a.

left gastro-epipolic a.

superior mesenteric a.

right gastroepiploic a.

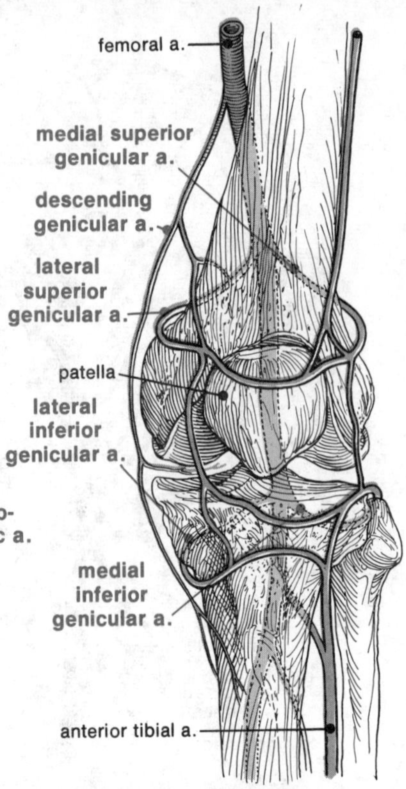

femoral a.

medial superior genicular a.

descending genicular a.

lateral superior genicular a.

patella

lateral inferior genicular a.

medial inferior genicular a.

anterior tibial a.

ARTERY	ORIGIN	BRANCHES	DISTRIBUTION
femoral circumflex a., lateral lateral circumflex a. of thigh *a. circumflexa femoris lateral*	deep femoral a.	ascending, descending, transverse	hip joint, thigh muscles
femoral circumflex a., medial medial circumflex a. of thigh *a. circumflexa femoris medial*	deep femoral a.	deep, ascending, transverse, acetabular	hip joint, thigh muscles
fibular a.	see peroneal artery		
frontal a.	see supraorbital artery		
gastric a., left *a. gastrica sinistra*	celiac a.	esophageal; hepatic (at times)	lesser curvature of stomach, abdominal part of esophagus; left lobe of liver (at times)
gastric a., right *a. gastrica dextra*	common hepatic a.		pyloric end of stomach
gastric a.'s, short vasa brevia *aa. gastricae breves*	splenic a.		greater curvature of stomach
gastroduodenal a. *a. gastroduodenalis*	common hepatic a.	right gastroepiploic, superior pancreaticoduodenal, retroduodenal	stomach, duodenum, pancreas, greater omentum
gastroepiploic a., left *a. gastroepiploica sinistra*	splenic a.	gastric, omental	stomach, greater omentum
gastroepiploic a., right *a. gastroepiploica dextra*	gastroduodenal a.	pyloric, ascending, descending, long ventral epiploic	stomach, greater omentum
genicular a., descending descending a. of the knee highest genicular a. *a. genus descendens*	femoral a.	saphenous, articular	knee joint and adjacent parts
genicular a., highest	see genicular artery, descending		
genicular a., lateral inferior *a. genus lateralis inferior*	popliteal a.		knee joint, gastrocnemius muscle
genicular a., lateral superior *a. genus lateralis superior*	popliteal a.		lower part of femur, knee joint, patella, contiguous muscles
genicular a., medial inferior *a. genus medialis inferior*	popliteal a.		proximal end of tibia, knee joint
genicular a., medial superior *a. genus medialis superior*	popliteal a.		femur, knee joint, patella, contiguous muscles

artery | artery

36

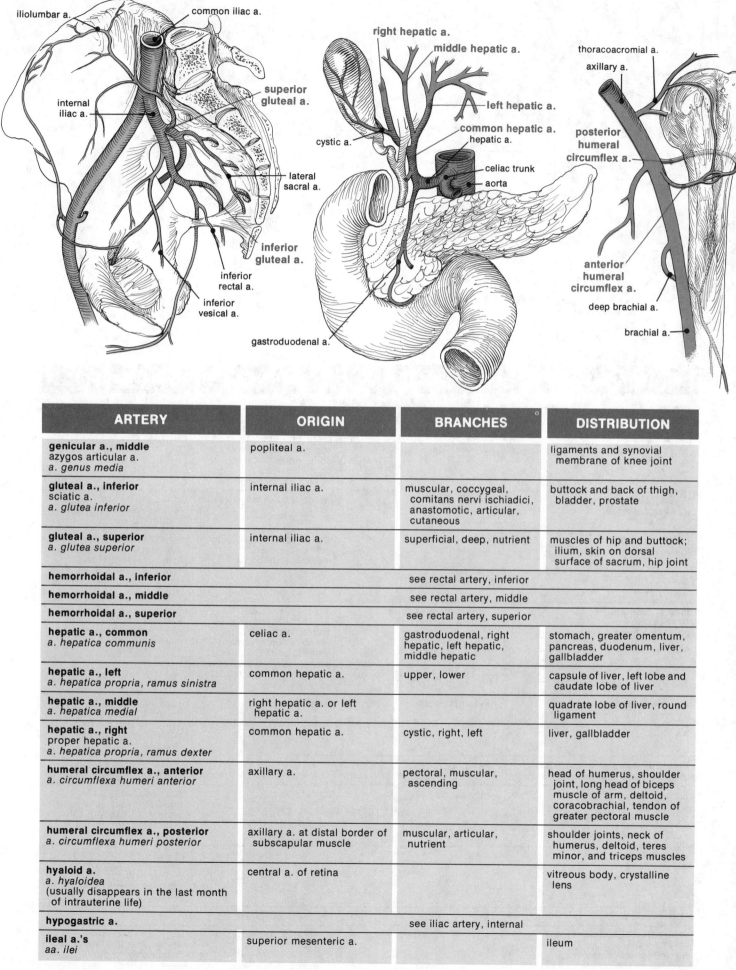

ARTERY	ORIGIN	BRANCHES	DISTRIBUTION
genicular a., middle azygos articular a. *a. genus media*	popliteal a.		ligaments and synovial membrane of knee joint
gluteal a., inferior sciatic a. *a. glutea inferior*	internal iliac a.	muscular, coccygeal, comitans nervi ischiadici, anastomotic, articular, cutaneous	buttock and back of thigh, bladder, prostate
gluteal a., superior *a. glutea superior*	internal iliac a.	superficial, deep, nutrient	muscles of hip and buttock; ilium, skin on dorsal surface of sacrum, hip joint
hemorrhoidal a., inferior		see rectal artery, inferior	
hemorrhoidal a., middle		see rectal artery, middle	
hemorrhoidal a., superior		see rectal artery, superior	
hepatic a., common *a. hepatica communis*	celiac a.	gastroduodenal, right hepatic, left hepatic, middle hepatic	stomach, greater omentum, pancreas, duodenum, liver, gallbladder
hepatic a., left *a. hepatica propria, ramus sinistra*	common hepatic a.	upper, lower	capsule of liver, left lobe and caudate lobe of liver
hepatic a., middle *a. hepatica medial*	right hepatic a. or left hepatic a.		quadrate lobe of liver, round ligament
hepatic a., right proper hepatic a. *a. hepatica propria, ramus dexter*	common hepatic a.	cystic, right, left	liver, gallbladder
humeral circumflex a., anterior *a. circumflexa humeri anterior*	axillary a.	pectoral, muscular, ascending	head of humerus, shoulder joint, long head of biceps muscle of arm, deltoid, coracobrachial, tendon of greater pectoral muscle
humeral circumflex a., posterior *a. circumflexa humeri posterior*	axillary a. at distal border of subscapular muscle	muscular, articular, nutrient	shoulder joints, neck of humerus, deltoid, teres minor, and triceps muscles
hyaloid a. *a. hyaloidea* (usually disappears in the last month of intrauterine life)	central a. of retina		vitreous body, crystalline lens
hypogastric a.		see iliac artery, internal	
ileal a.'s *aa. ilei*	superior mesenteric a.		ileum

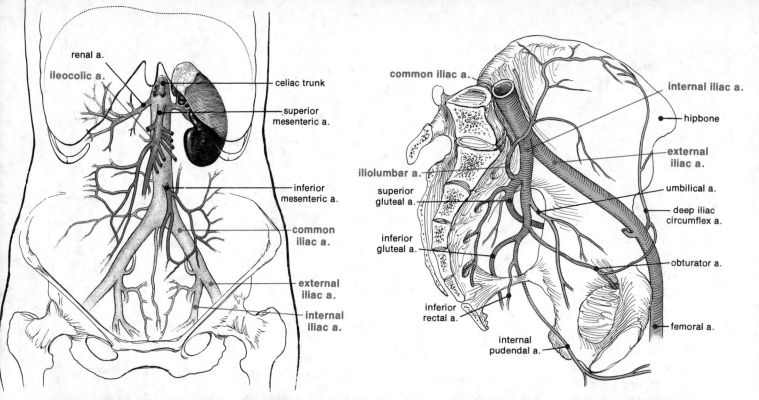

ARTERY	ORIGIN	BRANCHES	DISTRIBUTION
ileocolic a. *a. ileocolica*	superior mesenteric a.	superior branch (anastomoses with right colic a.), inferior branch (anastomoses with end of superior mesenteric a.), colic, anterior cecal, posterior cecal, appendicular, ileal	cecum, vermiform appendix, ascending colon, distal part of ileum
iliac a., common *a. iliaca communis*	abdominal aorta	internal and external iliac	pelvis, genital and gluteal regions, peritoneum, lower abdominal wall
iliac a., external *a. iliaca externa*	common iliac a.	inferior epigastric, deep iliac circumflex, muscular, glandular	lower part of abdominal wall, external genitals, psoas major, cremaster, ductus deferens in male, round ligament of uterus in female
iliac a., internal hypogastric a. *a. iliaca interna*	continuation of common iliac a.	visceral branches: umbilical, inferior vesical, middle rectal, uterine; ventral branch: obturator, internal pudendal; dorsal branch: iliolumbar, lateral sulcus, superior gluteal, inferior gluteal	wall and viscera of pelvis, external genitals, region of anus, medial aspect of thigh
iliac circumflex a., deep *a. circumflexa ilium profunda*	external iliac a.	muscular, cutaneous	psoas, iliac, sartorius, and neighboring muscles; overlying skin, oblique and transverse abdominal muscles
iliac circumflex a., superficial *a. circumflexa ilium superficialis*	femoral		skin of groin, superficial subinguinal lymph nodes
iliolumbar a. *a. iliolumbalis*	internal iliac a.	lumbar, iliac	greater psoas muscle, quadratus muscle of loins, gluteal, and abdominal muscles; ilium, cauda equina
infraorbital a. *a. infraorbitalis*	maxillary	orbital, alveolar, terminal	orbit, maxilla, maxillary sinus and teeth, lower eyelid, extrinsic eye muscles, cheek, side of nose
innominate a.	see brachiocephalic trunk		
intercostal a.'s, anterior intercostal a.'s *aa. intercostales anterior*	internal thoracic a.	pectoral, glandular	first five or six intercostal spaces, pectoral muscles, mammary gland

artery | artery

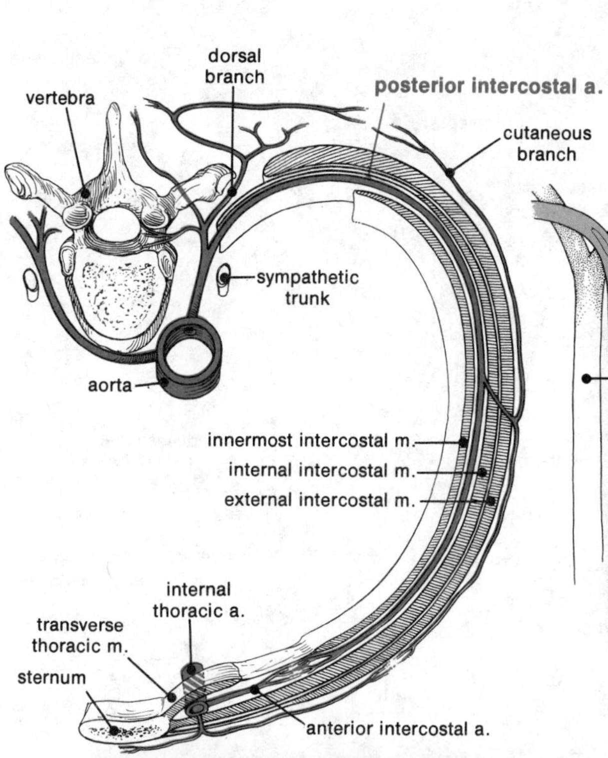

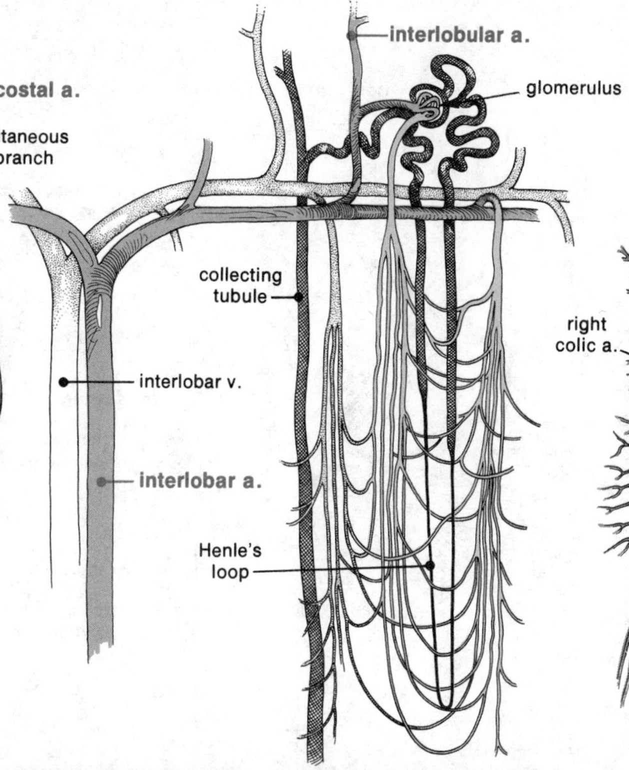

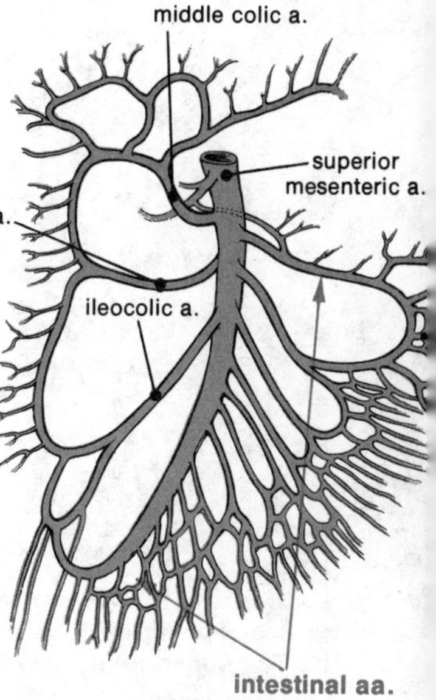

ARTERY	ORIGIN	BRANCHES	DISTRIBUTION
intercostal a.'s, highest *a. intercostalis suprema*	costocervical trunk	muscular, spinal	first and second intercostal spaces, spinal cord, back muscles
intercostal a.'s, posterior (usually nine pairs) aortic intercostals *aa. intercostales posterior*	thoracic aorta	collateral intercostal, muscular, lateral cutaneous, mammary	nine caudal intercostal spaces, pectoral and anterior serratus muscles, mammary gland
interlobar a.'s of kidney *aa. interlobares renis*	renal a.	arcuate	corticomedullary zone of kidney
interlobular a.'s of kidney *aa. interlobulares renis*	arcuate a.'s of kidney	afferent glomeruli	renal glomeruli
interlobular a.'s of liver *aa. interlobulares hepatis*	proper hepatic a.'s		between hepatic lobules
interosseous a., anterior volar interosseous a. *a. interossea anterior*	common interosseous a.	median, muscular, nutrient	deep parts of front of forearm; radius, ulna
interosseous a., common *a. interossea communis*	ulnar a., immediately distal to tuberosity of radius	dorsal interosseous, palmar metacarpal	forearm, radius, ulna
interosseous a., dorsal posterior interosseous a. *a. interossea dorsalis*	common interosseous a.	recurrent interosseous	deep parts of back of forearm
interosseous a.'s, palmar	see metacarpal arteries, palmar		
interosseous a., recurrent *a. interossea recurrens*	posterior interosseous a.		back of elbow joint
intestinal a.'s (12–15 in number) *aa. jejunales et ilei* *aa. intestinales*	superior mesenteric a.		jejunum, ileum
labial a., inferior *a. labialis inferior*	facial a. near angle of mouth		labial glands, mucous membrane, and muscles of lower lip
labial a., superior *a. labialis superior*	facial a.	septal, ala	upper lip, nasal septum, ala of nose
labyrinthine a. internal auditory a. *a. labyrinthi*	basilar a. or anterior inferior cerebellar a.	vestibular, cochlear	internal ear
lacrimal a. *a. lacrimalis*	ophthalmic a. close to optic foramen	lateral palpebral, zygomatic, recurrent, muscular, anterior ciliary	lacrimal gland, upper and lower eyelids, conjunctiva, superior and lateral recti muscles, cheek, ciliary processes

artery | artery

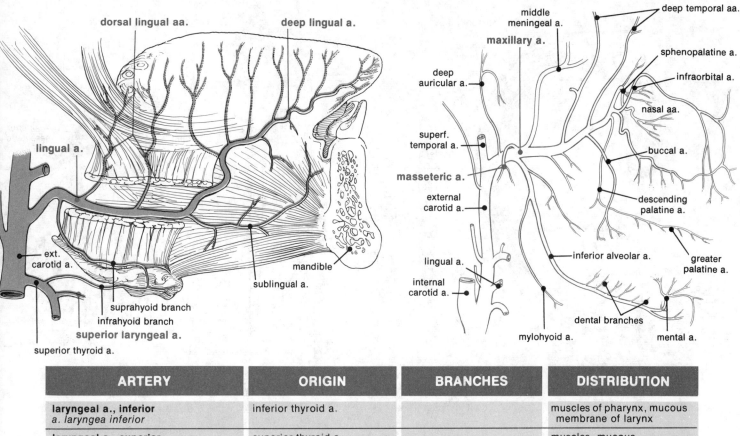

dorsal lingual aa.

deep lingual a.

lingual a.

ext. carotid a.

superior laryngeal a.

suprahyoid branch

infrahyoid branch

superior thyroid a.

mandible

sublingual a.

middle meningeal a.

deep temporal aa.

maxillary a.

sphenopalatine a.

deep auricular a.

infraorbital a.

nasal aa.

superf. temporal a.

buccal a.

masseteric a.

external carotid a.

descending palatine a.

lingual a.

inferior alveolar a.

greater palatine a.

internal carotid a.

dental branches

mylohyoid a.

mental a.

ARTERY	ORIGIN	BRANCHES	DISTRIBUTION
laryngeal a., inferior *a. laryngea inferior*	inferior thyroid a.		muscles of pharynx, mucous membrane of larynx
laryngeal a., superior *a. laryngea superior*	superior thyroid a. (occasionally from external carotid a.)		muscles, mucous membrane, and glands of larynx
lienal a.	see splenic artery		
lingual a. *a. lingualis*	external carotid a.	suprahyoid, dorsal lingual, sublingual, deep lingual	muscles and mucosa of tongue, sublingual gland, gingiva, soft palate, tonsil, epiglottis
lingual a., deep ranine a. *a. profunda linguae*	lingual a. (terminal portion)		intrinsic lingual muscles, genioglossus muscles, lingual mucosa
lingual a.'s, dorsal *a. dorsales linguae*	lingual a.		mucous membrane of posterior part of tongue; glossopalatine arch, tonsil, soft palate, epiglottis
lumbar a.'s (4–5 in number) *aa. lumbalis*	abdominal aorta	dorsal, spinal	lumbar vertebrae, back muscles, abdominal wall
lumbar a., lowest *a. lumbalis ima*	median sacral a.		sacrum, iliac muscle
malleolar a., anterior lateral external malleolar a. *a. malleolaris anterior lateral*	anterior tibial a.		outer side of ankle
malleolar a., anterior medial internal malleolar a. *a. malleolaris anterior medial*	anterior tibial a.		inner side of ankle
malleolar a., posterior medial internal malleolar a. *a. malleolaris posterior medial*	posterior tibial		inner side of ankle
mammary a., external	see thoracic artery, lateral		
mammary a., internal	see thoracic artery, internal		
mandibular a.	see alveolar artery, inferior		
masseteric a. *a. masseterica*	maxillary		masseter muscle
maxillary a. internal maxillary a. deep facial a. *a. maxillaris*	external carotid a.	mandibular portion: deep auricular, anterior tympanic, inferior alveolar, middle	ear, teeth, dura mater, trigeminal ganglion, temporal, masseter, buccinator, and eye

artery | artery

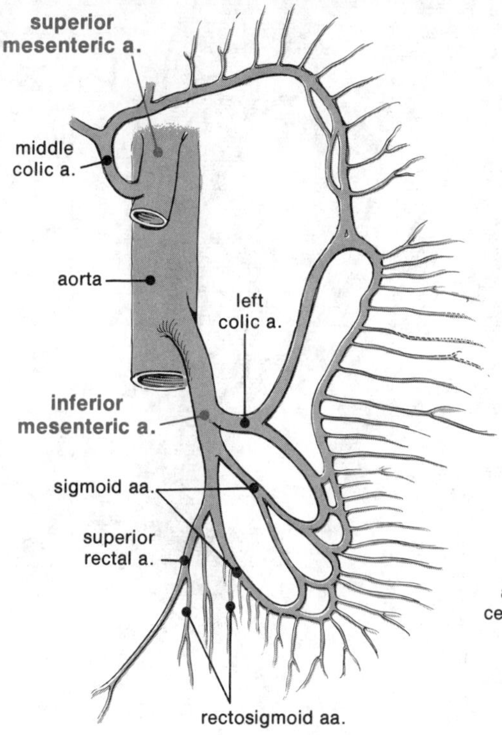

superior mesenteric a.

middle colic a.

aorta

left colic a.

inferior mesenteric a.

sigmoid aa.

superior rectal a.

rectosigmoid aa.

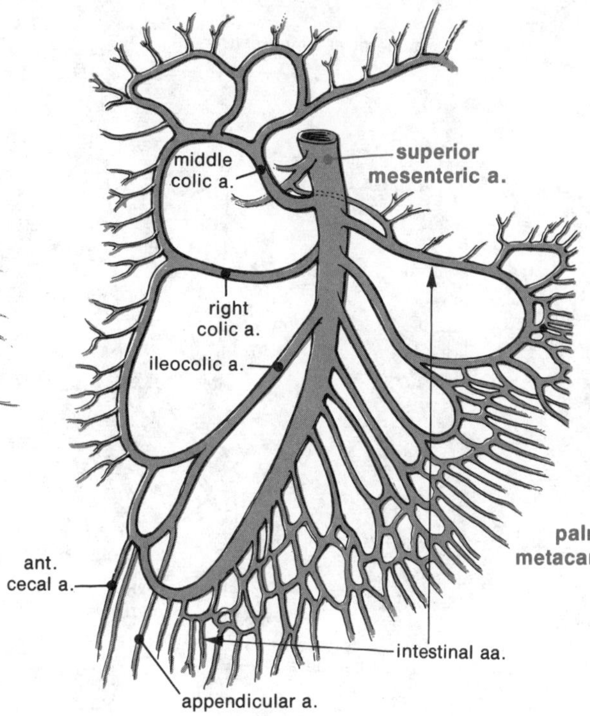

middle colic a.

superior mesenteric a.

right colic a.

ileocolic a.

ant. cecal a.

intestinal aa.

appendicular a.

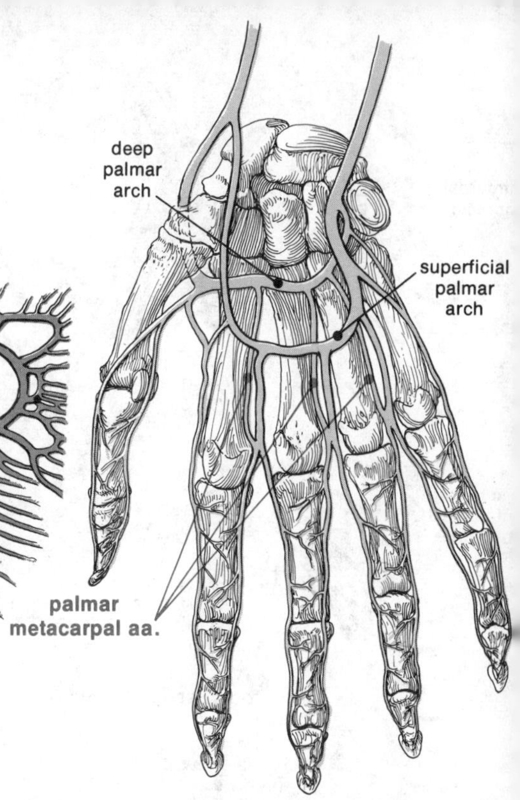

deep palmar arch

superficial palmar arch

palmar metacarpal aa.

ARTERY	ORIGIN	BRANCHES	DISTRIBUTION
		meningeal, accessory meningeal; pterygoid portion: deep temporal, ptyergoid, masseteric, buccal; pterygopalatine portion: posterior superior alveolar, infraorbital, greater palatine, artery of the pterygoid canal, pharyngeal, sphenopalatine	muscles, lacrimal gland, palatine tonsil, soft palate, upper pharynx, auditory tube, nasal cavity, sinuses
maxillary a., external	see facial artery		
maxillary a., internal	see maxillary artery		
median a. *a. mediana*	anterior interosseous a.		accompanies median nerve to palm
medullar a.'s *aa. medullaris*	vertebral a. and its branches		medulla oblongata
meningeal a., anterior *a. meningea anterior*	anterior ethmoidal a. or internal carotid a.		dura mater of anterior cranial fossa
meningeal a., middle *a. meningea media*	maxillary a.	anterior, posterior	cranial bones, dura mater, tensor tympani muscle, semilunar ganglion, orbit
meningeal a., posterior *a. meningea posterior*	ascending pharyngeal a.		dura mater of posterior and middle cranial fossae
mesenteric a., inferior *a. mesenterica inferior*	abdominal aorta	left colic, sigmoid, superior rectal	transverse, descending, and sigmoid colons, upper part of rectum
mesenteric a., superior *a. mesenterica superior*	abdominal aorta	inferior pancreaticoduodenal, intestinal, ileocolic, right colic, middle colic	small intestine, proximal half of colon
metacarpal a.'s, dorsal (three in number) *aa. metacarpeae dorsales*	radial a. (posterior carpal arch)	dorsal digital	back of second, third, and fourth fingers
metacarpal a.'s, palmar palmar interosseous a.'s *aa. metacarpeae palmares*	deep palmar arch		interosseous muscles, metacarpal bones, second, third, and fourth lumbrical muscles
metatarsal a., first dorsal *a. dorsalis hallucis*	dorsal a. of foot	branch to medial side of great toe, branch to adjoining sides of the second and great toes	medial border of great toe and adjoining sides of great and second toes

artery | artery

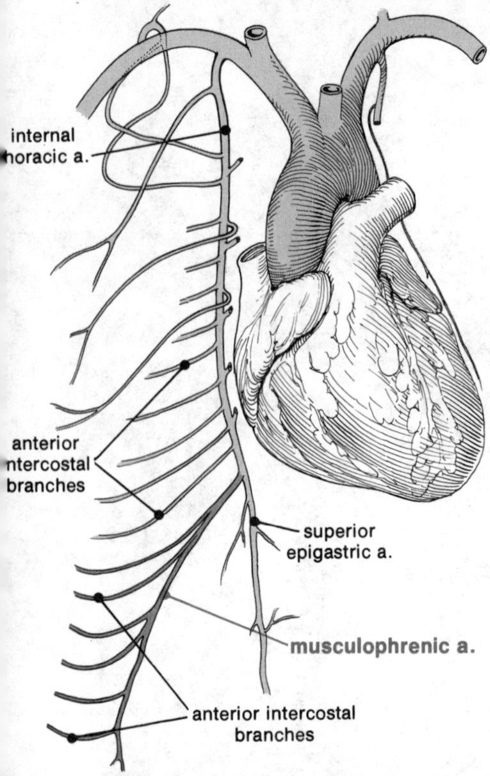

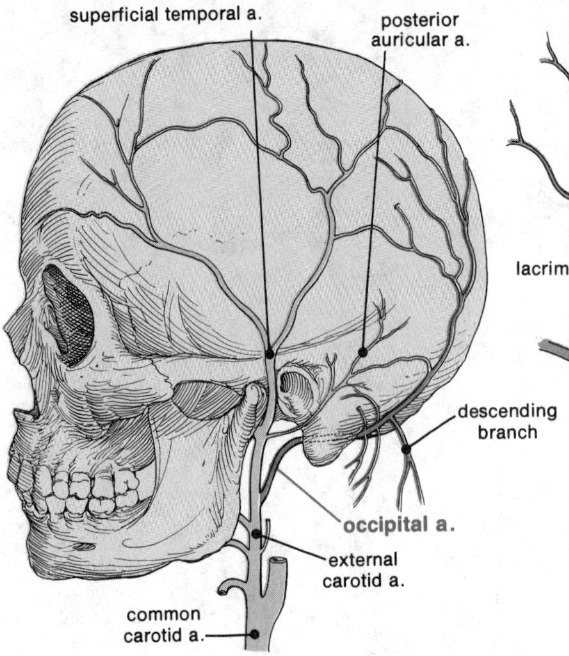

internal thoracic a.

anterior intercostal branches

superior epigastric a.

musculophrenic a.

anterior intercostal branches

superficial temporal a.

posterior auricular a.

descending branch

occipital a.

external carotid a.

common carotid a.

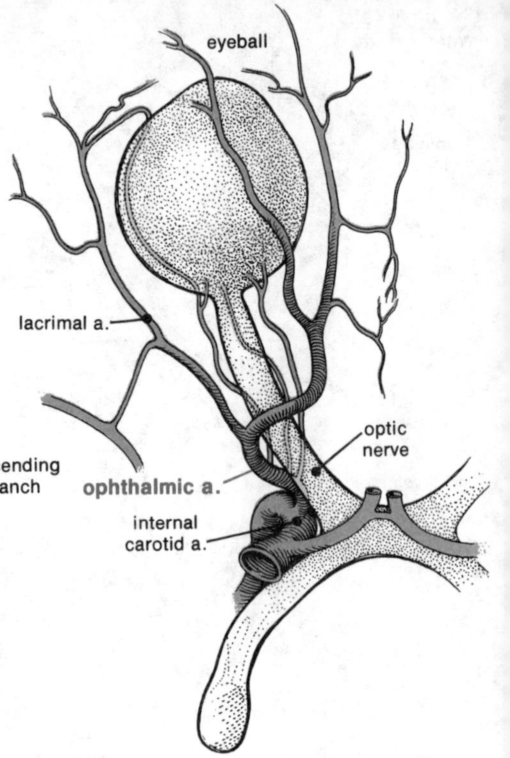

eyeball

lacrimal a.

ophthalmic a.

internal carotid a.

optic nerve

ARTERY	ORIGIN	BRANCHES	DISTRIBUTION
metatarsal a.'s, plantar (four in number) digital a.'s of foot, common *aa. metatarseae plantares*	plantar arch	common digital, anterior perforating	plantar surface and adjacent sides of toes
musculophrenic a. *a. musculophrenica*	internal thoracic a.	anterior intercostal, phrenic, muscular	diaphragm, seventh, eighth, and ninth intercostal spaces, pericardium
mylohyoid a. *a. mylohyoideus*	inferior alveolar a.		mylohyoid muscle
nasal a., dorsal *a. dorsalis nasi*	ophthalmic a.	lacrimal	skin of nose, lacrimal sac
nasal a., lateral *a. nasalis lateral*	maxillary a.		lateral nasal wall
nasal a., posterior *a. nasalis posterior*	maxillary a.		posterior parts of conchae and lateral nasal wall
nasal a., septal *a. nasalis septi*	maxillary a.		nasal septum
nutrient a. of fibula *a. nutricia fibulae*	peroneal a.		substance of fibula
nutrient a. of humerus *a. nutricia humeri*	brachial a., about middle of arm		substance of humerus
nutrient a. of tibia (largest nutrient a. of bone in body) *a. nutricia tibiae*	posterior tibial a.		substrate of tibia
obturator a. *a. obturatoria*	internal iliac a.	iliac, vesical, pubic, anterior branch, posterior branch, muscular, acetabular	bladder, ilium, pelvic muscles, hip joint
occipital a. *a. occipitalis*	external carotid a.	muscular, sternocleidomastoid, auricular, meningeal, descending, terminal	dura mater, diploë, mastoid cells, muscles of neck and scalp
ophthalmic a. *a. ophthalmica*	internal carotid a.	orbital portion: lacrimal, supraorbital, posterior ethmoidal, anterior ethmoidal, medial palpebral supratrochlear, dorsal nasal; ocular portion: central artery of the retina, short posterior ciliary, long posterior ciliary, anterior ciliary, muscular	orbit and surrounding parts

muscles and bulb of the eye |

artery | artery

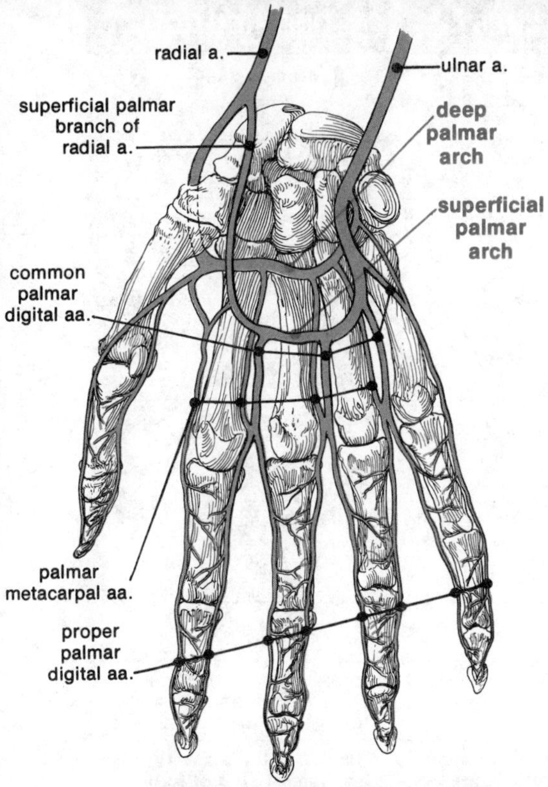

radial a.

ulnar a.

superficial palmar branch of radial a.

deep palmar arch

superficial palmar arch

common palmar digital aa.

palmar metacarpal aa.

proper palmar digital aa.

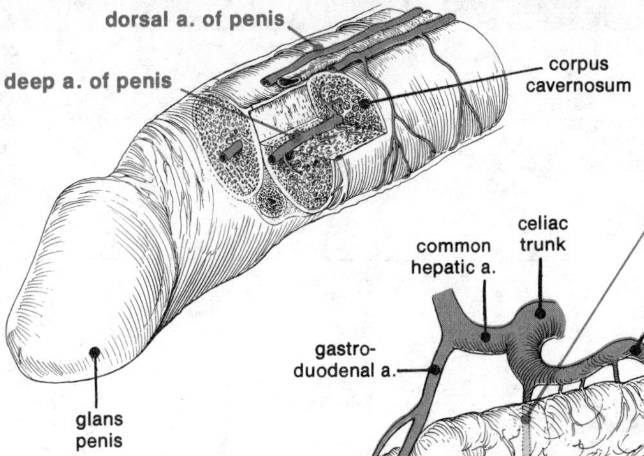

dorsal a. of penis

deep a. of penis

corpus cavernosum

glans penis

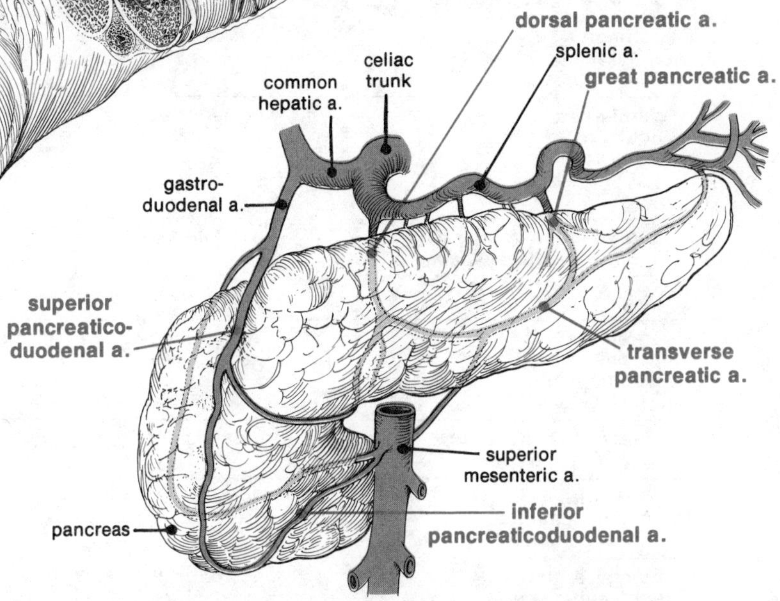

dorsal pancreatic a.

celiac trunk

splenic a.

common hepatic a.

great pancreatic a.

gastro-duodenal a.

superior pancreatico-duodenal a.

transverse pancreatic a.

superior mesenteric a.

inferior pancreaticoduodenal a.

pancreas

ARTERY	ORIGIN	BRANCHES	DISTRIBUTION
ovarian a.'s *aa. ovaricae*	ventral surface of abdominal aorta slightly below the renal a.'s	ureteric, uterine, ovarian; anastomose with uterine a.	ovary, ureter, uterus, round ligament, skin of labium major and groin
palatine a., ascending *a. palatina ascendens*	facial		soft palate, palatine glands, auditory tube
palatine a., descending *a. palatina descendens*	maxillary a.	greater palatine, lesser palatine	soft palate, hard palate, tonsil, gums
palatine a., greater *a. palatina major*	maxillary a.		hard palate, gums, palatine glands
palatine a.'s, lesser *aa. palatinae minores*	greater palatine a.		soft palate, palatine tonsil
palmar arch, deep *arcus palmaris profundus*	radial a.	palmar metacarpal; anastomoses with deep palmar branch of ulnar	carpal extremities of metacarpal bones, interosseous muscles
palmar arch, superficial *arcus palmaris superficialis*	ulnar a.	common palmar digital	palm
palpebral a.'s, lateral *aa. palpebrales laterales*	ophthalmic a. or lacrimal a.	superior, inferior	eyelids, conjunctiva
palpebral a.'s, medial *aa. palpebrales mediales*	ophthalmic a. near the pulley of the superior oblique muscle	superior, inferior	eyelids, conjunctiva, nasolacrimal duct
pancreatic a., dorsal *a. pancreatica dorsalis*	splenic a.	right, left (becomes transverse pancreatic a.)	pancreas
pancreatic a., great *a. pancreatica magna*	splenic a.		pancreas
pancreatic a., transverse *a. pancreatica transversalis*	dorsal pancreatic a.	long, short	pancreas, greater omentum
pancreaticoduodenal a., inferior duodenal a. *a. pancreaticoduodenalis inferior*	superior mesenteric a. or from its first intestinal branch		head of pancreas, descending and inferior parts of duodenum
pancreaticoduodenal a., superior *a. pancreaticoduodenalis superior*	gastroduodenal a.	ventral pancreaticoduodenal arcade	pancreas, three parts of duodenum
penis, deep a. of a. of corpus cavernosum *a. profunda penis*	internal pudendal a.		corpus cavernosum of penis
penis, dorsal a. of *a. dorsalis penis*	internal pudendal a.		glans and prepuce of penis, integument and fibrous sheath of corpus cavernosum

ARTERY	ORIGIN	BRANCHES	DISTRIBUTION
perforating a.'s *aa. perforantes*	deep femoral a.	first perforating, second perforating, third perforating	back of thigh, femur
pericardiacophrenic a. *a. pericardiacophrenica*	internal thoracic a.		diaphragm, pericardium, pleura
perineal a. superficial perineal a. *a. perinei*	internal pudendal a.	transverse perineal	perineum, external genitalia
peroneal a. fibular a. *a. peronea*	posterior tibial a.	muscular, nutrient (fibula), perforating, communicating, posterior lateral malleolar, lateral calcaneal	soleus and other deep calf muscles, lateral side and back of ankle and heel
pharyngeal a., ascending *a. pharyngea ascendens*	external carotid a.	pharyngeal, palatine, prevertebral, inferior tympanic, posterior meningeal	wall of pharynx, soft palate, tonsil, ear, meninges, muscles of back of head and neck
phrenic a.'s phrenic a.'s, inferior diaphragmatic a., inferior *aa. phrenicae*	abdominal aorta or celiac a.	medial, lateral, suprarenal	diaphragm, adrenal gland
phrenic a.'s, superior *aa. phrenicae superior*	thoracic aorta		diaphragm
plantar a., deep communicating a. *ramus plantaris profundus*	dorsal a. of foot	first plantar metatarsal; with lateral plantar a., forms plantar arch	undersurface and adjacent sides of first and second toes
plantar a., lateral *a. plantaris lateral*	posterior tibial a.	calcaneal, muscular, cutaneous; continues to form plantar arch by uniting with deep plantar branch of the dorsal artery of foot	muscles of foot, skin of toes and lateral side of foot
plantar a., medial internal plantar a. *a. plantaris medial*	posterior tibial a.	deep, superficial	flexor muscle of toes, abductor muscle of great toe, skin of inner side of sole
plantar arch	lateral plantar a.	perforating, plantar metatarsal	interosseous muscles, toes
popliteal a. *a. poplitea*	continuation of femoral a. at junction of middle and distal thirds of thigh	superior muscular, sural, cutaneous, medial superior genicular, lateral superior genicular, middle genicular, medial inferior genicular, lateral inferior genicular; it divides at the distal border of the popliteus and continues as anterior and posterior tibial arteries	muscles of thigh in region of knee, femur, patella, and tibia
princeps pollicis a.	see principal artery of thumb			
principal a. of thumb princeps pollicis a. *a. princeps pollicis*	radial a.	volar digital	sides of thumb, dorsal interosseous muscles of hand
profunda a., inferior	see collateral artery, superior ulnar			
profunda a., superior	see brachial artery, deep			
a. profunda brachii	see brachial artery, deep			
profunda femoris a.	see femoral artery, deep			
profunda linguae a.	see lingual artery, deep			
a. of pterygoid canal Vidian a. *a. canalis pterygoidei*	maxillary a.	pharyngeal, auditory, tympanic, muscular	upper part of pharynx, auditory tube, sphenoidal sinus, middle ear chamber, muscles of palate
pudendal a., deep external deep external pudic a. *a. pudenda externa profunda*	femoral a.	anterior scrotal or anterior labial; inguinal	skin of scrotum and perineum in male; labium major in female
pudendal a., internal *a. pudenda interna*	internal iliac a.	muscular, inferior rectal, perineal, artery of the bulb, urethral, deep artery of the penis, dorsal artery of the penis	penis, scrotum, clitoris, muscles of perineum, anal canal

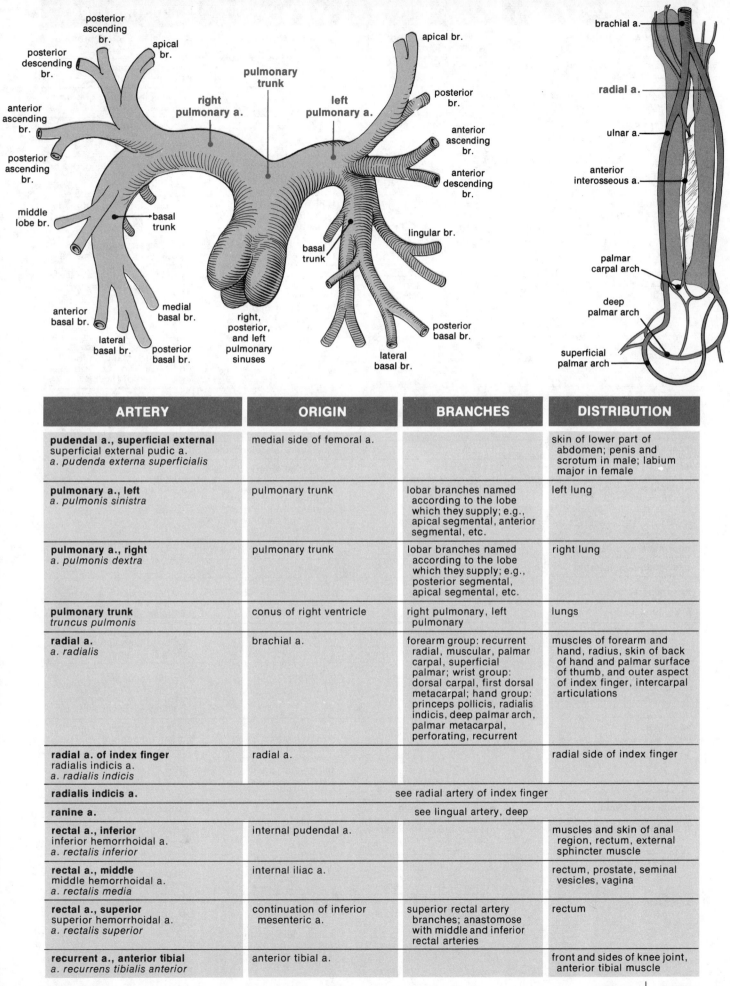

ARTERY	ORIGIN	BRANCHES	DISTRIBUTION
pudendal a., superficial external superficial external pudic a. *a. pudenda externa superficialis*	medial side of femoral a.		skin of lower part of abdomen; penis and scrotum in male; labium major in female
pulmonary a., left *a. pulmonis sinistra*	pulmonary trunk	lobar branches named according to the lobe which they supply; e.g., apical segmental, anterior segmental, etc.	left lung
pulmonary a., right *a. pulmonis dextra*	pulmonary trunk	lobar branches named according to the lobe which they supply; e.g., posterior segmental, apical segmental, etc.	right lung
pulmonary trunk *truncus pulmonis*	conus of right ventricle	right pulmonary, left pulmonary	lungs
radial a. *a. radialis*	brachial a.	forearm group: recurrent radial, muscular, palmar carpal, superficial palmar; wrist group: dorsal carpal, first dorsal metacarpal; hand group: princeps pollicis, radialis indicis, deep palmar arch, palmar metacarpal, perforating, recurrent	muscles of forearm and hand, radius, skin of back of hand and palmar surface of thumb, and outer aspect of index finger, intercarpal articulations
radial a. of index finger radialis indicis a. *a. radialis indicis*	radial a.		radial side of index finger
radialis indicis a.	see radial artery of index finger		
ranine a.	see lingual artery, deep		
rectal a., inferior inferior hemorrhoidal a. *a. rectalis inferior*	internal pudendal a.		muscles and skin of anal region, rectum, external sphincter muscle
rectal a., middle middle hemorrhoidal a. *a. rectalis media*	internal iliac a.		rectum, prostate, seminal vesicles, vagina
rectal a., superior superior hemorrhoidal a. *a. rectalis superior*	continuation of inferior mesenteric a.	superior rectal artery branches; anastomose with middle and inferior rectal arteries	rectum
recurrent a., anterior tibial *a. recurrens tibialis anterior*	anterior tibial a.		front and sides of knee joint, anterior tibial muscle

ARTERY	ORIGIN	BRANCHES	DISTRIBUTION
recurrent a., anterior ulnar *a. recurrens ulnaris, ramus anterior*	ulnar a., immediately distal to elbow joint		brachial and round pronator muscles
recurrent a., posterior tibial *a. recurrens tibialis posterior*	posterior tibial a.		tibiofibular joint, knee joint, popliteus muscle
recurrent a., posterior ulnar *a. recurrens ulnaris, ramus posterior*	ulnar a.		elbow joint and neighboring muscles and skin
recurrent a., radial *a. recurrens radialis*	radial a., immediately distal to elbow		elbow joint, supinator, brachioradial, and brachial muscles
renal a. *a. renalis*	abdominal aorta	inferior suprarenal, ureteral, perirenal, glandular	kidney, adrenal gland, ureter
retroduodenal a. *a. retroduodenalis*	gastroduodenal a., just above the duodenum	U-shaped dorsal pancreaticoduodenal arcade	all four parts of duodenum, head of pancreas, bile duct
sacral a.'s, lateral *aa. sacrales laterales*	internal iliac	superior and inferior spinal branches	muscles and skin on dorsal surface of sacrum; sacral canal
sacral a., middle *a. sacralis mediana*	dorsal side of aorta, slightly above its bifurcation	middle sacral artery branches; anastomose with lumbar branch of iliolumbar and lateral sacral arteries	rectum, sacrum, coccyx
scapular circumflex a. *a. circumflexa scapulae*	subscapular a.		subscapular, teres major, teres minor, and deltoid muscles; shoulder joint, long head of triceps
scapular a., descending transverse cervical a. *a. scapularis descendens*	thyrocervical trunk	superficial, deep	levator muscle of scapula, and trapezius; rhomboid, and latissimus dorsi muscles
scapular a., transverse		see suprascapular artery	
sciatic a.		see gluteal artery, inferior	
sigmoid a.'s *aa. sigmoideae*	inferior mesenteric	branches of sigmoid arteries; anastomose cranially with left colic artery and caudally with superior rectal artery	caudal part of descending colon, iliac colon, sigmoid (pelvic colon)
spermatic a., external		see cremasteric artery	
spermatic a.'s, internal		see testicular arteries	
sphenopalatine a. nasopalatine a. *a. sphenopalatina*	maxillary a.	posterior lateral nasal, posterior septal	frontal, maxillary, ethmoidal, and sphenoidal sinuses, nasal septum
spinal a., anterior ventral spinal a. *a. spinalis anterior*	vertebral a. near termination		anterior side of medulla oblongata and spinal cord, filum terminale, meninges
spinal a., posterior dorsal spinal a. *a. spinalis posterior*	vertebral a. at side of medulla oblongata	ascending	medulla oblongata, posterior part of spinal cord, and cauda equina, meninges, fourth ventricle
splenic a. lienal a. *a. lienalis*	celiac a.	pancreatic, left gastroepiploic, short gastric, splenic, dorsal pancreatic, caudae pancreatic, great pancreatic	spleen, pancreas, stomach, greater omentum
sternocleidomastoid a. sternomastoid a. *a. sternocleidomastoidea*	occipital a. close to its commencement (occasionally from external carotid a.)		sternocleidomastoid muscle
stylomastoid a. *a. stylomastoidea*	posterior auricular a.	mastoid, stapedial, posterior tympanic	middle ear chamber, stapes, stapedius muscle, mastoid cells, semicircular canals
subclavian a. *a. subclavia*	right side: brachiocephalic trunk; left side: arch of aorta	vertebral, thyrocervical, internal thoracic, costocervical, descending scapular; it becomes the axillary artery at the outer border of the first rib	neck, thoracic wall, muscles of upper arm and shoulder, spinal cord and brain

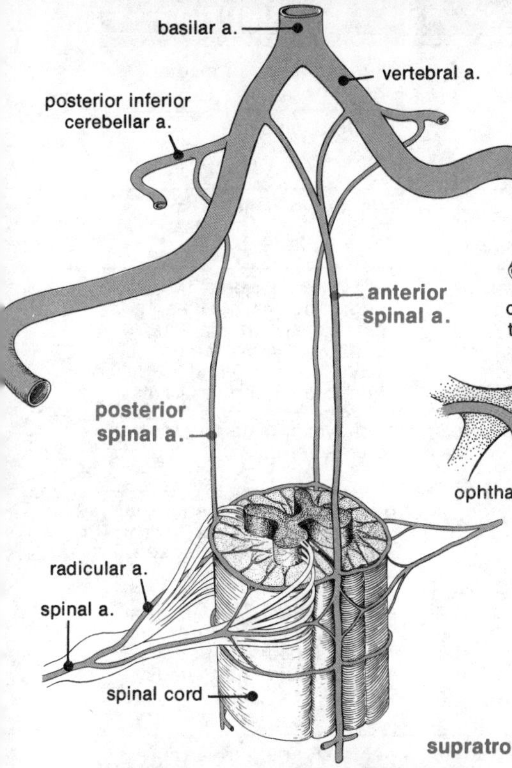

basilar a.
vertebral a.
posterior inferior cerebellar a.
anterior spinal a.
posterior spinal a.
radicular a.
spinal a.
spinal cord 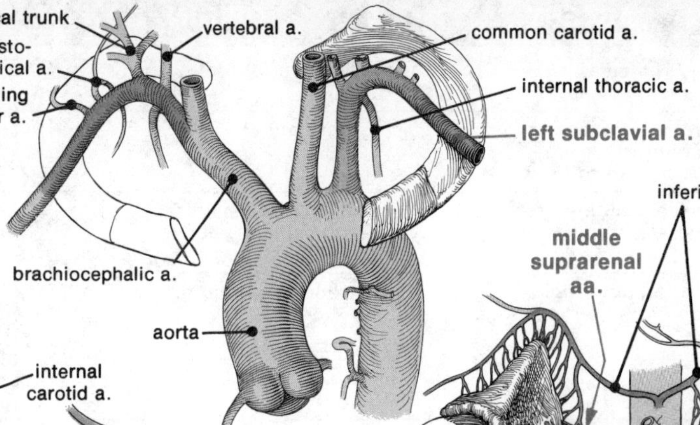
optic tract
internal carotid a.
ophthalmic a.
supraorbital a.
eyeball
supratrochlear a.
thyrocervical trunk
costo-cervical a.
descending scapular a.
vertebral a.
common carotid a.
internal thoracic a.
left subclavial a.
brachiocephalic a.
aorta
inferior phrenic aa.
middle suprarenal aa.
superior suprarenal aa.
renal a.
inferior suprarenal a.
kidney

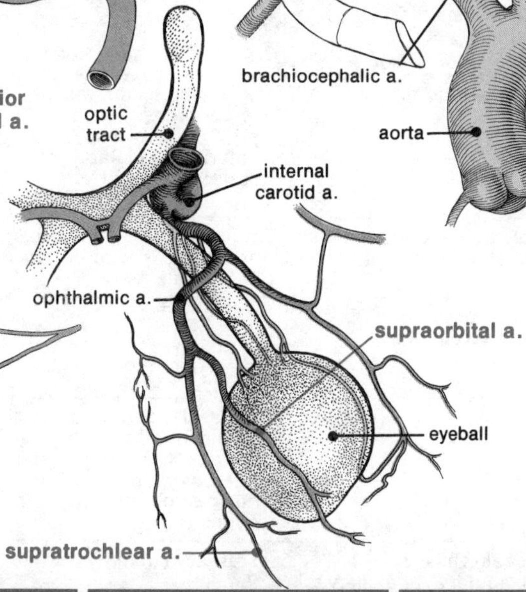

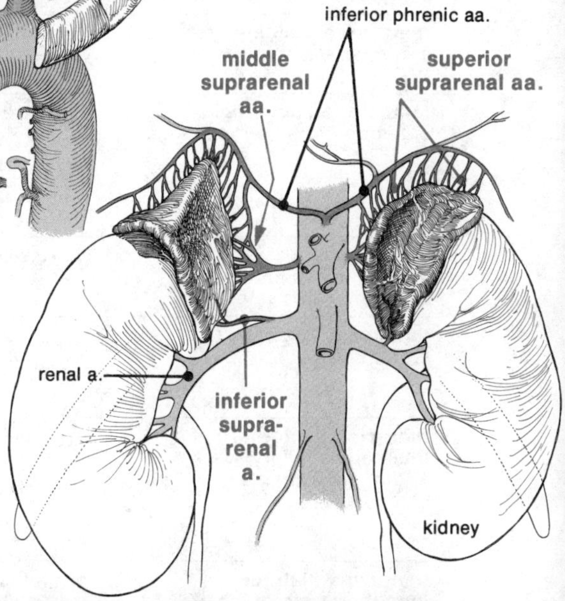

ARTERY	ORIGIN	BRANCHES	DISTRIBUTION
subcostal a. 12th thoracic a. *a. subcostalis*	thoracic aorta	dorsal, spinal	upper abdominal wall below 12th rib
sublingual a. *a. sublingualis*	lingual a.		sublingual gland, mylohyoid, geniohyoid, and genioglossus muscles, mucous membrane of mouth and gums
submental a. *a. submentalis*	facial a. (occasionally external maxillary a.)	superficial, deep	mylohyoid, digastric, and platysma muscles; sublingual salivary gland, skin under chin, lip
subscapular a. *a. subscapularis*	axillary a. (largest branch)	circumflex scapular, thoracodorsal	scapular region, shoulder joint
superficial perineal a.		see perineal artery	
supraorbital a. frontal a. *a. supraorbitalis*	ophthalmic a. as it crosses the optic nerve	superficial, deep	skin, muscles, and pericranium of forehead; superior rectus muscle of eyeball, levator muscle of upper eyelid, diplöe
suprarenal a., inferior *a. suprarenalis inferior*	renal a.		adrenal gland
suprarenal a.'s, middle middle capsular a.'s *aa. suprarenales mediae*	abdominal aorta, at level of superior mesenteric a.	anastomose with suprarenal branches of inferior phrenic and renal arteries	adrenal gland
suprarenal a., superior *a. suprarenalis superior*	phrenic a.		adrenal gland
suprascapular a. transverse scapular a. *a. suprascapularis*	thyrocervical trunk	acromial, suprasternal articular, nutrient	clavicle, scapula, skin of chest, skin over acromion, acromioclavicular and shoulder joints, supraspinous and infraspinous muscles
supratrochlear a. frontal a. *a. supratrochlearis* *a. frontalis*	ophthalmic a.		skin, muscles, and pericranium of forehead
sural a.'s inferior muscular a.'s *aa. surales*	popliteal a. opposite the knee joint		gastrocnemius, soleus, and plantar muscles, neighboring skin
tarsal a., lateral tarsal a. *a. tarsea lateralis*	dorsal a. of foot		muscles and articulations of tarsus

ARTERY	ORIGIN	BRANCHES	DISTRIBUTION
tarsal a.'s, medial *aa. tarseae medialis*	dorsal a. of foot		skin and joints of medial border of foot
temporal a.'s, deep (two in number) *aa. temporales profundae*	maxillary a.		temporal muscle
temporal a., middle *a. temporalis media*	superficial temporal a. immediately above zygomatic arch		temporal muscle
temporal a., superficial *a. temporalis superficialis*	external carotid a.	transverse facial, middle temporal, zygomaticoorbital, anterior auricular, frontal, parietal, parotid	temporal, masseter, frontal, and orbicular muscles, external auditory meatus, auricle, skin of face and scalp, parotid gland, temporomandibular joint
testicular a.'s spermatic a.'s, internal *aa. testiculares*	ventral surface of abdominal aorta, slightly caudal to the renal a.'s	branches of testicular a.'s; anastomose with ductus deferens a.	epididymis, testis, ureter, cremaster muscle
thoracic a., highest *a. thoracica suprema*	axillary a. or thoracoacromial a.		pectoral muscles, parietes of the thorax, anterior serratus and intercostal muscles
thoracic a., internal internal mammary a. *a. thoracica interna*	subclavian a.	pericardiacophrenic, mediastinal, thymic, sternal, anterior intercostal, perforating, musculophrenic, superior epigastric	anterior thoracic wall, diaphragm, structures in mediastinum such as pericardium and thymus gland
thoracic a., lateral long thoracic a. external mammary a. *a. thoracica lateralis*	thoracoacromial a. or subscapular a. or axillary a.	external mammary (in female)	pectoral, anterior serratus, subscapular muscles; axillary lymph nodes, mammary gland (in female)
thoracic a., twelfth	see subcostal artery		
thoracoacromial a. acromiothoracic a. *a. thoracoacromialis*	axillary a.	pectoral, acromial, lavicular, deltoid	pectoral, deltoid, and subclavius muscles; mammary gland, coracoid process, sternoclavicular joint, acromion
thoracodorsal a. *a. thoracodorsalis*	subscapular a.		subscapular, latissimus dorsi, anterior serratus, and intercostal muscles
thyrocervical trunk *truncus thyrocervicalis*	first portion of subclavian a.	inferior thyroid, suprascapular, transverse cervical	thyroid gland, scapular region, deep neck
thyroid a., inferior *a. thyroidea inferior*	thyrocervical trunk	inferior laryngeal, tracheal, esophageal, ascending cervical, muscular	larynx, trachea, esophagus, thyroid gland, neck muscles
thyroid a., lowest *a. thyroidea ima*	arch of aorta or brachiocephalic trunk		thyroid gland
thyroid a., superior *a. thyroidea superior*	external carotid a.	infrahyoid, sternocleidomastoid, superior laryngeal, cricothyroid	muscles and mucosa of larynx, pharynx, esophagus; thyroid gland, muscles attached to thyroid cartilage and hyoid bone, sternocleidomastoid and neighboring muscles and integument
tibial a., anterior *a. tibialis anterior*	popliteal a. at bifurcation	posterior tibial recurrent, fibular, anterior tibial recurrent, muscular, anterior medial malleolar, anterior lateral malleolar; continues as dorsal a. of foot at ankle joint	muscles of leg; knee joint, ankle, foot, skin of front of leg
tibial a., posterior *a. tibialis posterior*	popliteal a.	peroneal, nutrient (tibial), muscular, posterior medial malleolar, communicating, medial calcaneal, medial plantar, lateral plantar	muscles and bones of leg; ankle joint, foot
tibial recurrent a., anterior *a. recurrens tibialis anterior*	anterior tibial a.		anterior tibial muscle, knee joint, patella, long extensor muscle of toes
tibial recurrent a., posterior *a. recurrens tibialis posterior*	anterior tibial a.		popliteal muscle, knee joint, tibiofibular joint

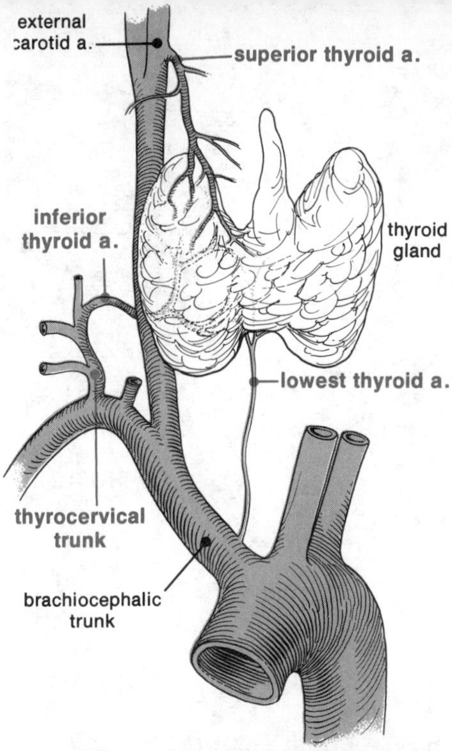

external carotid a. — superior thyroid a.

inferior thyroid a.

thyroid gland

lowest thyroid a.

thyrocervical trunk

brachiocephalic trunk

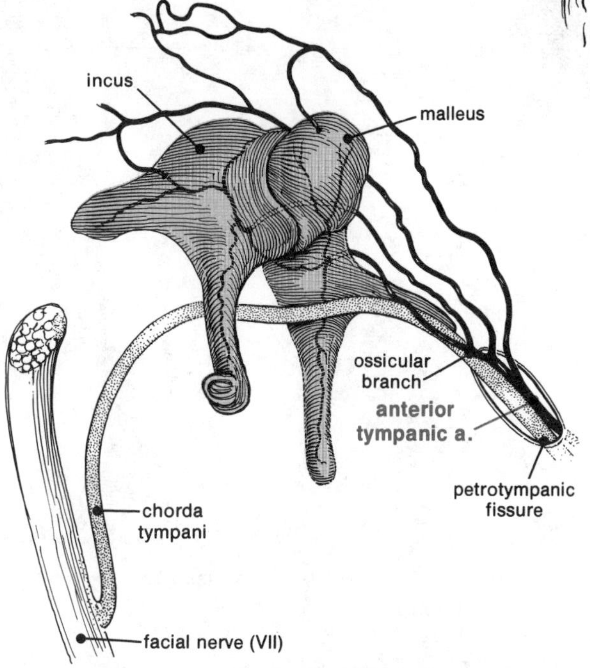

incus

malleus

ossicular branch

anterior tympanic a.

petrotympanic fissure

chorda tympani

facial nerve (VII)

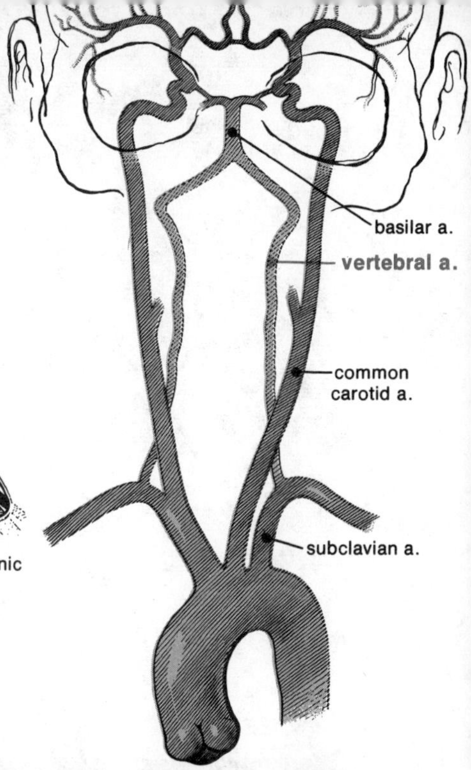

basilar a.

vertebral a.

common carotid a.

subclavian a.

ARTERY	ORIGIN	BRANCHES	DISTRIBUTION
tympanic a., anterior tympanic a. *a. tympanica anterior*	maxillary a.	posterior, superior, ossicular	tympanic membrane, middle ear chamber; ossicles
tympanic a., inferior *a. tympanica inferior*	ascending pharyngeal a.		medial wall of the middle ear chamber
tympanic a., posterior *a. tympanica posterior*	stylomastoid a.	mastoid, stapedial	middle ear chamber, posterior part of tympanic membrane
tympanic a., superior *a. tympanica superior*	middle meningeal a.	frontal, parietal	middle ear chamber, tensor tympani muscle
ulnar a. *a. ulnaris*	brachial a., a little distal to bend of elbow	forearm portion: anterior ulnar recurrent, posterior ulnar recurrent, common interosseous, muscular; wrist portion: palmar carpal, dorsal carpal; hand portion: deep palmar, superficial palmar arch, common palmar digital	hand, wrist, forearm
umbilical a. *a. umbilicalis*	internal iliac a.	ductus deferens, superior vesical; continues as lateral umbilical ligament	urinary bladder, ureter, testes, seminal vesicles, ductus deferens
urethral a. *a. urethralis*	internal pudendal		urethra, corpus cavernosum of penis
uterine a. fallopian a. *a. uterina*	medial surface of internal iliac	cervical, ovarian, tubal, vaginal, ligamentous, ureteric	uterus, uterine tube, round ligament, part of vagina, ovary
vaginal a. *a. vaginalis*	internal iliac a. or uterine a.	rectal, vesical, vestibular	vagina, fundus of urinary bladder, and part of rectum, vestibular bulb
vertebral a. *a. vertebralis*	subclavian a.	cervical portion: spinal, muscular; cranial portion: meningeal, posterior spinal, anterior spinal, posterior inferior cerebellar, medullary	bodies of vertebrae, deep muscles of neck, falx cerebelli, spinal cord, cerebellum, brain stem
vesical a., inferior *a. vesicalis inferior*	internal iliac a.		fundus of bladder, prostate, seminal vesicles
vesical a.'s, superior aa. vesicales superior	umbilical a.		ureter, bladder, urachus
Vidian a.	see pterygoid canal, artery of		
zygomaticoorbital a. *a. zygomatico-orbitalis*	superficial temporal a. (occasionally from the middle temporal a.)		orbicular muscle of eye

artery | artery

rheumatoid arthritis

epiglottis

thyroid cartilage

arytenoid

articulation

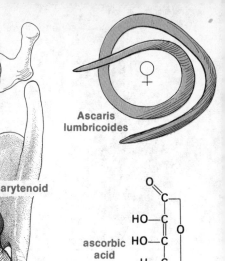
Ascaris lumbricoides

ascorbic acid

aspartic acid

$$HOOC—CH_2—\overset{\overset{\displaystyle NH_2}{|}}{\underset{\underset{\displaystyle H}{|}}{C}}—COOH$$

arthrospores
(culture of *Coccidioides immitis*)

arthral′gia. Pain in a joint; also called arthrodynia.
arthrec′tomy. Removal of a joint.
arthriti′ic. Relating to or suffering from arthritis.
arthri′tis. Inflammation of the joints.
  atrophic a., rheumatoid arthritis.
  degenerative a., see degenerative joint disease.
  gonococcal a., a form associated with gonorrhea, involving one or several joints, especially of the knees, ankles, and wrists; *Neisseria gonorrhoeae* can be isolated from the joint fluid.
  hypertrophic a., see degenerative joint disease.
  juvenile rheumatoid a., an uncommon, crippling disease of children involving the large joints and cervical spine with enlargement of lymph nodes, liver, and spleen; also called Still's disease.
  rheumatoid a., chronic disease of unknown cause involving most connective tissues of the body with predilection for small joints, especially those of the fingers; marked by proliferative inflammation of the synovial membranes leading to deformity, ankylosis, and invalidism; also called atrophic and chronic proliferative arthritis.
  suppurative a., purulent infection involving, as a rule, a single large joint; caused by any of several microorganisms, especially *Streptococcus hemolyticus, Staphylococcus aureus,* pneumococcus, and meningococcus; it usually follows injury to the affected joint; also called pyogenic arthritis.
  syphilitic a., a condition characterized by (1) mild chronic effusion into the knee joints (Clutton's joints) occurring during puberty in congenital syphilis; (2) painful, stiff, tender joints with transient swelling occurring with secondary syphilis; inflammation of adjacent periosteum usually occurs.
  tuberculous a., arthritis caused by a tuberculosis bacillus; usually mono-articular, involving any joint in the body, especially the knee, hip, and spine, with destruction of contiguous bone.
arthrocente′sis. Puncture of a joint followed by the withdrawal of fluid, usually by suction through the puncture needle.
arthrod′esis. Surgical fixation of a joint; also called artificial ankylosis.
arthro′dia. Gliding joint; one that permits a gliding motion, as between the articular processes of the vertebrae.
arthro′dial. Relating to arthrodia.
arthrodyn′ia. Arthralgia; pain in a joint.
arthrodyspla′sia. Malformation of a joint or joints.
arth′rogram. X-ray picture of a joint.
arthrog′raphy. 1. Roentgenography of a joint. **2.** A treatise on joints.
arthrogrypo′sis. Permanent or persistent flexure of a joint.

  a. multiplex congenita, congenital contraction of several joints of the extremities.
arthrono′sos. Disease of the joints.
arthrop′athy. Any disease of the joints.
  diabetic a., arthrosis occurring in diabetes as a result of disease of the trophic nerves innervating the joint.
  neuropathic a., any joint disease having a nervous origin.
  tabetic a., Charcot's disease; a form of neurophathic joint disease marked by a chronic, progressive degeneration and enlargement of a joint, with effusion of fluids into the synovial space.
ar′throplasty. Surgical restoration of joint function, either by repairing damaged joint surfaces or by inserting an artificial joint.
arth′ropod. Any of several invertebrate animals (phylum Arthropoda) having a segmented external covering and jointed limbs, e.g., scorpions, crabs, centipedes, etc.
arthropyo′sis. The production of pus within a joint; also called arthro-empyesis.
arthro′sis. 1. A joint. **2.** A degenerative condition of a joint.
ar′throspore. A sporelike cell produced by the fragmentation of any part of the segmented filamentous mycelium, as seen in *Coccidioides immitis.*
arthrosynovi′tis. Inflammation of the synovial membrane of a joint.
arthrot′omy. Incision into a joint.
artic′ular. Relating to an articulation or a joint.
artic′ulate. 1. To unite or connect by means of a joint. **2.** To utter distinct speech sounds. **3.** Having joints; jointed. **4.** Capable of speaking in clear, expressive language.
articula′tion. 1. A joint, as between bones. **2.** The process of producing a speech sound.
ar′tifact. Anything that has been artificially changed from its normal state, as a histologic tissue that has been mechanically altered.
aryt′enoid. 1. One of a pair of small pyramidal cartilages situated in the back of the larynx. **2.** Relating to the arytenoid cartilages.
arytenoidec′tomy. Surgical removal of an arytenoid cartilage in the larynx.
A.S. Abbreviation for Latin *auris sinistra.*
asbes′tos. An incombustible fibrous mineral form of magnesium and calcium silicate.
asbesto′sis. Fibrosis of the lungs caused by prolonged inhalation of asbestos particles and resulting in chronic shortness of breath; a pneumoconiosis.
ascari′asis. Infestation with the large roundworm *Ascaris lumbricalis,* characterized by a larval pulmonary stage and an adult intestinal stage.
ascaridi′asis. Ascariasis.

As′caris. A genus of roundworms (order Nematoda) that are intestinal parasites.
  A. lumbricoides, a species, reddish and tapered at both ends, found in the small intestines, especially of children.
asci′tes. Accumulation of free serous fluid in the abdominal cavity in clinically detectable amounts, seen sometimes as a result of cirrhosis of the liver, kidney disease, intraabdominal cancer, and severe congestive heart failure; also called hydroperitoneum and abdominal dropsy.
ascit′ic. Relating to ascites.
asco′mycete. Any of numerous fungi that contain spore-producing saclike structures (asci).
ascor′bic acid. A white crystalline substance, $C_6H_8O_6$; found in citrus fruits, green leafy vegetables, and tomatoes; used in the treatment and/or prevention of scurvy; also called vitamin C.
ASD. Abbreviation for atrial septal defect.
-ase. Suffix denoting an enzyme, e.g., lactase.
asep′sis. Absence of disease-causing microorganisms.
asep′tic. Not septic; free of contamination.
aseptic necrosis. See necrosis, aseptic.
asex′ual. Without sex.
asia′lia. Lack of saliva.
aspar′aginase. An enzyme that promotes the breakdown of asparagine to aspartic acid and ammonia.
aspar′agine. A nonessential amino acid found in asparagus shoots and other plants.
aspar′tase. An enzyme that promotes the conversion of aspartic acid to fumaric acid.
aspar′tic acid. A nonessential amino acid found mostly in sugar cane and sugar-beet molasses.
aspergillo′ma. A mass of fungus mycelium in a pulmonary cavity (intercavitary fungus ball) caused by fungi of the genus *Aspergillus.*
aspergillo′sis. The presence in the tissues of fungi of the genus *Aspergillus.*
  pulmonary a., a fungal infection of the lungs, from which it may spread to other organs; caused by the fungus *Aspergillus fumigatus.*
Aspergil′lus. A genus of fungi (family Ascomycetes); it contains several disease-causing species.
aspermatogen′ic. Failing to produce spermatozoa.
asphyg′mia. Temporary absence of pulse.
asphyx′ia. A state due to interference with the oxygen supply of the blood; suffocation.
  a. neonatorum, asphyxia occurring in the newborn.
asphyx′iant. Anything that causes asphyxia or suffocation.
asphyx′iate. 1. To cause asphyxia. **2.** To undergo

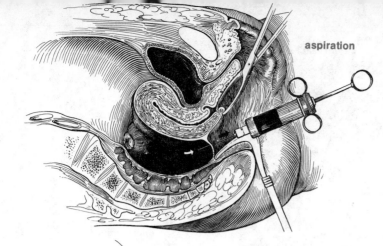

aspiration

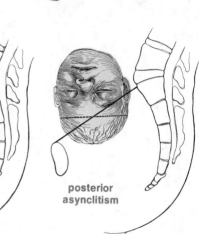

astrocyte
(protoplasmic
type)

capillary

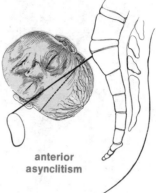

aspirator

asterion

anterior
asynclitism

posterior
asynclitism

asphyxia; to suffocate.

asphyxia′tion. Asphyxia.

aspi′dium. The rhizome and leaf of the male fern (*Dryopteris filix-mas*); formerly used in the treatment of tapeworm infestation.

as′pirate. To remove fluid from a bodily cavity by means of a suction device.

aspira′tion. 1. Intake of foreign material into the lungs during the act of breathing. **2.** Withdrawal, by suction, with an aspirator of fluid or gases from a body cavity.

as′pirator. An instrument for removing fluids from a body cavity by suction.

as′pirin. Common name for acetylsalicylic acid.

asporog′enous. Not propagating by spores.

assay′. 1. Analysis of a substance to determine its purity, potency, weight, etc. **2.** To examine.

assim′ilate. To consume and incorporate into the tissues.

assimila′tion. The process of converting food substances into tissues.

associa′tion. Relationship between persons or ideas.

asta′sia. Inability to stand, in the absence of organic disorders.

asteato′sis. Condition marked by deficient activity of the sebaceous glands.

   a. cutis, dry-scaly skin with scanty sebaceous gland secretion.

as′ter. See astrosphere.

astereogno′sis. Stereoanesthesia; failure to recognize objects or to appreciate their form by feeling them.

aste′rion. A craniometric point on either side of the skull at the junction of the lambdoid, occipitomastoid, and parietomastoid sutures.

asterix′is. A flapping movement or tremor, best seen in the outstretched hands, characteristic of certain metabolic disorders, particularly hepatic coma; also called liver flap.

asthe′nia. Loss of strength; weakness.

   neurocirculatory a., condition marked by breathlessness, palpitation, chest pain, giddiness, and fatigue, in absence of organic heart disease.

asthenocor′ia. Sluggish reaction of the pupil to light stimulus.

astheno′pia. General term denoting distress arising from the use of the eyes; eyestrain.

asthenosper′mia. Reduction of motility of spermatozoa.

as′thma. Disease characterized by an increased responsiveness of the trachea and bronchi to various stimuli, manifested by recurrent attacks of widespread narrowing of the airways, difficult breathing, wheezing, and cough; most commonly an allergic

reaction to some extrinsic allergen or may be triggered by infection (infectious asthma), or associated with emotional stress.

   atopic a., bronchial asthma.

   bronchial a., the common form of asthma characterized by spasm of the muscular walls of the small bronchial tubes, with swelling and edema of the mucous membrane; believed to be an allergic reaction.

   cardiac a., an attack simulating an asthmatic episode, caused by pulmonary congestion secondary to left heart failure.

   spasmodic a., a form caused by spasm of the bronchioles.

astigmat′ic. Relating to or marked by astigmatism.

astig′matism. 1. Faulty vision caused by imperfections in the curvature of the cornea which prevent light rays from focusing at a single point on the retina; instead they are focused separately; occasionally due to defects in the curvature of the crystalline lens; may accompany myopia or hyperopia. **2.** In an electron-beam tube, a focus defect in which electrons from a single source point of a specimen come to focus at different points; the main cause of image deterioration in electron microscopy. **3.** A refractive defect of an optical system, such as a lens or mirror, that prevents sharp focusing.

astigmom′eter, astigmatom′eter. An instrument for measuring the degree of astigmatism.

astrag′alus. See talus.

astrapopho′bia. A morbid fear of lightning.

astrin′gent. 1. Causing contraction of the tissues and arresting discharges. **2.** An agent that produces such an effect.

as′troblast. An immature astrocyte.

astroblasto′ma. A relatively rare, rapidly growing brain tumor made up of astroblasts; two-thirds of cases occur in the cerebrum of middle-aged adults; the cerebellum is the second most frequent site.

as′trocele. Centrosphere.

as′trocyte. The largest neuroglial cell having a star-shaped cell body with numerous processes radiating outward; many of the processes end on blood vessels as perivascular feet.

astrocyto′ma. A non-capsulated brain tumor arising from astrocytes.

astrocyto′sis. An increase in the number of astrocytes; usually occurring close to degenerative lesions, abscesses, or brain tumors.

astrog′lia. A cell of non-neuronal tissue (neuroglia cell) consisting of a small body and several long straight processes.

astrokinet′ic. Relating to the movements of the

centrosome in a dividing cell.

as′trosphere. A group of fibrillar cytoplasmic rays extending outward from the centrosome and centrosphere of a dividing cell; also called aster and attraction sphere.

asym′metry. Dissimilarity in corresponding parts.

asymptomat′ic. Free of symptoms.

asyn′clitism. In obstetrics, state in which the fetal head does not lie exactly between the sacral promontory and symphysis but is deflected either anteriorly, near the symphysis, or posteriorly, near the promontory, with its occipitofrontal plane oblique to any given maternal pelvic plane; formerly called obliquity.

   anterior a., anterior parietal presentation, deflection of the fetal head posteriorly; the sagittal suture approaches the sacral promontory and the anterior parietal bone presents itself to the examining fingers; formerly called Nägele's obliquity.

   posterior a., posterior parietal presentation, deflection of the fetal head anteriorly; the sagittal suture lies close to the symphysis and the posterior parietal bone presents itself to the examining fingers; formerly called Litzmann's obliquity.

asyner′gia, asyn′ergy. Lack of coordination among the parts that normally work together.

asy′stole. Absence of muscular contractions of the heart.

atactil′ia. Lack of the sense of touch.

atarac′tic. Tranquilizing; said of some drugs.

atarax′ia. Emotional tranquility.

at′avism. The reappearance of a trait in an individual after being absent for several generations.

atax′ia. Lack of muscular coordination.

   a. telangiectasia, hereditary, progressive cerebellar ataxia associated with recurrent pulmonary infections and ocular and cutaneous telangiectases (permanent dilatation of capillaries and small arteries).

   cerebellar a., ataxia resulting from disease of the cerebellum.

   Friedreich's a., hereditary spinal a., hereditary disease occurring in children, marked by degeneration of the dorsal and lateral columns of the spinal cord, attended by progressive ataxia, nystagmus, and absence or diminution of deep tendon reflexes.

   vasomotor a., disorder of the vasomotor centers, causing spasm of the smaller blood vessels.

atelec′tasis. A shrunken and airless state of the lung, or a portion of it, due to failure of expansion or resorption of air from the alveoli; it may be acute or chronic, complete or incomplete.

   primary a., failure of the lungs to expand adequately after birth; may be due to fetal hypoxia, prematurity, excessive intrapulmonary secretions,

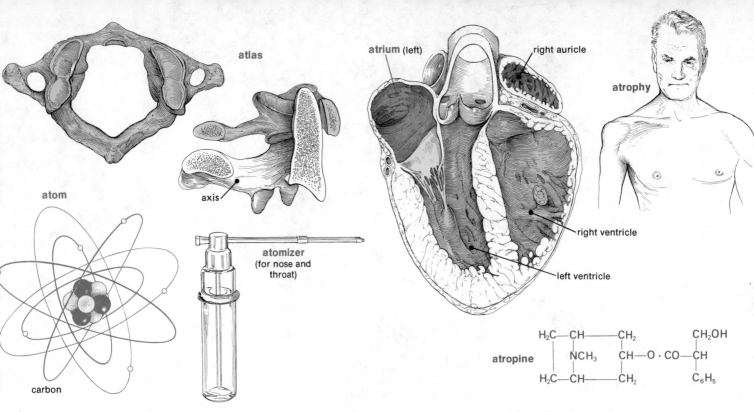

atlas

atom

carbon

axis

atomizer
(for nose and
throat)

atrium (left)

right auricle

atrophy

right ventricle

left ventricle

atropine

$$H_2C-CH \quad\quad CH_2 \quad\quad CH_2OH$$
$$NCH_3 \quad CH-O\cdot CO-CH$$
$$H_2C-CH \quad\quad CH_2 \quad\quad C_6H_5$$

or intercurrent pneumonia; lack of surfactant, especially in premature infants, is a prime cause.

secondary a., pulmonary collapse, especially of infants, due primarily to hyaline membrane disease.

atelio'sis. Incomplete development; also called infantilism.

atelocar'dia. Incomplete development of the heart.

atelochi'lia. Incomplete or defective development of the lip; also called harelip.

atelogna'thia. Defective development of the lower jaw.

atherogen'esis. The formation of atheroma in the arterial walls.

atherogen'ic. Having the capacity to contribute to the formation of atheroma.

athero'ma. A degenerative cholesterol-containing plaque in the inner layer of an artery.

athero'matous. Relating to atheroma.

atherosclero'sis. A form of arteriosclerosis marked by the deposition of lipids in the inner layer of arterial walls, resulting in the formation of elevated fatty-fibrous plaques (atheromas); the process usually begins during the first two decades of life and increases in severity with the rising age level.

ath'etoid. Resembling athetosis.

atheto'sis. Condition marked by constant, slow, involuntary writhing movements of the hands, fingers, and sometimes the feet.

athlete's foot. See tinea pedis.

athlet'ic support'er. A ventilated elastic cloth pouch attached to a body belt and leg straps that supports the male genitals; worn especially during strenuous physical activities.

athrep'sia. See marasmus.

athy'mia. 1. Lack of emotion. **2.** Absence of the thymus gland.

athy'roidism. Condition caused by absence, or deficient functioning, of the thyroid gland.

athyro'sis. Athyroidism.

atlantoax'ial. Relating to the atlas and the axis; as the articulation of these two vertebrae.

atlanto-occip'ital. Relating to the atlas and the occipital bone.

atlanto-odon'toid. Relating to the atlas (first cervical vertebra) and the odontoid process of the axis (second cervical vertebra).

at'las. The first cervical vertebra articulating with the occipital bone above and the second vertebra (axis) below.

at'mos. A unit of air pressure equal to one dyne per cm²; also called aer.

at'mosphere. 1. The layer of gases surrounding the earth; composed of 20.94 per cent oxygen, 0.04 per cent carbon dioxide, 78.03 per cent nitrogen,

and 0.99 per cent inert gases. **2.** A unit of air pressure.

ATN. Abbreviation for acute tubular necrosis.

ato'cia. Sterility in the female.

at'om. The smallest chemical unit, consisting of a cloud of electrons moving rapidly around a positively charged, dense, central nucleus composed of protons and neutrons; an atom is classified by the number of protons (proton or atomic number, Z) and the number of neutrons (neutron number, N) contained in its nucleus.

atomicity. 1. The state of being composed of atoms. **2.** The number of replaceable atoms or groups in the molecule of a substance.

atomiza'tion. The process of reducing a fluid to a spray.

at'omizer. A device for delivering a liquid as a fine spray.

ato'nia. See atony.

aton'ic. Lacking normal tone or strength; said of a muscle.

at'ony. Lack of normal tone; also called atonia.

uterine a., loss of muscular tone of the uterus, which may result in failure of progress of labor or postpartum hemorrhage.

atop'ic. Displaced; not in the usual or normal place.

atopogno'sis, atopogno'sia. Inability to localize tactile stimuli; loss of ability to correctly locate a sensation.

at'opy. Denoting an allergy characteristic of humans and tending to be inherited, e.g., hay fever and asthma.

ATP. Abbreviation for adenosine triphosphate.

ATPase. Abbreviation for adenosine triphosphatase.

atre'sia. Absence or closure of a normal body opening or canal.

a. ani, imperforate anus.

biliary a., a condition of infants who are born without functioning bile ducts; these children usually die after several years because of resultant cirrhosis.

esophageal a., congenital failure of the full esophageal lumen to develop.

tricuspid a., absence of the opening between the right atrium and right ventricle.

atre'sic. Imperforate; lacking an opening.

atreto-. Combining form meaning imperforation; without an opening.

atretoblepha'ria. Symblepharon.

a'trial. Relating to an atrium.

atrichia. Congenital or acquired absence of hair.

atricho'sis. Atrichia.

atriomeg'aly. Enlargement of an atrium.

atriosep'topexy. A heart operation to correct a defect in the interatrial septum.

atriot'omy. Surgical incision of an atrium.

atrioventric'ular. Relating to both an atrium and ventricle of the heart.

a'trium. 1. One of the two (right and left) upper chambers of the heart; after birth, in the normal human the right atrium receives blood from the vena cavae and the left atrium receives blood from the pulmonary veins; the blood passes from each atrium to the respective ventricle. **2.** A shallow depression in the nasal cavity; the anterior extension of the middle meatus, located above the vestibule.

At'ropa. A genus of herbs (family Solanacea).

A. belladonna, a poisonous plant commonly called nightshade from which belladonna and atropine are derived.

atro'phia. Atrophy.

a. cutis, see atrophoderma.

atroph'ic. Characterized by atrophy.

at'rophied. Wasted; shrunken.

atrophoder'ma. Atrophy of the skin; also called atrophia cutis.

a. pigmentosum, see xeroderma pigmentosum.

a. senile, the characteristic dry condition of the skin in old age.

at'rophy. A wasting, progressive degeneration and loss of function of any part of the body.

Leber's hereditary optic a., a hereditary condition of rapid onset, affecting primarily young adult males; marked by bilateral degeneration of the optic disk occasionally involving only the papillomacular bundle; also called Leber's disease.

peroneal muscular a., a hereditary disorder appearing during adolescence or adulthood; marked by degeneration of peripheral nerves and roots, resulting in weakness and wasting of the distal muscles of the extremities, especially the legs; the wasting does not extend above the elbows or above the middle third of the thighs; also called Charcot-Marie-Tooth disease.

Pick's a., localized atrophy of the cerebral cortex.

progressive muscular a., an inheritable disease, transmitted as an autosomal recessive trait, with an early onset and a progressive course; marked by degeneration of the anterior horn cells of the spinal cord, resulting in wasting and paralysis of the muscles of the extremities and trunk; also called Duchenne-Aran disease.

at'ropine. An alkaloid with antimuscarinic actions obtained from *Atropa belladonna;* used to dilate the pupil, as an antispasmodic, and to inhibit gastric secretion; other effects include inhibition of salivary, bronchial, and sweat secretion, increase in

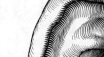

tooth

free gingiva

epithelial attachment

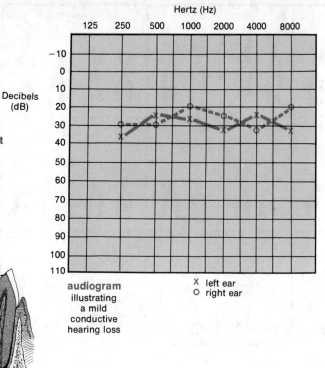

Hertz (Hz)
125 250 500 1000 2000 4000 8000

Decibels (dB)

audiogram
illustrating a mild conductive hearing loss

X left ear
O right ear

attrition

auricle

helix

tragus

concha

lobule

audiometer

---

heart rate, and inhibition of the urinary bladder.

at′ropinism. Poisoning caused by an overdose of belladonna derivatives (atropine and scopolamine) or by accidental ingestion of plants such as jimson weed.

attach′ment. A device by which something is stabilized; in dentistry, a mechanical device for the fixation of a dental prosthesis, such as a clasp, retainer, or cap.

  epithelial a., a collar of epithelial cells which adheres to the tooth, at the base of the gingival sulcus, and is continuous with the free marginal gingiva.

  precision a., one used in fixed and removable partial dentures, consisting of closely fitting male and female parts; the precise retention of the denture depends upon resistance between parallel walls of the two parts forming the attachment; also called internal, key-and-keyway, parallel, or slotted attachment.

attack′. The occurrence or establishment of a destructive process.

  drop a., sudden convulsions, occurring without warning.

  heart a., occlusion of an artery supplying the heart, usually accompanied by pain and frequently by irritability of the myocardium and/or congestive heart failure. See also myocardial infarction and coronary thrombosis.

  vagal a., condition characterized by slow pulse, labored breathing, and sometimes convulsions.

atten′uant. Any agent that (a) dilutes a fluid, (b) rarifies a gas, (c) reduces the virulence of a pathogenic microorganism, or (d) reduces the strength of a drug.

attenua′tion. 1. Dilution or weakening. **2.** Reduction of virulence of a microorganism.

at′titude. 1. Posture or position of the body; in obstetrics, relationship of the fetal parts to one another. **2.** A manner of behavior.

attrac′tion. The force acting between two bodies that draws them together.

  capillary a., the force that causes a fluid to move up and along a fine, hairlike tube.

  chemical a., the force causing atoms of different elements to unite.

  magnetic a., the force that tends to draw iron and steel toward a magnet and resist their separation.

  neurotropic a., the tendency of a regenerating axon to direct itself toward the motor end-plate.

attri′tion. Wearing away by friction; in dentistry, the normal wearing away of the biting surfaces of teeth due to mastication.

atyp′ical. Differing from the normal or usual type; not typical.

A.U. Abbreviation for Latin *aures unitas.*

Au. Chemical symbol of gold.

audiogen′ic. 1. Sound producing. **2.** Caused by sound.

au′diogram. A chart plotted from the results of hearing tests with the audiometer.

audiol′ogy. The study and measurement of hearing and the treatment of deafness.

audiom′eter. An instrument for determining the acuity of hearing.

audiom′etry. The measuring of hearing acuity with the audiometer.

  Bekesy a., testing of hearing with the audiometer while the patient controls the intensity of the tone.

audi′tion. 1. The sense of hearing. **2.** The act of hearing.

au′ditory. Relating to the special sense of hearing.

au′ra. The peculiar sensation that precedes an epileptic seizure, recognized by the individual.

  auditory a., noises or buzzing in the ears sometimes heard by a patient prior to an epileptic attack.

  olfactory a., olfactory sensation which sometimes precedes an epileptic seizure.

  visual a., flashes of light sometimes seen by an individual immediately prior to an attack of epilepsy.

au′ral. 1. Relating to the ear. **2.** Relating to an aura.

auriasis. See chrysiasis.

au′ric. Relating to gold.

au′ricle. 1. Pinna; the external portion of the ear. **2.** The pouchlike appendage projecting from the upper anterior portion of each atrium of the heart.

auric′ular. 1. Relating to the ear. **2.** Relating to an auricle of the heart.

auriculoventric′ular. Atrioventricular.

au′ris, *pl.* **au′res.** Latin for ear.

  a. dextra (A.D.), right ear.

  a. sinistra (A.S.), left ear.

  aures unitas (A.U.), both ears.

auscult′. To auscultate.

aus′cultate. To examine the chest or abdomen by listening.

auskulta′tion. The act of listening to the sounds made by the internal organs for diagnostic purposes.

auscul′tatory. Of or relating to auscultation.

au′tism. Emotional disturbance characterized by morbid self-absorption and inability to relate to other people, usually diagnosed in early childhood (early infantile autism).

autis′tic. Morbidly self-centered.

autoagglutina′tion. The spontaneous clumping together or agglutination of red blood cells.

autoagglu′tinin. A serum factor that causes the individual's own cellular elements (red blood cells,

---

platelets, etc.) to agglutinate.

autoanal′ysis. Self-analysis; the attempted analysis, or psychoanalysis, of one's own self.

autoan′tibody. Antibody that is produced in, and reacts with, an antigen in the same person or animal.

  cold a., an antibody that reacts at zero to 5°C.

  warm a., one that reacts best at 37°C.

autoantibody disease. Autoimmune disease.

autoan′tigen. An antigen which incites the production of autoantibodies.

au′toblast. A unicellular organism.

autocatal′ysis. A reaction that gradually accelerates due to the catalytic property of one of the products of the reaction.

autoch′thonous. Found in the part of the body in which it originates; not moved to a new site.

aut′oclave. 1. A container used for sterilization by pressurized steam. **2.** To sterilize in an autoclave.

autodiges′tion. Degeneration of tissues due to separation from blood supply; applied especially to spontaneous digestion of the walls of the stomach after death; also called autolysis and self-digestion.

autoer′otism, autoerot′icism. Self-arousal and self-gratification of sexual desire.

autog′amy. A process of fertilization within the cell, as in certain protozoans; the nucleus divides, giving rise to two pronuclei which immediately unite.

autog′enous. 1. Self-producing. **2.** Having its origin within the body.

au′tograft. Autogenous graft; see under graft.

autohemol′ysin. An antibody that acts upon the red blood cells of the individual in whose blood it was formed.

autohemol′ysis. Destruction of the red blood cells of an individual produced by the action of hemolytic agents in his blood.

autohemother′apy. Treatment by withdrawal and injection of the person's own blood.

autohypno′sis. Self-induced hypnosis; also called self-hypnosis.

autoimmune′ disease. Any disease characterized by tissue injury caused by an apparent immunologic reaction of the host with his own tissues; distinguished from autoimmune response, with which it may or may not be associated.

autoim′munize. To immunize an individual against his own antigens.

autoinfec′tion. Infection with organisms already present in the body; also called self-infection.

autoinocula′tion. The spread of an infection from one site of the body to another.

autointoxica′tion. A condition caused by absorption of waste products or any toxin produced by the

---

atropinism | autointoxication

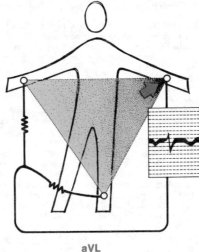

autosomes

augmented limb leads

aVR

aVL

aVF

body.

autol′ogous. Related to self; derived from the subject itself.

autol′ogy. Study of one's own self.

autol′ysis. See autodigestion.

au′tolyze. To cause the disintegration of tissues or cells within the organism in which the autolyzing agent is produced.

autom′atism. 1. Involuntary or automatic action. **2.** A condition in which activity is carried out by the patient without his conscious knowledge, often inappropriate to circumstances.

autonom′ic. Independent; self-controlling.
a. nervous system, see under system.

autopep′sia. Self-digestion, as of the gastric mucosa by its own secretion.

au′topsy. Examination of a dead body, usually to determine the cause of death; also called necropsy and postmortem diagnosis or examination.

autora′diograph. Image on photographic film produced by the emission of radioactive substances in tissues, showing the location and relative concentrations of these substances; made by placing the structure in close contact with photographic emulsion; also called radioautograph.

autoradiog′raphy. A cytochemical procedure for localizing sites of radioactivity within tissue sections.

autosen′sitize. To develop sensitivity to one's own serum or tissue.

au′tosome. Any member of the 22 pairs of nonsex chromosomes.

autotopagno′sia. The impaired recognition of any part of the body; may occur with lesions of the posteroinferior portion of the parietal lobe.

autotox′ic. Marked by autointoxication.

autotox′in. Any poison acting upon the body from which it originates.

autotransfu′sion. Transfusion of the patient's own blood.

autotransplanta′tion. The transferring of tissue from one part of the patient's body to another.

autovaccina′tion. Vaccination with vaccine prepared from the patient's own body.

autoxida′tion, auto-oxidation. The spontaneous combination of a substance with oxygen at ordinary temperatures and without a catalyst, as in the rusting of iron.

aux′otroph. A mutant microorganism that can be cultivated only by supplementing a minimal medium with growth factors or amino acids, not required by wild-type strains.

A-V. Abbreviation for (a) atrio-ventricular, as in A-V valve of the heart; (b) arteriovenous, as in A-V fistula.

avas′cular. Without blood vessels, normally or otherwise.

aVF. One of three unipolar augmented limb leads. See under lead.

avir′ulent. Not virulent; not causing disease.

avitamino′sis. Any condition caused by deficiency of one or more vitamins in the diet.

aVL. One of three unipolar augmented limb leads. See under lead.

avoirdupois′. A system of weight measurements in which 16 ounces make a pound.

AVP. Abbreviation for antiviral protein.

aVR. One of three unipolar augmented limb leads. See under lead.

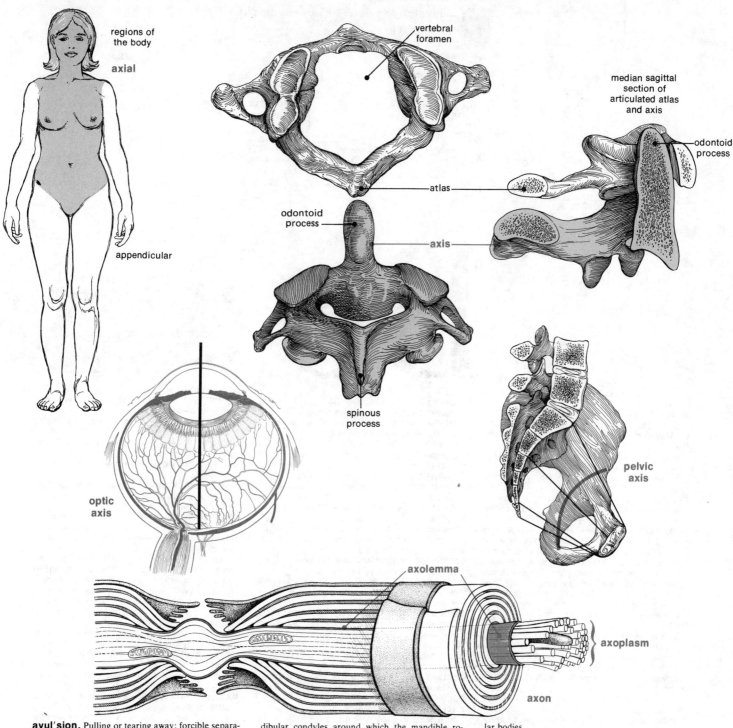

regions of
the body

axial

appendicular

vertebral
foramen

atlas

odontoid
process

axis

spinous
process

median sagittal
section of
articulated atlas
and axis

odontoid
process

optic
axis

pelvic
axis

axolemma

axoplasm

axon

avul′sion. Pulling or tearing away; forcible separation.

axen′ic. Germ free, said of animals reared in a bacteria-free environment; denoting a pure culture.

ax′ial. 1. Relating to or forming an axis. **2.** In dentistry, relating to the long axis of a tooth. **3.** Relating to or situated in the central part of the head, neck, and trunk. **4.** Denoting a region of the body that includes the head, neck, and trunk.

ax′illa. The pyramidal region between the junction of the arm and the chest; it contains the axillary vessels, lymphatics, brachial plexus, and muscles; also called armpit.

ax′illary. Of or relating to the axilla (armpit).

ax′is, *pl.* **ax′es. 1.** The second cervical vertebra; also called epistropheus. **2.** Any of the imaginary lines used as points of reference, about which a body or a part may rotate. **3.** Any of various centrally located structures, as the notochord of the embryo.

long a., a line passing through the center of a structure lengthwise.

mandibular a., a line passing through both man-

dibular condyles around which the mandible rotates.

optic a., (1) a line passing through the centers of the cornea and lens, or the closest approximation of this line; (2) in doubly refracting crystals, the direction in which light is not doubly refracted.

pelvic a., a hypothetical curved line passing through the center point of each of the four planes of the pelvis.

rotational a., fulcrum line; see under line.

visual a., see line, visual.

axoden′drite. A short process extending from the axon of a nerve cell.

axof′ugal. Directed away from an axon.

axolem′ma, axilem′ma. The thin sheath enclosing the axon of a nerve fiber.

ax′on. Neuraxon; the long cytoplasmic process of a neuron (nerve cell).

ax′onal. Of or relating to an axon.

axoneu′ron. A neuron of the cerebrospinal axis.

ax′oplasm. The cytoplasm of an axon containing mitochondria, microtubules, neurofilaments, agranular endoplasmic reticulum, and some multivesicu-

lar bodies.

azo-. Prefix denoting the presence of the nitrogen group −N:N− in a molecule.

azobiliru′bin. A red-violet pigment resulting from the condensation of diazotized sulfanilic acid and bilirubin in the van den Bergh reaction for determination of bilirubin.

az′ole. See pyrrole.

azoosper′mia. Absence of spermatozoa in the semen, causing sterility.

azote′mia. An excess of urea or other nitrogenous substances in the blood.

prerenal a., elevation of blood urea nitrogen resulting from primary alterations outside of the kidney, such as a reduction of renal blood flow due to congestive heart failure or hypotension, rather than renal disease per se.

azotifica′tion. The action of bacteria upon nitrogenous matter in the soil; also called nitrification.

az′otize. To combine with nitrogen.

az′ygos. A single or unpaired anatomical structure.

az′ygous. Unpaired.

Bb

Figure labels (top of page):

Bacillus subtilis

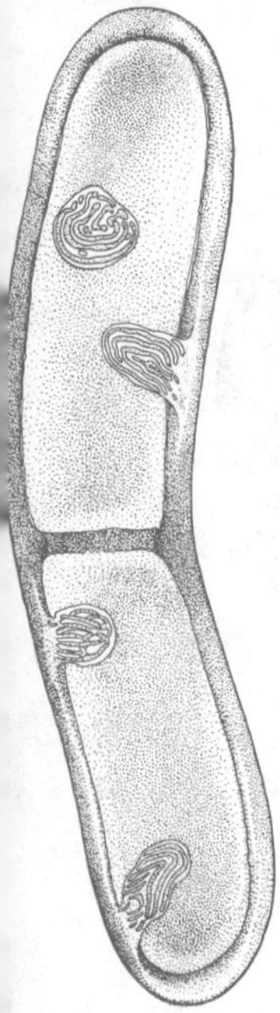

bacteriophage T4
- head — 950 Å
- core
- tail sheath
- tail fibers
- nucleic acid (in most cases double-stranded DNA)
- protein coat
- tail sheath contracts, forcing core through cell wall
- viral DNA entering bacterium
- cytoplasm of bacterium

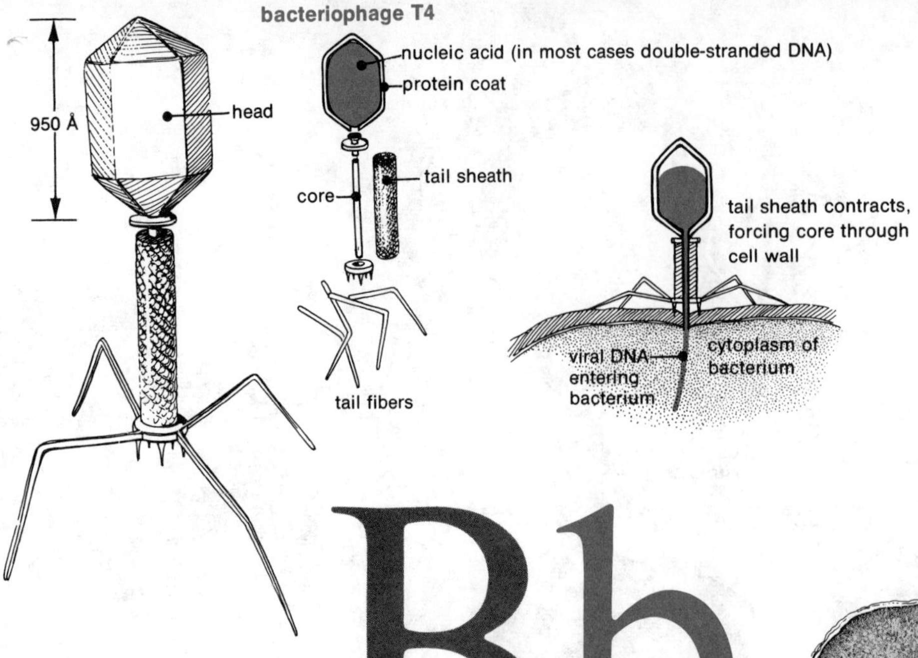

Douglas bag

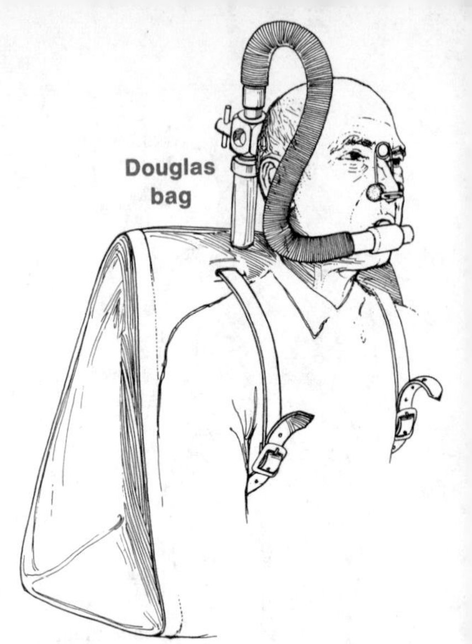

bacterium (Escherichia coli)

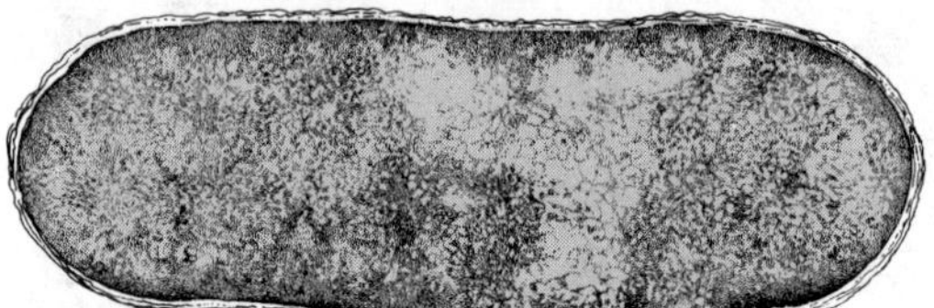

β. Beta. For terms beginning with β, see under specific term.

B. 1. Abbreviation for base (of prism). **2.** Symbol for (a) the element boron; (b) *Bacillus*.

b. Abbreviation for buccal.

Ba. The chemical symbol for the element barium.

Babe′sia. A genus (family Babesidae, order Haemosporidia) of irregularly shaped parasites of the red blood cells, causing babesiosis in most domestic animals.

babesi′osis. Any disease caused by a species of *Babesia* spread by ticks and afflicting many domestic animals.

Babinski′s sign. Extension of the large toe with fanning of the small toes upon stimulation of the sole of the foot, a normal response up to six months of age but abnormal thereafter; a positive response is pathognomonic of corticospinal disease; although upper extremity and head signs were also described by Babinski, the term is usually applied to the Babinski toe sign; also called Babinski′s reflex or phenomenon and extensor plantar response.

ba′by. An infant.

  blue b., an infant with a congenital heart defect in which the ductus arteriosus or foramen ovale of the heart fails to close, causing a mixing of venous and arterial blood in the left ventricle and a blood supply inadequate in oxygen; the skin usually has a bluish tint.

bacillary, bacillar. Relating to or caused by a bacillus.

bacille′mia. The presence of rod-shaped bacteria (bacilli) in the blood.

bacil′li. Plural of bacillus.

bacil′liform. Shaped like a bacillus; rod-shaped.

bacillu′ria. The passage of urine containing rod-shaped bacteria (bacilli).

Bacil′lus. A genus of rod-shaped bacteria (family Bacillaceae).

  B. anthracis, the causative agent of anthrax.

  B. botulinus, see *Clostridium botulinum.*

  B. cereus, a saprophytic, spore-forming bacillus with peritrichous flagella; thought to be responsible for some outbreaks of food poisoning.

  B. coli, see *Escherichia coli.*

  B. leprae, see *Mycobacterium leprae.*

  B. polymyxa, a saprophytic, gram-negative bacillus that produces the antibiotic polymyxin.

  B. subtilis, a widely distributed saprophytic, spore-forming, gram-positive bacillus found in soil and decomposing organic matter; a source of antibiotics; also called grass or hay bacillus.

  B. tetani, see *Clostridium tetani.*

  B. tuberculosis, see *Mycobacterium tuberculosis.*

bacil′lus, *pl.* **bacil′li.** Any of various rod-shaped bacteria.

  Bang′s b., see *Brucella abortus.*

  Ducrey′s b., see *Haemophilus ducreyi.*

  Friedländer′s b., see *Klebsiella pneumoniae.*

  gas b., see *Clostridium perfringens.*

  grass b., see *Bacillus subtilis.*

  Hansen′s b., see *Mycobacterium leprae.*

  Koch-Weeks b., see *Haemophilus influenzae.*

  Pfeiffer′s b., see *Haemophilus influenzae.*

  tubercle b. (t.b.), *Mycobacterium tuberculosis.*

  Weeks′ b., see *Haemophilus influenzae.*

  Welch′s b., see *Clostridium perfringens.*

bacitra′cin. An antibiotic substance obtained from a microorganism belonging to the *Bacillus subtilis* group; used as a topical application.

back. The posterior portion of the trunk.

back′ache. Pain in the back, especially in the lumbosacral or lower part of the back.

back′bone. 1. Vertebral column; see under column. **2.** Atoms in a polymer that are common to all its molecules.

back′ground. 1. The natural radiation of the earth and its atmosphere, and that coming from outer space. **2.** The presence of sound or radiation at a fairly constant low level.

back′ing. A metal support used in dentistry to attach a facing to a prosthesis.

bactere′mia. The presence of viable bacteria in the blood stream.

bacte′ria. Plural of bacterium.

bacte′rial. Relating to bacteria.

bacterici′dal. Capable of destroying bacteria.

bacter′icide. Any substance that destroys bacteria.

bacter′iform. Resembling bacteria; bacteroid.

bacteriolog′ic. Relating to bacteriology.

bacteriol′ogist. A specialist in bacteriology.

bacteriol′ogy. The branch of microbiology concerned with the study of bacteria, especially in relation to medicine and agriculture.

bacteriol′ysin. An antibody that combines with the bacterial cells (antigen) that caused its formation and later destroys the cells.

bacteriolyt′ic. Capable of dissolving bacteria.

bacte′riophage. A very delicate bacterial virus with considerable variation in structure which may attack and destroy bacterial cells under certain conditions; it contains a nucleic acid core (usually DNA, but may also be RNA) and a protein coat; it is the simplest replicating structure currently known to exist; also called phage.

bacteriopha′gia, bacteriopha′gy. The destruction of bacteria by any agent that causes disintegration.

bacteriop′sonin. An opsonin or antibody that acts upon bacteria.

bacteriosta′sis. The retardation of the growth and reproduction of bacteria.

bacte′riostat. Any chemical agent that inhibits bacterial growth.

bacteriostat′ic. Inhibiting the growth and reproduction of bacteria. Cf bactericidal.

bacteriother′apy. Treatment of disease by means of bacteria.

Bac′terium. A group of bacteria formerly classified as a genus of the family Bacteriaceae, later reclassified as *Acetobacter.*

bacte′rium, *pl.* **bacte′ria.** Any of various one-celled microorganisms of the plant kingdom, existing as free-living organisms or as parasites, multiplying by subdivision, and having a large range of biochemical (including pathogenic) properties; they are classified according to their shape into: (a) bacilli (rod-shaped), (b) cocci (spherical), (c) spirilla (spiral-shaped), and (d) vibrios (comma-shaped); they are further classified on the basis of staining characteristics, colony morphology, and metabolic behavior.

  enteric b., a bacterium indigenous to the intestines, usually a nonpathogenic gram-negative rod.

  L-forms of bacteria, small, filtrable bacterial forms with defective or absent cell walls (caused by antibiotics, specific antibodies, or lysosomal enzymes) which retain the ability to multiply.

bacteriu′ria. The presence of bacteria in the urine.

Bacteroi′des. A genus of bacteria (family Bacteroidaceae) composed of gram-negative, nonmotile, anaerobic bacilli normally inhabiting the mouth, intestinal tract, and genital organs of man; some species are pathogenic.

bad trip. Colloquialism for an unpredictable effect of psychedelic drugs which produces unpleasant or disastrous perceptual distortions; recurrent reactions may appear up to many months after the last use of the drug (flashback).

bag. 1. Pouch. **2.** The udder of a cow. **3.** Slang term for scrotum.

  Ambu b., a self-reinflating bag used to produce positive pressure respiration during resuscitation.

  b. of waters, the amniotic sac and fluid in which the fetus is suspended.

  Douglas b., a device for measuring oxygen consumption of an individual, consisting of a 100-liter canvas or plastic bag with an attached mouthpiece which houses inspiratory and expiratory valves; room air is breathed in and all expired air is collected in the bag for analysis of the oxygen and carbon dioxide content.

  ice b., rubber bag into which crushed ice is put to produce local cooling; available in a variety of

ballistocardiogram
in contrast to electrocardiogram recorded simultaneously

BCG

ECG

dental matrix band

Barton's bandage

spiral reverse bandage

spiral bandage

sarcomere

I band

A band   A band

omphalomesenteric band

shapes to fit specific parts of the body.

bagasso'sis. A chronic respiratory disorder caused by continued inhalation of the dust of bagasse (the crushed, juiceless residue of sugar cane).

BAL. Abbreviation for British antilewisite; see dimercaprol.

bal'ance. 1. A weighing device. **2.** A state of bodily stability produced by the harmonious functional performance of its parts. **3.** In chemistry, equality of the reacting components on each side of a chemical equation.

acid-base b., the normal ratio of acid and base elements in the blood plasma; also called acid-base equilibrium.

fluid b., state of the body in relation to the intake and loss of water.

nitrogen b., state of the body in relation to the intake and loss of nitrogen; positive nitrogen balance occurs when the amount of nitrogen excreted is smaller than the amount ingested, as during the growing age of children; negative nitrogen balance occurs when the amount of nitrogen excreted is greater than the amount ingested, as during malnutrition or febrile illnesses.

balani'tis. Inflammation of the glans penis.

balanoblennorrhe'a. Inflammation of the glans penis due to gonorrhea.

bal'anoplasty. Any reconstructive operation upon the glans penis.

balanoposthi'tis. Inflammation of the glans penis and the adjacent surface of the prepuce.

balanoprepu'tial. Relating to the glans penis and the prepuce.

bald'ness. Absence or decrease in the amount of hair; also called alopecia.

bal'lism, ballis'mus. 1. Violent or jerking movements as observed in chorea. **2.** Paralysis agitans.

ballistocar'diogram. A graphic record of the movements of the body with each cardiac contraction and ejection of blood from the ventricles; used as a noninvasive means to calculate cardiac output and examine cardiac dynamics.

ballistocar'diograph. A device for taking a ballistocardiogram, consisting of a recording system and a table suspended from the ceiling or an apparatus resting on the patient's body.

ballistocardiog'raphy. The making, study, and interpretation of ballistocardiograms.

balloon'. 1. To expand a cavity with air to facilitate its examination. **2.** To distend an organ or vessel with gas or fluid. **3.** A spherical, inflatable, nonporous sac, as the one near the tip of a Foley catheter.

ballot'tement. A method of physical examination to determine the size and mobility of an organ in the body, particularly in the presence of fluid; especially a method of diagnosis of pregnancy: the examining finger is inserted into the vagina and a sudden tap is given on the uterus; the fetus, if present, rises in the amniotic fluid and bounces back to its original position, striking the wall of the uterus which is felt by the examining finger.

balm. An ointment or a soothing application.

balneol'ogy. The branch of medical science dealing with mineral waters and their therapeutic use, especially as a bath.

balneotherapeu'tics, balneother'apy. The treatment of disease by means of baths of mineral waters.

bal'sam. The gummy exudate of some trees and shrubs, used in pharmacologic preparations.

band. 1. Any appliance or structure that encircles or binds another. **2.** Any ribbon-shaped anatomic structure.

A b., the broad, dark band produced by the thick (100 Å) myosin filaments which traverse the central part of the sarcomere.

I b., a light band extending toward the center of the sarcomere from each Z line of the striated muscle fibers, composed of thin (50 Å) longitudinally oriented actin filaments.

Maissiati's b., iliotibial tract; see under tract.

omphalomesenteric b., an abnormal persistent band from the intestine to the navel, a remnant of the embryonic omphalomesenteric (vitelline) duct that failed to obliterate; it occasionally results in small bowel obstruction when intestines loop around it.

orthodontic b., a thin strip of metal closely encircling the crown of a tooth in a horizontal plane.

Z b., see line, Z.

ban'dage. 1. A piece of gauze or other material used for protecting an injured part, for immobilizing an injured limb, for keeping dressings in place, etc. **2.** To cover by wrapping with a strip of material.

Barton's b., a figure-of-eight bandage for the support of the lower jaw.

capeline b., a double-headed roller bandage used to cover the head or an amputation.

elastic b., one made of an elastic material, used to exert mild continuous pressure.

figure-of-eight b., a roller bandage applied in such a way that the turns cross like the figure eight.

Galen's b., a broad head bandage with the ends split into three sections; the bandage is placed on the head; the anterior ends are tied behind the neck, the posterior ends, on the forehead, and the middle ends, under the chin.

plaster b., one that is impregnated with plaster of Paris; used for immobilization.

reverse b., one applied to a limb in such a way that the roller is half-twisted with each revolution.

spiral b., one applied spirally around a limb.

spiral reverse b., one that is folded on itself as it is applied around a limb, i.e., with alternate obverse and reverse turns.

T-b., one shapted like the letter T, generally used to keep dressings on the perineum.

Velpeau's b., one used to support the arm and hold it across the chest.

ban'daging. The application of a bandage.

Banti's syndrome. Chronic congestive splenomegaly; see under splenomegaly.

bar. 1. The international unit of pressure; one megadyne (10^6 dyne) per cm² or 0.987 atmosphere. **2.** A piece of metal connecting two or more parts of a removable partial denture.

Passavant's b., see ridge, Passavant's.

baragno'sis. Absence of the power to estimate the weight of objects held in the hand.

bar'ba. Latin for beard or a hair of the beard.

bar'bital. A colorless or white crystalline powder, $C_8H_{12}N_2O_3$; a barbituric acid derivative used as a sedative.

barbit'urate. 1. A salt of barbituric acid. **2.** Any derivative of barbituric acid used as a sedative.

barbitur'ic acid. A crystalline substance, $CH_2(CONH)_2CO$, not itself a sedative, but from which barbiturates (sedative drugs) are derived.

bar'biturism. Poisoning (chronic or acute) by any of the derivatives of barbituric acid.

bariatrician. A doctor who specializes in reducing the weight of obese patients, usually by the use of appetite-suppressing drugs; also called fat doctor.

bariat'rics. The branch of medicine that deals with the care and treatment of overweight people.

bar'ium. A soft silvery-white metallic element; symbol Ba, atomic number 56, atomic weight 137.36.

b. sulfate, a fine, white, almost insoluble powder, $BaSO_4$; used as a radiopaque contrast medium when given orally or as an enema for x-ray visualization of the gastrointestinal tract.

barocep'tor. See baroreceptor.

barorecep'tor. A sensory nerve terminal (sense organ) that responds to changes in pressure; also called stretch receptor, pressoreceptor, and baroceptor.

barosinusi'tis. See aerosinusitis.

barotrau'ma. Injury caused by pressure, generally to the middle ear or paranasal sinuses, due to the difference between atmospheric pressure and that within the affected cavity.

bar reader. A device that provides for the placement of a bar (opaque septum) between a printed

57

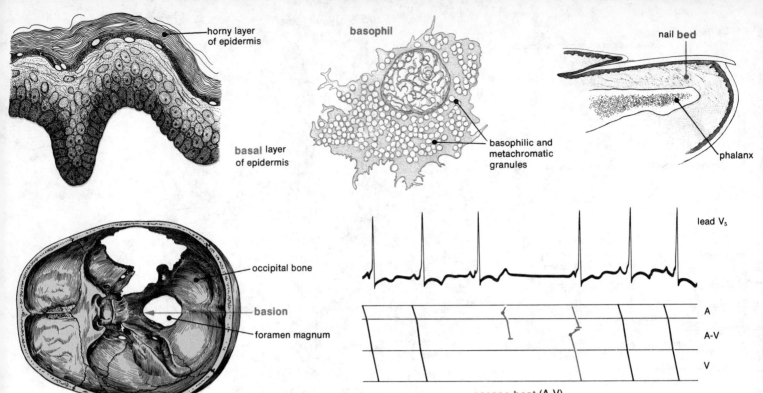

horny layer of epidermis

basal layer of epidermis

basophil

basophilic and metachromatic granules

nail bed

phalanx

occipital bone

basion

foramen magnum

lead V₅

A

A-V

V

escape beat (A-V)

page and the viewer's eyes so as to occlude different areas of the page for each of the eyes; used principally for the diagnosis and training of simultaneous binocular vision.

bar′rel. A cylinder or hollow shaft.

vaginal b., the vaginal cavity extending from the uterus to the vulva.

bar′ren. Sterile; denoting a woman who is incapable of producing offspring.

bar′rier. An impediment or obstacle.

blood-air b., the tissues in the lung, measuring about 0.2μ in thickness, separating the blood from the air and through which the exchange of gases occur; comprised of squamous endothelium (lining the capillary), a basal lamina layer, and an attenuated pneumocyte type I cell (squamous alveolar cell in contact with the air).

blood-brain b., the barrier of tissues interposed between the blood and the neurons in the brain; consists of the walls of the capillaries, the layers of the perivascular sheath, the neuroglia, and the ground substance of the brain; also called hemato-encephalic barrier.

blood-testis b., the tight junction barrier of the Sertoli cells in the seminiferous tubules of the testis that restricts substances from getting to the lumen where the spermatozoa (sperms) are developing, thereby protecting them, especially from the vascular supply.

hemato-encephalic b., see blood-brain barrier.

placental b., the semipermeable epithelial layer of the placenta separating the maternal blood from the fetal blood.

protective b., in radiology, material such as lead or concrete, used for absorbing ionizing radiation for protective purposes.

bartholini′tis. Inflammation of the greater vestibular glands (Bartholin's glands).

Bartonella bacilliformis. A species of gram-negative encapsulated bacillus that causes bartonellosis; transmitted to man by the bite of sandflies.

bartonello′sis. Disease occurring mainly in Peru, caused by an arthropod-borne bacillus (*Bartonella bacilliformis*), usually marked by a febrile stage with anemia (Oroya fever) followed several weeks later by a nodular cutaneous eruption (verruga peruana); occasionally one stage of the disease occurs without the other; also called Carrion's disease. See also Oroya fever (under fever) and verruga peruana.

Bartter's syndrome. Disorder marked by juxtaglomerular cell hyperplasia, secondary hyperaldosteronism, hypokalemic alkalosis, and a marked increase in plasma renin levels in the absence of hypertension.

ba′sal. Of or relating to a base.

base. 1. The foundation or supporting part of anything. **2.** The chief ingredient of a mixture. **3.** A substance that turns litmus indicators blue and combines with an acid to form a salt.

acrylic resin b., a denture base made of acrylic resin.

cement b., a dressing placed at the bottom of deep cavities to protect the dental pulp from thermal shock and to serve as a floor for a permanent filling.

denture b., saddle; the framework of a partial denture that rests on the ridge.

Basedow's disease. Disorder caused by the excessive production of thyroid hormones; also called thyrotoxicosis with exophthalmic goiter and Grave's disease.

base′plate. A temporary form corresponding to the base of a denture, used for making jaw relation plates, or for arranging artificial teeth; also called record, temporary, or trial base.

bas′ic. Of or relating to a base; also called basilar.

basicra′nial. Of or relating to the base of the skull.

bas′ilar. Of or relating to a base, as the basilar membrane of the cochlear duct.

basilat′eral. Relating to the base and side or sides of a structure.

ba′sion. The middle point on the anterior margin of the foramen magnum (occipital foramen).

ba′sis. Latin for base.

b. cordi, the base of the heart.

b. cranii, the base of the skull; the inner surface is called basis cranii interna; the outer surface is termed basis cranii externa.

Basle Nomina Anatomica (BNA). A system of anatomic nomenclature adopted by an anatomic association; it is superseded by *Nomina Anatomica*.

basocyto′sis. Abnormal increase in the number of basophils in the blood; also called basophilic leukocytosis.

ba′sophil. A cell, especially a white blood cell (basophilic leukocyte), containing large granules that stain readily with basic dyes.

basophil′ia. 1. Abnormal increase of basophilic leukocytes in the blood. **2.** The presence of basophilic red blood cells in the blood.

basophil′ic. Staining easily with basic dyes.

bath. 1. The immersion of the body, or part of it, in water or any other medium. **2.** The apparatus in which the body is immersed.

contrast b., the alternate immersion of a bodily part in hot and cold water (usually at half-hour intervals). for the purpose of increasing blood circulation to the part.

douche b., the local application of a stream of water.

Finnish b., sauna.

sitz b., one in which only the hips and buttocks of the patient are immersed in a tub of water.

tepid b., one in water at a temperature of approximately 86°F.

water b., (1) the immersion of the body, or part of it, in water; (2) the immersion in water of a liquid-containing vessel for the purpose of heating or cooling the liquid.

Batten-Mayou disease. Cerebral sphingolipidosis; see under sphingolipidosis.

battered child syndrome. Multiple injuries inflicted upon a child by an older individual, usually an adult and often a parent.

Battle's sign. Discoloration behind the ear, seen in fracture of the base of the skull.

BBB. Abbreviation for bundle-branch block.

BCG. Abbreviation for bacillus Calmette-Guèrin; see under vaccine.

Be. Chemical symbol for the element beryllium.

bead′ed. Having the appearance of a string of beads, as in rachitic rosary.

beak′er. A wide mouth glass cylinder with a pouring lip, used in laboratories for mixing and heating substances.

bearing down. The expulsion effort of a woman during the second stage of labor.

beat. 1. To pulsate. **2.** To strike. **3.** A pulsation, as of the heart.

apex b., the beat of the apex of the heart during ventricular systole; normally felt at the left fifth intercostal space, at the midclavicular line.

capture b., a conducted heart beat occurring after a period of atrioventricular (A-V) dissociation.

double b., coupled pulse; see under pulse.

dropped b., a nonconducted heart beat; one that fails to appear due to an atrioventricular (A-V) block.

ectopic b., a heart beat originating at some point in the heart other than the sinoatrial node.

escape b., an automatic heart beat following an interval longer than the dominant cycle, i.e., after the normal beat has defaulted.

fusion b., one arising from the simultaneous activation of either the atria or ventricles of the heart by two impulses from different sites.

premature b., an ectopic heart beat that depends on, and is coupled to, the preceding beat, occurring before the next dominant beat.

bed. 1. A piece of furniture for resting and sleeping. **2.** In anatomy, a base or layer of tissue upon which a structure rests.

capillary b., the total mass of capillaries and their volume capacity.

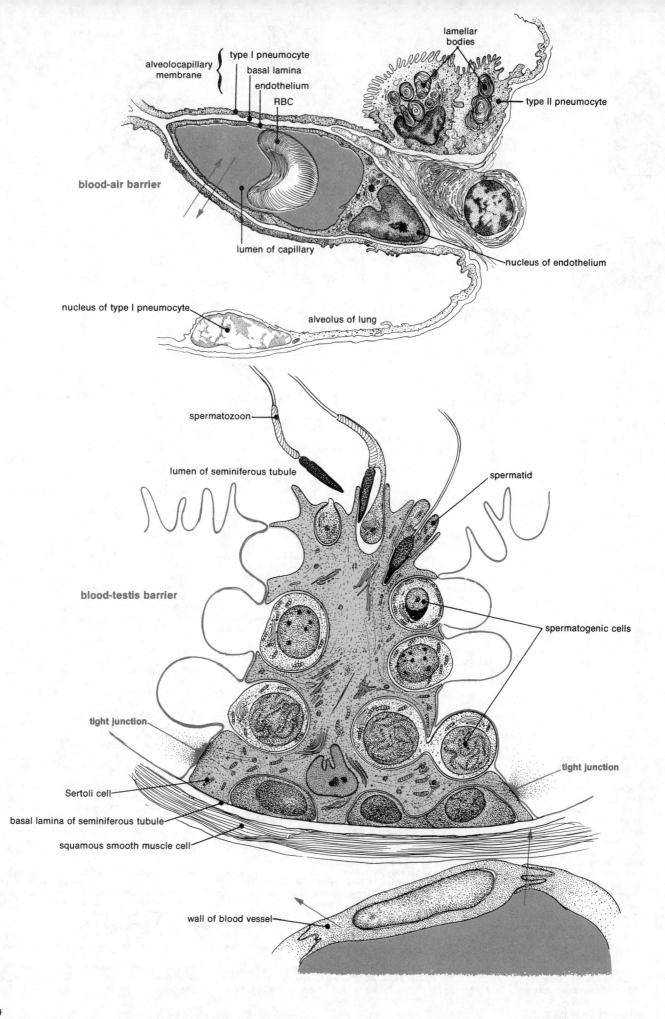

lamellar
bodies

alveolocapillary
membrane

type I pneumocyte

basal lamina

endothelium

RBC

type II pneumocyte

blood-air barrier

lumen of capillary

nucleus of endothelium

nucleus of type I pneumocyte

alveolus of lung

spermatozoon

lumen of seminiferous tubule

spermatid

blood-testis barrier

spermatogenic cells

tight junction

tight junction

Sertoli cell

basal lamina of seminiferous tubule

squamous smooth muscle cell

wall of blood vessel

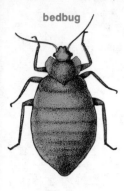

bedbug

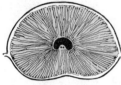

normal section

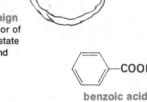

bladder

benign tumor of prostate gland

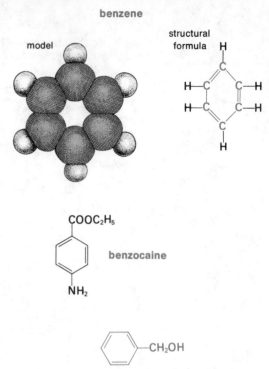

benzene

model

structural formula

$COOC_2H_5$

benzocaine

NH_2

—COOH

benzoic acid

—CH_2OH

benzyl alcohol

Gatch b., a hinged bed in which the patient's head and knees may be elevated.

bed′bug. A blood-sucking insect (family Cimicidae), about $1/8$-inch long when fully grown, with a flat, reddish-brown body and a disagreeable odor; its bite produces urticarial wheals with central hemorrhagic points; it often infests human dwellings and usually hides during the day in bed frames, torn mattresses, between floorboards, and under the edges of wallpaper.

bedewing, corneal. A swelling of the corneal epithelium characterized by irregular reflections from a multitude of droplets when seen with the slit lamp.

bed′pan. A pan with a wide flat rim which serves as a receptacle for the exreta of bedridden individuals.

bed′sore. Decubitus ulcer; ulcer of the skin, and sometimes of the muscles, occurring in pressure areas of bedridden patients who are allowed to lie in the same position for long periods of time.

bed-wet′ting. An involuntary release of urine during sleep, usually of concern if continued beyond the age of toilet training; may be of nervous or emotional origin, or due to faulty nutrition and infection or inflammation of the urinary tract; also called nocturnal enuresis.

bee. An insect of the genus *Apis,* of which the honeybee is the most common stinging insect; it leaves its stinger and venom sac attached to the victim.

bees′wax. Wax secreted by the honeybee; one of the ingredients of many dental waxes.

behav′ior. The manner in which a person acts or functions.

  automatic b., automatism.

  compensatory b., a behavior in which psychoneurotics who are intolerant of themselves often exhibit a compensatory attitude of intolerance of others.

behav′ioral. Relating to behavior.

  b. manifestation, b. disorder, neuropsychologic disorder; see under disorder.

behav′iorism. A school of psychologic theory concerned with the observable, tangible, and objective facts of behavior, rather than with subjective phenomena such as thoughts, emotions, or impulses.

Behçet's disease, Behçet's syndrome. Recurrent ulceration of the genitals and oral cavity with inflammation of the iris, ciliary body, and choroid and the formation of a puslike fluid in the anterior chamber of the eye; pyodermas are common and involvement of the central nervous system occurs in a variety of forms.

bej′el. Nonvenereal infection with a treponeme very similar to *Treponema pallidum;* occurs mainly in arid climates, especially among children of nomadic African tribes.

bel. A unit of sound intensity, being the logarithm to the base 10 of the ratio of two levels of sound; the difference in intensity between a sound that is barely audible and one 10 times louder is 1 bel; named after Alexander Graham Bell.

belch. To expel gas from the stomach through the mouth.

belladon′na. 1. A poisonous plant, *Atropa belladonna,* with purple flowers and black berries; also called deadly nightshade. **2.** An atropine preparation derived from the leaves and roots of the belladonna, used in the treatment of asthma and colic; the drug, whose name means beautiful woman in Italian, was onced used to dilate the pupils of the eyes and hence render the female morc attractive.

belle indifference. French term meaning a constant unjustified state of complacency and indifference, often seen in patients with conversion hysteria.

bel′ly. 1. Abdomen. **2.** The prominent fleshy part of a muscle.

bel′lyache. Colic.

bel′lybutton. Umbilicus; navel.

Bence Jones albumin, Bence Jones protein. See protein, Bence Jones.

bends. One of the manifestations of caisson disease (decompression sickness); symptoms include severe pain in the joints, abdominal pain, and weakness; caused by liberation in the tissues of gas bubbles. See also caisson disease.

benign′. Denoting a condition capable of disturbing the function of an organ, without endangering the life of the individual; not malignant.

benzalko′nium chlo′ride. A compound used as an antiseptic and germicide.

ben′zene. A thin, colorless, highly flammable liquid, C_6H_6; a coal-tar derivative, used in the manufacture of numerous chemical products; commonly called benzol.

  b. ring, see ring, benzene.

  methyl b., see toluene.

γ-ben′zene hexachlo′ride. See lindane.

benzimida′zole. A compound occurring as part of the vitamin B_{12} molecule.

ben′zoate. An ester or salt of benzoic acid.

ben′zocaine. A surface anesthetic of the skin and mucous membranes, widely used for relief of sunburn, pruritus, and burns; an ethyl ester of aminobenzoic acid.

benzo′ic. Of or relating to benzoic acid.

benzo′ic acid. A white crystalline acid occurring naturally in the resin benzoin; used in fungicides and dentifrices.

ben′zoin. A resin obtained as a gum from a tree, *Styrax benzoin,* sometimes used as an inhalant expectorant in the treatment of laryngitis and bronchitis; tincture of benzoin is also used as a base to provide a sticky surface for adhesive tape.

ben′zyl. A hydrocarbon radical.

  b. alcohol, $C_6H_5CH_2OH$; a substance used as a local anesthetic.

  b. benzoate, a colorless oily liquid.

ber′iber′i. Disease resulting from a dietary deficiency of thiamine (vitamin B_1).

  cardiovascular b., disease manifested principally by high output cardiac failure and edema; the acute fulminating form is called shoshin; also called wet beriberi.

  dry b., a chronic form in which polyneuropathy is prominent.

  infantile b., a form occurring during the first year of life, usually with prominent cardiovascular manifestations; most commonly occurs in the first months of life in small, breast-fed infants; reflects severe thiamine deficiency in the mother.

  wet b., see cardiovascular beriberi.

berk′elium. A synthetic, transuranium radioactive element; symbol Bk, atomic number 97, atomic weight 247; it has nine isotopes with half-lives from three hours to 1,380 years.

Bernheim's syndrome. Right heart failure without pulmonary congestion in the presence of left ventricular enlargement.

beryllio′sis. Condition caused by either inhalation of, or contact with, fumes or particles of beryllium salts; marked by granulomatous growths in the lungs or skin.

beryl′lium. A high melting point, corrosion-resistant metallic element; symbol Be, atomic number 4; atomic weight 9.013; used as a reflector in nuclear reactors and, in a copper alloy, for electrical contracts and nonsparking tools; formerly called glucinum.

bestial′ity. Sexual relations between a human and an animal.

be′ta. 1. The second letter of the Greek alphabet, β. **2.** The second item in a system of classification, as of chemical compounds. For terms beginning with beta see under specific term.

beta particle. See particle, beta.

be′tel. A climbing plant of East India, *Piper betle;* a species of pepper, the leaves and nuts of which are chewed to produce both stimulant and narcotic effects.

be′zoar. A hard mass found chiefly in the alimentary canal of ruminants and occasionally in man, composed of hair and/or vegetable fibers; it was

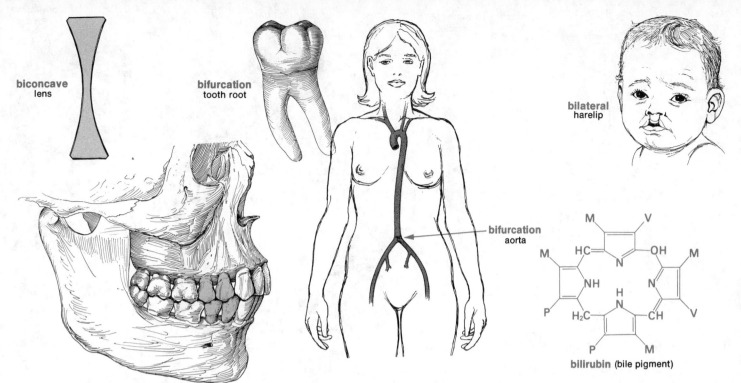

biconcave
lens

bifurcation
tooth root

bifurcation
aorta

bilateral
harelip

bilirubin (bile pigment)

bicuspids

formerly thought to have magical properties and was used as an antidote for poison.

BHN. Abbreviation for Brinell hardness number; see under number.

Bi. Chemical symbol for the element bismuth.

bi-, bin-. Prefixes meaning two or twice.

bi′as. 1. In statistics, the distortion in the results of a study arising from systematic errors in sampling or analysis. **2.** An unvarying voltage applied to an electrode.

biauric′ular. 1. Having two auricles. **2.** Relating to both auricles.

biba′sic. See dibasic.

bib′ulous. Absorbent.

bicam′eral. Composed of two chambers or cavities; said of an abscess.

bicar′bonate. A compound containing the radical group HCO_3.

bi′ceps. Denoting a muscle with two heads or points of origin.

bichlo′ride. See dichloride.

bicip′ital. 1. Having two heads. **2.** Of or relating to a biceps muscle.

bicon′cave. Having a depression on both sides or surfaces.

bicon′vex. Protruding on both sides or surfaces.

bicor′nous, bicor′nuate, bicor′nate. Having two horns or horn-shaped structures.

bicus′pid. Having two cusps or points, such as the premolars or the left atrioventricular (mitral) valve of the heart.

b.i.d. Abbreviation for Latin *bis in die.*

bi′fid. Divided into two parts, as a bifid ureter.

bifo′cal. Having two focal lengths.

bifo′cals. Eyeglasses in which each lens has two focal lengths, used for both distant and near vision.

bi′furcate. To divide or separate into two parts.

bifurca′tion. Division or separation into two parts or branches.

bigem′inal. Occurring in pairs.

bigem′iny. Doubling, especially the occurrence of two pulse beats in rapid succession followed by a pause before the next two beats; also written bigemini.

bilat′eral. Relating to or having two sides.

bile. A bitter, yellowish brown or brownish green liquid, secreted by the liver, stored in the gallbladder, and discharged into the duodenum; it aids in digestion mainly by emulsifying fats; also called gall.

Bilhar′zia. Former name for a genus of trematode worms or flukes now called *Schistosoma.*

bilharzi′asis, bilharzio′sis. See schistosomiasis.

bil′iary. Relating to bile and the bile ducts.

bilifus′cin. A dark green-brown pigment present in

bile and bile salts.

bil′ious. 1. Of, relating to, or containing bile; biliary. **2.** A vague popular term denoting a disturbed condition of the digestive system.

bil′iousness. A vaguely defined condition marked by indigestion, excessive gas, and often constipation and headache, popularly attributed to excessive secretion of bile.

biliru′bin. An orange-red pigment formed from hemoglobin during destruction of erythrocytes by the reticuloendothelial system; in the presence of liver disease or excessive destruction of red blood cells, accumulation of bilirubin in the blood and tissues causes jaundice.

bilirubine′mia. The presence of bilirubin in the blood, usually referring to an increased level.

bilirubinu′ria. The occurrence of the pigment bilirubin in the urine.

biliu′ria. The presence of bile or bile salts in the urine.

biliver′din, biliver′dine. A green bile pigment formed from the oxidation of bilirubin.

bilo′bate. Composed of two lobes.

bilob′ular. Having two lobules.

biman′ual. Performed with both hands, e.g., bimanual palpation.

bimo′dal. Having two distinct modes or peaks; said of a graphic curve.

bimolec′ular. Relating to or affecting two molecules.

bi′nary. Composed of two parts.

binau′ral. Relating to both ears.

bind. 1. To secure, as with ligature or band. **2.** To bandage. **3.** To unite molecules. **4.** To constipate.

bin′der. A broad abdominal bandage.

binoc′ular. 1. Relating to both eyes. **2.** Used by both eyes at the same time, as a microscope.

bino′mial. 1. Having two names. **2.** In mathematics, an expression pertaining to two terms connected by a plus or minus sign (as $m + n$ or $10 - 5$).

binu′clear, binu′cleate. Possessing two nuclei.

bio-. Combining form denoting a relationship to life.

bioassay′. The evaluation of a drug by comparing its effects on a test animal with those of a standard preparation.

bioastronau′tics. The study of the effects of space travel on living organisms.

bioavailabil′ity. The degree to which the active ingredient of a drug is absorbed by the body in the form which is physiologically active; it is an indication of both the relative amount of an administered drug that reaches the general circulation and the rate at which this occurs.

biocat′alyst. Enzyme.

biochem′istry. The chemistry of living matter or

organisms; also called biologic chemistry.

biodynam′ics. The science concerned with energy as it relates to living organisms and their environment.

bioenerget′ics. The study of energy changes produced within living tissues.

bioengineer′ing. Biomedical engineering; the application of engineering principles to solve biomedical problems, e.g., design and construction of devices, using suitable materials, for implantation within the body (plastic heart valves, metal pins and plates, electrodes, etc.), or of life-supporting apparatus for external use (heart-lung machine, artificial kidney, etc.).

bioequiv′alence. The application of the bioavailability concept whereby it can be assumed that a drug has the same therapeutic efficacy as another drug if it achieves the same maximum concentration, the same rate of absorption, and the same total amount of absorption as a recognized standard.

bioeth′ics. The branch of ethics concerned with the moral and social implications of practices and developments in medicine and the life sciences.

biofeed′back. A technique which uses electronic monitoring to give an individual immediate and continuing signals on changes in bodily functions of which he is not usually conscious, such as fluctuations in blood pressure; the subject endeavors to learn to control the function.

biogen′esis. Huxley's term given to the view that living things originate only from things already living, as opposed to spontaneous generation.

biokinet′ics. The study of the growth changes and movements within developing organisms.

biolog′ic, biolog′ical. Relating to biology.

biol′ogist. A specialist in biology.

biol′ogy. The science devoted to the study of living organisms, their structure, function, growth, etc.

  cell b., the science devoted to the study of the cell; it seeks an explanation of the physicochemical and metabolic processes of protoplasm; also called cytology.

biomed′ical. Relating to biomedicine.

  b. engineering, see bioengineering.

biomed′icine. The aspects of biologic sciences that relate to clinical medicine.

biometri′cian. A specialist in biometry.

biom′etry. The statistical study of biologic information.

biomi′croscope. A binocular microscope, used with a narrow beam of light (slit lamp) for examining the living eye.

biomicros′copy. 1. A microscopic inspection of the living tissues in the body. **2.** Inspection of the cornea or the lens by means of a slit lamp and

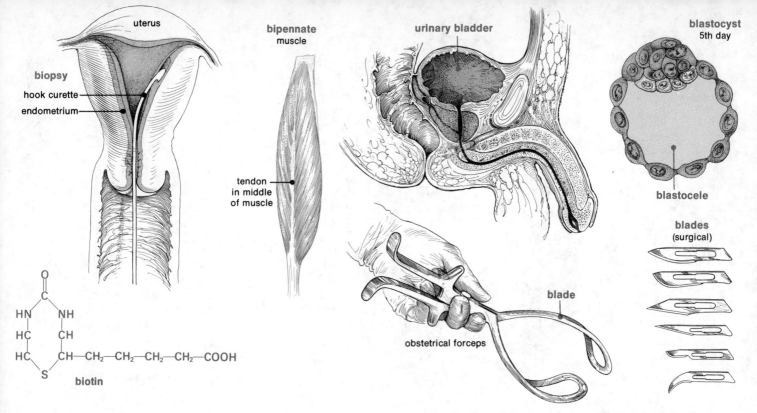

uterus

biopsy
hook curette
endometrium

bipennate
muscle

tendon
in middle
of muscle

urinary bladder

blastocyst
5th day

blastocele

blades
(surgical)

blade

obstetrical forceps

biotin

corneal microscope combination.

biomol'ecules. Molecules present in living matter.

bi'on. Any living organism.

bion'ics. The application of biologic principles to the design of electronic systems.

biono'sis. Any disease caused by living organisms.

biophys'ics. The science of the physical forces acting on the cells of the living body.

dental b., the relationship between the biologic behavior of the structures of the mouth and the physical action of a dental prosthesis.

bi'opsy. The removal and examination (gross and microscopic) of tissue from the living body for the purpose of diagnosis.

needle b., obtaining of biopsy material by aspiration through a needle.

surface b., examination of cells scraped from a surface, as from the cervix of the uterus.

surgical b., obtaining of biopsy tissue by surgery.

biorhyth'm. 1. The cyclic occurrence of a biologic process. **2.** A self-sustaining pattern of behavior that occurs in cycles, is relatively independent of the environment's ambient temperature, and which deviates (at least slightly) from the external geophysical cycle which it parallels.

biospectrom'etry. The determination of the quantity of various substances in living tissues by means of a spectroscope; also called clinical spectrometry.

biospectros'copy. Examination of specimens of living tissue with the spectroscope; also called clinical spectroscopy.

biostatis'tics. The study concerned with the acquisition, analysis, and interpretation of data relating to human mortality, morbidity, natality, and demography.

biosyn'thesis. The formation of chemical substances by or in living organisms.

biotechnol'ogy. The application of human and engineering data to problems relating to the adjustment of man and the machine; also called ergonomics.

biotelem'etry. The recording and measuring, without wires, of the vital processes of an organism located at a point remote from the measuring device.

biot'ic. Relating to the life processes; also called biologic.

bi'otin. A vitamin acting as a coenzyme, found chiefly in liver, yeast, and egg yolk; formerly called vitamin H.

biotox'in. Any toxic substance formed in the body tissues.

biotransforma'tion. The interaction between a drug and the living organism which results in a chemical change in the drug molecule; also called drug metabolism.

biotransport'. The translocation of a solute through a biologic barrier without being altered.

bi'otype. See physique.

bip'ara. Secundipara; a woman who has given birth twice.

bipari'etal. Relating to both parietal bones of the skull.

bip'arous. Having borne twins.

bi'ped. An animal with two feet.

bipen'nate, bipen'niform. Having a double feather arrangement; said of certain muscles from the arrangement of their fibers on each side of a tendon.

bipo'lar. 1. Having two poles. **2.** Relating to both ends of a cell.

bipos'itive. Having two positive charges or valences, as the calcium ion, Ca^{++}.

birefrin'gence. The splitting of light in two slightly different directions to form two rays; also called double refraction.

birth. The act of being born.

birth'mark. A circumscribed growth present at birth, as a hemangioma.

bis-. Prefix meaning two or twice.

bis'cuit. In dentistry (in association with porcelain), the fired article before it is glazed; referred to as low, medium, or high biscuit, depending on the stage of vitrification.

bisex'ual. Having the reproductive organs of both sexes; also called hermaphrodite.

bis in die. Latin for twice a day.

bishydroxycoum'arin. See dicumarol.

bis'muth. A crystalline, brittle metallic element; symbol Bi, atomic number 83, atomic weight 209.

b. subcarbonate, $(BiO)_2CO_3$; a white or pale yellow powder, used as an astringent and antacid; also called bismuth oxycarbonate.

bisul'fite. Any compound containing the inorganic acid group HSO_3.

bite. 1. To grip or tear with the teeth. **2.** To pierce the skin with the teeth or stinger. **3.** In dentistry, the term is generally used in relation to the amount of pressure produced in closing the jaws. See also record, interocclusal.

b. plane, see plane, bite.

close b., small interarch distance; see under distance.

open b., condition in which some of the apposing teeth (usually the anterior teeth) fail to make contact when the jaws are fully closed; also called apertognathia.

bitem'poral. Relating to both temples.

biuret paper, reagent, test. See under nouns.

biv'alence, biv'alency. Combining power double that of a hydrogen atom; valence 2.

biva'lent. 1. Having valence 2 or the combining power of two hydrogen atoms; also called divalent. **2.** In genetics, composed of two homologous chromosomes.

bi'venter. Having two bellies, said of some muscles, e.g., the digastric muscle.

black'head. Comedo; a plug of sebaceous material dilating or filling the orifice of a hair follicle.

black'out. Temporary loss of consciousness.

black widow. One of the world's most dangerous spiders, *Latrodectus mactans*; the extremely poisonous female is about one and a half inches long with a shiny black body and a red hourglass patch on its abdomen; the male is about one-fourth the size of the female and has yellow-brown markings; name acquired from the fact that the female eats its mate.

blad'der. 1. A distendable musculomembranous sac that serves as a receptacle for fluid, especially the urinary bladder. **2.** A blister.

atonic b., one that is unable to contract due to paralysis of the motor nerves that innervate it.

autonomic b., condition marked by periodic involuntary urination.

cord b., dysfunction of the bladder due to a lesion of its nervous supply.

gall b., see gallbladder.

ileal b., a surgically created bladder consisting of an isolated segment of ileum which is opened to the exterior through the abdominal wall and into which the ureters are attached.

nervous b., a constant desire to urinate, with incomplete emptying of the bladder.

urinary b., the reservoir for urine, which it receives from the kidneys through the ureters and discharges through the urethra.

blade. 1. The cutting end of an instrument. **2.** The long arm of instruments such as certain forceps.

shoulder b., the scapula.

blast. The immature stage in the development of a cell prior to attaining its definitive form.

-blast. A suffix indicating an immature or stem cell.

blasto-. A prefix relating to the process of budding, growth, or germination; e.g., blastoderm.

blas'tocele. The fluid-filled cavity of a blastocyst.

blas'tocyst. The embryo at the time of its implantation into the uterine wall, consisting of a single layer of outer cells (trophoblast), a fluid-filled cavity 2(blastocele), and a mass of inner cells (embryoblast); also called blastodermic vesicle.

blastogen'esis. 1. Reproduction by budding. **2.** The development of an embryo during cleavage and germ layer formation. **3.** The transformation of

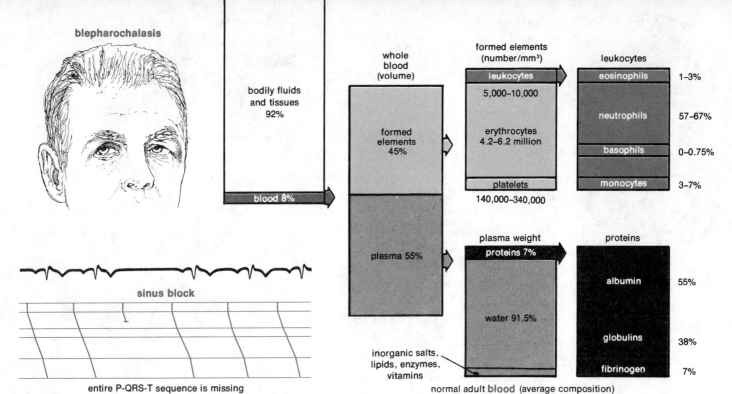

blepharochalasis

bodily fluids and tissues 92%

blood 8%

whole blood (volume)

formed elements 45%

plasma 55%

formed elements (number/mm³)

leukocytes 5,000–10,000

erythrocytes 4.2–6.2 million

platelets 140,000–340,000

leukocytes

eosinophils 1–3%

neutrophils 57–67%

basophils 0–0.75%

monocytes 3–7%

plasma weight

proteins 7%

water 91.5%

inorganic salts, lipids, enzymes, vitamins

proteins

albumin 55%

globulins 38%

fibrinogen 7%

normal adult **blood** (average composition)

sinus block

entire P-QRS-T sequence is missing

small lymphocytes of human blood in tissue culture into large blastlike cells capable of undergoing mitosis.

blas'tomere. One of the cells into which the fertilized egg divides.

Blastomy'ces. A genus of pathogenic fungi (family Moniliaceae).

  B. coccidivides, see *Coccidioides immitis.*

  B. dermatitidis, the cause of North American blastomycosis.

blastomyco'sis. A fungal infection of the skin and internal organs.

  North American b., a chronic disease caused by a yeastlike fungus (*Blastomyces dermatitidis*), originating in the respiratory system, especially the lungs, and disseminating to the skin and sometimes to bone and other organs.

  South American b., see paracoccidioidomycosis.

blas'topore. A small opening into the archenteron (primitive digestive cavity) of the embryo at the gastrula stage.

blas'tospore. A spore developed by budding from a fungal filament or hypha.

blas'tula. Early stage in the development of an embryo; a spherical structure consisting of a single layer of cells that enclose a fluid-filled cavity.

blastula'tion. The formation of the blastocyst or blastula.

bleach'ing. 1. The removal of color by menas of chemical agents. **2.** In dentistry, a method for returning a discolored tooth to its normal color.

  b. agent, any chemical used for brightening discolored teeth.

bleb. A blister.

bleed'er. A person afflicted with hemophilia or any other bleeding disease.

bleed'ing. The escape of blood.

  dysfunctional uterine b., bleeding from the uterus due to endocrine imbalance rather than a localized disorder.

blennadeni'tis. Inflammation of the mucous glands.

blennorrhe'a. A profuse mucous discharge from the vagina or urethra.

blennorrhe'al, blennorrhag'ic. Relating to blenorrhea.

blepharec'tomy. Surgical removal of all or a portion of an eyelid.

blephari'tis. Inflammation of the eyelids.

blepharochal'asis. Condition of the upper eyelids marked by excessive tissue which hangs over the lid margin when the eye is open; also called false ptosis.

blepharoconjuncti'vitis. Inflammation of the eyelid and of the conjunctiva, especially of the pal-

pebral conjunctiva.

bleph'aron. Eyelid.

blepharophimo'sis. A condition in which the aperture of the eyelids is narrow; also called blepharostenosis.

bleph'aroplasty. Tarsoplasty; any restorative surgical procedure of the eyelids.

blepharopto'sis. Drooping of the upper eyelid.

bleph'arospasm. Spasmodic winking, or contraction of the muscles of the eyelid.

blepharot'omy. An incision on an eyelid.

blind loop syndrome. Syndrome which may occur after operations of the small intestine which form a blind loop; stagnation of intestinal contents results in increased bacterial growth with malabsorption of vitamin B_{12}, fat, and other nutrients.

blind'ness. Lack or loss of sight.

  color b., inability to distinguish differences between some colors.

  day b., see hemeralopia.

  legal b., loss of vision to a degree as defined by legal statute to constitute blindness; maximal correction of acuity of 20/200 or less, and diameter of visual field of 20 degrees or less.

  letter b., a form of aphasia in which letters, though seen, relate no meaning to the mind.

  night b., nyctalopia; impaired vision in subdued light, generally due to a deficiency of vitamin A.

  snow b., temporary blindness caused by excessive exposure to sunlight reflected from snow.

  word b., inability to recognize written or printed words as conveyors of ideas.

blind spot. See spot, blind.

blink. To close and open the eyelids rapidly; an involuntary act by which the tears are spread over the conjunctivas, keeping them moist.

blis'ter. A common name for vesicle (2) and bulla.

bloat, bloat'ing. Distention of the abdomen with gas.

block. 1. To obstruct or to prevent passage through. **2.** To experience difficulty in recollection due to an unconscious emotional factor. **3.** An obstruction. **4.** In psychoanalysis, the difficulty in recollection due to an unconscious emotional factor.

  arborization b., a form of intraventricular block, thought to be due to widespread blockage in the Purkinje ramifications.

  atrioventricular (A-V) b., disorder of the atrioventricular bundle, causing disruption in the transmission of impulses from atria to ventricles; usually classified in three degrees: in first degree A-V block, conduction time of the impulses is prolonged but all impulses reach the ventricles; in second degree A-V block, some impulses are blocked and do not reach the ventricles so that ventricular beats are

dropped; in third degree A-V block, (complete block), no impulses can reach the ventricles.

  bundle-branch b. (BBB), a form of intraventricular block due to impaired conduction in one of the main branches of the atrioventricular bundle (bundle of His).

  heart b., atrioventricular block.

  intra-atrial b., impaired conduction through the atria.

  intraventricular (I-V) b., impaired conduction through the ventricles.

  peri-infarction b., delayed conduction through the myocardium at the site of an old myocardial infarct.

  sinus b., sinoatrial b., sinoauricular (S-A) b., failure of the nervous impulse to leave the sinus node.

blockade. 1. The intravenous injection of harmless material, such as colloidal dyes, for the purpose of rendering the reticuloendothelial cells temporarily functionless. **2.** The obstruction of nerve impulse transmission by a drug.

  adrenergic b., inhibition by a drug of the responses of effector cells to adrenergic sympathetic nerve impulses (sympatholytic), and to adrenaline (adrenolytic).

  cholinergic b., interruption by a drug of nerve impulse transmission at autonomic ganglionic synapses (ganglionic blockade), at myoneural junctions (myoneural blockade), and at postganglionic parasympathetic effector cells.

  ganglionic b., interruption by a drug of nerve impulse transmission at automatic ganglionic synapses.

blood. The fluid circulated by the heart through the vascular system of vertebrates; consisting of plasma (a pale yellow fluid) in which are suspended red and white blood cells and platelets; it carries oxygen and nutrients to all the body tissues and waste products to the excretory systems.

  occult b., blood in the feces in amounts too small to be seen but detectable by laboratory tests.

blood count. 1. The number of red or white blood cells in 1 mm³ of blood. **2.** The determination of these numbers.

  complete b. c. (CBC), one usually comprised of a hemoglobin determination, a hematocrit, a red blood cell count, a white blood cell count, and a differential white blood cell count.

  differential b. c., the percentage of various types of white blood cells in a specific volume of blood; also called differential white blood cell count.

blood group, blood type. Any of various immunologically distinct and genetically determined classes of human blood, identified clinically by char-

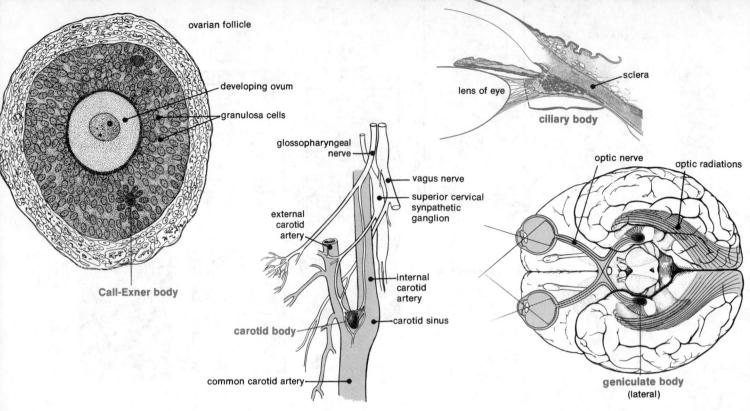

ovarian follicle

developing ovum

granulosa cells

Call-Exner body

lens of eye

sclera

ciliary body

glossopharyngeal nerve

vagus nerve

superior cervical synpathetic ganglion

external carotid artery

internal carotid artery

carotid sinus

carotid body

common carotid artery

optic nerve

optic radiations

geniculate body
(lateral)

acteristic agglutination reactions. For individual blood groups, see specific names.

blood grouping. The classification of blood samples according to their agglutinating characteristics.

blood′letting. The removal of blood from a vein for therapeutic purposes.

blood′shot. The reddish appearance of a part, as the conjunctiva, due to the congested state of the blood vessels.

blood substitute. Any of various fluid substances (human plasma, serum albumin, dextran solution, etc.) used for transfusion.

blood type. See blood group.

blood vessel. A tubular structure conveying blood.

Blount's disease. Condition, often unilateral, marked by a growth disturbance at the medial side of the proximal tibial epiphyses resulting in a severe bowing of the legs; also called tibia vara.

blue. A clear skylike hue; one of the primary colors evoked by radiant energy of wavelengths from 455 to 475 nanometers.

cresyl b., an oxazine dye with a strong affinity for nucleic acid, used mainly for staining blood to demonstrate reticulocytes and platelets.

Evans b., a diazo blue injected intravenously to determine blood or plasma volume by the method of dilution (the dye adheres to plasma proteins).

methylene b., methylthionine chloride, an aniline dye which when dissolved in water forms a deep blue liquid; formerly used as a urinary antiseptic; now used in the treatment of methemoglobinemia, as an antidote for cyanide poisoning, and as a staining agent, especially for demonstrating basophilic and metachromatic substances; also called toluidine blue.

toluidine b., methylene blue.

b.m. Abbreviation for bowel movement.

BMR. Abbreviation for basal metabolic rate; see metabolism, basal.

BNA. Abbreviation for *Basle Nomina Anatomica.*

BNDD. Abbreviation for Bureau of Narcotics and Dangerous Drugs.

bod′y. 1. The whole material structure of man or animal. **2.** The main part of anything.

adrenal b., adrenal gland.

aortic b.'s, small bilateral structures on a branch of the aorta near its arch; they contain chemoreceptors which are stimulated by decreases in blood oxygen tension.

Aschoff b.'s, the specific lesions of acute rheumatic carditis occurring as nodules within the connective tissue of the myocardium; a fully developed body consists of nonspecific phagocytes, myocardial histiocytes, multinucleated cells, and fibroblastic

proliferation; also called Aschoff nodules.

Auer b.'s, elongated structures found in the cytoplasm of immature myeloid cells in acute myelocytic leukemia.

Barr b., sex chromatin body.

Call-Exner b.'s, extracellular multilaminated bodies containing an accumulation of densely staining material; they are located among the granulosa cells in maturing ovarian follicles.

carotid b., one of two neurovascular ellipsoidal structures, three to six millimeters in diameter, situated on each side of the neck at the bifurcation of the common carotid artery; it is part of the visceral afferent system that helps to regulate respiration; it contains chemoreceptor endings that monitor the oxygen and carbon dioxide content of the blood circulating through the organ; also called carotid glomus.

chromaffin b.'s, see paraganglia.

ciliary b., the circular structure at the front of the eye between the outer edge of the iris and the ora serrata of the retina; it consists of six layers including the ciliary muscle (which, through the suspensory ligament, permits the lens to accommodate for near and far vision) and a layer of vessels and processes (the most vascular portion of the eye).

Councilman b., hyaline b., a globule formed from necrosis of a liver cell, seen in yellow fever; also called Councilman's lesion.

elementary b., (1) see particle, elementary (3); (2) blood platelet; (3) old term for a virion or virus particle.

geniculate b.'s, four paired oval masses located in the posteroinferior aspect of the thalamus (two lateral and two medial); the lateral are relay nuclei in the visual pathway; the medial serve as relay nuclei in the auditory pathway to the cerebral cortex.

Golgi b., see apparatus, Golgi.

Heinz b.'s, irregularly shaped, refractile granules in red blood cells (usually located at or close to the periphery of the cell), occurring as a result of polymerization and precipitation of denatured hemoglobin molecules.

hematoxylin b.'s, hematoxyphil bodies; relatively large, deeply staining bodies occasionally found lying free in the tissues in certain diseases, believed to be the remnants of an injured cell nucleus; the structures are so named because of their affinity for hematoxylin stain; found most commonly in systemic lupus erythematosus, especially in renal glomeruli and blood vessel walls; also called hematoxyphil bodies.

hematoxyphil b.'s, see hematoxylin bodies.

Howell-Jolly b.'s, small, round, well defined nu-

clear remnants commonly found near the periphery of red blood cells following splenectomy; occasionally present in megaloblastic anemia and leukemia.

hyaline b., see Councilman body.

hyaline b.'s of the pituitary, cells filled with hyaline material occasionally occurring in the posterior lobe of the hypophysis; also called herring bodies.

inclusion b.'s, structures frequently observed in either the nucleus or the cytoplasm (occasionally in both) of cells infected with certain viruses.

juxtaglomerular b., a group of cells around the renal glomerular arterioles containing cytoplasmic granules believed to be composed of renin.

ketone b.'s, acetoacetic acid, acetone, and β-hydroxybutyrate present in excess in the blood and urine of diabetics; also called acetone bodies and ketones.

Leishman-Donovan b.'s (L-D bodies), the ovoid, nonflagellated form of the parasite *Leishmania donovani,* usually packed in clusters within the cells of their mammalian host, causing visceral leishmaniasis (kala azar).

lipid b., see droplet, lipid.

Mallory b.'s, large accumulation of eosinophilic material in damaged liver cells; seen in certain diseases, especially those caused by alcoholism; also called alcoholic hyaline bodies.

malpighian b., renal corpuscle; see under corpuscle.

mammillary b., one of two small pea-shaped bodies of the hypothalamus located behind the infundibulum in the interpeduncular space; it receives fibers from the fornix and projects to the anterior thalamic nuclei; also called corpus mamillare.

Negri b.'s, bodies containing the rabies virus in the cytoplasm of nerve cells; also called Negri corpuscles.

Nissl b.'s, clusters of ribosomes and endoplasmic reticulum in the cell body and dendrites of a nerve cell; they stain deeply with basic dyes.

pacchionian b.'s, arachnoid granulations; see under granulation.

para-aortic b.'s, small masses of chromaffin tissue (derived from neural ectoderm) found near the sympathetic ganglia along the abdominal aorta; they secrete epinephrine; also called Zuckerkandl's bodies.

pineal b., a small gland-like structure, located on the roof of the third ventricle of the brain, overhanging the two superior quadrigeminal bodies; also called epiphysis cerebri and pineal gland.

pituitary b., see hypophysis.

polar b., one of the three cells formed by the ovum during its maturation.

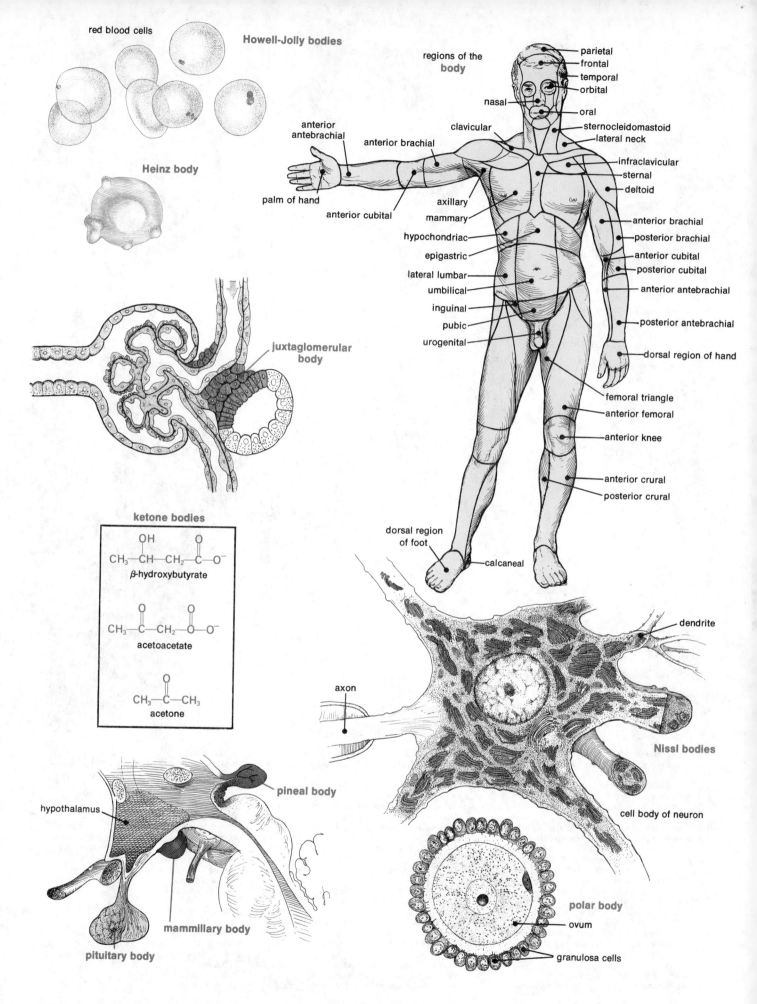

red blood cells

Howell-Jolly bodies

Heinz body

regions of the body

parietal
frontal
temporal
orbital
nasal
oral
clavicular
sternocleidomastoid
lateral neck
infraclavicular
sternal
deltoid

anterior antebrachial
anterior brachial
palm of hand
anterior cubital
axillary
mammary
hypochondriac
epigastric
lateral lumbar
umbilical
inguinal
pubic
urogenital

anterior brachial
posterior brachial
anterior cubital
posterior cubital
anterior antebrachial
posterior antebrachial
dorsal region of hand

femoral triangle
anterior femoral
anterior knee
anterior crural
posterior crural

dorsal region of foot
calcaneal

juxtaglomerular body

ketone bodies

$CH_3{-}CH{-}CH_2{-}C{-}O^-$
OH   O
β-hydroxybutyrate

$CH_3{-}C{-}CH_2{-}O{-}O^-$
O   O
acetoacetate

$CH_3{-}C{-}CH_3$
O
acetone

axon
dendrite
Nissl bodies
cell body of neuron

hypothalamus
pineal body
mammillary body
pituitary body

polar body
ovum
granulosa cells

65

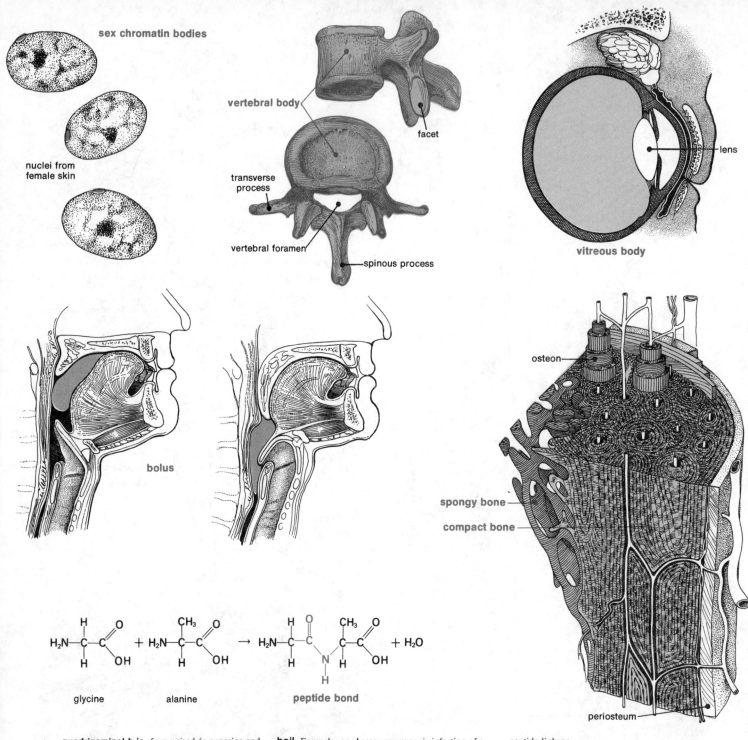

sex chromatin bodies

nuclei from female skin

vertebral body

facet

transverse process

vertebral foramen

spinous process

lens

vitreous body

bolus

osteon

spongy bone

compact bone

periosteum

$H_2N-\overset{\overset{\displaystyle H}{|}}{\underset{\underset{\displaystyle H}{|}}{C}}-\overset{\overset{\displaystyle O}{\parallel}}{C}-OH$ + $H_2N-\overset{\overset{\displaystyle CH_3}{|}}{\underset{\underset{\displaystyle H}{|}}{C}}-\overset{\overset{\displaystyle O}{\parallel}}{C}-OH$ → $H_2N-\overset{\overset{\displaystyle H}{|}}{\underset{\underset{\displaystyle H}{|}}{C}}-\overset{\overset{\displaystyle O}{\parallel}}{C}-\underset{\underset{\displaystyle H}{|}}{N}-\overset{\overset{\displaystyle CH_3}{|}}{\underset{\underset{\displaystyle H}{|}}{C}}-\overset{\overset{\displaystyle O}{\parallel}}{C}-OH$ + H_2O

glycine   alanine   peptide bond

quadrigeminal b.'s, four paired (a superior and an inferior pair) eminences forming the dorsal part of the midbrain; also called corpora quadrigemina.

residual b.'s, pockets of undigestible ingested material in a cell; e.g., aging pigments (lipofuscin).

restiform b., inferior cerebellar peduncle; see under peduncle.

sex chromatin b., a small, darkly stained mass of chromatin located almost always just inside the nuclear membrane; it appears in 40 to 80 per cent of the cells of a normal female and represents one of the two X chromosomes; also called Barr body.

trachoma b.'s, distinctive bodies found in cells of the conjunctiva of a trachomatous eye.

vertebral b., the cylindrical ventral portion of the vertebra; adjacent vertebral bodies are joined by fibrocartilaginous disks.

vitreous b., the transparent, gelatinous mass, of a consistency slightly firmer than egg white, filling the eyeball behind the lens; also called corpus vitreum and vitreous.

wolffian b., see mesonephros.

Zuckerkandl's b.'s, para-aortic bodies.

boil. Furuncle; an abscess or pyogenic infection of a sweat gland or hair follicle, usually caused by *Staphylococcus aureus*.

bo′lus. 1. A soft mass of food moved as a unit in the process of swallowing. **2.** A volume of material injected rapidly as a single unit into a fluid channel.

bomb. An apparatus containing a radioactive material for application of rays to a desired area of the body.

bombard′. To subject a specific area of the body to the action of rays.

bond. In chemistry, any of several forces holding atoms or ions together in a molecule.

covalent b., one resulting from the sharing of one, two, or three pairs of electrons by neighboring atoms.

ionic b., one formed by the transfer of one or more electrons from one kind of atom to another; characteristic of salts; also called electrovalent bond.

peptide b., a covalent bond linking two amino acids, formed when the carboxyl group of one is linked to the amino group of the other; also called

peptide linkage.

bone. The hard, semirigid, calcified connective tissue forming the skeleton of vertebrates. For specific bones, see table of bones.

alveolar b., the thin plate forming the walls of the tooth sockets.

cancellous b., spongy bone.

cheek b., zygomatic bone; see table of bones.

compact b., a type in which the bony substance is densely packed and the spaces and channels are narrow; also called dense bone.

dense b., compact bone.

elbow b., ulna.

heel b., see calcaneus.

hip b., see hipbone.

innominate b., see hipbone.

jaw b., mandible.

shin b., see tibia.

spongy b., bone having a latticework appearance and relatively large marrow spaces; also called cancellous bone.

tail b., coccyx.

thigh b., femur.

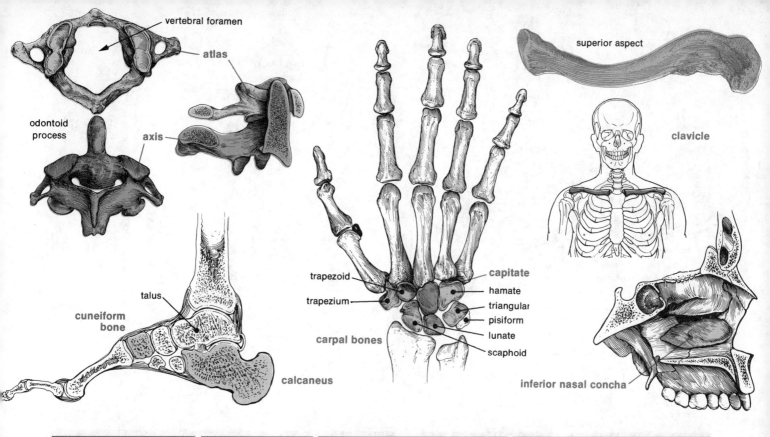

vertebral foramen

atlas

odontoid process

axis

talus

cuneiform bone

trapezoid

trapezium

carpal bones

calcaneus

capitate

hamate

triangular

pisiform

lunate

scaphoid

superior aspect

clavicle

inferior nasal concha

BONE	LOCATION	DESCRIPTION	ARTICULATIONS
ankle b.		see talus	
anvil b.		see incus	
astragalus		see talus	
Atlas *atlas*	neck	first cervical vertebra	occipital (above), axis (below)
axis epistropheus *axis*	neck	second cervical vertebra	atlas (above), third cervical vertebra (below)
backbones		see vertebrae	
calcaneus heel b. *calcaneus*	foot	largest of the tarsal bones, situated at back of foot, forming heel; somewhat cuboidal	talus, cuboid
capitate b. magnum b. *os capitatum*	wrist	largest of carpal bones, occupies center of wrist	second, third, and fourth metacarpal bones, lunate, trapezoid, scaphoid, hamate
carpal b.'s *ossa carpi*	wrist	eight in number, arranged in two rows: scaphoid, lunate, triangular, pisiform, trapezium, trapezoid, capitate, and hamate	
cheekbone		see zygomatic arch	
clavicle collar b. *clavicula*	shoulder	long curved b. placed nearly horizontally above first rib	sternum, scapula, cartilage of first rib
coccyx *os coccygis*	lower back	from three to five triangular rudimentary vertebrae with only the first not fused	sacrum
concha, inferior nasal inferior turbinate b. *concha nasalis inferior*	skull	thin, irregular scroll-shaped b. extending horizontally along lateral wall of nasal cavity	ethmoid, maxilla, lacrimal, palatine
cuboid *os cuboideum*	foot	pyramidal b. on lateral side of foot, proximal to fourth and fifth metatarsal b.'s	calcaneus, lateral cuneiform, fourth and fifth metatarsal b.'s, navicular
cuneiform b., intermediate second cuneiform b. *os cuneiforme intermedium*	foot	wedge-shaped; smallest of the three cuneiforms, positioned between the medial and lateral ones	navicular, medial cuneiform, lateral cuneiform, second metatarsal
cuneiform b., lateral external cuneiform b. *os cuneiforme lateral*	foot	intermediate-sized cuneiform located in the center of the front row of the tarsal b.'s	navicular, intermediate cuneiform, cuboid, second, third, and fourth metatarsals

bone | bone

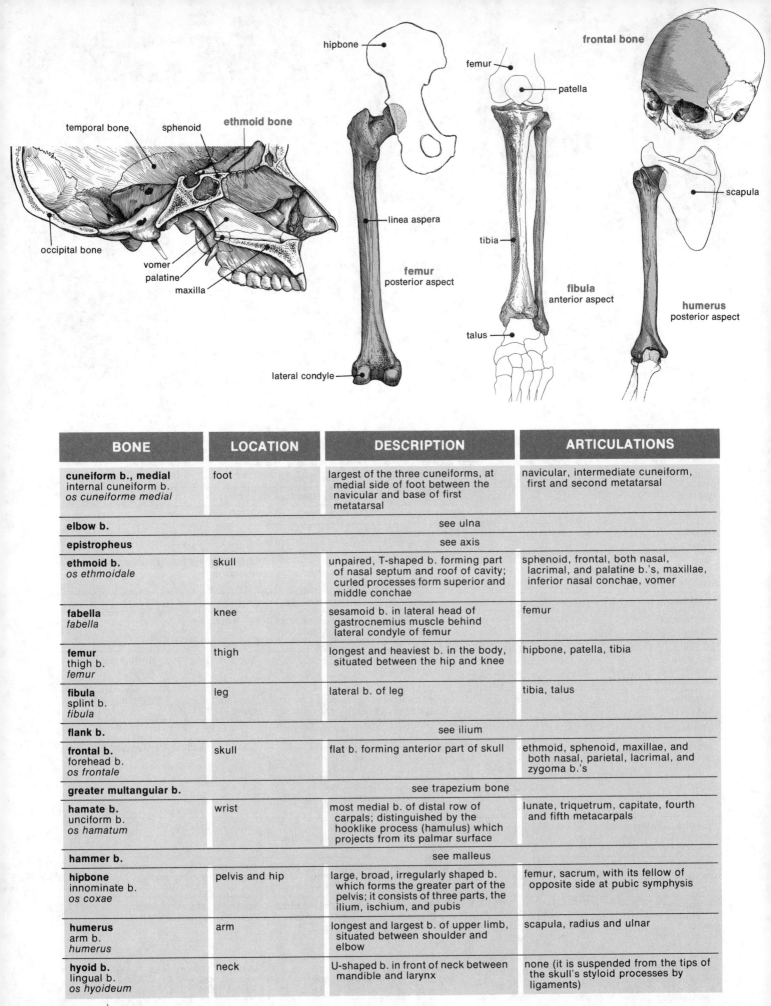

temporal bone　　sphenoid　　**ethmoid bone**

hipbone

femur

frontal bone

femur

patella

occipital bone

vomer
palatine
maxilla

femur
posterior aspect

linea aspera

lateral condyle

tibia

talus

fibula
anterior aspect

scapula

humerus
posterior aspect

BONE	LOCATION	DESCRIPTION	ARTICULATIONS
cuneiform b., medial internal cuneiform b. *os cuneiforme medial*	foot	largest of the three cuneiforms, at medial side of foot between the navicular and base of first metatarsal	navicular, intermediate cuneiform, first and second metatarsal
elbow b.	see ulna		
epistropheus	see axis		
ethmoid b. *os ethmoidale*	skull	unpaired, T-shaped b. forming part of nasal septum and roof of cavity; curled processes form superior and middle conchae	sphenoid, frontal, both nasal, lacrimal, and palatine b.'s, maxillae, inferior nasal conchae, vomer
fabella *fabella*	knee	sesamoid b. in lateral head of gastrocnemius muscle behind lateral condyle of femur	femur
femur thigh b. *femur*	thigh	longest and heaviest b. in the body, situated between the hip and knee	hipbone, patella, tibia
fibula splint b. *fibula*	leg	lateral b. of leg	tibia, talus
flank b.	see ilium		
frontal b. forehead b. *os frontale*	skull	flat b. forming anterior part of skull	ethmoid, sphenoid, maxillae, and both nasal, parietal, lacrimal, and zygoma b.'s
greater multangular b.	see trapezium bone		
hamate b. unciform b. *os hamatum*	wrist	most medial b. of distal row of carpals; distinguished by the hooklike process (hamulus) which projects from its palmar surface	lunate, triquetrum, capitate, fourth and fifth metacarpals
hammer b.	see malleus		
hipbone innominate b. *os coxae*	pelvis and hip	large, broad, irregularly shaped b. which forms the greater part of the pelvis; it consists of three parts, the ilium, ischium, and pubis	femur, sacrum, with its fellow of opposite side at pubic symphysis
humerus arm b. *humerus*	arm	longest and largest b. of upper limb, situated between shoulder and elbow	scapula, radius and ulnar
hyoid b. lingual b. *os hyoideum*	neck	U-shaped b. in front of neck between mandible and larynx	none (it is suspended from the tips of the skull's styloid processes by ligaments)

bone　|　bone

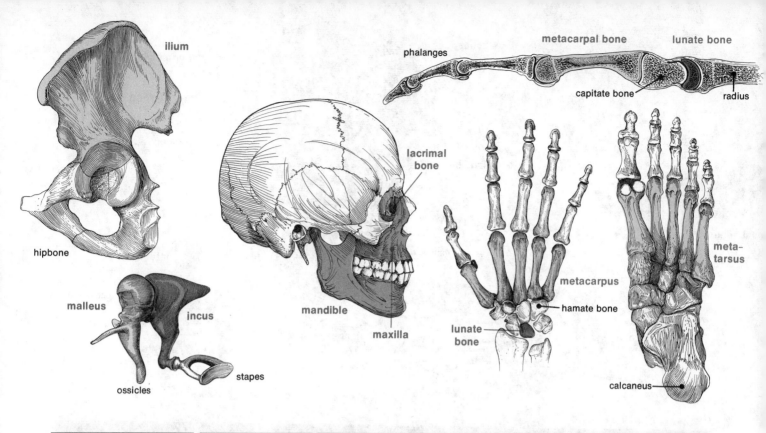

BONE	LOCATION	DESCRIPTION	ARTICULATIONS
ilium flank b. *os ilii*	pelvis	broad expanded upper part of the hipbone, divisible into two parts, the body and the ala	sacrum, femur, ischium, pubis
incus anvil b. *incus*	ear	middle b. of auditory ossicles	malleus, stapes
inferior turbinate b.		see concha, inferior nasal	
innominate b.		see hipbone	
ischium *os ischii*	pelvis	the inferior and dorsal part of the hipbone, divisible into a body and a ramus	femur, ilium, pubis
lacrimal b. *os lacrimale*	skull	the smallest and most fragile b. of the face; it resembles a fingernail and is situated in the anterior medial wall of orbit	ethmoid, frontal, maxilla, inferior nasal concha
lesser multangular b.		see trapezoid bone	
lunate b. semilunar b. *os lunatum*	wrist	in center of proximal row of the carpus between the scaphoid and triangular b.'s	radius, capitate, hamate, triquetrum, scaphoid
malar b.		see zygomatic bone	
malleus hammer b. *malleus*	ear	most lateral b. of auditory ossicles, somewhat resembling a hammer and consisting of a head, neck, and three processes	incus
mandible inferior maxillary b. *mandibula*	lower jaw	horseshoe-shaped b. containing the lower teeth	both temporal b.'s
maxilla maxillary b. *maxilla*	upper jaw	largest b. of the face excepting the mandible; it contains the upper teeth	frontal, ethmoid, nasal, zygomatic, lacrimal, vomer, inferior nasal concha, other maxilla
metacarpus metacarpal b.'s *ossa metacarpalia*	hand	five slender b.'s of the hand proper, each consisting of a body and two extremities, and numbered starting from the thumb side	base of first metacarpal with trapezium, base of other metacarpals with each other and with distal row of carpal b.'s, heads with corresponding phalanges
metatarsus metatarsal b.'s *ossa metatarsalia*	foot	five slender b.'s of the foot proper, each consisting of a body and two extremities (head and base) and numbered starting from the great toe side	distal tarsal b.'s, bases with each other, heads with corresponding phalanges

bone | bone

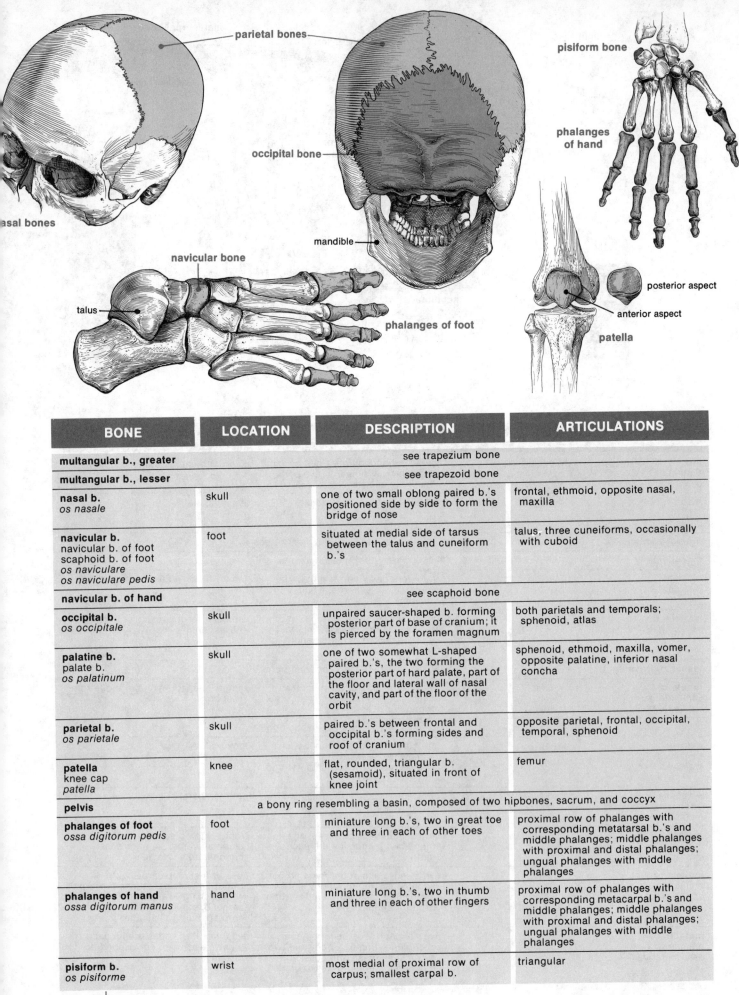

parietal bones

occipital bone

mandible

nasal bones

navicular bone

talus

phalanges of foot

pisiform bone

phalanges of hand

posterior aspect

anterior aspect

patella

BONE	LOCATION	DESCRIPTION	ARTICULATIONS
multangular b., greater	see trapezium bone			
multangular b., lesser	see trapezoid bone			
nasal b. *os nasale*	skull	one of two small oblong paired b.'s positioned side by side to form the bridge of nose	frontal, ethmoid, opposite nasal, maxilla
navicular b. navicular b. of foot scaphoid b. of foot *os naviculare* *os naviculare pedis*	foot	situated at medial side of tarsus between the talus and cuneiform b.'s	talus, three cuneiforms, occasionally with cuboid
navicular b. of hand	see scaphoid bone			
occipital b. *os occipitale*	skull	unpaired saucer-shaped b. forming posterior part of base of cranium; it is pierced by the foramen magnum	both parietals and temporals; sphenoid, atlas
palatine b. palate b. *os palatinum*	skull	one of two somewhat L-shaped paired b.'s, the two forming the posterior part of hard palate, part of the floor and lateral wall of nasal cavity, and part of the floor of the orbit	sphenoid, ethmoid, maxilla, vomer, opposite palatine, inferior nasal concha
parietal b. *os parietale*	skull	paired b.'s between frontal and occipital b.'s forming sides and roof of cranium	opposite parietal, frontal, occipital, temporal, sphenoid
patella knee cap *patella*	knee	flat, rounded, triangular b. (sesamoid), situated in front of knee joint	femur
pelvis	a bony ring resembling a basin, composed of two hipbones, sacrum, and coccyx			
phalanges of foot *ossa digitorum pedis*	foot	miniature long b.'s, two in great toe and three in each of other toes	proximal row of phalanges with corresponding metatarsal b.'s and middle phalanges; middle phalanges with proximal and distal phalanges; ungual phalanges with middle phalanges
phalanges of hand *ossa digitorum manus*	hand	miniature long b.'s, two in thumb and three in each of other fingers	proximal row of phalanges with corresponding metacarpal b.'s and middle phalanges; middle phalanges with proximal and distal phalanges; ungual phalanges with middle phalanges
pisiform b. *os pisiforme*	wrist	most medial of proximal row of carpus; smallest carpal b.	triangular

bone | bone

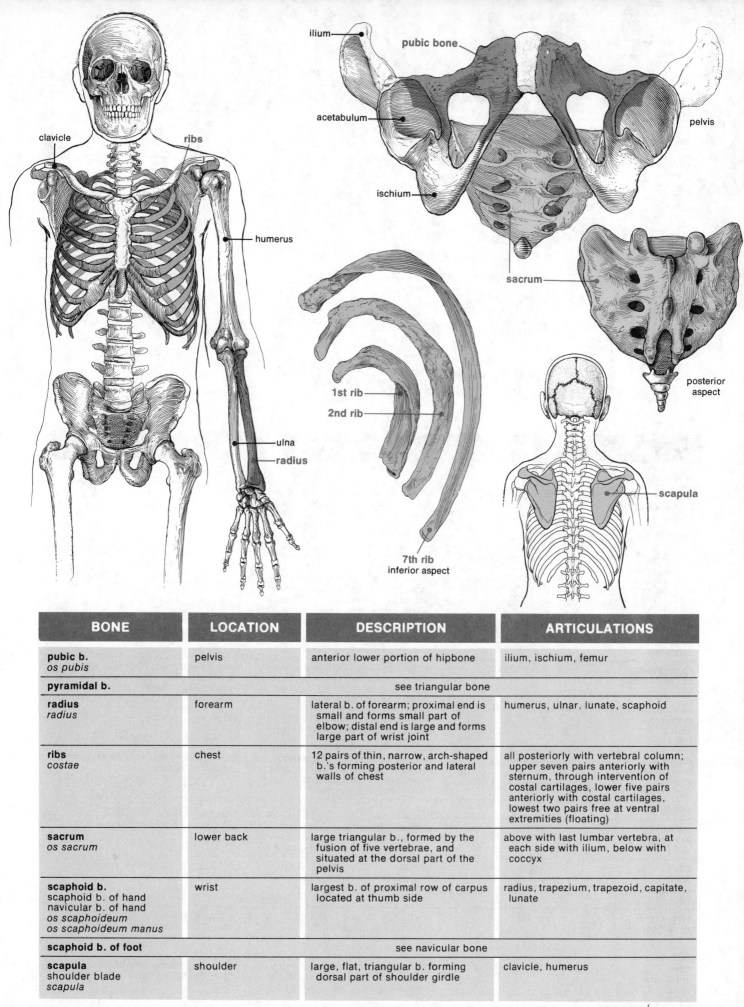

BONE	LOCATION	DESCRIPTION	ARTICULATIONS
pubic b. *os pubis*	pelvis	anterior lower portion of hipbone	ilium, ischium, femur
pyramidal b.	*see triangular bone*		
radius *radius*	forearm	lateral b. of forearm; proximal end is small and forms small part of elbow; distal end is large and forms large part of wrist joint	humerus, ulnar, lunate, scaphoid
ribs *costae*	chest	12 pairs of thin, narrow, arch-shaped b.'s forming posterior and lateral walls of chest	all posteriorly with vertebral column; upper seven pairs anteriorly with sternum, through intervention of costal cartilages, lower five pairs anteriorly with costal cartilages, lowest two pairs free at ventral extremities (floating)
sacrum *os sacrum*	lower back	large triangular b., formed by the fusion of five vertebrae, and situated at the dorsal part of the pelvis	above with last lumbar vertebra, at each side with ilium, below with coccyx
scaphoid b. scaphoid b. of hand navicular b. of hand *os scaphoideum* *os scaphoideum manus*	wrist	largest b. of proximal row of carpus located at thumb side	radius, trapezium, trapezoid, capitate, lunate
scaphoid b. of foot	*see navicular bone*		
scapula shoulder blade *scapula*	shoulder	large, flat, triangular b. forming dorsal part of shoulder girdle	clavicle, humerus

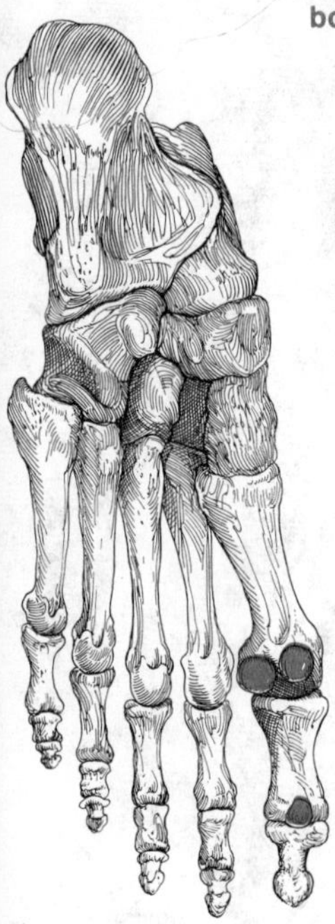

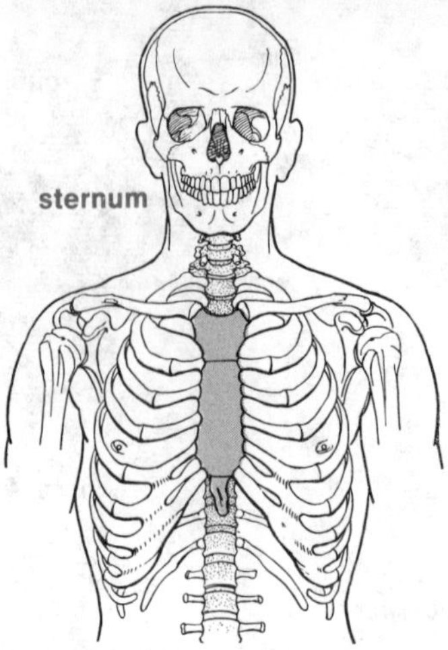

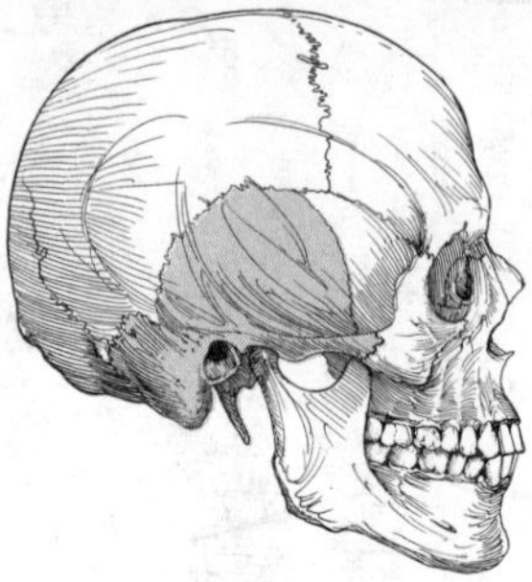

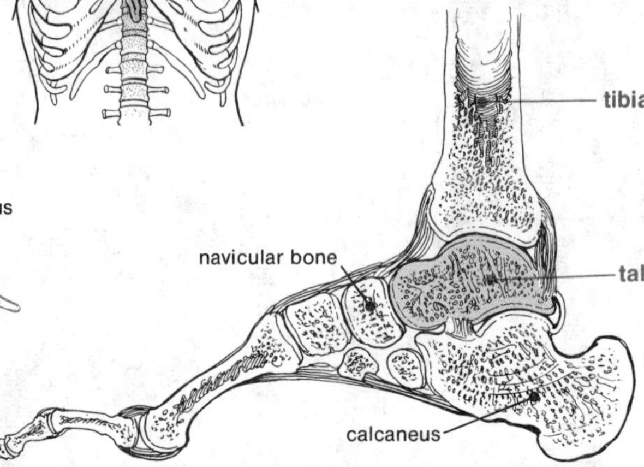

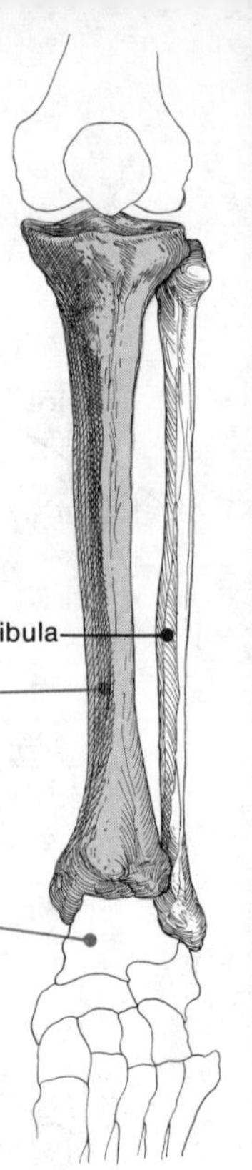

sphenoid bone

sternum

temporal bone

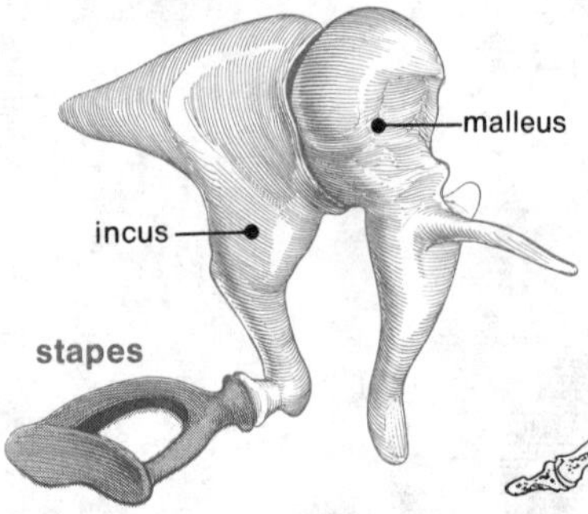

sesamoid bones

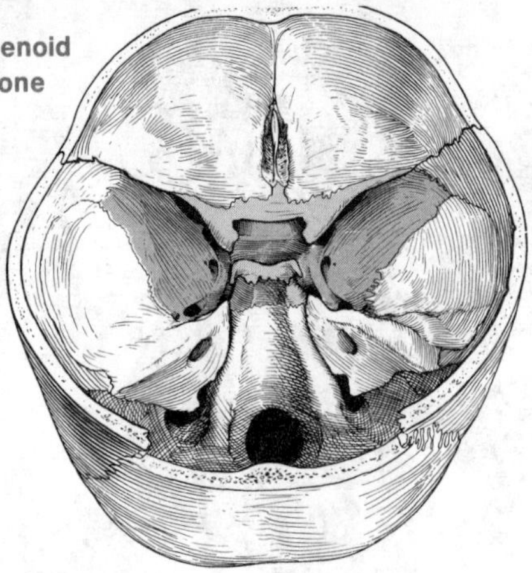

malleus

incus

stapes

navicular bone

fibula

tibia

talus

calcaneus

BONE	LOCATION	DESCRIPTION	ARTICULATIONS
semilunar b.		see lunate bone	
sesamoid b.'s *ossa sesamoidea*	extremities	small rounded b.'s embedded in certain tendons; some constant ones include the tendons of the quadriceps muscle of thigh (m. quadriceps femoris), short flexor muscle of great toe (m. flexor hallucis brevis), long peroneal muscle (m. peroneus longus), anterior tibial muscle (m. tibialis anterior), posterior tibial muscle (m. tibialis posterior), and greater psoas muscle (m. psoas major); the patela (kneecap) is the largest sesamoid bone.	
shinbone		see tibia	
sphenoid b. *os sphenoidale*	base of skull	unpaired, irregularly shaped b. forming anterior part of base of skull and portions of cranial, orbital, and nasal cavities	vomer, ethmoid, frontal, occipital, both parietals, both temporals, both zygomatics, both palatines; also articulates with tuberosity of maxilla
stapes stirrup *stapes*	ear	most medial b. of auditory ossicles, somewhat resembling a stirrup	incus, oval window
sternum breastbone *sternum*	chest	elongated, flattened, dagger-shaped b. forming ventral wall of thorax; consists of three parts: manubrium, body, xiphoid process	both clavicles and first seven pairs of costal cartilages
stirrup b.		see stapes	
sutural b.'s wormian b.'s	skull	irregular, isolated b.'s occasionally found along cranial sutures, especially the lambdoid suture	usually occipital and parietal b.'s
talus ankle b. astragalus *talus*	ankle	second largest of the tarsal b.'s, it supports the tibia and rests on the calcaneus	tibia, fibula, calcaneus, navicular
temporal b. *os temporale*	skull	irregularly shaped b. consisting of three parts: squama, petrous, and tympanic; it forms part of the side and base of the cranium	occipital, parietal, zygomatic, sphenoid, mandible
tibia shinbone *tibia*	leg	situated at the medial side of the leg between the ankle and knee joint; the second longest b. in the body	above with femur and fibula; below with fibula and talus

bone | bone

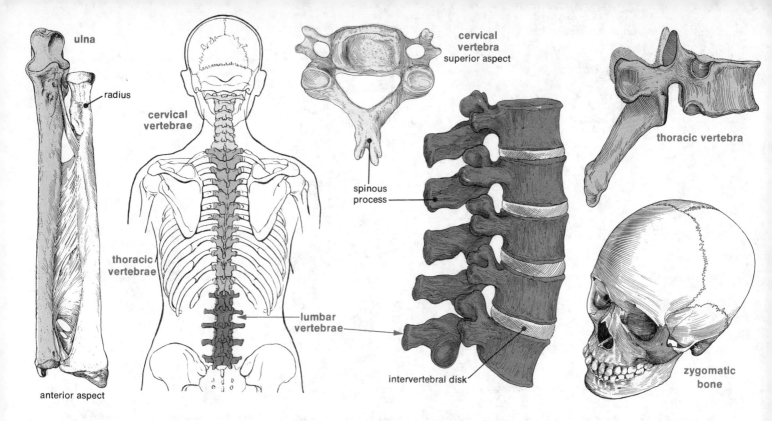

ulna

radius

cervical vertebrae

cervical vertebra superior aspect

spinous process

thoracic vertebrae

lumbar vertebrae

intervertebral disk

thoracic vertebra

zygomatic bone

anterior aspect

BONE	LOCATION	DESCRIPTION	ARTICULATIONS
trapezium b. greater multangular b. *os trapezium*	wrist	most lateral of four b.'s of distal row of carpus	scaphoid, first metacarpal, trapezoid, second metacarpal
trapezoid b. lesser multangular b. *os trapezoideum*	wrist	smallest b. in distal row of carpus	scaphoid, second metacarpal, trapezium, capitate
triangular b. pyramidal b. triquestral b. *os triquetrum*	wrist	pyramidal shape; second from little finger side of proximal row of carpus	lunate, pisiform, hamate, triangular articular disk
triquetral b.	see triangular bone		
turbinate b., inferior	see concha, inferior nasal		
turbinate b., middle	not a separate bone; see ethmoid bone		
turbinate b., superior	not a separate bone; see ethmoid bone		
ulna elbow b. *ulna*	forearm	medial b. of forearm; lies parallel with radius	humerus, radius
unciform b.	see hamate bone		
vertebrae, cervical backbones *vertebrae*	back of neck	seven segments of vertebral column; smallest of the true vertebrae; they possess a foramen in each transverse process	first vertebra with skull, all others with adjoining vertebrae
vertebrae, lumbar backbones *vertebrae*	lower back	five segments of vertebral column; the largest b.'s of movable part of vertebral column	with adjoining vertebrae; fifth vertebra with sacrum
vertebrae, thoracic backbones *vertebrae*	back	12 segments of vertebral column; they possess facets on the sides of all the bodies and the first 10 also have facets on the transverse processes	with adjoining vertebrae, heads of ribs, tubercles of ribs (except 11th and 12th)
vomer *vomer*	skull	thin, flat b. forming the posterior and inferior part of the nasal septum	ethmoid, sphenoid, both maxillae, both palatine bones; also articulates with septal cartilage of nose
wormian b.'s	see sutural bones		
zygomatic b. malar b. cheekbone *os zygomaticum*	skull	forms prominence of the cheek and lower, lateral aspects of orbit	frontal, sphenoid, temporal, maxilla

bone | bone

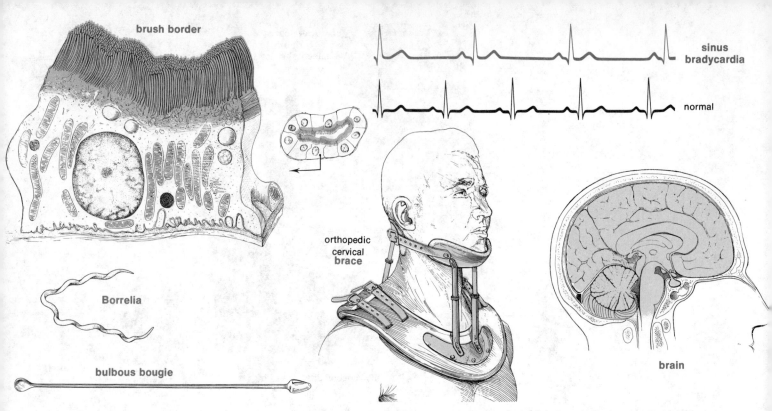

brush border

sinus bradycardia

normal

orthopedic cervical brace

Borrelia

bulbous bougie

brain

bo′rate. A salt of boric acid.

bo′rax. Sodium borate, $Na_2B_4O_7$; used in dentistry in the casting of fluxes and to retard the setting reaction of gypsum products.

borboryg′mus. Rumbling noise produced by movement of gas in the intestines.

bor′der. Edge or margin.

  brush b., a border of many fine, closely packed microvilli, as seen on the free surface of the cuboidal cells of the proximal convoluted tubules of the kidney.

  denture b., denture edge, (1) the boundary of a denture base; (2) the area of a denture base at the junction of the polished surface with the impression (tissue) surface.

  striated b., a border of many fine, closely packed microvilli on the free surface of the columnar absorptive cells of the intestine; it greatly increases the surface area of intestinal epithelium; also called striated free border.

  vermilion b., the exposed reddish portion of the upper and lower lips.

Bordetel′la. A genus of gram-negative pathogenic coccobacilli.

  B. pertussis, the causative agent of whooping cough in man; formerly called *Hemophilus pertussis*.

bor′ic acid. A white or crystalline compound, H_3BO_3; used as an antiseptic.

Bornholm disease. Epidemic pleurodynia; see under pleurodynia.

bor′on. A soft, brown nonmetallic element; symbol B, atomic number 5, atomic weight 10.82.

Borrel′ia. A genus of bacteria (family Teponemataceae), several species of which are the cause of relapsing fever throughout the world; formerly called *Spironema*, the organisms are now included by many authorities in the genus *Treponema*.

  B. vincentii, a species occurring along with *Fusobacterium fusiforme* in fusospirochetal pharyngitis; also called *Spirochaeta recta* and *Spirochaeta tenuis*.

boss. 1. A round swelling. 2. A hump on the back.

bossela′tion. Condition marked by the presence of one or more round protuberances or swellings.

Bothrioceph′alus. *Diphyllobothrium.*

bot′ryoid. Resembling a bunch of grapes.

botryomyco′sis. An infectious disease of cattle, horses, and swine, marked by the presence of granulomatous nodules on the skin and sometimes the viscera; it may be transmitted to man.

bot′tle. A receptacle with a narrow neck.

  wash b., (1) a fluid-containing bottle with two tubes passing through its cork, arranged in such a way that blowing through one tube forces a stream of fluid through the other; used for washing chemi-

cal materials; (2) a fluid-containing bottle with a tube passing to the bottom through which gasses are forced for the purpose of purifying them.

bot′ulism. Poisoning caused by the toxin of *Clostridium botulinum* in improperly preserved food.

bou′gie. A flexible cylindrical instrument used in the diagnosis and treatment of strictures of tubular structures, such as the esophagus or urethra; it also serves to measure the degree of narrowing.

  b. à boule, bulbous bougie.

  bulbous b., one with a bulb-shaped tip.

  filiform b., a very slender bougie.

bougienage′. Examination or treatment (dilation) of a tubular structure by means of a bougie or cannula.

bouillon′. 1. A clear thin broth. 2. A culture medium prepared from beef.

bouton′. A swelling or thickening.

  b. de Bagdad, cutaneous leishmaniasis; see under leishmaniasis.

  b. en chemise, abscesses of the intestinal mucosa, seen in amebic dysentery.

  b.'s termineaux, the numerous enlarged synaptic axon terminals of a neuron which make contact with the receptive end of another neuron (either with the cell body, a dendrite, or its axon); also called terminal buttons, synaptic knobs, and end-feet.

bo′vine. Relating to cattle.

bow′el. The intestine.

bowleg. See genu varum.

BP. Abbreviation for blood pressure.

brace. A device for supporting a bodily part.

  orthodontic b.'s, general term for orthodontic appliances designed to move teeth into a more esthetic and/or functional position; composed of bands fitted to the teeth with attachments or brackets to hold spring wires; often the wires are supplemented by rubber bands.

bra′chial. Relating to the arm.

  b. plexus, see table of nerves.

brachiot′omy. Incision into or amputation of an arm.

bra′chium, *pl.* **bra′chia.** 1. The arm, especially above the elbow. 2. Any armlike structure.

brachycephal′ic. Characterized by brachycephalism.

brachyceph′alism. A deformity in which the skull has an abnormally flattened anteroposterior plane, due to premature closure of the coronal suture.

brachydac′tyly. Abnormal shortness of fingers and toes.

brachyther′apy. Radiotherapeutic treatment applied with the x-ray source near the tissues being irradiated; also called plesiotherapy.

brack′et. In orthodontics, a small piece of metal fixed on the band surrounding a tooth; used to fasten the arch wire to the band.

bradycar′dia. Abnormal slowness of the heart beat, a rate usually less than 60 beats per minute.

  sinus b., bradycardia resulting from the sinus node originating impulses at a slow rate; usually due, in part at least, to vagal inhibition of the sinus node; seen often in patients with high vagal tone, in trained athletes, in hypothyroidism, and secondary to increased intracranial tension.

bradycrot′ic. Marked by a slow pulse.

bradykine′sia. Abnormal slowness of movement.

bradyki′nin. A potent vasodilator polypeptide hormone.

bradypne′a. Abnormally slow rate of breathing, as in shock.

braille. A system of writing and printing for the blind, consisting of raised dots representing letters and numerals; invented by Louis Braille, a French teacher of the blind.

brain. The portion of the central nervous system contained within the skull; composed of the cerebrum, cerebellum, pons, and medulla oblongata; also called encephalon.

  b. stem, the part of the brain connecting the forebrain (prosencephalon) and the spinal cord; it consists of the midbrain (mesencephalon), pons, and medulla oblongata.

bran′chia. The gills of water-living animals.

bran′chial. Relating to gills.

branch′ing. Dividing.

branchiogen′ic, branchiogen′ous. Originating from the embryonic branchial arches or the ridges between the branchial clefts.

breakdown, nervous. A vague popular euphemism for a mental disorder, usually implying an acute and marked change in behavior and inability to function.

breast. 1. Mammary gland. 2. Chest.

breast′bone. See sternum.

breath. 1. The inhaled and exhaled air in respiration. 2. The air exhaled, as evidenced by vapor.

  b. analyzer, a simple device for detecting whether or not a person is intoxicated. The subject blows into a balloon and if the proportion of alcohol in his breath is sufficiently high, a chemical reactant in the device changes color.

breath′ing. The act of taking in and expelling air from the lungs.

  intermittent positive pressure b. (IPPB), the intermittent inflation of the lungs with air or an oxygen mixture at an adjustable pressure and rate of flow.

  mouth b., the process of inhaling and exhaling air

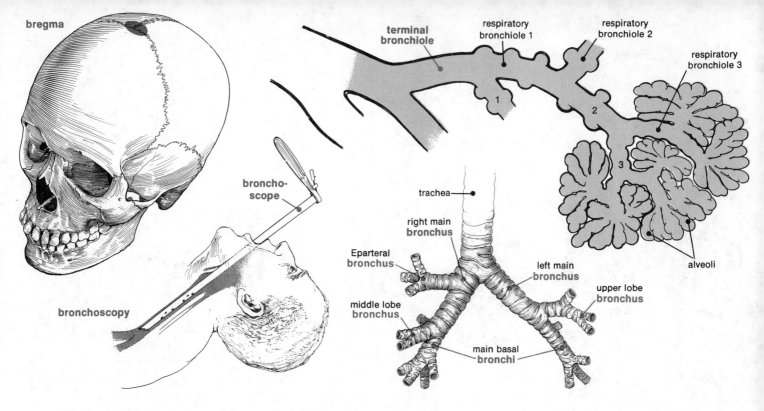

chiefly through the mouth rather than the nose.

mouth to mouth b., a form of resuscitation in which the resuscitator expands the lungs of the nonbreathing subject by blowing directly into the subject's mouth.

shallow b., a weak type of breathing, as seen in acute pulmonary disease.

breech. The buttocks.

breed. 1. To develop new or improved strains in animals or plants. **2.** A strain of animal or plant.

breg′ma. The point on the skull where the sagittal and coronal sutures meet; also called sinciput (2).

brei. A suspension of minced tissue, used especially in metabolic experimentation.

bridge. 1. In dentistry, a nonremovable prosthesis consisting of one or more artificial teeth suspended between and attached to abutments (terminal natural crowns or roots). **2.** The upper part of the human nose, between the eyes.

Wheatstone's b., an instrument used to measure electrical resistance.

bridge′work. Partial denture; see under denture.

Bright's disease, chronic. A name proposed for kidney failure caused by a group of progressive pathologic processes having a common pattern of deranged kidney excretory and regulatory function.

Brill's disease. See Brill-Zinsser disease.

Brill-Zinsser disease. The occurrence of typhus in persons who suffered an infection of primary epidemic typhus in the past; caused by *Rickettsia prowazekii* which, according to Zinsser, remain viable in the body of the patient and recrudescence or relapse occurs years after the original infection; also called Brill's disease and recrudescent typhus.

British antilewisite (BAL). See dimercaprol.

broach. A small instrument used in the examination or treatment of the root canal of a tooth.

Broadbent's sign. Pulsation observed in the left posterior axillary line, occurring synchronously with cardiac systole; a sign of adherent pericardium.

broad-spectrum. Widely effective. See also antibiotic, broad-spectrum.

bromcresol green. A slightly yellow crystalline compound, $C_{21}H_{14}Br_4O_5S$, slightly soluble in water; soluble in alcohol, ether, and ethyl alcohol; used as an indicator of pH: yellow at pH 3.8, blue-green at pH 5.4.

bromcresol purple. a pale yellow crystalline compound, $C_{21}H_{16}Br_2O_5S$; soluble in alcohol and dilute alkalis; used as an indicator of pH: yellow at pH 5.2, purple at pH 6.8.

brom′ic. Of or containing bromine.

bro′mide. A binary compound of bromine and another element or organic radical; a salt of hydrobromic acid.

bro′mine. A heavy, corrosive, reddish, volatile, nonmetallic liquid element, with a highly irritating vapor; symbol Br, atomic number 35, atomic weight 79.916.

bro′mism. Bromide poisoning marked by headache, skin eruptions, apathy, and muscular weakness.

bromphe′nol blue. An indicator of pH.

bron′chi. Plural of bronchus.

bron′chial. Relating to the bronchi.

bronchiec′tasis, bronchiecta′sia. An irreversible, abnormal dilatation of the bronchi or bronchioles; the extent of the disorder may range from a mild involvement of a single pulmonary segment to gross distortion of the entire bronchial tree.

bronchiogen′ic, bronchogen′ic. Of bronchial origin.

bron′chiole. Any of the thin-walled extensions of a bronchus.

terminal b., the last bronchiole without alveoli in its wall.

bronchiolec′tasis, bronchiolecta′sia. Chronic dilatation of the terminal bronchioles.

bronchioli′tis. Inflammation of the bronchioles.

acute obliterating b., a form of fibrosis of the lung due to fibrous induration of the walls of the terminal bronchioles.

bronchiolo-. Combining form pertaining to the bronchiole.

bronchiosteno′sis. Narrowing of the bronchi.

bronchi′tis. Inflammation of the mucous membrane of the bronchi.

bronchoalveo′lar. See bronchovesicular.

bronchocav′ernous. Relating to a bronchus and a pulmonary cavity.

bron′chocele. A circumscribed dilatation of a bronchus.

bronchoconstric′tor. An agent that causes narrowing of the lumen of a bronchus.

bronchodila′tor. An agent that causes dilatation of the lumen of a bronchus.

bronchoegoph′ony. An exaggerated egophony (bleating quality of voice heard in auscultation).

bronchogen′ic. Of bronchial origin.

bron′chogram. The radiogram obtained by bronchography.

bronchog′raphy. Radiographic examination of the bronchi after injection of a radiopaque material.

bron′cholith. Bronchial calculus (stone).

broncholithi′asis. Presence of bronchial calculi, often leading to inflammation or obstruction of the bronchi.

bronchomala′cia. Degeneration of the supporting tissues of the bronchi and trachea.

bronchomo′tor. An agent that changes the cali-

ber of bronchi.

bronchop′athy. Disease of the bronchial tubes.

bronchoph′ony. Exaggerated resonance of the voice heard in auscultation over a bronchus surrounded by consolidated lung tissue.

bron′choplasty. Surgical repair of a defect in the trachea or the bronchi.

bronchople′gia. Paralysis of the muscular fibers in the walls of the bronchi.

bronchopneumo′nia. Inflammation of the lungs, usually following infection of the bronchi; also called lobular or bronchial prenumonia.

bronchopul′monary. Relating to the bronchi and the lungs.

bronchorrhe′a. Copious discharge from the bronchial mucosa.

bron′choscope. A thin tubular instrument used for inspecting the interior of the trachea and bronchi.

bronchos′copy. The endoscopic examination and treatment of the tracheobronchial tree and lungs, by means of the bronchoscope used as a speculum.

bron′chospasm. Spasmodic constriction of the bronchial tubes; also called bronchoconstriction.

bronchospirog′raphy. The measuring of the airflow in one lung only, or one lobe of a lung.

bronchospirom′eter. A device for measuring separately the air capacity of each lung.

bronchospirom′etry. The determination of the respiratory capacity of a lung by the use of a bronchospirometer.

bronchosteno′sis. Narrowing of the lumen of a bronchial tube.

bronchovesic′ular. Relating to the bronchial tubes and air sacs in the lungs; also called bronchoalveolar.

bron′chus, *pl.* **bron′chi.** Either of two main branches of the trachea leading to the bronchioles and serving to convey air to and from the lungs.

brow. 1. Eyebrow. **2.** Forehead.

Brown-Séquard syndrome. Damage of a lateral half of the spinal cord, causing motor and sensory disturbances below the level of the lesion, i.e., motor paralysis and loss of joint position sense and vibration sense on the same side of the body and loss of pain and temperature sensation on the opposite side.

Brucel′la. A genus of bacteria (family Brucellaceae) composed of gram-negative, rod-shaped to coccoid parasitic cells; they cause primary infections of the genital organs, mammary glands, and respiratory and intestinal tracts.

B. abortus, Bang's bacillus, a species causing abortion in cattle and undulant fever (brucellosis) in man.

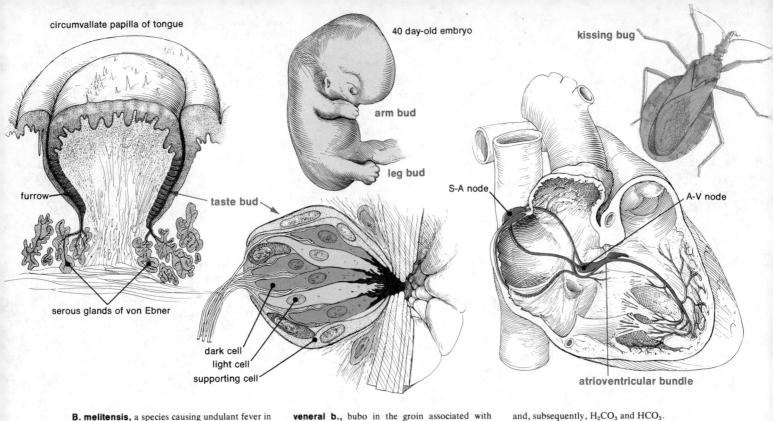

circumvallate papilla of tongue

furrow

taste bud

serous glands of von Ebner

dark cell
light cell
supporting cell

40 day-old embryo

arm bud

leg bud

kissing bug

S-A node

A-V node

atrioventricular bundle

B. melitensis, a species causing undulant fever in man and abortion in goats.

B. suis, a species resembling *Brucella melitensis*; the cause of abortion in swine and brucellosis in man.

brucello'sis. An infectious disease caused by bacteria of the *Brucella* genus and transmitted by animals; characterized by remittent fever, general weakness, aches, and pains, sometimes becoming chronic; also called undulant fever, Malta fever, Mediterranean fever (2), abortus fever, and melitensis.

Brudzinski's signs. 1. Brudzinski's neck sign; flexion of both legs and thighs upon forcible flexion of the neck. **2.** Brudzinski's contralateral leg sign, (a) flexion of one thigh at the hip causes a similar movement of the other thigh; (b) when one thigh and leg are flexed and the other extended, lowering of the flexed leg causes flexion of the extended one; Brudzinski's signs are seen in meningitis.

Bru'gia. A genus of parasitic filarial worms transmitted to man and other mammals by mosquitoes.

B. malayi, the species causing filariasis and elephantiasis in Southeast Asia; formerly called Malayan filaria and *Wuchereria malayi*.

bruise. Hematoma without laceration; usually a superficial lesion but can occur in deeper structures; a contusion.

bruit'. Sound or murmur, especially an abnormal one heard during auscultation.

aneurysmal b., a blowing murmur heard over an aneurysm.

b. de canon, cannon sound; the abnormally loud first heart sound heard intermittently in complete heart block.

b. de Roger, Roger's murmur; see under murmur.

diastolic b., bruit occurring during the diastolic phase of the heart cycle after the second heart sound; this usually connotes an abnormal valve function.

systolic b., bruit heard during the systolic phase of the heart cycle between the first and second heart sounds.

thyroid b., a vascular murmur heard over a hyperactive thyroid gland.

brux'ism. Forceful clenching and grinding of the teeth, especially during sleep.

bruxoma'nia. Unconscious grinding of the teeth while awake.

BSP. Abbreviation for Bromsulphalein®; see sulfobromophthalein sodium.

bu'bo. Enlargement and inflammation of a lymph node, especially in the groin or axilla.

malignant b., one associated with bubonic plague.

tropical b., see lymphogranuloma venereum.

veneral b., bubo in the groin associated with venereal disease.

buc'cal. Pertaining to the cheek.

buccoling'ual. 1. Denoting the plane of a posterior tooth from its buccal surface across to its lingual surface. **2.** Relating to the cheek and the tongue.

bucco-occlu'sal. Relating to the buccal and occlusal surfaces of a posterior tooth; usually denoting the line angle formed by the junction of the two surfaces.

buccopharyn'geal. Relating to both the mouth and pharynx.

buccover'sion. Malposition of a tooth toward the cheek.

bud. Any small organic part resembling a plant bud.

bronchial b., one of the outgrowths from the primordial bronchus, giving rise to the bronchial tree.

metanephric b., an outgrowth from the mesonephric duct, giving rise to the lining of the ureter, pelvis, and calyces of the kidney, and the straight collecting tubules.

taste b., gustatory caliculus, one of numerous flask-shaped minute organs, located on the tongue, the under surface of the soft palate, and the posterior surface of the epiglottis; composed of modified epithelial supporting cells which surround a mass of spindle-shaped gustatory cells and the fibrils of the nerves of taste (chorda tympani and glossopharyngeal); also called taste bulb.

tooth b., the primordial structures from which a tooth develops.

lung b.'s, two lateral outpocketings of the respiratory primordium of the foregut that gives rise to the tracheobronchial tree.

Budd-Chiari syndrome. Hepatic vein occlusion; see under occlusion.

bud'ding. See gemmation.

Buerger's disease. See thromboangiitis obliterans.

buf'fer. 1. Any substance that maintains the relative concentrations of hydrogen and hydroxyl ions in a solution by neutralizing any added acid or alkali. **2.** To add a buffer to a solution; to maintain body fluids at a relatively constant pH when acid or alkali is added to or lost from the body.

buf'fering. A process by which hydrogen ion concentration is maintained constant.

biologic b., ionic shifts between intra- and extracellular spaces which protect extracellular pH.

renal b., removal of excess acid or base by the kidney.

respiratory b., increases or decreases in respiratory rate which act to increase or decrease CO_2

and, subsequently, H_2CO_3 and HCO_3.

buf'fy coat. The upper, grayish layer of a blood clot, formed when coagulation is delayed and consisting mainly of coagulated plasma and white blood cells.

bug. Any of various insects of the order Hemiptera.

assassin b., kissing bug.

bed b., bedbug.

cone-nose b., kissing bug.

kissing b., an insect (family Reduviidae) similar to the ordinary bedbug but with a cone-shaped anterior end; usually found in bedrooms where it feeds at night on the blood of its sleeping and unsuspecting hosts; acquired its name because of its inclination to bite the lips of sleeping people; also called cone-nose or assassin bug.

red b., see chigger.

bulb. 1. Any globular structure. **2.** The medulla oblongata.

aortic b., a dilatation at the beginning of the aorta.

b. of the corpus spongiosum, see bulb of penis.

b. of penis, the expanded posterior portion of the corpus spongiosum penis.

carotid b., see sinus, carotid.

duodenal b., see cap, duodenal.

jugular b., a dilatation of the internal jugular vein just before it joins the subclavian vein.

Krause's end-b., Krause's corpuscle; a spherical sense organ located at the termination of some sensory nerve fibers; it responds to the sensation of cold.

olfactory b., the expanded anterior end of the olfactory tract.

taste b., see bud, taste.

bul'bar. 1. Relating to or resembling a bulb. **2.** Relating to the medulla oblongata.

bulbopon'tine. Relating to the part of the brain composed of the pons and the portion of the medulla oblongata over it.

bulboure'thral. Relating to the bulb of the urethra, the enlarged posterior portion of the corpus spongiosum of the penis.

bulim'ia. Insatiable hunger.

bulk'age. Any substance, such as agar, that stimulates peristalsis by increasing the bulk of the intestinal contents.

bul'la, *pl.* **bul'lae.** A blister or circumscribed elevation on the skin containing serous fluid, larger than one centimeter in size, e.g., as in a second degree burn. Cf vesicle.

bul'lous. 1. Characterized by the presence of blisters (bullae). **2.** Of the nature of bullae.

bun'dle. a group of nerve or muscle fibers.

atrioventricular (A-V) b., b. of His, a bundle of

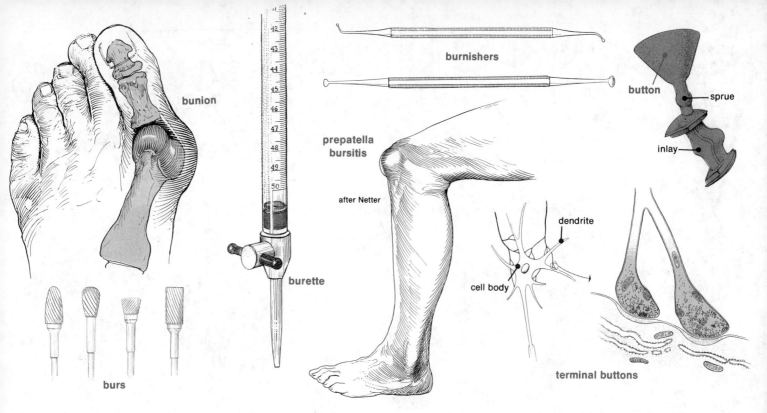

bunion

burnishers

button — sprue

inlay

prepatella bursitis

after Netter

burette

dendrite

cell body

terminal buttons

burs

specialized muscular fibers located in the membranous interventricular septum of the heart; the only direct muscular connection between the atria and the ventricles; it originates at the atrioventricular (A-V) node in the floor of the right atrium, extends downward in the septum, divides into right and left branches, and ends in numerous strands (Purkinje system) in the papillary and ventricular muscles; also called fasciculus atrioventricularis.

b. of His, see atrioventricular bundle.

b. of Kent, atrioventricular bundle.

posterior longitudinal b., medial longitudinal fasciculus; see under fasciculus.

bundle-branch block. See block, bundle-branch.

bun'ion. Painful condition of the big toe, marked by lateral angulation of the toe (hallux valgus), enlargement of the head of the metatarsal bone, and a swollen, inflamed overlying bursa; caused by poorly fitted shoes. Cf hallux valgus.

bunionett'e. A bursal enlargement over the angular projection of the fifth metatarsophalangeal joint of the foot; the counterpart of the bunion of the great toe.

buphthal'mos. A condition marked by an increase of intraocular fluid with enlargement of the eyeball and protrusion of the cornea; also called congenital glaucoma and hydrophthalmos.

bur. A rotary dental instrument with one cutting end designed in any of several shapes and a shaft at the other end which is inserted into a hand piece; used for excavating decay from a tooth, shaping cavity forms, or any surface reduction of tooth substance.

burett'e, buret'. A calibrated, uniform-bore glass tube with a stopcock at its lower end, used in the laboratory for accurate fluid dispensing.

burn. 1. To injure by fire, heat, or a chemical. **2.** The lesion thus produced.

brush b., injury to the skin by friction of a rapidly moving object; also called rope or mat burn.

chemical b., one caused by a caustic agent.

flash b., one caused by brief exposure to radiant heat of high intensity.

radiation b., one due to overexposure to x-rays, radium, ultraviolet rays, etc.

thermal b., one produced by contact with heat.

bur'ner. The part of a lamp or stove that is lighted to produce a flame.

Bunsen b., a gas burner used in the laboratory, consisting of a metal tube with adjustable air holes at the base.

Burnett's syndrome. See milk-alkali syndrome.

bur'nisher. A dental instrument with rounded edges for smoothing, polishing, or stretching the

metallic surface of a tooth restoration.

bur'sa, *pl.* **bur'sae.** A closed sac lined with specialized connective tissue and containing a viscid fluid; usually present over bony prominences, between and beneath tendons, and between certain movable structures; it serves to facilitate movement by diminishing friction.

Achilles b., see bursa of calcaneal tendon (tendo calcaneus).

adventitious b., an abnormal bursa developed as a result of irritation.

anserine b., one located at the medial aspect of the knee, under, and near the insertion of, the gracilis and semitendinous tendons.

b. of calcaneal tendon, b. of tendo calcaneus, one located at the heel, between the calcaneus bone and calcaneal tendon (Achilles tendon); also called Achilles bursa and retrocalcaneal bursa.

deep infrapatellar b., one located below the patella (kneecap) between the lower portion of the patellar ligament and the tibia.

deep trochanteric b., one located in the hip between the greater trochanter of the femur and the gluteus maximus muscle; also called trochanteric bursa of gluteus maximus muscle.

gastrocnemius b., one composed of two portions (lateral and medial) and located in the back of the knee, under the two heads of the gastrocnemius muscle; the medial portion is usually connected with the semimembranous bursa (of clinical importance because when distended with fluid, it is the usual cause of a popliteal cyst).

iliopectineal b., one located on the anterior surface of the hip joint capsule, between the iliofemoral and pubofemoral ligaments; it frequently communicates with the capsule of the joint.

ischiogluteal b., a large bursa separating the gluteus maximus muscle from the ischial tuberosity; chronic ischiogluteal bursitis is caused by prolonged sitting on hard surfaces and is commonly known as weaver's bottom.

olecranon b., one located at the elbow between the skin and the tip of the olecranon process of the ulna.

omental b., lesser sac of peritoneum; see under sac.

popliteal b., one located on the posterolateral portion of the knee, under the popliteus muscle; it is often a continuation of the synovial sac of the knee.

prepatellar b., one situated anterior to the lower part of the patella (kneecap); chronic irritation causes prepatellar bursitis (housemaid's knee).

quadriceps b., an extension of the synovial sac on the anterior aspect of the knee, between the

femur and the quadriceps tendon; also called suprapatellar bursa.

radiohumeral b., one located at the elbow, over the radiohumeral joint, between the extensor digitorum and supinator muscles.

semimembranous b., one located in the medial aspect of the knee, between the semimembranous tendon and the medial head of the gastrocnemius muscle. See also gastrocnemius bursa.

subacromial b., one located between the acromium and the capsule of the shoulder joint; usually connected with the subdeltoid bursa.

subdeltoid b., one located between the deltoid muscle and the capsule of the shoulder joint; usually combined with the subacromial bursa.

subscapular b., a bursa between the tendon of the subscapular muscle and the glenoid border of the scapula; it communicates with the shoulder joint.

superficial acromial b., one located at the shoulder between the acromium and the skin.

superficial prepatellar b., one on the anterior aspect of the knee, over the insertion of the patellar ligament into the tuberosity of the tibia; also called pretibial bursa.

bursec'tomy. Surgical removal of a bursa.

bursi'tis. Inflammation of a bursa.

prepatellar b., inflammation of the bursa in front of the patella (kneecap), usually due to repeated trauma; also called housemaid's knee.

bursot'omy. Incision into a bursa.

busul'fan. Tetramethylene salt of methanesulfonic acid; used in the treatment of myelocytic leukemia; Myleran®.

but'ter. 1. Milk fat churned into a coherent mass. **2.** Any substance having the consistency of butter.

but'tock. One of two protuberances formed by the gluteal muscles.

but'ton. 1. Any knob-shaped or disk-shaped structure, lesion, or device. **2.** A collection of cells obtained after centrifuging a fluid specimen containing a small number of cells. **3.** In dentistry, the excess metal remaining from casting; located at the end of the sprue.

peritoneal b., a device for draining ascitic fluid.

terminal b.'s, boutons terminaux; knoblike terminal enlargements of nerve endings; also called end-feet and synaptic knobs.

by'pass. Shunt.

byssino'sis. A form of chronic inflammatory and fibrotic disease caused by inhalation of dust in cotton, flax, and hemp mills; chief symptom is acute airway obstruction; also called cotton-mill fever.

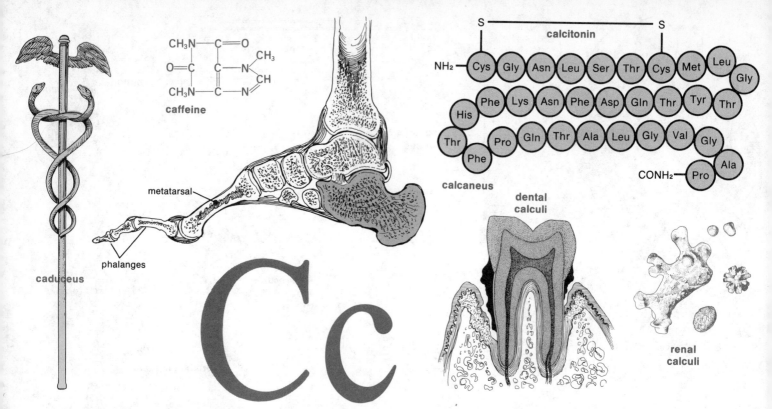

caffeine

metatarsal

phalanges

caduceus

calcitonin

calcaneus

dental calculi

renal calculi

Cc

C. Symbol for (a) large calorie; (b) the element carbon; (c) Celsius; (d) centigrade.

c. Abbreviation for (a) small calorie; (b) cylinder.

c̄. Abbreviation for Latin *cum*.

CA. Abbreviation for (a) cancer; (b) carcinoma.

Ca. 1. Symbol for the element calcium. **2.** Abbreviation for cathode.

ca. Abbreviation for Latin *circa*.

caca′o. An evergreen tropical tree, *Theobroma cacao*; also called chocolate tree.

  c. butter, a solid fat obtained from the seeds of the *Theobroma cacao,* used in the making of suppositories and other pharmaceutical preparations.

cachec′tic. Relating to cachexia.

cach′et. A wafer capsule formerly used by pharmacists to enclose unpalatable drugs.

cachex′ia. Severe malnutrition, weakness, and muscle wasting resulting from a chronic disease.

caco-, caci-, cac-. Combining forms meaning bad or ill.

cacos′mia. An olfactory hallucination; a perception of unpleasant odors that do not exist.

cadav′er. Corpse; a dead body.

cadav′erine. An amine, $C_5H_{14}N_2$, found in decomposing animal tissue.

cad′mium. A soft, bluish-white metallic element; symbol Cd, atomic number 48, atomic weight 112.40; found in nature associated chiefly with zinc; used in the manufacture of storage batteries, in plating, and in alloys; inhalation may produce pulmonary edema; excessive absorption may also produce interstitial nephritis.

cadu′ceus. The winged staff of Mercury, with two oppositely entwined serpents; emblem of the U.S. Army Medical Corps.

cafe au lait. French for coffee with milk; in dermatology, the term is used to express a shade of brown; see under spot.

caf′feine. A bitter alkaloid compound found in coffee, tea, and cola beverages; used medicinally as a stimulant and diuretic.

caf′feinism. The chronic results of excessive consumption of beverages containing caffeine, characterized by rapid beating of the heart, irritability, and insomnia.

cage. 1. Any enclosure used to confine. **2.** Any structure resembling a cage.

  Faraday c., one screened from external electrical waves, used in electroencephalography.

  thoracic c., the bones and musculature of the chest which enclose the thoracic organs.

CAH. Abbreviation for congenital adrenal hyperplasia.

ca′isson disease. A disorder occurring in divers, tunnel workers, or individuals exposed to increased atmospheric pressures; the high pressure causes the gases to dissolve in the blood and body tissues; when the individual returns too suddenly to normal pressure, the dissolved gases return to their original gaseous form and are trapped as bubbles within blood vessels and tissues; symptoms include pain in the joints, respiratory distress, and sometimes coma and death; also called the bends and decompression sickness.

cal′amine. 1. A mineral; hydrous zinc silicate. **2.** A powder composed of zinc oxide (not less than 98 per cent) with about 0.5 per cent of ferric oxide, used in lotions and ointments to relieve itching in inflammatory skin disorders. See also lotion, calamine.

calca′neal, calca′nean. Pertaining to the calcaneus (heel bone).

calca′neus. The quadrangular bone articulating with the talus above and the cuboid anteriorly; also called heel bone.

calca′reous. Chalky; resembling or containing calcium or limestone.

calcico′sis. A lung disease (pneumoconiosis) caused by prolonged inhalation of limestone dust; also called marble cutters' phthisis.

calcif′erol. See vitamin D_2.

calcif′erous. 1. Containing lime. **2.** Forming any of the salts of calcium.

calcif′ic. Caused by or producing calcification.

calcifica′tion. 1. The normal deposition of mineral salts in the bone and tooth tissues, thus contributing to their hardening and maturation. **2.** The pathologic hardening of organic tissue by deposits of calcium salts within its substance.

calcina′tion. The process of calcining.

cal′cine. To heat material to a high temperature causing loss of water, reduction, or oxidation; in dentistry, the removal of water of crystallization from gypsum by heating in order to produce plaster of Paris.

calcino′sis. A disorder marked by the deposition of calcium salts in the skin and subcutaneous tissues, and sometimes in the tendons and muscles.

  c. circumscripta, localized deposits of calcium salts in the skin and subcutaneous tissues.

  c. cutis, a calcium deposit on the skin, usually occurring secondary to a preexisting skin eruption.

  c. universalis, calcinosis involving widespread areas or the entire body.

calciphil′ia. Condition in which the tissues tend to absorb calcium salts from the blood, thus becoming calcified.

calcito′nin, thyrocalcito′nin. A thyroid gland hormone which regulates calcium metabolism; it is secreted in response to a high level of blood calcium and acts to lower the level by inhibiting bone resorption.

cal′cium. A silvery, moderately hard metallic element; symbol Ca, atomic number 20, atomic weight 40.08; together with phosphate and carbonate, it gives bone most of its structural properties; it is an essential nutrient in regulating blood coagulation, muscular contraction, conduction of nerve impulses, cell membrane function, enzyme action, and in assuring cardiac rhythmicity; several of the salts of calcium are used in medicine.

  c. carbonate, chalk; an antacid and astringent; $CaCO_3$; 40 per cent calcium by weight.

  c. fluoride, a compound occurring naturally in bones and teeth; CaF_2.

  c. gluconate, an odorless, tasteless, granular salt of calcium; eight per cent calcium by weight.

  c. hydroxide, slaked lime, used in dentistry as a topical stimulant for production of secondary dentin to reseal the pulp cavity; $Ca(OH)_2$.

  c. oxalate, a white, crystalline, insoluble calcium compound, CaC_2O_4; found as sediment in acid urine and in urinary stones.

cal′cium-45. A radioactive calcium isotope (^{45}Ca) having a half-life of 164 days; may be used as a tracer in the study of bone metabolism.

cal′ciuria. The urinary excretion of calcium; occasionally used as a synonym for hypercalciuria.

calcody′nia. Pain in the heel.

cal′culous. Relating to, resembling, or containing stones or calculi.

cal′culus, *pl.* **cal′culi.** Stone; an abnormal stony concretion usually composed of mineral salts and formed most frequently in the cavities of the body which serve as reservoirs for fluids.

  arthritic c., articular c., a deposit of urates in or near a joint; also called chalkstone.

  biliary c., gallstone.

  dental c., a yellow to brown concretion adhering to the surface of a tooth, made up of calcium salts, microorganisms, and other debris; also called tartar.

  mulberry c., one composed mainly of calcium oxalate, shaped like a mulberry, and deposited in the bladder.

  renal c., kidney stone; concretion in the kidney usually made up of calcium oxalate, calcium phosphate, or uric acid.

  salivary c., one in a salivary duct or gland.

  stag-horn c., one with several branches occurring in the kidney pelvis.

  subgingival c., a dental calculus occurring below the margin of the gum.

  supragingival c., a dental calculus adherent to the exposed surface of a tooth.

  urinary c., one in the kidney, ureter, bladder, or

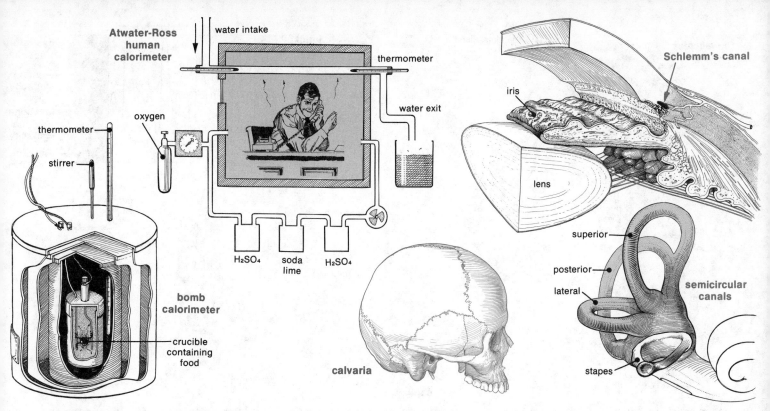

Atwater-Ross human calorimeter

water intake

thermometer

water exit

H_2SO_4 soda lime H_2SO_4

thermometer

stirrer

oxygen

bomb calorimeter

crucible containing food

Schlemm's canal

iris

lens

superior

posterior

lateral

semicircular canals

stapes

calvaria

urethra.

vesical c., a bladder stone; a urinary stone lodged in the bladder.

calefa′cient. Anything that produces a localized sensation of warmth.

calf, *pl.* **calves.** The muscular back portion of the human leg; formed by the bellies of the gastrocnemius and soleus muscles.

cal′iber. The diameter of a tube.

cal′ibrate. 1. To standardize systematically the graduations of a quantitative measuring apparatus. **2.** To determine the diameter of a tube.

calice′al, calyce′al. Relating to the calix.

calicec′tasis. See caliectasis.

cal′ices. Plural of calix.

calic′ulus. A cup-shaped structure.

gustatory c., taste bud; see under bud.

caliec′tasis. Distention of the pelvis and calices of a kidney; also called calicectasis.

cal′ipers, caliper. An instrument composed of two hinged legs, used for measuring diameters, such as the pelvic diameters, or intervals as on an electrocardiogram.

calisthen′ics. 1. A system of light gymnastic exercises to improve muscular tone and to improve physical well-being. **2.** The practice of such simple, systematic exercises.

ca′lix, *pl.* **cal′ices.** A cup-shaped cavity in an organ; also written calyx.

major renal c., one of two or three cup-shaped subdivisions of the pelvis of the kidney.

minor renal c., one of several (seven to 13) cup-shaped subdivisions of the major renal calices.

Calkins′ sign. In obstetrics, the morphologic change of the uterus at delivery from a discoid to ovoid shape; due to a separation of the placenta from the uterine wall.

callo′sal. Of or relating to the corpus callosum.

callos′ity. See callus (1).

cal′lous. Hard and toughened; relating to callus.

cal′lus. 1. Callosity; a circumscribed thickening of the skin. **2.** A hard bonelike substance which is formed between and around the fragments of broken bone and eventually accomplishes repair of the fracture.

central c., provisional callus formed within the medullary cavity of fractured bone.

definitive c., the exudate formed between fractured surfaces of a bone, which changes into true bone.

provisional c., callus formed between and around the fractured surfaces of a bone, keeping the ends of the bone in apposition and becoming absorbed after repair is completed.

ca′lor. Latin for heat.

calor′ic. 1. Relating to calories. **2.** Relating to heat.

cal′orie. Any of several units of heat.

large c. (Cal, kcal), the calorie used in metabolic studies as a measurement of energy-producing value of various foods according to the amount of heat they produce when oxidized in the body; specifically the amount of heat required to raise the temperature of one kilogram of water one degree centigrade (from 15° to 16°) at a pressure of one atmosphere; also called kilocalorie.

small c. (cal), the unit of heat equal to the amount of heat required to raise the temperature of one gram of water one centigrade at a pressure of one atmosphere; also called gram calorie.

calorif′ic. Heat generating.

calorigen′ic. Producing or increasing heat.

calorim′eter. An apparatus for measuring the amount of heat given off by an individual.

Atwater-Rosa human c., a large chamber in which an individual can reside for an extended period of time in order to measure the total output of bodily heat.

Benedict-Roth c., see apparatus, Benedict-Roth.

bomb c., a cyclindrical apparatus for determining the potential energy of food; the food is ignited and the heat of combustion is calculated from the rise in temperature in the calorimeter.

calorim′etry. The measurement of the amount of heat given off by the body.

calva′ria. The upper part of the skull.

calva′rium. Term used incorrectly instead of calvaria.

calx. 1. Lime or calcium oxide. **2.** The heel.

calyce′al. See caliceal.

calycec′tasis. See caliectasis.

cal′ycele. Caliculus.

calyc′ulus. Caliculus.

ca′lyx. See calix.

cam′era. 1. An apparatus used for recording images, either photographically or electronically. **2.** Any cavity of the body.

cam′phor. A solid, crystalline, volatile substance obtained from an evergreen tree, *Cinnamomum camphora,* or prepared synthetically; used medicinally as an expectorant, stimulant, and diaphoretic.

canal′. A tubular structure; a channel.

adductor c., An aponeurotic canal in the middle third of the thigh; it contains the femoral artery and vein, and the saphenous nerve; also called Hunter's canal.

Alcock's c., see pudendal canal.

alimentary c., the mouth, esophagus, stomach, and intestines.

auditory c., external auditory meatus; see under

meatus.

birth c., the cavity of the uterus and vagina through which a child passes at birth; also called parturient canal.

c. of Arantius, venous duct; see under duct.

carotid c., a passage through the petrous part of the temporal bone, transmitting the internal carotid artery.

central c., one extending throughout the entire length of the spinal cord.

femoral c., the medial and smallest of the three compartments of the femoral sheath; it contains some lymphatic vessels and a lymph gland.

Hunter's c., see adductor canal.

incisive c., incisor c., one of two canals opening on either side of the midline in the hard palate, just behind the incisor teeth; through each pass the terminal branches of the descending palatine artery and of the nasopalatine nerve.

inferior dental c., see mandibular canal.

inguinal c., an obliquely directed passage through the layers of the lower abdominal wall on either side, through which passes the spermatic cord in the male and the round ligament of the uterus in the female.

mandibular c., the canal within the mandible containing the inferior alveolar vessels and nerves, from which terminal branches reach the mandibular teeth; also called inferior dental canal.

Müller's c., paramesonephric duct; see under duct.

parturient c., birth canal.

pterygoid c., the canal which passes through the root of the pterygoid process of the sphenoid bone.

pudendal c., the fibrous tunnel within the obturator fascia that lines the lateral wall of the ischiorectal fossa; it transmits the pudendal vessels and nerves; also called Alcock's canal.

root c., pulp c., the portion of the pulp cavity within the root of a tooth which leads from the apex to the pulp chamber and contains the pulp tissue.

Schlemm's c., a ringlike canal in the anterior edge of the sclera, encircling the cornea; it serves as a flow drainage of the excess aqueous humor of the anterior chamber of the eye; also called venous sinus of the sclera.

semicircular c.'s, the three bony canals (superior, lateral, and posterior) in the internal ear in which the membranous semicircular ducts are located.

spinal c., vertebral c., canal formed by the vertebrae, containing the spinal cord.

tympanic c., see scala tympani.

vertebral c., see spinal canal.

vestibular c., see scala vestibuli.

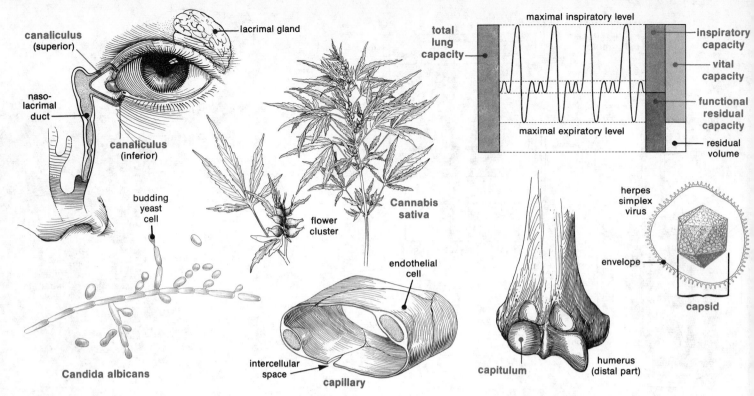

canaliculus (superior) — lacrimal gland

naso-lacrimal duct

canaliculus (inferior)

budding yeast cell

Candida albicans

flower cluster — **Cannabis sativa**

endothelial cell

intercellular space — **capillary**

total lung capacity — maximal inspiratory level — **inspiratory capacity** — **vital capacity** — **functional residual capacity** — maximal expiratory level — **residual volume**

herpes simplex virus — **envelope** — **capsid**

capitulum — **humerus (distal part)**

canalic'ular. Relating to a small canal or canaliculus.

canaliculiza'tion. The formation of small canals in a tissue.

canalic'ulus, *pl.* **canalic'uli.** A minute channel or canal.

  canaliculi dentales, dental tubules; see under tubule.

  lacrimal c., one of two fine channels leading from the medial ends of the eyelids to the lacrimal sac.

cana'lis, *pl.* **cana'les.** Latin for canal or channel.

can'cellated. Having a netlike or spongelike structure, such as the spongy bone between the cortical plates and the alveolar bone proper of the mandible.

can'cellous. Denoting the spongy or honeycomb structure of some bone tissue, such as the ends of long bones.

can'cer. General term for any malignant tumor.

  scirrhous c., see carcinoma, scirrhous.

cancerici'dal. Capable of destroying carcinomas.

canceropho'bia. Abnormal fear of acquiring a malignant growth.

can'cerous. Relating to or of the nature of a malignant neoplasm.

can'croid. 1. Like cancer. **2.** A tumor of moderate malignancy.

can'crum. An ulcer that spreads rapidly, occurring usually in the mucosa of the mouth or nose.

candel'a (cd). The unit of luminous intensity equal to the luminous intensity of five mm² of platinum at its solidification point (1773.5°C); also called new or international candle.

Can'dida. Yeastlike fungi.

  C. albicans, the saprophyte which most commonly is responsible for monilial infections, such as thrush, vaginitis, and sometimes systemic infection.

candidi'asis. Infection with microorganisms of the genus *Candida*.

can'dle. Old term for the unit of luminous intensity; preferred term is candela.

cane. A device used primarily for balance in walking.

ca'nine. 1. Relating to a dog. **2.** Relating to a cuspid (canine tooth).

can'ker. Aphthous stomatitis; see under stomatitis.

can'nabis. The dried flowering tops of the *Cannabis sativa* plants, commonly known as marijuana and hashish.

can'nabism. Condition caused by overuse of hashish or Indian hemp; marked by hallucinations and other subjective symptoms.

can'nula. A tube inserted into the body to withdraw or deliver fluid; it is used in conjunction with a metal rod (trocar) which is fitted into its lumen to puncture the wall of the cavity or vessel and then withdrawn, leaving the cannula in place.

cannula'tion. The insertion of a cannula into a bodily cavity or vessel.

Cantelli's sign. See doll's eye sign.

can'tharis, *pl.* **canthar'ides.** Toxic preparation from the dried beetle *Cantharis vesicatoria*; mistakenly believed to have aphrodisiac qualities; formerly used as a counterirritant and to promote blister formation; also called Spanish fly.

canthec'tomy. Surgical excision of a canthus.

canthi'tis. Inflammation of a canthus.

canthoplas'ty. Plastic surgery of the canthus of the eye.

canthor'rhaphy. Suturing of the eyelids, usually at the outer canthus, to shorten the palpebral fissure.

canthot'omy. The surgical slitting of the canthus, usually for widening the space between eyelids; also called cantholysis.

can'thus. The angle (nasal or temporal) formed by the junction of the upper and lower eyelids.

cap. 1. Abbreviation for Latin *capiat*, let him take. **2.** Any structure that serves as a cover. **3.** Abbreviation for capsule.

  acrosomal c., a thin covering over the anterior two-thirds of the nucleus of sperm.

  cradle c., the grayish-yellow crust formed on the scalp of an infant, caused by seborrhea; also called milk crust.

  duodenal c., the first portion of the duodenum, extending four to five cm from the pylorus; also called bishop's cap, pileus ventriculi, and duodenal bulb.

  enamel c., the enamel organ covering the top of a growing tooth papilla.

  knee c., see patella.

  metanephric c., one of the masses of mesodermal cells adhering to the ureteral bud of an embryo and developing into the uriniferous tubules of the kidney.

capacitance. The quantity of electric charge that may be stored in a body; formerly called capacity.

capacita'tion. The series of physiologic and biochemical events through which spermatozoa become fertilizable when coming in contact with various fluids of the uterus and uterine tube.

capac'itor. An electric circuit element capable of temporarily holding a charge of electricity; formerly known as a condenser.

capac'ity. 1. The maximum potential amount a cavity or receptacle can contain. **2.** A measure of ability.

  cranial c., the cubic content of the skull.

  functional residual c. (FRC), the amount of air remaining in the lungs during normal quiet respiration.

  heat c., the quantity of heat needed to raise the temperature of a substance 1°C.

  inspiratory c., the maximal volume of air that can be inspired after a normal expiration; formerly called complemental air.

  maximum breathing c., the volume of air breathed when a person breathes as deeply and as quickly as possible for 15 seconds.

  residual c., former name for residual volume; see under volume.

  total lung c. (TLC), the amount of air contained in the lungs at the end of a maximal inspiration; the vital capacity plus residual volume; formerly called total lung volume.

  vital c. (VC), the greatest volume of air that can be exhaled forcefully following maximal inspiration; also called breathing capacity and respiratory capacity.

capetel'lum. A small rounded end or head, as the elbow end of the humerus.

capillar'iomotor. Causing dilatation or constriction of the capillaries.

cap'illarity. The interaction between surfaces of a liquid and solid that causes the liquid to rise or fall as in capillary tubes.

cap'illary. A blood vessel intermediate between the arteriole and venule, whose walls consist of a single layer of cells; oxygen and chemicals filter through the capillary into the tissues, while carbon dioxide and other metabolic wastes pass from the tissue into the capillary.

capil'lus, *pl.* **capil'li.** A hair of the head.

capit'ulum. A small head-shaped eminence or rounded articular extremity of a bone.

Caplan's syndrome. Pulmonary nodules due to lesions which appear to be a combination of rheumatoid arthritis and pneumoconiosis.

capping. Covering.

  pulp c., the procedure of placing a covering over the exposed vital pulp of a tooth.

cap'sid. Protein coat of a virus.

cap'sule. 1. A small, soluble, gelatinous container used to enclose a dose of an oral medicine. **2.** A fibrous or membranous sac surrounding a part, an organ, or a tumor. **3.** A mucopolysaccharide layer surrounding certain bacteria.

  Bowman's c., glomerular capsule.

  c. of the lens, a transparent, brittle but highly elastic membrane closely surrounding the lens of the eye.

  Crosby c., an attachment at the end of a flexible tube, used to obtain a peroral biopsy of intestinal

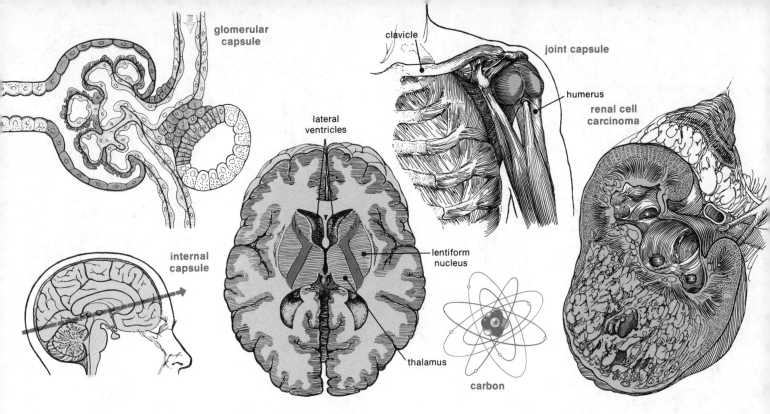

glomerular capsule

clavicle

joint capsule

humerus

renal cell carcinoma

lateral ventricles

internal capsule

lentiform nucleus

thalamus

carbon

---

mucosa.

Glisson's c., former name for the fibrous capsule of liver; a thin layer of loose connective tissue enveloping the bile duct, hepatic artery, and portal vein.

glomerular c., a double walled membranous envelope surrounding a minute mass of non-anastomosing capillaries (glomerulus); it is the invaginated pouchlike beginning of a renal tubule.

internal c., a broad band of white fibers located in each cerebral hemisphere, between the caudate nucleus and thalamus on the medial side and the lentiform nucleus on the lateral side; generally divided into an anterior limb, a genu, a posterior limb, a retrolentiform part, and a sublentiform part; along with the caudate and lentiform nuclei, it forms the corpus striatum, an important unit of the extrapyramidal system.

joint c., a saclike structure enclosing the cavity of a synovial joint, composed of an outer fibrous layer and an inner synovial membrane.

capsuli'tis. Inflammation of the capsule of an organ or part.

capsulot'omy. The surgical cutting of a capsule, as of the capsule of the crystalline lens in a cataract operation.

cap'ut, *pl.* **cap'ita. 1.** The head. **2.** Any headlike prominence of an organ or structure.

car'amel. Burnt sugar, used in pharmacology as a flavoring agent.

carbam'ide. An isomer of urea in anhydrous form; see urea (1).

carbaminohemoglo'bin. Carbon dioxide in combination with hemogloblin in the blood.

car'bamoyl. The organic group NH_2CO-.

carbamoylglutamic acid. An intermediate in the carbamoylation of ornithine to citrulline in the urea cycle.

car'barsone. A crystalline odorless acid, containing 28.85 per cent arsenic in its anhydrous state; used in the treatment of protozoan infections such as amebiasis.

carbohy'drases. A general term for enzymes that promote the digestion of carbohydrates.

carbohy'drates. Any of the group of organic compounds composed of carbon, hydrogen, and oxygen, with a 2 to 1 ratio of hydrogen to oxygen; e.g., sugars, starches, and cellulose.

carbol'ic. Relating to phenol.

car'bon. A tetravalent organic element; symbol C, atomic number 6, atomic weight 12.011.

c. dioxide, CO_2; the product of the combustion of carbon with a large supply of air; also called carbonic acid gas.

c. monoxide, CO; a colorless, odorless poisonous gas with a strong affinity for hemoglobin; formed by the imperfect combustion of carbon with a limited supply of air.

c. tetrachloride, CCl_4; tetrachloromethane; a colorless oily liquid; formerly used as a local anesthetic, anthelmintic, and cleaning agent but no longer recommended because of its toxicity to the liver and kidney; commonly called carbon tet.

car'bon-12. An isotope of carbon, ^{12}C; its atomic weight, 12.000, was adopted in 1961 as the atomic weight unit (awu).

car'bon-14. A radioactive carbon isotope with atomic weight 14 and a half-life of 5600 years.

carbon'ic. Relating to carbon.

car'bonize. To convert into charcoal; to char.

car'bonyl. The organic bivalent radical $=CO$, characteristic of the ketones and aldehydes.

carbotriamine. See guanidine.

carboxyhemoglo'bin. Carbon monoxide in combination with oxygen, present in the blood in carbon monoxide poisoning.

carboxyhemoglobine'mia. The presence of carboxyhemoglobin in the blood.

carbox'yl. The characteristic univalent group $-COOH$ of nearly all organic acids.

carbox'ylase. An enzyme that catalyzes the removal of carbon dioxide from the carboxyl group (COOH) of organic acids.

carboxypep'tidase. An enzyme of intestinal juice that acts on the peptide bond of amino acids having a free carboxyl.

carbun'cle. Painful infection of the skin and subcutaneous tissues with production and discharge of pus and dead tissue, similar to a boil (furuncle) but more severe, and with multiple sinus formation; usually caused by *Staphylococcus aureus*.

renal c., an abscess in the cortex of the kidney, usually resulting from the union of several smaller abscesses; it may occasionally rupture into the collecting system or it may rupture through the renal capsule, causing perirenal abscess.

carbun'cular. Relating to carbuncles.

car'cinogen. A cancer-producing agent.

carcinogen'esis. The formation of cancer.

carcinogen'ic. Anything that causes cancer.

car'cinoid. A small yellow tumor occurring in the intestinal tract, chiefly in the appendix, and in the lungs; also called argentaffinoma.

carcinoid syndrome. A group of symptoms associated with carcinoid tumors, chiefly skin flushes, diarrhea, lesions of the heart valves, and bronchial constriction; caused by release from the tumor of one or more biologically active substances.

carcino'ma. A malignant cellular tumor which tends to invade surrounding tissues and/or spread to other parts of the body by metastasis, causing eventual death.

alveolar cell c., terminal bronchiolar c., a rare type of carcinoma derived either from the lining cells of the pulmonary alveoli or from the terminal bronchioles; occurring in the peripheral parts of the lung in the form of single nodules or multiple nodules that coalesce to form a diffuse mass.

basal cell c., a malignant tumor derived from the basal layer of the skin or from structures derived from basal cells; it invades locally but rarely metastasizes and occurs most frequently on the face and scalp; also called basal cell epithelioma.

bronchogenic c., carcinoma arising from a bronchus; the most common form of carcinoma of the lung.

clear cell c. of kidney, the predominant form of renal cell carcinoma; composed of cells having unstainable cytoplasm.

colloid c., mucinous c., a form of adenocarcinoma in which the degenerative process results in the formation of several areas of mucinous or hyaline material.

embryonal c., a highly malignant neoplasm of the testis appearing as a small grayish-white nodule or mass, sometimes associated with hemorrhage and necrosis.

epidermoid c., squamous cell carcinoma.

in situ c., carcinoma that is still confined to its site of origin, before it spreads to other tissues.

intraductal c., malignant neoplasm consisting of proliferating epithelial cells of a duct, especially in the breast, which eventually fill the lumen.

medullary c., a soft, fleshy, usually large tumor consisting chiefly of epithelial cells with little fibrous stroma; also called medullary or encephaloid cancer.

melanotic c., malignant melanoma; see under melanoma.

mucinous c., see colloid carcinoma.

oat cell c., a small-celled carcinoma usually originating in a bronchus; also called small cell carcinoma.

primary c., carcinoma at the site of origin.

renal cell c., the most common malignant tumor of the kidney; also called hypernephroma.

scirrhous c., a stony-hard tumor having a great amount of fibrous tissue, usually occurring in the breast; also called scirrhous cancer and fibrocarcinoma.

squamous cell c., a malignant epithelial tumor which may originate from normal epithelium, probably made susceptible by chronic radiodermatitis, senile keratosis, burn scars, or leukoplakia; squamous cell carcinomas of the skin occur more frequently in persons over 40 years old; also called

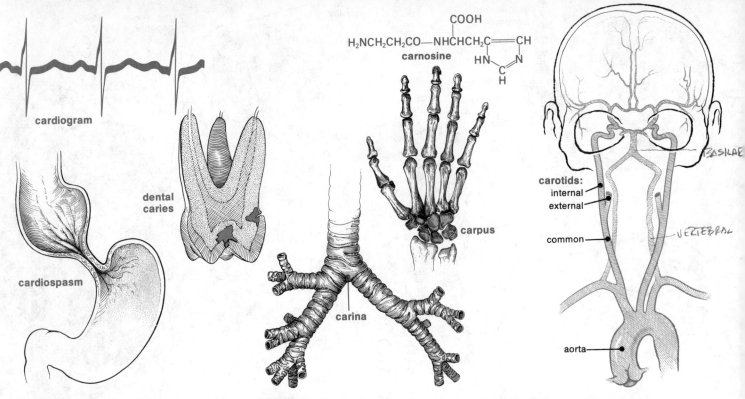

cardiogram

dental caries

cardiospasm

carnosine

$H_2NCH_2CH_2CO-NHCHCH_2C-CH$
COOH
HN   N
    C
    H

carina

carpus

carotids:
internal
external
common
aorta

BASILAE
VERTEBRAL

epidermoid or prickle cell carcinoma.

terminal bronchiolar c., see alveolar cell carcinoma.

transitional c., a malignant neoplasm derived from transitional epithelium; usually occurring in the bladder, ureters, renal pelves, and nasopharynx.

carcino′matoid. Resembling a carcinoma.

carcinomato′sis. Condition resulting from the spread of carcinoma to multiple sites in the body.

carcino′matous. Having characteristics of carcinoma.

car′dia. The esophageal opening of the stomach.

car′diac. 1. Pertaining to the heart. **2.** Relating to the esophageal opening of the stomach. **3.** A person with heart disease.

cardiate′lia. Incomplete development of the heart.

cardiecta′sia. Enlargement of the heart.

cardiec′tomy. Surgical removal of the cardiac portion of the stomach.

cardiecto′pia. Development of the heart in a position other than the normal.

cardio-, cardi-. Combining forms meaning heart.

cardioaccel′erator. An agent that hastens the heart's action.

cardioac′tive. Having an influence upon the heart.

cardiocente′sis. Surgical puncture of the heart.

cardiodynam′ics. The study of the movements and forces involved in the action of the heart.

cardiogen′ic. Originating in the heart.

car′diogram. A graphic record of the activity of the heart, made with the cardiograph; the term is commonly used instead of electrocardiogram.

car′diograph. Instrument used to record graphically the movements of the heart.

cardiog′raphy. The recording of the heart movements with a cardiograph.

cardioinhib′itory. Retarding the action of the heart.

cardiokinet′ic. Having an influence on the action of the heart.

cardiolip′in. A substance obtained from beef heart muscle; used as an antigen in tests for syphilis.

car′diolith. A calculus within the heart.

cardiol′ogist. A specialist in the diagnosis and treatment of diseases of the heart.

cardiol′ogy. The branch of medicine concerned with the heart and its diseases.

car′diomeg′aly. Enlargement of the heart; also called megalocardia.

cardiomyolipo′sis. Fatty degeneration of the muscle of the heart.

cardiomyop′athy. Disease of the muscular wall of the heart; also called myocardiopathy.

cardiomyot′omy. Cardiotomy.

cardionecro′sis. Necrosis of the heart.

cardioneuro′sis. Cardiac neurosis; see under neurosis.

cardiop′athy. Any disease of the heart.

cardiopericar′diopexy. The operative procedure of spreading sterile magnesium silicate within the pericardial sac for the purpose of creating adhesive pericarditis, thus increasing the blood supply of the heart muscle.

car′diophone. A stethoscope for listening to the heart sounds.

cardioplas′ty. Plastic surgery of the junction of the esophagus and stomach for the relief of spasm of the esophagus or upper end of the stomach (cardio- spasm).

cardiople′gia. Temporary interruption of the heart's activity for the purpose of performing surgery upon the heart.

cardiopul′monary. Relating to the heart and lungs.

cardiore′nal. Relating to the heart and kidneys; also called cardionephric and nephrocardiac.

cardiorrhex′is. Rupture of the heart wall.

car′diospasm. Spasmodic constriction of the distal portion of the esophagus, at its junction with the stomach, with accompanying dilatation of the rest of the esophagus; also called achalasia cardia.

cardiot′omy. 1. Surgical incision into the heart wall. **2.** Incision into the esophageal opening (cardia) of the stomach.

cardioton′ic. Having a favorable or tonic effect on the heart; strengthening the heart action.

cardiotox′ic. Having a toxic effect on the heart.

cardiovas′cular. Relating to the heart and blood vessels.

cardiover′sion. The restoration of the heart's normal rhythm by means of electrical shock; the technique is used for treatment in selected cases of supraventricular tachycardia, ventricular tachycardia, and atrial fibrillation.

car′dioverter. Device used to administer electrical countershock to restore the normal heart rhythm.

cardi′tis. Inflammation of the heart.

ca′ries. Molecular death and breakdown of a bone.

central c., abscess in the bone marrow.

contact c., caries occurring in the proximal surface of the tooth adjacent to the restoration.

dental c., localized, progressive decay of the teeth that starts on the surface and, if untreated, extends to the pulp with subsequent infection.

spinal c., tuberculosis of the vertebrae.

cari′na. Any ridgelike structure, as the central ridge formed by the bifurcation of the trachea.

cario-. Combining form meaning caries.

cariogen′esis. The process of caries formation.

cariogen′ic. Producing caries; said of certain foods.

cariostat′ic. Anything that inhibits the progress of dental caries.

ca′rious. Relating to or having caries.

car′neous. Fleshy.

Carniv′ora. An order of flesh-eating mammals.

car′nosine. A nitrogenous base made up of alanine and histadine, found in skeletal muscle.

Caroli's disease. A disorder characterized by segmental saccular dilatation of the intrahepatic bile ducts, a marked predisposition to biliary calculous disease, cholangitis, and lung abscesses; the disease is familial and is probably inherited as a Mendelian recessive.

car′otene. A provitamin capable of conversion into vitamin A; the yellow pigment in carrots and other yellow foods.

carotene′mia. Increased carotene in the blood causing a yellowish pigmentation of the skin; also called carotinemia, xanthemia, and pseudojaundice.

carot′id. 1. Either of the two principal arteries of the neck (carotid artery). **2.** Relating to either of the carotid arteries.

carotid sinus syndrome. Fainting with occasional convulsions caused by overstimulation of the carotid sinus.

carotine′mia. See carotenemia.

car′pal. Relating to the bones of the wrist (carpus).

carpal tunnel syndrome. A complex of symptoms caused by any condition (usually thickening of the synovia of the flexor tendons) that compresses the median nerve in the carpal tunnel of the wrist; marked by pain and numbness in the area of the hand innervated by the median nerve; the duration and degree of nerve compression determine the patient's complaints; in late stages there is atrophy of thenar muscles.

carpometacar′pal. Relating to the wrist bones and the metacarpus (the five bones between the wrist and fingers).

carpope′dal. Relating to the wrists and feet, as the spasm of tetany.

car′pus. The wrist; the eight bones of the wrist.

car′rier. 1. An individual who, although showing no symptoms of disease, harbors infectious organisms in his body and spreads the infection to others. **2.** An individual who carries a normal gene and an abnormal recessive gene which is not expressed obviously, although it may be detectable by appropriate laboratory tests. **3.** A substance in a cell which is capable of accepting an atom or a

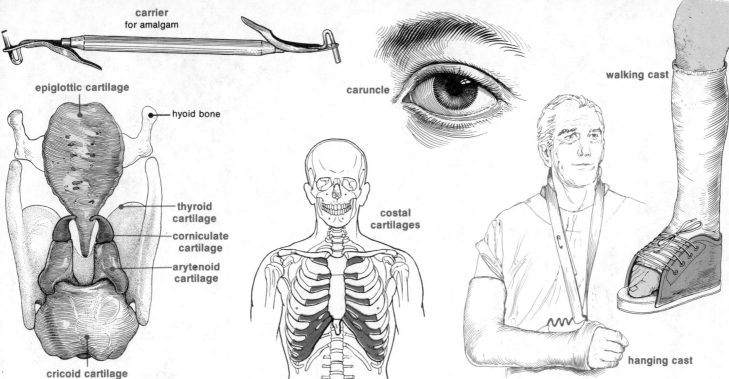

carrier
for amalgam

epiglottic cartilage

hyoid bone

thyroid
cartilage

corniculate
cartilage

arytenoid
cartilage

cricoid cartilage

caruncle

costal
cartilages

walking cast

hanging cast

subatomic particle, thus facilitating transport of organic solutes. **4.** In dentistry, an instrument for carrying plastic amalgam to the cavity into which it is inserted.

c. state, an individual in a carrier condition.

chronic c., a person who harbors disease-producing organisms for some time after recovery.

passive c., one who harbors infectious organisms without having had the disease.

Carrion's disease. See bartonellosis.

car′tilage. A tough, nonvascular connective tissue making up most of the fetal skeleton and present in the adult in the articular parts of bones and certain tubular structures; there are three main varieties: hyaline cartilage (most widely distributed type), elastic cartilage, and fibrous cartilage.

accessory c.'s of nose, see lesser alar cartilages.

articular c., a type of hyaline cartilage forming a thin sheet upon the joint surface of bones.

arytenoid c., one of two triangular cartilages located in the back of the larynx.

c. of nasal septum, a somewhat quadrilateral plate of cartilage completing the separation of the nasal cavities in front.

corniculate c., one of two minute cones of yellow elastic cartilage in the larynx, located at the apex of each arytenoid cartilage.

costal c., one of 24 bars of hyaline cartilage serving to prolong the ribs anteriorly and contribute to the elasticity of the chest wall.

cricoid c., the ring-shaped and lowermost of the cartilages of the larynx.

cuneiform c., one of two small rod-shaped laryngeal cartilages on either side in the aryepiglottic fold.

elastic c., yellow fibrocartilage, a variety of cartilage containing bundles of yellow elastic fibers with little or no white fibrous tissue; found chiefly in the external ear, the auditory tube, and some laryngeal cartilages.

epiglottic c., a thin leaflike lamina of yellow fibrocartilage located behind the root of the tongue and the body of the hyoid bone, forming the central portion of the epiglottis.

epiphyseal c., the layer of cartilage between the shaft and the epiphysis of a long bone, present during the growing years; then the cartilage ossifies and growth in length ceases.

fibrous c., fibrocartilage.

greater alar c.'s, two cartilaginous plates supporting the nostrils; also called lower lateral cartilages of nose.

hyaline c., an elastic bluish-white translucent type of cartilage; covered with a membrane (perichondrium) except when coating the articular ends of

bones.

lateral c., upper lateral c., one of two triangular plates of cartilage located below the inferior margin of the nasal bone.

lesser alar c.'s, two to four cartilages located posterior to the greater alar cartilage on either side; also called accessory cartilages of nose.

lower lateral c.'s of nose, see greater alar cartilages.

thyroid c., the largest of the cartilages of the larynx; its anterior prominence is also called Adam's apple.

tracheal c., one of from 16 to 20 incomplete cartilaginous rings forming the trachea.

upper lateral c., see lateral cartilage.

cartilag′inous. Consisting of cartilage.

car′uncle. A small fleshy protuberance.

lacrimal c., a small reddish protuberance at the medial junction of the eyelids.

urethral c., a small, fleshy, painful growth, occurring at the orifice of the female urethra.

car′ver. A dental instrument used to shape wax or amalgam.

cascar′a sagra′da. The dried bark of a tree, *Rhamnus purshiana* or buckthorn; used as a laxative.

case. An instance or occurrence of disease.

casea′tion. Necrosis of tissues into a cheeselike mass.

ca′sein. The chief protein of milk.

casein′ogen. The precursor of casein; a substance present in milk which, when activated by rennin, is converted into casein.

ca′seous. Resembling cheese, as certain necrotic tissue.

cassett′e. 1. A light-proof camera cartridge or metal plate holder for daylight loading of x-ray or photographic film. **2.** A cartridge containing magnetic tape designed for automatic use in a tape player or recorder. **3.** A cartridge containing both a film loop and a synchronized magnetic tape, usually used for self-study purposes.

cast. 1. A solid mold of a hollow, usually tubular, structure of the body. **2.** A rigid dressing, usually made of gauze and plaster of Paris, used for immobilization of a bodily part.

blood c., one composed of a thick material containing various elements of blood, formed in kidney tubules or bronchioles and caused by bleeding into the structures.

cellular c., a renal cast containing red and white blood cells or epithelial cells.

epithelial c., one containing cells from the inner lining of renal tubules, found in the urine.

false c., see cylindroid.

fatty c., a renal cast composed chiefly of fat globules.

granular c., a colorless renal cast composed of particles of cellular debris.

hanging c., a plaster cast applied to immobilize a fracture as well as deliver a traction force via the weight of the cast; commonly used for the treatment of fractures of the lower part of the humerus.

hyaline c., a relatively transparent renal cast consisting mainly of precipitated protein.

leukocyte c., a renal cyclindrical plug of tightly packed leukocytes.

mucous c., see cylindroid.

red blood cell c., a renal cast containing red blood cells due to bleeding in the glomeruli or the upper parts of the nephron.

renal c., urinary cast.

urinary c., one discharged in the urine.

walking c., a plaster cast extending from below the knee to the toes with an added attachment, such as a boot, to allow a natural gait

waxy c., a light yellow cylinder with a tendency to split transversely, found in the urine in cases of oliguria or anuria.

cas′trate. 1. To remove the testes or the ovaries. **2.** One from whom the gonads have been removed.

castra′tion. Removal of the testes or ovaries.

functional c., atrophy of the gonads by prolonged treatment with sex hormones.

CAT. Abbreviation for computer-assisted tomography.

catabol′ic. Promoting or exhibiting catabolism.

catab′olism. The breakdown of chemical compounds into more elementary principles by the body; an energy-producing metabolic process, the reverse of anabolism.

catab′olite. A product of catabolism.

catac′rotism. Anomaly of the pulse marked by one or more minor expansions of the artery following the main beat.

cat′alepsy. A trance-like condition with rigidity of muscles permitting the body (including extremities) to assume a position for an indefinite period of time.

cat′alyst. A substance, usually present in small amounts, that influences the rate of a chemical reaction without being changed in the process.

negative c., one that retards a chemical reaction.

organic c., an enzyme that catalyzes specific reactions.

positive c., one that accelerates a chemical reaction.

cat′alyze. To modify the rate of a chemical reaction; to act as a catalyst.

catamne′sis. A patient's medical history follow-

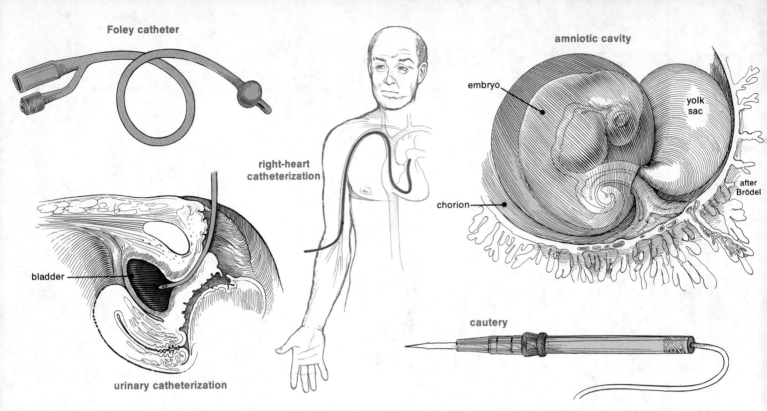

Foley catheter

right-heart catheterization

bladder

urinary catheterization

amniotic cavity

embryo

yolk sac

chorion

after Brödel

cautery

---

ing an illness; the "follow-up" history.

cataphasia. A speech disorder consisting of involuntary repetition of the same word.

cataplasia, cataplasis. Degenerative reversion of cells or tissues to an embryonic state.

cataplexy. A sudden and temporary loss of muscle tone and of postural reflexes, causing limpness of the body or a part, usually triggered by an emotional surge, such as gales of laughter, sudden elation, anger, etc.

　narcolepsy c., transient loss of muscle tone in conjunction with intermittent attacks of uncontrollable sleep.

cataract. Loss of transparency of the lens of the eye and/or its capsule, resulting in partial or total blindness.

　immature c., an early stage of a cataract.

　mature c., one in which the entire lens substance has become opaque and can be easily separated from its capsule.

　radiation c., one caused by continued exposure to radioactive materials.

　senile c., one occurring in old age.

　stationary c., one that has ceased to progress.

　traumatic c., one caused by an injury or foreign body.

catarrh'. Inflammation of a mucous membrane, especially of the nose and throat, with a discharge.

catatonia. A type of schizophrenia characterized by generalized inhibition, mutism, stupor, negativism, or waxy flexibility (withdrawn type), or occasionally by excessive and sometimes violent motor activity and excitement (excited type).

cat-cry syndrome. See cri-du-chat syndrome.

catechol. A chemical compound, 1,2-dihydroxybenzene, $C_6H_6O_2$; of interest mainly because of the importance of its aminated derivatives.

catecholamines. Amine compounds derived from catechol, such as epinephrine and norepinephrine, which have sympathomimetic activity and are concerned with nervous transmission, vascular tone, and many metabolic activities.

catgut. A tough, thin thread made from the dried intestines of sheep, used as absorbable surgical ligatures and sutures.

catharsis. 1. Purging or cleansing, especially of the bowels. **2.** A method of treating mental illness by means of which the patient is made to recall a forgotten traumatic experience.

cathartic. 1. A drug that promotes evacuation of intestinal contents in a more or less fluid state by increasing motor activity of the intestine, either directly or reflexly; distinguished from a laxative which produces a milder effect; also called purgative. **2.** Relating to a catharsis.

cathepsin. Any intracellular protein-splitting enzyme that acts on the interior peptide bonds of a protein, causing its decomposition; cathepsins are widely distributed in animal tissues, especially the liver, kidney, and spleen.

cathepsis. Protein hydrolysis by the action of cathepsins.

catheter. A slender, flexible tube made of rubber, metal, or plastic; used to introduce or remove fluids from a bodily channel or hollow organ.

　Fogarty c., one having an inflatable balloon near the tip; used to remove thrombi from large veins and stones from the biliary ducts.

　Foley c., one equipped with a small balloon near the tip which can be inflated to retain the catheter in place.

catheterization. The introduction of a catheter into a bodily passage.

　cardiac c., passage of a catheter into the heart by way of a blood vessel; first attempted by Forsmann on himself in 1928.

　left-heart c., the introduction of a radiopaque catheter into the brachial or femoral artery and passage in a retrograde direction, through the artery to the aorta and, frequently, across the aortic valve into the left ventricle.

　right-heart c., the passage of a radiopaque flexible catheter into a vein, usually the basilic; the catheter is manipulated under fluoroscopic control through the venous system to the right atrium, and eventually into the right ventricle and pulmonary artery.

　urinary c., withdrawal of urine from the bladder with a urethral catheter.

catheterize. To introduce a catheter into a bodily canal or passage.

cathexis. The attachment of emotional energy and significance to a person, object, or idea.

cathode. The negatively charged electrode of an electron tube, galvanic cell (primary cell) or storage battery (secondary cells); also called negative electrode.

cation. A positively charged ion that is characteristically attracted to the negatively charged cathode; indicated as a plus sign, e.g., H^+.

cat-scratch disease. Regional inflammation of lymph nodes of unknown origin, frequently following the scratch or bite of a cat; also called cat-scratch fever.

cauda, *pl.* **caudae.** A tail or tapered end of a structure.

　c. equina, the bundle of nerves (sacral and coccygeal) in which the spinal cord ends.

cauda equina syndrome. Dull pain and anesthesia of the buttocks, genitalia, and/or thigh with impaired bladder and bowel function; caused by compression of the spinal nerve roots.

caudad. Directed posteriorly or toward the tail.

caudal. Near the tail; posterior.

caudate. Possessing a tail or a tail-like appendage.

　c. nucleus, see nucleus, caudate.

caul. The portion of fetal membranes surrounding the head of the fetus at birth when the membranes remain intact until completion of delivery.

causalgia. A painful, burning sensation, accompanied by trophic changes in the skin and nails, due to a peripheral nerve injury, usually the median or sciatic nerves.

caustic. Corrosive; capable of burning.

cauterization. The act of cauterizing; the application of a caustic substance or electric current for the purpose of scarring or destroying aberrant tissue.

cauterize. To apply a cautery.

cautery. An agent used for scarring or destroying tissue.

caval. Of or relating to the vena cava.

caveolae. Minute vesicles that develop by invagination of the plasmalemma of the cell surface; they usually pinch off to form free vesicles within the cytoplasm and serve as a mechanism for cell ingestion.

cavern. A cavity, especially one caused by disease, as seen in tuberculous lungs.

cavernitis. Inflammation of a corpus cavernosum penis.

　fibrous c., see Peyronie's disease.

cavernous. Relating to or having cavities.

cavernous sinus syndrome. A syndrome caused by thrombosis of the cavernous sinus, characterized by edema of eyelids and conjunctivae, protrusion of the eyeball (proptosis), and paralysis of the third, fourth, and sixth cranial nerves; also called Foix's syndrome.

cavitary. 1. Relating to or having cavities. **2.** Any parasite having a body cavity and living inside the host's body.

cavitation. Formation of cavities, as in the lungs in pulmonary tuberculosis.

cavity. 1. A hollow space within the body; a chamber. **2.** Loss of tooth structure due to decay.

　abdominal c., the bodily cavity between the diaphragm above and the pelvis below.

　amniotic c., the space within the amnion.

　body c., the cavity of the body containing the organs.

　buccal c., (1) the space between the lips and the gums and teeth; (2) decay on the buccal surface of a tooth.

　c. preparation, the final step in the excavation of

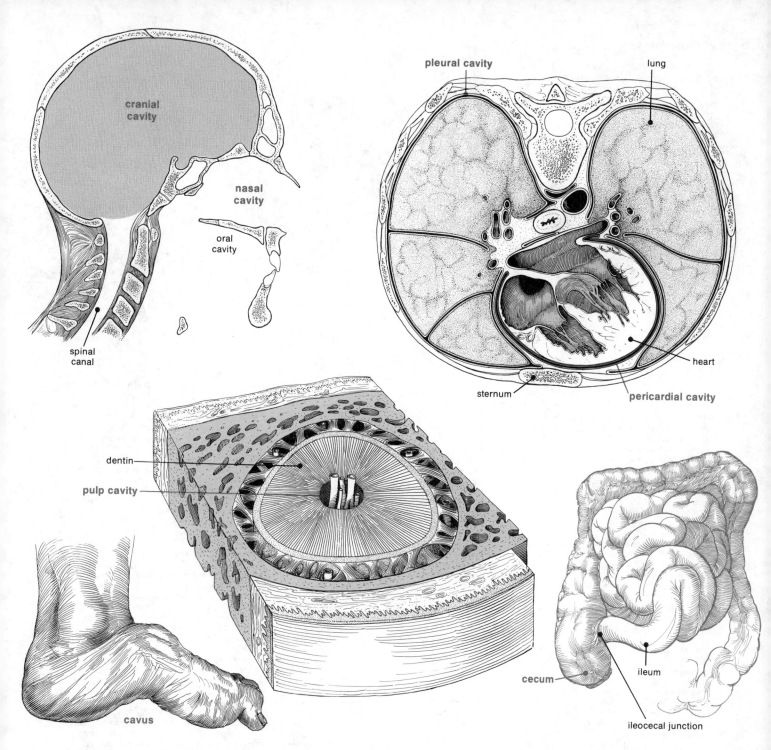

cranial cavity

nasal cavity

oral cavity

spinal canal

pleural cavity

lung

sternum

heart

pericardial cavity

dentin

pulp cavity

cavus

cecum

ileum

ileocecal junction

a tooth prior to the insertion of a restoration.

compound c., one involving two or more surfaces of a tooth.

cranial c., the space within the skull.

distal c., one located on the surface of a tooth away from the midline.

glenoid c., glenoid fossa; see under fossa.

medullary c. of bone, the elongated cavity within the shaft of a long bone.

nasal c., an irregular space extending from the base of the cranium to the roof of the mouth and divided in two by a thin vertical septum (nasal septum).

oral c., the cavity of the mouth.

pelvic c., the short, wide, curved canal within the bony framework of the minor pelvis; it contains the pelvic colon, rectum, bladder, and some of the organs of reproduction.

pericardial c., the potential cavity between the two layers of the membrane enveloping the heart (pericardium).

pleural c., the potential space between the two layers of the pleura (parietal and visceral).

proximal c., one occurring on the mesial or distal surface of a tooth.

pulp c., the central chamber of a tooth containing blood vessels, lymphatic vessels, and nerve fibers; the entire space occupied by the pulp.

splanchnic c., one of the three major cavities of the body: cranial, thoracic, or abdominal.

tympanic c., the cavity of the middle ear, located in the temporal bone and containing the ear ossicles.

visceral c., splanchnic cavity.

cav′ogram. A roentgenogram of the vena cava.

ca′vosurface. Relating to a prepared cavity and the surface of a tooth.

c. angle, the angle formed by the junction of the wall of a prepared cavity and the surface of a tooth.

ca′vum. Latin for cavity or hollow.

cav′us. The condition in which the longitudinal arch of the foot is exaggerated, due to contraction of the plantar fascia or to a deformed bony arch.

Cb. Chemical symbol of the element columbium.

CBC. Abbreviation for complete blood count.

CC. Abbreviation for *cum* correction.

C.C. Abbreviation for chief complaint.

cc., c.c. Abbreviation for cubic centimeter.

CCU. Abbreviation for coronary care unit.

Cd. Chemical symbol of the element cadmium.

CDC. Abbreviation for Center for Disease Control.

Ce. Chemical symbol of the element cerium.

cec-, ceco-. Combining forms denoting cecum.

cecos′tomy. Surgical creation of an opening into the cecum through the abdominal wall.

ce′cum. The cul-de-sac that forms the beginning of the large intestine; the blind gut.

ce′liac. Relating to the abdominal cavity.

ce′liac disease. Disorder characterized by intolerance to gluten (a protein present in the grains of wheat, rye, oats, and barley), abnormal structure of the small intestine, and poor absorption of food; also called nontropical sprue, gluten-induced enteropathy, and sprue. Cf tropical sprue.

celiohysterec′tomy. Surgical removal of the uterus through an incision in the abdomen; also called abdominal hysterectomy.

celios′copy. See laparoscopy.

celiot′omy. See laparotomy.

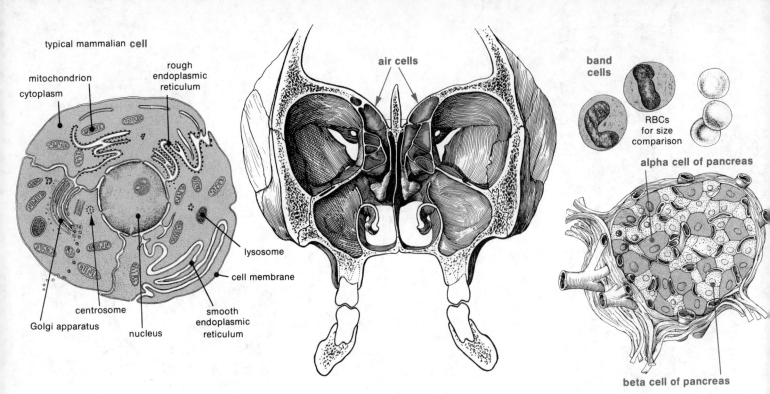

typical mammalian **cell**

mitochondrion

cytoplasm

rough endoplasmic reticulum

lysosome

cell membrane

centrosome

Golgi apparatus

nucleus

smooth endoplasmic reticulum

air cells

band cells

RBCs for size comparison

alpha cell of pancreas

beta cell of pancreas

cell. 1. The smallest unit of living matter capable of independent functioning, composed of protoplasm and surrounded by a semipermeable plasma membrane. **2.** A receptacle.

acidophilic c., a cell whose cytoplasm or its granules have an affinity for acid dyes such as eosin.

acinar c., one of the secreting cells lining an acinus or alveolus of a compound acinous gland, such as the pancreas; also called acinous cell.

adipose c., see fat cell.

air c., an air-containing space of one of the air sinuses of the skull.

alpha c. of pancreas, a cell of the islet of Langerhans (islet of pancreas) marked by fine cytoplasmic granules; believed to produce glucagon (hyperglycemic-glycogenolytic factor); it stains red with phloxine.

alveolar c.'s, (1) thin epithelial cells lining the alveoli of the lungs; (2) cells lining a secretory alveolus.

amacrine c., a special inhibitory retinal cell, regarded as a modified nerve cell.

anaplastic c., an undifferentiated cell characteristic of carcinoma.

aneuploid c., a cell with an unbalanced number of chromosomes.

antigen-sensitive c., see immunocompetent cell.

argentaffin c.'s, cells having an affinity for silver salts and therefore capable of being stained by them; located throughout the gastrointestinal tract.

B c.'s, bone marrow-derived lymphocytes.

band c., any granulocytic leukocyte in which the nucleus has a simple, nonlobulated, elongated shape, resembling a band; it represents a normal stage prior to the development of a mature segmented granulocytic leukocyte (polymorphonuclear white blood cell); also called stab cell.

basal c., one appearing in the deepest layer of a stratified epithelium; an early keratinocyte.

basophil c. of anterior lobe of hypophysis, the beta cell of the anterior lobe of the hypophysis (pituitary gland).

beta c. of anterior lobe of hypophysis, one that contains basophil granules and is thought to furnish the gonadotrophic hormones.

beta c. of pancreas, the predominant cell of the islet of Langerhans (islet of pancreas), marked by coarse cytoplasmic granules that represent precursor of insulin; it stains blue with the Gomori stain.

Betz c.'s, the large pyramidal cells of the fifth layer of the motor cortex.

bipolar c., a neuron having two processes (afferent and efferent), as those in the retina.

blast c., (1) an immature precursor cell (e.g., erythroblast, lymphoblast, neuroblast); a primitive cell, the least differentiated of a line of blood-forming elements; (2) a leukemic cell of indeterminable type.

blood c., one of the formed elements of the blood; an erythrocyte or leukocyte.

burr c., an elongated erythrocyte with multiple long, sharp, spinelike projections from the cell surface; seen in uremia and in diseases of the stomach such as carcinoma and peptic ulcer; essentially a subclass of schistocytes.

cartilage c.'s, cells situated in the smooth walled spaces or lacunae of cartilage; also called chondrocytes.

chief c. of parathyroid gland, the principal cell of the parathyroid gland.

chief c. of stomach, an enzyme-producing cell of a gastric gland in the stomach; also called zymogenic cell.

chromaffin c., a cell whose cytoplasm exhibits fine brown granules when stained with a dichromate; occurring in the adrenal medulla and paraganglia of the sympathetic nervous system and some other tissues.

cleavage c., a blastomere.

columnar c., a cell in which the height is significantly greater than the width, usually epithelial; it may be a tall columnar or low columnar.

committed c., any cell committed to the production of antibodies specific for a given antigen-determinant, such as primed cell, memory cell, and antibody-producing cell.

cone c. of retina, one of the visual receptors sensitive to color.

cuboid c., a cell which resembles a cube, i.e., all its diameters are approximately the same size.

daughter c., any cell resulting from the division of a parent cell.

dentin c., odontoblast.

dust c., alveolar macrophage; see under macrophage.

endothelial c., one of the thin, flat cells (squamous) forming the lining (endothelium) of the blood and lymph vessels and the inner layer of the endocardium.

epithelial c., one of the numerous varieties of cells that form epithelium, which covers all free surfaces of the body except the synovial membranes and bursae of joints.

eukaryotic c., a cell with a true nucleus; a cell with a nuclear membrane.

fat c., a very large connective tissue cell (60 to 80 μ) in which neutral fat is stored; the cytoplasm is usually compressed into a thin envelope, with the nucleus at one point in the periphery; also called adipose cell.

fibroblast c., a spindle-shaped connective tissue cell responsible for elaborating collagen and reticular fibers; the most common cell type found in connective tissue.

foam c., a macrophage exhibiting a peculiar vacuolated appearance due to the presence of lipids in a multitude of small vacuoles; notably seen in xanthoma; also called xanthoma cell.

fusiform c.'s of cerebral cortex, spindle-shaped cells in the sixth layer of the cerebral cortex.

ganglion c., a large nerve cell in a ganglion peripheral to the central nervous system; also called gangliocyte.

Gaucher c., a round or polyhedral, pale reticular cell (20 to 80 μ) containing a fibril network in the cytoplasm caused by glucocerebroside deposition.

germ c., the ovum or spermatozoon.

germinal c.'s, cells from which other cells are derived or proliferated, especially the dividing cells in the embryonic neural tube.

ghost c., (1) a dead cell in which the outline remains visible, but without cytoplasmic structures or stainable nucleus; (2) a red blood cell after loss of its hemoglobin.

gitter c., a honeycombed, compound granule cell; a microglial cell.

glitter c., a large leukocyte seen in the urine exhibiting brownian movement in the cytoplasm; associated with urinary tract infection.

goblet c.'s, unicellular mucous glands found in the epithelium of certain mucous membranes, especially of the respiratory and intestinal tracts.

Golgi's c.'s, type I: nerve cells with very long axons that leave the gray matter of the central nervous system to terminate in the periphery; also called Golgi type I neuron; type II: nerve cells with short axons that ramify in the gray matter and terminate near the cell body; also called Golgi type II neuron.

granule c., one of many small cells in the granular layer of the cerebellar cortex.

granulosa c.'s, special epithelial cells displaying high mitotic activity which surround the ovum in a primary follicle and, in a vesicular follicle, form the stratum granulosum, corona radiata, and cumulus oophorus; they secrete a refractile substance that forms the protective zona pellucida around the ovum; during the early stages of follicular maturation, they secrete an inhibitory substance (polypeptide) that maintains the primary oocyte in an arrested stage of meiotic prophase; also called follicular cells.

granulosa lutein c.'s, giant, glandular cells that comprise the major part of the wall of a ruptured vesicular follicle (corpus luteum) in the ovary; formed by hypertrophy of the follicular granulosa

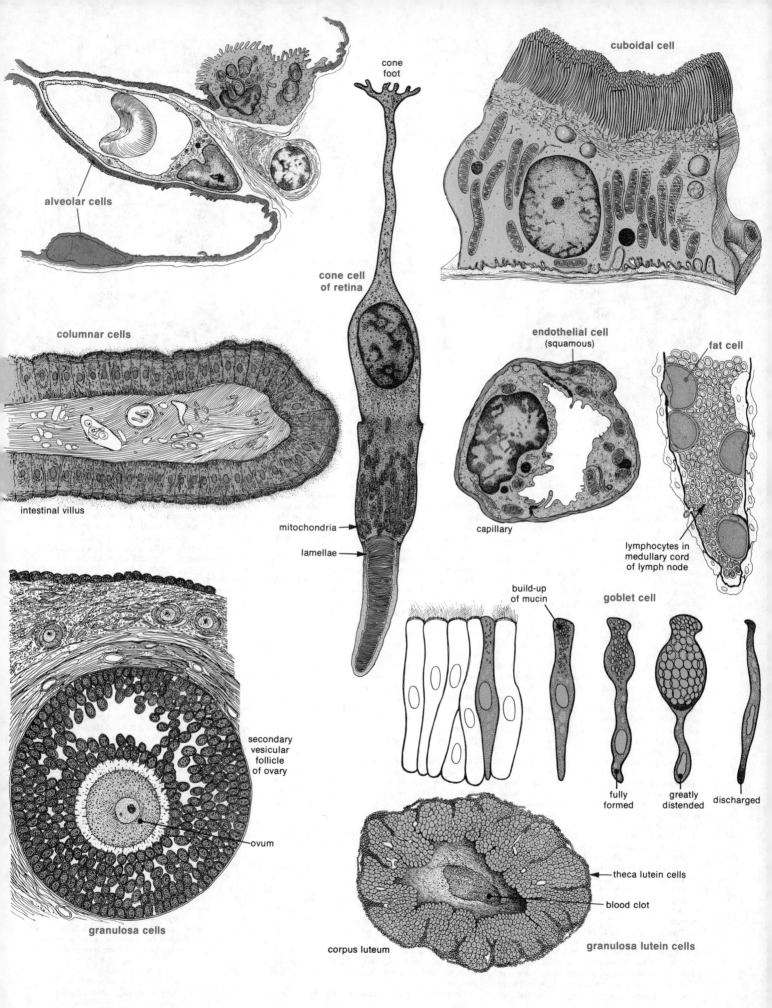

alveolar cells

cuboidal cell

cone foot

cone cell of retina

columnar cells

intestinal villus

mitochondria

lamellae

endothelial cell (squamous)

capillary

fat cell

lymphocytes in medullary cord of lymph node

secondary vesicular follicle of ovary

ovum

granulosa cells

build-up of mucin

goblet cell

fully formed

greatly distended

discharged

corpus luteum

theca lutein cells

blood clot

granulosa lutein cells

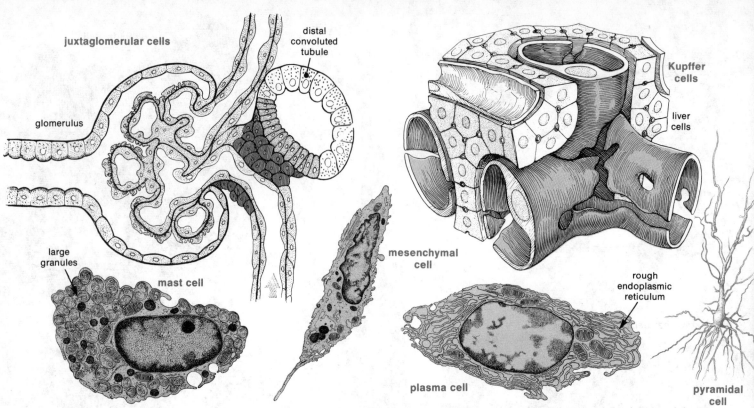

juxtaglomerular cells

distal convoluted tubule

glomerulus

Kupffer cells

liver cells

large granules

mast cell

mesenchymal cell

rough endoplasmic reticulum

plasma cell

pyramidal cell

cells of the old vesicular follicle;'they produce the sex steroid progesterone; also called follicular lutein cells.

great alveolar c., type II pneumocyte; see under pneumocyte.

hair c.'s, pear-shaped epithelial cells with delicate hairlike microvilli (stereocilia) one to 100 μ in length on the free surface; they are present in the neuroepithelial sensory areas of the utricle, saccule, ampullae, and the spiral organ of Corti.

HeLa c.'s, the first documented, continuously cultured human malignant cells, derived from a cervical carcinoma; used in the cultivation of viruses.

helmet c., an irregular, contracted, somewhat triangular erythrocyte; seen in microangiopathic anemia.

Hürthle c., an enlarged, granular thyroid follicular epithelial cell with acidophilic cytoplasm, as seen in Hashimoto's disease.

immunocompetent c., any cell which can form antibodies or elaborate cells which form antibodies when stimulated by antigen; e.g., inducible cell; also called antigen-sensitive cell.

inducible c., an unprimed cell which can become a primed cell or an antibody-producing cell when stimulated by antigen; also called virgin lymphocyte and antigen-inducible cell.

interstitial c.'s, the cells of the connective tissue of the ovary or testis which are believed to produce internal secretion of those structures; in the seminiferous tubules of the testis they are also known as Leydig's cells.

islet c., one of the cells in the islet (island) of Langerhans of the pancreas.

juxtaglomerular c.'s, a group of secretory cells forming the middle layer of the wall of the afferent arteriole just before it enters the glomerulus in the kidney; thought to play a role in production of the hormone renin.

Kulchitsky c.'s, the argentaffin cells of the intestinal glands; also called cells of Kultschitzsky.

Kupffer c.'s, reticuloendothelial cells of the liver; fixed macrophages or reticuloendothelial cells lining the capillary system which conveys blood from the interlobular branches of the portal vein to the central vein; they are phagocytic in character and are active in freeing the blood stream of foreign particles.

Langhans' giant c.'s, (1) multinucleated giant cells in tuberculosis and other granulomas; the nuclei are located in an arciform manner at the periphery of the cells; (2) cytotrophoblast cells.

L.E. c., abbreviation for lupus erythematosus cell; a leukocyte containing an amorphous round body which is a phagocytosed nucleus from another cell

which has been traumatized and exposed to serum antinuclear globulin; a large purple-red homogenous inclusion body is seen occupying most of the cytoplasm of the phagocytosing cell; L.E. cells are formed in vitro in the blood of individuals with systemic lupus erythematosus, or by the action of the individual's serum on normal leukocytes.

lepra c.'s, large mononuclear phagocytes (macrophages) with foamlike cytoplasm; associated with lepromatous lesions which contain the acid-fast organisms of leprosy.

Leydig's c., an endocrine interstitial cell located between the seminiferous tubules of the testis.

lupus erythematosus c., see L.E. cell.

lymph c., lymphoid c., lymphocyte.

Marchand's c.'s, the phagocytes in the adventitia of blood vessels; also called adventitial cells.

mast c.'s, large cells with coarse cytoplasmic granules containing heparin (anticoagulant) and histamine (vasodilator) occurring in most loose connective tissue, especially along the path of blood vessels; the cells act as mediators of inflammation on contact with antigen; sometimes called tissue mast cells or histogenous mast cells to distinguish them from the hematogenous mast cells (basophilic leukocytes) circulating in the blood.

memory c.'s, short-memory and long-memory cells which can mount an accelerated antibody response to antigen.

mesangial c., an intercapillary cell of the renal glomerulus located mostly near that part of the capillary facing the center of the glomerulus; it borders directly on the endothelial cell.

mesenchymal c.'s, a cell present in mesenchyme and capable of differentiating into any of the special types of connective tissue or supporting tissues, smooth muscle, vascular endothelium, or blood cells.

mesothelial c., one of the flat cells of the simple squamous epithelium (mesothelium) lining the pleural, pericardial, peritoneal, and scrotal cavities.

mother c., see parent cell.

myeloid c., any young cell that develops into a mature granulocyte.

myoepithelial c., one of the smooth muscle cells of ectodermal origin, with processes that spiral around some of the epithelial cells of sweat, mammary, lacrimal and salivary glands; their contraction forces the secretion of the glands toward the ducts.

nerve c., see neuron.

neuroglial c., any of the nonneuronal cells of nervous tissue including the oligodendroglia, astrocytes, microglia, and ependymal cells; also called glial cell.

neurosecretory c., a nerve cell that elaborates a

chemical substance, as those of the hypothalamus.

olfactory c., one of the slender sensory nerve cells surmounted by sensitive hairs, present in the olfactory mucous membrane at the roof of the nose; the receptor for the sense of smell.

oxyphilic c.'s, (1) parietal cells; (2) acidophilic cells present in the parathyroid glands; they increase in number with age.

Paneth's c.'s, pyramidal-shaped cells occurring in small groups near the base of the crypts of Lieberkühn; believed to secrete digestive enzymes throughout the small intestine.

parent c., a cell which gives rise to a new generation of daughter cells by cell division; also called mother cell.

parietal c., one of the cells present in the periphery of the gastric glands; it lies upon the basement membrane covered by the chief cells and secretes hydrochloric acid which reaches the lumen of the gland through fine channels.

plasma c., a cell that stores and releases antibody and is believed to be of primary importance in antibody synthesis; characterized by RNA-rich cytoplasm and an eccentrically placed nucleus; the cytoplasm contains an extensive system of endoplasmic reticulum studded with ribosomes; the cell is derived embryologically from a bursal equivalent tissue and is therefore also referred to as a B cell; in certain diseases, such as chronic lymphocytic leukemia, there is a proliferation of this cell type.

primed c., one which has been primed by antigen for antibody production.

prokaryotic c., cell in which the nuclear substance, lacking an envelope (plasmalemma), is in direct contact with the rest of the protoplasm; includes most viruses and bacteria.

Purkinje's c.'s, the large nerve cells of the cerebellar cortex with flask-shaped bodies forming a single cell layer between the molecular and granular layers; their dendrites are arranged in the molecular layer in a plane transverse to the folia, and their axons penetrate the granular layer to form the only pathways out of the cerebellar cortex; they terminate in the central cerebellar nuclei; also called Purkyně cells.

pus c., a neutrophilic leukocyte; a necrotic granulocyte characteristic of suppurative inflammation.

pyramidal c., a nerve cell of the cerebral cortex; usually somewhat triangular with an apical dendrite directed toward the surface of the cortex and several smaller dendrites at the base; the axon is given off at the base of the cell and descends to deeper layers.

red blood c., see erythrocyte.

Renshaw c., an inhibitory interneuron in the ventral horn of the spinal cord that acts as a

cell | cell

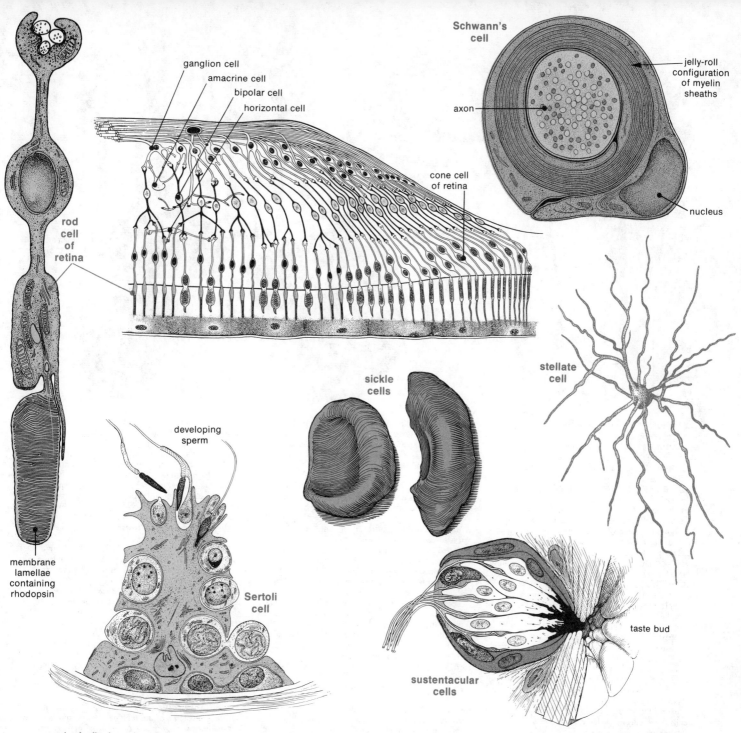

ganglion cell
amacrine cell
bipolar cell
horizontal cell

cone cell
of retina

Schwann's
cell

jelly-roll
configuration
of myelin
sheaths

axon

nucleus

rod
cell
of
retina

stellate
cell

membrane
lamellae
containing
rhodopsin

developing
sperm

sickle
cells

Sertoli
cell

sustentacular
cells

taste bud

negative feedback monitor of motorneurons.

respiratory c., type I pneumocyte; see under pneumocyte.

reticular c., a primitive mesenchymal cell affording the framework of such structures as bone marrow, lymph nodes, and spleen.

reticuloendothelial c., phagocytic cell similar to the leukocyte, but attached to vascular and lymphatic channels rather than being circulatory.

rod c. of retina, one of the visual photoreceptor cells of the retina sensitive to gray shades.

Schwann's c., a special cell which surrounds a peripheral axon forming a myelin sheath.

septal c., type II pneumocyte; see under pneumocyte.

Sertoli c.'s, the elaborate nonspermatogenic sustentacular cells in the seminiferous tubules of male gonads (testes) extending from the basal lamina to the lumen; they house the developing spermatogenic cells in deep recesses and produce sex hormone-binding globulin and androgens.

sickle c., an abnormal crescent-shaped red blood cell; the shape is due to the presence of hemoglobin S; also called drepanocyte and meniscocyte.

smudge c., any leukocyte that becomes so degen-

erated that the cytoplasm disappears leaving a naked nucleus that stains poorly and exhibits no characteristic chromatin pattern; rarely found in normal blood but seen in large numbers in acute myeloblastic and lymphoblastic anemia and in chronic lymphatic leukemia.

sperm c., a spermatozoon.

squamous c., a flat, scalelike epithelial cell.

squamous alveolar c., type I pneumocyte; see under pneumocyte.

stab c., see band cell.

stellate c.'s of the cerebral cortex, a star-shaped interneuron cell located in the second, third, and fourth layers of the cortex of the brain.

stem c.'s, cells that can produce cells that are able to differentiate.

sustentacular c., one of the supporting cells of an epithelium, as seen in the spiral organ of Corti, taste bud, and olfactory epithelium.

T c.'s, thymus-derived lymphocytes.

target c., an abnormal erythrocyte, characteristic of target cell anemia, which when stained shows a dark center surrounded by a light band which is encircled by a darker ring, resembling a bull's eye target; also called Mexican hat cell.

tart c., a granulocyte which has an engulfed nucleus of another cell that is still well preserved.

taste c., a neuroepithelial cell that perceives gustatory stimuli, situated at the center of a taste bud.

theca lutein c.'s, lutein cells located within the folds of the glandular corpus luteum of the ovary and derived from the theca interna; they produce estrogens; also called paraluteal cells.

Tiselius electrophoresis c., the cell or container in a Tiselius apparatus containing the solution to be electrophoretically analyzed; the cell is divided into cubicles which permit isolation of the components separated by the electric current.

transitional c., (1) a monocyte; (2) any cell thought to represent a phase of development from one form to another.

type I c., type I pneumocyte; see under pneumocyte.

type II c., type II pneumocyte; see under pneumocyte.

wasserhelle c.'s, the water-clear cells of the parathyroid gland.

white blood c.'s, formed elements in the blood that include granular leukocytes, lymphocytes, and monocytes.

cell | cell

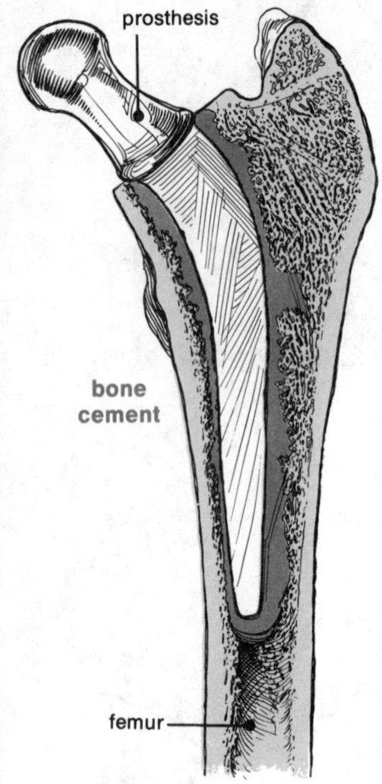
prosthesis
bone
cement
femur

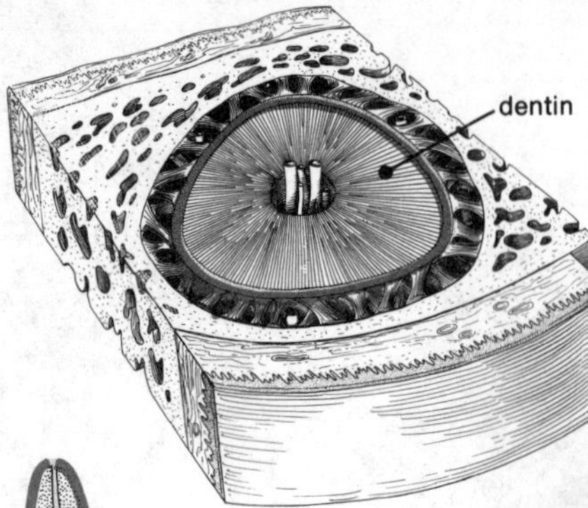
dentin

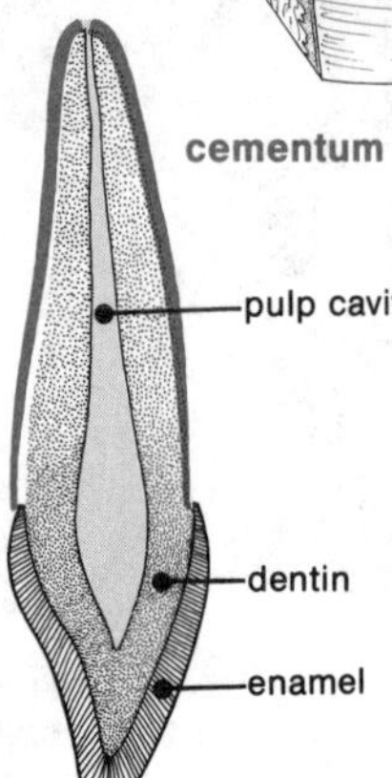
cementum
pulp cavity
dentin
enamel

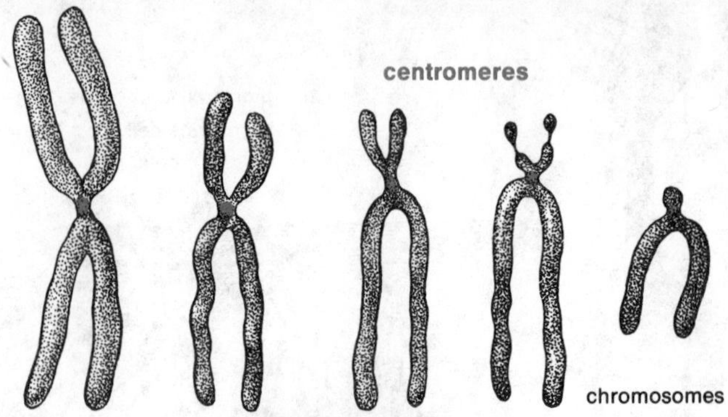
centromeres
chromosomes

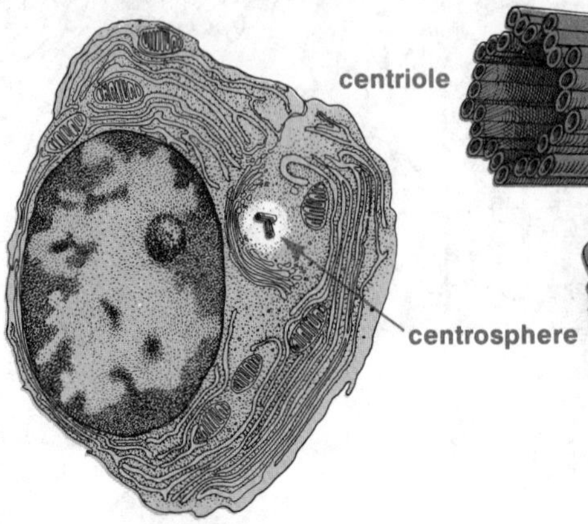
centrosphere

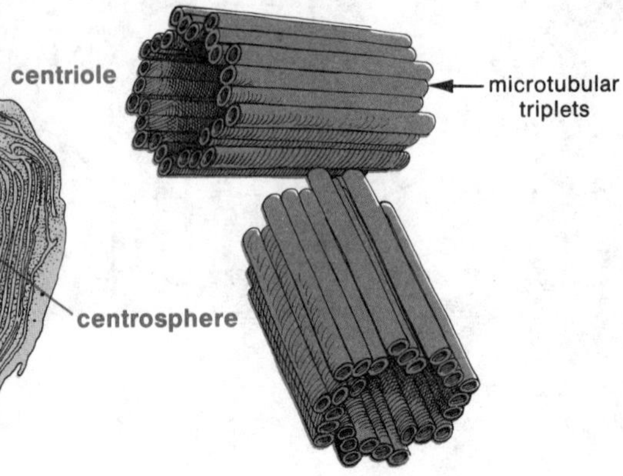
centriole
microtubular
triplets

cel'lular. Relating to, resembling, composed of, or derived from cells.

cellular'ity. The number and quality of the cells constituting a tissue.

cel'lule. 1. A small cavity or compartment. 2. A minute cell.

celluli'tis. A diffuse spreading infection, especially of the subcutaneous tissue.

cel'lulose. A carbohydrate polymer, $C_6H_{10}O_5$; the main constituent of the cell walls of plants; an important source of bulk in the diet because it is not affected by the digestive enzymes.

ce'lom. The body cavity of the embryo, between the two layers of the mesoderm after one unites with the ectoderm and the other with the endoderm.

celom'ic. Relating to the body cavity or celom.

Cel'sius (C). Denoting a temperature scale that indicates the freezing point of water as 0°C and the boiling point as 100°C under normal atmospheric pressure; also called centigrade.

cement'. 1. Cementum. 2. Any of several materials used in dentistry, neurosurgery, and orthopedic surgery as luting and sealing agents, temporary restorations, and bases.

bone c., a luting agent for filling interstices of bone; it is widely used in the fixation of hip and knee implants.

intercellular c., a substance holding together cells, especially epithelial cells.

muscle c., see myoglia.

cemen'toblast. One of the cells active in the formation of cementum.

cemen'tocyte. A cell occupying a lacunar space in the cementum of a tooth; it generally possesses protoplasmic processes that radiate from the cell body into the canaliculi of the cementum; derived from cementoblasts trapped within newly formed cementum.

cemento'ma. Periapical ossifying fibroma, an asymptomatic periapical lesion marked by the proliferation of fibrous connective tissue at the apex of a tooth; it is generally replaced by a calcified mass resembling cementum.

cemen'tum. A specialized, bonelike fibrous tissue covering the anatomic roots of human teeth, which serves primarily as an attachment area of the tooth to its surrounding structures; it is more resistant to resorption than bone, thus making orthodontic movement of teeth possible.

cellular c., cementum possessing cementocytes, primarily located in the apical portion of the tooth.

cen'sor. In Freudian psychoanalytic theory, the part of the unconscious self that prevents the emergence of repressed thoughts and wishes into consciousness.

cen'ter. 1. The middle; the central part of an organ or structure; also called core. 2. A specialized region in which a process, such as ossification, begins. 3. A collection of neurons governing a particular function.

cell c., see centrosome.

germinal c., a light staining oval mass in the center of a secondary lymphatic nodule consisting primarily of large lymphoid cells; a site of antibody synthesis.

ossification c., any region in which the process of ossification first begins in a tissue.

reflex c., any part of the nervous system where the reception of a sensory impression is automatically followed by a motor impulse.

respiratory c.'s, regions in the medulla and pons which coordinate the activity of respiration.

speech c., a unilateral area in the inferior frontal gyrus, associated with articulate speech.

vomiting c., a center in the lower part of the medulla oblongata, stimulation of which may cause vomiting.

cente'sis. The puncturing of a cavity.

centi-, cent-. Combining forms meaning one-hundredth.

cen'tibar. A unit of atmospheric pressure; one-hundredth of a bar.

cen'tigrade. 1. Divided into or consisting of 100 gradations. 2. Denoting a temperature scale in which the interval between the freezing and boiling points of water is divided into 100 degrees; normal human body temperature is approximately 37°C; also called Celsius.

cen'timeter. A unit of length; one-hundredth of a meter.

cen'trad. 1. A unit of ophthalmic prism strength, corresponding to the arc formed by a deviating light ray; equal to one-hundredth of the radius of the circle; symbolized by an inverted delta (∇). 2. Toward the center.

cen'trage. Condition in which the center of the various refracting and reflecting surfaces of an optical system lie on a straight line.

central core disease. A congenital myopathy usually manifested before the first month of life; characterized by proximal muscle weakness, most severe in the lower limbs, resulting in delayed walking; on biopsy the central core of muscle fibers stains abnormally.

cen'tric. Of or relating to a center.

centrif'ugal. Directed away from a center or axis; efferent.

cen'trifuge. 1. An apparatus which, by means of centrifugal force, separates substances of different densities or simulates gravitational effects. 2. To separate substances by a centrifuge.

centrilob'ular. Occurring at or near the center of a lobule.

cen'triole. Any of two short, cylindrical organelles (usually at right angles to each other) containing nine pairs of parallel microtubules about a central cavity, located in the centrosome and considered to play an important role in cell division; usually associated with the Golgi apparatus in a nondividing cell; sometimes called attraction particle.

centrip'etal. Directed toward a center or axis; afferent.

cen'tromere. The constricted part of the chromosome to which the spindle fibers attach during mitosis; chromosome movement occurs about this point; also called kinetochore.

cen'trosome. Two associated centrioles, which play an important role in cell division (mitosis); also called cell center.

cen'trosphere. A clear, gel-like zone of a cell which contains the centrosome.

cen'trum, *pl.* **cen'tra.** The center of an anatomical structure.

cephal-, cephalo-. Combining forms indicating head.

ceph'alad. Toward the head.

cephalal'gia. See headache.

cephalhemato'ma. Accumulation of blood under the periosteum of the skull of a newborn infant; it usually occurs over one or both parietal bones, appears hours or days after delivery, increases in size, and disappears after a few weeks; caused by injury to the periosteum during labor.

cephal'ic. Relating to the head.

ceph'alin. A member of a large group of lipids known as phospholipids; found in most animal tissues, especially the brain and spinal cord; important in the blood clotting process.

cephaliza'tion. 1. The gradual evolutionary concentration in the brain of important functions of the nervous system. 2. The concentration of growth tendency at the anterior end of the embryo.

cephalocente'sis. The draining of fluid from the brain by means of a hollow needle or trocar and cannula.

cephalodyn'ia. Headache.

cephalogy'ric. Referring to circular movements of the head.

cephalomeg'aly. Abnormal enlargement of the head.

cephalome'nia. Bleeding from the nose and other structures of the head during menstruation.

cer'amide. General term used to designate any *N*-acyl fatty acid derivative of a sphingosine.

ceratal'gia. Keratalgia.

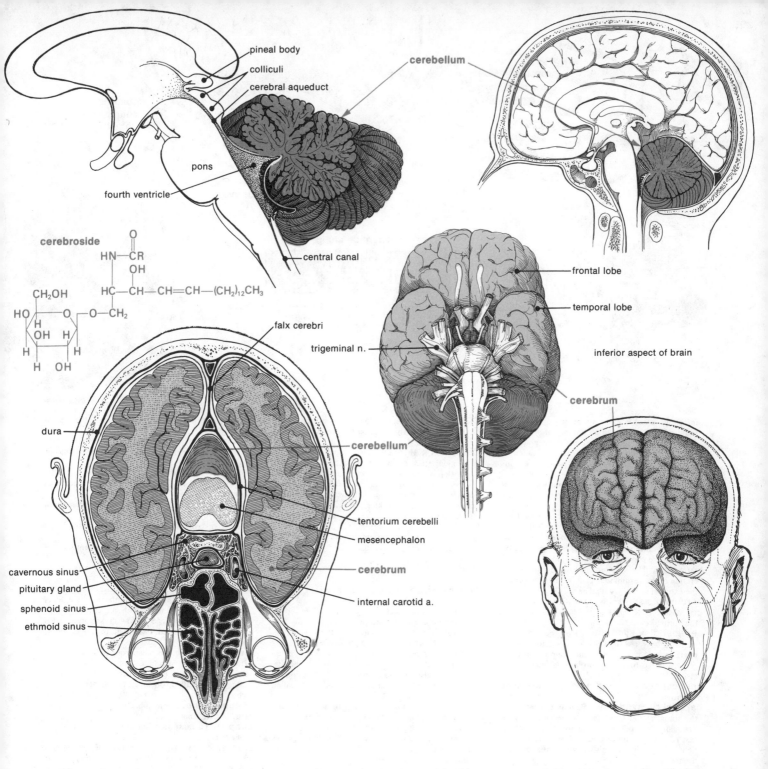

pineal body
colliculi
cerebral aqueduct
pons
fourth ventricle
central canal

cerebellum

cerebroside

frontal lobe
temporal lobe
inferior aspect of brain
cerebrum

falx cerebri
trigeminal n.
cerebellum

dura

tentorium cerebelli
mesencephalon
cerebrum
internal carotid a.

cavernous sinus
pituitary gland
sphenoid sinus
ethmoid sinus

cerea flexibilitas. The characteristic "waxy flexibility" of catatonic schizophrenia in which the patient holds his limbs for an indefinite period of time in the position in which they are placed.

ce′real. 1. An edible grain, the plant producing it, or the food prepared from it. **2.** Of or relating to such grain.

cerebel′lar. Of or relating to the cerebellum.

cerebellar syndrome. Cerebellar deficiency manifested chiefly by slurred speech, slow and clumsy movement of the limbs, and staggering gait.

cerebellopon′tile. Relating to both the cerebellum and pons.

cerebelloru′bral. Relating to the cerebellum and the red nucleus.

cerebel′lum. The part of the central nervous system situated below and posterior to the cerebrum and above the pons and medulla; it has a somewhat

oval shape and is morphologically divided into two lateral hemispheres and a middle portion; its function is to maintain equilibrium and coordination.

cerebr-. Combining form indicating the brain.

cere′bral. Of or relating to the brain.

cerebra′tion. Conscious or unconscious mental activity.

cerebromeningi′tis. Inflammation of the brain and its membranes (meninges).

cer′ebron. See phrenosin.

cerebrop′athy. See encephalopathy.

cerebropsycho′sis. Mental disorder caused by, or associated with, a lesion of the brain.

cerebrosclero′sis. Sclerosis of the brain substance; also called encephalosclerosis.

cer′ebrose. A hexose (monosaccharide having six carbon atoms) present in brain tissue.

cer′ebroside. A phosphorous-free glycolipid con-

taining galactose (occasionally glucose), an unsaturated amino-alcohol, and a fatty acid.

cerebrospi′nal. Relating to the brain and spinal cord.

cerebrot′omy. 1. Surgical incision of the brain substance. **2.** Anatomy of the brain.

cerebrovas′cular. Denoting the blood supply of the brain.

cer′ebrum. The brain, excluding the medulla, pons, and cerebellum.

ce′rium. A metallic element; symbol Ce, atomic number 58, atomic weight 140.25.

certifi′able. 1. Applied to any disease required by law to be reported to the health authorities. **2.** Denoting a person exhibiting sufficiently severe psychotic behavior to require hospitalization. **3.** Having satisfied the requirements for certification.

certifica′tion. 1. The notification of reportable

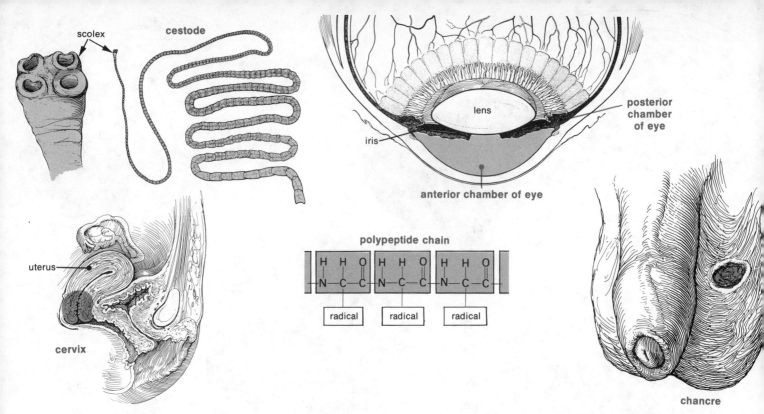

scolex

cestode

lens

posterior chamber of eye

iris

anterior chamber of eye

uterus

cervix

polypeptide chain

H	H	O	H	H	O	H	H	O
N	C	C	N	C	C	N	C	C

radical radical radical

chancre

infectious disease cases to health authorities as required by law. **2.** The attainment of a document attesting that a person may officially practice in certain professions; verification of qualifications. **3.** The court procedure by which a patient is committed to an institution.

ceruloplas′min. A plasma protein which carries more than 95 per cent of the body's circulating copper; it is thought that the copper carried by ceruloplasmin goes into the cellular manufacture of cytochrome oxidase, which is the terminal enzyme in the chain of events that constitutes cellular oxygen consumption; ceruloplasmin is deficient in Wilson's disease (hepatolenticular degeneration).

ceru′men. The soft brownish-yellow waxlike secretion of the ceruminous glands lining the canal of the external ear; also called earwax.

cerumino′sis. Excessive formation of earwax.

cer′vical. 1. Relating to the neck. **2.** Relating to the uterine cervix.

cervical disk syndrome. Pain, numbness, and muscular spasm of the neck, radiating to the shoulders, caused by irritation and compression of the cervical nerve roots by a protruding intervertebral disk.

cervical fusion syndrome. See Klippel-Feil syndrome.

cervical rib syndrome. Pain and tingling along the forearm and hand due to pressure upon the brachial plexus and subclavian artery by a rudimentary cervical rib, fibrous band, first thoracic rib, or tight scalene muscle; also called Naffziger's syndrome.

cervicec′tomy. Amputation of the uterine cervix; also called trachelectomy.

cervici′tis. Inflammation of the uterine cervix.

  cystic c., cervix containing multiple nabothian cysts.

cervicobra′chial. Relating to the neck and the arm.

cer′vix. Any neck-shaped anatomic structure, as the narrow end of the bladder.

  uterine c., The neck of the uterus; the lower part of the uterus extending from the isthmus into the vagina.

cesa′rean. See under section.

cesarean hysterectomy. See under hysterectomy.

Cesto′da. A class of Platyhelminthes or flatworms, which includes the tapeworm; term derived from the Latin *cestoda*, meaning ribbon shaped.

ces′tode. A tapeworm.

CF. Abbreviation for (a) citrovorum factor; (b) cystic fibrosis.

Cf. Chemical symbol of the element californium.

CG. Abbreviation for chorionic gonadotropin.

C.G.S., c.g.s. Abbreviation for centimeter-gram-second unit.

Chaddock's signs. Reflexes usually obtained in pyramidal tract lesions. **1.** Chaddock's toe sign; extension of the toe on stroking the lateral malleolus and the lateral dorsum of the foot. **2.** Chaddock's wrist sign; flexion of the wrist with fanning of the fingers upon stroking the wrist on the side of the little finger.

Chadwick's sign. Dark bluish discoloration of the lining of the vagina and cervix; considered an early sign of pregnancy; also called Jacquemier's sign.

chafe. 1. To irritate or wear away by rubbing. **2.** Irritation.

Chagas' disease. Disease characterized by great enlargement of the heart, which becomes very heavy but rather feeble in action, and by apical aneurysms; caused by the protozoan parasite *Trypanosoma cruzi* and transmitted by the kissing bug; the parasite multiplies in the gut of the kissing bug and is discharged in the feces, and man is infected through contamination of the bite wound; the disease may also be transmitted by transfusion or inoculation with contaminated blood; also called American trypanosomiasis.

chain. 1. In chemistry, a group of atoms bonded together in a linear fashion. **2.** In bacteriology, a group of microorganisms attached end-to-end.

  closed c., one formed by atoms linked together in the shape of a ring.

  lateral c., see side chain.

  polypeptide c., a repeating peptide chain formed by amino acids, each of which contributes an identical group to the backbone of the chain plus a distinguishing radical as a side group.

  side c., lateral c., a group of atoms linked to a closed chain.

chala′sia, chala′sis. The relaxation of a group of muscles, especially muscles that work together.

chala′zion. A cyst in a tarsal (meibomian) gland that is seen merely as a lump in an otherwise normal eyelid; also called meibomian cyst.

chalmoo′gra, chalmu′gra. Any of several trees of Asia, especially *Taraktogenos kurzi* and *Hydnocarpus wightiana,* the ripe seeds of which yield an oil used in the treatment of leprosy.

chal′one. A substance that inhibits cell division and is synthesized by mature cells of the tissue upon which it acts.

cham′ber. A closed space.

  anterior c. of the eye, the space between the cornea and the iris; it is filled with aqueous humor.

  hyperbaric c., one in which the air pressure may

be raised to higher than normal atmospheric pressure.

  ionization c., a gas-filled enclosure fitted with electrodes between which an electric current passes when the gas is ionized by radiation.

  posterior c. of the eye, the space between the iris and the crystalline lens; it is filled with aqueous humor.

  pulp c., the space in the crown or body of a tooth occupied by the pulp; principally the area of the pulp cavity within the coronal portion of the tooth and into which the root canals open.

  Thoma's counting c., Thoma-Zeiss hemocytometer; see under hemocytometer.

  vitreous c., the cavity of the eyeball behind the lens containing the vitreous body.

chan′cre. The first lesion of syphilis present at the site of entrance of the syphilitic infection; it appears as a hard, reddish ulcer with an eroded center which is covered by a yellowish secretion; also called hard, Hunterian, indurated, or ture chancre, and hard sore.

  soft c., simple c., see chancroid.

chan′croid. An infectious, nonsyphilitic, pus-discharging, venereal ulcer caused by *Haemophilus ducreyi*; also called soft or simple chancre and soft sore.

change of life. See menopause.

chan′nel. Canal.

chap. 1. To cause the skin to crack or split. **2.** A split or crack.

char′acter. 1. The combination of features or traits that distinguishes an individual or object from another. **2.** One such feature, attribute, or trait.

char′coal. A black porous material obtained by burning wood with a restricted amount of air.

  activated c., medicinal charcoal, charcoal that has been treated to increase its adsorptive power; used as an antidote and to reduce hyperacidity.

Charcot-Marie-Tooth disease. Peroneal muscular atrophy; see under atrophy.

Charcot's disease. Tabetic arthropathy; see under arthropathy.

char′leyhorse. A popular name for a cramp or stiffness of muscles, especially of the leg or arm following injury or excessive activity.

chart. 1. Information or data depicted in the form of graphs or tables. **2.** The health record of a patient. **3.** To enter information into the patient's record or to record data in graphic form.

Ch.D. Abbreviation for *Chirurgiae Doctor,* Doctor of Surgery.

Chediak-Higashi syndrome. A rare hereditary condition found in infants; symptoms include decreased pigmentation of the skin, hair, and eyes,

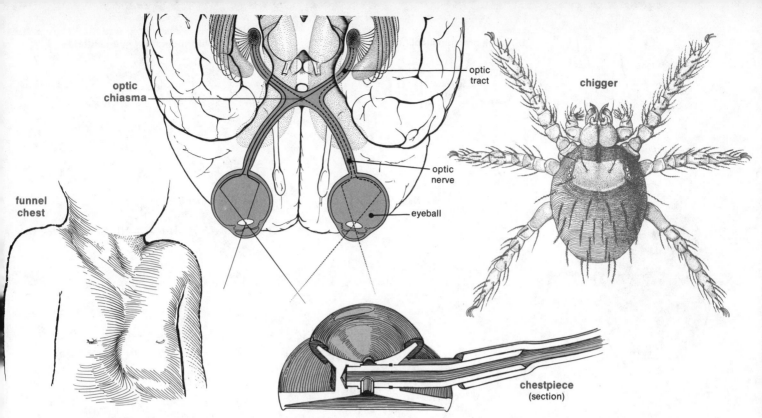

optic chiasma

optic tract

optic nerve

eyeball

chigger

funnel chest

chestpiece
(section)

cytoplasmic inclusions of the leukocytes, and susceptibility to pyogenic infections; early death is common.

cheek. A fleshy protuberance on either side of the face, forming the lateral walls of the mouth; also called bucca and mala.

  c. biting, the interposing of cheek tissue between the teeth of the upper and lower dentitions, occasionally resulting in hyperkeratotic lesions and irritations of the buccal mucosa.

cheek′bite. Interocclusal record; see under record.

cheek′bone. Zygomatic bone; see table of bones.

cheil-, cheilo-. Combining forms denoting lips.

cheilion. The corner or angle of the mouth.

cheili′tis. Inflammation of the lip.

  actinic c., solar c., inflammation of the lip characterized by a scaly crust on the vermillion border, usually due to overexposure to sunlight.

cheilec′tomy. 1. Surgical removal of a portion of the lip. **2.** Cutting away of bony irregularities on the rim of a joint cavity.

cheilectro′pion. A turning outward of the lips.

cheilogna′thouragnos′chisis. Congenital malformation consisting of a cleft that extends from the palate, through the gum, to the upper lip.

chei′loplasty. Plastic surgery of the lips; also called labioplasty.

cheilos′chisis. See harelip.

cheilo′sis. A noninflammatory condition of the lip marked by fissuring and chapping; characteristic of riboflavin deficiency.

cheir′oscope. A binocular instrument used for antisuppression training of the eyes in strabismus.

che′late. 1. A compound containing a metal ion connected by coordinate bonds to two or more nonmetal ions in the same molecule. **2.** To effect chelation.

chela′tion. The coordinate bond formation between a metal ion and two or more nonmetal ions in the same molecule.

chem′ical. 1. Relating to chemistry. **2.** A substance produced by the interaction of elements.

chemise′. A piece of linen used to secure a tampon around a catheter that has been inserted into a wound.

chem′istry. The science concerned with the atomic and molecular composition of the different types of matter and the laws that govern their mutual reactions.

  analytic c., the breaking up of compounds to determine and study their composition.

  biologic c., see biochemistry.

  inorganic c., the branch of chemistry concerned with substances not containing carbon.

  organic c., the study of substances containing carbon.

  physiologic c., see biochemistry.

chemobiot′ic. Denoting a compound containing an antibiotic and another therapeutic chemical.

chemocau′tery. The destruction of tissue by the application of a caustic substance.

che′moceptor. See chemoreceptor.

chemodecto′ma. A tumor of the chemoreceptor system, such as the carotid body, glomus jugulare, and aortic arch bodies.

chemodectomato′sis. The occurrence in the lungs of multiple minute tumors of the chemoreceptor type.

chemodifferentia′tion. Differentiation at the molecular level which usually precedes and controls morphologic differentiation of cells in the developing embryo.

chemokine′sis. Increased activity of an organism stimulated by a chemical substance.

chemolumines′cence. 1. Light produced by the transformation of chemical energy. **2.** Radiation producing chemical action.

chemol′ysis. Chemical decomposition.

chemopallidec′tomy. Injection of a chemical substance in the globus pallidum in the brain; an operation performed for the relief of rigidity in Parkinsonism.

chemopal′lidothalamec′tomy. Destruction of portions of brain tissue (globus pallidus and thalamus) by injection of a chemical.

chemoprophylax′is. The prevention of a specific disease by the use of a chemical.

chemorecep′tor. An end organ, such as a taste bud, or sense organ, such as the carotid body, sensitive to chemical stimuli; also called chemoceptor.

chemosen′sitive. Sensitive to changes in the chemical composition of substances.

chemo′sis. Eye disorder marked by swelling of the conjunctiva around the cornea.

chemosur′gery. The use of chemical substances to destroy tissues.

chemotax′is. The movement of an organism toward or away from a chemical substance, especially the unidirectional migration of white blood cells toward an attractant.

chemotherapeu′tics. The branch of therapeutics dealing with the treatment of disease with chemicals.

chemother′apy. Treatment or prevention of disease by means of chemical substances.

chenodeoxychol′ic acid. One of the acids present in bile which participate in digestive processes.

cher′ubism. The characteristic facial features of individuals affected with familial fibrous dysplasia

of the jaws: chubbiness and upturned eyes.

chest. The thorax.

  barrel c., short and round chest with ribs in a horizontal position; seen in cases of advanced emphysema.

  flail c., one with an unstable chest wall due to multiple rib fractures causing a paradoxical motion (moving inward on inspiration and outward on expiration); also called flapping chest wall.

  funnel c., a developmental deformity marked by depression of the sternum and rib cartilages; caused by a short central tendon of the diaphragm; also called pectus excavatum.

chest′piece. The portion of the stethoscope placed against the patient's body for the determination and study of sounds within the body.

Chiari-Frommel syndrome. Condition characterized by prolonged milk secretion and atrophy of the uterus following pregnancy.

chias′ma, chi′asm. An X-shaped crossing.

  optic c., the point of crossing of the fibers of the optic nerves.

chick′enpox. An acute contagious disease, usually of young children, caused by a virus and marked by a skin eruption, fever, and mild constitutional symptoms; incubation period is from 11 to 24 days; also called varicella.

chig′ger. Any of various six-legged larvae of mites; the most common is *Trombicula alfreddugesi*; the chigger usually attaches itself to parts of the body that are snugly clothed, such as the waist and ankles; itching generally begins three to six hours after it has attached; also called red bug and harvest mite.

chig′oe. The small tropical sand flea, *Tunga penetrans*; the egg-carrying female burrows under the skin of man, causing intense itching.

chil-, chilo-. Combining forms denoting lip.

chil′blain. Condition resulting from excessive exposure to cold temperature, marked by inflammatory swelling of hands and feet accompanied by severe itching and burning sensations, and sometimes ulceration; usually affects individuals with a history of cold limbs in summer as well as in winter; also called pernio. Cf frostbite.

child. A young person between the periods of infancy and adolescence.

  battered c., a child who has been subjected to physical abuse, usually by parents, with resulting injuries.

  hyperactive c., one who is characterized by excessive energy, emotional instability, and short attention span, usually related to minimal brain dysfunction.

child′bearing. Pregnancy and parturition.

child′birth. Parturition; labor.

chloramphenicol

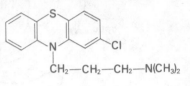

chlordiazepoxide

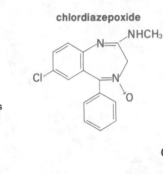

chlorpromazine hydrochloride

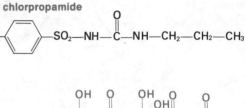

chlorpropamide

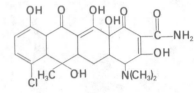

Cl—◯—SO₂—NH—C—NH—CH₂—CH₂—CH₃

Chlamydomonas

flagellum

contractile vacuole

eye spot

nucleus

pyrenoid

cell wall

chlorothiazide

chlortetracycline

---

natural c., a concept in the management of parturition in which prenatal education, exercises, and psychologic conditioning largely replace anesthesia and surgical intervention at the time of labor; also called physiologic childbirth.

chill. 1. A moderate sensation of coldness. **2.** A feeling of coldness accompanied by shivering and fever.

Chilomas'tix. A genus of protozoa parasitic in the intestines; one species, *Chilomastix mesnili,* is believed to cause diarrhea.

chime'ra. 1. In experimental embryology, an organism developed from combined portions of different embryos. **2.** An individual who has received a genetically different transplant.

chin. The central anterior prominence of the lower jaw; also called the mentum.

  double c., loose fatty flesh under the chin.

  galoche c., an extremely long pointed chin.

Chinese restaurant syndrome. Transient syndrome consisting of chest pains, throbbing of the head, and feelings of tightness of facial muscles after ingesting monosodium L-glutamate, which is used in Chinese food; occurs in individuals who are unusually sensitive to this additive.

chirognos'tic. Capable of distinguishing between right and left.

chirokinesthe'sia. The subjective sensation of motions of the hand.

chi'roplasty. Plastic surgery of the hand.

chirop'odist. See podiatrist.

chirop'ody. See podiatry.

chiroprac'tic. A philosophy of therapy in which disease is attributed to mild dislocations of the vertebral column, causing pressure on the nerves; the preferred method of treatment is by manipulation of the vertebrae.

chiroprac'tor. One who practices chiropractic.

chis'el. A metal instrument with a beveled cutting edge designed after the carpenter's chisel; used in dentistry for cutting or cleaving enamel.

chi'tin. A transparent, horny organic substance (polysaccharide), constituting the chief component of insect exoskeletons, crustacean shells, and the cell walls of certain fungi.

chitobi'ose. The disaccharide present in chitin.

chito'samine. See glucosamine.

chlamyd'iae. A large group of nonmotile, gram-negative intracellular parasites, including some human and animal pathogens; they were once considered viruses because of their intracellular parasitism but are now viewed as bacteria (genus *Chlamydia*).

Chlamydom'onas. A genus (phylum Chlorophyta) of single-celled algae that can reproduce both sexually and asexually; used in genetic studies.

Chlamydozo'a. A name formerly given to the chlamydiae.

chloas'ma. The occurrence of irregularly shaped brownish spots or patches on the skin; commonly known as the mask of pregnancy when appearing on the face and neck of a pregnant woman and as liver spots in elderly people, although there is no association with disease of the liver.

chlor-. Combining form meaning (a) green; (b) a relationship to chlorine.

chlorac'ne. A skin eruption, resembling acne, caused by constant contact with certain chlorinated compounds.

chlor'al. A colorless oily liquid of pungent odor, CCl₃CHO; produced by the action of chlorine gas on alcohol.

  c. hydrate, a colorless crystalline compound, soluble in water and alcohol; used as a hypnotic and sedative.

chlo'ralism. Condition caused by the constant use of chloral as an intoxicant.

chlo'ralose. A crystalline substance used as a general anesthetic in laboratory animals.

chloram'bucil. A derivative of nitrogen mustard which retards proliferation and maturation of lymphocytes used in the treatment of chronic lymphocytic leukemia and some lymphomas; Leukeran®.

chloramphen'icol. A broad-spectrum antibiotic originally obtained from *Streptomyces venezuellae* but now produced synthetically; effective against many strains of gram-positive and gram-negative pathogenic microorganisms; used selectively because of the occurrence (infrequently) of aplastic anemia. Chloromycetin®.

chlordiazepox'ide. The nonproprietary name for Librium®, a drug widely used for treating anxiety, tension, and psychoneuroses.

chlore'mia. 1. See chlorosis. **2.** The presence of large amounts of chloride in the blood.

chlorhy'dria. The presence of abnormally large amounts of hydrochloric acid in the stomach.

chlor'ic. Of or containing chlorine.

chlor'ide. Any compound of chlorine.

chloridom'eter. An apparatus used in the turbidimetric analysis of chlorides.

chloridu'ria. The presence of chloride in the urine.

chlo'rinate. To combine with chlorine or a chlorine compound.

chlo'rinated. Containing chlorine.

chlor'ine. A greenish yellow, irritating, gaseous element; symbol Cl, atomic number 17, atomic weight 34.45; used as a disinfectant and bleaching agent.

chlor'ite. Any salt of chlorous acid.

chloroeth'ane. See ethyl chloride.

chlo'roform. A colorless, volatile, heavy liquid of sweetish taste, CHCl₃; formerly used as a general anesthetic.

chloro'ma. A tumor arising from myeloid tissue and containing a pale green pigment; most frequently found in the periosteum and ligamentous structures of the skull; seen usually in children and young adults; commonly called green cancer.

chlorom'etry. The quantitative study of chlorine.

p-chlorophenoxyisobutyrate. See clofibrate.

chloroph'illins. Substances derived from chlorophyll, capable of absorbing odorous molecules and thus acting as deodorants.

chlo'rophyll, chlo'rophyl. Any of a group of green pigments in plant cells that absorb light during the food making process of photosynthesis.

chlor'oplast. A cytoplasmic organelle of all green plant cells; it contains chlorophyll.

chlorop'sia. Green vision; condition in which all objects appear to have a tint of green.

chloroquine phosphate. Quinoline diphosphate; an agent used in the treatment of malaria, hepatic amebiasis, and certain skin diseases.

chloro'sis. A form of anemia occurring in adolescent girls; marked by a moderate reduction in red blood cells and a great reduction in hemoglobin content; attributed to insufficient intake of iron; also called green sickness and chloremia.

chlorothi'azide. A commonly prescribed diuretic and antihypertensive drug; it inhibits renal tubular reabsorption of sodium and is used in treating hypertension and edema due to congestive heart failure, liver disease, and pregnancy; Diuril®.

chlorot'ic. Relating to chlorosis.

chlorpromazine hydrochloride. A phenothiazine derivative used orally, muscularly, or intravenously to depress conditioned reflexes and the hypothalamic centers; used as a major tranquilizer in psychoses, and in the management of postoperative nausea and in radiation sickness; Thorazine Hydrochloride®.

chlorpro'pamide. An oral hypoglycemic agent in the sulfonylurea class; Diabinese®.

chlortetracy'cline. An antibiotic substance obtained from *Streptomyces aureofaciens;* active against hemolytic streptococci, staphylococci, typhoid bacilli, brucellae, and certain viruses; it has been supplanted in use by other tetracycline compounds with fewer side effects; Aureomycin®.

chlorure'sis. The presence of chloride in the urine.

chloruret'ic. Relating to an agent that promotes an increase of chloride excretion in the urine.

cho'ana. The funnel-like opening of the nasal

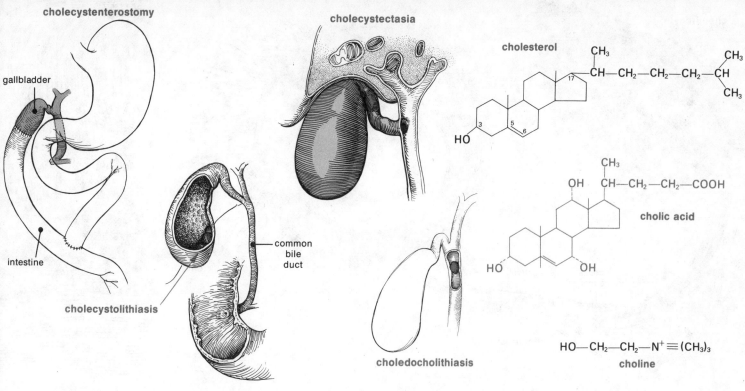

cholecystenterostomy

gallbladder

intestine

cholecystolithiasis

cholecystectasia

common
bile
duct

choledocholithiasis

cholesterol

cholic acid

choline

cavity into the nasopharynx on either side; the posterior naris.

cho'anal. Of or relating to a choana.

choke. To interfere with or terminate breathing by obstructing or breaking the trachea.

chol-, chole-, cholo-. Combining forms denoting bile.

chol'agogue. Any agent that promotes the flow of bile.

cholangiecta'sis. Dilation of the bile duct.

cholangiocarcino'ma. Malignant tumor of the liver originating in the epithelium of the intrahepatic bile ducts; also called cholangioma.

cholangioenteros'tomy. Surgical union of the bile duct to the intestine.

cholangiog'raphy. Radiologic examination of the bile ducts after ingestion of a radiopaque substance.

cholan'giole. One of the minute terminal branches of the bile duct.

cholangio'ma. See cholangiocarcinoma.

cholangios'tomy. The surgical creation of a fistula into a bile duct.

cholangiot'omy. Surgical incision into a bile duct.

cholangi'tis. Inflammation of the bile duct.

cholanopoie'sis. The synthesis by the liver of cholic acid or its conjugates, or of natural bile salts.

cholecalcif'erol. See vitamin D_3.

cholechromopoie'sis. The synthesis of bile pigments by the liver.

cho'lecyst. Gallbladder.

cholecystagog'ic. Tending to stimulate gallbladder activity.

cholecyst'agogue. An agent that stimulates gallbladder activity.

cholecystecta'sia. Dilatation of the gallbladder.

cholecystec'tomy. Surgical removal of the gallbladder.

cholecystenteros'tomy. Surgical joining of the gallbladder and the intestine.

cholecys'tic. Relating to the gallbladder.

cholecys'tis. Gallbladder.

cholecysti'tis. Inflammation of the gallbladder.

cholecystoduodenos'tomy. Surgical creation of a direct connection between the gallbladder and the duodenum.

cholecystog'raphy. X-ray visualization of the gallbladder after administration of a radiopaque substance, which is excreted by the liver and concentrated by the gallbladder.

cholecystojejunos'tomy. Surgical establishment of a connection between the gallbladder and the jejunum.

cholecystokin'ase. An enzyme that promotes

the breakdown of cholecystokinin.

cholecystokinet'ic. Causing release of the gallbladder contents.

cholecystoki'nin. A hormone secreted by the mucosa of the upper intestinal tract which stimulates contraction of the gallbladder.

cholecystolithi'asis. The presence of one or more stones in the gallbladder.

cholecystor'raphy. Suturing of the bladder.

cholecystos'tomy. Surgical formation of an opening into the gallbladder with insertion of a drainage tube through the abdominal wall.

cholecystot'omy. Surgical incision into the gallbladder.

cho'ledoch. Common bile duct.

choledoch'al. Of or relating to the common bile duct.

choledochec'tomy. Surgical removal of a portion of the common bile duct.

choledochen'dysis. Ideal choledochotomy, removal of a gallstone directly from the common bile duct.

choledochi'tis. Inflammation of the common bile duct.

choledocho-, cholodoch-. Combining forms denoting a relationship to the common bile duct.

choledochoduodenos'tomy. Surgical anastomosis between the common bile duct and the duodenum.

choledochoenteros'tomy. The surgical formation of a connection between the common bile duct and any part of the intestine.

choled'ocholith. Stone in the common bile duct.

choledocholithi'asis. The presence of stones in the common bile duct.

choledocholithot'omy. Incision into the common bile duct for the removal of a stone.

choledochoplas'ty. Reparative surgery of the common bile duct.

choledochor'raphy. Suturing of the common bile duct.

choled'ochoscope. A device for inspecting the lumen of the common bile duct.

choledochos'copy. Visual examination of the common bile duct by means of a choledochoscope.

choledochos'tomy. Surgical formation of an opening into the common bile duct for drainage.

choledochot'omy. Surgical incision into the common bile duct.

choled'ochous. Containing or conveying bile.

choled'ochus. Common bile duct; see under duct.

cho'lelith. Gallstone.

cholelithi'asis. The presence of gallstones.

cholelithot'omy. Surgical removal of a gallstone.

choleme'sia, cholem'esis. The vomiting of bile.

chole'mia. The presence of bile in the blood.

cholem'ic. Relating to the presence of bile in the blood.

choleperitoni'tis. Inflammation caused by the presence of bile in the peritoneal cavity.

cholepoie'sis. The formation of bile.

chol'era. An acute infectious disease of man caused by the bacteria *Vibrio cholerae*; characterized by severe diarrhea, vomiting, cramps, and loss of huge amounts of fluid and electrolyte from the body; occurs endemically and epidemically in Asia; also called Asiatic cholera.

cholere'sis. The secretion of bile by the liver, distinguished from the expulsion of bile by the gallbladder.

cholerrha'gia. Excessive secretion of bile.

cholesta'sis, cholesta'sia. Suppression or arrest of the flow of bile.

cholesta'tic. Tending to arrest the flow of bile.

cholesteato'ma. A misnomer for a cystic mass in the middle ear composed of a lining of stratified squamous epithelium filled with material containing blood and cholesterol; associated with chronic middle ear infection.

cholestere'mia. Increased amounts of cholesterol in the blood.

choles'terol. A white, waxy, crystalline organic alcohol; a universal tissue constituent, present in all animal fats and oils, in bile, brain tissue, blood, and egg yolk; it constitutes a large portion of the most common type of gallstone and is found in deposits in the vessel walls in atherosclerosis.

cholesterolo'sis. The focal deposits of cholesterol in the tissues, especially the gallbladder mucosa.

chol'ic. Relating to the bile.

cholic acid. A digestive acid present in bile.

cho'line. A compound synthesized by the body and found in most animal tissues; important in fat metabolism; a precursor of acetylcholine.

choliner'gic. 1. Stimulated by or capable of liberating acetylcholine; parasympathomimetic. 2. Simulating the effects of acetylcholine.

chol'inester. An ester of choline.

cholines'terase. An enzyme present throughout the body tissues that promotes the hydrolysis of acetylcholine to form acetic acid and choline; it acts to remove acetylcholine discharged at the neuromuscular junction and prevent it from re-exciting the muscle; also called acetylcholinesterase.

cholinomimet'ic. Producing an effect similar to that of acetylcholine.

cholorrhe'a. Excessive secretion of bile.

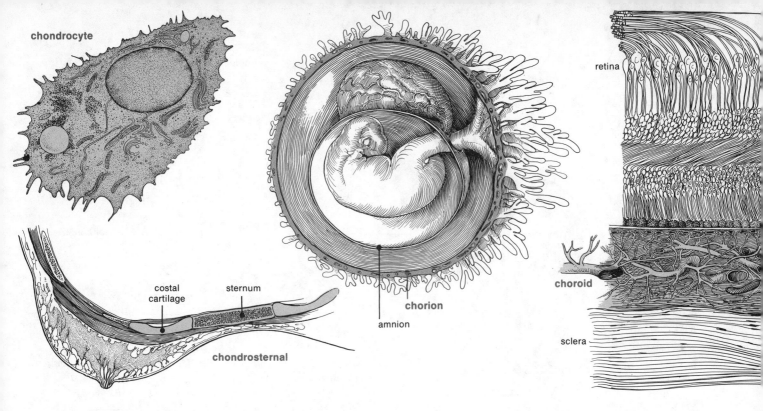

chondrocyte

retina

costal
cartilage

sternum

chorion

amnion

chondrosternal

choroid

sclera

---

cholylcoen'zyme A. A condensation product of choline and coenzyme A.

chon'dral. Relating to cartilage.

chondral'gia. Pain in a cartilage; also called chondrodynia.

chondrec'tomy. Removal of a cartilage.

chondrifica'tion. Conversion into cartilage.

chon'drin. A gelatin-like protein obtained from cartilage by boiling.

chondri'tis. Inflammation of cartilage.

  costal c., costochondritis, painful inflammation of the costal cartilages, occasionally mistaken for pain of cardiac origin.

chondro-, chondrio-. Combining forms meaning (a) cartilage and (b) granular.

chon'droblast. A cartilage-producing cell.

chondroblasto'ma. A benign tumor of long bones occurring in children under the age of 20; it consists of tissue resembling fetal cartilage.

chon'droclast. A giant cell concerned with the absorption of cartilage.

chondrocos'tal. Relating to the cartilage of the ribs.

chondrocra'nium. The embryonic skull.

chon'drocyte. A cartilage cell; since the cartilage has no blood vessels, the chondrocyte receives its nutrition by diffusion from the capillaries of the perichondrium.

chondrodermati'tis nodular'is chron'ica hel'icis. The presence of painful nodules on the helix of the ear.

chondrodyn'ia. Chondralgia; pain in a cartilage.

chondrodystro'phia, chondrodys'trophy. See achondroplasia.

chondrogen'esis. The formation of cartilage.

chondro'itin. A mucopolysaccharide present in chondrin; upon hydrolysis it yields acetic acid, glucuronic acid, and galactosamine.

chondro'ma. A benign tumor composed of cartilage.

chondromala'cia. Abnormal softening of cartilage.

chondromato'sis. The presence of multiple cartilaginous growths (chondromas).

chon'dro-os'seous. Relating to cartilage and bone.

chondrop'athy. Any disease of cartilage.

chon'drophyte. A cartilaginous growth at the articular surface of a bone.

chon'droplasty. Reparative surgery of cartilage.

chondro'samine. See galactosamine.

chondrosarco'ma. A malignant bone tumor derived from cartilage cells which erodes the bone and invades adjacent soft tissues.

chondroster'nal. Relating to (a) a sternal carti-

lage; (b) the rib cartilages and the sternum.

chon'drotome. A surgical knife used for cutting cartilage.

chor'da, *pl.* **chor'dae. 1.** A tendon. **2.** A stringlike anatomic structure.

  c. tendineae, tendinous strands extending from the papillary muscles to the leaflets of the atrioventricular valves of the heart.

  c. tympani, a branch of the facial nerve that inner- vates the submandibular and sublingual glands and the anterior two-thirds on the tongue.

Chorda'ta. The phylum that includes all animals having a notochord at some developmental stage.

chor'date. Any animal of the phylum Chordata.

chordee'. Downward curvature of the penis due to fibrous bands on the undersurface of the corpora.

chordi'tis. Inflammation of a chorda.

chordo'ma. A rare tumor believed to arise from remnants of notochordal tissue; occurring along the vertebral column, especially the sacrococcygeal area and at the base of the skull.

chore'a. Any of a group of disorders characterized by brief, rapid, involuntary movements of the limbs, face, trunk, and head.

  acute c., Syndenham's c., St. Vitus' dance; a symptom complex occurring in children, marked by muscle weakness, incoordination, and involuntary movements intensified by voluntary effort; associated with acute rheumatic fever; also called infectious chorea.

  hereditary c., chronic progressive c., Huntington's c., a hereditary, progressive, degenerative disease of the brain beginning in adult life and causing mental deterioration; characterized by involuntary jerky movements, usually of the trunk, shoulders, and lower limbs.

  senile c., mild involuntary, usually unilateral, movements of the limbs occurring in the aged.

chore'ic. Of or relating to chorea.

chore'iform. Resembling chorea (a spasmodic nervous disorder).

choreatheto'sis. Abnormal involuntary movements of the body, a combination of choreic and athetoid patterns as twitching, writhing, contortions of face, heel walking, and bizarre postures.

chorioadenoma destruens. A cellular, locally invasive tumor of the outermost fetal membrane (chorion); it penetrates and sometimes perforates the wall of the uterus, extending into adjacent tissues.

chorioamnioni'tis. Inflammation of the fetal membranes.

chorioangio'ma. A rare benign tumor arising from placental capillaries which appears as a solitary nodule in the placenta.

choriocarcino'ma. A malignant tumor arising from the outermost of the fetal membranes (chorion); rarely coexisting with the pregnancy but usually developing immediately afterward; it may result from either ectopic or normal pregnancies; formerly called chorionepithelioma.

choriomeningi'tis. Inflammation of the cerebral membranes (meninges) with involvement of the choroid plexuses, especially of the third and fourth ventricles.

  lymphocytic c., a rare viral disease prevalent in mice, sometimes transmitted to man.

cho'rion. The outermost membrane enclosing the fetus.

chorionepithelio'ma. See choriocarcinoma.

chorion'ic. Relating to the outermost of the fetal membranes (chorion).

chorion'ic gonadotro'pin (CG). A substance that originates in the chorionic tissue which has a stimulating effect on the gonads; usually obtained from the urine of pregnant women (human chorionic gonadotropin, HCG).

chorioretini'tis. Inflammation of the middle layer of the eye (choroid) and the retina; also called Jensen's disease and retinochoroiditis.

choristo'ma. A growth composed of normal tissue occurring in abnormal locations.

cho'roid. 1. The middle, vascular layer of the eyeball. **2.** Resembling the chorion membrane enclosing the fetus.

choroidere'mia. A hereditary disease marked by progressive degeneration of the vascular layer of the eye (choroid); the earliest symptom is night blindness followed by loss of peripheral vision and eventual total blindness.

choroidi'tis. Inflammation of the vascular coat of the eye.

choroidocycli'tis. Inflammation of the vascular coat of the eye and the ciliary body.

Christmas disease. Hemophilia B. See also factor IX.

chrom-, chromat-, chromato-, chromo-. Combining forms denoting color.

chro'maffin. 1. Readily staining yellow or brown with chromium salts. **2.** Denoting certain cells present mostly in the medulla of the adrenal glands and to a lesser extent along the ganglionated sympathetic chain (paraganglia) and the abdominal aorta (organs of Zuckerkandl).

chromaffino ma. A tumor composed of chromaffin tissues.

chromaffinop'athy. Any disease of the chromaffin tissues.

chro'mate. A salt of chromic acid.

chromat'ic. Of or relating to color.

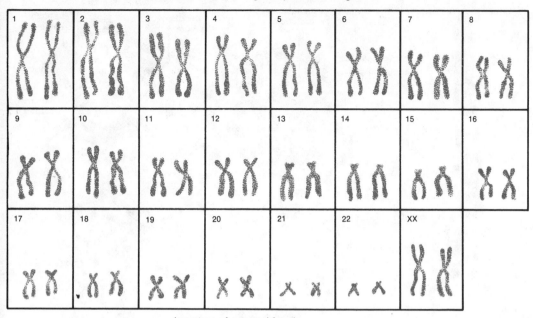

chromosomes arranged in pairs according to size

1	2	3	4	5	6	7	8
9	10	11	12	13	14	15	16
17	18	19	20	21	22	XX

karyotype of a normal female

acrocentric chromosome

chromosome satellite

metacentric chromosome

submetacentric chromosome

---

chro′matids. Two daughter strands joined by a single centromere, formed by the splitting of a chromosome in the prophase stage of mitosis; eventually each chromatid becomes a chromosome.

chro′matin. The portion of the cell nucleus that is easily stained by dyes, consisting of nucleic acids and proteins.

chro′matism. 1. Abnormal pigmentation. **2.** Color distortion in an image produced by a lens; also called chromatic aberration.

chromatog′enous. Producing pigmentation or color.

chromat′ogram. The absorbent column containing the stratified constituents separated from a solution by chromatography.

chromatog′raphy. A method of chemical analysis by means of which substances in solution are separated into constituent layers of different colors as they pass through an adsorbent (paper or powder) at different velocities; also called adsorption analysis and chromatographic analysis.

  gas c., differential separation of complex mixtures by vaporizing and diffusing the substance along with a carrier gas through an adsorbent.

  paper c., partition chromatography in which one of the substances being separated adheres to, and forms a film on, filter paper; used in biochemistry to estimate traces of complex organic compounds; also called paper partition chromatography.

  partition c., the separation of similar substances by repeated divisions between immiscible liquids.

  thin-layer c. (TLC), chromatography through a thin layer of an inert material (e.g., cellulose) supported on a glass or plastic plate.

chromatol′ysis. 1. The dissolution of the chromidial (chromophilic) substance (Nissl bodies) in the neuron following injury to the cell body or to the axon. **2.** The destruction of the body of the cell by a specific lysin, leaving only the cell membrane.

chromat′omere. A group of membrane-limited round granules containing a substance thought to have lysosomal properties.

chromatom′eter. See chromometer.

chromat′ophore. A pigment-containing cell.

chromatop′sia. Color vision, abnormal condition in which all objects appear tinged with one particular color; also called chromopsia.

chromatoptom′etry. See chromometry.

chromesthe′sia. 1. Condition in which colors are seen when other senses are stimulated. **2.** The perception of other sensations, such as taste or smell, when colors are seen. **3.** The color sense.

chromid′ium, *pl.* **chromid′ia.** A granule in the cell cytoplasm that stains deeply with basic dyes.

chro′mium. A steel-gray metallic element; symbol

Cr, atomic number 24, atomic weight 52.01.

Chromobacte′rium. A genus of gram-negative flagellated bacteria (family Rhizobiaceae); it produces a violet pigment.

chro′moblast. An embryonic pigment cell.

chromoblastomyco′sis, chromomyco′sis. A chronic infection caused by *Phialophora* or *Cladosporium*, principally in the tropics; the lesion is usually a slow-growing nodule which ulcerates and becomes purplish red to gray and wartlike.

chro′mocyte. A pigmented cell.

chromocytom′eter. An instrument for determining the amount of hemoglobin in red blood cells.

chro′mogen. 1. A substance capable of chemically changing into a pigment. **2.** A pigment-producing organelle.

chromogen′esis. The production of pigment.

chromom′eter. A scale used for testing color perception; also called chromatometer.

chromom′etry. The measuring of color perception; also called chromatoptometry.

chromomyco′sis. See chromoblastomycosis.

chromone′ma, *pl.* **chromone′mata.** A coiled filament which extends the entire length of a chromosome and contains the genes.

chro mophil, chro′mophile. 1. A cell or tissue that stains readily. **2.** Chromaffin.

chromophil′ia. The property of being readily stained; said of certain cells.

chromophil′ic, chromoph′ilous. Staining readily.

chro′mophobe, chromophob′ic. Denoting a cell or tissue that resists staining.

chromopho′bia. 1. Resistance to stains. **2.** Morbid dislike of colors.

chro′mophore. Color radical, a molecular group which is capable of selective absorption of light, resulting in coloration of certain substances.

chromopro′tein. A compound, such as hemoglobin, composed of a pigment and a simple protein.

chromop′sia. See chromatopsia.

chro′moscope. An instrument or scale used in the study and testing of color phenomena as related to color perception.

chro′mosome. One of a group of threadlike structures contained in the nucleus of a cell, composed primarily of genes, or the genetic material DNA; human cells normally have 46, or 23 pairs of chromosomes; one of each pair is contributed by the mother, the other by the father at conception.

  acrocentric c., a chromosome with the centromere placed very close to one end so that the shorter arm is very small.

  c. satellite, a small chromosomal segment separated from the main body of the chromosome by a

secondary constriction; in man usually associated with the short arm of an acrocentric chromosome.

  metacentric c., a chromosome with a centrally placed centromere that divides the chromosome into two arms of approximately equal length.

  Philadelphia (Ph¹) **c.,** an abnormal minute chromosome probably derived from a small acrocentric chromosome (no. 21 or 22) by loss of a large part of the long arm; found in cultured leukocytes of many patients afflicted with chronic myelocytic leukemia.

  sex c.'s, chromosomes responsible for the determination of sex; normally females have two X chromosomes, males have one X and one Y.

  submetacentric c., a chromosome with the centromere so placed that it divides the chromosome into two arms of unequal length.

  telocentric c., a chromosome with a terminal centromere; such chromosomes are unstable and arise by misdivision or breakage within the centromere region.

chromosome aberration. A departure from the normal number of chromosomes; e.g., in Down's syndrome there are 47 chromosomes, in Turner's syndrome there are 45.

chro′naxie, chro′naxy, chro′naxia. The unit which serves as the quantitative index of electric excitability; the time required by an electric current (of twice the minimum strength needed to elicit a threshold response) to pass through a motor nerve and cause a contraction in the associated muscle.

chron′ic. Denoting a disease of slow progress and persisting over a long period of time; opposite of acute.

chronic brain syndrome. Impairment of brain function, usually permanent, manifested by faulty memory, judgement, comprehension, and orientation; secondary to other conditions such as alcoholism, senility, cerebrovascular disease, etc.

chronic granulomatous disease. A congenital hereditary susceptibility to severe infection caused by the inability of polymorphonuclear leukocytes to destory bacteria; also called congenital dysphagocytosis.

chronobio′logy. The study of the duration of life and ways of prolonging it; see also geriatrics and gerontology.

chronogno′sis. Perception of the passage of time.

chron′ograph. An instrument used for graphically recording short periods of time, as the duration of an event or episode.

chronopho′tograph. One of a series of photographs showing motion.

chronotarax′is. Confusion relating to the passage of time.

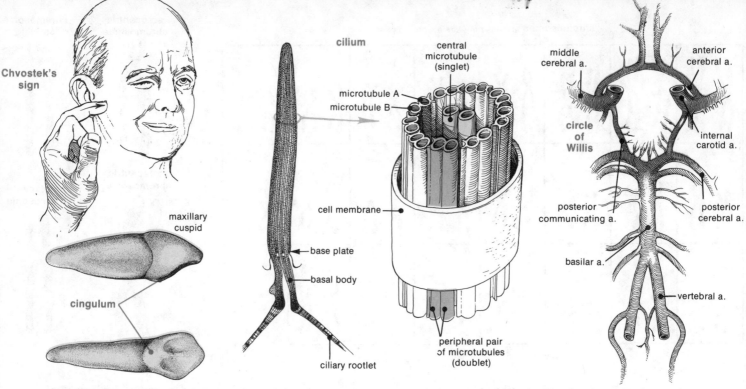

Chvostek's sign

maxillary cuspid

cingulum

cilium

central microtubule (singlet)

microtubule A
microtubule B

cell membrane

base plate

basal body

ciliary rootlet

peripheral pair of microtubules (doublet)

middle cerebral a.

anterior cerebral a.

circle of Willis

internal carotid a.

posterior communicating a.

posterior cerebral a.

basilar a.

vertebral a.

chronot′ropism. Modification of the rate of a regular periodic movement, as of the heart beat.

chrysi′asis. Deposition of gold in the tissues following administration of gold salts; also called auriasis.

chryso-, chrys-. Combining forms denoting gold.

chrysother′apy. The therapeutic administration of gold salts; also called aurotherapy.

Chvostek's sign. A unilateral spasm of facial muscles elicited by a slight tap over the facial nerve; seen in tetany; also called Weiss' sign.

chyle. A milky fluid composed of lymph and digested fat, absorbed into the lymphatic capillaries (lacteals) from the intestine during digestion; it is transported by the thoracic duct to the left subclavian vein where it becomes mixed with the blood.

chylo-, chyl-. Combining forms denoting a relationship to chyle.

chylomi′crons. Minute fat particles (about one μ in size) present in lymph which normally are quickly cleared from the blood.

chylomicrone′mia. Increased number of microscopic particles of fat (chylomicrons) in the blood.

chylopericar′dium. A milky effusion into the pericardium due to injury or to obstruction of the thoracic duct.

chyloperitone′um. Accumulation of a milky liquid in the peritoneal cavity; also called chylous ascites.

chylopoie′sis. The formation of chyle.

chylotho′rax. The collection of a milky fluid of lymphatic origin (chyle) in the pleural cavity.

chylu′ria. The presence of chyle or lymph in the urine, giving it a white, turbid appearance.

chyme′. The semifluid mass of food passed from the stomach to the duodenum.

chymopoie′sis. The conversion of food into chyme, also called chymification.

chy′mosin. See rennin.

chymotryp′sin. A digestive enzyme (proteinase) present in pancreatic juice; proposed for use in the treatment of inflammation and edema caused by trauma.

chymotrypsin′ogen. Pancreatic enzyme that gives rise to chymotrypsin.

Ci. Abbreviation for curie.

μCi. Abbreviation for microcurie.

cicatrec′tomy. Surgical removal of a scar.

cica′trix. The fibrous tissue formed during the healing of a wound; also called scar.

cicatriza′tion. The formation of scar tissue.

cil′ia. Plural of cilium.

ciliarot′omy. An incision through the peripheral region of the anterior surface of the iris (ciliary zone).

cil′iary. Relating to (a) any hairlike process; (b) the eyelashes; (c) certain structures of the eye.

cil′iated. Having hairlike processes.

cilioreti′nal. Relating to the ciliary body and the retina.

cil′ium, pl. **cil′ia. 1.** A microscopic hairlike projection on a cell surface capable of vibratory or lashing movements. **2.** Eyelash.

cillo′sis. Twitching of the eyelids; also called ciliosis.

cim′bia. A band of white fibers across the ventral surface of the cerebral peduncle.

cincho′na. Any of various trees of the genus *Cinchona,* found in South America, whose bark contains quinine and a number of alkaloids.

cin′chonism. Toxic condition resulting from an overdose of cinchona or its alkaloids, marked by headache, deafness, giddiness, and ringing in the ears; also called quininism.

cine-. Combining form meaning movement; for words beginning thus and not found here see kin- and kine-.

cineangiocardiog′raphy. The production of motion picture films showing, fluoroscopically, contrast medium passing through the heart chambers and great vessels.

cineangiog′raphy. The production of motion picture films of the passage of a radiopaque substance through blood vessels.

cinefluorog′raphy. The production of motion picture film of fluoroscopic observations.

cinegastros′copy. Motion pictures of the interior of the stomach.

cinemicrog′raphy. The producing of motion picture films through a microscope.

cineradiog′raphy. The production of motion picture films of sequential images appearing on a fluoroscopic screen; also called cineroentgenography.

cineroentgenog′raphy. See cineradiography.

cinesal′gia. Kinesalgia.

cin′gulum. 1. A band of association fibers in the brain that partly encircle the corpus callosum. **2.** A U-shaped enamel ridge on the lingual surface of incisor teeth.

cingulumot′omy. Creation of a precisely placed leukotome lesion in the cingulum of the frontal lobe to relieve intractable pain and emotional anguish.

cir′ca (ca). Latin for approximately.

circa′dian. Denoting the rhythm of biologic phenomena that cycle approximately every 24 hours; e.g., in persons who sleep at night ACTH (and cortisol) secretion begins to rise in the early morning hours, peaks at the time of awakening, and falls to low values in the evening.

cir′cinate. Ring-shaped.

cir′cle. A ring-shaped anatomic structure.

  c. of Willis, a circle of anastomosing arteries at the base of the brain; also called circulus arteriosus.

cir′cuit. The path followed by an electric current.

circula′tion. Movement through a circular course, as of the blood through bodily vessels.

  collateral c., circulation of blood taking place through small anastomosing vessels when the main course is obstructed.

  coronary c., circulation taking place through the system of blood vessels supplying the heart muscles.

  fetal c., blood supply to the fetus during intrauterine life through the placenta and umbilical cord.

  lymph c., The flow of lymph through lymphatic vessels and glands.

  placental c., the flow of blood through the placenta which transfers oxygen and nutritive materials from mother to fetus and carbon dioxide and waste products from fetus to mother.

  portal c., circulation of blood through capillaries in the liver from the portal to the hepatic veins.

  pulmonary c., the flow of blood from the heart, through the pulmonary artery and lungs, and back to the heart through the pulmonary veins.

  systemic c., general circulation, circulation throughout the whole body.

cir′culus, pl. **cir′culi.** Latin for circle.

circum-. Prefix meaning around or on all sides.

circumci′sion. The removal of a circular portion of the foreskin or prepuce.

circumduc′tion. The circular movement of a part, as of a limb or eye.

cir′cumflex. Denoting certain arched anatomic structures.

circumnu′clear. Surrounding a nucleus.

circumoc′ular. Surrounding the eye.

circumo′ral. Around the mouth.

cir′cumscribed. Confined within bounds; encircled.

circumval′late. Any structure surrounded by a raised ring.

circumvol′ute. Coiled or twisted around a central axis.

cirrho′sis. A chronic disease of the liver marked by a loss of normal lobular architecture, with nodular regeneration of parenchymal cells separated by fibrous septa, and by vascular derangement and anastomoses; these structural abnormalities interfere with liver function and circulation, and ultimately cause death.

  alcoholic c., variable fatty change of liver cells in small, uniform, regenerative nodules which replace the lobular architecture of the entire liver; each nodule is surrounded by thin septa of connective tissue; the color varies between brown and yellow,

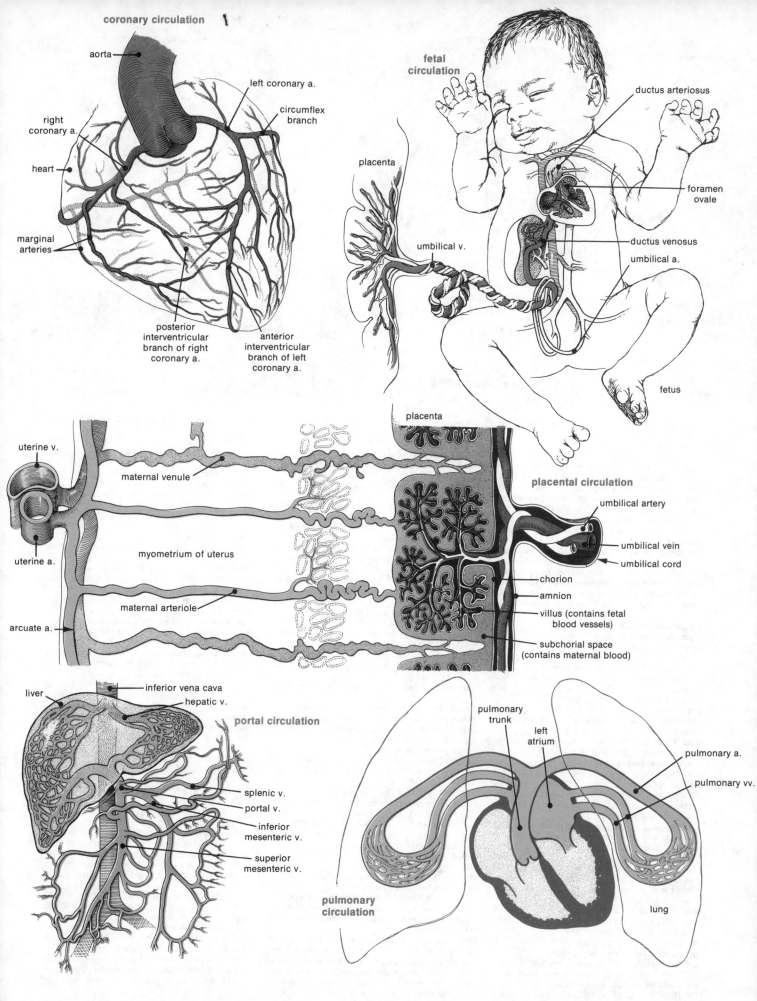

coronary circulation

aorta

left coronary a.

circumflex branch

right coronary a.

heart

marginal arteries

posterior interventricular branch of right coronary a.

anterior interventricular branch of left coronary a.

fetal circulation

placenta

umbilical v.

ductus arteriosus

foramen ovale

ductus venosus

umbilical a.

fetus

uterine v.

maternal venule

myometrium of uterus

uterine a.

maternal arteriole

arcuate a.

placenta

placental circulation

umbilical artery

umbilical vein

umbilical cord

chorion

amnion

villus (contains fetal blood vessels)

subchorial space (contains maternal blood)

liver

inferior vena cava

hepatic v.

portal circulation

splenic v.

portal v.

inferior mesenteric v.

superior mesenteric v.

pulmonary trunk

left atrium

pulmonary a.

pulmonary vv.

pulmonary circulation

lung

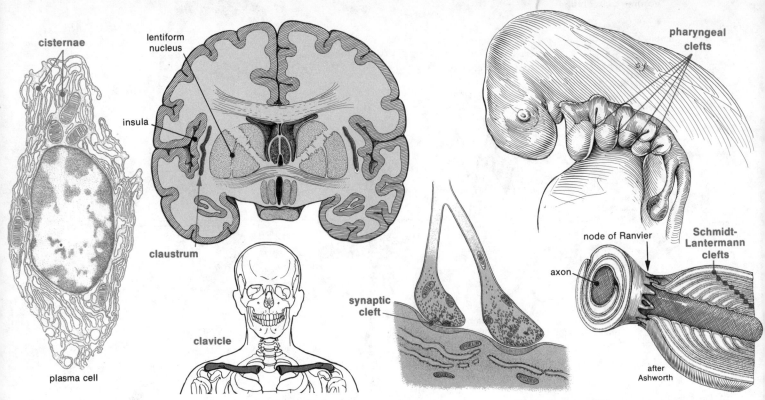

cisternae

lentiform nucleus

insula

claustrum

clavicle

plasma cell

pharyngeal clefts

node of Ranvier

axon

synaptic cleft

Schmidt-Lantermann clefts

after Ashworth

determined by the amount of fatty deposition; also called Laënnec's or portal cirrhosis.

biliary c., any of several morphologically and etiologically different types of cirrhosis which have in common a long history of extra- or intra-hepatic suppression of bile flow, and an enlarged, firm, finely granular liver with a green hue; extensions of connective tissue septa into the lobular parenchyma are sparse; regenerative nodules are rare.

cardiac c., an extensive centrilobular fibrotic reaction, as in chronic passive hepatic congestion from any cause.

cryptogenic c., cirrhosis in which nodularity and distribution of fibrous tissue is more variable than in alcoholic cirrhosis; functional derangement is the same as other types, and fatty change is rare; cause is often unknown, but may result from chronic or recurrent viral hepatitis or from autoimmune liver disease.

Laënnec's c., see alcoholic cirrhosis.

portal c., see alcoholic cirrhosis.

postnecrotic c., cirrhosis caused by massive necrosis involving multiple lobules, with collapse of the reticular framework to form large scars alternating with large nodules of regenerated or residual liver.

cirrho′tic. Affected with cirrhosis.

cis-. Prefix meaning location on the same or the near side. For terms beginning with *cis*, see under specific term.

cister′na. Any dilatation or enclosed space serving as a reservoir for lymph or other body fluid.

c. cerebellomedullaris, see cisterna magna.

c. chyli, the triangular dilatation at the beginning of the thoracic duct, situated in front of the second lumbar vertebra; it receives two lumbar lymphatic trunks and the intestinal lymphatic trunk; also called receptaculum chyli.

c. magna, c. cerebellomedullaris, the large subarachnoid space between the medulla oblongata and the under side of the cerebellum.

subarachnoid c., one of several intercommunicating spaces at the base of the brain formed by the separation of the arachnoid from the pia mater.

cister′nal. Relating to any fluid-containing sac or cavity in the body.

cis′tron. The smallest hereditary unit of function; the section of the DNA molecule that specifies a particular biochemical function.

cit′rate. A salt of citric acid.

cit′rated. Containing a salt of citric acid.

cit′ric acid. A colorless crystalline acid, $C_6H_8 \cdot O_7H_2O$, present in the juice of citrus fruits.

citrovorum factor. See folinic acid.

Ciuffini-Pancoast syndrome. See Pancoast's

syndrome.

clamp. An instrument used to compress a part.

clap. Slang expression for gonorrhea.

clarif′icant. Any agent that clears a turbid liquid.

class. A biologic category ranking below a phylum and above an order.

classifica′tion. A systematic grouping into categories.

Angle's c., a list of the several forms of malocclusion grouped into four main classes.

Caldwell-Moloy c., a classification of the different types of the female pelvis.

Duke's c., classification of the degree of spread of operable carcinoma of the large intestine in surgical specimen.

Lancefield's c., the division of streptococci into several categories by means of specific precipitin reactions.

clast′ic. Having a tendency to break or divide.

claudica′tion. Limping.

intermittent c., condition marked by cramplike pains and weakness of legs induced by walking, and the disappearance of all discomfort when at rest; caused by sclerosis with narrowing of the arteries of the legs.

claustropho′bia. A morbid fear of confined spaces.

clau′strum. An anatomic structure resembling a barrier, as the thin layer of grey matter on the lateral surface of the external capsule of the brain, separating the insula from the lentiform nucleus.

c. virginale, the hymen.

cla′va. The swelling on the back side of the medulla oblongata, which contains the gracile nucleus; also called gracile tubercle.

clav′icle. Either of two long, curved bones extending from the sternum to the acromion and forming the anterior half of the shoulder girdle; its medial end articulates with the sternum and the first rib and is the only bony attachment between the upper extremity and the trunk; also called collarbone.

clavicot′omy. Surgical division of a clavicle.

cla′vus. Latin for corn.

claw′foot. A disabling deformity of the foot in which the longitudinal arch is extremely high, the toes are clawed, and the forefoot is dropped; it may be congenital or acquired (from polio or diseases of the central nervous system); also called pes cavus and cavus foot.

clear′ance. 1. Removal of a substance from the blood by an excretory organ such as the kidney, usually expressed in terms of the milliliters of blood that would contain the amount of substance removed per minute; a virtual volume per unit of time; the standard clearance formula is $C = UV/P$;

C = clearance in milliliters per minute; U = urine concentration of a substance; P = plasma concentration of the substance; V = urine flow in milliliters per minute. **2.** The space existing between apposed structures.

creatinine c., the renal clearance of creatinine, used clinically as an indicator of the glomerular filtration rate and usually based on the clearance of endogenous creatinine; in some experimental situations exogenous creatinine may be infused to raise creatinine levels and provide greater accuracy in the determination.

immune c., clearance of antigen from the blood resulting from complexing with antibodies.

inulin c., the most precise of the commonly used measures of glomerular filtration rate, since inulin is freely filtered but neither secreted nor reabsorbed by the tubules; requires infusion of inulin since this substance occurs naturally only in plants.

occlusal c., in dentistry, condition in which the upper and lower teeth pass one another horizontally without contact or interference.

osmolar c., the volume of blood which would contain the number of osmolar particles excreted by the kidney in one minute.

PAH c., an approximate measure of renal blood flow; when combined with the extraction ratio, a more precise value is obtained.

urea c., the volume of blood which would be cleared of urea by one minute's excretion of urine; formerly a standard procedure for assessment of renal function; maximum urea clearance is approximately 60 per cent of inulin clearance.

cleav′age. 1. The first stages of cell division after the egg is fertilized. **2.** The splitting up of a molecule into two or more simpler ones.

cleft. A fissure.

branchial c., see pharyngeal clefts.

c. palate, see palate, cleft.

pharyngeal c.'s, a series of ectodermal grooves on the surface of an embryo, along the lateral walls of the pharyngeal gut, corresponding to the pharyngeal pouches; they usually appear during the fourth or fifth weeks of development; also called branchial clefts.

synaptic c., the space, usually 200 to 300 Å, between the presynaptic terminal knob and the apposing postsynaptic neuron.

Schmidt-Lantermann c., the funnel-shaped intrusion of cytoplasm in the myelin lamellae around the axon of a nerve cell; thought to play a role in the transport of nutrients through the supporting cell.

clenched fist sign. The gesture of a patient with angina pectoris; he presses his chest with his clenched fist.

cirrhosis | clenched fist sign

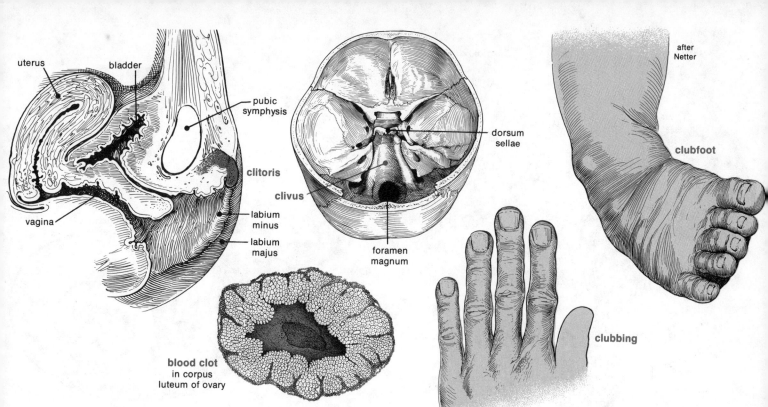

uterus
bladder
pubic symphysis
clitoris
vagina
labium minus
labium majus

dorsum sellae
clivus
foramen magnum

after Netter
clubfoot

clubbing

blood clot
in corpus
luteum of ovary

cle′oid. A dental carving instrument.
click. A sharp sound.
  ejection c., a sharp cardiac sound heard in early systole over the area of the aorta or the pulmonary artery when these vessels are dilated.
  mitral c., the opening sound of the mitral valve.
  systolic c., a sharp cardiac sound heard during systole; a midsystolic click (whether or not followed by a late systolic murmur) often seems to indicate a floppy mitral valve leaflet.
cli′dal. Of or relating to a clavicle.
clidarthri′tis. 1. Gouty pain in the clavicle. **2.** Inflammation of the articular portions of the clavicle.
clidocos′tal. Pertaining to the clavicle and ribs.
clidot′omy. Surgical division of the clavicles of a dead fetus to facilitate its delivery.
climac′ter. See climacteric.
climac′teric. A critical period of life when physiologic changes take place; known as menopause for women and male climacteric for men; also called climacterium and climacter.
climacte′rium. See climacteric.
climatol′ogy. The study of climate in relation to health and disease.
climatother′apy. Treatment of disease by moving the patient to a suitable climate.
cli′max. 1. The height or crisis of a disease. **2.** Orgasm.
clin′ic. 1. An institution where treatment is given to patients not requiring hospitalization. **2.** Medical instruction given to students in which patients are examined and treated in their presence. **3.** An establishment run by medical specialists working cooperatively.
clin′ical. 1. Relating to the bedside observation of the course and symptoms of a disease. **2.** Relating to a clinic.
clinician. A practicing physician.
clinicopathologic′ic. Relating to the signs and symptoms of a disease and the laboratory study of specimens obtained through biopsy or autopsy.
  c. conference (CPC), a teaching conference in which the patient's case is discussed followed by the presentation of pathologic data.
clinoceph′aly. Congenital deformity marked by flatness or concavity of the upper part of the skull; also called saddle head.
clinodac′tyly. Permanent deviation (lateral or medial) of one or more fingers.
cli′noid. Resembling a bed; said of certain anatomic structures, as the clinoid process of the sphenoid bone.
cli′noscope. Instrument to measure cyclophoria (tendency of one eye to deviate).

clithropho′bia. Abnormal fear of being locked in.
clitoridec′tomy. Surgical removal of the clitoris.
clit′oris. A small, cylindric organ situated at the anterior part of the vulva, homologous with the penis.
clit′orism. 1. Prolonged, usually painful, erection of the clitoris. **2.** Abnormally large clitoris.
clitoromeg′aly. Enlargement of the clitoris.
cli′vus. The internal slope at the base of the skull, from the front of the foramen magnum to the dorsum sellae and formed by the basilar portion of the occipital bone and the body of the sphenoid bone; it supports the pons and the medulla oblongata.
cloa′ca. 1. The cavity into which the intestinal, urinary, and genital tracts open in certain animals. **2.** The combined intestinal and urogenital opening in the embryo.
clofi′brate. p-Chlorophenoxyisobutyrate; a lipid-lowering drug used in the treatment of hyperlipidemia; Atromid-S®.
clon′al. Of or relating to a clone.
clone, clon. A colony of genetically identical cells derived from a single cell by asexual division.
clon′ic. Characterized by alternate contraction and relaxation of muscles.
clonicoton′ic. Characterized by rapid alternate contraction and relaxation (clonic) and continued tension (tonic); said of certain muscular spasms.
clonorchio′sis. Disease, prevalent in the Far East, caused by invasion of the bile ducts by Clonorchis sinensis; transmitted to man by ingestion of raw or undercooked freshwater fish infected with larvae.
Clonor′chis. A genus of flukes (family Opisthorchiidae) having both sets of sex organs in the same worm, in which self-fertilization often occurs; some species are parasitic in the liver of man.
  C. sinensis, the cause of clonorchiosis; also called Chinese liver fluke.
clon′us. A spasm in which contraction and relaxation of a muscle alternate in rapid succession.
Clostrid′ium. A genus of bacteria (family Bacillaceae) characterized by gram-positive, motile (occasionally nonmotile), anaerobic, or aerotolerant rods; some species produce putrefaction of proteins.
  C. bifermentans, a species found in putrid meat, gaseous gangrene, and soil; some strains are pathogenic.
  C. botulinum, a species that produces botulinum toxin, the cause of food poisoning (botulism); there are five types (A to E), each of which elaborate an immunologically distinct form of exotoxin; the toxins of types A, B, and E cause human illness, with type A toxin being responsible for the severest and most common intoxications; formerly called Bacillus botulinus.

  C. haemolyticum, a species producing a hemolytic toxin; found in cattle afflicted with icterohemoglobinuria or red-water disease.
  C. novyi, a species producing a powerful exotoxin; pathogenic for man and animals; classified into three immunologic types, A, B, and C.
  C. perfringens, a species consisting of short encapsulated rods; the chief cause of gas gangrene; also the cause of enterotoxemia in cattle, sheep, and man; found in soil and milk; also called Clostridium welchii and gas bacillus; formerly called Welch's bacillus.
  C. septicum, a species producing a lethal and hemolytic exotoxin; found in the intestines and in manured soil.
  C. tetani, a species consisting of motile rods with a drumstick shape, producing an exotoxin with affinity for motor nerve centers; the cause of tetanus or lockjaw; found in soil and wounds; formerly called Bacillus tetani.
  C. welchii, see Clostridium perfringens.
clo′sure. 1. The act of closing or the state of being closed. **2.** The conclusion of a reflex pathway.
clot. 1. A thrombus. **2.** To coagulate.
  blood c., a solidified elastic mass of fibrin enmeshing platelets, red blood cells, and white blood cells; produced when whole blood coagulates.
club′bing. Broadening and thickening of the soft tissues of the ends of fingers or toes.
club′foot. One of the most common congenital deformities of the foot in which only the outer portion of the ball of the foot touches the ground; the ankle is plantar flexed, the foot is inverted, and the anterior half of the foot is directed toward the midline; also called talipes equinovarus.
clump. 1. To aggregate; to form a cluster. **2.** A mass so formed.
clump′ing. The clustering of bacteria or other cells suspended in a liquid.
-clysis. Combining form denoting injection.
clysis. Infusion of fluid into the body.
Cm. Chemical symbol of the element curium.
cm. Abbreviation for centimeter.
CMP. Abbreviation for cytidine monophosphate.
CMV. Abbreviation for cytomegalovirus.
CN. The cyanide radical.
CNS. Abbreviation for central nervous system.
Co. Chemical symbol of the element cobalt.
Co I. Abbreviation for coenzyme I; currently called NAD.
Co II. Abbreviation for coenzyme II; currently called NADP.
Co III. Abbreviation for coenzyme III.
CoA. Abbreviation for coenzyme A.
coagglut′inin. A substance that causes agglutina-

cleoid | coagglutinin

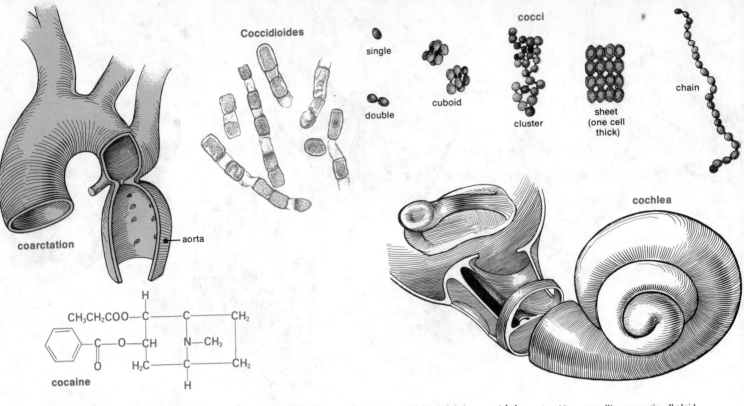

single

double

cuboid

cocci

cluster

sheet
(one cell
thick)

chain

Coccidioides

cochlea

coarctation

aorta

$CH_3CH_2COO-C \quad C \quad CH_2$

cocaine

tion of antigen only in the presence of univalent antibody; by itself it does not cause agglutination.

coag′ulable. Capable of clotting.

coag′ulant. 1. Causing coagulation or clotting. **2.** A substance that causes clotting.

coag′ulase. In microbiology, an extracellular enzyme or complex that promotes plasma coagulation and is clinically associated with disease production.

coag′ulate. 1. To cause the conversion of a fluid into a semisolid mass. **2.** To become such a mass.

coag′ulation. 1. Clotting; the conversion of a fluid into a jellylike solid. **2.** A clot.

coag′ulative. Causing coagulation.

coag′ulin. An antibody that causes coagulation of its antigen.

coagulop′athy. A disease affecting the blood-clotting process.

consumption c., condition marked by great reduction in the circulating levels of platelets and of certain coagulation factors; due to utilization of platelets in excessive blood clotting throughout the body.

coag′ulum, *pl.* **coag′ula.** A clot; a curd.

coapta′tion. The fitting together of parts, as the ends of a broken bone.

coarct′. To press together; to constrict.

coarcta′tion. A narrowing or constriction, as of a blood vessel.

coat. A membrane or layer of tissue.

cobal′amin. A general term for a member of the vitamin B_{12} group.

co′balt. A hard, brittle, steel-gray metallic element; symbol Co, atomic number 27, atomic weight 58.94; cobalt ingestion has been associated with cardiomyopathy.

co′balt-60. A radioactive isotope of cobalt, used in radiotherapy.

cobral′ysin. The substance in cobra venom that destroys red blood cells.

co′ca. A tree, *Erythroxylon coca*, with leaves that contain cocaine and other alkaloids.

cocaine′. A crystalline narcotic alkaloid, colorless or white, extracted from coca leaves; used as a local anesthetic; also called coke and snow (street expressions).

co′cainism. The habitual use of cocaine.

co′cainize. To anesthetize by the administration of cocaine.

cocarbox′ylase. See thiamine pyrophosphate.

cocarcin′ogen. An agent that increases the activity of a carcinogen.

coc′ci. Plural of coccus.

Coccid′ia. An order of protozoans, some of which are pathogenic and parasitic in the epithelium of the small intestine.

Coccidioi′des. A genus of zygomycetous fungi, some of which are parasitic in man.

C. immitis, a species of fungi causing coccidioimycosis; also called *Blastomyces coccidioides*.

coccidioidomyco′sis. A disease caused by the fungus *Coccidioides immitis,* affecting primarily the lungs; it is frequently asymptomatic and rarely disseminated; the disease is endemic in desert areas of the United States; one benign form is known as desert or San Joaquin Valley fever.

coccidio′sis. Disease of certain vertebrates caused by any protozoans of the order Coccidia; in man, the infection is self-limiting and accompanied by nausea and diarrhea.

coccobacil′lus. An oval-shaped microorganism.

coc′coid. Resembling a spherical bacterium (coccus).

coc′cus, *pl.* **coc′ci.** A bacterium of round or oval shape.

coccyal′gia. See coccydynia.

coccydyn′ia. Pain in the coccygeal region, frequently caused by a fall upon the buttocks; also called coccygodynia and coccyalgia.

coccyg′eal. Relating to or located in the proximity of the coccyx.

coccygec′tomy. Surgical removal of the coccyx.

coccygodyn′ia. See coccydynia.

coc′cyx, *pl.* **coc′cyges.** Three or four small, fused, rudimentary vertebrae, forming the caudal extremity of the vertebral column.

coch′lea. The spiral cavity in the internal ear; the essential organ of hearing containing the membranous cochlear duct in which the spiral organ of Corti with its nerve endings is located.

coch′lear. Of or relating to the cochlea.

cochleare magnum (coch. mag.) Latin for tablespoonful.

cochleovestib′ular. Relating to the cochlea and the vestibule of the ear.

cochli′tis. Inflammation of the cochlea.

coch. mag. Abbreviation for Latin *cochleare magnum.*

code. 1. A systematic collection of rules. **2.** A system of symbols used for transmitting information.

genetic c., the pattern of three adjacent nucleotides in a DNA molecule that controls protein synthesis.

codecarbox′ylase. A coenzyme of various amino acid decarboxylases; also called pyridoxal phosphate.

codehy′drogenase I. See nicotinamide adenine dinucleotide.

codehy′drogenase II. See nicotinamide adenine dinucleotide phosphate.

co′deine. A white, crystalline narcotic alkaloid obtained from opium or morphine, used for the relief of cough and as an analgesic.

co′don. A group of usually three adjacent nucleotides that code or specify the insertion of a specific amino acid during protein synthesis.

coefficient. A numerical measure of the effect or change produced by variations of specified conditions, or of the ratio between two quantities.

c. of absorption, (1) the milliliters of a gas that will saturate 100 ml of liquid, at standard temperature and pressure; (2) in radiology, the constant for radiation of a given wavelength, the value of which depends on the atomic number of the substance through which the radiation passes.

c. of relationship, the probability that two persons with a common ancestor have a common gene that came from that ancestor.

correlation c., a measure of the closeness of the relationships between variables; a value of 1 represents perfect correlation and 0 represents no relationship; the sign of the correlation coefficient is positive when the variables move in the same direction (height vs. weight) and negative when they move in opposite directions (life expectancy vs. weight).

distribution c., the constant ratio in which a substance, soluble in two immiscible solvents, distributes itself in equilibrium between the two solvents; the basis of many chromatographic separation procedures; also called partition coefficient.

partition c., see distribution coefficient.

phenol c., see Rideal-Walker coefficient.

Poiseuille's viscosity c., the ratio of the shearing force per unit area between two parallel layers of a liquid in motion, to the velocity gradient between the layers; a numerical measure of the viscosity as determined by the capillary tube method; usually symbolized by η.

Rideal-Walker c., the ratio of bactericidal effectiveness of a germicide compared to that of phenol as a standard; the disinfecting power of the substance is obtained by dividing the figure indicating the degree of dilution of the germicide that destroys a microorganism in a given time by that indicating the degree of dilution of phenol which destroys the same organism in the same time under the same conditions; also called phenol coefficient.

temperature c., the fractional change in any physical property per degree rise in temperature.

coe′lom. Celom.

coen′zyme. A nonprotein organic compound, produced by living cells, which plays an intimate and frequently essential role in the activation of enzymes; e.g., thiamine, riboflavin, etc.

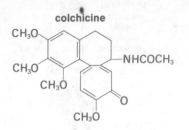

colchicine

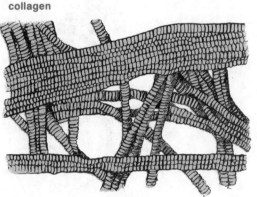

collagen

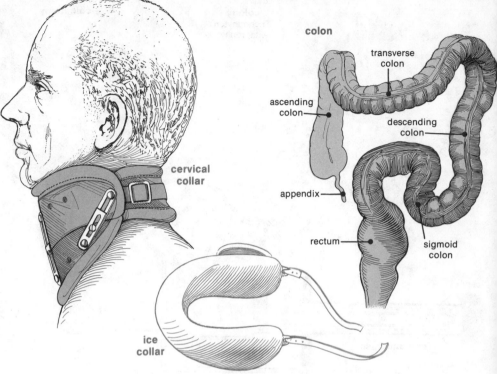

cervical collar

ice collar

colon

transverse colon

ascending colon

descending colon

appendix

rectum

sigmoid colon

---

c. III (ColII), a nucleotide containing nicotinamide which functions in oxidation of cysteine.

c. A (CoA), the "active" acetate.

coeur. French for heart.

c. en sabot, the characteristic x-ray appearance of the heart in tetralogy of Fallot; it vaguely resembles a wooden shoe.

co'factor. A substance that is essential to bring about the action of an enzyme.

cogni'tion. 1. The intellectual process by which knowledge is acquired, as opposed to emotional processes. **2.** The product of this process; also called comprehension; judgment; perception.

cohe'sion. The mutual attraction by which the molecules of a substance are held together.

coin-counting. A sliding movement of the tips of thumb and index finger against each other, occurring in paralysis agitans.

co'ition. Coitus.

co'itus. Copulation; sexual intercourse.

c. interruptus, sexual intercourse intentionally interrupted by withdrawal immediately prior to ejaculation; also called interrupted or incomplete coitus.

c. reservatus, sexual intercourse in which ejaculation is purposely suppressed; also called reserved coitus.

co'la. See kola.

col'chicine. An alkaloid obtained from colchicum; used in the treatment of acute gout.

cold. Common cold; a symptom complex due to a viral infection of the respiratory tract; marked by nasal discharge, sneezing, some malaise, and usually without fever.

chest c., bronchitis.

head c., coryza; rhinitis.

cold sore. A small lesion, usually on the lips, caused by the virus herpes simplex; often accompanies a fever or cold or exposure to the sun; also called fever blister.

cold turkey. Slang for the withdrawal from an addiction to a narcotic drug by abruptly discontinuing rather than tapering the dosage or substituting another drug; the name is derived from the goose bumps that appear on the body making the skin resemble that of a plucked fowl.

colec'tomy. Surgical removal of the colon, or a segment of it.

colibacillu'ria. The presence of *Escherichia coli* in a urine specimen that has been aseptically obtained; also called coliuria.

col'ic. 1. Relating to the colon. **2.** Acute abdominal pain. **3.** A symptom complex seen in infants under three months of age, characterized by paroxysmal abdominal pain and frantic crying.

biliary c., severe pain caused by the passage of a gallstone through the bile duct.

intestinal c., more or less severe pain caused by spasm of smooth muscle, as in gallstones, appendicitis, lead poisoning, or air-swallowing.

lead c., abdominal pain caused by lead poisoning.

renal c., one caused by the impaction or passage of a stone along the ureter or renal pelvis.

ureteral c., severe pains caused by obstruction of the ureter.

co'liform. Resembling the colon bacillus (*Escherichia coli*).

coli'tis. Inflammation of the colon.

granulomatous c., a disease of the colon which produces lesions involving all layers, resembling the changes produced in the ileum by regional enteritis (inflammation of the intestine).

mucous c., irritable colon; see under colon.

spastic c., irritable colon; see under colon.

ulcerative c., a chronic disease of unknown cause marked by ulceration of the mucosa and submucosa of the colon with bleeding and malnutrition.

coliuria. See colibacilluria.

col'lagen. The supportive protein component of connective tissue, bone, cartilage, and skin; converted into gelatin by boiling.

collag'enase. An enzyme that promotes the breakdown of collagen.

collagen diseases. A group of diseases having in common such histologic features as inflammatory damage to connective tissues and blood vessels with deposition of fibrinoid material; included in this group are such disorders as systemic lupus erythematosus, polyarteritis nodosa, dermatomyositis, scleroderma, and rheumatoid arthritis; also called connective tissue diseases.

collageno'sis. Collagen diseases.

collapse. 1. A state of extreme prostration. **2.** The act of caving in.

col'lar. 1. A band or device, usually one encircling the neck. **2.** An encircling anatomic structure.

cervical c., a device generally used to support, stabilize, immobilize, or hyperextend the neck in cases where a rigid cast or bracing is not indicated.

ice c., a rubber bag designed to be filled with crushed ice and placed on the neck to produce cooling, as in postoperative care of tonsillectomies.

col'larbone. See clavicle.

collat'eral. Secondary, auxiliary, or alternate.

collic'ulus, *pl.* **collic'uli.** A small elevation, as in the roof of the midbrain.

collig'ative. In physical chemistry, denotes dependence on the number of particles (molecules, atoms, or ions) present in a given space, rather than on their nature; applied to solutions.

collima'tion. The controlling of the size of x-ray beam spread by use of lead plates placed in front of the primary roentgen ray beam.

collima'tor. An apparatus, often consisting of a pair of lead plates, used to confine a beam of radiation within a specific area.

colliqua'tion. The degeneration of tissue with subsequent conversion into a liquid-like form (liquefaction).

ballooning c., liquefaction of the cell protoplasm leading to edematous swelling and softening; also called ballooning degeneration.

colliq'uative. 1. Denoting an excessive watery discharge. **2.** Characterized by liquefaction of tissues.

collo'dion. A colorless, flammable, syrupy solution of pyroxylin or gun cotton in ether and alcohol; used as a protective coat for cuts and surgical dressings and as a support film on copper grids in election microscopy; also called collodium.

collo'dium. See collodion.

col'loid. 1. A gluelike substance, such as gelatin, consisting of a suspension of submicroscopic particles in a continuous medium. **2.** A yellowish, gelatinous material present in the tissues as a result of colloid degeneration.

col'lum. 1. Latin for neck. **2.** Any necklike structure.

c. anatomicum humeri, anatomic neck of the humerus; a narrow groove separating the head of the humerus from its tubercles; it affords attachment to the capsular ligament of the shoulder-joint.

c. chirurgicum humeri, surgical neck of the humerus; the constriction below the tubercles of the humerus; a frequent site of fractures.

c. femoris, a more or less conical portion of bone separating the head and shaft of the femur; also called neck of femur.

c. tali, a constriction separating the head from the body of the ankle bone (talus); also called neck of talus.

colobo'ma. Any defect in which a portion of a structure, especially of the eye, is absent; it may be congenital, pathologic, or artificial.

colocol'ic. Denoting a surgical joining of one part of the colon to another.

colol'ysis. Freeing the colon from adhesions.

co'lon. Portion of the large intestine extending from the cecum to the rectum.

ascending c., the part of the colon extending upward on the right side of the abdomen from the cecum to the hepatic flexure.

descending c., the part of the colon extending downward on the left side of the abdomen from the splenic flexure to the sigmoid colon.

irritable c., a condition marked by abdominal

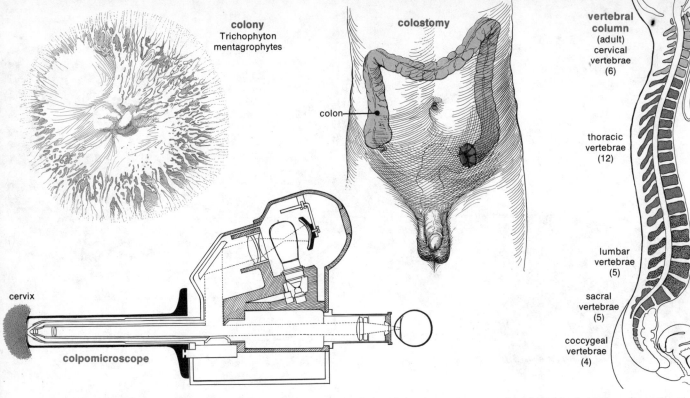

colony
Trichophyton mentagrophytes

colostomy

colon

vertebral column
(adult)
cervical vertebrae (6)

thoracic vertebrae (12)

lumbar vertebrae (5)

sacral vertebrae (5)

coccygeal vertebrae (4)

cervix

colpomicroscope

pain, gas, constipation or diarrhea, and the passage of mucus; it usually starts in adolescence or early adult life, and the attacks frequently coincide with emotional stress; also called irritable bowel syndrome, spastic or mucous colitis, and spastic colon.

lead pipe c., a term applied to the radiologic appearance of a scarred, contracted, and rigid colon, usually the consequence of advanced ulcerative colitis.

sigmoid c., the S-shaped part of the colon in the pelvis between the descending colon and rectum.

spastic c., see irritable colon.

transverse c., the portion of the colon which crosses the abdomen from the hepatic flexure to the splenic flexure.

colon'ic. Of or relating to the colon.

coloniza'tion. 1. Innidiation; metastasis. **2.** The act of forming compact groups or colonies, e.g., the developing of colonies of the same type of microorganisms, or grouping and caring for individuals with a common disease, as leprosy.

colonorrha'gia. See colorrhagia.

colonorrhe'a. See colorrhea.

colonos'copy. Examination of the upper portion of the rectum with an endoscope.

col'ony. A visible group or growth of microorganisms on a solid medium, presumably arising from a single microorganism.

M-type c., mucoid c., a usually virulent colony marked by a well developed carbohydrate capsule which may act as a defense mechanism.

R-type c., rough c., a nonvirulent or slightly virulent colony having a granular growth, irregular margins, and flat surface.

S-type c., smooth c., a colony presenting a round, even, smooth surface; some capsule-forming species have a degree of virulence.

co'lopexy, colopex'ia. Shortening of an elongated gastrocolic omentum by means of sutures for the purpose of supporting a prolapsed transverse colon; a supplementary procedure in the correction of a prolapsed stomach.

coloproc'titis. Inflammation of the colon and rectum; also called proctocolitis and rectocolitis.

col'or. A visual perception characterized by the attributes of brightness, hue, and saturation, arising from stimulation of the retina by light.

c. blindness, see blindness, color.

complementary c.'s, (1) two colors in which the direct perception of one produces an afterimage of the other; **(2)** two primary colors which, when mixed, produce light gray or white.

monochromatic c., see pure color.

primary c.'s, a set of three colors (red, blue, and yellow) from which all other colors can be produced

by mixing.

pure c., color produced by one wavelength; also called monochromatic color.

colorim'etry. 1. The quantitative analysis of color, either in terms of hue, saturation, and brightness, or by comparison with known standards. **2.** The quantitative chemical analysis of a solution by color comparison with a standard solution.

colorrha'gia. Abnormal discharge from the colon; also called colonorrhagia.

colorrhe'a. Diarrhea thought to originate in the colon, also called colonorrhea.

colos'tomy. Surgical establishment of a permanent opening into the colon through the abdominal wall.

colostrorrhe'a. A copious secretion of colostrum (first milk secreted at the end of pregnancy).

colos'trum. A thin, sticky secretion of the breasts occurring a few days before and after childbirth; also called foremilk.

colot'omy. Incision of the colon.

colpal'gia. Pain in the vagina.

colpatre'sia. Occlusion of the vagina.

colpec'tomy. Surgical removal of the vagina.

colpi'tis. Vaginitis.

c. emphysematosa, emphysematous vaginitis; see under vaginitis.

c. mycotica, mycotic vaginitis; see under vaginitis.

colpo-, colp-. Combining forms denoting vagina.

col'pocele. 1. A hernia into the vagina; also called elytrocele and vaginocele. **2.** Colpoptosis.

colpoclei'sis. Surgical closure of the vaginal lumen.

colpocys'tocele. Prolapse of the bladder into the vagina.

colpody'nia. Neuralgic vaginal pain; also called vaginodynia.

colpohysterec'tomy. Removal of the uterus through the vagina.

colpohysterot'omy. Incision into the uterus through the vagina.

colpomi'croscope. A high-powered microscope with a built-in light source for direct visual examination of a stained cervix; it facilitates a histologic diagnosis in vivo.

colpomicros'copy. Examination of cells of the cervix and vagina in situ with the aid of a colpomicroscope.

colpoperineor'rhaphy. Surgical repair of an injured vagina and torn perineum; also called vaginoperineorrhaphy.

col'popexy. Suture of a prolapsed vagina to the abdominal wall; also called vaginofixation.

col'poplasty. Reparative surgery of the vagina;

also called vaginoplasty.

colpopoie'sis. Surgical construction of an artificial vagina.

colpopto'sis, colpopto'sia. Prolapse of the walls of the vagina.

colpor'rhaphy. Surgical repair of a tear in the vagina.

colporrhex'is. The partial or total tearing loose of the uterine cervix from its vaginal attachment; an uncommon injury occurring during childbirth.

col'poscope. A low-powered microscope with a built-in light source for direct visual inspection of the uterine cervix and vagina; also called vaginoscope.

colpos'copy. Examination of the uterine cervix and vagina by means of a colposcope.

col'pospasm. Spasm of the vaginal wall.

colposteno'sis. Narrowing of the vagina.

colpot'omy. Incision through the vaginal wall, usually for the purpose of draining a pelvic abscess.

colpoxero'sis. Abnormal dryness of the vaginal mucosa.

colum'bium. An element, symbol Cb, now known as niobium.

columel'la. 1. A small column. **2.** The lower portion of the nasal septum.

col'umn. A pillar-shaped anatomic structure.

anterior c., the anterior (ventral) portion of the gray matter on either side of the spinal cord.

enamel c., one of the groups of fibers which make up the tooth enamel.

lateral c., the portion of gray matter of the spinal cord, extending between the anterior and posterior columns; present only in the thoracic and upper lumbar regions.

posterior c., the posterior (dorsal) portion of the gray matter on either side of the spinal cord.

spinal c., see vertebral column.

vertebral c., the columnar arrangement of vertebrae, from the skull through the coccyx, which encloses and supports the spinal cord; also called spinal column, backbone, and spine.

co'ma. A state in which psychologic and motor responses to stimulation are impaired.

deep c., one in which responses are completely lost.

moderately deep c., one in which only rudimentary responses of a reflex nature are present; e.g., corneal reflex.

semi-c., one in which responses are present, but elicited only by painful stimuli, e.g., vigorous shaking.

co'matose. In a condition of coma.

combust'ion. Burning; oxidation or other chemical change accompanied by the production of heat

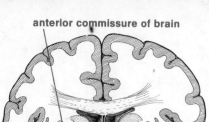

anterior commissure of brain

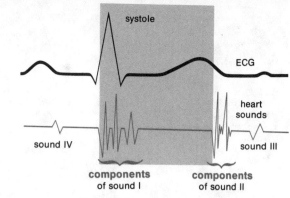

systole
ECG
sound IV
heart sounds
sound III
components of sound I
components of sound II

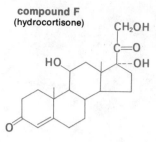

compound F
(hydrocortisone)

atrial complex

ventricular complex

ECG

element	O	C	H	N	Ca	P	K	Total
composition by weight (%)	65	18	10	3	1.5	1.0	0.35	98.85

and light.

heat of c., see under heat.

com'edo, *pl.* **comedo'nes.** A plug of dried sebaceous material retained in the orifice of a hair follicle; commonly called blackhead.

comedocarcino'ma. Carcinoma of the breast filling the ducts with a necrotic cheesy material which can be extruded with slight pressure.

co'mes, *pl.* **com'ites.** A companion blood vessel of another vessel or nerve.

commen'sal. Denoting two non-parasitic organisms that live together, one benefiting from the association while the other is neither benefited nor harmed.

com'minuted. Denoting a bone broken into several fragments.

comminu'tion. The process of breaking into small pieces.

com'missure. 1. Joining together; in the brain or spinal cord, bundles of nerve fibers crossing the midline from side to side. **2.** A line formed by the junction of two bones in the skull. **3.** The angle or corner of the eye, the lips, or the labia.

anterior c. of brain, a bundle of white fibers crossing the midline in front of the third ventricle.

posterior c. of brain, a bundle of white fibers crossing the midline posterior to the third ventricle, at its junction with the cerebral aqueduct.

commissurot'omy. Surgical division of the bands of a commisure.

mitral c., surgical division of the fibrous band of the mitral valve in the heart to relieve mitral stenosis.

commun'icable. Capable of being transmitted or communicated; denoting the ease with which infection is transmitted from one person to another.

commu'nicans. Denoting a nerve that connects two others.

commu'nis. Latin for common; belonging to more than one.

compac'tion. In dentistry, the progressive insertion and compression of a filling material into a prepared cavity.

compat'ible. 1. In pharmacology, denoting two or more substances that are capable of being mixed without undergoing undesirable chemical changes or loss of therapeutic properties. **2.** Describing two samples of blood in which the serum of each does not agglutinate the red blood cells of the other; blood that causes no reaction when transfused.

compensat'ed. Counteracted; counterbalanced.

compensa'tion. 1. The act of offsetting a functional or structural defect. **2.** A defense mechanism in which the individual, consciously or unconsciously, strives to make up for real or imagined

deficiencies.

compen'satory. Serving to counterbalance or make up for.

com'petence. 1. The tight closure of a normal heart valve; also called integrity. **2.** The quality or condition of being capable. **3.** The ability of a group of embryonic cells to react to a given morphogenic stimulus with resulting differentiation.

complaint'. 1. An expression of pain or discomfort. **2.** A malady or a disease.

chief c., the symptom primarily reported by the patient as responsible for his seeking medical attention.

com'plement. A multifactorial immune system consisting of eleven discrete proteins, characterized by their capacity to participate in certain antigen-antibody reactions which subsequently mediate a number of biologic consequences, thus strengthening the antibody defense activity; also called alexin.

complex. 1. A group of interrelated parts or factors. **2.** In psychiatry, a group of associated ideas (largely unconscious), having a strong emotional tone and influencing the personality. **3.** In electrocardiography, a group of deflections corresponding to a base in the cardiac cycle.

atrial c., the P wave in the electrocardiogram; also called auricular complex.

auricular c., see atrial complex.

brain wave c., a combination of fast and slow electrical activities of the brain, recurring often enough to be identified as a discrete phenomenon.

castration c., see anxiety, castration.

Electra c., Oedipus complex.

Eisenmenger's c., congenital heart condition consisting of a ventricular septal defect with pulmonary hypertension, resulting in right-to-left shunt through the defect; it may or may not be associated with overriding aorta.

inferiority c., feelings of inferiority due to real or imagined physical or social inadequacies; may be manifested by extreme shyness or timidity or by overcompensation through excessive ambition or aggressiveness.

melanosome c., two or more pigment granules (melanosomes) embedded in a supporting matrix.

Oedipus c., the strong attachment and desire that a child (usually between the ages of three and six) develops for the parent of the opposite sex; the feelings are largely repressed because of fear of punishment by the parent of the same sex, who is regarded as a rival; resolution centers on identification with the same sex parent; in girls, the complex is technically called the Electra complex.

persecution c., the feeling that others have evil intentions against one's well-being.

QRS c., an electrocardiographic display of ventricular contraction.

spike and wave c., in electroencephalography, one consisting of a dart and dome wave, usually seen in petit mal seizures.

superiority c., exaggerated aggressiveness, an overcompensation for feelings of inferiority.

ventricular c., the QRST wave in the electrocardiogram.

vitamin B c., a group of water-soluble compounds found together in foodstuffs; some are believed to be chiefly concerned with release of energy from food (e.g., nicotinamide, riboflavin, thiamine, and biotin), others with the formation of red blood cells (e.g., vitamin B_{12} and folic acid).

complex'ion. The appearance and general condition of the skin.

compli'ance. The quality of yielding; the tendency of a hollow organ (e.g., the bladder) to distend.

lung c., change of volume per change of pressure, an index of the mechanical properties of the lung.

compo'nent. A constituent part.

composition. 1. The act of combining parts or elements to form a whole. **2.** In chemistry, the group of atoms that forms the molecule of a substance.

com'pos men'tis. Latin term meaning of sound mind.

com'pound. 1. A substance consisting of two or more chemical elements or parts in union. **2.** In pharmacy, a preparation containing a mixture of drugs. **3.** In dentistry, a molding or impression material that softens when heated and solidifies without chemical change when cooled. **4.** To prepare a pharmaceutical mixture.

acyclic c., aliphatic c., see open chain compound.

aromatic c., a cyclic compound with conjugated double bonds within the ring; e.g., benzene.

azo c., an organic compound containing the azo (—N═N—) group; also called diazo compound.

binary c., a compound whose molecule is composed of two elements or atoms of different kinds; e.g., HCl.

closed chain c., see cyclic compound.

c. A, the adrenal hormone 11-dehydrocorticosterone.

c. B, the adrenal hormone corticosterone.

c. E, the adrenal hormone cortisone (DOC).

c. F, the adrenal hormone hydrocortisone; also called cortisol.

c. S, the adrenal hormone 11-deoxycortisol.

cyclic c., any organic compound that has atoms linked together in the form of a ring; also called

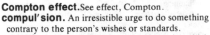

ring compound

helix

concha of auricle

tragus

superior nasal concha

middle nasal concha

light microscope

phase microscope

electron microscope

compression of bladder by anteflexed uterus

inferior nasal concha

condensers

* specimen

closed chain compound.

endothermic c., one whose formation involves the absorption of heat.

exothermic c., one whose formation involves the emission of heat.

heterocyclic c., an organic compound that contains rings composed of dissimilar elements.

impression c., modeling c., one used to secure an imprint of negative likeness of oral tissues.

inorganic c., any compound that does not contain carbon.

modeling c., see impression compound.

nonpolar c., one composed of molecules possessing asymmetrical distribution of charge so that no positive or negative poles exist; e.g., hydrocarbons.

open chain c., an organic compound in which the carbon atoms are linked in a linear fashion; also called acyclic, aliphatic, paraffin, or fatty compound.

organic c., any compound containing carbon.

quaternary c., one which contains four elements.

ring c.'s, a group of compounds in which the molecules are structured in such a way that the ends of the chain of carbon atoms are linked together in a closed ring.

saturated c., one in which all the atoms of the molecules are united by single bonds.

substitution c., a compound formed when elements of a molecule are replaced by other elements or radicals.

ternary c., tertiary c., a compound whose molecules contain three elements.

tray c., an impression-like compound which is more viscous when soft and more rigid when cooled.

unsaturated c., an organic compound containing $C=C$ or $C\equiv C$ combinations, capable of becoming saturated by the addition of other atoms.

com′press. A pad of gauze or other soft material used as a dressing or applied to a part of the body where localized pressure is necessary.

graduated c., one made of several layers of cloth gradually increasing in number so that it is thickest in the center.

wet c., one moistened with an antiseptic solution or with hot or cold water.

compres′sion. Pressing together.

cerebral c., pressure on the brain by tumor, hemorrhage, depressed fracture of the skull, etc.

digital c., pressure applied with the fingers over a blood vessel to check bleeding.

c. molding, in dentistry, the pressing of a plastic material to the negative form of a mold.

external cardiac c., closed chest massage; see under massage.

compression syndrome. See crush syndrome.

Compton effect. See effect, Compton.

compul′sion. An irresistible urge to do something contrary to the person's wishes or standards.

cona′tion. The volitional aspect of behavior which includes impulse, drive, and purposive striving; one of three elements of behavior, the other two being cognition (thinking) and affect (feeling).

con′ative. Denoting the basic strivings of a person as expressed by the volitional aspects of behavior, distinct from the cognitive and affective aspects.

concamera′tion. A series of connecting cavities.

concat′enate. Connected in a chainlike series.

con′cave. Having a hollowed surface.

concav′ity. A depression.

concavocon′vex. 1. Concave on one side and convex on the opposite. **2.** Denoting a lens with greater concave than convex curvature.

concentra′tion. 1. The quantity of a specified substance in a unit amount of another substance. **2.** A preparation that has had its strength increased by evaporation.

concen′tric. Having a common center.

concep′tion. 1. The act of forming an idea. **2.** The fertilization of an ovum or the act of becoming pregnant.

concep′tus. The product of conception; also called embryo.

con′cha, *pl.* **con′chae.** A shell-shaped structure such as the external ear or a turbinated bone in the nose.

bony inferior nasal c., a thin, spongy, curved bony plate forming the lower part of the lateral wall of the nasal cavity; it articulates with the ethmoid, maxilla, palatine, and lacrimal bones; also called inferior turbinate bone.

bony superior nasal c., the upper and smaller of the two curved bony plates projecting from the inner wall of the ethmoid in the nasal cavity; also called superior turbinate bone.

c. of auricle, the large shell-shaped hollow of the external ear, between the tragus and antihelix.

c. bullosa, distention of the nasal conchae, especially of the middle one, seen in some cases of chronic rhinitis.

inferior nasal c., the bony inferior nasal concha and its overlying mucous membrane.

middle nasal c., the bony middle nasal concha and its overlying mucous membrane.

sphenoidal c., a thin curved bony plate forming part of the roof of the nasal cavity; also called sphenoturbinal bone.

superior nasal c., the bony superior nasal concha and its overlying mucous membrane.

conchoi′dal. Shell-like in shape.

con′crement. Concretion.

concres′cence. The growing together of normally separate parts, as the roots of a tooth.

concre′tion. An aggregation of solid material; a calculus.

concus′sion. 1. A violent jarring or shaking of a part of the body, as caused by a fall or a blow. **2.** The morbid condition resulting from such a jarring.

brain c., the immediate and temporary disturbance of brain function as manifested by dizziness, cold perspiration, visual disturbances, and loss of consciousness.

condensa′tion. 1. The act of making more compact. **2.** The changing of a gas to a liquid or a liquid to a solid. **3.** In psychoanalysis, the representation of several ideas by a single dream-image or symbol. **4.** In dentistry, compaction.

condense. To compress, such as the restorative material into the prepared cavity of a tooth.

conden ser. 1. A device for cooling a gas to a liquid, or a liquid to a solid. **2.** A dental instrument designed to compress restorative material into the prepared cavity of a tooth. **3.** A simple or compound lens used to gather light rays and focus them on an object to be illuminated.

achromatic c., one used in a microscope for bright field work and corrected for both spherical aberration and chromatic aberration.

dark-field c., an optical system used in microscopes, by means of which light is collected and directed upon the specimen while the remainder of the field is dark.

phase contrast c., one that transmits light through rings so as to work in conjunction with a phase-altering pattern in the objective.

substage c., a lens or group of lenses which converges the illuminating beam for proper passage of light through the microscope.

condition. In psychology, to train to respond to a specific stimulus in a specific way.

conditioning. The process of training an individual or organism to respond to a specific stimulus in a specific way, usually by simultaneous presentation of unrelated stimuli one of which evokes the desired response.

instrumental c., see operant conditioning.

operant c., instrumental c., the procedure whereby a stimulus, once having evoked a response that produces a reward (or removes or prevents a punishment), is thereafter more likely to evoke that response.

physical c., improvement in strength or efficiency of muscular performance by exercise.

con′dom. A sheath, usually made of thin rubber, used to cover the penis during sexual intercourse to prevent conception or infection.

compound | **condom**

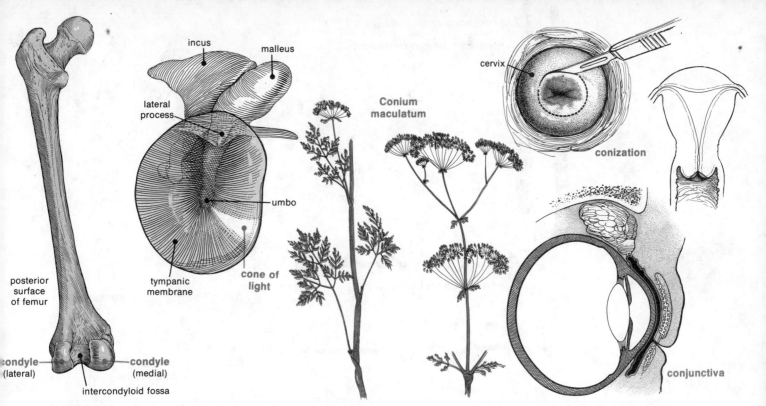

incus
malleus
lateral process
cervix
Conium maculatum
conization
umbo
posterior surface of femur
cone of light
tympanic membrane
condyle (lateral)
condyle (medial)
intercondyloid fossa
conjunctiva

conduc'tance. A measure of the readiness with which a substance allows an electric charge to pass through it.

conduc'tion. The transmitting of energy (heat, electricity, etc.) or nerve stimuli from one point to another.

  aberrant ventricular c., abnormal spread of a supraventricular impulse in the ventricle, caused by delayed activation of one of the branches of the atrioventricular bundle (His); also called ventricular aberration.

  accelerated c., the partial or complete bypass of the normal conduction pathways by the sinus impulse, resulting in early activation of the ventricular muscle.

  air c., the transmission of sound to the internal ear through the external auditory canal and the middle ear.

  bone c., the transmission of sound to the internal ear through the bones of the skull.

  concealed c., the partial transmission of an impulse through the A-V junction, which depolarizes only a portion of the junction, thus causing abnormal conduction of the next impulse.

  delayed c., first degree atrioventricular (A-V) heart block; see under block.

  intraventricular c., conduction of the cardiac impulse through the ventricular muscle; also called ventricular conduction.

  nerve c., transmission of an impulse through a nerve.

  retrograde c., transmission of an impulse through the cardiac muscle or the conduction system in a manner opposite to that of the normal impulse; also called reconduction and ventriculoatrial conduction.

  saltatory c., conduction in which the nerve impulse jumps from one node of Ranvier to the next.

  synaptic c., the propagation of a nerve impulse through a synapse.

  ventricular c., see intraventricular conduction.

  ventriculoatrial c., see retrograde conduction.

conductiv'ity. The ability to transmit or convey heat, electricity, sound, etc.

conduc'tor. 1. Any substance capable of transmitting heat, electricity, sound, etc. **2.** A grooved probe for guiding a surgeon's knife.

con'dylar. Of or relating to a condyle.

condylarthro'sis. A joint in which an ovoid surface (condyle) fits into an elliptical cavity.

con'dyle. A rounded knoblike prominence at the end of a bone by means of which it articulates with another bone.

condylec'tomy. Surgical removal of a condyle.

condylo'ma. A venereal wartlike growth at the junction of skin and mucous membrane of the anus, vulva, or the glans penis.

  c. acuminatum, moist wart; see under wart.

  c. latum, a flat raised lesion of secondary syphilis appearing in moist areas such as the lips, the female genitalia, or the perianal region.

condylo'matous. Of or relating to a condyloma.

condylot'omy. Division of a condyle.

cone. A figure or anatomic structure tapering to a point from a circular base.

  c. of light, the triangular reflection of light seen on inspection of the tympanic membrane.

  medullary c., the tapered end of the spinal cord.

  retinal c., one of about six or seven million photoreceptor cells which, with the rod cells, form the second of the 10 layers of the retina.

confabula'tion. The replacement of memory lapses with detailed fabrications of imaginary experiences; sometimes occurring in organic brain diseases in which intellectual impairment takes place.

confec'tion. A sweetened pharmaceutical preparation; also called confectio and electuary.

configura'tion. 1. The shape or outline of something as determined by the arrangement of its parts. **2.** The spatial grouping of atoms in a molecule.

confinement. The period of childbirth.

con'flict. The struggle between two opposing emotions, thoughts, needs, or courses of action.

confluence of the sinuses, confluens sinuum. The junction of the sinuses of the dura mater (superior sagittal, straight, occipital, and two transverse), located in a slight depression at one side of the internal protuberance of the occipital bone.

confluens sinuum. See confluence of the sinuses.

con'fluent. Running together, as the skin lesions of certain diseases which are not distinct but become merged.

conforma'tion. The spatial arrangement of atoms in a molecule achieved by rotation of groups about single, covalent bonds, without breaking any covalent bonds.

conform'er. A mold or shell fitted in a cavity to preserve its shape, as in the eye socket after removal of the eye prior to insertion of an artificial eye.

confu'sion. Mental state in which a person is disoriented in regard to his environment; impaired capacity to think clearly and with customary speed.

con'gener. 1. A drug which is part of a group of chemical compounds sharing the same parent compound. **2.** One of two or more muscles with the same function.

congen'ital. Present at birth.

congest'ed. Containing an abnormally large amount of blood.

conges'tion. Abnormal accumulation of blood in a part.

  hypostatic c., accumulation of blood in the lowest part of an organ due to the action of gravity when the circulation is feeble.

  passive venous c., congestion of a part due to partial stagnation of blood in the capillaries and venules, resulting from faulty venous drainage or failure of the right ventricle of the heart.

conglutina'tion. 1. Abnormal adhesion. **2.** Agglutination or clumping of red blood cells in the presence of serum (complement).

conglu'tinin. A nonantibody protein with the capability of combining with the carbohydrate portion of complement and thus capable of clumping particles covered by the complement; found in normal bovine serum.

conid'iophore. A spore-bearing, specialized hyphal filament in fungi.

conid'iospore. A fungal spore produced on a specialized conidiophore.

conid'ium, *pl.* **conid'ia.** The reproductive spore of fungi produced asexually.

coniofibro'sis. Abnormal formation of fibrous tissue caused by the presence of dust.

conio'sis. Any disease caused by dust.

Conium maculatum. A notoriously poisonous large herb of the carrot family; also called poison hemlock and spotted parsley.

coniza'tion. The removal of a conical piece of tissue, as from the cervix.

con'jugase. An enzyme, present in the liver and kidney of mammals, that splits folic acid conjugates into pteroylglutamic acid and glutamic acid.

con'jugate. Paired.

conjuga'tion. 1. Sexual reproduction of unicellular organisms whereby the two cells exchange genetic material. **2.** In chemistry, the combination of large molecules (e.g., proteins) with those of another substance.

conjuncti'va. The thin transparent mucous membrane lining the inner surface of the eyelids (palpebral conjunctiva) and the exposed surface of the anterior sclera up to the border of the cornea (bulbar conjunctiva); the epithelial layer of the conjunctiva is continuous with the corneal epithelium.

conjunctivi'tis. Inflammation of the conjunctiva resulting from bacterial, viral, or allergic agents; e.g., acute catarrhal conjunctivitis is caused by a bacterium (usually pneumococcus), epidemic keratoconjunctivitis is caused by a virus (adenovirus 8), vernal catarrh is caused by hypersensitivity to exogenous allergens.

connective tissue diseases. See collagen diseases.

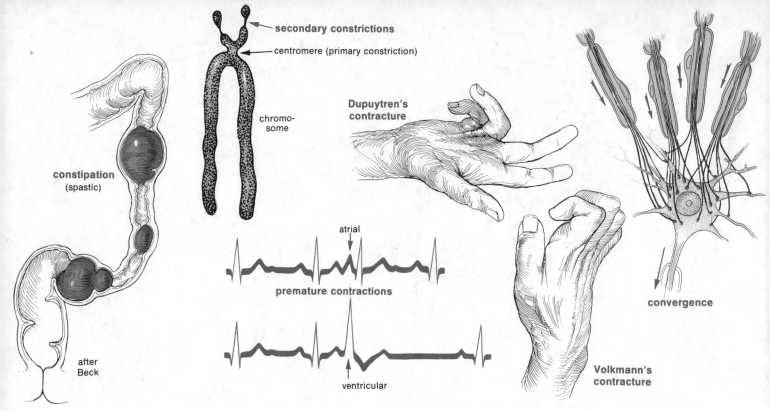

secondary constrictions

centromere (primary constriction)

chromo-
some

Dupuytren's
contracture

constipation
(spastic)

atrial

premature contractions

after
Beck

ventricular

convergence

Volkmann's
contracture

connec'tor. In dentistry, the part of a fixed partial denture which unites its component parts; e.g., an artificial tooth.

Conn's syndrome. Primary aldosteronism (1); excessive secretion of the hormone aldosterone due to a tumor in the cortex of the adrenal gland; the typical findings include hypertension, hypokalemic alkalosis, weakness, and low plasma renin.

consanguin'eous. Related by blood.

con'scious. Being aware of one's existence, actions, and environment.

con'sciousness. State of awareness of and responsiveness to environment.

consciousness-raising. A method of making individuals realize their potentials, in order to bring about change.

consen'sual. Denoting an involuntary act; also called reflex.

conser'vative. Applied to a cautious method of treatment.

consolida'tion. 1. Solidification into a dense mass; applied especially to the inflammatory solidification of the lung in pneumonia. **2.** The mass so formed.

con'stant. A quantity which, under stated conditions, does not vary with changes in the environment.

   decay c., the mathematical expression for the number of atoms of radionuclide which will decay in a unit of time.

   dissociation c., in chemistry, the constant that depends upon the equilibrium between the dissociated and undissociated forms of a compound.

   gas c. (R), the universal constant of proportionality, appearing in the equation of the general gas law, equal to the pressure of the gas times its volume divided by its temperature.

   Michaelis-Menten c. (K_m), one that expresses the concentration of the substrate at which half the maximum velocity of a reaction is achieved.

   Plank's c. (h), a constant expressing the ratio of the energy possessed by a quantum of energy to its frequency; its value is approximately 6.625×10^{-27} erg-sec.

   transformation c., the quantity of radioactive material that disintegrates (decays) each second.

constella'tion. In psychiatry, a set of related ideas.

const'ipate. To slow the action of the bowels.

constipa'tion. A decrease in the frequency of bowel movements, accompanied by a difficult prolonged effort in passing a very hard stool, followed by a sensation of incomplete evacuation.

constitu'tion. The physical make-up and state of health of the body.

constric'tion. 1. A narrowing; a binding. **2.** A subjective sensation of being tightly bound or squeezed.

   secondary c., the slender heterochromatic area of a chromosome which separates the satellite from the rest of the chromosome (the primary constriction is at the centromere).

constric'tor. Denoting a muscle that narrows a canal or opening.

consul'tant. A physician who is called in an advisory capacity.

consulta'tion. A conference of two or more physicians to evaluate the diagnosis and treatment of the disease in a particular patient.

consump'tion. Wasting away of tissues; previously a popular name for pulmonary tuberculosis.

con'tact. 1. The point at which two adjacent bodies touch one another. **2.** A person who has been exposed to the virus of an infectious disease.

conta'gion. Transmission of a disease by direct or indirect contact.

conta'gious. Transmissible by direct or indirect contact; also called catching.

conta'gium. The causative agent of an infectious disease.

contam'inant. That which contaminates; an impurity.

contamina'tion. 1. The process of soiling, as with infectious matter or unwanted radioactive matter. **2.** In an experiment, allowing the variable that is to be validated to influence the variable used for validation. **3.** An error of speech characterized by the fusion of part of one word with that of another.

con'tent. 1. That which is contained in an enclosed space. **2.** The amount of a specified substance.

contigu'ity. The state of being adjacent in time or space; immediately preceding or following.

con'tinence. Self-restraint, especially from sexual activity.

con'tour. 1. Surface configuration **2.** To shape into a desired form, as a denture or a broken tooth.

contra-. Prefix meaning against.

contracep'tion. The prevention of conception.

contracep'tive. Any agent or device used for the prevention of conception.

contract'. To pull together; to reduce in size or increase tension by drawing together.

contrac'tile. Able to contract.

contractil'ity. The ability to shorten or increase tension, applied to a muscle.

contrac'tion. 1. The shortening or increase in tension of functioning muscle **2.** A heart beat. **3.** A shrinkage or reduction in size.

   Braxton-Hicks c.'s, Braxton-Hicks sign, painless irregular contractions of the pregnant uterus,

beginning during the first trimester and increasing in frequency as pregnancy advances; occasionally observed in hematometria and cases of soft myomas.

   hourglass c., the narrowing of the middle of a hollow organ.

   premature c., a premature heart beat.

contrac'ture. A permanent contraction due to tonic spasm, muscle atrophy, or scars.

   Dupuytren's c., shortening of the palmar fascia producing permanent flexion of one or more fingers.

   Volkmann's c., contraction of the fingers and sometimes wrist following a severe injury or improper use of a tourniquet.

contraindica'tion. Any condition that renders undesirable the use of a medication or surgical procedure.

contralat'eral. Located on the opposite side.

contrastim'ulant. 1. Counteracting the effects of a stimulant. **2.** Any agent producing such an effect.

contrecoup. Occurring on the opposite side, as the fracture of a portion of the skull opposite to the point of impact.

control'. 1. To verify a scientific experiment by comparing with a standard or by conducting a parallel experiment, conditions being equal except for one factor. **2.** A standard against which the results of an experiment are checked.

   birth c., limitation of the number of children conceived by the voluntary use of contraceptive measures.

contu'sion. A superficial injury or bruise.

   brain c., a localized injury to the surface of the brain, usually attended by extravasation of blood and sometimes swelling; symptoms vary according to the extent and location of the injury.

co'nus, pl. **co'ni.** A cone-shaped structure.

   c. arteriosus, the upper, anterior portion of the right ventricle of the heart, ending in the pulmonary artery; also called arterial cone.

   c. medullaris, the tapered end of the spinal cord; also called medullary cone.

convales'cence. A stage in recovery between the abatement of a disease or injury and complete health.

convec'tion. Heat transfer in liquids or gases by the movement of heated particles.

conver'gence. 1. The turning toward or approaching a common point from different directions; e.g., the coordinated movement of the two eyes toward a near point, or the movement of the peripheral cells of the blastula toward the center during the gastrulation stage of the embryo. **2.** The synapsing of several presynaptic neurons with one postsynaptic neuron.

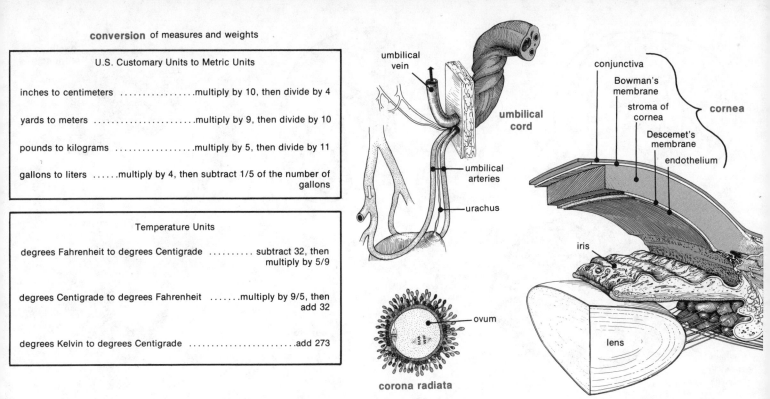

U.S. Customary Units to Metric Units
inches to centimeters ....multiply by 10, then divide by 4
yards to meters ....multiply by 9, then divide by 10
pounds to kilograms ....multiply by 5, then divide by 11
gallons to liters ......multiply by 4, then subtract 1/5 of the number of gallons

Temperature Units
degrees Fahrenheit to degrees Centigrade .... subtract 32, then multiply by 5/9
degrees Centigrade to degrees Fahrenheit ....multiply by 9/5, then add 32
degrees Kelvin to degrees Centigrade ....add 273

umbilical cord

corona radiata

cornea

---

negative c., outward deviation of the visual axes; also called divergence.

positive c., inward deviation of the visual axes; also called convergent squint.

conver′gent. Moving or inclined toward a common point.

conver′sion. 1. The act of changing. **2.** In psychiatry, the symbolic physical manifestation of a psychic conflict.

conver′tin. See factor VII.

con′vex. An outwardly curved surface.

convexocon′cave. Denoting a lens that has a greater convex than concave curvature.

con′voluted. Rolled, coiled, or twisted.

convolu′tion. A twisting or infolding of an anatomic part upon itself; see also gyrus.

convul′sant. Causing convulsions.

convul′sion. A violent involuntary muscular contraction, or a series of such contractions producing jerking movements.

Cope′s sign. A sign of appendicitis: (1) tenderness over the area of the appendix on extending the thigh; (2) tenderness on compressing the femoral artery in the femoral (Scarpa′s) triangle.

copol′ymer. A plastic composed of two or more chemically different monomers or base units.

copolymeriza′tion. The chemical joining of different monomers to form a compound of a high molecular weight.

cop′per. A malleable, reddish-brown metallic element; symbol Cu, atomic number 29, atomic weight 63.54.

coproan′tibodies. Antibodies present in the intestinal contents.

coprola′lia. The involuntary use of obscene words.

cop′rolith. A mass of inspissated feces.

copropor′phyrin. A porphyrin compound normally present in feces; a decomposition product of bilirubin; also called stercoporphyrin.

copula′tion. Sexual intercourse; coitus.

cor. Latin for heart.

c. biloculare, a more or less two-chambered heart due to the absence or incomplete development of the interatrial and interventricular septa.

c. bovinum, an abnormally large heart; also called bucardia.

c. pulmonale, enlargement of the right ventricle of the heart, secondary to a disorder of the substance or blood vessels of the lung.

c. triloculare, a three-chambered heart due to absence of either the interatrial or the interventricular septum.

coracoacro′mial. Relating to the coracoid and acromial processes of the scapula (shoulder blade).

coracobra′chial. Relating to the coracoid process of the scapula and the arm.

coracoclavic′ular. Relating to the coracoid process of the scapula and the clavicle.

coracohu′meral. Relating to the coracoid process of the scapula and the humerus.

cor′acoid. Shaped like a raven′s beak; denoting the thick, curved process at the superior border of the scapula (shoulder blade).

cord. Any flexible, stringlike structure.

spermatic c., the structure that extends from the internal inguinal ring to the testis.

spinal c., the elongated portion of the central nervous system which is enclosed by the vertebral column.

umbilical c., the structure connecting the placenta with the umbilicus of the fetus; it contains two arteries and one vein coiled around each other; in the newborn it measures about two feet in length and one-half inch in diameter.

vocal c., one of the four membranous bands in the larynx; the upper pair is called false vocal cords, the lower pair the true vocal cords (those that enter into voice production).

cor′date. Heart-shaped.

cordec′tomy. Surgical removal of a cord, as of a vocal cord.

cord′opexy. Surgical fixation of a cord, especially a vocal cord.

cordot′omy. Severing of the sensory tracts of the spinal cord for the relief of intractable pain.

core. 1. The central mass of a boil. **2.** A metal casting designed to retain in position the artificial crown of a tooth. **3.** A section of a mold used to record and maintain the relationships of parts, such as teeth or metallic restorations.

coreclei′sis, corecli′sis. Obliteration of the pupil.

corec′tasis. Pathologic dilatation of the pupil.

corecto′pia. Abnormal position of the pupil to one side of the center of the iris.

coreom′eter. An instrument for measuring the size of the pupil; also called pupillometer.

coreom′etry. Measurement of the pupil of the eye; also called pupillometry.

co′repressor. A small molecule, usually a product of a specific enzyme pathway, capable of combining with the inactive repressor to form an active complex which combines with the operator and prevents mRNA synthesis; a homeostatic mechanism for regulating enzyme production in repressible enzyme systems.

coresteno′ma. A narrowing or partial closing of the pupil.

co′rium. See dermis.

corn. A circumscribed induration and thickening of the skin.

hard c., one over a toe joint caused by friction and/or pressure from ill-fitting shoes.

seed c., a wart on the foot.

soft c., a thickening of the skin between two toes caused by pressure and kept soft by moisture.

cor′nea. The transparent anterior part of the outer coat of the eyeball which serves as the major refracting medium; it consists of five layers; eye banks are now common to preserve donated corneas for transplantation.

conical c., see keratoconus.

cor′neal. Relating to the cornea.

cornei′tis. See keratitis.

corneoscle′ra. The cornea and sclera considered as a unit which forms the outer layer of the eyeball.

cor′neous. Hornlike.

cor′neum. Stratum corneum; the superficial layer of the skin.

cornic′ulate. Having the shape of a small horn.

cornifica′tion. Conversion into horny tissue or keratin.

cor′nu, *pl.* **cor′nua. 1.** A horn-shaped structure. **2.** Any structure composed of bony tissue.

coro′na. Any structure resembling a crown.

c. radiata, an investment of follicular cells remaining attached to the ovum when released by the ovary; formerly the cumulus oophorus around the developing oocyte.

corona′lis. Coronal, relating to the coronal suture or plane.

cor′onary. 1. Encircling in the manner of a crown, as the vessels supplying the heart muscle. **2.** Coronary occlusion; a heart attack.

c. care unit, see under unit.

cor′oner. An official whose duty is to investigate any death thought to be of other than natural causes.

coro′nion. A craniometric point at the tip of the lower jaw.

cor′onoid. 1. Shaped like a crow′s beak; denoting certain processes of bones, as the coronoid process of the mandible (lower jaw). **2.** Crown-shaped.

cor′pora. Plural of corpus.

corpo′real. 1. Relating to or characteristic of the body. **2.** Relating to a corpus.

cor′pulence, cor′pulency. Obesity.

cor′pus, *pl.* **cor′pora.** Body; the main portion of a structure.

c. albicans, a mass of white, collagenous scar tissue formed in the ovary after discharge of the ovum; it represents the remnants of a corpus luteum, either of the menstrual cycle or of pregnancy, and eventually disappears.

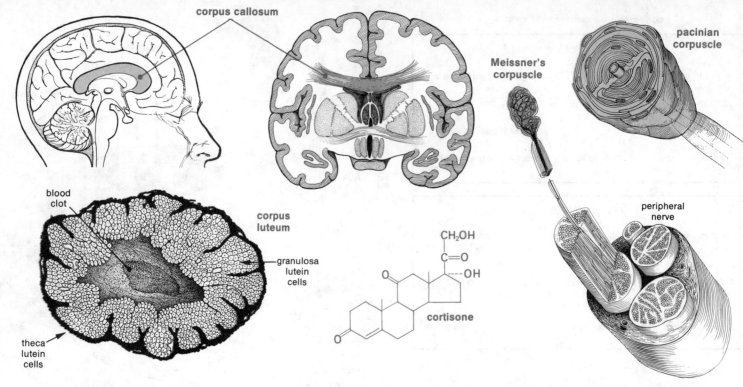

corpus callosum

pacinian corpuscle

Meissner's corpuscle

blood clot

corpus luteum

granulosa lutein cells

peripheral nerve

CH₂OH
C=O
OH

cortisone

theca lutein cells

c. callosum, a mass of transverse fibers connecting the two hemispheres of the brain.

c. cavernosum, one of the two parallel columns of erectile tissue of the penis or of the clitoris.

c. ciliare, ciliary body; see under body.

c. geniculatum laterale, lateral geniculate body; see under body.

c. geniculatum mediale, medial geniculate body; see under body.

c. luteum, an endocrine body producing the hormone progesterone; it is composed of a mass of large cells containing a yellow pigment (lutein) and develops in the ovary, at the site of a ruptured ovarian follicle and discharge of the ovum; if pregnancy does not occur, the corpus luteum retrogresses to a mass of scar tissue (corpus albicans) which eventually disappears; if pregnancy occurs, it continues to grow until the 13th week before slowly retrogressing.

c. mamillare, mamillary body; see under body.

corpora quadrigemina, quadrigeminal bodies; see under body.

c. spongiosum, the median column of erectile tissue of the penis, situated between and inferior to the corpora cavernosa and surrounding the urethra.

c. striatum, the caudate and lentiform nuclei and the internal capsule considered as a whole situated in front and lateral to the thalamus in each hemisphere of the brain; also called striate body.

c. vitreum, vitreous body; see under body.

cor′puscle. 1. A small body or mass. **2.** A cell capable of moving freely in the body. **3.** A primary particle such as a photon or electron.

blood c., any blood cell.

colostrum c., one of numerous large, round bodies containing fat droplets, present in colostrum; thought to be modified leukocyte; also called galactoblast.

giant c., cell, giant.

Golgi-Mazzoni c., an encapsulated sensory nerve found in the subcutaneous tissue of the pulp of the fingers; similar to a pacinian corpuscle but with a thinner capsule and with axons that ramify more extensively and end in flat expansions.

Krause's c., a spherical sense organ located at the termination of some sensory nerve fibers; it responds to the sensation of cold; also called Krause's end-bulb.

malpighian c., see renal corpuscle.

Meissner's c., a small, oval, encapsulated receptor organ present in the dermal papillae of the skin, particularly prevalent on the palmar and plantar surfaces; signals fine, discriminative touch sensations; also called tactile corpuscle of Meissner.

pacinian c., an encapsulated receptor organ that

signals mechanical deformations as touch or vibratory sensations; characterized by an unmyelinated terminal axon covered by numerous concentric layers of connective tissue; found in subcutaneous tissue, fascial planes around joints and tendons, and in the mesentery about the pancreas; especially numerous in the palm of the hand, sole of the foot, and genital organs; it responds to deep pressure and vibrations.

phantom c., a red blood cell that is devoid of color due to losing its hemoglobin; also called shadow corpuscle and achromocyte.

Purkinje's c.'s., see cell, Purkinje's.

red blood c., see erythrocyte.

renal c., one of many invaginated pouchlike commencements of a renal tubule (glomerular or Bowman's capsule) with a central tuft of vessels (glomerulus); also called malpighian body or corpuscle.

Ruffini's c.'s, Ruffini's nerve endings; see under ending.

shadow c., see phantom corpuscle.

terminal c., any specialized encapsulated nerve ending such as the pacinian corpuscle.

white blood c., see cell, white blood.

correspon′dence. The state of being in harmony.

retinal c., the faculty of vision of which an object seen with the two eyes (thus forming two retinal images) is perceived as one due to the coordinate functioning of retinal receptors.

corro′sive. Caustic; denoting an agent that causes a gradual wearing away or disintegration of a substance by chemical alteration.

cor′tex. The external portion of an organ, such as the brain, kidney, or adrenal gland.

cortexone. See deoxycorticosterone.

cor′tical. Relating to a cortex.

corticif′ugal. Conducting impulses away from the cerebral cortex.

corticip′etal. Conducting impulses toward the cerebral cortex.

cor′ticoid. Corticosteroid.

corticotro′ntine. Relating to the cerebral cortex and pons.

corticospi′nal. Relating to the cerebral cortex and spinal cord.

cortico′steroid. Any of the hormones of the adrenal cortex or any synthetic substitute.

cortico′sterone. See cortisone.

corticothalam′ic. Relating to the cerebral cortex and thalamus.

corticotro′pin, adrenocorticotrophin (ACTH). **1.** A hormone produced by the anterior lobe of the pituitary gland that stimulates the secretion of cortisone and other hormones of the adrenal

cortex. **2.** A pharmaceutical preparation made synthetically or extracted from the anterior pituitary of mammals, used to stimulate the activity of the adrenal cortex.

corticotropin-releasing-factor (CRF). A factor released by the hypothalamus in response to a low plasma cortisol level, capable of causing secretion of ACTH by the anterior pituitary gland.

cor′tisol. 17-Hydroxycorticosterone; a steroid hormone isolated from the adrenal cortex or produced synthetically; of the naturally occurring adrenal cortical hormones, cortisol is most capable of correcting by itself the effects of adrenalectomy; provides resistance to stresses and maintains a number of enzyme systems; also called hydrocortisone.

cor′tisone. A hormone from the adrenal cortex active in regulating carbohydrate metabolism and the nutrition of connective tissue; its release is regulated by the action of the adrenocorticotropic hormone (ACTH) of the pituitary gland; an excess of cortisone activity is responsible for Cushing's syndrome; also called corticosterone.

Corynebacte′rium. A genus of irregularly staining, gram-positive bacteria having a club shape and causing disease in plants and animals.

C. diphtheriae, the species that causes diphtheria in man; produces a powerful exotoxin; found in the mucous membrane of the upper respiratory tract of infected persons.

cory′za. Acute inflammation of the nasal mucosa, attended by a discharge.

cosme′sis. Concern for the appearance of the patient, especially in surgical operations.

cosmet′ic. Denoting any preparation or operative procedure intended to improve the appearance of a person.

cos′ta, *pl.* **cos′tae.** Latin for rib.

cos′tal. Relating to a rib.

costec′tomy. Surgical removal of a rib.

cos′tive. 1. Relating to or causing constipation. **2.** Constipated.

costocen′tral. See costovertebral.

costochon′dral. Relating to a rib and its cartilage.

costoclavic′ular. Relating to the ribs and a clavicle.

costoclavicular syndrome. Vascular disorders of the upper limb due to intermittent compression of the neuromuscular bundle between the clavicle and the first rib; also called Falconer-Weddell syndrome.

costophren′ic. Relating to the ribs and the diaphragm.

costoscap′ular. Relating to the ribs and a scapula.

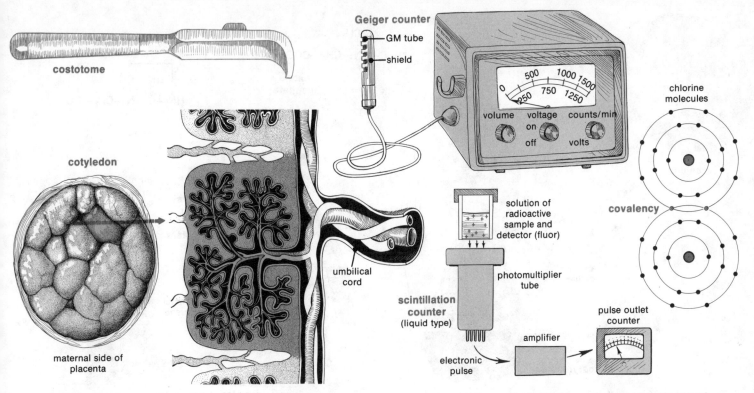

costotome

cotyledon

maternal side of placenta

umbilical cord

Geiger counter — GM tube — shield

volume — voltage on off — counts/min volts

solution of radioactive sample and detector (fluor)

photomultiplier tube

scintillation counter (liquid type)

amplifier

pulse outlet counter

electronic pulse

chlorine molecules

covalency

costoster'nal. Relating to the ribs and the sternum.

cos'totome. An instrument used for cutting through a rib.

costot'omy. Division of a rib or costal cartilage.

costover'tebral. Relating to the ribs and the thoracic vertebrae; also called costocentral.

cot'ton. 1. Any of various plants of the genus *Gossypium*. **2.** The soft, white fiber covering the seeds of the cotton plant.

  absorbent c., cotton from which fatty matter and impurities have been removed.

cotyle'don. One of 15 to 20 irregularly shaped compartments (lobes) into which the maternal surface of the placenta is divided; it houses numerous small villi.

cough. A forceful and sudden expulsion of air from the lungs.

  whooping c., an acute respiratory illness of infants and young children usually caused by *Bordetella pertussis*, a gram-negative coccobacillus; also called pertussis.

cou'lomb. A unit of electrical quantity equal to the amount of charge transferred in one second by a steady current of one ampere.

coun'seling. A professional service that provides an individual with a better understanding of his problems and potentialities.

  genetic c., a service by individuals knowledgeable in human genetics that provides information about inherited disorders so that people can make informed choices about family planning.

count. 1. To list one by one in order to calculate a total. **2.** The formulation of a total obtained by examining a sample.

  Arneth c., the percentage of distribution of polymorphonuclear neutrophils according to the number of lobes their nuclei contain.

  blood c., see blood count.

  complete blood c., see blood count, complete.

  differential blood c., see blood count, differential.

coun'ter. A computer or any apparatus for counting.

  Geiger c. (GM counter), an instrument used to detect, measure, and record the emission of radioactive particles; it consists of a negatively charged metallic cylinder in a vacuum tube containing a positively charged wire; also called Geiger-Müller counter.

  scintillation c., device used to detect and count radioactive particles; also called scintillator.

counterdepres'sant. 1. Preventing or antagonizing the depressing action of a drug. **2.** Any agent producing this effect.

coun'terdrug. A drug that counteracts or neutralizes an opposing agent.

counterexten'sion. Countertraction.

counterir'ritant. A substance applied locally to produce superficial irritation in order to relieve a deep seated inflammation.

coun'tero'pening. A second opening made opposite to another (e.g., in an abscess) to facilitate drainage; also called contra-aperture and counterpuncture.

coun'terpulsa'tion. A procedure used to aid the failing heart by automatically removing arterial blood just before and during ventricular ejection and returning it to the circulation during diastole.

coun'tershock. Electric shock applied to the heart to correct a disturbance of its rhythm.

coun'terstain. A second stain, usually of a contrasting color, applied to a microscopy specimen to color parts not affected by the first stain.

countertrac'tion. A traction or pull which is antagonistic to the action of another traction; a back-pull.

countertransfer'ence. The psychiatrist's emotional reaction to his patient; it may be conscious or unconscious.

coup. French for stroke or blow.

coup'le. To copulate; said of lower animals.

coup'ling. Bigeminal rhythm; heart beats occurring in pairs; a normal sinus beat followed by a premature beat.

  constant c., see fixed coupling.

  fixed c., the occurrence of several premature beats with a constant interval between each of them and the preceding normal beat; also called constant coupling.

  variable c., the occurrence of several premature beats with different intervals between each of them and the preceding normal beat.

Courvoisier's sign. See law, Courvoisier's.

cova'lency. In chemistry, a bond marked by the sharing of electrons (usually in pairs) by two atoms in a chemical compound.

cov'er glass, cov'erslip. A piece of thin glass used to cover a mounted specimen for examination under the microscope.

cow'pox. See vaccinia (1).

cox'a, *pl.* **cox'ae.** Latin for hipbone and hip joint.

coxal'gia. Pain in the hip joint.

Coxiel'la burnet'ii. The species of *Coxiella* that causes Q fever in man.

coxodyn'ia. Coxalgia; pain in the hip joint.

coxsack'ievirus. A member of the picornavirus group of viruses, having pathologic effects on the brain, heart, muscle, respiratory epithelium, and skin of man; the name is derived from the town of Coxsackie, New York, where it was discovered while an outbreak of poliomyelitis was being investigated.

c.p. Abbreviation for chemically pure.

CPC. Abbreviation for clinicopathologic conference.

CPK. Abbreviation for creatine phosphokinase.

CPR. Abbreviation for cardiopulmonary resuscitation.

cps. Abbreviation for cycles per second.

Cr. Chemical symbol of the element chromium.

cramp. 1. A painful spasm. **2.** Intestinal colic. **3.** An occupational neurosis.

  heat c., pain in the abdomen and/or legs occurring in persons working in extreme hot weather.

  tailor's c., spasm and neuralgic pain of the fingers, hand, and forearm; also called tailor's spasm.

  writer's c., spastic pain of the muscles of the thumb and two adjoining fingers induced by excessive writing; also called mogigraphia and graphospasm.

cra'nial. Of or relating to the skull.

craniec'tomy. Surgical removal of a portion of the skull.

cranio-, crani-. Combining forms meaning skull.

cra'niocele. See encephalocele (3).

craniofa'cial. Relating to both the skull and the face.

craniol'ogy. The scientific study of the skull, especially human, in all its aspects.

craniomala'cia. Thinning and softening of the bones of the skull.

craniom'eter. An instrument used to measure skulls.

craniomet'ric. Relating to skull measurement.

craniom'etry. Measurement of the skull, especially human, after removal of the soft tissues.

craniop'athy. Any disease of the skull.

craniopharyngio'ma. The second most frequent type of tumor of the pituitary gland, arising from remnants of the embryonic hypophyseal stalk (Rathke's pouch) and having a cystic or a solid form, frequently with calcium deposits; also called Rathke's pouch tumor.

craniopunc'ture. Puncture of the skull.

craniorrhachis'chisis. Congenital fissure of the skull and vertebral column.

craniosa'cral. Relating to the origins of the parasympathetic nervous system.

cranios'chisis. Congenital defect of the skull in which it fails to close completely, leaving a fissure.

cranioscle'ro'sis. Abnormal thickening of the skull.

craniosteno'sis. Congenital malformation of the

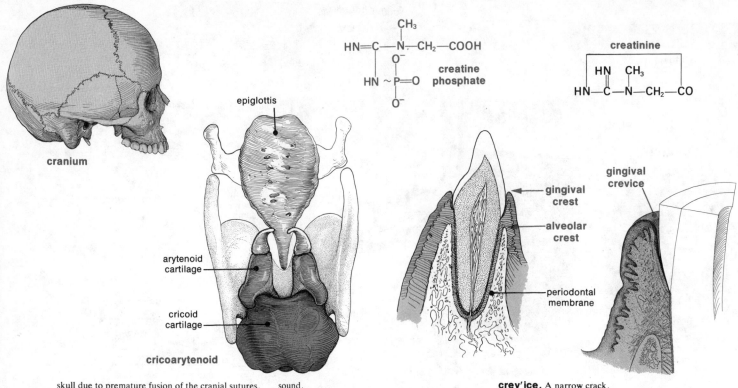

cranium

epiglottis

arytenoid cartilage

cricoid cartilage

cricoarytenoid

$$HN=C-N-CH_2-COOH$$
with CH_3, O^-, $HN \sim P=O$, O^-

creatine phosphate

creatinine

$$HN=C-N-CH_2-CO$$
with HN, CH_3

gingival crest

alveolar crest

periodontal membrane

gingival crevice

---

skull due to premature fusion of the cranial sutures.

craniosto′sis. Premature ossification of the skull.

cra′niotabes. Localized softening of an infant's skull, usually due to severe rickets.

cra′niotome. An instrument used for perforation and crushing of the skull of a fetus.

craniot′omy. 1. Surgical opening into the skull. **2.** In obstetrics, puncturing of the head of a dead fetus and evacuation of the contents to facilitate its delivery.

cra′nium. The skull; the bones of the head in general; specifically, the bones enclosing the brain.

cra′ter. The most depressed area of an ulcer.

crater′iform. Hollowed like a bowl; in bacteriology, denoting a type of liquefaction of gelatin by bacteria in a stab culture.

cra′zing. The formation of fine cracks on the surface of a structure, such as an artificial tooth, induced by release of internal stress.

cream. 1. The fatty constituent of milk that tends to accumulate at the surface on standing. **2.** Any of various substances resembling cream.

cre′atine, cre′atin. A nitrogenous compound found mainly in muscle tissue.

 c. phosphate, phosphocreatine; a creatine phosphoric acid compound; a source of energy in muscle contraction.

 c. phosphokinase (CPK), an enzyme that promotes the formation of ATP (adenosine triphosphate) from phosphocreatine and ADP (adenosine diphosphate); essential to muscle contraction.

creat′inine. A normal metabolic waste, a product of creatine metabolism; excreted in the urine, primarily by filtration; since it is generally produced at a constant rate, the clearance rate and the serum level are widely used as an index of kidney function.

 c. clearance, rate at which the kidney removes endogenous or exogenous creatinine from the blood plasma; an approximate measure of glomerular filtration rate.

creatinu′ria. The presence of increased amounts of creatine in the urine; usually a sign of a decrease in muscle mass, as in muscular dystrophy.

cremas′ter. See table of muscles.

cre′nate, cre′nated. Notched.

cre′nocyte. An abnormal red blood cell with scalloped or notched edges.

crep′itant. Crackling.

crepita′tion. 1. A grating sound like that produced when rubbing hair between the fingers, heard in certain diseases such as pneumonia. **2.** Noise made by friction of the two ends of a fractured bone. **3.** Sensation felt when palpating over an area in which there is subcutaneous gas.

crep′itus. 1. Crepitation. **2.** A dry, crackling sound.

crescent, malarial. A gametocyte of the malarial parasite *Plasmodium falciparum*, characterized by its crescentic shape; also called sickle form.

cre′sol. Any of three isomeric phenols (ortho-cresol, meta-cresol, and para-cresol); poisonous, colorless liquid or crystals, used as disinfectant.

crest. A bony ridge.

 alveolar c., the margin of the bone surrounding each tooth.

 c. of scapular spine, the border of the spine of the scapula (shoulder blade).

 ethmoidal c., one located in the medial side of the maxilla which articulates with the middle concha.

 ganglionic c., see neural crest.

 gingival c., the edge of the free gingiva separating the gingival sulcus from the external gingiva.

 iliac c., the long curved upper border of the ileum.

 infundibuloventricular c., see supraventricular crest.

 intertrocanteric c., the ridge between the greater and lesser trochanters of the femur, marking the junction of the neck and shaft of the bone.

 nasal c., the ridge along the middle of the floor of the nasal cavity.

 neural c., a band of ectodermal cells dorsolateral to the embryonic neural tube which gives origin to ganglia of the cranial and spinal nerves; also called ganglionic crest.

 pubic c., the rough anterior border of the pubic bone.

 spiral c., the serrated edge of the osseous spiral lamina of the cochlea.

 supraventricular c., the muscular ridge separating the conus arteriosus from the remaining cavity of the right ventricle of the heart; also called infundibuloventricular crest.

cre′tin. A mentally retarded dwarf due to congenital thyroid deficiency; one afflicted with cretinism.

cret′inism. Condition characterized by stunted growth, apathy, distended abdomen, protruding swollen tongue, and arrested mental development, resulting from an inadequate production of thyroid hormones in early infancy.

cre′tinoid. Exhibiting symptoms similar to those of cretinism.

Creutzfeldt-Jakob disease. A spongiform encephalopathy characterized by dementia accompanied by myoclonus; the dementia progresses so rapidly that deterioration is usually seen daily; the individual afflicted with the disease moves inevitably from good health to total helplessness or death within a year; believed to be caused by a transmissible agent (slow virus); also called Jakob-Creutzfeldt disease.

crev′ice. A narrow crack.

 gingival c., the space between the enamel of a tooth and the margin of the gums; in cases in which the gums have receded, between the gums and the cementum.

CRF. Abbreviation for corticotropin-releasing factor.

crib death. See sudden infant death syndrome.

crib′riform. Sievelike; perforated.

cricoaryte′noid. Relating to both the cricoid and arytenoid cartilages.

cri′coid. Ring-shaped, denoting the cartilage at the lower end of the larynx.

cricoidec′tomy. Surgical removal of the cricoid cartilage.

cricothy′roid. Relating to the cricoid and thyroid cartilages.

cricotracheot′omy. Division of the cricoid cartilage and upper trachea.

cri-du-chat syndrome. Hereditary condition marked by abnormal smallness of the head and jaw, severe mental deficiency, and a characteristic high-pitched catlike cry; caused by deletion of the short arm of chromosome 5; also called cat-cry syndrome.

Crigler-Najjar disease. See Crigler-Najjar syndrome.

Crigler-Najjar syndrome. An inherited disease of infants, usually fatal, associated with deficiency of the bilirubin enzyme glucuronyl transferase in the liver; also called Crigler-Najjar disease.

crinogen′ic. Causing increased glandular secretion.

crip′ple. 1. One who is partially or completely disabled. **2.** To render disabled.

cri′sis. 1. A sudden change in the course of an acute disease; a disease that terminates by crisis is one in which a change for the better occurs suddenly. **2.** A paroxysmal attack of pain or distress in an organ as seen in tabes dorsalis.

 anaphylactoid c., symptoms resembling those of life-threatening allergic reactions (e.g., to penicillin) arising from a breaking up of the body's colloid equilibrium; produced by injecting a variety of substances, such as peptones, into the body.

 Dietl's c., severe abdominal pain caused by a kinked ureter, occurring in individuals with a floating kidney.

 oculogyric c., one in which the eyeballs become fixed in one position (usually upward) for a length of time; occurring in encephalitis lethargica.

 thyroid c., see thyrotoxic crisis.

 thyrotoxic c., a sudden increase of the symptoms of thyrotoxicosis: rapid pulse, fever, nausea, diarrhea, a rise in the basal metabolic rate, and coma; also called thyroid crisis and thyroid storm.

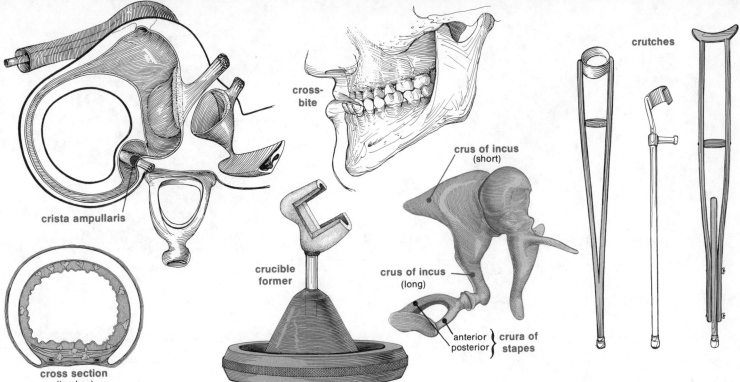

crista ampullaris

cross section
(trachea)

cross-bite

crucible former

crus of incus
(short)

crus of incus
(long)

anterior
posterior } crura of
stapes

crutches

cris′ta, *pl.* **cris′tae.** A sharp upstanding ridge or crest.

  c. ampullaris, an elevation on the inner surface of the ampulla of each semicircular duct which contains innervated hair cells responsive to movement of the endolymph.

  c. galli, the cock's comb; a perpendicular bony ridge on the upper surface of the ethmoid in the anterior cranial fossa projecting above the level of the cribriform plate; the anterior end of the falx cerebri is attached to it.

  c. iliaca, iliac crest; see under crest.

cristo′balite. A form of crystalline silica used in dental casting investment; it has a high thermal expansion.

crocodile tears syndrome. Spontaneous secretion of tears occurring simultaneously with normal salivation during eating, caused by a lesion of the facial nerve; usually follows partial recovery from facial paralysis.

Crohn's disease. Regional enteritis; see under enteritis.

cross′bite. Condition in which the normal labiolingual or bucco-lingual relationship between the upper and lower teeth is reversed (the lower teeth are anterior and/or buccal to the upper teeth).

  anterior c., condition in which the upper incisors are locked lingual to the lower incisors.

cross′breed. 1. Hybrid. **2.** To produce a hybrid by the mating of animals or plants of different breeds of varieties; also called hybridize.

crossing over. See under gene.

cross match′ing. Cross-agglutination test; see under test.

cross sec′tion. A section through an organ, usually at right angles to an axis.

croup. A term commonly used to denote any kind of laryngitis with laryngeal spasm in children; marked by a hoarse, barking cough (croupy cough), and difficult breathing.

  c. kettle, a vessel with a long spout used to boil water and convey steam to a sick room.

croup′y. Of the nature of croup.

crown. The topmost part of a structure, as of the head or tooth.

  anatomical c., the portion of a tooth covered by enamel.

  artificial c., a restoration of the major part or of the entire coronal part of a tooth which is affixed to the remains of a natural tooth structure; usually made of gold, porcelain, or plastic.

  clinical c., the portion of a tooth visible in the oral cavity, beyond the margin of the gums; also called physiologic crown.

  dowel c., a crown replacing the entire coronal part of a tooth secured with the aid of a retention post extending into a filled root canal.

  face c., a crown with a veneer for esthetics.

  partial c., a crown that does not cover all the surfaces of a tooth; used as a retainer or single unit restoration.

crown and bridge. The branch of prosthodontics which deals with crown restorations and the fixed type of tooth-borne partial denture prosthesis.

crown′ing. The stage of childbirth in which the head of the baby is visible, its largest diameter being encircled by the stretched vulva.

cru′ciate. Shaped like a cross; overlapping or crossing.

cru′cible. A vessel or receptacle made of porcelain or graphite, used for melting materials at very high temperatures.

  c. former, a stand which holds a sprued wax pattern of a dental restoration; it forms the base for the casting ring.

cru′ra. Plural of crus.

cru′ral. Relating to the leg or thigh.

crus, *pl.* **cru′ra. 1.** Latin for leg. **2.** Any leglike structure.

  common membranous c., the short canal formed by the united ends of the posterior and superior semicircular ducts.

  common osseous c., the short canal formed by the union of the posterior and superior semicircular canals.

  c. cerebri, cerebral peduncle; see under peduncle.

  c. of the diaphragm, either of two fibromuscular bands (right and left) that connect the diaphragm with the lumbar vertebrae; the two crura encircle the aorta.

  c. of the incus, either of two processes (short and long) of the incus.

  c. of penis, the tapering posterior portion of the corpus cavernosum penis.

  c. of the stapes, either of two limbs (anterior and posterior) of the stapes.

crush. To press between two bodies so as to cause injury.

crush syndrome. Shock and renal failure following a severe crushing injury causing soft tissue trauma; acute tubular necrosis is thought to result from the myoglobin released from the damaged muscles; also called compression syndrome.

crust. 1. A hard outer layer or covering. **2.** A scab; the dried exudate of a lesion.

Crusta′cea. A class of predominantly aquatic animals (phylum Arthropoda) having segmented bodies covered with an exoskeleton; it includes lobsters, crabs, shrimps, barnacles, wood lice, etc.

crusta′cean. Belonging or relating to the class Crustacea.

crutch. A supporting device, used singly or in pairs, designed to aid those who need help in walking.

Cruveilhier-Baumgarten syndrome. Intrahepatic portal vein obstruction, usually due to cirrhosis of the liver, associated with patency of the umbilical vein, varicose paraumbilical veins, and a venous hum or thrill.

cry. 1. An inarticulate expression of distress. **2.** To utter such a sound.

  epileptic c., a vocal sound sometimes made by a person at the onset of an epileptic convulsion.

cryanesthe′sia. Loss of the ability to feel cold.

cryesthe′sia. Sensitiveness to cold temperatures.

cryo-. Combining form meaning cold.

cryoaerother′apy. The use of cold air in the treatment of disease.

cryobiol′ogy. The study of the effect of low temperatures on living organisms.

cryocau′tery. Destruction of tissue by freezing with substances such as liquid air or carbon dioxide snow.

cryoextrac′tion. The removal of a cataract by the use of an instrument that is supercooled to make frozen contact with the lens of the eye.

cryoextrac′tor. A copper pencil-shaped instrument with a small ball in its end′that is placed in a freezing substance and used in the removal of a cataractous lens of the eye.

cryogen′ic. Relating to the production and use of very low temperatures.

cryogen′ics. The branch of physics concerned with the production and effects of very low temperatures.

cryoglob′ulin. Abnormal γ-globulin which precipitates when exposed to low temperatures (less than 37°C).

cryoglobuline′mia. The presence of cryoglobulin (abnormal protein) in the blood plasma.

cryom′eter. An instrument for measuring very low temperatures.

cryop′athy. Any condition caused by cold.

cryopro′tein. A blood protein that precipitates from solution when cooled.

cry′oscope. An instrument used to determine the freezing point of solutions.

cryos′copy. The determination of the freezing point of a solution compared with that of distilled water; based on the principle that the freezing point is depressed according to the concentration and nature of the solute.

cry′ostat. Apparatus used to maintain low-temperature environments so that certain procedures (e.g., sectioning frozen tissues) may be carried out.

cryosur′gery. Surgery performed by the applica-

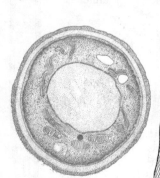

Cryptococcus
neoformans

cryptorchidism

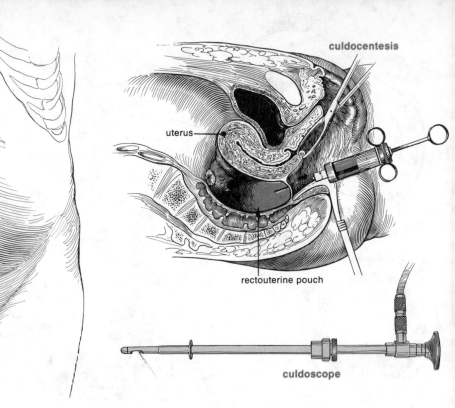

culdocentesis

uterus

rectouterine pouch

culdoscope

tion of extreme cold temperatures.

cryothalamec'tomy. Destruction of the thalamus by extreme cold temperatures for the treatment of Parkinson's disease.

cryother'apy. The therapeutic use of extremely low temperatures, as of liquid nitrogen in the treatment of chronic cervicitis.

crypt. A glandular sac or pitlike depression.

anal c., one of the furrows separating the folds of mucous membrane in the upper anal canal.

c.'s of Leiberkühn, simple tubular glands in the mucous membrane of the intestines, believed to be concerned with the secretion of digestive enzymes and of some hormones; also called intestinal glands.

dental c., the space filled by a developing tooth.

tonsillar c., one of several pits on the surface of the palatine tonsil.

crypti'tis. Inflammation of a crypt or a follicle.

anal c., inflammation of the mucous membrane of an anal crypt, especially painful during bowel movements.

urethral c., inflammation of the mucous follicles of the external orifice of the female urethra.

crypto-, crypt-. Combining form meaning (a) hidden; (b) follicle or pit.

cryptoco'ccin. An antigen derived from the fungus *Cryptococcus neoformans.*

cryptococco'sis. A chronic disseminated disease caused by the fungus *Cryptococcus neoformans;* it causes a respiratory infection often overlooked until it spreads to other areas of the body, particularly the central nervous system where it causes meningitis; also called torulosis.

Cryptococ'cus. A genus of yeastlike fungi (family Cryptococcaceae).

C. neoformans, species commonly found in pigeon droppings and causing cryptococcosis in man; formerly called *Saccharomyces neoformans.*

cryptogen'ic, cryptogenet'ic. Of obscure origin.

cryp'tolith. A calculus in a crypt or pit of a structure.

cryptomenorrhe'a. Monthly occurrence of the signs of menstruation without a flow of blood, as in imperforate hymen.

cryp'tomerorachis'chisis. See spina bifida occulta.

cryptophthal'mos. Congenital anomaly marked by the absence of eyelids; the skin is continuous from the forehead to the cheek over a rudimentary eye.

cryptor'chid. 1. Relating to an undescended testis. **2.** An individual whose testis or testes have not descended into the scrotum.

cryptorchidec'tomy. Surgical removal of an un-

descended testis.

cryptor'chidism, cryptor'chism. Condition in which the descent of a testis is arrested at some point in its normal path into the scrotum; the testis may be situated anywhere between the renal and scrotal areas.

cryptozo'ite. A stage in the cycle of the malarial parasite, when it exists in bodily tissue, usually the liver parenchyma, prior to entering the red blood cell.

crys'tal. 1. A solid substance composed of atomic groupings (unit cells) having a geometric form which is characteristic for different compounds. **2.** One unit cell of such a substance.

Charcot-Leyden c.'s, Charcot-Neumann crystals; elongated crystalline structures formed from eosinophils, found in the sputum of patients with bronchial asthma.

Charcot-Neumann c.'s, see Charcot-Leyden crystals.

crys'talline. 1. Transparent; clear. **2.** Relating to or made of crystal or composed of crystals.

crystalliza'tion. Spontaneous grouping of the molecules of a substance into an orderly repetitive pattern; change in form to a solid phase, as when a solute precipitates from solution.

crystallog'raphy. The study of the structure and phenomena of crystals.

x-ray c., a technique for the three-dimensional mapping of substances, too small to be viewed even through an electron microscope, through the use of x-ray diffraction techniques.

crys'talloid. 1. Resembling a crystal. **2.** A noncolloidal substance which, when in solution, can diffuse through a semipermeable membrane, and is generally capable of being crystallized.

c. of Charcot-Böttcher, a slender crystal-shaped inclusion peculiar to the Sertoli cell of the seminiferous epithelium.

crystallu'ria. The presence of crystals in the urine.

CS. Abbreviation for conditioned stimulus.

Cs. Chemical symbol for cesium.

CSF. Abbreviation for cerebrospinal fluid.

CT. Abbreviation for connective tissue.

Cu. Chemical symbol of copper (cuprum).

cu'bital. Of or relating to the forearm or to the ulna.

cu'bitus. The elbow; the joint between the arm and forearm.

cu'boid. Cube-shaped.

cue. A perceived stimulus to which a person responds.

cuirass'. A piece of armor to protect the chest; the term is used in medical terminology to indicate a relationship to the chest.

cul-de-sac', pl. culs-de-sac'. A pouch or sac.

c. of Douglas, the peritoneal cavity between the posterior wall of the uterus and the anterior wall of the rectum; currently called rectouterine pouch.

conjunctival c., the recess, upper or lower, formed by the junction of the ocular and palpebral conjunctiva.

culdocente'sis. Aspiration of pus or any fluid from the rectouterine pouch (cul-de-sac of Douglas) through a transvaginal puncture.

cul'doscope. A lighted instrument used for the visual examination of the pelvic cavity and its contents.

culdos'copy. Viewing of the pelvic cavity and organs by introduction of an instrument (culdoscope) through the posterior wall of the vagina.

Cu'lex. A genus of mosquitoes including some species which carry and transmit several disease-causing agents.

C. pipiens, the common house mosquito.

C. tarsalis, mosquito that transmits St. Louis and western equine encephalomyelitis.

cu'licide. Any agent that kills mosquitoes.

culicifuge. An agent that drives away mosquitoes and gnats.

Cullen's sign. Blue discoloration of the skin around the navel as a result of intraperitoneal hemorrhage, as in ruptured ectopic pregnancy.

cul'ture. 1. The propagation of microorganisms in a nutrient medium. **2.** A colony of microorganisms grown in a nutrient medium.

pure c., one in which all the microorganisms are of one species.

tissue c., the growth and maintenance of tissue cells in vitro after removal from the body.

culture medium. See medium (3).

cum (c̄). Latin meaning with; used in prescription writing.

c. correction (CC), Latin for with correction; in ophthalmology, wearing prescribed lenses.

cumulus oophorus. A mass of granulosa (follicular) cells surrounding the developing ovum in the ovarian follicle.

cu'neate. Wedge-shaped.

cune'iform. Wedge-shaped.

cu'neus, pl. cu'nei. The posterior portion of the occipital lobe of each cerebral hemisphere.

cunic'ulus. The burrow made in the skin by the itch mite.

cunnilin'gus. Oral stimulation of the vulva or clitoris.

cun'nus. Latin for vulva.

cup. A cuplike structure.

eye c., a small oblong cup that fits on the orbit; used for the application of a medicated liquid or

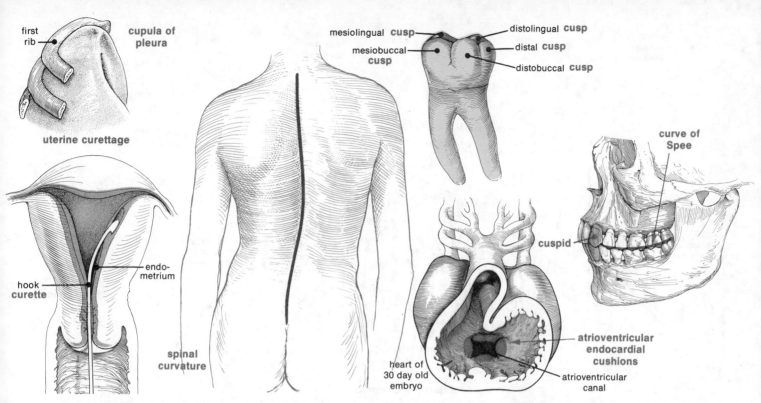

first rib

cupula of pleura

uterine curettage

hook curette

endo-metrium

spinal curvature

mesiolingual **cusp**

mesiobuccal **cusp**

distolingual **cusp**

distal **cusp**

distobuccal **cusp**

curve of Spee

cuspid

heart of 30 day old embryo

atrioventricular endocardial cushions

atrioventricular canal

---

wash to the eye; also called eye bath.

glaucomatous c., a deep depression of the optic disk, occurring in glaucoma due to increased intraocular pressure.

physiologic c., a normal depression on the surface of the optic disk.

cu'pola. See cupula.

cup'ping. 1. Formation of a cup-shaped depression. **2.** Application of a cupping glass (glass vessel from which air has been exhausted) to the skin in order to draw blood to the surface.

c. of the optic disk, exaggerated depression at the center of the optic disk, as seen in glaucoma.

cu'pric. Relating to or containing divalent copper.

c. sulfate, deep blue crystals used as irritant, astringent, and fungicide; also called copper sulfate and blue vitriol.

cu'pula. A dome-shaped structure; also called cupola.

c. cristae ampullaris, a gelatinous mass over the crista of the ampulla of the semicircular canal containing tufts of cilia from the underlying hair cells.

c. of pleura, the domelike peak of the pleural sac covering the apex of the lung and located near the neck; also called cervical pleura.

cura're. A resinous substance obtained from *Strychnos toxifera* and other plants, used as a poison on arrows; death results from paralysis of the muscles of respiration unless artificial respiration is provided; used medicinally, it is administered systemically as an effective muscle relaxant, acting by blocking nerve impulses at the myoneural junction.

curariza'tion. The administration of curare or related compounds to produce muscular relaxation or paralysis.

cu'rarize. To administer curare or related compounds to induce motor, but not sensory, paralysis.

cur'ative. 1. Serving to cure. **2.** A remedy.

curd. The coagulated part of milk.

cure. 1. To restore to health. **2.** A method of treatment or a remedy. **3.** In dentistry, the procedure by which a plastic material (as that of a denture base) is hardened.

faith c., psychotherapy based upon prayer.

radical c., one that completely eradicates a condition.

rest c., the treatment of a mental disorder by rest and change of environment.

curet. See curette.

cu'rettage. Surgical scraping of the interior of a cavity with a curette to remove growths or diseased tissue, or to obtain tissue for examination (biopsy).

fractional c., separate curettage of the uterine lining (endometrium) and the endocervix for diagnostic evaluation.

periapical c., removal of diseased tissue surrounding the root of a tooth.

uterine c., curettage of the uterus. See also D and C.

curett'e. A spoon-shaped surgical instrument used to scrape the walls of a body cavity; also written curet.

cu'rie (Ci). A unit of radioactivity expressed in terms of particles emitted per second; one curie of a radioactive substance emits 37,000,000,000 particles per second; this value was established from what was originally thought to be the disintegration rate of one gram of radium.

cu'rium. A synthetic radioactive element; symbol Cm, atomic number 96, atomic weight 247.

cur'rent. A steady onward movement, as of water or electricity.

alternating c. (AC), an electric current that reverses direction of flow at regular intervals.

c. of injury, the current that passes through a conductor connecting the injured and the uninjured portions of a nerve or other excitable tissue.

direct c. (DC), an electric current that flows in one direction only.

high frequency c., an alternating electric current having a frequency of at least 10,000 cycles per second.

stabile c., a current applied with both electrodes placed in a fixed position.

cur'vature. A bending or curving.

greater c. of the stomach, the left and inferior borders of the stomach.

lesser c. of the stomach, the right border of the stomach.

spinal c., deviation of the spine.

curve. 1. A line that deviates from a straight course in a smooth, continuous, nonangular manner. **2.** A line representing plotted data on a graph.

c. of Spee, one formed by the upper dental arch meeting with the lower dental arch viewed bucally from the first bicuspid to the last molar.

distribution c., a curve in which the number of individuals is plotted along the ordinate and the property under investigation is plotted along the abscissa.

dye-dilution c., indicator-dilution curve; a curve indicating the serial concentrations of a dye.

frequency c., one representing an approximation of the rate of occurrences of a periodic event; also called gaussian or probability curve.

gaussian c., see frequency curve.

indicator-dilution c., see dye-dilution curve.

Price-Jones c., one representing variations in the diameters of red blood cells.

probability c., see frequency curve.

Starling c., one indicating cardiac output against atrial pressure.

strength-duration c., one indicating the relationship between the intensity of an electrical stimulus and the time it must flow to be effective.

stress-strain c., one showing the ratio of deformation to load during testing of a material under tension.

Traube-Hering c.'s, slow oscillations in blood pressure usually extending through several respiratory cycles; also called Traube-Hering waves.

Cushing's disease. Adrenocortical overactivity caused by excessive secretion of pituitary adrenocorticotropic hormone (ACTH).

Cushing's syndrome. A metabolic disorder caused by chronic excess of glucocorticoids; characterized by a round face, central obesity, prominent dorsal fat pad, florid complexion, abdominal striae, hypertension, and impaired carbohydrate tolerance among other findings.

cush'ion. Any anatomic structure resembling a pad.

atrioventricular canal c.'s, see atrioventricular endocardial cushions.

atrioventricular endocardial c.'s, a pair of apposing masses of mesenchymal tissue in the embryonic heart; they appear at the superior and inferior borders of the atrioventricular canal in a six-mm embryo; they grow together and fuse, dividing the canal into right and left atrioventricular orifices; also called atrioventricular canal cushions.

Passavant's c., see ridge, Passavant's.

cusp. 1. One of the triangular segments of a heart's valve. **2.** A pronounced elevation on the occlusal surface (grinding surface) of a tooth.

cus'pid. A tooth having one cusp or point; one of the four anterior teeth situated between the upper and lower incisors and bicuspids; used primarily for biting and tearing; the longest and most stable tooth in the mouth; also called canine or dog tooth; an upper cuspid is also called eye tooth.

cus'pidor. In dentistry, a bowl-shaped vessel adjacent to a dental chair, used for spitting into; also called spittoon.

cut. 1. To dilute; to reduce or adulterate the strength of, such as to adulterate heroin with milk sugar (lactose) or quinine. **2.** Medical colloquialism meaning to operate.

cuta'neous. Relating to the skin.

cu'ticle. 1. The epidermis. **2.** The thin fold of skin overlying the base of a fingernail or toenail.

cuticulariza'tion. The formation of skin over an abraded area.

cutis vera. True skin or dermis; also called corium.

cuvet', cuvett'e. A glass container in which

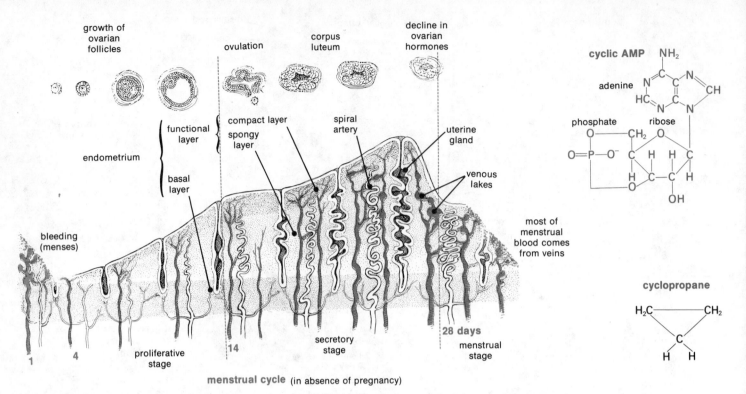

menstrual cycle (in absence of pregnancy)

solutions are placed for photometric study.

CVA. Abbreviation for cerebrovascular accident.

cy'anate. A salt of cyanic acid.

cy'anide. Any of a group of compounds of hydrocyanic acid containing the radical –CN or ion $(CN)^-$.

mercuric c., an extremely poisonous compound, $Hg(CN)_2$; used as an antiseptic.

potassium c., an extremely poisonous compound, KCN; used as a reagent, fumigant, and insecticide.

cyanmethemoglo'bin. Cyanide methemoglobin; a compound of cyanide with methemoglobin.

cyano-, cyan-. 1. Combining forms meaning a blue coloring. **2.** In chemistry, denoting the presence of the cyanide group, CN, in a molecule.

cyanocobal'amin. Vitamin B_{12}; a substance having hematopoietic properties; used in the treatment of pernicious anemia.

cy'anophil, cy'anophile. Any cell or tissue element readily stainable with blue dyes.

cyanop'sia. A defect of vision in which all objects seem to be tinted blue.

cyanop'sin. A photosensitive substance, thought to have a spectral sensitivity similar to that of the cones of the retina of some animals.

cyanose tardive. Term applied to the potentially cyanotic group of congenital heart diseases with an abnormal communication between systemic and pulmonary circulation; cyanosis is absent while the shunt is from left to right, but if the shunt reverses, as after exercise or late in the course of the disease, cyanosis appears; also called delayed cyanosis.

cyano'sis. Bluish discoloration of the skin, lips, and nail beds caused by insufficient oxygen in the blood; it appears when the reduced hemoglobin in the small vessels is 5 g per 100 ml or more.

cyanot'ic. Relating to or characterized by cyanosis.

cybernet'ics. The comparative study of biologic and mechanoelectric systems of automatic control, such as the nervous system and electronic computers, for the purpose of explaining the nature of the brain.

cycl-. Combining form denoting (a) circle or cycle; (b) the ciliary body.

cyclarthro'dial. Of or relating to a rotary joint.

cyclarthro'sis. A rotary joint.

cy'cle. A time interval in which a regularly repeated sequence of events takes place.

anovulatory c., a sexual cycle in which no ovum is produced.

brain wave c., the complete series of changes in amplitude of a wave of the electroencephalogram before repetition occurs.

carbon dioxide c., carbon c., the natural processes through which carbon in the atmosphere, in the form of carbon dioxide, is converted into carbohydrates by photosynthesis, metabolized by living organisms, and ultimately returned to the atmosphere, again as carbon dioxide.

cardiac c., the complete round of events that occur in the heart with each beat.

citric acid c., see tricarboxylic acid cycle.

estrous c., the periodic series of physiologic changes that occur under the influence of sex hormones in higher animals.

exogenous c., the phase in the development of a parasite spent in the body of the invertebrate host, as of the malarial parasite in the body of a mosquito.

Krebs c., see tricarboxylic acid cycle.

life c., the entire life of an organism.

menstrual c., the periodic changes that take place in the female reproductive organs; the period in which an ovum matures, is ovulated, and enters the lumen of the uterus through the uterine tube; ovarian hormonal secretions effect endometrial changes such that, if fertilization occurs, nidation will be possible; in the absence of fertilization, ovarian secretions wane, the endometrium sloughs, and menstruation begins.

nitrogen c., the continuous process in which nitrogen is deposited in the soil, assimilated by bacteria and plants, transferred to animals, and returned to the soil.

ovarian c., the normal periodic changes that take place in the ovary during the production and discharge of an ovum.

reproductive c., the series of physiologic changes that takes place in the female reproductive organs from the time of conception to delivery.

tricarboxylic acid c., a series of enzymatic reactions involving the complete oxidation of acetyl units, providing the main source of energy in the mammalian body and taking place mostly during respiration; also called Krebs or citric acid cycle.

urea c., the series of chemical reactions that occur in the liver, resulting in the production of urea.

cyclec'tomy. Surgical removal of a portion of the ciliary body.

cy'clic. Occurring periodically.

cy'clic AMP. Adenosine-3',5'-cyclic monophosphate; ubiquitous in nature and the mediator of hormone actions in mammals; also called genetic regulator.

cy'clic GMP. 3',5'-Guanosine cyclic monophosphate; a nucleotide that serves as a second messenger, playing a role complementary to cyclic AMP's in regulating intracellular processes, one nucleotide promoting those the other inhibits; when the cyclic GMP level goes up the cyclic AMP level goes down

and vice versa.

cycli'tis. Inflammation of the ciliary body.

plastic c., severe cyclitis with exudation of a material rich in fibrin that accumulates in the anterior and posterior chambers.

purulent c., acute cyclitis with a copious discharge of pus, usually involving the iris and choroid.

serous c., simple cyclitis with a relatively fluid discharge.

cyclizine hydrochloride. An antihistamine used in preventing and relieving symptoms of motion sickness and postoperative nausea and vomiting; also relieves vertigo and other symptoms caused by vestibular disorders of the ear; Marezine®.

cyclochoroidi'tis. Inflammation of the ciliary body and the choroid layer of the eye.

cyclodial'ysis. The surgical creation of an opening between the anterior chamber of the eye and the suprachoroidal space to reduce intraocular pressure in glaucoma.

cyclodiather'my. The partial destruction of the ciliary body by the application of heat for the reduction of intraocular pressure in the treatment of glaucoma.

cy'cloid. 1. In psychiatry, a personality characterized by alternating states of elation and depression. **2.** Resembling cyclothymia.

cyclokerati'tis. Inflammation of the ciliary body and the cornea.

cyclopho'ria. Tendency of one eye to deviate on its anteroposterior axis.

cyclophorom'eter. Instrument used to measure cyclophoria.

cyclophos'phamide. A white crystalline powder used as an antitumor agent; Cytoxan®.

cyclople'gia. Paralysis of the ciliary muscle and loss of the power of accommodation.

cyclople'gic. 1. Relating to paralysis of the ciliary muscle of the eye. **2.** An agent that causes paralysis of the ciliary muscle.

cyclopro'pane. A colorless, inflammable, explosive gas, C_3H_6; used as a general anesthetic; also called trimethylene.

cyclothy'mia. Cyclic fluctuations of mood between elation and mild depression.

cyclot'omy. Surgical incision of the ciliary muscle of the eye.

cy'clotron. A circular accelerator capable of producing high energy ions (protons and deuterons) under the influence of an alternating magnetic field.

cye'sis. Pregnancy.

cyl. Abbreviation for (a) cylinder (b) cylindrical lens.

cyl'inder. 1. A cylindrical lens. **2.** A rodlike renal

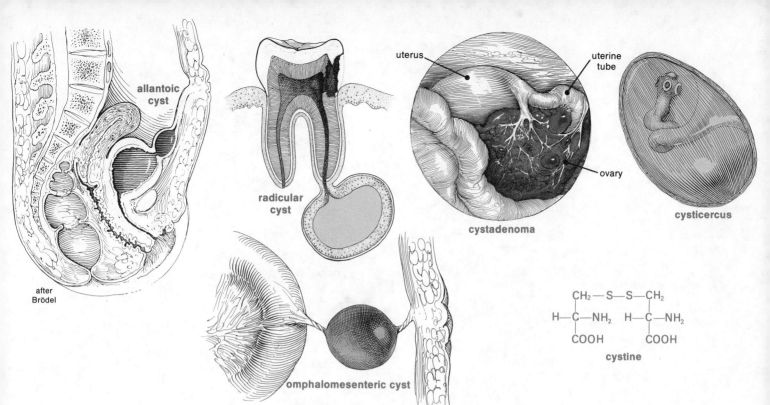

allantoic cyst

after Brödel

radicular cyst

uterus · uterine tube · ovary

cystadenoma

cysticercus

$$CH_2-S-S-CH_2$$
$$H-C-NH_2 \quad H-C-NH_2$$
$$COOH \quad COOH$$

cystine

omphalomesenteric cyst

cast.

cyl'indroid. A cylindrical mass in the urine resembling a hyaline cast; also called false or mucous cast.

cylindro'ma. A relatively benign epithelial tumor appearing as multiple nodules, especially on the scalp and face.

cylindru'ria. The presence of casts in the urine.

cynopho'bia. Exaggerated fear of dogs.

cypridop'athy. Any venereal disease.

cypridopho'bia. Abnormal fear of venereal disease or of sexual intercourse.

cyst-, cysto-. Combining forms denoting a relationship to a bladder or to a cyst.

cyst. 1. An abnormal sac within the body containing air or fluid. **2.** A bladder.

   allantoic c., a cystic dilation of the urachus; also called urachal cyst.

   alveolodental c., one associated with an unerupted tooth, occurring either in the surrounding tissues (extracapsular) or within the developing tooth (intracapsular); also called odontocele.

   Baker's c., a collection of escaped synovial fluid in the tissues outside the knee joint.

   branchial c., cyst resulting from the nonclosure of a bronchial cleft.

   Bartholin-gland c., the most common cyst of the vulva, resulting from retention of glandular secretions due to a blocked duct.

   bursal c., a retention cyst in a bursa.

   chocolate c., cyst of the ovary containing a thick dark brown tenacious fluid; often seen in endometriosis; also called Sampson cyst.

   corpus luteum c., cyst in the ovary formed from corpus luteum that remains cystic with excessive fluid content instead of regressing normally; commonly associated with disturbance of or delay in menstruation.

   dermoid c., a common tumor of the ovary, usually bilateral, consisting of displaced ectodermal tissues; it has thick, bluish white, smooth walls with sebaceous and hairy contents.

   dilatation c., see retention cyst.

   distention c., see retention cyst.

   echinococcus c., hydatid cyst.

   ependymal c., a cystic dilatation of the central canal of the spinal cord or of the cerebral ventricles; also called neural cyst.

   hydatid c., one formed, usually in the liver, by the larval stage of the tapeworm.

   lacteal c., milk cyst; a retention cyst in the breast resulting from obstruction of a lactiferous duct.

   meibomian c., see chalazion.

   milk c., see lacteal cyst.

   mother c., the main echinococcus cyst containing smaller daughter cysts.

   mucous c., retention cyst resulting from closure of the duct of a mucous gland.

   nabothian c., retention cyst resulting from obstruction of a mucous gland of the uterine cervix; also called nabothian follicle.

   neural c., see ependymal cyst.

   omphalomesenteric duct c., a cystic dilatation along the remnant of the embryonic omphalomesenteric (vitelline) duct.

   ovarian c., cystic tumor of the ovary.

   periapical c., see radicular cyst.

   piliferous c., dermoid cyst containing hair.

   pilonidal c., a hair-containing cyst in the dermis or subcutaneous tissues, usually connected to the surface of the skin by a sinus tract; generally situated in the sacrococcygeal region; also called sacrococcygeal cyst.

   pseudomucinous c., one containing a gelatinous material.

   radicular c., one around the root of a nonvital tooth; also called root or periapical cyst.

   retention c., one resulting from obstruction of the duct of a gland; also called dilatation, distention, or secretory cyst.

   root c., see radicular cyst.

   Sampson's c., see chocolate cyst.

   sebaceous c., tumor resulting from retention of the excretion of a sebaceous gland; also called wen, steatoma, steatocystoma, sebocystoma, and sebaceous tumor.

   secretory c., see retention cyst.

   serous c., one containing clear serous fluid.

   solitary bone c., cyst lined with a thin layer of connective tissue and containing serous fluid; usually seen in the shaft of a long bone of a child; also called unicameral cyst and osteocytoma.

   sublingual c., see ranula.

   subsynovial c., distention of a synovial follicle.

   unicameral c., see solitary bone cyst.

   urachal c., see allantoic cyst.

cystadenocarcino'ma. A malignant tumor derived from glandular epithelium, most frequently occurring as a partially solid mass with a cystic pattern; seen chiefly in the ovaries.

cystadeno'ma. A cystic neoplasm lined with epithelial cells and filled with retained secretions.

   papillary c. lymphomatosum, a rare benign tumor of salivary gland origin; seen chiefly in the region of the parotid gland; also called Warthin's tumor and adenolymphoma.

cystal'gia. Pain in the bladder.

cystathi'onine. An intermediate in the conversion of methionine to cysteine.

cystathioninu'ria. A rare, inherited disorder of amino acid metabolism resulting in an excessive secretion of cystathionine in the urine; associated with mental retardation.

cystecta'sia, cystec'tasy. Dilatation of the bladder.

cystec'tomy. Surgical removal of a portion of the urinary bladder.

cys'teine. An amino acid, $C_3H_7NO_2S$, present in most proteins.

cys'tic. 1. Relating to a cyst. **2.** Relating to the gallbladder or urinary bladder.

cystic disease of breast. See fibrocystic disease of breast.

cystic disease of renal medulla. The presence of multiple cysts in the medulla of the kidney, seen primarily in two clinical syndromes: uremic medullary cystic disease (nephrophthisis) and sponge kidney (non-uremic medullary cystic disease); the former is an inherited disease in which medullary cysts are associated with glomerulosclerosis, interstitial fibrosis, and renal failure, often appearing in childhood; the latter is a relatively benign condition, usually diagnosed by intravenous pyelography, which may be associated with calculi or infections.

cysticerco'sis. Infestation with the larvae of the cestode *Taenia solium* (pork tapeworm).

cysticer'cus. The cystic or larval form of the tapeworm, consisting of a scolex or head enclosed in a fluid-filled sac or cyst.

cystic fibrosis of pancreas. Congenital hereditary disease marked by dysfunction of any of the exocrine glands, resulting in a striking increase in the sodium and potassium concentration of sweat and overproduction of viscid mucus, which causes obstruction of the structures involved (pancreatic and bile ducts, intestines, and bronchi); it affects principally infants and children; common forms include meconium ileus in the newborn and chronic pulmonary disease and pancreatic insufficiency in older children; also called mucoviscidosis and fibrocystic disease of pancreas.

cysticot'omy. Surgical incision into the cystic duct.

cys'tiform. Resembling a cyst.

cys'tine. A sulfur-containing amino acid present in many proteins.

cystino'sis. Failure of normal cystine (amino acid) metabolism due to a genetically determined enzyme deficiency; the cystine accumulates and precipitates widely in many tissues, including the renal tubular epithelium and the bone marrow; one of many causes of the Fanconi syndrome; a milder form is seen in the adult in which cystine is deposited in the cornea but not in the kidney.

cystinu'ria. 1. The presence of cystine in the

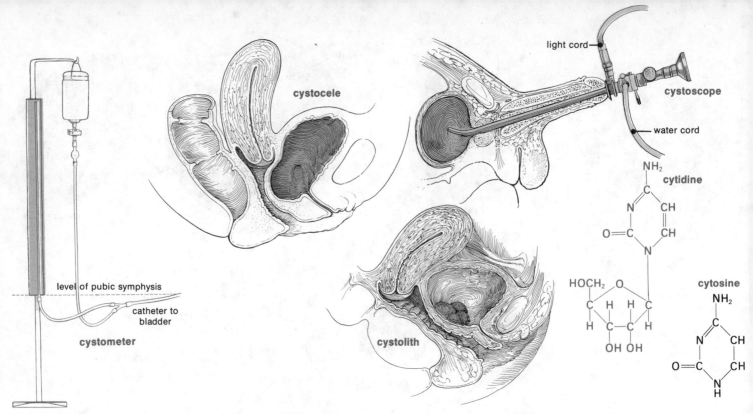

cystocele

cystoscope

light cord

water cord

cytidine

cytosine

cystolith

cystometer

level of pubic symphysis

catheter to bladder

urine. **2.** A hereditary defect in renal tubular reabsorption of the amino acids cystine, lysine, arginine, and ornithine, resulting in recurrent kidney stone formation.

cysti'tis. Inflammation of the urinary bladder.

cystit'omy. 1. Capsulotomy. **2.** Cystotomy. **3.** Cholecystotomy.

cys'tocele. Hernia formed by the downward and forward displacement of the urinary bladder toward the vaginal orifice, due most commonly to weakening of the musculature during childbirth; also called vesicocele.

cys'togram. X-ray picture of the bladder, obtained after instilling radiopaque fluid into it through a catheter.

cystog'raphy. Roentgenography of the bladder after introduction of a radiopaque fluid.

cys'toid. 1. Resembling a cyst. **2.** A collection of soft material resembling a cyst but without an enclosing capsule.

cys'tolith. A bladder stone.

cystolithec'tomy. Surgical removal of a bladder stone; erroneously used when referring to the removal of a gallbladder stone; also called cystolithotomy.

cystolithi'asis. The presence of bladder stones.

cystolith'ic. Of or relating to a bladder stone.

cystolithot'omy. See cystolithectomy.

cysto'ma. A tumor containing cysts.

cystom'eter. A diagnostic device that measures the tone of the detrusor muscle in the wall of the urinary bladder in relation to the volume of fluid in the bladder.

cystomet'rogram. A graphic record of the pressure within the urinary bladder.

cystom'etry. The continuous recording of the pressures within the urinary bladder by means of a cystometer; the procedure is used for determining the tone of the bladder when neurologic disturbance of the bladder wall is suspected.

cys'topexy. Surgical fixation of the urinary bladder or gallbladder to wall of abdomen.

cys'toplasty. Surgical repair of the bladder.

cystople'gia. Paralysis of the bladder.

cystopto'sia, cystopto'sis. Prolapse of a portion of the mucous membrane of the bladder into the urethra.

cystopyeli'tis. Inflammation of the bladder and of the pelvis of the kidney.

cystorrha'gia. Bleeding from the bladder.

cystorrhe'a. Discharge of mucus from the bladder; also called vesical catarrh.

cys'toscope. A tubular instrument fitted with a light for examining the interior of the urinary bladder.

cystos'copy. Visual examination of the interior of the urinary bladder by means of a cystoscope.

cys'tospasm. Spasmodic contraction of the bladder.

cystos'tomy. A temporary opening made into the bladder in order to divert urine from the urethra.

cystot'omy. Surgical incision of the urinary bladder; also called vesicotomy.

cystoureteri'tis. Inflammation of the bladder and a ureter or ureters.

cystourethri'tis. Inflammation of the bladder and urethra.

cy'tidine. A nucleoside consisting of cytosine attached through a β-glycosidic linkage to ribose.

cytoan'alyzer. A machine used to screen smears containing cells suspected of malignancy.

cytoar'chitecture. The arrangement of cells in a tissue, especially of the cerebral cortex.

cytobiol'ogy. Cell biology.

cytocen'trum. Centrosome.

cytochem'istry. A branch of cell biology devoted to the chemical and physicochemical analysis of living matter.

cy'tochrome. A respiratory enzyme capable of undergoing alternate reduction and oxidation; chemically related to hemoglobin.

  c. oxidase, the terminal enzyme in the chain of events that constitutes cellular oxygen consumption.

cy'tocide. Destructive to cells.

cytoc'lasis. The fragmentation of cells.

cy'tocyst. The remains of a cell enclosing a schizont (malarial parasite undergoing asexual division).

cytoden'drite. Dendrite.

cytodiagno'sis. Diagnosis of disease based on the study of cells.

cytogen'esis. The origin of cells.

cytogenet'icist. A specialist in cytogenetics.

cytogenet'ics. The combined study of heredity and the structure and function of cells.

cytol'ogy. Cell biology; the science concerned with the study of cells.

  exfoliative c., examination, for the purpose of diagnosis, of cells recovered from secretions, exudate, or washings of a tissue, such as sputum, vaginal secretion, gastric washings, etc.

cytol'ysin. An antibody that is capable of causing the dissolution of an animal cell.

cytol'ysis. The destruction of a cell.

cytomeg'alic. Characterized by greatly enlarged cells.

cytomegalic inclusion disease. A viral infection presenting symptoms according to the organs affected; formerly believed to affect only children, but seen now in adults with debilitating diseases;

caused by a cytomegalovirus of the herpesvirus group; also called salivary gland virus disease.

cytomegalovi'rus. One of a group of highly host-specific herpesviruses which cause intranuclear inclusions and enlargement of cells of various organs; in man it causes cytomegalic inclusion disease; it has a special affinity for salivary glands and thus is also termed salivary gland virus.

cytom'eter. A device used for counting and measuring blood cells.

cytomorphol'ogy. The study of the configuration of cells.

cy'ton. The body of a nerve cell; also called soma.

cytopath'ic. Characterized by a diseased condition of cells.

cytopathogen'ic. Capable of producing a diseased condition in cells.

cytopathol'ogy. The study and interpretation of cellular changes as an aid in diagnosing disease.

cytopem'phis. Movement of substances completely through a cell, especially within vesicles formed from the cell membrane, without their being utilized by the cell.

cytope'nia. Diminution of the cellular elements in the blood.

cytoph'agy. The devouring or ingestion of cells by other cells (phagocytes).

cy'toplasm. The protoplasm or substance of a cell surrounding the nucleus, carrying structures within which most of the life processes of the cell take place.

cytopoie'sis. The development of cells.

cytopy'ge. The orifice that serves as the anus in certain complex protozoa.

cy'tosine. A pyrimidine base, $C_4H_5N_3O$; a disintegration product of nucleic acid.

cyto'sis. 1. The presence of more than the usual number of cells. **2.** Term used with a prefix to denote certain characteristics of cells.

cy'tosmear. Cytologic smear; see under smear.

cy'tosol. The soluble portion of the cytoplasm after all the particles, such as mitochondrial and endoplasmic reticular components, are removed.

cy'tosome. The cell body without the nucleus.

cy'tostome. The opening which serves as a mouth in certain complex protozoa.

cytotax'is, cytotax'ia. The movement of a cell toward or away from another cell in response to a specific stimulus.

cytotox'ic. Damaging to cells; also called cytolytic.

cytotox'in. An antibody that destroys or inhibits the functions of cells.

cytotrop'ic. Having an affinity for cells.

cytozo'ic. Living in a cell.

cytozo'on. A protozoan parasitic in a cell.

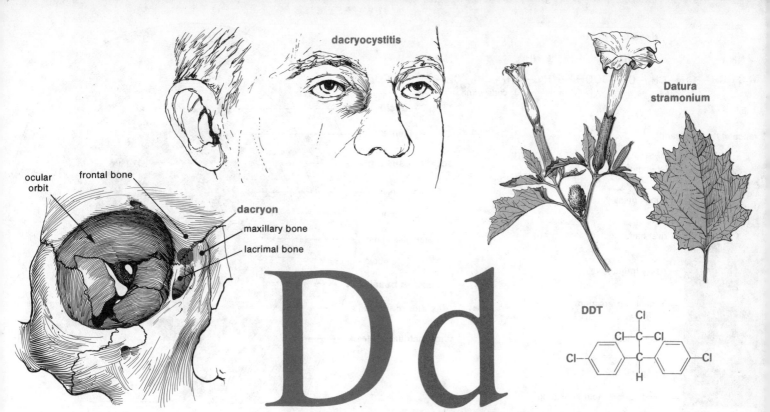

dacryocystitis

ocular
orbit

frontal bone

dacryon

maxillary bone

lacrimal bone

Datura
stramonium

DDT

D d

δ. Delta. For terms beginning with δ, see under specific term.

D. 1. Abbreviation for (a) deciduous; (b) density of gases; (c) *dexter* (right); (d) diopter. **2.** Symbol for (a) deuterium; (b) dose.

d. Abbreviation for deuteron.

d-. Prefix indicating dextrorotatory; said of a chemical compound.

dacry-, dacryo-. Combining forms denoting tears or referring to the lacrimal gland or duct.

dacryadeni'tis. See dacryoadenitis.

dac'ryagogue. 1. Promoting the flow of tears. **2.** Any agent that induces the lacrimal gland to secrete tears.

dacryoadenal'gia. Pain or discomfort in a lacrimal gland.

dacryoadeni'tis. Inflammation of the lacrimal gland; also called dacryadenitis.

dacryoblennorrhe'a. A chronic discharge of mucus from the lacrimal ducts, as in chronic dacryocystitis; also called dacryocystoblennorrhea.

dac'ryocyst. The lacrimal sac.

dacryocystal'gia. Pain or discomfort in a lacrimal sac.

dacryocystec'tomy. Surgical removal of the lacrimal sac.

dacryocysti'tis. Inflammation of the lacrimal sac, usually due to obstruction of the nasolacrimal duct; most often seen in infants or in menopausal women.

dacryocys'tocele. Protrusion of the lacrimal sac; also called dacryocele.

dacryocys'togram. An x-ray picture of the lacrimal apparatus obtained after injection with a radiopaque substance.

dacryocystorhinosteno'sis. Narrowing of the nasolacrimal duct, obstructing the normal flow of tears to the nasal cavity.

dacryocystorhinos'tomy. The operative creation of a passage between the lacrimal sac and the nose to effect the drainage of tears when the nasolacrimal duct is occluded.

dacryocystot'omy. Surgical incision of the lacrimal sac.

dacryohemorrhe'a. The shedding of tears mixed with blood.

dac'ryolith. A calculus or stone in the lacrimal apparatus (tear-forming and tear-conducting structures); also called tear stone.

dacryolithi'asis. The presence of calculi (dacryoliths) in the lacrimal passage.

dacryo'ma. 1. A cyst caused by obstruction of the lacrimal duct. **2.** A tumor of the lacrimal apparatus.

dac'ryon. A cranial point where the lacrimal, frontal, and maxillary bones meet, at the angle of the ocular orbit.

dac'ryops. 1. A watery condition of the eye; the constant presence of excess tear fluid on the eye due to poor drainage caused by constriction of the lacrimal punctum. **2.** Dilatation of a lacrimal duct by contained fluid.

dacryopyorrhe'a. The shedding of tears containing pus.

dacryopyo'sis. The formation or discharge of pus in the lacrimal sac or duct.

dacryorrhe'a. An excessive flow of tears.

dacryosoleni'tis. Inflammation of the lacrimal or nasal duct.

dacryosteno'sis. Stricture of any lacrimal passage.

dactinomy'cin. An antineoplastic agent used in the treatment of Wilm's tumor in children and trophoblastic disease in women.

dac'tyl. A digit; a finger or toe.

dactylal'gia. Pain in the fingers or toes.

dactylede'ma. Edema of a finger.

dactyli'tis. Inflammation of a digit.

dactylo-, dactyl-. Combining forms denoting finger or toe.

dactylocamp'sis. Permanent flexion or bending of the fingers or toes.

dactylog'raphy. The study of fingerprints.

dactylogrypo'sis. Contraction of the fingers or toes.

dactyloid. Finger-shaped.

dactylol'ogy. The use of the finger alphabet as a means of communication, as by deaf-mutes.

dactylol'ysis. 1. Surgical correction of fused or webbed fingers or toes. **2.** Loss of a finger or toe.

  d. spontanea, the spontaneous loss of a digit; thought to be associated with the sickle-cell trait.

dactylomeg'aly. Macrodactylia; a condition in which fingers or toes are abnormally large.

dactylos'copy. The examination of fingerprints for purposes of personal identification.

dac'tylospasm. Spasmodic contraction of the fingers.

dac'tylus. A finger or a toe; usually a toe, as distinguished from digitus, a finger.

Dalrymple's sign. Abnormal wideness of the palpebral fissures, occurring in exophthalmic goiter.

dal'ton. A unit of molecular weight equivalent to the weight of a hydrogen atom; a water molecule weighs 18 daltons and a hemoglobin molecule weighs 64,500 daltons.

dam. A barrier preventing the flow of fluid; especially a thin rubber sheet used in dentistry and surgery to isolate the operative field from the access of bodily fluid; also called rubber-dam.

  coffer d., a thin sheet of rubber stretched around the neck of a tooth to keep it dry during dental

restoration.

D and C. Abbreviation for dilatation and curettage; dilatation of the uterine cervix and scraping of the lining of the uterus (endometrium) with a curette.

D and E. Abbreviation for dilatation and evacuation.

dan'druff. Common name for the mild form of seborrheic dermatitis; see under dermatitis.

Dandy-Walker syndrome. Congenital hydrocephalus in infants due to obstruction or atresia of the median aperture of the fourth ventricle (foramen of Magendi) and the lateral aperture of the fourth ventricle (foramen of Luschka).

dap'sone. A compound used in the treatment of leprosy and tuberculosis.

Datu'ra stramo'nium. A narcotic-poisonous annual herb; also called jimsonweed and thorn apple.

datu'rine. See hyoscyamine.

D.C. Abbreviation for (a) direct current; (b) Doctor of Chiropractic.

DC. Abbreviation for Dental Corps.

DCA. See DOCA.

D.D.S. Abbreviation for Doctor of Dental Surgery.

DDT. Abbreviation for dichlorodiphenyltrichloroethane, a colorless, toxic insecticide.

deacidifica'tion. The act of removing or neutralizing an acid.

deactiva'tion. The process of rendering inactive; making harmless or ineffective.

dead. Lifeless.

deaf. Afflicted with deafness; unable to hear.

deafferenta'tion. The suppression or loss of afferent nerve impulses from a portion of the body.

deaf-mute. An individual who can neither hear nor speak.

deafmu'tism. Inability to speak due to congenital or early deafness.

deaf'ness. Inability to hear, partial or complete.

  acoustic trauma d., loss of hearing caused by prolonged exposure to excessive noise.

  cerebral d., deafness caused by a lesion in the auditory area of the brain.

  conductive d., loss of hearing caused by disease of, or injury to, the tympanic membrane or ear ossicles.

  nerve d., deafness caused by damage to the cochlear division of the vestibulocochlear nerve.

  sudden d., a sudden loss of hearing, thought to be related to systemic diseases including fat metabolism and hypercoagulation (diseases that block the circulation).

  toxic d., loss of hearing caused by certain chemical agents.

  word d., acoustic or auditory aphasia; inability to understand the spoken word.

decarboxylase

$$H_2C-CH_2-CH_2-CH_2-\overset{NH_2}{CH}-COOH \rightarrow H_2C-CH_2-CH_2-CH_2-CH_2 + CO_2$$

with NH_2 groups

lysine   cadaverine

range of human hearing
in
decibels

130	— jet engine
120	— punch press
110	
100	— rivet hammer
90	
80	— heavy traffic
70	
60	— normal conversation
50	
40	— quiet office
30	
20	— whisper
10	
0	— standard threshold of hearing

decidua vera
uterine cavity
decidua capsularis
chorionic villi
amnion
umbilical cord
embryo
decidua basalis
decidua marginalis
myometrium of uterus

dealcoholiza′tion. The removal of alcohol from a substance.

deam′idate, desam′idate, deam′idize. To remove the amido group from an organic compound.

deam′inase. An enzyme that promotes the removal of the amino group from amino compounds such as amino acids.

deam′inate. To remove, usually by hydrolysis, an amino group from an organic compound.

deamina′tion. The removal of an amino group (NH_2) from an organic compound; also called deaminization.

death. The cessation of life.
  apparent d., see death trance.
  black d., the worldwide epidemic of the 14th century, believed to be pneumonic plague.
  crib d., popular name for sudden infant death syndrome.
  maternal d., the death of a woman from any cause while pregnant or within 42 days of termination of pregnancy, irrespective of the duration and the site of pregnancy.
  rapid d., see sudden death.
  sudden d., death most commonly caused by myocardial infarction, subarachnoid hemorrhage secondary to ruptured aneurysm, intracerebral hemorrhage, rupture of the aorta or other great vessel secondary to trauma, or extradural hematoma; also called rapid death.

death rattle. The gurgling noise rarely heard in the throat of a dying person caused by loss of the cough reflex and accumulation of mucus.

death struggle. The rare symptoms of the final moments of death; a twitching or convulsion; also called agony, death throe, and psychorrhagia.

death trance. Unconsciousness and feeble respiration; also called apparent death.

debil′itate. To make weak or feeble; to enervate.

debil′ity. The condition of abnormal bodily weakness; lack or loss of strength.

debouch′. 1. To open or empty into another part. 2. An outlet.

debridement′. The excision of devitalized tissue and the removal of all foreign matter from a wound surface.

deca-, deka-. Combining forms meaning ten.

dec′agram (dag). Ten grams.

decalcifica′tion. 1. The loss of calcium salts from bones or teeth. 2. The removal of calcium ions from the blood to prevent or delay coagulation.

decal′cify. To remove calcium salts, especially from bones or teeth.

decal′cifying. 1. Denoting any agent or process that removes calcium salts from bones or teeth. 2.

Denoting an agent that removes calcium ion from blood to render it incoagulable.

dec′aliter. A measure of 10 liters; 2.64 gallons; roughly 10 quarts.

decant′. 1. To pour off the upper clear portion of a fluid without disturbing the sediment. 2. To pour fluid from one bottle into another.

decap′itate. To remove the head; to behead.

decapsula′tion. The removal of a capsule or enveloping membrane.

decarbox′ylase. Any enzyme that accelerates the removal of carbon dioxide (CO_2) from the carboxyl group of a compound, especially from α-amino acids; e.g., lysine decarboxylase.

decarboxyla′tion. Replacing of a carboxyl group from an organic compound, usually with hydrogen.

decay′. 1. The decomposition of organic compounds as a result of bacterial or fungal action. 2. In physics, spontaneous, progressive decrease of the number of atoms in a radioactive substance.

decelera′tion. Decrease in velocity.

decer′ebrate. 1. To remove the portion of the brain above the lower border of the quadrigeminal bodies. 2. Said of an experimental animal so prepared. 3. A person who has sustained a brain injury which renders him physiologically comparable to a decerebrate animal.

decerebra′tion. Removal of a portion of brain in experimental animals.

decer′ebrize. To remove the brain.

deci-. Combining form meaning one-tenth.

decibel (db). A unit for measuring the ratio of two powers or intensities (electric or acoustic power); in measurement of acoustic intensities, it is equal to 10 times the common logarithm of the ratio of two levels of intensity, or to the smallest degree of loudness that is ordinarily heard by the human ear; at a distance of about four feet, an ordinary conversation produces a level of approximately 60 db (on a scale from 1 to 130).

decid′ua. The mucous membrane (endometrium) lining the uterus that undergoes modification in preparation for and during pregnancy and is cast off at parturition and during menstruation.
  d. basalis, d. serotina, the endometrium between the implanted chorionic vesicle and the myometrium of the uterus; it becomes the maternal part of the placenta.
  d. capsularis, d. reflexa, the endometrium that seals the implanted chorionic vesicle from the uterine cavity; it undergoes rapid regression from about the fourth month of pregnancy.
  d. marginalis, the junction between the decidua basalis and the decidua capsularis.
  d. menstrualis, the hyperemic endometrial mu-

cosa of the nonpregnant uterus during the menstrual period.
  d. parietalis, see decidua vera.
  d. reflexa, see decidua capsularis.
  d. serotina, see decidua basalis.
  d. vera, d. parietalis, the entire endometrium lining the uterus, except the parts surrounding the chorionic vesicle.

decidua′tion. The casting off of endometrial tissue during menstruation.

deciduo′ma. A mass of decidual tissue in the uterus.

decid′uous. Temporary; not permanent; denoting that which falls off at the end of a stage of development; in dentistry, used to designate the primary dentition.

dec′iliter (dl). A measure of one-tenth (10^{-1}) of a liter.

dec′imeter (dm). A linear measure of one-tenth (10^{-1}) of a meter.

decinor′mal (0.1 N). One tenth of normal; denoting a solution having one-tenth of the normal strength. See also solution, normal.

decip′ara (para X). A woman who has borne 10 children.

declina′tion. 1. A sloping; a bending downward. 2. In ophthalmology, rotation of the eye about an anteroposterior axis.

decline. 1. The stage of abatement of symptoms of an acute disease. 2. A period of involution. 3. A wasting disease.

declive. Latin for hill or slope.
  d. cerebelli, the sloping portion of the vermis of the middle lobe of the cerebellum, bounded anteriorly by the primary fissure and posteriorly by the postclival fissure; also called clivus monticuli.

decoc′tion. 1. The process of boiling down or concentrating by boiling. 2. A medicine prepared by boiling.

decompensa′tion. Failure of the heart to maintain adequate circulation in certain cardiac and circulating disorders.

decompose′. 1. To decay. 2. To separate a compound into its basic elements.

decomposi′tion. 1. Organic decay; disintegration; lysis. 2. The separation of compounds into constituents by chemical reaction.

decompres′sion. The removal of pressure.
  cerebral d., removal of a section of the skull, with puncture of the dura mater, to relieve intracranial pressure.
  bowel d., relief of a distended portion of the intestine by passage of a long tube connected to suction or by establishing a direct opening, such as a cecostomy.

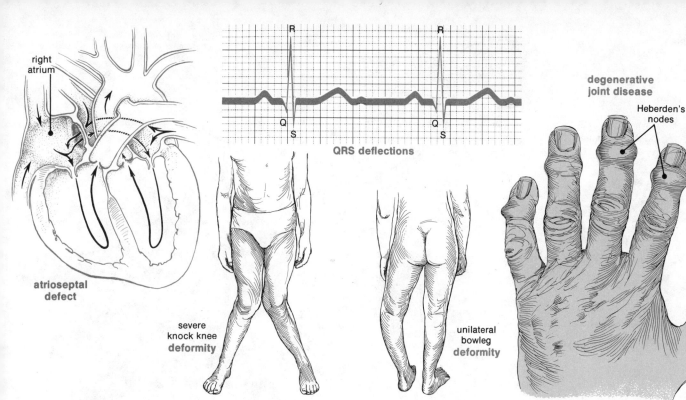

right atrium

atrioseptal defect

QRS deflections

severe knock knee **deformity**

unilateral bowleg **deformity**

degenerative joint disease

Heberden's nodes

---

cardiac d., surgical incision into the pericardium for the release of accumulated fluid from the pericardial sac; also called pericardial decompression.

orbital d., removal of bone from the orbit to relieve pressure behind the eyeball, as in exophthalmus.

pericardial d., see cardiac decompression.

deconges'tant. Any agent that reduces congestion or swelling.

deconges'tive. Reducing congestion or swelling.

decontamina'tion. 1. Making safe by eliminating or neutralizing harmful agents (noxious chemicals, radioactive material). **2.** Removal of contamination.

decor'ticate. To surgically remove the cortex of an organ or structure.

decortica'tion. Removal of the cortical substance (external layer) of an organ or structure, as the brain or kidney.

decrudes'cence. Abatement of the intensity of symptoms of disease.

decu'bital. Relating to a decubitus ulcer (bedsore).

decu'bitus. The act of reclining; lying down.

decus'sate. 1. To cross or intersect so as to form an X. **2.** Crossed like the letter X.

decussa'tion. A point of crossing, especially of nerve tracts.

dedifferentia'tion. 1. The reversion of specialized cellular forms to a more primitive condition. **2.** The process in which specialized tissues are the site of origin of primitive elements of the same type.

defeca'tion. The discharge of feces from the bowels.

de'fect. Malformation.

atrial septal d., defect in the septum between the atria of the heart.

birth d., congenital malformation; see under malformation.

filling d., any abnormality in the contour of the digestive tract, as seen in an x-ray picture.

ventricular septal d., defect in the septum between the ventricles of the heart.

defec'tive. Denoting a person deficient in some physical or mental attribute.

defemina'tion. The loss or decrease of feminine characteristics.

de'fense mech'anism. An unconscious process through which a person seeks relief from anxiety.

def'erent. Carrying down or away; also called efferent.

deferentec'tomy. See vasectomy.

deferenti'tis. Inflammation of the ductus deferens; also called vasitis and spermatitis.

deferves'cence. The disappearance or subsid-

ence of fever.

defibrilla'tion. The arrest of quivering movements of cardiac muscle fibers (fibrillation).

defi'brillator. 1. Anything that arrests ventricular fibrillation and restores the normal heart beat. **2.** An apparatus capable of delivering an electric shock to arrest ventricular fibrillation.

defibrina'tion. The removal of fibrin from the blood to prevent it from clotting.

deficiency. The state of being insufficient; a lack; a shortage.

antitrypsin d., hereditary disorder that in its severe form is frequently associated with emphysema.

pseudocholinesterase d., hereditary disorder manifested by an excessive reaction to drugs that are usually hydrolyzed by serum pseudocholinesterase, especially some of the agents used to achieve muscular relaxation during anesthesia, such as succinylcholine.

pyruvate kinase d., hereditary disorder marked by lack of pyruvate kinase, causing hemolytic anemia.

definition. 1. The power of an optical system to produce a sharp image. **2.** The maximum ability of the eye to discriminate between two points.

deflec'tion. 1. The act of turning aside, as of a light ray toward an opaque body. **2.** A wave of the electrocardiogram.

intrinsicoid d., in electrocardiography, the sudden downstroke from maximum positivity.

deflora'tion. The act of rupturing the hymen; also called deflowering.

deflores'cence. Disappearance of the skin eruption of any eruptive disease.

deflu'vium. Hair loss.

deforma'tion. 1. A change of form from the normal. **2.** A deformity; a bodily disfiguration or malformation.

defor'mity. Any bodily disfigurement.

gunstock d., displacement of the forearm to one side resulting from condylar fracture at the elbow.

lobster-claw d., a hand or foot with the middle digits fused or missing.

defunda'tion. Surgical removal of the fundus of the uterus.

defurfura'tion. The falling off or shedding of fine scales from the skin; also called branny desquamation.

degen'erate. 1. Marked by deterioration. **2.** A person who is morally degraded.

degenera'tion. 1. Deterioration of physical, mental, or moral characteristics. **2.** The deterioration of tissues with corresponding functional impairment as a result of injury or disease; the process may advance to an irreversible stage and eventually

cause death of the tissues (necrosis).

atheromatous d., localized accumulation of lipid material (atheroma) in the inner layers of the arterial walls.

ballooning d., liquefaction of the cell protoplasm leading to edematous swelling and softening; also called ballooning colliquation.

basophilic d., blue staining of connective tissue by the hematoxylin-eosin stain in conditions such as lupus erythematosus and senile skin.

cerebromacular d., cerebral sphinoglipidosis; see under sphingolipidosis.

fatty d., any abnormal accumulation of fat within the parenchymal cells of organs or glands; also called fatty change and fatty metamorphosis.

fibrinoid d., the formation of a dense, homogeneous, acidophilic substance in the tissues.

hepatolenticular d., an inherited disorder characterized by abnormal metabolism of copper causing accumulation of the metal in the liver and in the lenticular nucleus of the brain, accompanied by deposition of a brown pigment at the corneal margins; also called Wilson's disease.

heredomacular d., see macular degeneration.

hyaline d., a regressive process in which cellular cytoplasm becomes glossy and homogeneous due to injury that causes coagulation and denaturation of proteins.

hydropic d., a reversible form of intracellular edema with accumulation of water within the cell.

macular d., a hereditary condition marked by progressive degeneration of the macula and loss of vision; also called Best's disease and heredomacular degeneration.

mucoid medial d., cystic medial necrosis; see under necrosis.

reaction of d., the abnormal reaction of a degenerated nerve or muscle to an electric stimulus.

secondary d., see Wallerian degeneration.

senile d., the normal degeneration of tissues in old age.

Wallerian d., dissolution and resorption of the distal stump of a sectioned peripheral nerve; also called secondary degeneration.

Zenker's d., a form of hyaline degeneration in which the cytoplasm of striated muscle cells becomes clumped, homogeneous, and waxy; occurs in patients dying of febrile illnesses, as typhoid fever and diphtheria.

degenerative joint disease (DJD). A chronic disorder marked by degeneration of articular cartilage and hypertrophy of bone, accompanied by pain which appears with activity and subsides with rest; a common form of chronic joint disease in the middle-aged and the elderly; also called osteoarthritis and

decompression | degenerative joint disease

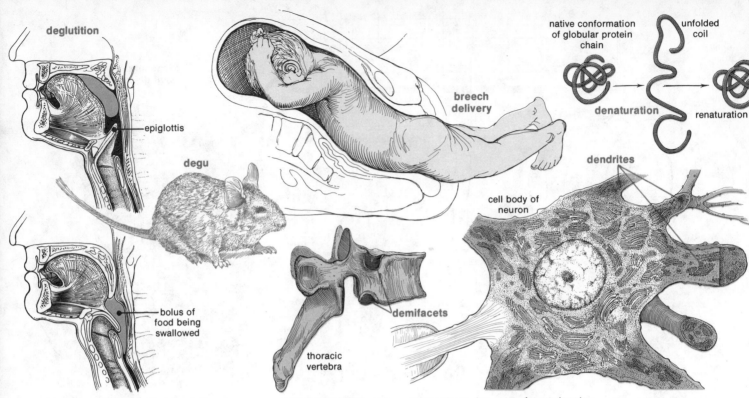

deglutition

epiglottis

degu

bolus of food being swallowed

breech delivery

native conformation of globular protein chain

unfolded coil

denaturation

renaturation

dendrites

cell body of neuron

demifacets

thoracic vertebra

degenerative or hypertrophic arthritis.

degluti'tion. The act of swallowing.

degranula'tion. The loss of granules, as in the disappearance of the neutrophilic granules in a leukocyte immediately following particle ingestion.

degree'. 1. A division of a temperature scale. **2.** A unit of angular measure equal to 1/360 of the circumference of a circle. **3.** Severity; extent.

degu. A ratlike animal from Chile possessing two anatomically separate thymus glands (cervical thymus and mediastinal thymus); used extensively by immunologists to study the thymus, which, in early life, sets up the immune defense mechanisms for the body; also called trumpet-tailed rat.

degusta'tion. The act or sense of tasting.

dehal'ogenase. Enzyme present in the thyroid gland that promotes the removal of iodine from mono- and diiodotyrosines.

dehis'cence. A rupturing or bursting, as the coming apart of the sides of a wound.

dehy'drate. To extract water from the body or from any substance; to make anhydrous.

dehydra'tion. Diminution of water content of the body or tissues.

dehydro-, dehydr-. Combining forms denoting a chemical compound from which hydrogen has been removed.

dehydrog'enase. An enzyme that catalyzes the removal of hydrogen from a substrate and the transfer of the hydrogen to an acceptor.

dehydrogena'tion. To remove hydrogen from a compound; also called dehydrogenization.

dehyp'notize. To awaken from a hypnotic state.

déjà vu. A feeling that a new experience or situation has happened before; also called déjà vu phenomenon.

dejec'tion. 1. A state of mental depression; also called melancholy. **2.** Defecation.

delacta'tion. Weaning.

delamina'tion. A division into layers or laminae; specifically the splitting of blastoderm into ectoderm and entoderm.

de-lead. To remove lead from bodily tissues.

delete'rious. Harmful.

delimita'tion. The process of putting bounds; preventing the spread of a disease.

deliques'ce. To become damp; to melt.

deliques'cent. Denoting a solid substance that becomes liquified by absorbing moisture from the atmosphere.

delir'ious. In a state of mental confusion and excitement.

delir'ium. A condition of temporary mental excitement and confusion, marked by hallucinations, delusions, anxiety, and incoherence.

d. tremens (DT's), acute mental disturbance due to withdrawal from alcohol, marked by sweating, tremor, anxiety, precordial pain, and both visual and auditory hallucinations.

deliv'er 1. To assist a woman in birth. **2.** To remove; e.g., a tumor.

deliv'ery. Childbirth; labor.

abdominal d., delivery of a child by cesarean section.

breech d., extraction of an infant whose pelvis or lower extremity is the presenting part.

forceps d., delivery in which an instrument is placed on the fetal head to exert traction on its body; classified according to the level of the head of the fetus at the time the instrument is applied, as follows: (1) high forceps, the application of forceps before engagement has taken place; (2) low forceps, the application of forceps when the head of the fetus has reached the perineal floor and is visible, and the sagittal suture of the fetal skull is in the anteroposterior diameter of the pelvis; (3) midforceps, the application of forceps after engagement has taken place but before the criteria of low forceps have been met.

postmortem d., delivery of a child after death of its mother.

premature d., expulsion of a fetus before full term, after the 28th week of gestation.

delouse'. To rid of infestation with lice.

del'ta. 1. The fourth letter of the Greek alphabet, Δ, δ; used to denote the fourth in a series. **2.** Any triangular anatomic space. **3.** In chemistry, the capital (Δ) denotes a double bond between carbon atoms; the lower case (δ) denotes the location of a substituent on the fourth atom from the primary functional group in an organic molecule. **4.** Symbol (Δ) for change. For terms beginning with delta see under specific term.

del'toid. Triangular; shaped like the Greek letter delta, Δ. See table of muscles.

delu'sion. A false belief, maintained even against contradictory evidence or logical argument.

d. of grandeur, exaggerated belief in one's importance.

d. of persecution, a false belief that one is being persecuted.

demarca'tion. The marking of boundaries.

line of d., an inflamed area separating gangrenous and healthy tissue.

demasculiniza'tion. The loss of male characteristics.

dement'ed. Afflicted with dementia or loss of reason.

demen'tia. Deterioration of intellectual function due to organic factors; formerly used to denote

madness or insanity.

d. praecox, obsolete term for schizophrenia.

senile d., mental deterioration caused by atrophy of the brain due to aging.

demi-. A prefix indicating half; e.g., demifacet.

demifac'et. The half of a facet on the side of some thoracic vertebrae for articulation with the head of a rib; also called costal facet.

dem'ilune. 1. Crescent; semilunar. **2.** The gametocyte of *Plasmodium falciparum*.

serous d., five to 10 serous cells capping the terminal end of a mucous, tubuloalveolar secretory unit of mixed salivary glands; also called crescent of Gianuzzi.

demineraliza'tion. A reduction of the mineral constituent of the tissues through excessive elimination.

demipenn'iform. Feather-shaped on one side only; said of certain muscles with a tendon on one side.

demog'raphy. The study of human populations, especially their growth, geographical distribution, and vital statistics.

dem'onstrator. A person who supplements the teachings of a professor by instructing small groups, preparing dissections, etc.

demopho'bia. Morbid fear of crowds.

demul'cent. 1. Soothing; allaying irritation. **2.** Any gummy or oily substance having such properties.

demyelina'tion, demyeliniza'tion. Destruction or loss of myelin from the sheath of a nerve.

denar'cotize. To remove or separate narcotic properties from an opiate.

denatura'tion. Loss of characteristic biologic activity in protein molecules due to extremes of pH or temperature.

dena'tured. Changed in nature; adulterated.

den'driform. Branched like a tree; tree-shaped.

den'drite. One of the cytoplasmic branches of nerve cells (neurons) which conducts the impulses received from the terminations of other neurons toward the cell body; also called dendritic process.

dendrit'ic. Relating to or resembling dendrites or protoplasmic processes of the nerve cells.

dendro-, dendri-, dendr-. Combining forms denoting tree-shaped.

den'droid. Branched; treelike.

dener'vate. To remove or sever the nerve supply to a bodily part.

den'gue. 1. An endemic disease of tropical and subtropical regions caused by a dengue virus and transmitted by *Aedes* mosquitoes; it is marked by severe headache, intense pain of the back and joints, high fever, and a spotty rash; after three or

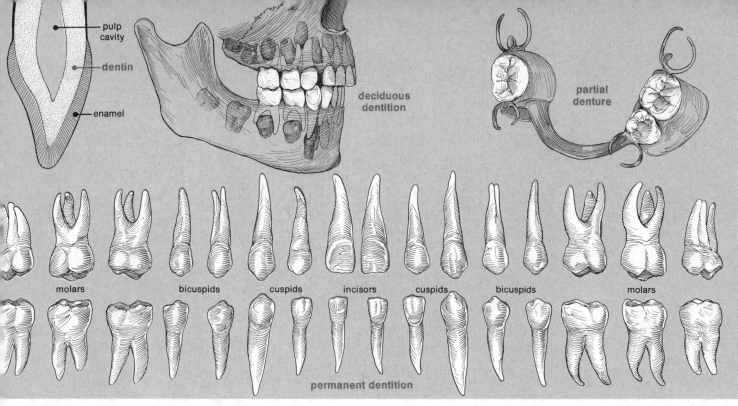

pulp cavity
dentin
enamel

deciduous dentition

partial denture

molars   bicuspids   cuspids   incisors   cuspids   bicuspids   molars

permanent dentition

four days, all symptoms subside, only to reappear 24 hr later with a characteristic skin eruption; also called break-bone, 7-day, or dandy fever. **2.** A virus of the arbovirus group B.

deni′al. An unconscious defense mechanism, in which consciously intolerable thoughts, wishes, feelings, or needs are rejected or blocked out.

denida′tion. Disintegration and expulsion of the superficial uterine mucosa.

deni′trify. To remove nitrogen from a compound.

dens, *pl.* **den′tes. 1.** Latin for tooth. **2.** A toothlike structure, as the odontoid process of the axis (second vertebra).

densim′eter. An instrument for determining the density of a fluid.

densitom′eter. A type of densimeter for determining the degree of bacterial growth in a fluid by means of its turbidity.

  photon d., a device used to measure the density of bone by passage of a beam of photons through the bone to be measured; also called bone-mineral analyzer.

densitom′etry. Technique for measuring the density of a substance, especially bone.

  bone d., the use of a densitometer to pass a beam of photons through bone; the attenuation of the beam is the measure of the density of the bone.

den′sity. 1. The state of compactness. **2.** The amount of matter per unit volume expressed in grams per cubic centimeter. **3.** The measure of the degree of resistance to the speed of a transmission.

  count d., see photon density.

  optical d., the light-absorbing quality of a translucent substance.

  photon d., in radioisotope scanning, the number of counted events per square centimeter or per square inch of imaged area; also called count density.

  vapor d., the ratio of the weight of a vapor or gas to an equal volume of hydrogen.

den′tal. Of or relating to teeth.

dental floss. Waxed thread of nylon or silk used to remove loose debris from interproximal spaces.

dental′gia. Toothache.

den′tate. Notched; having toothlike projections.

den′ticle. A calcified body in the pulp chamber of a tooth; also called pulp stone.

dentic′ulate. Having toothlike projections.

den′tiform. Shaped like a tooth; also called odontoid and dentoid.

den′tifrice. A compound, such as a paste or powder, used in conjunction with a toothbrush for cleaning the teeth.

dentig′erous. Containing teeth, as certain cysts.

den′tin. The hard tissue forming the main substance of teeth; it surrounds the tooth pulp and is covered by enamel on the crown and by cementum on the roots.

  primary d., dentin formed before the eruption of a tooth.

  secondary d., highly irregular dentin formed after tooth eruption due to irritation from caries or injuries, or the normal wearing down of the teeth.

den′tinal. Relating to dentin.

den′tine. Dentin.

dentino′ma. An extremely rare encapsulated tumor composed of connective tissue and masses of dentin.

den′tinum. Latin for dentin.

den′tist. One who practices dentistry.

den′tistry. The science and art concerned with the diagnosis, prevention, and treatment of diseases of the tissues comprising the mouth, especially the restoration or replacement of defective teeth.

denti′tion. The arrangement of the natural teeth in the dental arch.

  deciduous d., primary d., set of 20 teeth that begin to erupt when the child is about six months old.

  primary d., see deciduous dentition.

  retarded d., delayed eruption or growth of one or more teeth, deciduous or permanent.

  permanent d., set of 32 teeth that begin to erupt when the child is about 6 years old.

  transitional d., dentition containing deciduous and permanent teeth.

den′tulous. Possessing natural deciduous or permanent teeth.

den′ture. An artificial substitute for missing natural teeth and surrounding tissues.

  complete d., a dental prosthesis which replaces all the natural teeth and associated structures of one jaw.

  d. base, the part of the denture to which teeth are attached.

  fixed partial d., a partial denture that is supported by the teeth or roots and cannot be readily removed; often designated as a fixed bridge.

  immediate d., one made before the anterior teeth are extracted and inserted immediately after extraction for cosmetic reasons.

  partial d., a dental prosthesis replacing one or more teeth and held in place by remaining teeth and underlying tissues; may be removable or fixed.

denu′cleated. Deprived of a nucleus.

denu′dation. To make bare; to divest of covering.

deo′dorant. An agent that counteracts undesirable odors.

deossifica′tion. Removal of the mineral elements of bone.

deoxida′tion. Removal of oxygen from a compound; also called reduction.

deox′idize. To remove oxygen from a chemical compound; to reduce.

deoxy-, desoxy-. Combining forms denoting a chemical compound that is derived from another compound by the removal of one oxygen atom.

deoxycorticos′terone. A steroid hormone occurring in the adrenal cortex; a precursor of corticosterone; also called deoxycortone and cortexone.

  d. acetate (DOCA, DCA), a salt-retaining steroid.

deoxycor′tone. See deoxycorticosterone.

deox′ygenate. To deprive of oxygen.

deox′yribonu′clease (DNase, DNAase). An enzyme that breaks down deoxyribonucleic acid (DNA) to nucleotides.

deox′yribonucle′ic acid (DNA). The molecular basis of heredity, present in chromosomes; it is the largest biologically active molecule presently known and is responsible for the replication of the key substances of life, proteins and nucleic acid; it consists of two very long chains of alternate sugar (with attached base) and phosphate groups twisted into a double helix.

deox′yribonucleopro′tein. A nucleoprotein that yields deoxyribonucleic acid (DNA) on hydrolysis.

deox′yribonu′cleoside. A compound consisting of a purine or pyrimidine base combined with deoxyribose (a DNA sugar); also called pulp stone.

deox′yribonu′cleotide. A substance composed of a purine or pyrimidine base bonded to deoxyribose (a DNA sugar), which in turn is bound to a phosphate group.

deoxyri′bose. The pentose sugar constituent of deoxyribonucleic acid (DNA).

deox′ysugar. Any of several sugars containing less oxygen atoms than carbon atoms in the molecule, resulting in one or more carbons lacking an attached hydroxyl group.

deoxyvi′rus. DNA virus; see under virus.

depan′creatize. To remove the pancreas.

depersonaliza′tion. A condition in which a person loses his sense of personal identity or feels his body to be unreal.

dephosphoryla′tion. The removal of a phosphate group from a compound through the action of an enzyme.

depigmenta′tion. Partial or complete loss of pigment.

dep′ilate. To remove hair, usually from the surface of the body.

depila′tion. The removal of hair.

depil′atory. 1. An agent that removes or destroys

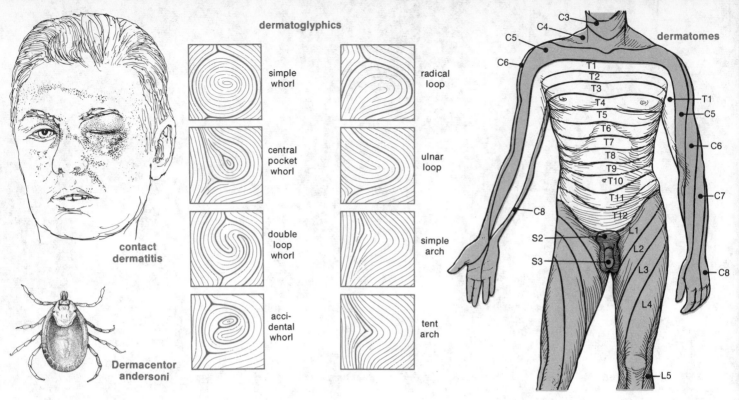

contact dermatitis

Dermacentor andersoni

dermatoglyphics

simple whorl

central pocket whorl

double loop whorl

acci- dental whorl

radical loop

ulnar loop

simple arch

tent arch

dermatomes

hair from the body. **2.** Capable of removing hair.

deplete. To exhaust; to empty.

deple'tion. 1. The process of emptying. **2.** Exhausted condition caused by excessive loss of bodily fluids. **3.** Excessive loss of bodily constituents necessary for normal functioning.

depluma'tion. Abnormal loss of the eyelashes.

depolariza'tion. The elimination or neutralization of polarity.

depos'it. Sediment.

deprav'ity. 1. Moral deterioration or corruption. **2.** A perverse act.

depres'sant. Serving to reduce functional activity.

depressed'. 1. Sunk below level of surrounding parts. **2.** Below normal functional level. **3.** Dejected.

depres'sion. 1. Emotional dejection; morbid sadness accompanied by loss of interest in surroundings and lack of energy. **2.** Area lower than the surrounding level.

  anaclitic d., impairment of an infant's development (physical, intellectual, and social) which sometimes follows a sudden separation from its mother or mother substitute.

depressomo'tor. 1. Serving to retard motor activity. **2.** Anything that causes such an effect.

depres'sor. 1. Anything that depresses or reduces functional activity, as certain nerves, muscles, or chemicals. **2.** An instrument or device used to push structures out of the way during an examination or operation.

  tongue d., a broad wooden blade used to push the tongue against the floor of the mouth during examination of the throat.

depriva'tion. Loss or absence of stimuli, nurture, organs, powers, or attributes that are needed.

  sensory d., a diminution of sensory stimuli.

depth. A dimension downward or inward.

  d. of focus, the variation of the distance between an object and a lens or optical system without causing objectionable blurring.

depuliza'tion. The destruction of fleas carrying the plague bacillus.

dep'urant. 1. Anything that purifies. **2.** An agent that promotes the excretion of waste matter.

derange'ment. 1. Mental disorder. **2.** Disarrangement of the regular order; disorder.

deriva'tion. 1. The source from which something originates. **2.** The diversion of fluids from one part of the body to another.

deriv'ative. 1. In chemistry, a compound obtained from another and containing some of the elements of the original substance. **2.** Resulting from derivation.

dermabra'sion. Operative procedure used to remove acne or chicken pox scars, tattoos, and superficial foreign bodies acquired during road or industrial accidents; the most popular method consists of freezing the skin, followed by mechanical removal of the epidermis and upper dermis with a high-speed rotary steel brush; also called skin planing and surgical planing.

Dermacen'tor. A genus of ticks (family Ixodidae).

  D. andersoni, the wood tick, a transmitter of Rocky Mountain spotted fever and tularemia and the cause of tick paralysis.

  D. variabilis, the American dog tick, the transmitter of spotted fever and tularemia.

der'madrome. Any syndrome that includes cutaneous and internal symptoms.

der'mal. Of or relating to the skin.

dermalax'ia. Softening of the skin.

dermametrop'athism. A method of diagnosing certain skin disorders by observing the markings when a blunt instrument is drawn across the skin.

dermati'tis, *pl.* **dermatit'ides.** Inflammation of the skin.

  actinic d., a sensitivity reaction of the skin produced by exposure to sunlight, distinguished from sunburn.

  atopic d., any dermatitis caused by allergy; also called atopic eczema.

  chemical d., dermatitis produced by contact with chemicals.

  contact d., dermatitis caused by contact with material to which a person is hypersensitive.

  d. exfoliativa infantum, d. exfoliativa neonatorum, a pustular dermatitis with abundant flaking and red coloration of the skin accompanied by fever, malaise, and occasionally gastrointestinal symptoms; it affects young infants and is frequently fatal; also called Ritter's disease.

  d. herpetiformis, chronic disorder marked by an eruption of itchy, burning clusters of vesicles and papules occurring mostly on the forearms and abdomen; also called Duhring's disease and hydroa herpetiforme.

  d. medicamentosa, an allergic reaction to medications taken internally or applied locally, manifested by the eruption of a rash.

  d. venenata, edematous, vesicular eruption caused by contact with a sensitizing substance such as poison ivy, cosmetics, etc.

  exfoliative d., generalized exfoliation, redness, and severe scaling of the skin with constitutional symptoms; also called Wilson's disease.

  industrial d., any dermatitis caused by contact with materials used in industry.

  ivy d., see poison ivy (2).

  seborrheic d., a condition of unknown cause with a predilection for the scalp but also seen on the eyebrows, behind the ears, the chest, back, and pubic area; characterized by varying degrees of redness, scaling, and sometimes itching; commonly known in its mild form as dandruff and seborrhea.

  solar d., dermatitis produced in persons allergic to sun's rays.

dermato-, derm-, derma-, dermat-. Combining forms meaning skin.

Dermato'bia. A genus of flies (family Oestridae) which includes the parasitic botflies.

der'matocele. A localized loose condition of the skin.

dermatoconio'sis. Occupational dermatitis caused by irritation of the skin by dust.

dermatofibro'ma. A benign skin tumor believed to be a capillary hemangioma that has become indurated, cellular, and fibrous; also called sclerosing hemangioma and histiocytoma.

dermatofibrosarco'ma protu'berans. A skin tumor composed of several small nodules covered with dark reddish blue skin; it tends to recur after removal.

dermatoglyph'ics. 1. The variety of pattern configurations of epidermal ridges on the volar aspect of the hands and feet; the ridge configuration may be altered in some disorders. **2.** The study of skin patterns, especially of the palms of the hands and soles of the feet.

dermatog'raphy, dermatog'raphism. See dermographia.

der'matoid. Resembling skin.

dermatol'ogist. A specialist in disorders of the skin and related systemic diseases; also called skin specialist.

dermatol'ogy. The medical specialty concerned with the diagnosis and treatment of skin diseases.

der'matome. 1. Surgical instrument used in cutting thin slices of skin for grafting. **2.** In embryology, the dorsolateral wall of a somite from which the skin is derived. **3.** A skin area supplied by sensory fibers of a single spinal nerve.

dermatomeg'aly. Congenital defect consisting of an excessive amount of skin which hangs in folds.

dermatomyco'sis. Any cutaneous fungal infection.

dermatomyosi'tis. A form of polymyositis; a painful inflammation of the skin, subcutaneous tissue, and muscle; the muscles most affected are those of the pelvic and shoulder girdles and pharynx; in 15 to 20 per cent of cases there is an associated neoplasm.

dermatonosol'ogy. The classification of skin dis-

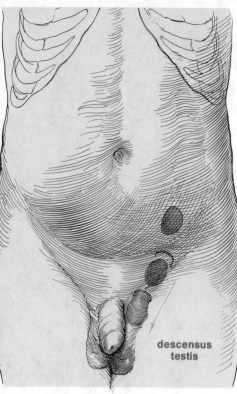

descensus testis

tooth designation

apical region of contact between two intestinal cells

micro-villi

zonula occludens

zonula adherens

desmosome

eases; also called dermonosology.

dermatopathol'ogy. The study of skin diseases.

dermatop'athy. Any disease of the skin.

der'matophyte. Any fungus capable of causing skin disease.

dermatoph'ytid. Secondary skin eruption, usually on the fingers and hands, following sensitization to fungi; often called id. See also reaction, id.

dermatophyto'sis. Any superficial fungal infection of the skin; e.g., athlete's foot.

der'matoplasty. Skin grafting to correct defects or replace loss of skin.

dermato'sis, *pl.* **dermato'ses.** Any skin eruption.

dermatoskeleton. See exoskeleton (2).

dermatother'apy. The treatment of skin diseases.

dermatotrop'ic, dermotrop'ic. Acting selectively on the skin.

dermatroph'ia, dermat'rophy. Thinning or atrophy of the skin.

der'mis. The broad, dense connective tissue layer of the skin positioned snugly under the epidermis and composed mostly of collagenous fibers with some elastic and reticular fibers; it contains blood vessels, lymphatic channels, nerves, sebaceous glands, hair follicles, and sweat glands; also called corium, true skin, and curtis vera.

der'moblast. One of the mesodermal cells that develops into the true skin or corium.

dermograph'ia. A sensitive condition of the skin in which wheals are formed by lightly drawing a pencil or blunt instrument over it; also called dermography, dermatography, dermatographia, and dermatographism.

  white d., blanching of the skin on stroking.

der'moid. 1. Resembling skin. **2.** A congenital cyst or saclike growth containing fluid and hair, skin, teeth, or other dermal structures.

dermoskeleton. See exoskeleton (2).

dermosto'sis. Bony formations on the skin.

dermotox'in. A substance that causes pathologic changes in the skin.

dermotrop'ic. See dermatotropic.

DES. Abbreviation for diethylstilbestrol.

desam'idate. See deamidate.

descementi'tis. An apparent inflammation of the posterior limiting (Descemet's) membrane of the cornea.

descen'sus. Falling; descent.

  d. testis, descent of the testis from the abdomen into the scrotum shortly before the end of intrauterine life.

desensitiza'tion. 1. See immunotherapy (3). **2.** In psychotherapy, the act of eliminating or reducing

an emotional complex.

desen'sitize. See hyposensitize.

desex'. To castrate.

des'iccant. 1. An agent possessing a high affinity for water, used to absorb moisture; a drying agent. **2.** Promoting dryness.

des'iccate. To dry.

des'iccator. A closed vessel containing a dehydrating agent (calcium chloride, sulfuric acid, etc.) in which a substance or an apparatus is placed for drying and to be kept free from moisture.

designa'tion. Distinguishing name.

desmi'tis. Inflammation of a ligament.

desmo-, desm-. Combining forms denoting a ligament, bond, or fibrous connection.

des'moid. A nodule resulting from the proliferation of fibrous tissue of muscle sheaths, especially of the abdominal wall; usually occurring in women following pregnancy; also called desmoid tumor.

des'molase. An enzyme capable of breaking a carbon-to-carbon bond in a molecule and taking part in oxidation-reduction reactions; it is not involved in hydrolysis.

desmopex'ia. Shortening of the round ligaments of the uterus by suturing them to the abdominal wall for the correction of uterine displacement.

desmopla'sia. Disproportionate formation of fibrous tissue.

desmoplas'tic. 1. Causing or forming adhesions. **2.** Causing fibrosis in the vascular stroma of a neoplasm.

des'mosome. Two apposed, small, ellipsoidal plates, about 0.5 μ in diameter, along the interfaces between the plasma membrane of adjacent cells; it serves as a site of adhesion; visible only by electron microscopy; also called macula adherens.

  half-d., a plate on one cell without a companion plate butting up against it, as found at the basal plasma membrane in some epithelia; also called hemidesmosome.

desoxy-. See deoxy-.

despuma'tion. The removal of impurities or scum from the surface of a liquid.

des'quamate. To cast off or shed the outer layer of a surface, as the scaling off of the epidermis.

desquama'tion. The shedding or peeling of the superficial layer of the skin (epidermis) in flakes or scales.

det. Abbreviation for the Latin *detur*.

detach'ment. 1. The state of being separated; e.g., the separation of the retina from its normally attached choroid. **2.** In psychiatry, the condition of being free from emotional or social involvement.

deteriora'tion. Worsening; in psychiatry, the chronic, progressive impairment of emotional and

intellectual functions.

determina'tion. The estimation of the extent, quality, or character of anything.

deter'minism. The doctrine that any event is the inevitable consequence of prior influences and hence can be completely explained by its antecedents.

De Toni-Fanconi syndrome. See Lignac-De Toni-Fanconi syndrome.

detox'icate. To remove the effects or counteract the toxic properties of a poison.

detoxica'tion. 1. The process of neutralizing the toxic properties of a substance. **2.** The recovery from the toxic effects of a substance.

detumes'cence. The return to the flaccid state or to the normal size of a swollen organ or part.

  d. of penis, the return of the penis to the flaccid state from an erection.

detur. Latin for let there be given; used in prescription writing.

deuterano'pia. A form of color blindness in which red, orange, yellow, and green cannot be differentiated when their brightnesses and saturations are equal; similarly, blue, violet, and blue-purple appear to differ only in brightness and saturation, but not in hue; a sex-linked hereditary defect, occurring in about one per cent of males and only rarely in females.

deuter'ium (D, ^{2}H). An isotope of hydrogen having an atomic weight of 2.0141, consisting of one proton and one neutron in the nucleus; also called hydrogen-2 and heavy hydrogen.

  d. oxide (D_2O), see heavy water.

deutero-, deuti-, deuto. Combining forms meaning second or secondary.

deu'teron. A subatomic particle consisting of a proton and a neutron; the nucleus of deuterium (heavy hydrogen); also called deuton and diplon.

deu'toplasm. The nonliving material in the cytoplasm, especially reserve food substance or yolk in the ovum.

Deutschländer's disease. March foot; see under foot.

devasculariza'tion. Removal of blood vessels from a part.

de'viance. A difference or departure from a norm or rule.

  psychiatric d., divergence from accepted norms of mental health.

  role d., see social deviance.

  sexual d., departure from accepted sexual norms; formerly called perversion.

  social d., departure from accepted social behavior; also called role deviance.

devia'tion. 1. A turning aside. **2.** Departure from

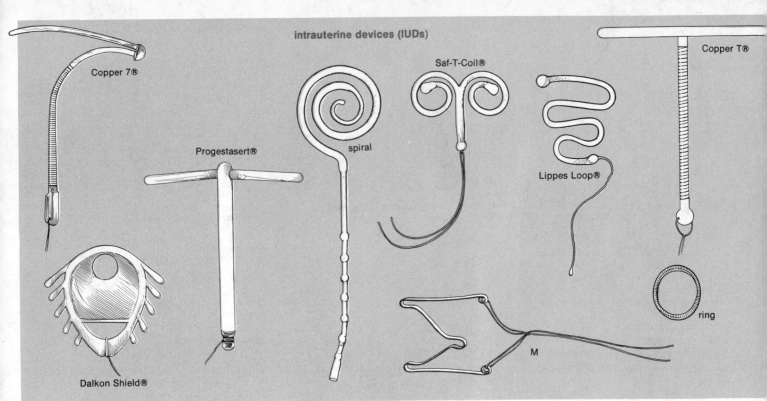

intrauterine devices (IUDs)

Copper 7®
Progestasert®
Dalkon Shield®
Saf-T-Coil®
spiral
Lippes Loop®
Copper T®
ring
M

an accepted course of behavior.

axis d., deflection of the electrical axis of the heart to the right or left.

parallel conjugate d., (1) normally, the joint and equal movement of the two eyes in the same direction when shifted from one object to another; (2) pathologically, failure of both eyes to turn to one side; the defect is compensated by rotating or tilting the head.

primary d., in strabismus, the deviation of the defective eye when the normal eye is fixed on an object.

secondary d., in strabismus, the deviation of the normal eye when the defective eye is made to fixate on an object.

skew d., special form of vertical imbalance of both eyes.

standard d., in statistics, a measure of dispersion or variation in a distribution.

device'. Something made or constructed for a particular purpose.

intrauterine d. (IUD), a stainless steel or plastic loop or spiral inserted into the uterus to prevent conception.

Devic's disease. See neuromyelitis optica.

devil's grip. Epidemic pleurodynia; see under pleurodynia.

devitaliza'tion. In dentistry, the destruction of the pulp of a tooth.

devi'talized. Without vitality; dead.

devolu'tion. 1. Degeneration; catabolism. **2.** The opposite of evolution.

dex'ter (D). Latin for right.

dex'trad. Toward the right.

dex'tral. 1. Of, related to, or located on the right side. **2.** Right-handed.

dex'tran. Any of various large polymers of glucose, used in solution as a plasma substitute.

dex'trans. Polysaccharides of glucose obtained from yeast and bacteria in which the glucose residues are bound in α-1,6 linkages; the linkage at the branch point (1, 2, 1, 3, 1, 4) and the spacing between the branch points is characteristic of the species of the organism from which the dextran was obtained; used as plasma substitutes.

dextrau'ral. Having better hearing with the right ear than with the left.

dex'trin. A soluble carbohydrate formed by the hydrolysis of starch, the first stage in the formation of glucose; commercial dextrin is a white or yellow powder, used in solution as an adhesive.

dextrin 6-glucosyltransferase. Dextran dextrinase, a bacterial enzyme that promotes the synthesis of dextrans from dextrins.

dextroamphetamine sulfate. A sympathomi-metic agent; a stimulant to the central nervous system and appetite depressant; Dexedrine®.

dextrocar'dia. Abnormal location of the heart on the right side of the chest.

dextroc'ular. 1. Relating to the right eye. **2.** Denoting a condition in which better vision exists in the right eye.

dextroposi'tion. Abnormal right-sided location of an organ normally located in the left side.

d. of heart, condition either congenital or acquired (as in collapse of the right lung), in which the major position of the heart lies on the right side.

dextroro'tatory. Turning the plane of polarization to the right; bending rays of light clockwise; said of some crystals and solutions.

dex'trose. See glucose.

dextrothyroxin sodium. d-Thyroxine, a thyroid hormone analog used to reduce the cholesterol content in the tissues.

dextrover'sion. Displacement or turning toward the right.

di-. Prefix meaning two.

dia-. Prefix meaning through or throughout.

diabe'tes. A disease characterized by excessive excretion of urine; when used alone the term refers to diabetes mellitus.

alloxan d., the production of diabetes mellitus in experimental animals by the administration of alloxan, an agent that damages the insulin-producing cells of the pancreas.

brittle d., diabetes in which there is an irregular pattern of tolerance for carbohydrates and need for insulin.

bronzed d., hemochromatosis; a disorder of iron metabolism marked by deposits of iron in the tissues, especially skin, pancreas, and liver; deposition in the skin causes a bronzed pigmentation; deposits in the pancreas lead to diabetes.

d. insipidus, a comparatively rare form of diabetes marked by excessive thirst and the passage of large amounts of dilute urine, due to inadequate production of antidiuretic hormone by the posterior pituitary gland. Cf nephrogenic diabetes insipidus.

d. mellitus, the most common form of diabetes; a chronic systemic disease marked by (1) disorders in the metabolism of insulin (a hormone produced by the pancreas) and of carbohydrate, protein, and fat and (2) disorders in the structure and function of blood vessels, referred to as "complication of diabetes;" the primary manifestation of the disease is high concentration of sugar in the blood; spillover of sugar into the urine leads to excessive urination, thirst, and loss of weight; mellitus is Latin for honeyed; referring to the presence of sugar in the urine.

juvenile d., a form of severe brittle diabetes occurring in children during the first two decades of life; also called juvenile or growth-onset diabetes mellitus.

latent d., a mild form of diabetes mellitus with no obvious symptoms.

maturity-onset d., a mild form of diabetes mellitus occurring in obese individuals over age 35.

nephrogenic d. insipidus, diabetes insipidus caused by inability of the kidney tubules to reabsorb water; it does not respond to the administration of antidiuretic hormone; also called vasopressin-resistant diabetes.

vasopressin-resistant d., see nephrogenic diabetes insipidus.

diabet'ic. 1. Relating to diabetes. **2.** An individual afflicted with diabetes.

diabetogen'ic. Causing diabetes.

diacetylmor'phine. See heroin.

diadochokine'sia, diadochokine'sis. The normal ability of alternating opposite muscular actions, such as extension and flexion of a limb.

diagnose'. To identify the nature of a disease; to make a diagnosis.

diagno'sis. The determination of the nature of a disease.

clinical d., one based on the signs and symptoms of a disease.

d. by exclusion, one made by excluding all but one of the disease processes thought to be possible causes of the symptoms being considered.

differential d., the determination of which of two or more diseases with similar symptoms is the one with which the patient is afflicted; consideration or listing of diseases possibly responsible for a patient's illness, based on information available at the time, e.g., symptoms, signs, physical findings, and laboratory data.

laboratory d., one made by a chemical, microscopic, bacteriologic, or biopsy study of secretions, discharges, blood, or tissue.

pathologic d., (1) a diagnosis (sometimes a postmortem diagnosis) made from a study of the lesions present; (2) a diagnosis of the pathologic conditions present, determined by a study and comparison of the symptoms.

physical d., one based on information obtained through physical examination of the patient, using the techniques of inspection, palpation, percussion, and auscultation.

postmortem d., autopsy; examination of a dead body, usually to determine the cause of death.

diagnosti'cian. One who is experienced in determining the nature of diseases; formerly used to apply to physicians with extensive training and ex-

deviation | **diagnostician**

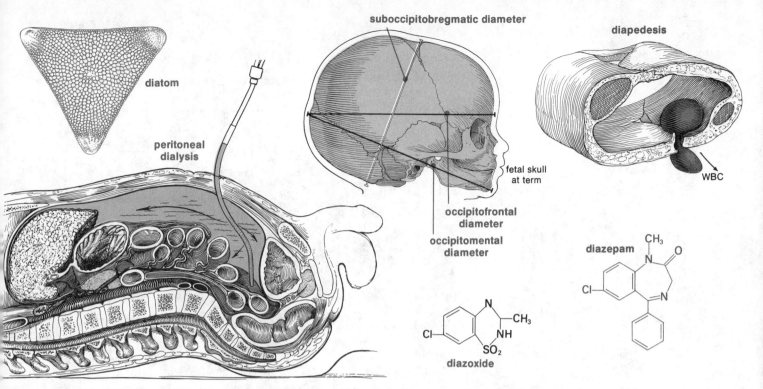

diatom

peritoneal dialysis

suboccipitobregmatic diameter

occipitofrontal diameter

occipitomental diameter

fetal skull at term

diapedesis

WBC

diazepam

diazoxide

perience in medicine, comparable to internists of today.

diakine′sis. The terminal part of the prophase stage in meiosis during which the spireme threads break up into shorter and thicker chromosomes, and the nucleolus and nuclear membrane disappear.

dialy′sance. The amount of blood (measured in milliliters) completely cleared of a substance by a dialyzing membrane in a period of time, usually one minute.

dial′ysate. Fluid used in dialysis.

dial′ysis. The separation of smaller molecules (crystalloids) from larger molecules (colloids) in a solution by selective diffusion through a semipermeable membrane.

   peritoneal d., one in which sterile dialyzing fluid is introduced into the abdominal cavity; the peritoneum acts as the semipermeable membrane.

dialysis disequilibrium syndrome. Nausea, vomiting, hypertension, and central nervous system signs occasionally occurring within hours after starting hemodialysis for kidney failure; thought to be due to removal of metabolites (especially urea) from the extracellular fluid and blood at a much greater rate than from the brain cells, with subsequent cerebral edema.

di′alyze. To separate a substance from a solution by dialysis; to subject to dialysis.

di′alyzer. A semipermeable membrane used in dialysis.

diam′eter. 1. A straight line passing through the center of a circle and terminating at opposite points of its periphery. **2.** The distance along such a line. **3.** The thickness or width of any structure or opening.

   biparietal d., the greatest transverse diameter of a fetal skull at term; it extends from one parietal bone to the other and usually measures 9.25 cm.

   occipitofrontal d., the diameter of a fetal skull at term which follows a line extending from the root of the nose to the most prominent portion of the occipital bone.

   occipitomental d., the diameter of a fetal skull at term from the chin to the most prominent portion of the occipital bone; it usually measures 11.5 cm.

   suboccipitobregmatic d., the diameter of a fetal skull at term which follows a line drawn from the middle of the large fontanel to the under surface of the occipital bone just where it joins the neck; it usually measures 9.5 cm.

di′amine. An organic compound containing two amino groups; e.g., $NH_2CH_2CH_2NH_2$, ethylene diamine.

di′apause. A period of biological dormancy, as the suspension of growth and decreased metabolism in insects during a specific stage in their life cycle.

diapede′sis. 1. The passage of blood or any of its corpuscles through the pores of blood vessels. **2.** The process by which phagocytic cells leave the blood and accumulate at extravascular sites of tissue injury.

diaphoret′ic. 1. An agent that causes sweating, especially profuse sweating. **2.** Perspiring.

di′aphragm. 1. The musculomembranous structure which separates the thoracic and abdominal cavities. **2.** Any dividing membrane.

   contraceptive d., a flexible ring covered with rubber or other plastic material, fitted over the cervix of the uterus to prevent pregnancy.

   d. flutter, rapid contractions of all or part of the diaphragm.

   pelvic d., the part of the pelvic floor formed by the paired levator ani and coccygeus muscles and their fasciae.

   urogenital d., a deep musculomembranous fascia extending between the ischiopubic rami and surrounding the urogenital ducts.

diaph′ysis. The shaft of a long bone.

diaphysi′tis. Inflammation of the body or shaft of a long bone.

diaplacen′tal. Passing through the placenta.

diapoph′ysis. The upper articular surface of a transverse vertebral process.

diarrhe′a. Abnormally frequent passage of loose stools; the evacuation of a single loose stool does not constitute diarrhea.

   nocturnal d., diarrhea occurring primarily at night; seen in diabetes mellitus.

   traveler's d., diarrhea affecting travelers usually during the first week of a trip and lasting one to three days.

diar′thric. Of or relating to two joints; also called biarticular.

diarthro′sis. Abarthrosis; diarthrodial joint; one that permits relatively free movement.

dias′chisis. A sudden functional disorder caused by a focal disturbance of the brain.

diastal′sis. The type of peristalsis of the small intestine in which a wave of inhibition precedes the wave of contraction.

di′astase. A mixture of amylolytic or starch-splitting enzymes that convert starch into dextrin and maltose; present in some germinating grains such as malt.

dias′tasis. Separation of two bones normally joined together without existence of a true joint, as in separation of the epiphysis from the shaft of a long bone.

   d. recti, separation of the abdominal rectus muscles from the midline, usually seen after pregnancy or abdominal surgery.

diaste′ma. Excessive space between two adjacent teeth.

dias′tole. The rhythmic relaxation of the muscles of the heart chambers during which time they fill with blood.

diastol′ic. Relating to a diastole.

diatax′ia. Loss of muscular coordination on both sides of the body.

diather′my. Local generation of heat in the body tissues by a high frequency electric current.

   medical d., the production of sufficient heat to warm the tissues without destroying them.

   short wave d., the heating of tissues by means of an oscillating current of high frequency, used in physiotherapy to relieve pain.

   surgical d., high frequency diathermy used for the destruction of diseased tissues (electrocoagulation), cauterization, etc.

diath′esis. An inherited or congenital bodily predisposition to a disease, or metabolic or structural abnormality; susceptibility to certain disorders.

   cystic d., a predisposition to the formation of cysts in an organ.

   gouty d., a predisposition to gout; goutiness.

   hemorrhagic d., a predisposition to spontaneous hemorrhage.

di′atom. A microscopic, unicellular alga with a hard silica-containing cell wall.

diatoma′ceous. Consisting of the siliceous skeletons or shells of the unicellular diatoms.

diatom′ic. 1. Consisting of two atoms. **2.** Dibasic.

diaz′epam. A benzodiazepine derivative, $C_{16}H_{13}ClN_2O$; used primarily as an antianxiety agent, e.g., for sedation prior to cardiac catheterization, endoscopy, and air encephalography; also a useful adjunct in the treatment of muscular spasms in individuals with acute musculoskeletal disorders and certain acute and chronic neurologic disorders, e.g., cerebral palsy and multiple sclerosis; Valium®.

diaz′o-. Combining form applied to a compound containing the $-N=N-$ or $-N\equiv N-$ group.

diaz′otize. To treat an amine with nitrous acid.

diazox′ide. A nondiuretic thiazide derivative used in the treatment of hypertensive crises; Hyperstat®.

diba′sic. Having two replaceable hydrogen atoms; denoting a compound with two hydrogen atoms replaceable by a monovalent metal; also called bibasic.

dibenzopyr′idine. See acridine.

Dibothrioceph′alus. See *Diphyllobothrium*.

DIC. Abbreviation for disseminated intravascular coagulation.

dicen′tric. Having two centromeres, as certain abnormal chromosomes.

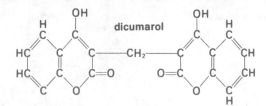

dicumarol

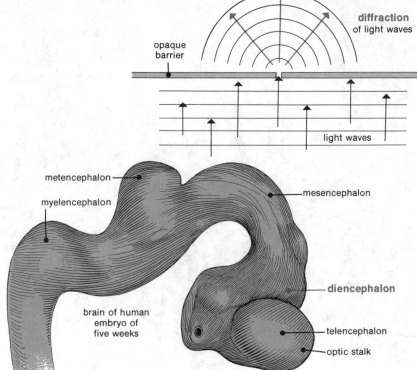

diffraction of light waves

opaque barrier

light waves

metencephalon

myelencephalon

mesencephalon

diencephalon

telencephalon

optic stalk

brain of human embryo of five weeks

dental stone **die** of a cavity prepared for an inlay

dichlo′ride. A chemical compound containing two chloride atoms per molecule; also called bichloride.

dicho′rial, dichorion′ic. Having two chorions (outermost fetal membrane).

dichot′omy. Division or cutting into two parts.

di′chroism. The property of exhibiting two colors, as certain crystals when seen from different directions, or certain solutions in varying degrees of concentration.

dichro′mate. A chemical compound containing the radical $Cr_2O_7=$; also called bichromate.

dichromat′ic. 1. Having two colors. **2.** Relating to the visual defect dichromatism.

dichro′matism. A defect in color perception; the spectrum is seen as comprised of only two colors separated by an achromatic or colorless band; also called dichromatopsia, parachromatopsia, and partial color blindness.

dichro′mophil, dichro′mophile. Denoting tissues that take both acid and basic stains but in different areas.

dicrot′ic. Double beat, denoting a pulse with two beats for each heart beat.

dictyokine′sis. The division of the Golgi apparatus of a cell during mitosis.

dictyo′ma. Tumor of the retina.

dicu′marol. A coumarin derivative that inhibits the formation of prothrombin in the liver; a long-acting anticoagulant agent; also called bishydroxycoumarin.

didac′tic. Intended to instruct by means of lectures or textbooks rather than by clinical demonstrations with patients.

didac′tylism. Having two fingers on a hand or two toes on a foot.

didym-, didymo-. Combining forms indicating a relationship to the testis (didymus).

-didymus, -dymus. Infrequently used combining form denoting a conjoined twin; the first part of the word specifies the part of the twins that remains unfused.

did′ymus. A testis; from the Greek word *didymos*, meaning twin.

die. A specialized model made from an impression, as the positive reproduction of a prepared tooth; usually made of metal or super hard dental stone.

dienceph′alon. The portion of the embryonic brain between the mesencephalon and the telencephalon from which develop the thalamus, metathalamus, epithalamus, subthalamus, and hypothalamus; it encloses the third ventricle; together with the telencephalon it makes up the prosencephalon.

die′ner. A laboratory assistant.

di′et. 1. Bodily nourishment. **2.** Regulated nourishment, especially as prescribed for medical reasons.

3. To follow a specific dietary plan, especially for reduction of body weight by limitation of caloric intake.

   balanced d., a diet containing the essential ingredients in proper proportion for adequate nutrition; also called adequate diet.

   bland d.'s, regular diets modified to be free from roughage or spicy foods; smooth, nonirritating, and bland in taste; progressive regimen (bland 1, 2, 3, or 4), generally used in treatment of upper gastrointestinal disturbances.

   clear liquid d., one used postoperatively for individuals unable to tolerate full liquids or solid food.

   diabetic d.'s, any of nine balanced diets recommended by the American Diabetes Association for diabetic individuals; they are free of sugar and high carbohydrate foods and have caloric levels from 1200 to 3500; they are commonly divided in fifths, generally consisting of three meals and two snacks.

   elimination d., a diet omitting foods suspected of causing allergic reactions; usually eliminated are eggs, milk, and wheat, less frequently, nuts, chocolate, and fish.

   full liquid d., one composed of foods which are in liquid form at body temperature; it basically serves as a pre- or postoperative diet, and as a transition to a more liberal soft regimen.

   Giordano-Giovannetti d., a renal diet providing 20–30g of high biologic value protein; also called Giovannetti diet.

   high potassium d.'s, diets for individuals undergoing vigorous diuretic therapy; they provide approximately 100 mEq of potassium per day.

   Kempner rice-fruit d., one consisting chiefly of rice and fruits with addition of minerals and vitamins and restriction of sodium; prescribed originally for arterial hypertension or chronic kidney disease.

   low calcium d., a daily diet of from 100 to 200 mg of calcium; used in the treatment of hyperparathyroidism and urinary calcium stones, or as a test diet to determine urinary calcium excretion; diets of 250 mg of calcium are used in the treatment of certain individuals with hypercalcemia and/or hypercalciuria.

   low cholesterol d., see low saturated fat diet.

   low fat d., one containing minimal amounts of fats (40–50 g per day), as lean meat, fish, skimmed milk, cottage cheese, and cereal products; the caloric level may be varied through changes in protein and carbohydrate levels.

   low residue d., a diet low in cellulose content, as fruits, vegetables, and unrefined cereals; vegetables are pureed to change the consistency of the cellulose.

   low saturated fat d., a diet high in polyunsaturated fatty acids of vegetable origin with restrictions on foods high in cholesterol and saturated fatty acids, such as eggs, butter, and meat; also called cholesterol-lowering or low cholesterol diet.

   low sodium d.'s, diets providing low levels of sodium for the treatment of congestive heart failure, and other conditions associated with edema; four levels of low sodium diets are used: 250 mg, 500 mg, 1000 mg, and 2000 mg of sodium (a regular diet without added salt provides two to four g of sodium).

   reduction d.'s, diets for weight reduction, with caloric levels of 800, 1000, 1200, 1500, and 1800, that are adequate in protein and restricted in carbohydrate and fat; a level should be selected which allows for approximately one pound of weight loss per week.

   regular d., one adequate to meet recommended daily allowances of the National Research Council; it contains approximately 80–100 g of protein, four g of sodium, 83 mEq of potassium, and 2000 cal.

   renal d.'s, diets low in protein, sodium, and potassium; used in the treatment of renal failure. Cf Giordano-Giovannetti diet.

   salt-free d., low sodium diet.

   Sippy d., bland diet.

   soft d., a regular diet modified to include foods easily digested, excluding those high in indigestible cellulose and gas-forming fruits and vegetables; it contains approximately 75 g of protein, four g of sodium, 72 mEq of potassium, and 2000 cal.

dietet′ic. 1. Of or relating to diet. **2.** Specially prepared or processed food for regulated diets.

dietet′ics. The study of diet in relation to health and disease.

dieth′ylstilbes′trol. See stilbestrol.

dietit′ian. A specialist in dietetics.

dietogenet′ics. The study of the relationship between the genetic constitution of an individual, his diet, and various food requirements.

dietother′apy. The treatment of disease by a regulated selection of food.

dif′ference. 1. A specific variation. **2.** The amount by which one quantity varies from another.

   arteriovenous oxygen d., the difference in the oxygen content of the arterial blood entering and the venous blood leaving a specified area or organ.

differen′tial. Relating to, showing, or dependent on a difference or distinction.

differentia′tion. 1. In biology, the process of developing into specialized organs; said of embryonic tissues. **2.** The act of distinguishing one disease from another; also called differential diagnosis.

diffrac′tion. The interaction of matter with any wave motion (light and sound waves and all electro-

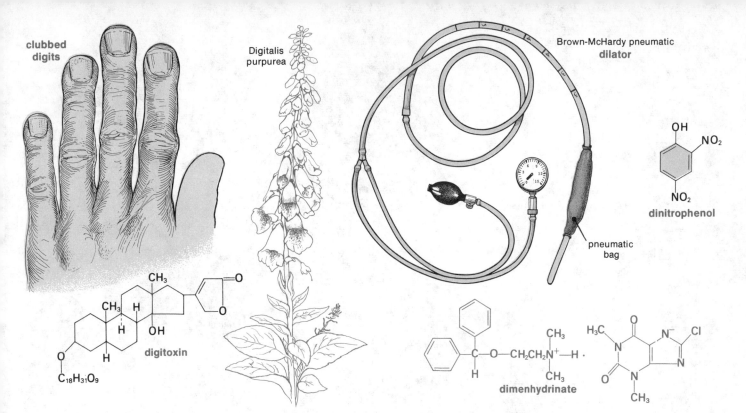

clubbed
digits

Digitalis
purpurea

Brown-McHardy pneumatic
dilator

dinitrophenol

pneumatic
bag

digitoxin

$C_{18}H_{31}O_9$

dimenhydrinate

magnetic waves); e.g., the tendency of light rays to bend in the direction of an obstacle.

diffuse′. 1. Spread out; not circumscribed, localized, or limited. **2.** To move by diffusion.

diffu′sion. 1. The process of uniformly spreading out or scattering; the passage of the molecules of one substance between the molecules of another to form a mixture of the two substances. **2.** Dialysis.

digas′tric. Having two bellies, as the digastric muscle.

Dige′nea. A subclass of flatworms or flukes (class Trematoda); parasitic in man and other mammals.

diGeorge's syndrome. Congenital thymic aplasia; see under aplasia.

digest′. 1. To break up food into simpler, assimilable compounds by the muscular and chemical action of the digestive tract. **2.** To absorb mentally.

diges′tant. An agent that aids the process of digestion.

diges′tion. The process taking place in the alimentary canal whereby the nutritive components of food are converted into substances that can be absorbed by the intestine; the decomposition of materials into simpler compounds.

diges′tive. Relating to digestion.

dig′it. A finger or toe.

clubbed d.'s, a bulbous enlargement of the fingertips, seen in some cases of heart disease and certain pulmonary disorders; also called drumstick or clubbed fingers.

dig′ital. 1. Pertaining to, performed by, or resembling a digit or digits, especially a finger. **2.** Possessing digits.

digital′is. 1. Foxglove, a plant of the genus *Digitalis*. **2.** Digitalis (USP), a drug obtained from the dried leaves of *Digitalis purpurea*, used in the treatment of heart disease, especially for congestive heart failure and some supraventricular tachyarrhythmias.

digitaliza′tion. The treatment of an individual with digitalis or a related cardiac glycoside, to achieve a desired therapeutic effect.

dig′itate. Having fingerlike processes.

digita′tion. A finger-like process.

digitox′in. A glycoside obtained from *Digitalis purpurea*; used in the treatment of congestive heart failure.

dig′itus, *pl.* **dig′iti.** Latin for finger.

digox′in. A glycoside obtained from the leaves of *Digitalis lanata*; used in the treatment of congestive heart failure.

DiGuglielmo's syndrome. Erythremic myelosis; see under myelosis.

dihy′drate. A compound having two molecules of water.

dihydro-. Combining form denoting the addition of two hydrogen atoms.

dihydroergot′amine (D.H.E. 45). A crystalline compound produced by the hydrogenation of ergotamine; used in the treatment of migraine headache.

dihydrostreptomy′cin. Compound made by the hydrogenation of streptomycin and having antibiotic properties.

dihydrotachys′terol (AT 10). A synthetic sterol that produces effects similar to those of vitamin D.

diiodoty′rosine (T_2, DIT). A precursor of the thyroid hormone thyroxin; also called iodogorgoic acid.

dil. Abbreviation for dilute or diluted.

dilata′tion. 1. The condition of being enlarged, occurring normally, artificially, or as a result of disease; said of a tubular structure, a cavity, or an opening. **2.** Dilation (1).

gastric d., acute distention of the stomach with fluid and air; commonly seen following surgery or trauma.

dila′tion. 1. The act of stretching or dilating. **2.** Dilatation (1).

di′lator. Instrument for enlarging a passage or cavity.

dil′do, dil′doe. An object having the approximate size and shape of an erect penis; used to produce sexual pleasure by vaginal insertion.

dil′uent. A substance which reduces the concentration of a solution.

dilu′tion. 1. The process of reducing the concentration of a solution or substance. **2.** A weakened solution or substance; an attenuated mixture.

dimenhy′drinate. Drug used in preventing and treating motion sickness; Dramamine®.

dimen′sion. Any measurable distance.

vertical d., in prosthodontics, the distance between two points on the face, one above and one below the mouth, usually in the midline; it may be measured when the opposing occlusal surfaces are in maximum contact (occlusal vertical dimension) or in rest position, when the jaws are not in contact (rest vertical dimension).

di′mer. A chemical compound composed of molecules that consist of two identical simpler molecules.

dimercap′rol. (BAL). A compound used as an antidote for lewisite and other arsenic poisoning; also called British antilewisite.

dimeth′yl sulfox′ide (DMSO). An industrial solvent occasionally used in medicine as a skin penetrant to facilitate absorption of medications from the skin; also called methyl sulfoxide.

dimor′phism. The property of occurring in two forms.

dinitrophe′nol (DNP). A drug which causes an increase in rate of metabolism by interruption of the coupling of oxidation and phosphorylation; not used clinically because of its toxicity.

dinu′cleotide. One of the compounds into which nucleic acid splits on hydrolysis; it may split into two mononucleotides.

diop′ter. The unit used to designate the refractive power of a lens or an optical system.

dioptom′eter. An instrument for measuring refraction and accommodation of the eye; also called dioptrometer.

diop′tric. 1. Relating to the unit of refractive power of lenses. **2.** Refractive.

diop′trics. The science of the refraction of light.

dioptrom′eter. See dioptometer.

dio′tic. In audiology, denoting an arrangement in which each ear receives the same signal.

diox′ide. An oxide containing two atoms of oxygen per molecule.

dipep′tidase. One of the protein-splitting enzymes that causes the breakdown of a dipeptide into its two constituent amino acids.

dipep′tide. Two amino acids linked by a peptide bond.

diphenhy′dramine hydrochlo′ride. An antihistamine used in the prevention and treatment of motion sickness, postoperative nausea, nausea and vomiting of pregnancy, and some allergies; Benadryl®.

diphenylhydan′toin. An anticonvulsant agent, used primarily to treat epilepsy; Dilantin®.

diphos′phonates. Synthetic substances similar to the pyrophosphates in structure but not biologically hydrolyzed; in vitro they prevent hydroxyapatite crystal formation; it has been suggested that they coat the bone surface and prevent bone resorption.

diphosphopyr′idine nu′cleotide (DPN). Old term for nicotinamide adenine dinucleotide (NAD).

diphthe′ria. An acute contagious disease caused by a bacillus, *Corynebacterium diphtheriae*; marked by inflammation of the upper respiratory tract, fibrin formation (false membrane) of the mucous membranes, and elaboration of soluble exotoxin which acts on the heart and cranial or peripheral nerve cells.

diph′theroid. 1. Resembling diphtheria. **2.** A bacterium resembling the organism that causes diphtheria.

diphyllobothri′asis. Infestation with *Diphyllobothrium latum* (broadfish tapeworm), caused by ingestion of inadequately cooked, infected fish.

Diphyllobothri′rium. A genus of tapeworms (family Diphyllobothriidae); formerly called *Dibothriocephalus*.

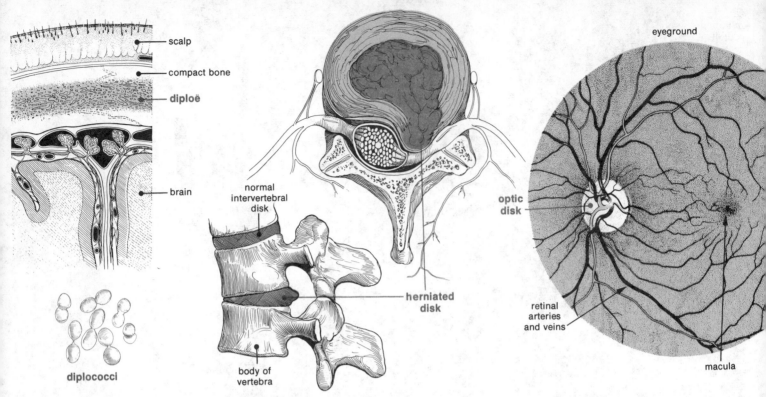

scalp

compact bone

diploë

brain

normal
intervertebral
disk

herniated
disk

body of
vertebra

diplococci

eyeground

optic
disk

retinal
arteries
and veins

macula

D. latum, intestinal parasite transmitted to man by ingestion of undercooked infected fresh water fish; also called fish tapeworm.

diplacu'sis. Condition in which one sound is heard differently by the two ears, resulting in the perception of two sounds instead of one.

diple'gia. Paralysis of corresponding parts on both sides of the body; also called bilateral paralysis.

  congenital facial d., see Möbius' syndrome.

diplo-, dipl-. Combining forms meaning double; e.g., diploid.

diplobacte'ria. Bacteria linked in pairs.

Diplococ'cus. Former name for a genus of bacteria.

  D. gonorrhoeae, see *Neisseria gonorrhoeae.*

  D. pneumoniae, see *Streptococcus pneumoniae.*

diplococ'cus, *pl.* **diplococ'ci.** Any of various spherical or ovoid bacteria joined together in pairs.

dip'loë. The spongy (cancellous) bone with a limited marrow cavity between the two tables of the cranial bones.

dip'loid. Having two sets of chromosomes, the total number of chromosomes being twice that of a gamete.

diplo'pia. Double vision.

dip'lotene. In meiosis, the fourth of five stages of prophase in which the intimately paired homologous chromosomes begin to separate, forming a characteristic chiasma or X appearance; at this stage, blocks of genes are exchanged between homologous chromosomes.

dip'sia. A great thirst.

dipsoma'nia. An insatiable, uncontrollable desire for alcoholic drinks.

dipso'sis. Abnormally excessive thirst.

Dirofila'ria. A genus (superfamily Filarioidea) which includes some species that are parasitic in man.

  D. immitis, the dog heartworm; a parasite in the pulmonary arteries of dogs.

disabil'ity. 1. A legal loss of function and earning power. **2.** Incapacity. **3.** Any handicap.

  learning d. (LD), a complex of symptoms that involves impairment of some or all of the following functions; learning, language, perception, memory, and concentration; neurologic examination usually yields minor abnormalities, if any; diagnosis rests on psychological assessment of cognitive function.

disa'blement. 1. A legal incapacity without loss of earning power. **2.** Incapacitation.

disac'charide. A class of sugars, including sucrose, lactose, and maltose, which yield two monosaccharides on hydrolysis.

disarticula'tion. Amputation of a limb by separating the bones at the joint.

disc. See disk.

discec'tomy. Surgical removal of an intervertebral disk.

discharge'. 1. Material which is released as an excretion or a secretion. **2.** To pour forth; to emit. **3.** The activation of a nerve cell.

discis'sion. Surgical procedure in which the capsule of the lens of the eye is either punctured or cut.

disco-, disc-, disko-. Combining forms indicating a relationship or similarity to a disk.

discogen'ic. Referring to a disorder originating in an intervertebral disk.

discog'raphy. See diskography.

dis'coid. 1. Having the shape of a disk. **2.** A dental disk-shaped carving and excavating instrument.

discop'athy. Disease of a disk, especially of an intervertebral disk.

discrete'. Denoting certain lesions of the skin which are separate, not joined or confluent.

discu'tient. Denoting an agent that causes the dispersal of a tumor or any pathologic accumulation.

dis'ease. Any abnormal condition, affecting either the whole body or any of its parts, which impairs normal functioning. For individual diseases, see specific names.

  communicable d., any disease transmissible by infection or contagion directly or through a carrier of the pathogen.

  congenital d., one present at birth.

  contagious d., one transmissible by direct or indirect contact.

  deficiency d., one due to a prolonged lack of vitamins, minerals, or any other essential dietary component.

  endemic d., one present in a specific locality more or less continuously.

  functional d., one occurring without an apparent physical cause.

  hereditary d., one transmitted genetically from a parent to offspring.

  infectious d., one caused by the presence of a pathologic microorganism.

  local d., disorder confined to a specific part or organ, usually without generalized involvement.

  mental d., see disorder, mental.

  occupational d., one caused by the environment of a particular occupation.

  organic d., one in which structural changes in the body take place.

  periodic d., any disease that recurs regularly.

  social d., popular and incorrect term for venereal diseases, especially gonorrhea and syphilis.

  systemic d., one affecting several organs or the entire body.

  venereal d., any disease acquired through sexual intercourse, as gonorrhea, syphilis, chancroid, etc.

disengage'ment. In obstetrics, the emergence of the presenting part of the fetus from the vulva.

disequilib'rium. Lack of balance or stability.

disinfec'tant. Any agent that kills disease-causing microorganisms; generally used on inanimate objects.

disinfec'tion. The destruction of infectious agents by chemical or physical means directly applied.

  terminal d., one in which the infectious agent is eliminated from personal clothing and possessions in the immediate environment of the patient.

disintegra'tion. 1. Breakdown or separation of component parts. **2.** Disorganization of mental processes.

disk. Any platelike structure; also written disc.

  articular d., a circular fibrocartilaginous pad present in some synovial joints and attached to the joint capsule; e.g., the articular disk of the temporomandibular joint, which separates the cavity of the capsule into two separate compartments, thus reducing friction between the articulating surfaces of the bones.

  dental d., a small disk of paper or plastic, coated with cuttle-fish bone, emery, garnet, or sand; used in dentistry to cut, smooth, or polish teeth and dental restorations.

  herniated d., posterior rupture of the inner portion of an intervertebral disk, causing pressure on the nerve roots with resulting pain; occurring most commonly in the lower back; also called slipped, ruptured, or prolapsed disk.

  intercalated d., the double membrane separating cells of cardiac muscle fibers.

  intervertebral d., the fibrocartilaginous tissue between the bodies of adjacent vertebrae, consisting of a jellylike center surrounded by a fibrous ring.

  optic d., the pinkish white oval or circular area of the retina, which is the site of entrance of the optic nerve; also called blind spot.

  ruptured d., see herniated disk.

  slipped d., see herniated disk.

  tactile d., the saucer-shaped termination of specialized sensory nerve fibers in contact with a modified cell in the deep layers of the epidermis; also called meniscus tactus.

diskec'tomy. The surgical removal, in part or whole, of an intervertebral disk.

diski'tis. Inflammation of a disk, especially of one between the vertebrae.

diskog'raphy. Radiographic visualization of intervertebral disk space after injection of a radiopaque substance; also written discography.

disk syndrome. Pain in the lower back, radiating

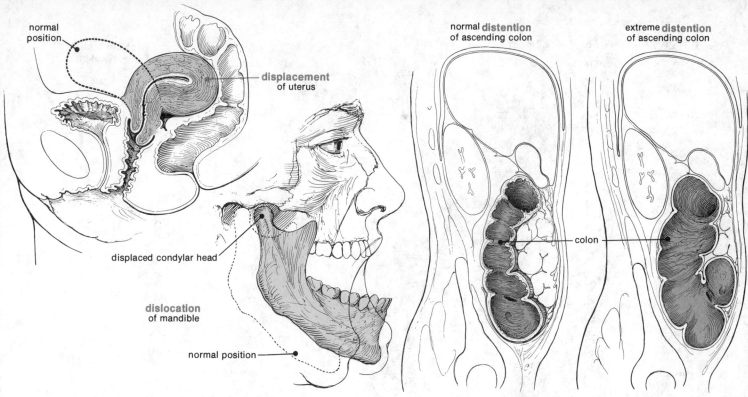

normal
position

displacement
of uterus

displaced condylar head

dislocation
of mandible

normal position

normal **distention**
of ascending colon

extreme **distention**
of ascending colon

colon

to the thigh with occasional loss of ankle and knee reflexes, resulting from compression of spinal nerve roots by an intervertebral disk.

dis'locate. To shift from the usual or normal position, especially to displace a bone from its socket; to luxate.

disloca'tion. Displacement of a limb or organ from the normal position; specifically, a displacement of a bone from its socket or joint.

dismem'ber. To remove a limb.

disor'der. A disturbance of function or health.

  affective d., manic-depressive psychosis; see under psychosis.

  autosomal dominant d., one occurring when only one abnormal gene is present and the corresponding gene (allele) on the homologous chromosome is normal; also called autosomal dominant disease.

  autosomal recessive d., one that is apparent only when both corresponding genes (alleles) in homologous chromosomes are abnormal; also called autosomal recessive disease.

  character d., deeply ingrained, maladaptive patterns of behavior unaccompanied by subjective feelings of anxiety or guilt.

  emotional d., mental disorder.

  functional d., mental disorder not caused by organic disease.

  genetic d., one in which the genetic component expresses itself in a predictable manner without much influence from the environment.

  immunoproliferative d., proliferation of cells of the lymphoreticular system associated with autoallergic disturbances or γ-globulin abnormalities.

  mental d., any psychiatric disorder listed in the *Standard Nomenclature of Diseases and Operations* of the American Medical Association, or in the *Diagnostic and Statistical Manual for Mental Disorders* of the American Psychiatric Association; also called mental illness or disease.

  neuropsychologic d., impairment of mental function due to a lesion in the brain; it may have a sudden onset and a short duration (acute) or it may be prolonged (chronic).

  personality d., general term used to denote any long-standing maladaptive pattern of behavior; distinguished from neurotic and psychotic symptoms.

  psychophysiologic d., psychosomatic d., disturbances of visceral functioning secondary to long-continued emotional attitudes.

  sleep d., any disturbance of sleep, such as somnambulism.

disorganiza'tion. Destruction or breakdown of tissues with resulting loss of function.

disorienta'tion. Loss of the sense of direction or

location.

dispen'sary. 1. An office in any institution (hospital, school, etc.) from which medical supplies and medicines are distributed. **2.** A public institution that dispenses free medical aid. **3.** An outpatient department of a hospital.

dispen'satory. A book describing the sources, preparation, contents, and uses of medicines.

dispense'. To prepare and distribute medicines to the sick.

disperse'. To scatter.

disper'sion. 1. The process of dispersing or the state of being dispersed. **2.** A suspension of solid, liquid, or gaseous particles of colloidal size in another medium.

  coarse d., a suspension of relatively large particles in a liquid.

  molecular d., one in which the dispersed particles are individual molecules; a true solution.

displace'ment. 1. The condition of being moved from a normal position. **2.** In chemistry, a reaction in which an atom, molecule, or radical group is removed from a compound and replaced with another. **3.** The weight of a fluid expelled by a floating body or by another fluid of greater density. **4.** A defense mechanism in which an emotion, such as anger, is unconsciously directed to an object or person other than the direct cause of frustration; e.g., an angry individual beating the wall with his fist.

dissect'. To cut apart, especially in the study of anatomy.

dissec'tion. 1. The act of dissecting. **2.** A tissue that has been dissected.

dissem'inated. Widely distributed throughout an organ, tissue, or the body; scattered; dispersed.

dissimula'tion. The act of feigning health by a sick person.

dissocia'tion. 1. Separation. **2.** Change of a complex chemical compound into a simple one.

  albuminocytologic d., increase in the protein content of the cerebrospinal fluid without increase in cell count.

  atrioventricular d., independent action of the atria and ventricles of the heart.

  complete A-V d., (1) atrioventricular dissociation not interrupted by ventricular captures; (2) complete atrioventricular block; independent beating of atria and ventricle caused by failure of impulses to reach the ventricles.

  incomplete A-V d., atrioventricular dissociation interrupted by ventricular captures.

  electromechanical d., electrical activity in the heart without resulting mechanical contraction, as in cardiac rupture.

  interference d., atrioventricular dissociation occasionally interrupted by ventricular captures.

dissolu'tion. 1. Decomposition into component parts; disintegration. **2.** A dissolving. **3.** Autolysis.

dissolve'. 1. To cause a substance to change from a solid to a dispersed state by placing it in contact with a solvent fluid. **2.** To melt; to reduce to a liquid state.

dissol'vent. Solvent; capable of dissolving another substance.

dis'tad. Toward the periphery.

dis'tal. 1. Farthest from a point of reference. **2.** In dentistry, the location most distant from the median line of the jaw.

  d. end, the posterior part of a dental appliance.

dis'tance. The space between two points.

  interocclusal d., free-way space; the distance or space between the occlusal surfaces of the mandibular and maxillary teeth when the mandible is in the physiologic rest position.

  small interarch d., a small space between the upper (maxillary) and lower (mandibular) dental arches; also called close bite.

distem'per. An infectious viral disease in certain mammals, especially young dogs, characterized by loss of appetite, dullness, fever, and a catarrhal discharge from the eyes and nose; often resulting in paralysis and death; also called Carre's disease.

distensibil'ity. The ability to stretch.

disten'tion, disten'sion. The state of being stretched or distended.

distill'. To subject a liquid mixture to vaporization and subsequent condensation with collection of components by differential cooling.

distilla'tion. The vaporization of a liquid mixture by heat followed by separation of its components by condensation of the vapor.

distobuc'cal. Relating to the distal and buccal surfaces of a posterior tooth; usually denoting the line angle formed by the junction of the two surfaces.

distobucco-occlu'sal. Relating to the distal, buccal, and occlusal surfaces of a posterior tooth; usually denoting the point angle formed by the junction of the three surfaces.

distolabioinci'sal. Relating to the distal, labial, and incisal surfaces of an anterior tooth; usually denoting the point angle formed by the junction of the three surfaces.

distoling'ual. Relating to the distal and lingual surfaces of a tooth; usually denoting the line angle formed by the junction of the two surfaces.

distolinguoinci'sal. Relating to the distal, lingual, and incisal surfaces of an anterior tooth; usually denoting the point angle formed by the junction

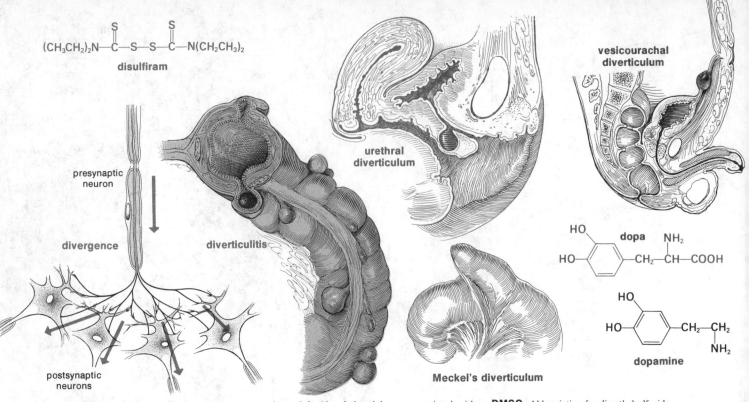

$$(CH_3CH_2)_2N-\underset{\underset{S}{\|}}{C}-S-S-\underset{\underset{S}{\|}}{C}-N(CH_2CH_3)_2$$

disulfiram

presynaptic
neuron

divergence

diverticulitis

postsynaptic
neurons

urethral
diverticulum

vesicourachal
diverticulum

Meckel's diverticulum

dopa

$$HO-\bigcirc-CH_2-\underset{\underset{NH_2}{|}}{CH}-COOH$$

$$HO-\bigcirc-CH_2-\underset{\underset{NH_2}{|}}{CH_2}$$

dopamine

of the three surfaces.

distolinguo-occlu'sal. Relating to the distal, lingual and occlusal surfaces of a posterior tooth; usually denoting the point angle formed by the junction of the three surfaces.

distomi'asis. Condition caused by the presence of flukes in the organs or tissues.

disto-occlu'sal. Relating to the distal and occlusal surfaces of a posterior tooth; usually denoting the line angle formed by the junction of the two surfaces.

distor'tion. 1. A deformed image caused by irregularities in a lens. **2.** A mechanism aiding in the disguising or repression of unacceptable thoughts.

distrac'tion. 1. Mental or emotional disturbance. **2.** Separation of joint surfaces without fracture or dislocation. **3.** In orthodontics, unusually large distance of structures, such as teeth, from the median plane.

distribu'tion. 1. The arrangement of blood vessels and nerves in the different bodily parts. **2.** The areas of the body supplied by the terminal branches of such structures.

disul'firam. A counterdrug that produces an aversion to alcohol; Antabuse®.

DIT. Abbreviation for diiodotyrosine.

diure'sis. Discharge of increased amounts of urine.

  alcoholic d., production of unusually large quantities of urine after consumption of alcoholic beverages.

  osmotic d., diuresis due to concentration in the kidney tubules of substances that limit the reabsorption of water.

  solute d., diuresis caused by increased concentration of solute in the blood or resulting from excretion of increased amounts of solute in the urine.

  water d., diuresis caused by diminution of antidiuretic hormone resulting in excretion of increased amounts of urine without a marked change in the excretion of solute.

diuret'ic. 1. Tending to promote the excretion of urine. **2.** An agent that increases the amount of urine.

diva'lent. See bivalent (1).

diver'gence. 1. The act or state of spreading apart from a common point. **2.** The spreading of branches of a presynaptic neuron to form synapses and cause activity with a number of postsynaptic neurons.

diverticu'lar. Of or relating to a diverticulum.

diverticulec'tomy. Surgical removal of a diverticulum or diverticula.

diverticuli'tis. Inflammation and infection of a diverticulum; the most common symptom of intestinal diverticulitis is a crampy pain usually in the

lower left side of the abdomen, associated with nausea and fever.

diverticulo'sis. A condition, usually producing no symptoms and requiring no treatment, marked by the presence of diverticula in the intestines, especially in the colon; it results from herniation of the mucosa through defects in the muscular wall, usually at the site of entry of blood vessels.

divertic'ulum, *pl.* **divertic'ula.** A saccular dilatation protruding from the wall of a tubular organ.

  hypopharyngeal d., one located in the hypopharynx between the inferior constrictor muscle and the cricopharyngeal muscle; also called Zenker's diverticulum and pharyngoesophageal diverticulum.

  intestinal d., a herniation of the mucous membrane through a defect in the muscular layer of the intestinal wall.

  Meckel's d., a congenital sacculation or appendage of the ileum.

  pulsion d., one formed by pressure from within, usually causing herniation of mucosa though a muscular layer.

  traction d., one formed by the pulling force of adhesions, occurring mainly in the esophagus.

  urethral d., a saccular dilatation of the female urethra in size from three mm to eight cm in diameter; when large, the diverticulum may be buried along the entire length of the urethra.

  vesicourachal d., a diverticulum of the bladder into the urachus resulting from persistent patency of part of the allantoic duct which prenatally extends from the bladder to the umbilical cord.

  Zenker's d., see hypopharyngeal diverticulum.

divis'ion. Separation.

  heterotypic d., the first reduction division of meiosis.

  homotypic d., the second reduction division of meiosis.

  indirect nuclear d., mitosis.

divulse'. To separate by tearing.

divul'sicn. The removal of a part by tearing or pulling apart.

dizygot'ic. Relating to twins derived from two separate zygotes.

dizy'gous. Fraternal (nonidentical) twins; twins derived from two separate zygotes.

diz'ziness. An abnormal sensation of unsteadiness characterized by a feeling of movement within the head without actual motion.

diz'zy. 1. Feeling a tendency to fall. **2.** Bewildered.

DJD. Abbreviation for degenerative joint disease.

dl. Abbreviation for deciliter.

dm. Abbreviation for decimeter.

D.M.D. Abbreviation for Doctor of Dental Medicine.

DMSO. Abbreviation for dimethylsulfoxide.

DNA. Abbreviation for deoxyribonucleic acid.

D.O. Abbreviation for (a) Doctor of Optometry; (b) Doctor of Osteopathy; (c) disto-occlusal.

D.O.A. Abbreviation for dead on arrival.

DOC. Abbreviation for (a) deoxycorticosterone; (b) 7-deoxycholic acid (deoxycholate).

DOCA, DCA. Abbreviations for deoxycorticosterone acetate.

doc'tor. 1. A person holding a doctorate degree awarded by a college or university in any specialized field, as in music. **2.** A person trained in and licensed to practice the healing arts, as a physician, dentist, or veterinarian. **3.** To treat medically.

dodecano'ic acid. See lauric acid.

dilicho-. Combining form meaning long.

dolichocephal'ic, dolichoceph'alous. Longheaded; having a disproportionately long head; denoting a skull with a cephalic index of below 80, or an individual with such a skull.

dolichoceph'alism, dolichoceph'aly. The state of being long-headed.

dolichoco'lon. An abnormally long colon.

dolichopel'lic, dolichopel'vic. A disproportionately long pelvis, with a pelvic index above 95.

doll's eye sign. Movement of the eyes in a direction opposite to a sudden movement of the head, caused by a lesion in the central mechanism for voluntary eye movement; also called doll's head phenomenon and Cantelli's sign.

do'lor. Latin for suffering.

  d. capitis, headache.

dom'inant. In genetics, capable of expression to the exclusion of a contrasted (recessive) character.

do'nor. 1. One who donates or contributes tissue, such as blood or an organ for transfusion or transplant. **2.** In chemistry, a substance that donates part of itself to another substance.

  methyl d.'s, compounds that, in living tissue, can supply methyl groups for transfer to other compounds.

do'pa. 3,4-Dihydroxyphenylalanine, a crystalline amino acid; a precursor of norepinephrine, epinephrine, and melanin.

do'pamine. A compound produced by the decarboxylation of dopa; in Parkinsonism, there is a depletion of dopamine in the basal ganglia of the brain, particularly in the caudate nucleus and putamen; also called *o*-hydroxytyramine.

dope. 1. An informal term denoting any narcotic drug used by addicts. **2.** To administer or to take such a drug.

dor'nase. Streptodornase.

  pancreatic d., a deoxyribonuclease preparation made from beef pancreas, used as an inhalation to

calculation of children's dosage

age	fraction of adult dosage
1 month	1/20
2 months	1/15
6 months	1/10
9 months	1/9
1 year	1/7
2 years	1/6
3 years	1/5
4 years	1/4
5–6 years	1/3
7–8 years	1/2
10–12 years	2/3
13–15 years	3/4

cigarette drain

Jackson-Pratt drain

Down's syndrome

three chromosomes in group 21

reduce the tenacity of thick secretions.

dor'sal. Relating to the back or to the posterior part of an anatomic structure.

dorsiflex'ion. Flexion or turning upward, as of the foot or toes.

dorso-, dorsi-, dors-. Combining forms indicating a relationship to the dorsal area or to the back of the body.

dorsolum'bar. Relating to the back of the body in the region of the lower thoracic and upper lumbar vertebrae.

dor'sum. The back or the upper or posterior surface.

d. sellae, the portion of the sphenoid bone that forms the posterior boundary of the sella turcica.

do'sage. 1. The giving of medication in prescribed amounts. **2.** The determination of the proper amount of a dose.

dose. 1. A specified quantity of medication to be taken or administered at one time or stated intervals. **2.** The amount of radiation administered to, or absorbed accidentally by, the tissues at one time.

booster d., a supplementary dose given sometime after the initial dose to maintain immunity.

curative d., the amount of a substance required to cure a disease or correct a deficiency.

daily d., the total amount of a medicine taken within 24 hours.

divided d., fractional portions of a medicine administered at short intervals so that the full dose is given within a definite period.

erythema d., the minimal safe amount of radiation required to produce redness of the skin within 10 days to two weeks; represented by the Sabouraud meter as the B tint, the Holzknecht as 5(5H), the Hampson as 4, and the Kienbock as 10.

initial d., the first, relatively large dose given at the beginning of a treatment.

maintenance d., the amount of a medicine administered to keep the patient under the influence of the drug after larger previous amounts.

maximal permissible d. (MPD), the greatest amount of radiation to which a person may be exposed without causing harmful effects.

mimimal infecting d. (MID), the smallest amount of infectious material that produces infection.

minimal lethal d. (MLD, mld), the smallest amount of a toxin required to kill an experimental animal.

sensitizing d., anaphylaxis.

skin d., the quantity of radiation received on the skin surface.

dosim'etry. Determination of correct dosage.

do'tage. The mental weakness or senility of old age.

double blind study. In clinical investigations, the coding of therapeutic agents so that neither patient nor physician knows what is being administered.

doub'let. 1. A combination of two similar structures, as a combination of two joined microtubules in a cilium or flagellum. **2.** A pair of lenses mounted together to form a single lens system.

douche. A stream of liquid, vapor, or gas directed into a cavity of the body, particularly the rinsing of the vagina with a liquid.

dove'tail. In dentistry, a fanned-out prepared cavity resembling the tail of a dove, made deliberately to prevent displacement of the restoration.

dow'el. A pin, usually made of metal, fitted into the root canal of a natural tooth to give support to an artificial crown.

Down's syndrome. Congenital defect caused by a chromosomal abnormality; the affected person has three chromosomes (trisomy) instead of the normal two for the pair designated Number 21; marked by various degrees of mental retardation and characteristic physical features such as short flattened skull, slanting eyes, thickened tongue, broad hands and feet, and other anomalies; also called mongolism and trisomy 21.

D.P. Abbreviation for (a) Doctor of Pharmacy; (b) Doctor of Podiatry; (c) displaced person.

D.P.H. Abbreviation for Doctor of Public Health.

D.P.M. Abbreviation for Doctor of Podiatric Medicine.

DPN. Abbreviation for diphosphopyridine nucleotide; now called nicotinamide adenine dinucleotide (NAD).

DPNH. Abbreviation for reduced diphosphopyridine nucleotide; now called reduced nicotinamide adenine dinucleotide (NADH).

draconti'asis. Infection with *Dracunculus medinensis*.

Dracun'culus. A genus of nematodes resembling the true filaria worms but having a crustacean rather than an insect as an intermediate host.

D. medinensis, threadlike, yard-long worm infecting the subcutaneous tissues of man and domestic animals in India, Africa, and Arabia; its larvae are discharged through ulcers that are formed in the skin; also called guinea, Medina, or serpent worm.

drain. 1. To draw off the fluid from a bodily cavity, especially to provide for its exit as soon as it is formed. **2.** To discharge. **3.** A device (tube or wick) used to remove fluid from a wound.

cigarette d., a cigarette-shaped gauze wick enclosed in a thin-walled rubber tube.

Jackson-Pratt d., a flexible silicon rubber suction drain with small intraluminal ridges which prevent collapse of its lumen and with a radiopaque marker

incorporated in the side; used to drain the subdural space after removal of a subdural hematoma; also called subdural brain drain.

Penrose d., cigarette drain.

stab d., one passed through a puncture wound some distance from the operative incision.

subdural brain d., see Jackson-Pratt drain.

sump d., one composed of two tubes, a larger one containing a slender tube which is attached to a suction pump.

drain'age. 1. The continuous withdrawal of fluids from a cavity or wound. **2.** The material withdrawn or discharged.

capillary d., one effected by means of a wick of gauze, strands of hair, or other material.

closed d., drainage of chest cavity carried out with protection against the entrance of outside air into the cavity.

open d., drainage of chest through an opening in the chest wall without sealing off the outside air.

tidal d., drainage of a paralyzed urinary bladder by an irrigation apparatus.

dram. 1. An avoirdupois unit of weight equal to 27.34 grains or 0.062 ounce. **2.** An apothecary unit of weight equal to 60 grains or 1/8 ounce.

drawer sign. One elicited from a patient lying on his back with his knee flexed at 90 degrees while the examiner grasps the upper part of the patient's leg with both hands and pulls the head of the tibia; a forward movement indicates rupture of the anterior cruciate ligament; if the tibia can be pushed under the femoral condyle, the posterior cruciate ligament is ruptured; also called Rocher's sign.

dream. A series of images experienced during sleep, usually with a definite sense of reality.

wet d., a dream, usually erotic, accompanied by emission of semen during sleep.

drepan'ocyte. Sickle cell; see under cell

drepanocyto'sis. Sickle cell anemia; see under anemia.

dress. To apply a dressing.

dres'sing. 1. Material or preparation applied to a wound or lesion for the purpose of preventing external infection, absorbing discharges, etc. **2.** The application of such materials.

occlusive d., one that covers and seals a wound completely.

drib'ble. To flow in drops, as the urine from a distended bladder.

drill. A cutting instrument for boring holes in bones or teeth by rotary motion.

drip. 1. To fall in drops. **2.** A liquid that falls in drops. **3.** Colloquial expression referring to a discharge.

intravenous d., the continuous intravenous injec-

cross section of
smooth muscle

lipid droplet

mitochondria
between
myofibrils

Drosophila
melanogaster
(fruit fly)

drumstick

polymorphonuclear
leukocyte

right
hepatic
duct

left
hepatic
duct

common
hepatic
duct

gallbladder

cystic
duct

common
bile
duct

small
intestine
(duodenum)

tion of a substance a drop at a time.

postnasal d., excessive discharge of mucus from
the posterior nares.

dro′mic. Denoting nerve impulses conducted in a
normal direction.

dromotrop′ic. Affecting conductivity of nerves.

drop. 1. The smallest possible quantity of a liquid
heavy enough to fall in a pear-shaped globule. **2.** To
fall in drops or to let fall in drops.

foot d., see footdrop.

hanging d., a drop of a fluid on the undersurface
of the object glass examined under the microscope.

toe d., see footdrop.

wrist d., wristdrop.

drop′let. A very small drop.

lipid d., a spherical body of lipid occurring freely
in the cytoplasm of cells; it is not ordinarily membrane bound and is generally surrounded by mitochondria; also called lipid body or inclusion.

drops. Popular name for any liquid medicine administered with a dropper.

eye d., ophthalmic solution; see under solution.

knock-out d., popular name for chloral alco-
holate; made by mixing chloral hydrate with any
alcoholic drink and given with criminal intent to
produce rapid unconsciousness.

drop′sy. 1. See hydrops. **2.** Obsolete term used to
describe heart failure, chronic renal disease, and
other fluid-retaining states.

Drosoph′ila. A genus of flies containing about 900
species, including the fruit fly (*D. melanogaster*),
which is used extensively in genetic studies.

drowse. To be partially asleep.

drug. 1. Any substance used as a medicine in the
treatment or prevention of disease. **2.** A narcotic or
hallucinogen, whether or not used for medical purposes, employed usually illegally for altering mood,
perception, or consciousness.

crude d., any medicinal material before refining.

d. dependence, condition in which the user of a
drug considers the effects it produces, or the conditions associated with its use, essential to maintain an
optimal state of well being.

d. misuse, the inappropriate use of medicine
either in improper dosages or for purposes for which
it was not intended.

psychedelic d., a drug, usually self-administered,
that causes marked changes in mood.

psychotropic d., any drug that influences psychic
functions, behavior, or experiences, such as chlorpromazine (Thorazine®).

sulfa d., any of a group of synthetic organic compounds, related to sulfonamide, used as antibacterial agents.

drug-fast. Relating to microorganisms that resist

the action of a chemical.

drum′stick. A minute protrusion from the nucleus
of a polymorphonuclear leukocyte, present in about
two per cent of these cells when two X chromosomes are present, as in normal females (XX) or in
patients with Klinefelter's syndrome who have an
extra sex chromosome (XXY).

drunkenness. Acute alcoholism; see under alcoholism.

dru′sen. Small, circular, yellow or white hyaline or
colloid nodules occurring in the innermost layer of
the vascular coat of the eye (choroid); usually they
do not interfere with vision.

DTPA. Abbreviation for diethylenetriaminepentaa-
cetic acid.

DT's. Abbreviation for delirium tremens.

Dubin-Johnson syndrome. Congenital familial
defect in the excretory function of the liver resulting
in mild jaundice, the presence of large amounts of
bilirubin in the blood, and frequently a dark pigment in the liver cells; also called chronic idiopathic
jaundice.

Duchenne-Aran disease. Progressive muscular
atrophy; see under atrophy.

duct. A tube or channel, usually for conveying the
product of a gland to another part of the body.

accessory pancreatic d., the smaller of the two
pancreatic ducts which enter the duodenum; also
called duct of Santorini.

Bartholin's d., see major sublingual duct.

cochlear d., a spirally arranged membranous tube
within the cochlea of the internal ear.

common bile d., the duct formed by union of the
hepatic duct and cystic duct; it conveys bile to the
duodenum.

common hepatic d., the duct formed by the
union of the right and left hepatic ducts.

cystic d., the duct leading from the gallbladder to
the common bile duct.

deferent d., the duct that conveys sperm from the
epididymis to the ejaculatory duct; also called vas
deferens, ductus deferens and spermatic duct.

ejaculatory d., the canal formed by the union of
the deferent duct (vas deferens) and the excretory
duct of the seminal vesicle; it opens into the prostatic urethra.

endolymphatic d., a duct in the labyrinth of the
ear which connects the endolymphatic sac with the
utricle and saccule.

excretory d. of the seminal vesicle, the duct
that drains the seminal vesicle and leads to the
ejaculatory duct.

lactiferous d., one of about eighteen ducts which
drain milk from the lobes of the mammary gland
and open at the nipple; also called milk duct.

major sublingual d., the duct that drains the
sublingual salivary gland and opens at the sublingual
papilla in the floor of the mouth; also called Bartholin's duct.

mesonephric d., an embryonic duct which develops, in the male, into the deferent duct; in the
female it is obliterated; also called wolffian duct.

milk d., see lactiferous duct.

mullerian d., see paramesonephric duct.

nasolacrimal d., one conveying tears from the
lacrimal sac to the nasal cavity.

omphalomesenteric d., a narrow yolk stalk connecting the midgut of the embryo with the yolk sac;
also called vitelline duct and yolk-stalk.

pancreatic d., the main excretory duct of the
pancreas; it opens into the duodenum.

papillary d. of Bellini, one of numerous ducts in
the inner part of the renal medulla, formed by a
succession of junctions of about seven straight collecting tubules.

paramesonephric d., either of the two embryonic tubes that develop, in the female, into the
uterine tubes, vagina, and uterus; it disappears in
the male; also called mullerian duct and Müller's
canal.

paraurethral d., one of several ducts of the
paraurethral (Skene's) glands; also called Schüler's
ducts.

parotid d., the duct that conveys saliva from the
parotid gland to the mouth at the level of the upper
second molar.

perilymphatic d., a minute canal connecting the
perilymphatic space of the cochlea with the subarachnoid space.

semicircular d., one of three membranous tubes
within the semicircular canal of the internal ear; it
contributes to balance and orientation.

spermatic d., see deferent duct.

sublingual d., major, the duct that drains the
sublingual gland and opens into the submandibular
duct.

sublingual d.'s, minor, the ducts (10 to 30) that
drain the sublingual gland and open along the fold
of mucous membrane (plica sublingualis) in the
mouth; also called Walther's ducts.

submandibular d., a duct about five centimeters
long that drains the submandibular gland and opens
at the tip of the sublingual papilla on the floor of the
mouth adjacent to the frenulum of the tongue; also
called Wharton's duct.

sudoriferous d., one leading from the body of a
sweat gland to the surface of the skin; also called
sweat duct.

thoracic d., the largest lymphatic channel in the
body; it conveys lymph into the left subclavian vein.

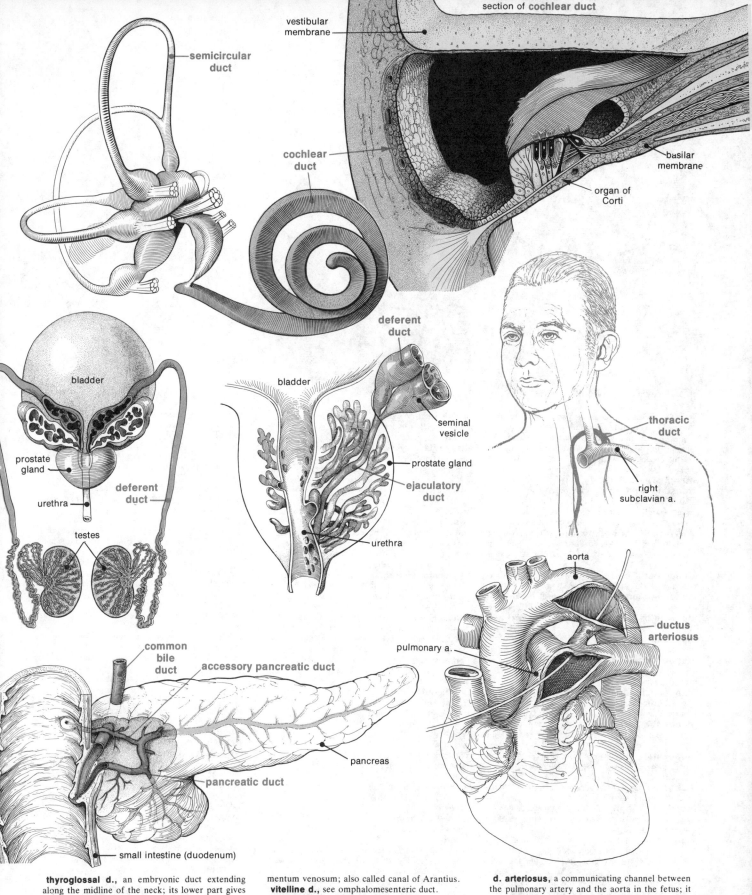

section of **cochlear duct**

vestibular membrane

cochlear duct

basilar membrane

organ of Corti

semicircular duct

deferent duct

bladder

prostate gland

urethra

testes

deferent duct

bladder

seminal vesicle

prostate gland

ejaculatory duct

urethra

thoracic duct

right subclavian a.

aorta

ductus arteriosus

pulmonary a.

common bile duct

accessory pancreatic duct

pancreas

pancreatic duct

small intestine (duodenum)

thyroglossal d., an embryonic duct extending along the midline of the neck; its lower part gives rise to the isthmus of the thyroid gland; normally the remainder disappears but occasionally it persists in the adult and forms a cyst or a fistula.

utriculosaccular d., one located in the internal ear extending from the utricle and joining the endolymphatic duct.

venous d., in the fetus, the continuation of the umbilical vein through the liver to the inferior vena cava; it obliterates after birth, becoming the liga-

mentum venosum; also called canal of Arantius.

vitelline d., see omphalomesenteric duct.

Wharton's d., see submandibular duct.

wolffian d., see mesonephric duct.

duc'tile. Capable of being made into wire or hammered into thin plates, as certain metals; capable of being shaped or molded, as plastic.

duc'tion. The movement of an eye by the extrinsic muscles.

duc'tus, *pl.* **duc'tus.** Latin for duct, a tubular structure.

d. arteriosus, a communicating channel between the pulmonary artery and the aorta in the fetus; it normally obliterates shortly after birth.

d. deferens, deferent duct; see under duct.

patent d. arteriosus, a ductus arteriosus that does not obliterate but remains patent after birth.

Duhring's disease. See dermatitis herpetiformis.

dull. 1. Not sharp; said of an instrument, pain, or sound. **2.** Lacking mental alertness.

dul'lness, dul'ness. The quality of sound elic-

duct | **dullness**

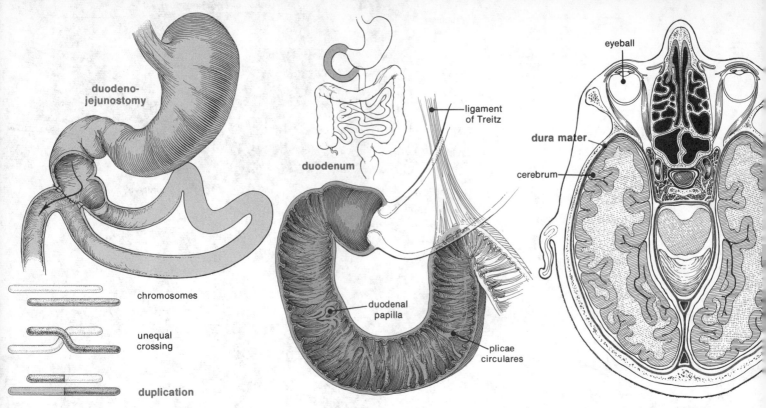

duodeno-jejunostomy

chromosomes

unequal crossing

duplication

ligament of Treitz

duodenum

duodenal papilla

plicae circulares

eyeball

dura mater

cerebrum

---

ited by percussion over a solid part or organ, characterized by very little resonance.

shifting d., dull sound produced by percussion, usually of the abdominal cavity, that shifts location as the patient is moved; indicative of the presence of free fluid.

dumb. Mute; lacking the faculty of speech.

dumping syndrome. Symptoms occurring within 30 minutes after the end of a meal, including nausea, warmth, sweating, palpitation, pallor, headache, diarrhea, pain in the upper abdomen, and weakness; caused by excessively rapid emptying of the stomach, usually following loss of the pylorus in stomach resection; also called postgastrectomy syndrome.

duode′nal. Of, relating to, or situated in the duodenum.

duodenec′tomy. Surgical removal of the duodenal portion of the small intestine, total or partial.

duodeni′tis. Inflammation of the duodenal portion of the small intestine.

duodeno-. Combining form relating to the duodenal portion of the small intestine.

duodenocholecystos′tomy. The surgical formation of a passage between the gallbladder and the duodenum.

duodenocholedochot′omy. Surgical incision into the common bile duct and the adjoining portion of the duodenum.

duodenoenteros′tomy. The surgical formation of a passage between the duodenum and another part of the small intestine.

duodenojejunos′tomy. The surgical formation of a passage between the duodenum and the jejunum.

duodenol′ysis. The operation of freeing the duodenum from adhesions.

duodenor′rhaphy. Suturing of the duodenum.

duodenos′copy. Visual observation of the duodenum's interior by means of an endoscope.

duodenos′tomy. The surgical formation of an orifice or passage into the duodenum.

duodenot′omy. Surgical incision into the duodenum.

duode′num. The first portion of the small intestine; shaped like a horseshoe; it starts at the lower end of the stomach and extends to the jejunum; the term comes from the Latin *duodeni* (twelve), because this portion of the intestine is about 12 fingerbreadths (25–30 cm) in length.

duplica′tion. In genetics, a chromosome aberration consisting of the presence of an extra piece of chromosome, usually originated by unequal exchange of fragments between homologous chromosomes; the other chromosome has a segment miss-

ing (deletion).

du′ra See dura mater.

du′ral. Relating to the dura mater.

dura mater. A tough, fibrous, whitish membrane; the outermost of the three membranes covering the brain and spinal cord; also called dura.

D.V.M. Abbreviation for Doctor of Veterinary Medicine.

dwarf. An abnormally small person; also called nanus.

dwarf′ism. In a broad sense, failure to achieve full growth potential; may be induced by ecological factors (e.g., dietary intake or systemic disease), by genetic factors, or by endocrine factors; lack of height is only one of the resulting features.

achondroplastic d., a form caused by congenital abnormality in the process of ossification of cartilage; affected individuals have a relatively elongated trunk, short extremities, and a large head.

pituitary d., dwarfism accompanied by sexual infantilism and decreased function of the thyroid and adrenal glands; caused by lesions of the anterior portion of the pituitary gland early in childhood.

primordial d., inadequate term designating a condition characterized by insufficient growth with normal functional development.

dy′ad. 1. A pair. **2.** A bivalent element or radical. **3.** One pair of chromosomes after the disjunction of a tetrad at the first meiotic division.

dye. Any coloring substance.

dynam′ics. 1. The science of the relationship between motion and the forces causing it. **2.** The emotional forces determining patterns of behavior.

dynamo-. Combining form meaning power or energy.

dynamom′eter. An apparatus for measuring the force of muscular contraction under controlled conditions.

dyne. A unit of force equal to the force required to give a body of 1 g an acceleration of 1 cm per second squared.

dys-. Combining form indicating faulty, difficult, painful, diseased, or bad; e.g., dysplasia, disphasia; the opposite of eu-.

dysacu′sis, dysacu′sia. 1. Defect of hearing marked by inability to discriminate between sounds; distinguished from lack of sensitivity to sound. **2.** Pain in the ear caused by sound.

dysar′thria. Impairment of articulation of speech.

dysarthro′sis. 1. Malformation of a joint. **2.** Impairment of articulation. **3.** A false joint.

dysautono′mia. Dysfunction of the autonomic nervous system.

familial d., congenital nerve disorder affecting infants and children; characterized by indifference to

pain, inability to shed tears, emotional instability, drooling, excessive sweating, and poor motor control; also called Riley-Day syndrome.

dys′barism. General term denoting physiologic changes resulting from changes in barometric pressure, such as the effects of rapid decompression.

dysba′sia. Difficult or distorted walking; it may be organically or psychically determined.

dyscepha′lia, dyscepha′ly. Malformation of the head and face.

dysche′zia. Difficult or painful defecation.

dyschi′ria. Disorder in which the individual is unable to tell which side of his body has been touched.

dyschondrogen′esis. Defective development of cartilage.

dyschondropla′sia. See Ollier's syndrome.

dyschro′mia. Any abnormality in the pigmentation (color) of the skin or hair.

dyscor′ia. Irregularly shaped pupil.

dyscra′sia. A general morbid condition of the body.

bleeding d., a pathologic condition due to abnormal hemostasis, as hemophilia.

plasma cell d., general term to describe various pathologic conditions and biochemical abnormalities of cells that normally produce γ-globulin; e.g., the proliferative disorders of plasma cells.

dysdiadochokine′sia. Inability to make alternating movements in rapid succession, such as extending and flexing a limb.

dysene′ia. Defective articulation arising from defects in hearing.

dys′entery. Disease marked by frequent watery stools containing blood and mucus, attended by abdominal pain, dehydration, and sometimes fever.

amebic d., dysentery due to infection with *Entamoeba histolytica*, which may cause ulceration of the colon; symptoms vary from slight abdominal discomfort and diarrhea alternating with constipation to profuse bleeding and discharge of mucus and pus.

bacillary d., dysentery caused by bacteria of the genus *Shigella*.

dyser′ethism. A slow response to stimuli.

dyser′gia. Motor incoordination.

dysesthe′sia. 1. Impairment or partial loss of sensation. **2.** Painful or disagreeable sensation produced by ordinary stimuli.

dysfunc′tion. Abnormal or impaired functioning of an organ or bodily system.

minimal brain d. (MBD), condition manifested by one or several of the following: short attention span, poor modulation of emotions, reading and/or writing disabilities, hyperactivity, poor coordination, and impulsiveness.

dysgammaglobuline′mia. Disorders or abnor-

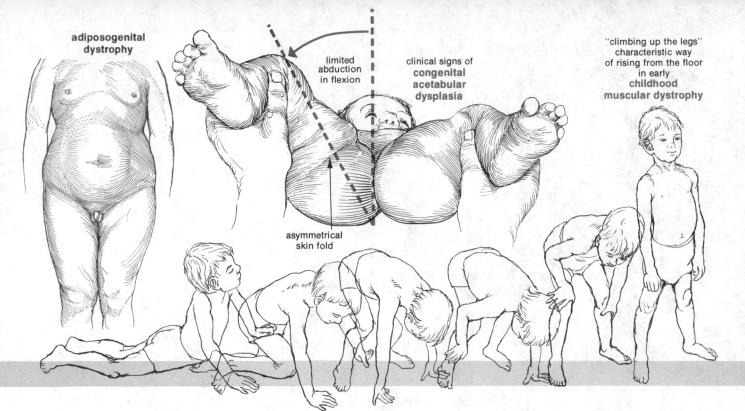

adiposogenital
dystrophy

limited
abduction
in flexion

clinical signs of
**congenital
acetabular
dysplasia**

"climbing up the legs"
characteristic way
of rising from the floor
in early
**childhood
muscular dystrophy**

asymmetrical
skin fold

malities of γ-globulins in the blood serum.

dysgen'ic. Applying to factors which cause the deterioration of hereditary qualities; the opposite of eugenic.

dysgen'ics, dysgen'esis. The study of the factors causing defective or deficient embryonic development; also called cacogenics.

gonadal d., defective gonadal development.

seminiferous tubule d., see Klinefelter's syndrome.

dysgermino'ma. A rare malignant ovarian tumor composed of undifferentiated germinal epithelium; the counterpart of seminoma of the testis; also called ovarian seminoma.

dysgeu'sia. A general term describing any distortion of normal taste perception.

dysgna'thia. Any abnormality of the maxilla or mandible.

dysgno'sia. Any disorder of the intellect.

dysgraph'ia. 1. Difficulty in writing, usually due to ataxia, tremor, or motor neurosis. **2.** Writer's cramp; see under cramp.

dyshematopoie'sia, dyshemopoie'sis. Defective or imperfect blood formation.

dyshidro'sis, dysidro'sis. 1. An abnormality of sweat production. **2.** A deep eruption of blisters occurring primarily on the hands and feet, accompanied by intense itching; also called pompholyx.

trichophytic d., Tinea pedis.

dyskerato'ma. Skin tumor containing cells that display abnormal keratinization.

warty d., a benign skin tumor with a central keratoic plug, occurring on the scalp, face, or neck.

dyskine'sia. Difficulty in performing voluntary movements.

dyslal'ia. Impairment of speech due to defective speech organs.

dyslex'ia. Impaired ability to learn to read.

dyslo'gia. Impairment of the thought processes and of speech.

dysmegalop'sia. A disordered visual perception of the size of objects; called micropsia when objects seem smaller, and macropsia when larger.

dysme'lia. Congenital absence of a portion of one or more limbs.

dysmenorrhe'a. Painful menstrual periods.

functional d., primary dysmenorrhea.

primary d., dysmenorrhea caused by a functional disturbance.

secondary d., dysmenorrhea caused by inflammation, tumor, infection, or anatomic factors.

dysmet'ria. Inability to stop a muscular movement at a desired point.

dysmor'phism. 1. Abnormality of shape. **2.** Allomorphism.

dysontogen'esis. Abnormal development.

dysos'mia. A general term describing any distortion of normal smell perception.

dysosto'sis. Defective bone formation.

craniofacial d., ocular hypertelorism; see under hypertelorism.

mandibulofacial d., hereditary abnormalities of the palpebral fissures, mandible and zygomatic bones, and lower lids, with malposition and malocclusion of teeth, low-set malformed ears, and high or cleft palate; called Franceschetti's syndrome when complete, and Treacher Collins' syndrome when partial.

d. multiplex, see Hurler's syndrome.

dyspareu'nia. Painful intercourse.

dyspep'sia. Indigestion.

dyspha'gia. Difficulty in swallowing; also called aphagia.

dyspha'sia. Impairment of coordination in speech and inability to arrange words in their proper order, usually associated with brain injury.

dyspho'nia. Difficulty or pain in speaking.

dyspho'ria. An emotional state characterized by depression, restlessness, and malaise, usually accompanied by poor self-esteem.

dyspla'sia. Abnormal development of bodily tissue.

chondroectodermal d., inherited disorder marked by short extremities with normal trunk, polydactyly, and abnormal development of teeth and nails; frequently associated with congenital heart defects; also called Ellis-van Creveld syndrome.

congenital acetabular d., congenital dislocation of the hip; a complete or partial displacement of the femoral head out of the acetabulum; not related to trauma or to other musculoskeletal disease.

dentinal d., hereditary abnormality of dentin formation marked by disarrangement of dentin tubules by masses of collagneous matrix, poorly developed tooth roots, and absence of pulp canals and chambers.

ectodermal d., general term denoting abnormal development of tissues derived from ectoderm.

fibrous d. of bone, condition in which the marrow of one or more bones is replaced by fibrous tissue.

fibromuscular d., nonatherosclerotic disease of arteries, especially the renal arteries, causing constriction.

hereditary renal-retinal d., inherited disorder marked by retinitis pigmentosa, diabetes insipidus, and progressive uremia.

polyostotic fibrous d., the occurrence of fibrous dysplasia in several bones, usually on one side of the body.

dysplas'tic. Relating to or marked by abnormality of development.

dysp'nea. Difficult or labored breathing usually associated with serious disease of the heart or lungs.

paroxysmal nocturnal d. (PND), acute dyspnea occurring suddenly at night, caused by pulmonary congestion and edema.

dysprax'ia. Impaired functioning of an organ or part.

dysproteine'mia. Abnormality in blood proteins.

dyssta'sia. Difficulty in standing.

dyssylla'bia. Syllable stumbling.

dyssyner'gia, dyssyner'gy. Disturbance of muscular coordination.

dysto'cia. Difficult childbirth.

fetal d., difficult labor due to abnormalities of position or size of the fetus.

maternal d., difficult labor due to uterine inertia or deformities of the birth canal.

dysto'nia. Abnormal tonicity of musculature.

dystontogen'esis. Abnormal development and differentiation of tissues.

dysto'pia. Malposition.

dystop'ic. Out of place.

dys'trophy. Disorder caused by faulty nutrition or by lesions of the pituitary gland and/or brain.

adiposogenital d., condition caused by lesions of the pituitary gland and the hypothalamus, marked by increase in fat, especially about the abdomen, hips, and thighs, with underdeveloped genital organs and loss of hair; usually manifested during puberty and often mistaken for obesity; also called Fröhlich's syndrome.

cerebrooculorenal d., see oculocerebrorenal syndrome.

childhood muscular d., an inherited disorder affecting boys usually between two and five years of age; the first symptoms and signs appear in the muscles of the pelvis and lower extremities; it is rapidly progressive and usually fatal by the third decade; also called Duchenne's dystrophy.

Duchenne's d., see childhood muscular dystrophy.

muscular dystrophy, inherited disease of muscles marked by progressive weakness and deterioration.

myotonic d., see myotonia atrophica.

progressive muscular d., progressive, gradual muscular deterioration of unknown cause.

pseudohypertrophic d., pseudomuscular d., degenerative disease of childhood, marked by enlargement and weakness, followed by wasting, of the muscles of the shoulder girdle and sometimes of the pelvic girdle.

dysu'ria. Difficulty or pain in urination.

dysgenic | dysuria

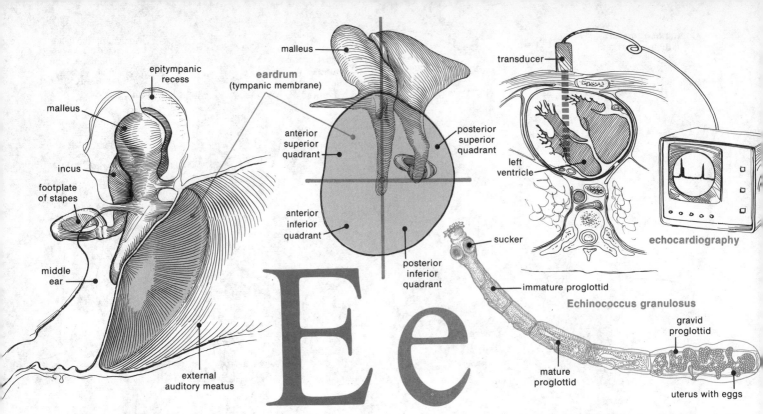

epitympanic recess

malleus

eardrum (tympanic membrane)

malleus

transducer

incus

footplate of stapes

middle ear

external auditory meatus

anterior superior quadrant

posterior superior quadrant

anterior inferior quadrant

posterior inferior quadrant

left ventricle

echocardiography

sucker

immature proglottid

Echinococcus granulosus

gravid proglottid

mature proglottid

uterus with eggs

E. 1. Abbreviation for emmetropia. **2.** Symbol for (a) electromotive force; (b) the element erbium.

e. Symbol for (a) electron; (b) the natural logarithm that has a numerical value of 2.7.

Eo⁺, Eo. Symbol for oxidation-reduction potential.

ear. The compound organ of hearing and equilibrium; it is sensitive to sound waves, to the effects of gravity, and to motion; the organ consists of the external ear, which includes the auricle (pinna) and the external auditory meatus, the middle ear or tympanic cavity, which contains the ossicles, and the internal ear, which includes the semicircular canals, vestibule, and cochlea.

  aviator's e., see aerotitis media.

  cauliflower e., boxer's ear, a thickened, deformed ear caused by injury to the tissues due to repeated blows.

  darwinian e., one with a protrusion on the helix.

  glue e., serous otitis media with very thick fluid in the middle ear chamber, characterized by a marked conductive hearing loss.

ear'ache. Pain in the ear; also called otalgia.

ear'drum. The tympanic membrane; a flattened cone-shaped fibrous sheet which separates the external auditory meatus from the middle ear chamber.

earth. 1. Soil; the loose, friable substances forming the ground. **2.** An amorphous pulverizable mineral. **3.** A metallic oxide characterized by a high melting point; e.g., alumina, which was formerly classed as an element.

  alkaline e., any oxide of the elements in the family to which calcium and magnesium belong.

  diatomaceous e., purified siliceous earth composed mainly of shell wall remains of minute aquatic unicellular diatoms; used as an inert filler in many dental materials and as a mild abrasive and polishing agent; also called infusorial earth.

  infusorial e., diatomaceous earth.

  rare e., those rare elements with atomic numbers from 57 to 71 that closely resemble one another chemically.

earth-eating. The practice of eating dirt or clay.

ear'wax. Cerumen; the soft brownish-yellow wax-like secretion of the ceruminous glands lining the canal of the external ear.

eat. 1. To chew and swallow solid food taken into the mouth. **2.** To erode.

Eaton agent pneumonia. Mycoplasma pneumonia; see under pneumonia.

Eaton-Lambert syndrome. Myasthenia syndrome usually associated with tumor, especially oat cell carcinoma of the lung; characterized by weakness and pain in the limbs with peculiarly slow movements and curare sensitivity; electromyogra-

phy is diagnostic.

eb'ullism. 1. The formation of water vapor in the tissues due to extreme reduction in barometric pressure occurring at altitudes above 60,000 feet. **2.** The bubbling of a fluid; a boiling. **3.** A sudden emotional outpouring, as of violence.

e'bur. Resembling ivory.

eburna'tion. The transformation of bone into a dense ivory-like substance.

ecbol'ic. 1. Accelerating childbirth; producing abortion. **2.** An agent that induces labor or abortion by stimulating uterine contractions.

eccen'tric. 1. Situated away from the center. **2.** Deviating from the established norm. **3.** One who deviates markedly from normal or conventional conduct or speech; abnormal in emotional reactions and in general behavior, with no intellectual defect; an erratic person.

eccentrochondropla'sia. Abnormal ossification, especially in long bones, in which osseous tissue is formed from areas other than the epiphysial cartilage.

ecchondro'ma. A benign cartilaginous tumor; an outgrowth of normally situated cartilage projecting through the shaft of a bone; also called ecchondrosis.

ecchondro'sis. See ecchondroma.

ecchymo'ma. A slight hematoma due to a bruise.

ecchymo'sis. A bruise; a "black and blue spot" on the skin caused by escape of blood from injured vessels.

ecchymot'ic. Relating to an ecchymosis.

ec'crine. See exocrine.

eccrinol'ogy. The study of secretions and excretions.

ec'crisis. 1. The excretion of a waste product. **2.** Any waste product.

eccrit'ic. Anything that promotes the excretion of waste products.

eccye'sis. Ectopic pregnancy or gestation.

ecdem'ic. Indicating a disease brought into an area from without; not endemic.

ec'dysis. Molting; desquamation or shedding of an outer covering.

ec'esis. The successful adjustment and growth of an organism in a new environment.

ECF. Abbreviation for extracellular fluid.

ECG. Abbreviation for electrocardiogram; also abbreviated EKG.

echin-, echino-. Combining forms denoting spiny.

echinococco'sis. Infection caused by the larval form of *Echinococcus granulosus* or *Echinococcus multilocularis*, producing expanding cysts in the liver or lungs; anaphylactic reaction may occur from

rupture of cyst fluid into the pleural or peritoneal cavity; also called hydatid disease.

Echinococcus granulosus. A species of tapeworm occurring in the adult form in dog's intestines; the larval forms occur in man, forming hydatid cysts in the liver and other tissues.

Echinoder'mata. A phylum of radially symmetrical invertebrates often having a'body covered with spines; it includes starfishes, sea urchins, sea lilies, etc.

echo. Repetition of a sound; reflection of a sound wave to its point of origin.

echocardiog'raphy. The use of an ultrasonic apparatus that sends sound impulses toward the walls of the heart, which in turn bounce or echo the sounds back; the patterns produced are graphically displayed for interpretation; used for determining the movement patterns of the heart and its valves, chamber size, wall thickness, and the presence of pericardial fluid.

echoencephalog'raphy. A method of examing the brain by recording the reflection of high frequency (ultrasonic) sound waves; it is used to obtain a safe, rapid, and painless estimate of the position of the midline of the third ventricle; useful in evaluating patients with suspected subdural or epidural hemorrhage or other conditions which might cause a brain shift.

echola'lia. Compulsive or involuntary echo-like repetition of another's words or phrases.

echoloca'tion. The method by which certain animals, as bats and dolphins, orient themselves, i.e., by means of reflected sound waves produced by the high-frequency sounds that they emit.

echop'athy. A syndrome characterized by the senseless imitation of speech (echolalia) or gestures and postures (echopraxia) of others; may be seen during the catatonic phase of schizophrenia.

echopho'nia, echoph'ony. The echo of the voice sometimes heard in auscultation of the chest.

echoprax'ia. The involuntary and meaningless imitation of movements made by another; also called echomatism.

echovi'rus. A member of the picornavirus group of viruses associated with aseptic meningitis and gastroenteritis in man; the term is an acronym of enteric cytopathogenic human orphan virus.

eclamp'sia. An acute disorder peculiar to pregnant and puerperal women, marked by convulsions during which there is a loss of consciousness usually followed by more or less prolonged coma; associated with hypertension, edema, and/or proteinuria; in most cases clinical manifestations occur after the 24th week of gestation and disappear after delivery; a phase of toxemia of pregnancy; also called

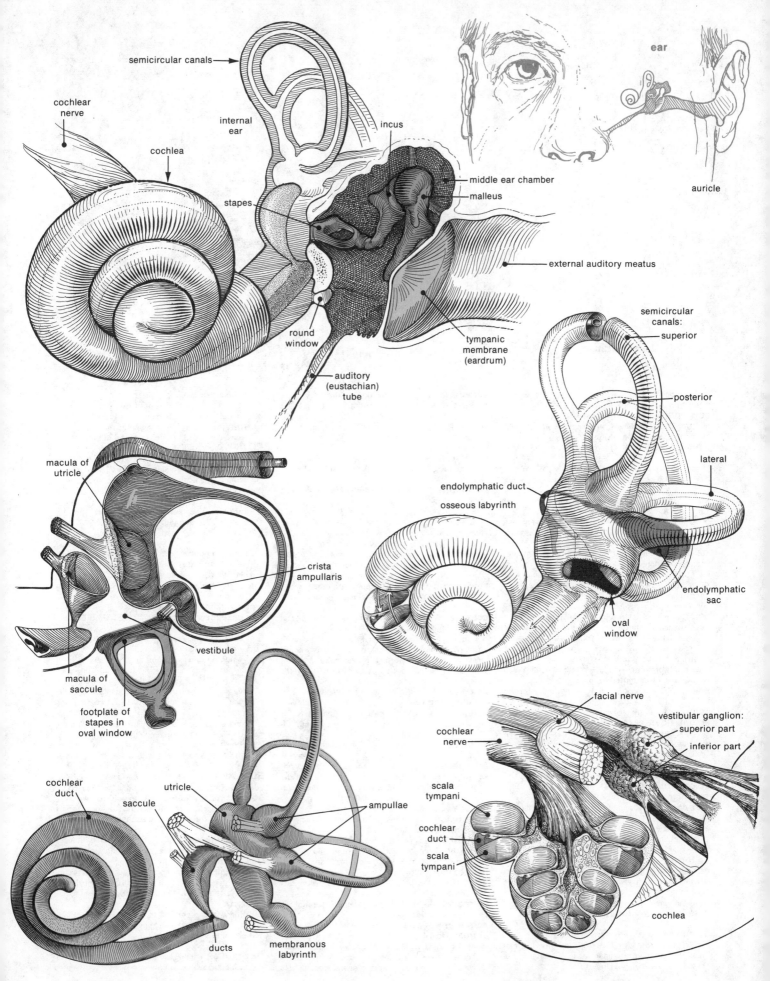

semicircular canals

cochlear nerve

internal ear

incus

ear

cochlea

stapes

middle ear chamber

malleus

auricle

external auditory meatus

round window

tympanic membrane (eardrum)

auditory (eustachian) tube

semicircular canals:

superior

posterior

lateral

macula of utricle

endolymphatic duct

osseous labyrinth

crista ampullaris

vestibule

macula of saccule

endolymphatic sac

footplate of stapes in oval window

oval window

facial nerve

vestibular ganglion:
superior part
inferior part

cochlear nerve

cochlear duct

utricle

saccule

ampullae

scala tympani

cochlear duct

scala tympani

ducts

membranous labyrinth

cochlea

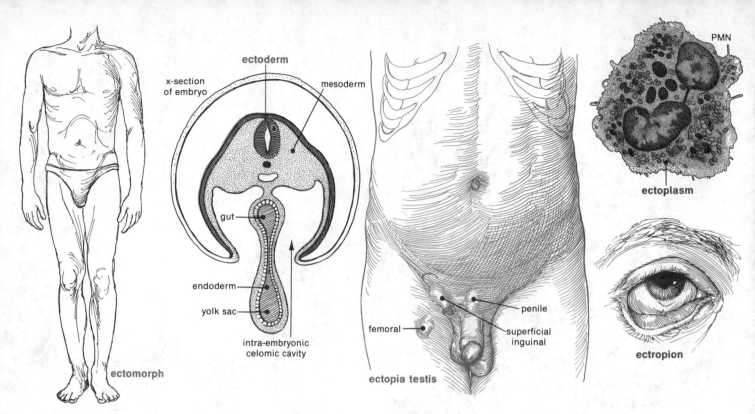

x-section of embryo
ectoderm
mesoderm
gut
endoderm
yolk sac
intra-embryonic celomic cavity

ectomorph

ectopia testis
femoral
penile
superficial inguinal

PMN
ectoplasm

ectropion

eclamptogenic toxemia.

 puerperal e., eclampsia occurring after delivery.

eclamp´tic. Relating to eclampsia.

eclamptog´enous. Convulsant; denoting anything that causes convulsions.

ecmne´sia. Inability to remember recent events only.

E. co´li. Abbreviation for *Escherichia coli*.

ecol´ogy. The science of the relationship between organisms and their environment.

econ´omy. The functional arrangement of organs and structures within the body.

e´cosite. A parasite to which the host is immune under normal conditions; also called ecoparasite.

ec´osystem. An ecological system; a community of organisms, together with its physical environment, considered as an entity.

ECT. Abbreviation for electroconvulsant therapy.

ecta´sia, ec´tasis. Dilatation of a hollow organ or a tubular structure; also used as a suffix to denote expansion, as in bronchiectasis.

ectat´ic. Characterized by ectasia.

ecthy´ma. A pustular eruption, usually seated upon a shallow ulcer, that evolves into a firm crust or scab; caused by staphylococci or streptococci; scarring is a characteristic sequela.

 e. contagiosum, orf; a viral disease of sheep occasionally transmitted to man.

ecti´ris. The anterior or outer endothelium of the iris.

ecto-, ect-. Prefixes meaning outer or external.

ectoan´tigen, exoan´tigen. 1. Any exciter of antibody formation, separate from its source. **2.** An antigen formed from the ectoplasm of bacterial cells.

ec´toblast. The ectoderm.

ectocar´dia. Abnormal position of the heart.

ectochoroi´dea. The suprachoroid; the outer part of the choroid layer of the eye.

ectocor´nea. The anterior or outer epithelium of the cornea.

ec´tocrine. 1. A substance, synthesized or resulting from the decomposition of organisms, that affects plant life. **2.** Ectohormone.

ec´tocyst. The outer layer of a hydatid cyst.

ec´toderm. The outermost of the three germ layers of the embryo; it gives rise to the nervous system and to the epidermis and its derivatives, such as hair and the lens of the eye.

ectoder´mal, ectoder´mic. Relating to the ectoderm.

ectodermato´sis. See ectodermosis.

ectodermo´sis. A disorder arising from the maldevelopment of any organ or tissue derived from the ectoderm; also called ectodermatosis.

ectog´enous. Originating outside the body.

ec´tohormone. A substance that is secreted by an organism into its immediate environment and modifies the functional activity of some distant organism; a parahormonal mediator of ecological importance; also called ectocrine.

ec´tomere. Any one of the cells into which the fertilized egg divides which takes part in the formation of ectoderm.

ec´tomorph. 1. In the somatotype, an individual exhibiting linear and fragile features; a person with a lean and slightly muscular body. **2.** A body build in which tissues that originated from the ectoderm predominate.

ectomor´phic. Slender and not muscular.

-ectomy. Combining form indicating removal of an organ or part by surgery; e.g., hysterectomy, appendectomy.

ectopa´gia. The lateral fusion of conjoined twins.

ectopar´asite. A parasite that lives on the surface of the body of its host.

ecto´pia. A congenital displacement or abnormal position of an organ.

 e. testis, a condition in which a testicle has strayed from the path of normal descent into the scrotum; it may be due to an abnormal connection of the distal end of the gubernaculum testis which leads the gonad to an abnormal position.

ectop´ic. Located in a place other than normal.

ectopic pregnancy. See pregnancy, ectopic.

ectopic ACTH syndrome. Secretion of ACTH by nonendocrine tumors producing hypokalemic alkalosis and weakness.

ectoplacen´tal. Outside or surrounding the placenta.

ec´toplasm. Clear, thin cytoplasm at the periphery of a cell; it is more gelled than the rest of the cytoplasm in the cell; the clarity is due to the exclusion of all organelles except filaments.

ec´topy. Ectopia.

ectosto´sis. Formation of bone beneath the perichondrium or the periostium.

ec´tothrix. Denoting a type of fungal infection in which the hyphae grow both within and on the surface of the hair shaft. Cf endothrix.

ectotox´in. Exotoxin.

ectozo´on. Any parasitic animal living on the surface of the host.

ectodact´ylism, ectodact´yly. Congenital absence of a digit or of digits.

ectrog´eny. Congenital absence of a part.

ectrome´lia. 1. Congenital absence of one or more limbs. **2.** A viral disease of mice causing, among other symptoms, gangrene and loss of feet; it causes high mortality in laboratory mouse colonies; also

called mousepox.

ectro´pion. Eversion or outward displacement of the margin of an eyelid.

ectrosyndac´tyly. A congenital absence of one or more digits and the fusion of the others.

ECW. Abbreviation for extracellular water.

ec´zema. General term for a group of acute or chronic inflammatory skin disorders characterized by redness, thickening, oozing, and the formation of papules, vesicles, and crusts; often accompanied by itching and burning.

 allergic e., one caused by an allergic reaction.

 atopic e., see dermatitis, atopic.

 e. herpeticum, a generalized widespread infection of the skin caused by the herpes simplex virus, occurring in persons with atopic dermatitis who are exposed to the virus for the first time.

 e. infantile, one occurring in infants.

 e. madidans, a moist eruption; also called weeping eczema.

 e. marginatum, see tinea cruris.

 e. pustulosum, one in which the lesions become covered with pus crusts.

 e. rubrum, one presenting excoriated oozing lesions accompanied by redness.

 e. vesiculosum, an eruption of vesicles.

 nummular e., eruption of coin-sized and coin-shaped patches of vesicular dermatitis, usually affecting the extensor surfaces of the hands, arms, and legs; also called nummular dermatitis and orbicular eczema.

 stasis e., eczema of the legs, frequently with ulceration, caused by impaired circulation.

 weeping e., see eczema madidans.

eczem´atous. Affected with or of the nature of eczema.

ED₅₀. Abbreviation for the dose which produces the desired effect in 50 per cent of the subjects tested.

edath´amil. Ethylenediaminetetraacetic acid.

ede´ma. Swelling of any part of the body due to collection of fluid in the intercellular spaces of tissues.

 angioneurotic e., recurrent local edema due to increased vascular permeability of allergic or nervous origin; affecting most commonly the eyelids, lips, tongue, lungs, larynx, or extremities and occurring in persons having a variety of allergies; also called angioedema, Quincke's disease, and giant urticaria.

 Berlin's e., edema of the macular area of the retina, giving it a white appearance, caused by a severe blow to the eyeball; also called concussion edema.

 cardiac e., edema caused by heart disease with resulting increase in venous pressures.

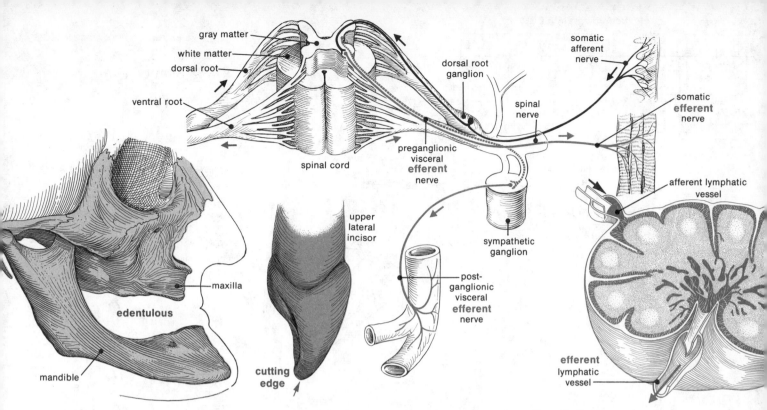

gray matter
white matter
dorsal root
ventral root
spinal cord
dorsal root ganglion
spinal nerve
preganglionic visceral efferent nerve
somatic afferent nerve
somatic efferent nerve
afferent lymphatic vessel
sympathetic ganglion
post-ganglionic visceral efferent nerve
efferent lymphatic vessel

maxilla
edentulous
mandible

upper lateral incisor
cutting edge

cerebral e., edema of the brain caused by tumors, infarction, generalized edema due to heart or kidney disease, or certain toxic conditions.

concussion e., see Berlin's edema.

e. neonatorum, a generalized, usually fatal, edema in the newborn.

famine e., see nutritional edema.

hydremic e., edema occurring in cases of pronounced hydremia (abnormally high plasma content of the blood); also called marantic edema.

idiopathic e., recurrent sodium and fluid retention and swelling occurring in women in the absence of cardiac, hepatic, or renal disease; it occurs most commonly in obese, premenopausal adults; the etiology is not known, although altered capillary and/or lymphatic permeability have been suggested as causes.

menstrual e., the increase in weight and retention of water occurring during or just before menstruation.

nutritional e., swelling caused by prolonged dietary deficiency; usually due at least in part to hypoproteinemia; also called famine edema.

pitting e., condition in which pressure on edematous area causes indentations which remain for a time after pressure is released.

pulmonary e., escape of fluid into the air sacs and interstitial tissue of the lungs; causes include left ventricular failure, mitral stenosis, and chemicals which are pulmonary toxins.

edem′atous. Characterized or affected by edema.

eden′tate. 1. Lacking teeth. **2.** Relating to or belonging to the order Edentata.

eden′tulous. Toothless.

edge. 1. A rim, margin, border, or ridge. **2.** The sharpened side of a blade.

cutting e., (1) the beveled, knifelike working angle of a dental hand instrument; (2) the incisal edge of an anterior tooth.

e. strength, in dentistry, the ability of a fine margin to resist fracture.

EDTA. Abbreviation for ethylenediaminetetraacetic acid.

educ′tion. The process of coming out, as the emerging from general anesthesia.

EEG. Abbreviation for electroencephalogram.

E.E.N.T. Abbreviation for eye, ear, nose, and throat.

EFA. Abbreviation for essential fatty acids, polyunsaturated fatty acids indispensable for nutrition.

effect′. A result; something brought about by a force or an agent.

Bohr e., the effect of carbon dioxide (CO_2) on the oxygen affinity of blood, i.e., CO_2 in the tissues facilitates the removal of oxygen from hemoglobin,

resulting in a greater availability of oxygen to the tissues.

Compton e., a change in wavelength of a bombarding photon with the displacement of an orbital electron.

cumulative e., cumulative action; the sudden pronounced effect resulting after several ineffective doses.

Doppler e., the apparent change in frequency of sound or light waves when the observer and the source are in relative motion; the frequency increases when they approach one another and decreases when they move away; also called Doppler phenomenon.

Pasteur's e., the slowing down of fermentation by oxygen, first observed by Pasteur.

side e., an effect other than that for which a drug or therapy is administered, especially an undesirable secondary effect.

toxic e., a drug-produced harmful effect on some biologic mechanism.

effec′tor. An end organ that, upon receiving a nerve impulse, distributes it, activating either secretion of a gland or contraction of a muscle.

allosteric e., any small molecule that modifies enzyme activity by binding at sites other than the catalytically active sites.

ef′ferent. Conveying a fluid or a nerve impulse away from a central organ or area.

effervesce′. To emit gas bubbles to the surface, as a carbonated liquid.

efferves′cent. 1. Bubbling; giving off gas. **2.** Producing effervescence.

ef′ficacy. The ability to produce a desired effect; effectiveness.

efficiency. The ability of accomplishing a desired effect or producing results with a minimum of unnecessary effort; competency.

visual e., a rating used in determining compensation for ocular injuries based on measurable functions of central acuity, field vision, and ocular motility.

effleurage′. A light stroking movement, as used in massage.

effloresce′. 1. To lose water upon exposure to a dry atmosphere, thus becoming a powder. **2.** To become covered with a powdery substance.

efflores′cent. Denoting a substance that gives up water on exposure to air at ordinary temperature.

efflu′vium. 1. An exhalation, especially one that is foul-smelling or noxious. **2.** An outflowing or shedding, especially subtle, as rising vapor or shedding of hair. **3.** Gaseous waste.

effuse′. Spread out widely and thinly on a surface; denoting the surface character of a bacterial culture;

spreading profusely.

effu′sion. 1. The escape of fluid into a body cavity. **2.** The fluid effused.

pleural e., fluid filling the membranous sac covering the lung and lining of the chest.

egg. 1. The female reproductive cell of birds and reptiles, expelled from the maternal body prior to the development of the embryo, or sometimes without fertilization. **2.** Ovum; also called oocyte.

e′gilops. An abscess at the inner canthus of the eye.

e′go. The awareness of the existence of the self as different from others; in psychoanalytic theory, all those functions of the personality which enable it to experience itself and act in self-fulfilling yet socially acceptable fashion; it mediates between the other two parts of the personality structure (id and superego) and reality.

ego-dystonic, denoting those aspects of the personality which are alien or unacceptable to the self.

ego-syntonic, denoting those aspects of the personality which are acceptable to the self.

egocen′tric. Marked by constant or extreme preoccupation with one's self.

egoma′nia. Pathologic preoccupation with one's self.

egoph′ony. A form of bronchophony; the bleating nasal quality of voice heard over an area of compressed lung above a pleural effusion or an area of consolidation; transmission of the spoken voice is altered so that long e ($\bar{e}$) sounds like long a ($\bar{a}$).

Ehlers-Danlos syndrome. Inherited disorder marked by hyperelasticity of the skin, fragility of cutaneous blood vessels, overextension of joints, and the formation of pigmented nodules (raisin tumors) at the site of skin injury.

eidet′ic. 1. Relating to the ability to produce voluntarily photographic, vivid images of objects previously seen or imagined. **2.** A person having this ability.

eikonom′eter. Any instrument used to measure the difference in sizes of the images seen by the two eyes (aniseikonia).

einstei′nium. A synthetic radioactive element; symbol Es, atomic number 99, atomic weight 254; first produced in 1955.

Eisenmenger's syndrome, Eisenmenger's complex. Strictly defined, a ventricular septal defect, overriding aortic right ventricular hypertrophy, and a normal or dilated pulmonary artery; because these terms have been frequently used to describe cases with right to left shunt without all of the above components, they are not regarded as useful terms by cardiologists.

ejac′ulate. To expel abruptly, especially to dis-

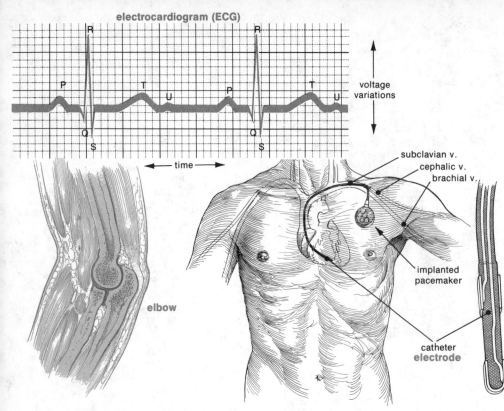

electrocardiogram (ECG)

voltage variations

time

subclavian v.
cephalic v.
brachial v.

implanted pacemaker

elbow

catheter electrode

electroencephalograms (EEG)

frontal-central
L
R

central-occipital
L
R

frontal-temporal
L
R

temporal-occipital
L
R

50 μV
1 second

charge semen in orgasm.

ejacula′tion. Emission of the semen.

  premature e., emission of the semen prior to or immediately upon engaging in sexual intercourse.

ejac′ulatory. Of or relating to ejaculation.

ejec′tor. Anything that removes any material forcefully.

  saliva e., a device containing a perforated suction tube used to remove fluids from the mouth.

EKG. Abbreviation for electrocardiogram; derived from the German Elektrokardiogramm; also written ECG.

EKY. Abbreviation for electrokymogram.

elas′tance. A measure of a structure's ability to return to its initial or original form following deformation; e.g., the measure of the ability of a hollow organ, such as the bladder, to revert toward its original dimensions upon removal of the distending force (urine).

elas′tic. 1. Capable of being stretched, bent, or deformed in any way, and then return to original form. **2.** A rubber band used in orthodontics to apply force to the teeth.

  intermaxillary e., a rubber band placed between orthodontic appliances of upper and lower jaws to cause tooth movement as the jaw opens and closes.

  intramaxillary e., one placed within an orthodontic appliance.

elas′tica. A general term for elastic tissue, such as the elastic layer in the wall of an artery.

elas′ticin. Elastin.

elastic′ity. The quality of being elastic.

  modulus of e., a measure of elasticity or stiffness of a material determined by dividing the stress by the corresponding strain value.

elas′tin. A yellow scleroprotein present in elastic fibers which allows them to stretch about one and one-half times their original length.

elas′tomer. Any of various polymers that can be stretched like rubber, and that will relax to their original dimensions when unstressed.

elastom′eter. A device for measuring the elasticity of bodily tissues.

elasto′sis. Degeneration of the elastic tissues.

  e. dystrophica, angioid streaks of the retina due to degeneration of the basal lamina of the choroid; a manifestation of pseudoxanthoma elasticum.

  e. perforans serpiginosa, circinate group of asymptomatic keratotic papules, marked by thickened epidermis around a central keratin plug overlying an accumulation of elastic tissue.

  senile e., a dermatosis marked by degeneration of elastic tissue in the skin of the elderly or in those afflicted with chronic actinic effect.

el′bow. The joint between the arm and the fore-arm.

  bend of the e., cubital fossa; see under fossa.

  miner's e., inflammation of the bursa over the elbow (olecranon bursitis) caused by pressure.

  point of the e., see olecranon.

  tennis e., lateral epicondylitis; soreness of the lateral aspect of the elbow and muscles of the forearm usually caused by excessive rotatory motions of the forearm as in tennis playing.

  tip of the e., see olecranon.

electroanal′ysis. Quantitative separation of metals by means of an electric current.

electroanesthe′sia. Anesthesia induced by an electric current.

electrobio′logy. The study of electrical phenomena in the living organism.

electrocar′diogram (ECG, EKG). A graphic record of the electric current produced by the contraction of the heart, obtained with an electrocardiograph; the voltage variations, resulting from the depolarization and repolarization of the heart muscle and producing electric fields, are plotted against time on paper tape.

electrocar′diograph. An instrument for recording the electric currents produced by heart muscle in the process of contraction; a galvanometer which records voltage variations; developed by Wilhem Einthoven in 1906.

electrocardiog′raphy. A method of recording the electric current generated by the activity of the heart muscle by means of an electrocardiograph.

  fetal e., electrocardiography of a fetus while in the uterus.

electrocar′dioscope. An oscilloscope for the continuous monitoring of the electrocardiogram (ECG).

electrocauteriza′tion. Cauterization by means of an electrically heated platinum wire.

electrocau′tery. An instrument for cauterizing tissue in which a platinum wire is heated by a current of electricity.

electrochem′istry. The science of chemical reactions produced by electricity; study of the electrical aspects of chemical reactions.

electrocoagula′tion. The hardening of diseased tissues induced by high frequency currents; a form of surgical diathermy.

electrocontractil′ity. The capability of muscle tissue to contract in response to an electric stimulation.

electroconvul′sant. Denoting a type of therapy for emotional disorders in which an electric current is passed through the head of the patient to produce convulsions; See also therapy, electroshock.

electrocor′ticogram (ECoG). A record of electrical activity emanating from the cerebral cortex; obtained by placing electrodes in direct contact with the cortex.

elec′trocute. To cause death by passing a high voltage electric current through the body.

elec′trode. A conductor of electricity through which current enters or leaves a medium such as gas, vacuum, nonmetallic solid, etc.

  central terminal e., in electrocardiography, one in which the wire connections (to the right and left arms and to the left leg) are fastened together at one end and connected to the electrocardiograph to form the indifferent electrode.

  exploring e., in unipolar electrocardiography, one which is placed on the chest near the heart region and paired with an indifferent electrode.

  glass e., one made of a thin-walled glass bulb containing a platinum wire and filled with a standard buffer solution mixed with a little quinhydrone; used in determining hydrogen ion (pH) concentrations.

  hydrogen e., an electrode considered the ultimate standard of reference in all hydrogen ion (pH) determinations; made by partly immersing platinum black in platinum and allowing it to absorb hydrogen to saturation.

  indifferent e., in unipolar electrocardiography, an electrode having multiple terminals.

  negative e., see cathode.

  positive e., see anode.

electrodesicca′tion. Destruction of tissue by dehydration using monopolar electric current through a needle electrode.

electrodial′ysis. Dialysis by the application of an electric field across the semipermeable dialysis membrane, used especially to separate electrolytes.

electroenceph′alogram (EEG). A graphic record of the electric activity of the brain obtained by means of the electroencephalograph.

  depth e., an electroencephalogram obtained by placing electrodes directly on subcortical structures.

  low voltage e., one in which no activity larger than 20 μv can be recorded between any two points on the scalp.

electroenceph′alograph. An instrument used to record the electric currents produced in the brain.

electroencephalog′raphy. The recording of the electric currents generated by the activity of the brain, especially the cerebral cortex, by means of an electroencephalograph.

electrogas′trograph. An instrument for recording the bioelectrical potentials associated with gastrointestinal activity.

elec′trogram. Any electrically produced graph or tracing; e.g., the recording of the electrical activity

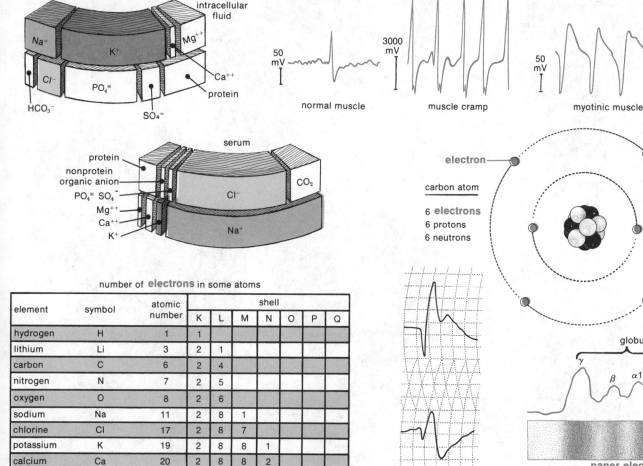

electrolyte composition

intracellular fluid

electromyograms

50 mV — normal muscle

3000 mV — muscle cramp

50 mV — myotinic muscle

300 mV — muscular dystrophy

serum

protein
nonprotein organic anion
$PO_4^=$ $SO_4^=$
Mg^{++}
Ca^{++}
K^+

electron

carbon atom

6 **electrons**
6 protons
6 neutrons

albumin

globulins

γ β $\alpha1$ $\alpha2$

paper electrophoresis

electroretinogram (ERG)

number of **electrons** in some atoms

element	symbol	atomic number	K	L	M	N	O	P	Q
hydrogen	H	1	1						
lithium	Li	3	2	1					
carbon	C	6	2	4					
nitrogen	N	7	2	5					
oxygen	O	8	2	6					
sodium	Na	11	2	8	1				
chlorine	Cl	17	2	8	7				
potassium	K	19	2	8	8	1			
calcium	Ca	20	2	8	8	2			
mercury	Hg	80	2	8	18	32	18	2	
radium	Ra	88	2	8	18	32	18	18	2

of the heart made with the recording electrode placed directly on the surface of the cardiac muscle.

His bundle e., an electrogram usually made by placing a catheter electrode in the right ventricle; it records the A-V junctional electrical activity.

electrog′raphy. The production of graphic records by means of electricity.

atrioventricular bundle e., electrography of the atrioventricular bundle during cardiac catherization.

His bundle e., atrioventricular bundle electrography.

electroky′mogram. A graphic record of the heart's movements obtained by electrokymography.

electrokymog′raphy. 1. The registered recording of the movements of the heart and great vessels by means of the electrokymograph. **2.** The science of interpreting electrokymograms.

electrolar′ynx. A vibrating mechanism that makes it possible for a person to speak intelligibly after his larynx has been surgically removed.

electro′lysis. 1. Chemical decomposition of a compound produced by passing a current of electricity through it. **2.** Decomposition or destruction of specific tissues of the body by means of electricity.

elec′trolyte. Any substance which, when in solution, dissociates into ions, thus becoming capable of conducting an electric current.

electrolyt′ic. 1. Relating to or produced by electrolysis. **2.** Relating to an electrolyte.

elec′trolyze. To cause a chemical decomposition by means of an electric current.

electromy′ogram (EMG). A graphic record obtained by electromyography of the somatic electric currents associated with muscle activity.

electromyog′raphy. The recording of the electric currents generated by muscular activity.

elec′tron. An elementary, subatomic particle of nature; it has a negative charge of one and a mass of 9.1×10^{-28} g.

valence e., an electron in an atom capable of participating in the formation of chemical bonds with other atoms.

electronarco′sis. The passing of an electric current through the brain to produce narcosis or unconsciousness.

electroneg′ative. 1. Possessing a negative electric charge. **2.** Referring to those elements whose unchanged atoms have a tendency to attract electrons and become anions; e.g., oxygen and chlorine.

elec′tron gun. An electrode, as in a cathode-ray tube, that emits a controlled beam of accelerated electrons.

electron′ic 1. Of, relating to, or conducting electrons. **2.** Relating to electronics.

electron′ics. The study of electronic phenomena.

elec′tron-volt (ev). The energy imparted to an electron by a potential of one volt; equal to 1.6×10^{-12} erg.

electronystagmog′raphy (ENG). The electronic recording of eye movements in nystagmus.

elec′tro-oc′ulogram (EOG). A record of eye positions made by an electro-oculograph.

elec′tro-oculog′raphy. The production of records of eye position (electro-oculograms) by recording, during eye movement, the difference in electrical potential between two electrodes placed on the skin at either side of the eye.

electrophore′sis. The movement of charged particles in an electric field toward either the anode or the cathode; used as a means of separating substances in a medium.

paper e., the migration of charged particles along a strip of filter paper, saturated with a few drops of an electrolyte, when a potential gradient is placed across the paper.

thin-layer e. (TLE), the movement of charged particles through a thin layer of an inert material such as cellulose.

electrophysiol′ogy. The study of electrical phenomena related to physiologic processes.

elec′troplate. To plate or coat with a thin layer of metal by electrolysis or electrodeposition; in dentistry, impressions are plated to form metalized working dies.

electropos′itive. 1. Relating to or possessing a positive electric charge. **2.** Denoting an element whose atoms tend to release electrons to form a chemical bond; e.g., sodium, potassium, or calcium.

electroretin′ogram (ERG). The electrical potential of the retina recorded by a galvanometer from the surface of the eyeball and originated by a pulse of light; it depicts the integrity of the neuro-epithelium of the retina.

elec′troscope. An instrument for detecting the presence of electric charges.

elec′troshock. See therapy, electroshock.

electrosteth′ograph. An electrical instrument for recording the respiratory and cardiac sounds of the chest.

electrother′apy, electrotherapeu′tics. The treatment of disease by means of electricity.

electrother′mal. Relating to electricity and heat; especially, the production of heat electrically.

el′ement. 1. A substance made up of atoms having the same number of protons in each nucleus. **2.** An irreducible substance or indivisible constituent of a composite entity.

electronegative e., one having more than four valence electrons and tending to gain electrons in a chemical combination.

electropositive e., one having less than four valence electrons and tending to release electrons in a chemical combination.

radioactive e., any element having an atomic number above 82 and disintegrating spontaneously, with emission of rays.

trace e.'s, elements present in the body in minute amounts.

eleo-. Combining form denoting oil.

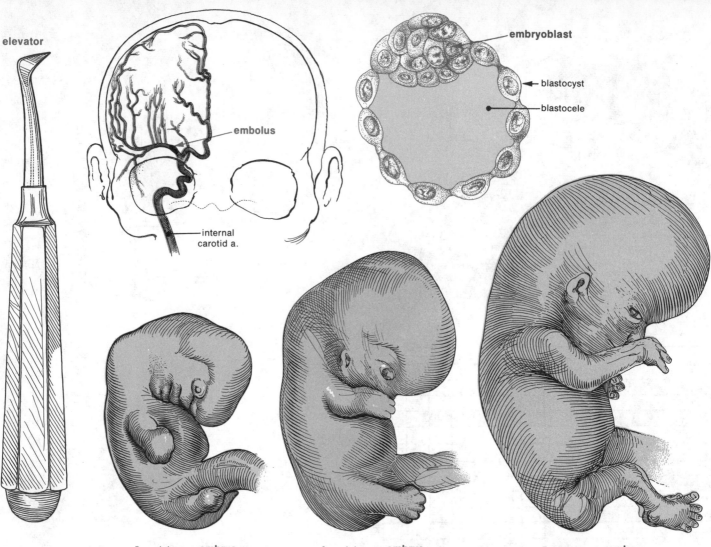

elevator

embolus

internal carotid a.

embryoblast

blastocyst

blastocele

5 week human **embryo**   6 week human **embryo**   7 week human **embryo**

eleothor'ax. See oleothorax.

elephanti'asis. Hypertrophy and inflammation of the skin and subcutaneous tissues, especially of the legs and scrotum, due to obstructed lymphatic circulation, usually caused by a nematode worm (*Wuchereria bancrofti*).

el'evator. 1. An instrument used as a lever to pry up a depressed bone fragment. **2.** An instrument for extracting teeth and roots that cannot be grasped with a forceps.

elim'inant. An agent that promotes the excretion or removal of waste.

elimina'tion. The expulsion of waste material from the body.

elix'ir. A clear, sweetened solution of alcohol and water, used as a vehicle for medicine taken orally.

ellip'soid. Any anatomic structure having an oval shape, especially (a) any one of the oval masses of cells surrounding the second part of the penicillate artery of the spleen, and (b) the outer portion of the inner rod segment of the retina.

elliptocyto'sis. Inherited disorder in which a large number of red blood cells (25 to 90 per cent) have an oval or elliptical shape; also called ovalocytosis.

Ellis type 1 nephritis. Ellis type 1 glomerulonephritis; see under glomerulonephritis.

Ellis type 2 nephritis. Ellis type 2 glomerulonephritis; see under glomerulonephritis.

Ellis-van Creveld syndrome. Chondroectodermal dysplasia; see under dysplasia.

elonga'tion. 1. The act of increasing in length, or the condition of being lengthened. **2.** A measure of the ability of a metal to increase in length before breaking; indicates the ductility of a metal.

el'uate. The material separated by elution.

elu'ent. The liquid used in elution.

elu'tion. Separation of substances by washing.

elutria'tion. The process of purifying, separating, or removing by washing, decanting, and settling.

elytro-. Combining form meaning vagina.

elytroclei'sis. Obliteration of the vaginal barrel, as with adhesions.

EM. Abbreviation for (a) electron microscope; (b) electron micrograph.

emacia'tion. Excessive wasting of the body; extreme leanness.

emacula'tion. The removal of blemishes from the skin.

email'loblast. See ameloblast.

emana'tion. 1. The act of giving off; exhalation. **2.** The gaseous product of disintegration of a radioactive substance.

emancipa'tion. In embryology, the gradual separation or segregation of different areas of the embryo into fields of specialized developmental potentialities.

emascula'tion. Castration.

embalm'. To treat a dead body with preservatives to prevent its decay.

embed'. To surround a tissue specimen with a firm substance, such as wax, to facilitate the cutting of thin slices.

embolec'tomy. Surgical removal of an embolus.

em'boli. Plural of embolus.

embol'ic. Of or relating to an embolus or to embolism.

embol'iform. Resembling an embolus or a wedge.

em'bolism. The sudden obstruction of a blood vessel by a clot or any foreign material (embolus) formed or introduced elsewhere in the circulatory system and carried to that point by the bloodstream.

  air e., the presence of air bubbles in the heart or blood vessels; also called pneumathemia and gas embolism.

  crossed e., see paradoxical embolism.

  fat e., the presence of fat globules in the blood; also called oil embolism.

  gas e., see air embolism.

  oil e., see fat embolism.

  paradoxical e., the presence in an artery of an embolus that originated in a vein, having passed to the arterial circulation through a septal defect in the heart; also called crossed embolism.

  pulmonary e., (PE), the plugging of pulmonary arteries with fragments of a thrombus, most frequently from the leg after an operation.

  septic pulmonary e. the lodging in a pulmonary artery of an infected thrombus that has become detached from its site of origin.

emboliza'tion. The introduction of certain substances into the circulation for the therapeutic occlusion of vessels.

embolola'lia. The involuntary insertion of meaningless words in a sentence.

em'bolus. A plug within a vessel (a blood clot or other substance such as air, fat, or a tumor) which is carried in the blood stream from another site until it lodges and becomes an obstruction to circulation.

  riding or straddling e., one located at the bifurcation of an artery and blocking both branches.

embra'sure. The space produced by the diverging surfaces of adjacent teeth; it may be labial, buccal, lingual, incisal, occlusal, or gingival.

embroca'tion. 1. The rubbing of the body with liquid medication. **2.** The liquid used.

em'bryo. An organism in the earliest stage of development; in man, from the time of conception to the end of the second month in the uterus.

em'bryoblast. An aggregation of cells which stick together and collect at the embryonic pole of the blastocyst and which give rise to the tissues of the embryo; also called inner cell mass.

embryogen'esis. The development of the embryo from the fertilized egg.

embryogen'ic, embryogenet'ic. Producing an embryo; relating to the origin of an embryo.

embryog'eny. The origin of the embryo.

embryol'ogist. A scientist who specializes in embryology.

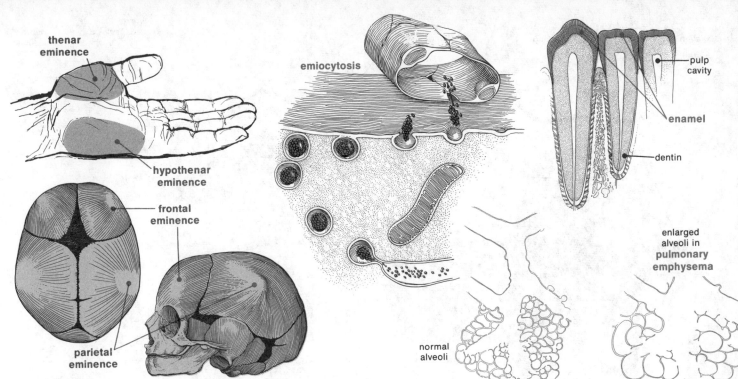

thenar eminence

hypothenar eminence

frontal eminence

parietal eminence

skull of newborn

emiocytosis

normal alveoli

pulp cavity

enamel

dentin

enlarged alveoli in pulmonary emphysema

embryol'ogy. The science concerned with the formation and development of living organisms from the fertilization of the ovum until birth; the study of the development of the embryo; also called developmental anatomy.

embryomor'phous. Relating to or similar to the structure of the embryo.

embryon'ic. 1. Of or relating to an embryo. **2.** Undeveloped; rudimentary.

embryoniza'tion. Reversion of any tissue to a primitive or embryonic stage.

embryop'athy. A morbid condition in the embryo or fetus resulting from interference with normal development.

em'bryophore. A membrane around the embryo of a tapeworm forming the inner layer of the egg shell.

embryot'omy. Any mutilating operation on the fetus to facilitate its removal when delivery is not possible.

embryotox'on. A congenital opacity in the deep layers of the peripheral part of the cornea.

em'bryotroph. 1. The nutriment supplied to the embryo. **2.** The fluid adjacent to the blastodermic vesicle of deciduate placental mammals during implantation.

emer'gency. A serious situation, developing suddenly and unexpectedly, and requiring immediate medical attention.

emer'gent. 1. Developing suddenly and unexpectedly, and requiring prompt action. **2.** Coming out; leaving a bodily cavity or other part.

em'ery. A fine-grained abrasive composed of an extremely hard mineral; aluminum oxide combined with iron, magnesia, or silica.

em'esis. Vomiting.

emet'ic. Causing vomiting.

emetine'. A bitter-tasting alkaloid, $C_{29}H_{40}N_2O_4$; used parenterally as an amebicide.

emetocathar'tic. 1. Both emetic and cathartic. **2.** Any agent that induces vomiting and purging.

EMF. Abbreviation for electromotive force.

EMG. Abbreviation for electromyogram.

-emia, -hemia. Combining forms indicating blood.

emigra'tion. The passage of white blood cells through the wall of a small blood vessel.

em'inence. A circumscribed, elevated area or prominence, especially of a bone.

frontal e., the rounded elevation on the skull on either side just above the eye.

hypothenar e., the prominence on the ulnar side (medial part) of the palm produced by the short muscles of the little finger; one of three muscle divisions of the hand.

parietal e., the prominence on either side of the skull just above the superior temporal line.

thenar e., the elevation on the radial side (lateral part) of the palm of the hand produced by the short muscles of the thumb; one of three muscle divisions of the hand.

emiocyto'sis. Ejection of material from a cell; e.g., ejection of insulin from the β-cells of the pancreas: the membranous sac containing insulin granules migrates to the periphery of the cell; when it comes into contact with the cell's plasma membrane, they fuse; rupture occurs at the site of fusion and insulin passes out of the cell and into the blood stream via the extracellular space; also called exocytosis.

emis'sion. A discharge.

nocturnal e., discharge of semen during sleep.

emmen'agogue. 1. Increasing or producing menstrual flow. **2.** Any agent producing such an effect.

emme'nia. Menses.

emmetro'pia. The normal condition of the refractive system of the eye in which the light rays entering the eyeball focus exactly on the retina.

emol'lient. 1. Soothing. **2.** An agent that softens and soothes the skin or mucous membranes.

emo'tion. Any strong feeling (joy, anger, fear).

emo'tional. 1. Relating to an emotion. **2.** Easily affected with emotions.

empath'ic. Relating to or marked by empathy.

em'pathy. The intimate understanding of, and identification with, the feelings of another person.

emphyse'ma. A swelling due to the abnormal presence of air in tissues or cavities of the body; the term usually refers to a condition of the lungs.

centrilobular e. (CLE), emphysema in which the alveoli occupying the central area of each acinus become dilated and destroyed; generally more prominent in the upper lobes, but extending to all lung areas; commonly seen in chronic bronchitis.

compensating e., dilatation of a portion of a lung when another portion is unable to function properly.

mediastinal e., the presence of air in the mediastinal tissue.

panlobular e., emphysema marked by enlarged lungs with loss of vascular lung markings in areas of radiologic hyperlucency in the lower lobes; seen in individuals with homozygous α-1-antitrypsin deficiency.

paraseptal e., emphysema with blebs and bullae that are largely localized subpleurally.

pulmonary e., lung disease characterized by enlargement of the alveoli (air spaces distal to the terminal bronchioles) with loss of elastic fibers and rupture of their walls.

subcutaneous e., the presence of air or gas in the subcutaneous tissues.

empir'ical, empir'ic. Based upon practical experience.

empir'icism. The view that experience serves as a guide to medical practice or to the therapeutic use of any remedy; reliance on experience as the only source of knowledge.

empye'ma. Pus in a body cavity, especially the pleural cavity.

em'pyocele. Accumulation of pus in the scrotum; also called suppurating hydrocele.

emu. Abbreviation for electromagnetic unit.

emul'sify. To convert into an emulsion.

emul'sion. A preparation composed of two liquids which do not mix, one being dispersed in the other in the form of small globules.

emul'sive. A substance that can be emulsified or by which a fat or resin can be emulsified.

emul'soid. A dispersion in which the dispersed particles are relatively liquid and absorb some of the liquid in which they are dispersed; also called emulsion colloid.

en-. Prefix meaning in, into, or within; used as em- before b, p, or m.

enam'el. The hard, vitreous substance that covers the anatomic crown of a tooth.

mottled e., defective structure of enamel due to excessive ingestion of fluoride during tooth formation; the affected teeth may have white, yellow, or brown spots which sometimes are pitted.

enamelo'ma. Enamel pearl; spherical nodule of enamel attached to a tooth, usually on the root.

enan'them, enanthe'ma. Eruption on a mucous membrane, especially one accompanying an eruptive fever.

enan'tiomer. One of a pair of molecules that are mirror images of each other; although they have the same chemical properties, certain of the physical and essentially all the physiologic properties are different.

enantiom'erism. In chemistry, isomerism in which the molecules in the configuration are related to one another like an object and its mirror image, thus not superimposable.

enan'tiomorph. A crystal that is similar in form but with the mirror image of another.

enantiop'athy. 1. Treating with antidotes or substances that produce effects opposite to those of the morbid state being treated. **2.** The mutual antagonism of two morbid states.

enarthro'dial. Relating to a ball and socket joint (enarthrosis).

enarthro'sis. Ball and socket joint; one that per-

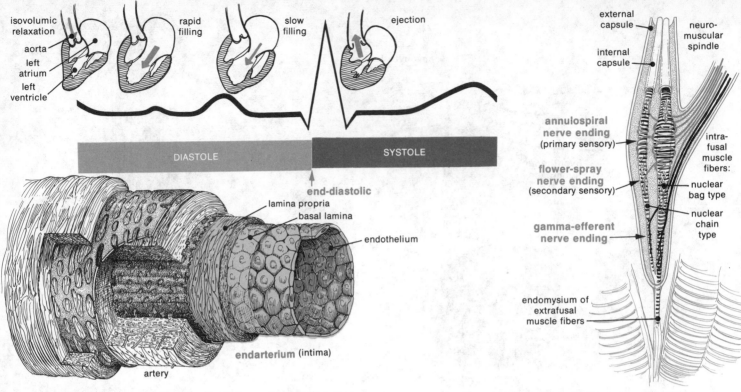

isovolumic relaxation
aorta
left atrium
left ventricle
rapid filling
slow filling
ejection

DIASTOLE | SYSTOLE

end-diastolic

lamina propria
basal lamina
endothelium

endarterium (intima)

artery

external capsule
internal capsule
neuro-muscular spindle

annulospiral nerve ending (primary sensory)
flower-spray nerve ending (secondary sensory)
gamma-efferent nerve ending

intra-fusal muscle fibers:
nuclear bag type
nuclear chain type

endomysium of extrafusal muscle fibers

---

mits extensive movement in almost any direction, as seen in the hip and shoulder.

encan'this. 1. A small tumor at the inner canthus of the eye. **2.** Inflammation of the lacrimal caruncle (the pink fleshy mound at the medial canthus).

encap'sulated. Encased in a capsule.

enceinte'. French for pregnant; from Late Latin *incincta*, without a girdle.

encephale'mia. Congestion of the brain.

encephal'ic. 1. Of or relating to the brain. **2.** In the skull.

encephalit'ic. Relating to or afflicted with inflammation of the brain.

encephali'tis. Inflammation of the brain, classified when possible by reference to the etiologic agent or pathogenic mechanism (e.g., Japanese B encephalitis caused by a group B arbovirus); headache, nausea, vomiting, fever, and lethargy are common initial symptoms.

e. periaxialis diffusa, a rapidly progressive disease occurring chiefly in children; marked by widespread demyelinization of the cerebral cortex, with convulsions, mental symptoms, motor and sensory disturbances, and gradual loss of sight; death usually occurs within three years after onset; also called Schilder's disease.

enceph'alo-, encephal-. Combining forms meaning brain.

enceph'alocele. 1. The cranial cavity. **2.** The ventricles of the brain. **3.** Protrusion of brain tissue through a congenital defect of the skull; also called craniocele.

enceph'alogram. An x-ray picture of the head.

echo e., the recording of the return of sound waves directed at the head in order to locate the various densities in the head.

encephalog'raphy. Roentgenography of the brain. Cf echoencephalography.

enceph'alolith. A cerebral calculus; a calculus in the brain.

enceph'alomalacia. Softening of the brain.

encephalomeningi'tis. See meningoencephalitis.

encephalomyeli'tis. Acute inflammation of the brain and spinal cord; also called myeloencephalitis.

benign myalgic e., epidemic neuromyosthemia; see under neuromyosthemia.

encephalomyel'ocele. Congenital bone defect of the occipital area with herniation of the meninges, medulla, and spinal cord.

encephalomyelop'athy. Any disease of the brain and spinal cord.

encephalomyeloradiculop'athy. Disease involving the brain, spinal cord, and roots of spinal nerves.

enceph'alon. See brain.

encephalop'athy. Any disease of the brain; also called cerebropathy.

encephalopsycho'sis. Any psychosis caused by physical damage to the brain.

enchondro'ma. A benign tumor composed of cartilaginous tissue and occurring within the interior of a bone.

enchondrosarco'ma. A malignant bone tumor arising from a preexistent benign cartilaginous tumor within the bone (enchondroma).

en'clave. A mass of tissue totally enclosed within another.

encli'tic. Denoting the relation of the planes of the fetal head to those of the pelvis of the mother.

encopre'sis. Unintentional passage of feces.

encye'sis. A normal pregnancy in the uterus.

encys'ted. Enclosed in a cyst or a membranous sac.

Endamoe'ba. A genus of amebae not parasitic in man; the term is sometimes used incorrectly for *Entamoeba*.

endarterec'tomy. Surgical removal of atheromas with the lining of an artery.

endarte'rial. Within an artery; relating to the intima or inner layer of the arterial wall.

endarteri'tis. Inflammation of the inner layer of an artery; also called endoarteritis.

endarte'rium. The intima or inner layer of the arterial wall.

endaur'al. 1. Within the ear. **2.** Through the ear canal.

endaxoneu'ron. A neuron of the cerebrospinal axis (axoneuron) that sends no process outside the spinal cord.

end-bulb, end-bud. One of the minute spherical bodies located at the termination of a sensory nerve fiber; present in certain parts of the skin, mucous membranes, muscles, joints, and connective tissue of internal organs.

Krause's e-b., Krause's corpuscle; see under corpuscle.

end-diastolic. 1. Occurring at the termination of diastole, just before the next systole, as in end-diastolic pressure. **2.** Interrupting the final stage of diastole, barely premature, as in end-diastolic extrasystole.

endem'ic. Relating to any disease prevalent continually in a particular locality.

endergon'ic. Indicating a chemical reaction that is accompanied by an absorption of free energy, regardless of the form of energy involved.

ender'mic, endermat'ic. Through the skin, as the action of certain medicines when absorbed through the skin.

end-feet. Terminal buttons; see under button.

end'ing. A termination, as of a nerve.

annulospiral nerve e., a coiled nerve ending around the nuclear region of a muscle fiber; sensitive to stretch.

flower-spray nerve e.'s, intricate series of nerve branches on the contractile part of the intrafusal muscle fibers; sensitive to increased tension.

free nerve e.'s, network of nerve endings found throughout the body, in skin, mucous membranes, and deep tissues; their fibers are both myelinated and non-myelinated.

gamma-efferent nerve e.'s, the terminal part of motor fibers that innervate the intrafusal muscle fibers near their ends.

nerve e., any one of the specialized terminations of sensory or motor nerve fibers.

Ruffini's nerve e.'s, sensory nerve endings that serve as joint receptors, mechanoreceptors, receptors for position sense, and skin receptors; characterized by whorls of fine fibers that end as numerous knobs; also called Ruffini's corpuscles.

endo-, end-. Prefixes denoting inside or within.

endoarteri'tis. See endarteritis.

endoausculta'tion. Auscultation of the heart or stomach by passing a stethoscopic tube or electronic amplifier into the esophagus or heart.

endobron'chial. Intrabronchial; within the bronchial tubes.

endocar'dial. 1. Relating to the endocardium. **2.** In the heart.

endocardiog'raphy. Recording of the electric currents traversing the heart muscle, prior to a heartbeat, with the exploring electrode within the heart chambers.

endocardi'tis. A disease caused by infection of the lining membrane of the cardiac chambers, or of the intima of a great vessel.

abacterial thrombotic e., see nonbacterial thrombotic endocarditis.

atypical verrucous e., see Libman-Sacks syndrome.

bacterial e., endocarditis due to bacteria or other microorganisms, causing deformity of the valve leaflets; it may be acute, usually caused by pyogenic organisms such as staphylococci, or subacute (chronic), usually due to *Streptococcus viridans* or *Streptococcus faecalis*.

marantic e., a nonbacterial type with deposition of clots.

nonbacterial thrombotic e., abacterial thrombotic endocarditis; terminal endocarditis; endocarditis associated with verrucous lesions and clots, occurring in the last stages of many chronic infections and wasting diseases.

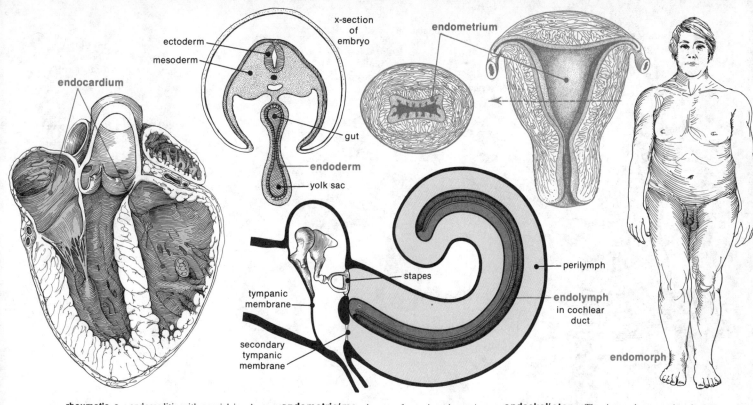

Labels in figure: ectoderm, mesoderm, x-section of embryo, endometrium, gut, endoderm, yolk sac, endocardium, stapes, perilymph, endolymph in cochlear duct, tympanic membrane, secondary tympanic membrane, endomorph

rheumatic e., endocarditis with special involvement of the valves associated with rheumatic fever.
terminal e., see nonbacterial thrombotic endocarditis.
vegetative e., verrucous e., a type associated with the formation of fibrinous clots on the ulcerated valves.
endocar'dium. The serous membrane that lines the chambers of the heart.
endoce'liac. In any of the cavities of the body; also called intracelial.
endocer'vical. Within the uterine cervix; also called intracervical.
endocervici'tis. Inflammation of the mucous membrane of the uterine cervix.
endochon'dral. Within cartilage; also called intracartilaginous.
endocra'nial. 1. Within the skull. **2.** Relating to the skull.
en'docrine. Secreting internally; denoting a gland whose secretions are discharged into the blood or lymph.
endocrinol'ogy. The branch of science dealing with endocrine glands and their secretions.
endocrinop'athy. Any disease of the endocrine glands.
endocrinother'apy. Treatment of disease with extracts of endocrine glands.
endoc'rinous. Of or relating to any internal secretion.
en'doderm. The innermost of the three germ layers of the embryo; it gives rise to the lining of the gastrointestinal tract from pharynx to rectum and to neighboring glands such as the liver, pancreas, thyroid, etc; also called entoderm.
endodon'tics. The branch of dentistry concerned with the diagnosis and treatment of diseases of the tooth pulp and/or infection of the root canal and periapical areas.
endodon'tist. A specialist in endodontics.
endoen'zyme. An enzyme that is retained by and acts within the cell that produced it.
endog'enous. Originating within the body.
endointoxica'tion. Poisoning by a toxin produced within the organism.
endolaryn'geal. Within the larynx.
Endoli'max. A genus of nonpathogenic amebae.
E. nana, a species parasitic in the large intestine of man, other primates, and pigs.
en'dolymph. The fluid contained in the membranous labyrinth of the internal ear; an isotonic solution which is of high potassium and low sodium concentration.
endome'trial. Relating to or containing endometrium.

endometrio'ma. A mass of ectopic endometrium in endometriosis.
endometrio'sis. An abnormal condition in which the uterine mucous membrane invades other tissues in the pelvic cavity; the uterus and ovaries are the most common sites; other areas include the intestines, umbilicus, bladder, and ureters.
endometri'tis. Inflammation of the membrane lining the interior of the uterus.
endome'trium. The mucosal layer lining the cavity of the uterus; its structure changes with age and with the mentrual cycle.
endomito'sis. See endopolyploidy.
en'domorph. A person having a body build characterized by prominence of the abdomen and other parts developed from the embryonic endodermal layer; also called brachytype.
endomys'ium. The microscopic sheath of delicate connective tissue that surrounds and separates individual muscle fibers.
endoneu'rium. The delicate connective tissue sheath surrounding and separating individual nerve fibers; also called Henle's sheath and connective tissue sheath of Retzius.
endonu'clease. A nuclease (phosphodiesterase) that cleaves polynucleotides into poly- or oligonucleotide fragments of varying size.
endopar'asite. A parasite that lives within the body of its host.
endopep'tidase. A proteolytic enzyme that is capable of hydrolyzing a peptide linkage at points within the chain, not near the ends; e.g., pepsin, trypsin, and ribonuclease.
endophlebi'tis. Inflammation of the inner layer of a vein.
endophthalmi'tis. Inflammation of the internal structures of the eye.
en'doplasm. The internal cytoplasm; it is less viscous than the ectoplasm.
endopol'yploidy. The reproduction of nuclear elements without accompanying spindle formation or cytoplasmic division, resulting in a polyploid nucleus; also called endomitosis.
end-organ. See organ, end.
endor'phin. One of a group of low-molecular weight peptides normally found in the brain, capable of producing effects similar to those of opiates.
endosal'pinx. The mucous membrane that lines the interior of a uterine tube.
en'doscope. An instrument used to examine the interior of a hollow organ or a cavity; e.g., gastroscope, proctoscope, and cystoscope.
endos'copy. Inspection of the interior of a canal or any air or food passage by means of an endoscope.

endoskel'eton. The internal supporting bony skeleton of vertebrates.
endosmo'sis. The passage of a fluid through a membrane into a cavity or a cell containing fluid of a lesser density; osmosis in a direction toward the interior of a cell or a cavity.
en'dospore. 1. A small, resistant, asexual spore, as that formed within the vegetative cells of some bacteria, particularly those belonging to the genera *Bacillus* and *Clostridium*. **2.** The innermost layer of the wall of a spore.
endostei'tis, endosti'tis. Inflammation of the tissue lining the medullary cavity of a bone (endosteum).
endosteo'ma. A benign tumor in the medullary cavity of a bone.
endos'teum. The membrane lining bone cavities.
endosti'tis. See endosteitis.
endothelio'ma. Any tumor, benign or malignant, derived from the endothelial tissue of blood vessels, lymphatic vessels, or serous membranes.
endothe'lium. A thin layer of cells lining serous cavities, blood vessels, and lymph vessels.
endother'mic. Denoting a chemical reaction that produces heat absorption.
endother'my. Diathermy.
en'dothrix. Within the hair shaft; denoting a type of fungal infection in which the hyphae grow only within the hair shaft, where they form long, parallel rows of arthrospores. Cf ectothrix.
endotox'in. A toxin produced and retained by bacterial cells and released only by destruction or death of the cells; also called intracellular toxin.
endotra'cheal. Within the trachea.
end'-plate. The terminal part of a motor nerve fiber that transmits nerve impulses to muscle.
end-prod'uct. A chemical product that represents the final sequence of metabolic reactions.
-ene. A suffix applied to a chemical name denoting the presence of a carbon-carbon double bond; e.g., propene.
enedi'ol. Compound characterized by two carbon atoms joined by a double bond (the ene group) with a hydroxyl group attached to each of the double bonded carbons.
en'ema. 1. The infusion of a fluid into the rectum for cleansing or other therapeutic purposes. **2.** The liquid so infused.
energet'ics. The physics of energy and its changes.
en'ergy. The exertion of power to effect physical change; dynamic force; the capacity to do work, taking the forms of kinetic energy, potential energy, rest energy, electrical energy, etc.
binding e., the energy released in binding a group

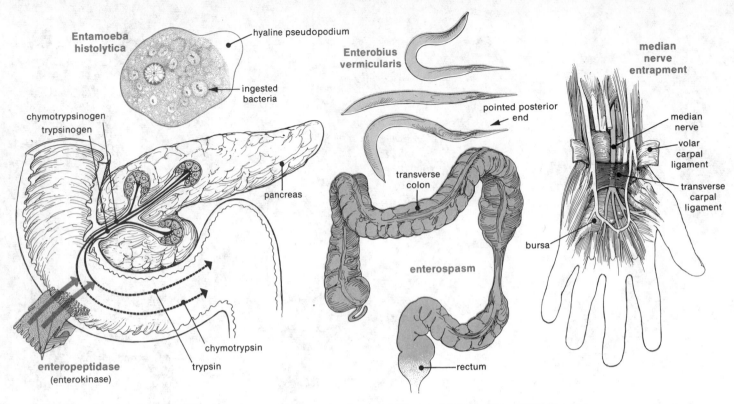

Entamoeba histolytica
hyaline pseudopodium
ingested bacteria

chymotrypsinogen
trypsinogen
pancreas

Enterobius vermicularis
pointed posterior end

transverse colon

enterospasm

rectum

enteropeptidase
(enterokinase)
chymotrypsin
trypsin

median nerve entrapment
median nerve
volar carpal ligament
transverse carpal ligament
bursa

of protons and neutrons into an atomic nucleus.

bond e., the amount of energy necessary to break a bond.

chemical e., energy emanating from a chemical reaction or absorbed in the formation of a chemical compound.

conservation of e., the principle that the total amount of energy remains constant, none being lost or created in the conversion of one type of force into another.

e. of activation, the amount of energy needed by molecules in order to initiate a reaction.

free e., a thermodynamic function, symbolized as ΔG, that expresses the maximum amount of work that can be obtained from a chemical reaction; also called Gibbs free-energy function.

nuclear e., the energy given off by a nuclear reaction, especially by fission, fusion, or radioactive deterioration; the energy stored in the formation of an atomic nucleus.

potential e., the energy existing in a particle or system of particles by virtue of its position or state of existence, which is not being exerted at the time.

psychic e., in psychoanalysis, a hypothetical mental force considered as analogous to the physical concept of energy.

en'ervate. To weaken; to debilitate; to deprive of strength.

enerva'tion. Lack of energy and vigor; lassitude; weakness.

E.N.G. Abbreviation for electronystagmography.

engorged'. Congested or filled to excess; distended with blood or other fluid.

e'nol. An organic compound containing a hydroxyl group (alcohol) attached to a doubly bonded (ethylenic) carbon atom; the name is derived as an abbreviation of ethyl*ene* alco*hol*.

enophthal'mos. Backward displacement of the eyeball causing it to recede within the orbit.

enosto'sis. A bony growth within a bone.

en'siform. Swordlike; said of certain bones, as the xiphoid process.

E.N.T. Abbreviation for ear, nose, and throat.

Entamoe'ba. A genus of protozoan parasites.

E. coli, a nonpathogenic form found in the intestines; also called amoeba coli.

E. gingivalis, a species occurring in the mouth.

E. histolytica, a species that inhabits the intestines of man and causes amebic dysentery; it may also invade the liver.

en'teral. Within the intestine.

enterec'tomy. Surgical removal of a segment of the intestine.

enter'ic. Relating to the intestines.

enteri'tis. Inflammation of the intestines.

regional e., a chronic recurrent disease, mainly of young adults, caused by inflammation of segments of the small intestine; characterized by abdominal pain, diarrhea, and frequently by fever and weight loss; similar lesions are occasionally found in the large bowel, where the process is referred to as granulomatous colitis; etiology is unknown; also called regional or terminal ileitis and Crohn's disease.

entero-, enter-. Combining forms denoting a relationship to the intestinal tract; e.g., enterostomy.

enterobi'asis. Infestation of the intestines with *Enterobius vermicularis,* a short roundworm commonly called pinworm; also called pinworm infestation.

Entero'bius. A genus of nematode worms, formerly called *Oxyuris.*

E. vermicularis, the pinworm, a species that infests the intestines.

en'terocele. 1. Any hernia of the intestine. **2.** Herniation through the rectouterine pouch (cul-de-sac of Douglas); also called posterior vaginal, rectovaginal, cul-de-sac, or Douglas' pouch hernia.

enteroclei'sis. Occlusion of the intestinal tract.

omentum e., the operative use of omentum to close an opening in the intestine.

enteroc'lysis. Enema directed into the colon; also called high enema.

enterococ'cus. Any streptococcus which inhabits the intestinal tract.

enterocoli'tis. Inflammation of the mucous membrane of the small intestine and colon.

enterocolos'tomy. Operative creation of an opening between the small intestine and any part of the colon.

en'terocyst. A cyst of the intestinal wall.

enteroenteros'tomy. Operative connection of any two noncontinuous segments of intestine; also called enteroanastomosis and intestinal anastomosis.

enterogas'trone. One of the gastrointestinal hormones released during digestion; it is secreted by the upper intestinal mucosa, when a significant amount of gastric contents reaches the upper intestine, and inhibits secretion and movements of the stomach.

enteroki'nase. See enteropeptidase.

enterokinet'ic. Stimulating contraction of the gastrointestinal tract.

en'terolith. Any concretion or calculus in the intestine.

enterol'ogy. The branch of medicine concerned with the intestinal tract.

en'teron. The intestinal tract, especially the small intestine.

enteroni'tis. Enteritis.

enteropar'esis. Weakness and relaxation of the intestinal walls.

enterop'athy. Any disease of the intestines.

gluten-induced e., see celiac disease.

enteropep'tidase. An enzyme secreted by the duodenal mucosa that converts trypsinogen (pancreatic secretion) to trypsin (protein-splitting enzyme); also called enterokinase.

enteropex'y. Fixation of a portion of the intestine to the abdominal wall.

enteropto'sia, enteropto'sis. Downward displacement of the intestines in the abdominal cavity, as observed sometimes in obese individuals.

en'terospasm. Intestinal spasm or colic.

enterosteno'sis. Narrowing or stricture of the intestinal lumen.

enteros'tomy. The establishment of an opening into the intestine, temporary or permanent, through the abdominal wall.

enterot'omy. Incision into the intestine.

enterotox'in. A cytotoxin specific for the cells of the mucous membrane of the intestine.

enterovi'rus. Any of a group of viruses that enter the body through, and multiply chiefly in, the gastrointestinal tract.

enterozo'on. An intestinal parasite.

enthesi'tis. Irritation of the attachments of muscle or tendons to bone, as in tennis elbow, shin splints, and glass arm of baseball pitchers.

en'toderm. See endoderm.

entomo-. Combining form relating to the insect; e.g., entomology.

entomol'ogy. The study of insects.

entomopho'bia. Abnormal fear of insects.

entop'ic. Occurring or located in the normal site; opposed to ectopic.

entop'tic. Located within the eyeball.

entozo'on, pl. entozo'a. A parasitic animal living in any of the internal organs of its host.

entrap'ment. The act or process of catching in, as if in a trap.

abdominal cutaneous nerve e. syndrome, the entrapment of cutaneous nerves when they pass through the abdominal muscles en route to the skin, resulting in neuromuscular compression and pain.

lateral femoral cutaneous e., compression of the lateral femoral cutaneous nerve in the fascia lata, resulting in a sensory neuropathy (meralgia paresthetica) characterized by pain and numbness over the lateral aspect of the thigh.

median nerve e., compression of the median nerve at the wrist beneath the transverse carpal ligament, causing pain and numbness in the palmar surface of the hand and the first three fingers (carpal

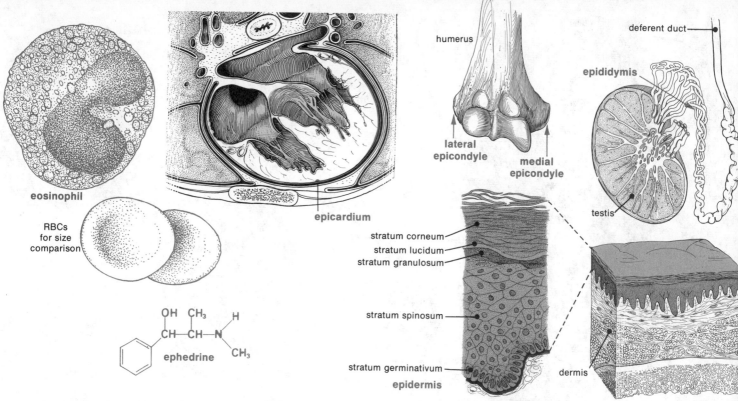

eosinophil

RBCs for size comparison

ephedrine

epicardium

humerus

lateral epicondyle

medial epicondyle

deferent duct

epididymis

testis

stratum corneum
stratum lucidum
stratum granulosum

stratum spinosum

stratum germinativum

epidermis

dermis

tunnel syndrome).

entro'pion. Inversion or inward displacement of the margin of an eyelid.

en'tropy. 1. That fraction of energy not available during a chemical reaction for the performance of work, because it has gone to increasing the random motion of the atoms or molecules in a system. **2.** A measure of the ability of a system to undergo spontaneous change.

enu'cleate. 1. To remove whole, as in shelling out a nut. **2.** To destroy or remove the nucleus.

enuclea'tion. The surgical removal of a tumor or of an organ, such as the eyeball, in its entirety, without rupture.

enure'sis. Involuntary discharge of urine.
    nocturnal e., see bed-wetting.

envi'ronment. The collection of physical or external conditions affecting the growth and development of organisms.

enzoot'ic. Indicating a disease of animals which is indigenous to a specific locality, analogous to an endemic disease among men.

enzymat'ic. Relating to an enzyme.

en'zyme. A protein secreted by the body which acts as a catalyst by promoting or accelerating a chemical change in other substances while remaining unchanged in the process.
    activating e., an enzyme that activates an amino acid by attaching it to the corresponding transfer ribonucleic acid.
    adaptive e., one that is detected in a culture of microorganisms only after the addition of a particular substance (inducer) to the culture medium and that can act on the inducer.
    digestive e., one that promotes the hydrolysis of protein, carbohydrate, and fat in the digestive tract prior to absorption.
    induced e., one produced by the addition of its specific substrate to cells that normally do not metabolize that substrate.
    proteolytic e., protease; an enzyme that acts upon the peptide bonds of proteins and peptides; a protein-splitting or hydrolyzing enzyme.
    reducing e., see reductase.
    transferring e., transferase; enzyme that catalyzes the tranfer of a chemical grouping from one substance to another.
    yellow e., riboflavin 5'-phosphate (flavin mononucleotide).

enzym'ic. Enzymatic.

enzymol'ogy. The branch of science concerned with the study of enzymes, their structure and function.

enzymol'ysis. The chemical decomposition brought about by an enzyme.

EOG. Abbreviation for electro-oculography.

e'osin. A crystalline product of coal tar, used in solution to stain cells for microscopic study.

eosin'oblast. A young granular white blood cell (myeloblast) that develops into an eosinophil.

eosinope'nia. Deficiency of eosinophilic leukocytes in the blood.

eosin'ophil. A cell, especially a white blood cell (eosinophilic leukocyte), that stains easily with eosin dye.

eosinophil'ia. The presence of an abnormally large number of eosinophils in the blood.

eosinophil'ic. Easily stained with eosin dyes; also called oxyphilic.

eosinophilic endomyocardial disease. See Löffler's disease.

epen'dyma. The lining membrane of the cerebral ventricles and the central canal of the spinal cord.

ependymo'ma. A brain tumor derived from cells of the membrane lining the ventricles (ependyma); occurring most frequently in children and young adults and constituting approximately one to three per cent of all intracranial tumors.

ephed'rine. A sympathomimetic amine obtained from species of *Ephedra* or produced synthetically; it dilates the bronchi and is used in the prevention and treatment of bronchial asthma; it acts, in part, by releasing catecholamines from their storage vesicles.

ephe'lis, *pl.* **ephe'lides.** A freckle.

epi-. Prefix meaning upon.

epican'thus. A skin fold extending from the root of the nose to the inner termination of the eyebrow, covering the inner angle (canthus) of the eye; normal in individuals of the Mongolian race; in children under the age of 10 with Down's syndrome, a fold is common, but confined to the inner angle; also called epicanthal fold and plica palpebronasalis.

epicar'dia. The portion of the esophagus from the diaphragm to the stomach.

epicar'dium. The visceral or inner layer of the pericardium that is in contact with the heart.

epicon'dyle. The bony prominence situated above or upon a smooth articular eminence of a long bone.
    lateral e., (1) of the femur, a prominence situated above the lateral condyle; it gives attachment to the fibular collateral ligament of the knee-joint; (2) of the humerus, a small tuberculated eminence situated at the lower end of the bone; it gives attachment to the radial collateral ligament of the elbow-joint, and to a tendon common to the origin of the supinator and some of the extensor muscles.
    medial e., (1) of the femur, a large convex eminence located above the medial condyle to which the tibial collateral ligament of the knee-joint is attached; (2) of the humerus, a large projection situated above and medial to the condyle; it gives attachment to the ulnar collateral ligament of the elbow-joint, to the pronator teres, and to a common tendon of origin of most of the forearm's flexor muscles.

epicondyli'tis, lateral. Pain and tenderness of the tendons near the lateral epicondyle of the humerus; a syndrome affecting the midportion of the upper extremity, usually due to repetitive rotatory motions of the forearm (believed to cause microscopic tears and subsequent chronic tendinitis); also called tennis elbow.

epicra'nium. The scalp; the structures (muscle, aponeurosis, and skin) covering the skull.

epicri'sis. A crisis occurring after the first crisis of a disease; a secondary crisis.

epicrit'ic. Denoting sensory nerve fibers in the skin and oral mucosa that perceive slight variations of touch and temperature.

epidem'ic. The outbreak and rapid spread of a disease in a community, affecting many people at the same time.

epidemiog'raphy. A treatise of one or several epidemic diseases.

epidemiol'ogist. A person who specializes in epidemiology.

epidemiol'ogy. The scientific study of epidemics and epidemic diseases, especially of the factors that influence the incidence, distribution, and control of infectious diseases; the study of disease occurrence in human populations.

epider'mal. Relating to or resembling the epidermis.

epidermatoplas'ty. Skin grafting.

epider'mis. The outer, thinner layer of the skin, consisting of layers of stratified squamous epithelium; it is devoid of blood vessels and contains a limited distribution of nerve endings. See also skin.

epidermi'tis. Inflammation of the superficial layer of the skin.

epider'moid. 1. Resembling epidermis. **2.** A tumor containing aberrant epidermal cells.

Epidermoph'yton. A genus of fungi causing skin disorders.

epididymec'tomy. Surgical removal of the epididymis.

epidid'ymis. A tortuous C-shaped cordlike structure; the first part of the excretory duct of the testis, lying along its posterior surface, in which the spermatozoa are stored; it consists of a head, a body, and a tail which is continuous with the deferent duct.

epididymi'tis. Inflammation of the epididymis.

epididymo-orchi'tis. Inflammation of both the

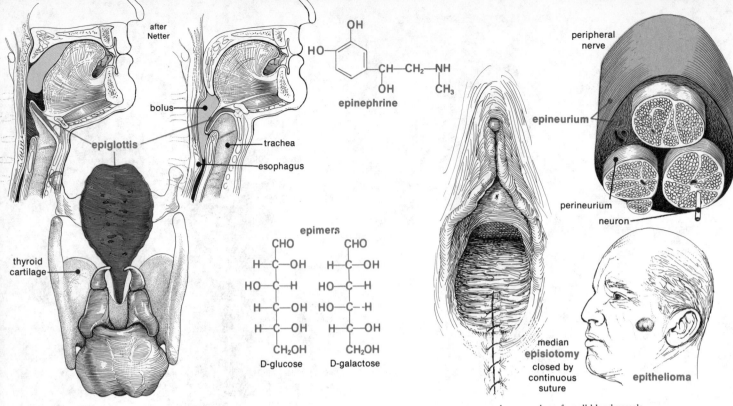

after Netter

bolus

epiglottis

trachea

esophagus

thyroid cartilage

epinephrine

epimers

CHO | CHO
D-glucose | D-galactose

peripheral nerve

epineurium

perineurium

neuron

median **episiotomy** closed by continuous suture

epithelioma

---

epididymis and testis.

ep'ididymot'omy. Surgical incision into the epididymis, usually for relief of tension and pain in epididymitis.

epididymovasos'tomy. The surgical joining of the epididymis and the deferent duct, usually for the purpose of bypassing an obstruction in the deferent duct.

epidu'ral. Situated upon or over the dura mater.

epigas'trium. The upper central area of the abdomen; pit of the stomach.

epigen'esis. The concept that an organism develops by the new formation of structures, as opposed to the old theory of preformation, i.e., that an organism develops by the growth of structures already existing in miniature in the egg.

epiglot'tis. The leaf-shaped cartilage that covers the aperture of the larynx during the act of swallowing to prevent food from entering the trachea.

epiglotti'tis. Inflammation of the epiglottis; it may cause respiratory obstruction, especially in children.

epila'tion. The removal of hairs with their roots.

epilem'ma. Endoneurium.

ep'ilepsy. A chronic neurologic disease, marked by sudden alterations in consciousness and frequently by convulsions.

activated e., seizures induced by drugs or electric shock for the purpose of observation.

generalized e., a seizure marked by loss of consciousness and spasms of the trunk and extremities, followed by generalized clonic jerking; also called grand mal or major epilepsy.

grand mal e., see generalized epilepsy.

laryngeal e., attacks precipitated by violent coughing.

major e., see generalized epilepsy.

musicogenic e., reflex epilepsy characterized by seizures precipitated by listening to a certain type of music.

petit mal e., brief or mild seizures, lasting from five to 30 seconds, characterized by a sudden cessation of activity and blank stare.

psychomotor e., disorder in which the seizure activity originates in or involves the temporal lobe, producing altered, bizarre activity and behavior; also called temporal lobe epilepsy.

sleep e., see narcolepsy.

temporal lobe e., see psychomotor epilepsy.

epilep'tic. 1. Relating to epilepsy. **2.** One who is afflicted with epilepsy.

epilep'toid. Resembling epilepsy; said of certain convulsions.

epiloi'a. Tuberous sclerosis; see under sclerosis.

epimandib'ular. On the lower jaw.

epimenorrhe'a. Menstruation occurring at excessively short intervals.

ep'imerase. One of a group of enzymes that promote epimeric changes.

ep'imers. Two sugars that differ from one another only in the configuration around a single carbon atom; e.g., glucose and galactose.

epimi'croscope. Opaque microscope, a microscope with a condenser around the objective; used for observing opaque or translucent specimens.

epimorpho'sis. Regeneration of a cut part of an organism.

epimys'ium. A sheath of connective tissue surrounding individual muscles.

epineph'rine, adren'aline. 1. Hormone produced by the medulla of the adrenal gland; it stimulates the sympathetic nervous system. **2.** A crystalline compound, $C_9H_{13}NO_3$, extracted from the adrenal glands of some mammals or produced synthetically; it produces cardiac stimulation, constriction or dilation of blood vessels, and bronchial relaxation; used as a heart stimulant and in the treatment of bronchial asthma and acute allergic disorders, and as a local vasoconstrictor.

epineu'ral. Located upon a neural arch.

epineu'rial. Relating to the connective tissue surrounding a nerve trunk.

epineu'rium. The connective tissue covering of a peripheral nerve.

epiphar'ynx. Nasopharynx.

epiphenom'enon. A symptom occurring during the course of a disease but not necessarily associated with it.

epiph'ora. Persistent overflow of tears onto the cheek, due to obstruction of the tear-conducting passages, eversion of the margin of the lower lid, or excessive secretion of tears.

epiphysiod'esis, epiphyseod'esis. An operation creating a permanent premature closure of an epiphysial plate, resulting in cessation of bone growth.

epiphysiol'ysis. The separation of an epiphysis from the shaft of the bone.

epiph'ysis, pl. **epiph'yses.** The end of a long bone, developed separately, and initially separated from the shaft by cartilage.

e. cerebri, pineal body; see under body.

epiphysi'tis. Inflammation of an epiphysis.

epiplo-. Combining form meaning omentum.

epip'locele. Hernia of the omentum.

epiploec'tomy. Surgical removal of the omentum.

epiplo'ic. Relating to the omentum.

epip'lopexy. See omentopexy.

episcle'ra. The loose connective tissue that constitutes the external surface of the sclera and contains

a large number of small blood vessels.

episcleri'tis. Inflammation of the connective tissue of the eye between the sclera and the conjunctiva.

episioperineoplas'ty. Reparative surgery of the vulva and perineum.

episioperineor'rhaphy. Suturing of a lacerated vulva and perineum.

epis'ioplasty. Surgical repair of a defect of the vulva.

episior'rhaphy. Suturing of a lacerated vulva.

episiot'omy. Incision of the perineum during childbirth, done to prevent vaginal, vulvar, or perineal tear by controlled enlargement of the vaginal orifice, to shorten the second stage of labor, and to prevent undue pressure on the fetal skull during delivery; the two most commonly used incisions are the mediolateral and median (midline); also called perineotomy.

ep'isome. A class of genetic elements of bacteria that may exist either as autonomous entities, replicating in the host independent of the bacterial chromosome, or as segments of the bacterial chromosome, replicating with it.

epispa'dias, epispa'dia. A rare congenital defect in the male in which the urethra opens on the dorsal surface of the penis; also a similar defect in the female in which a fissure is present in the upper wall of the urethra.

epispas'tic. Anything that causes blistering.

epispi'nal. On the vertebral column, spinal cord, or any spinelike structure.

epispleni'tis. Inflammation of the capsule of the spleen.

epis'tasis. 1. The film formed on the surface of a bodily discharge such as urine. **2.** The nonreciprocal interaction of nonallelic genes in which one suppresses the action of another.

epistax'is. See nosebleed.

epister'nal. Situated over or on the sternum; also called suprasternal.

epistro'pheus. Axis; the second cervical vertebra.

epithal'amus. A small area of the diencephalon consisting of the trigonum habenulae, the pineal body, and the posterior commissure.

epithe'lial. Relating to or composed of epithelium.

epithelializa'tion. The final stage in the healing of a surface injury in which epithelium is formed over the denuded area; also called epithelization.

epithe'lioid. Resembling epithelium.

epithelio'ma. A malignant tumor consisting of epithelial cells and arising mainly in the skin and mucous membrane.

Malherbe's calcifying e., see pilomatrixoma.

simple squamous **epithelium**

simple cuboidal **epithelium**

strata: skin
disjunctum
corneum
lucidum
granulosum
spinosum — prickle cell
germinativum
stratified squamous **epithelium** — basal cell

simple columnar **epithelium**
basal lamina

ciliated pseudostratified columnar **epithelium**
columnar cell
goblet cell
intermediate cell
basal cell

transitional **epithelium**
binucleate dome cell
basal lamina
lamina propria

equivalent measures and weights

US Customary Unit (Avoirdupois)	US Equivalents	Metric Equivalents
LENGTH		
inch	0.083 foot	2.54 centimeters
foot	1/3 yard or 12 inches	0.3048 meters
yard	3 feet or 36 inches	0.9144 meters
CAPACITY		
fluid ounce	8 fluid ounces	29.573 milliliters
pint	16 fluid ounces	0.473 liter
quart	2 pints	0.946 liter
gallon	4 quarts	3.785 liters
WEIGHT		
grain	0.036 dram	64.798 milligrams
dram	27.344 grains	1.772 grams
ounce	16 drams	28.350 grams
pound	16 ounces	453.592 grams

Apothecary Weight Unit	US Customary Equivalents	Metric Equivalents
scruple	20 grains	1.296 grams
dram	60 grains	3.888 grams
ounce	480 grains	31.103 grams

epithe'lium. The nonvascular cellular layer that covers the internal and external surfaces of the body.

germinal e., specialized peritoneal mesothelium (low cuboidal) that forms a continuous covering over the ovary; it was once thought to give rise to primordial germ cells (oogonia).

epitheliza'tion. See epithelialization.

ep'itope. The part of the surface of an antigen to which an antibody attaches. Cf paratope.

epizo'ic. Living as a parasite on the surface of the host's body.

epizo'on, *pl.* **epizo'a.** An animal parasite living on the exterior of the host's body.

eponych'ia. Infection at the groove of the nail.

eponych'ium. 1. The fold of skin overlying the root of the nail; its free, cornified margin forms the cuticle. **2.** The horny epidermis at the site of the future nail in the embryo.

ep'onym. The name of a disease, structure, or surgical procedure which includes the name of a person; e.g., Pott's disease.

eponym'ic. Named after a particular person.

epooph'oron. The vestiges of the mesonephros (wolffian body) consisting of rudimentary tubules located in the mesosalpinx between the ovary and the ovarian tube; also called pampiniform body and organ of Rosenmüller.

epox'y. In chemistry, an oxygen atom bound to two linked carbon atoms.

EPSP. Abbreviation for excitatory postsynaptic potential; see under potential.

epu'lis. A tumor of the gums.

e. gravidarum, tumor of the gums occurring during pregnancy.

equa'tion. A mathematical or chemical representation as a linear array of symbols expressing the quality of two things, separated into left and right sides by an equal sign.

Arrhenius' e., an equation relating chemical reaction rate with temperature.

Bohr's e., the equation for calculating the volume of the dead space gas in the respiratory tract by measuring the expired air and subtracting it from the alveolar gas volumes.

Einthoven's e., see law, Einthoven's.

Hasselbalch's e., see Henderson-Hasselbalch equation.

Henderson-Hasselbalch e., an equation for determining the pH of a buffer solution such as blood plasma; $pH = pK_1 - \log (BHCO_3)/(H_2CO_3)$; also called Hasselbalch's equation.

equa'tor bul'bi oc'uli. Equator of the eyeball; an imaginary circle around the eyeball at the same distance from both poles.

equicalor'ic. Having the same heat value.

equilibra'tion. 1. The act of bringing about or maintaining equilibrium. **2.** In dentistry, the equalization of pressure.

equilib'rium. 1. Condition in which all acting forces cancel each other, resulting in a stable unchanging system. **2.** In chemistry, a stable condition created by two reactions occurring at equal speed in opposite directions. **3.** Mental or emotional stability. **4.** A state of bodily balance.

Donnan e., the condition that exists when two solutions are separated by a semipermeable membrane (i.e., permeable only to some of the ions of the solutions); the unequal distribution of ions between the two solutions causes an electrical potential between the two sides of the membrane.

dynamic e., the condition of balance between the varying forces of living processes.

equimo'lar. Containing the same number of moles or having equal molarity.

equimolec'ular. Denoting solutions that contain an equal number of molecules.

equi'nus. Talipes equinus.

equiv'alence, equiv'alency. 1. In chemistry, the relative combining powers of a set of atoms or radicals. **2.** Valence.

equiv'alent. 1. Equal in any way (substance, value, force, etc.). **2.** Having similar or equal effects.

chemical e., see gram equivalent.

epileptic e., the occurrence of manifestations such as cough, severe headaches, abdominal pain, etc. instead of a typical seizure, usually observed in psychomotor epileptics.

gram e., (1) the weight (usually in grams) of a substance which can combine with, or displace, a unit weight of hydrogen from a compound or its equivalent of another substance; (2) the atomic or molecular weight in grams of an atom or group of atoms involved in a chemical reaction divided by the number of electrons donated, taken up, or shared by the atom or group of atoms in the course of that reaction; (3) the weight of a substance contained in one liter of one normal solution; also called chemical equivalent, equivalent weight, and combining weight.

ER. Abbreviation for endoplasmic reticulum.

rough ER, abbreviation for rough (granular) endoplasmic reticulum.

smooth ER, abbreviation for smooth (agranular) endoplasmic reticulum.

Er. Chemical symbol of the element erbium.

er'bium. A soft, malleable, silvery rare earth element; symbol Er, atomic number 68, atomic weight 167.27.

Erb's spastic paraplegia. Syphilitic inflammation of the inner coat of the arteries supplying the spinal cord, causing degeneration of the pyramidal tracts.

erec'tile. Able to be erected; relating to vascular tissue, as in the penis, which is capable of filling with blood and becoming somewhat rigid.

erec'tion. 1. The state of erectile tissue when filled with blood. **2.** An erect penis.

erec'tor. Something which raises or makes erect; denoting specifically certain muscles that hold up or cause the erection of a body part.

er'ethism. An exaggerated degree of irritability or excitability, either general or in any part of the body, accompanied by mental changes such as instability, memory loss, lack of attention, decrease in intellect, and shyness; may be associated with chronic poisoning.

ERG. Abbreviation for electroretinogram.

erg. A unit of energy equal to the force capable of moving a weight of one gram a distance of one centimeter.

ergas'toplasm. The basophilic component of the cytoplasm of certain cells that produce protein substances.

ergocalcif'erol. See vitamin D_2.

ergodynam'ograph. An instrument used to record the degree of muscular force and the amount of work accomplished by muscular contraction.

er'gograph. An instrument for recording the work capacity of a muscle.

ergom'eter. Dynamometer.

ergonom'ics. See biotechnology.

ergos'terol. A crystalline sterol present in plant and animal tissues, which, under ultraviolet irradiation, is converted to vitamin D_2; derived from ergot, yeast, and other fungi.

er'got. 1. Any fungus (genus *Claviceps*) which attacks cereal plants. **2.** The blackish mass which replaces the grain of rye infected with the fungus; it has vasoconstrictor and oxytocic properties and yields drugs of clinical usefulness.

ergot'amine. An alkaloid derived from ergot that stimulates smooth muscle, especially of the blood vessels and uterus.

er'gotism. Poisoning by ergot-infected grain such as rye, in which constriction of the arterioles leads to lameness and necrosis of the extremities.

erg-second. A unit of work or energy multiplied by time; equal to the amount of energy required to move a weight of one gram a distance of one centimeter in one second.

erog'enous, erogen'ic. Producing sexual desire.

ero'sion. 1. A gradual wearing away. **2.** In den-

eruption of deciduous teeth

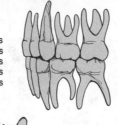

central incisors	6–8 months
lateral incisors	7–9 months
cuspids	16–18 months
first molars	12–14 months
second molars	20–24 months

refractive error

nearsightedness

corrected by a lens

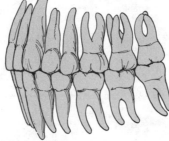

eruption of permanent teeth

central incisors	6–8 years
lateral incisors	7–9 years
cuspids	9–12 years
first bicuspids	10–12 years
second bicuspids	10–12 years
first molars	6–7 years
second molars	11–13 years
third molars	17–21 years

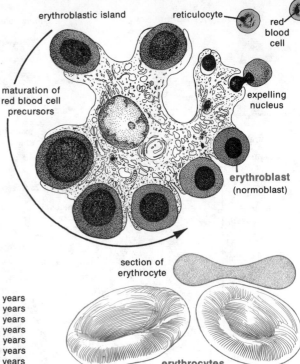

erythroblastic island · reticulocyte · red blood cell

maturation of red blood cell precursors

expelling nucleus

erythroblast (normoblast)

section of erythrocyte

erythrocytes

---

tistry, the progressive loss of tooth substance by a chemical process without the aid of bacteria, producing a hard, polished, smooth depression on the surface of the tooth.

erot'ic. Relating to or tending to arouse sexual desire.

erot'icism, erot'ism. 1. Erotic character. **2.** A state of sexual excitement.

erotogen'ic. Producing sexual excitement.

ERPF. Abbreviation for effective renal plasma flow.

errat'ic. 1. Denoting symptoms that do not follow a usual pattern. **2.** Unconventional.

er'ror, refrac'tive. Defect in the refractive system of the eye that prevents light rays from being brought to a focus on the retina.

erubes'cence. A flushing or reddening of the skin; a blush.

eructa'tion. The act of belching.

erupt'. To break or pierce through; said of a tooth.

erup'tion. 1. The act of breaking out, as the appearance of lesions on the skin. **2.** Redness or blemishing of the skin or mucosa as a manifestation of disease. **3.** Cutting of a tooth; the passage of a tooth through the gum.

ERV. Abbreviation for expiratory reserve volume.

erysip'elas. An acute contagious disease caused by *Streptococcus pyogenes*, marked by a circumscribed red eruption on the skin, chills, and fever.

erysip'eloid. Infection of the hands with the bacillus *Erysipelothrix rhysiopathiae*, marked by red lesions and occurring in persons handling infected fish or meat.

Erysip'elothrix. A genus of bacteria (family Corynebacteriaceae) containing gram-positive, rod-shaped organisms which have a tendency to form long filaments; parasitic on mammals, birds, and fish.

erysipelotox'in. A toxin produced by *Streptococcus pyogenes*, species of bacteria causing erysipelas.

erys'iphake. An operative instrument (a suction cup attached to an aspiration apparatus) for the removal of a cataractous crystalline lens by suction.

erythe'ma. Redness of the skin.

e. marginatum, a type of erythema multiforme in which the lesions have a disc shape with elevated edges.

e. multiforme, an acute inflammatory skin disease, marked by the symmetrical eruption of macules, papules, or vesicles of various shapes presenting a multiform appearance; may be an allergic reaction; severe cases may have a fatal termination; in mild cases (Hebra's disease) the eruption usually recurs.

e. multiforme bullosum, a blister-like eruption on the lips, tongue, and mucous membrane of the mouth.

e. multiforme exudativum, a rare severe form of erythema multiforme characterized chiefly by eruptive, ulcerative lesions of the skin, oral mucosa, and eyes; frequently the genitalia, lungs, and joints are affected; also called Stevens-Johnson syndrome.

e. nodosum, a skin disease, probably a hypersensitivity reaction, characterized by bright red, painful nodules on the shins and frequently on the anterior thighs and extensor surfaces of the forearms.

e. venenata, erythema due to contact with some sensitizing substance.

toxic e., a diffuse eruption of the skin due to an allergic reaction to a toxic substance.

erythral'gia. A state of painful redness of the skin.

erythras'ma. A contagious skin disease caused by the bacterium *Corynebacterium minutissimum;* marked by an eruption of reddish brown patches in the armpits and groin which glow under Wood's light.

erythrede'ma. See acrodynia.

erythre'mia. See polycythemia vera.

eryth'rityl tetrani'trate. A compound used in a diluted form in the treatment of angina pectoris and hypertension.

erythro-, erythr-. Combining forms denoting a relationship to red.

eryth'roblast. A young red blood cell in its immature, nucleated stage.

acidophilic e., see orthochromatic erythroblast.

basophilic e., the second stage in the development of the erythroblast, following the proerythroblast; also called basophilic normoblast, prorubricyte, and early erythroblast.

orthochromatic e., the last stage in the development of the erythroblast in which 80 per cent of the hemoglobin is synthesized; also called metarubricyte, orthochromatic normoblast, late erythroblast, and acidophilic erythroblast.

polychromatophilic e., the third stage in the development of the erythroblast; also called polychromatic normoblast and rubricyte.

erythroblaste'mia. The presence of nucleated red blood cells (erythroblasts) in the peripheral blood; may be seen in a variety of pathologic conditions.

erythroblastope'nia. Deficiency in bone marrow of erythroblasts (red blood cells in an early stage of development).

erythroblasto'sis. Excessive number of immature red blood cells (erythroblasts) in the blood.

e. fetalis, erythroblastosis of the fetus and newborn associated with Rh-factor incompatibility between mother and child; often accompanied by enlargement of the spleen and liver; also called hemo-

lytic disease of the newborn.

erythrochro'mia. A red coloration.

erythroc'lasis. Fragmentation of red blood cells.

erythrocu'prein. A copper-containing protein present in human red blood cells.

erythrocyano'sis. Swollen and reddish condition of the limbs upon exposure to cold, but not freezing, temperatures.

eryth'rocyte. A mature red blood cell or corpuscle which transports oxygen to the tissue by means of the hemoglobin it contains; normally it is a yellowish, non-nucleated, biconcave disk, measuring approximately from 7.2 to 8.6 μ in diameter; the thickness at the center is slightly less than 1 μ and at the rim approximately 2 μ; in a normal human adult, 2,500,000 erythrocytes are formed every second; their life span is about 120 days.

erythrocythe'mia. Polycythemia; excessive number of red blood cells in the blood.

erythrocyt'ic. Relating to a red blood cell.

erythrocytol'ysin. A substance capable of causing dissolution of red blood cells.

erythrocytol'ysis. See hemolysis.

erythrocytom'eter. See hemocytometer.

erythrocytope'nia. See erythropenia.

erythrocytorrhex'is. The partial escape of protoplasm from red blood cells, causing changes in the shape of the cells; also called plasmorrhexis.

erythrocyto'sis. Excessive formation of red blood cells.

erythrocytu'ria. Red blood cells in the urine.

erythroder'ma. A nondescriptive term denoting abnormal redness of the skin, especially over large areas of the body.

erythrodon'tia. Reddish discoloration of the teeth.

erythrogen'esis imperfec'ta. Congenital hypoplastic anemia; see under anemia.

erythrogen'ic. 1. Causing a rash. **2.** Producing red blood cells.

eryth'rogenin. An enzymatic factor (renal erythropoietic factor) produced by the kidney which converts a precursor, erythropoietinogen, in plasma to ESF (erythropoiesis-stimulating factor).

erythrogo'nium, pl. erythrogo'nia. Denoting tissues from which red blood cells develop.

eryth'roid. Reddish.

erythrokinet'ics. The maintenance of a steady number of circulating red blood cells in the normal individual by the balance achieved between the amount removed from and the amount delivered to the peripheral blood per unit of time.

erythroleuke'mia. Proliferation of immature red and white blood cells.

erythrol'ysin. Hemolysin.

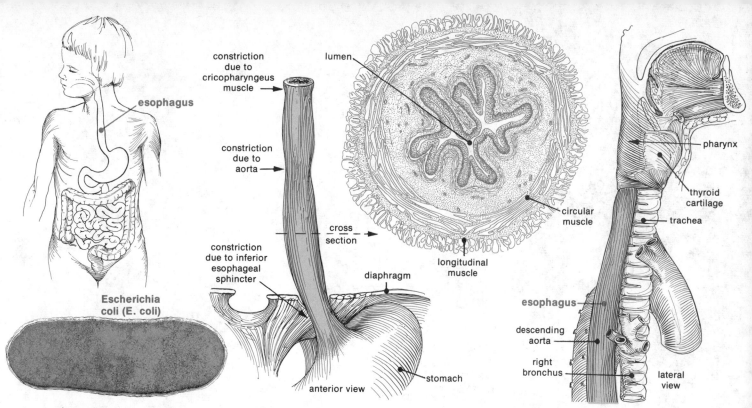

esophagus

constriction due to cricopharyngeus muscle

constriction due to aorta

cross section

constriction due to inferior esophageal sphincter

diaphragm

anterior view

stomach

Escherichia coli (E. coli)

lumen

circular muscle

longitudinal muscle

pharynx

thyroid cartilage

trachea

esophagus

descending aorta

right bronchus

lateral view

erythromelal'gia. A circulatory disorder causing a burning sensation of the hands and/or feet, sometimes involving the whole extremity and lasting minutes or hours; also called erythermalgia.

erythrome'lia. Diffuse atrophy of the skin.

erythromy'cin. An antibiotic substance obtained from a strain of *Streptomyces erythreus*; Ilotycin®.

eryth'ron. The total mass of erythropoietic cells and circulating erythrocytes, viewed as a functional, though dispersed, organ.

erythroneocyto'sis. Presence in the peripheral blood of regenerative forms of red blood cells.

erythrope'nia. Deficiency of red blood cells; also called erythrocytopenia.

erythropha'gia. Erythrophagocytosis.

erythrophagocyto'sis. The ingestion and digestion of red blood cells by other cells such as monocytes and polymorphonuclear leukocytes.

erythro'pia, erythrop'sia. Red vision, the subjective sensation that all objects are covered with a red tint.

erythropoie'sis. The formation of red blood cells.

erythropoie'tic. Relating to the origin of red blood cells.

erythropoi'etin. Erythropoiesis-stimulating factor (ESF); a hormone produced principally in the kidney which stimulates red blood cell production; also called erythropoietic factor and hematopoietin.

erythroprosopal'gia. Burning pain and redness of the face, believed to indicate organic disease of the nervous system.

erythropykno'sis. Degeneration of red blood cells; which become dark and shrunken (brassy bodies); occurs in malaria.

erythrorrhex'is. Fragmentation of red blood cells.

erythru'ria. The passage of red urine.

escape. The assumption of pacemaker activities by a lower pacemaker when a higher pacemaker defaults or atrioventricular (A-V) conduction fails.

 nodal e., escape with the A-V node as pacemaker.

 ventricular e., escape with an ectopic ventricular focus as pacemaker.

es'char. A scab or slough.

escharot'ic. Caustic.

Escheri'chia. A genus of bacteria (family Enterobacteriaceae) containing short, gram-negative rods; the motile species are covered with flagella; they ferment glucose and lactose with acid and gas formation, are present in feces, and may cause disease in man.

 E. coli, a motile variety normally present in the intestines of humans; formerly called *Bacillus coli.*

escutch'eon. A shield-shaped surface, as the pattern of distribution of the pubic hair.

es'erine. See physostigmine.

 e. salicylate, see physostigmine salicylate.

ESF. Abbreviation for erythropoiesis-stimulating factor (erythropoietin).

esocatapho'ria. Tendency of the eyes to turn down and in; a combination of esophoria and cataphoria.

esodevia'tion. The inward deviation of one or both eyes in convergent strabismus or in esophoria.

esod'ic. Denoting sensory nerves that conduct impulses toward the brain or spinal cord.

esophagal'gia. Pain in the esophagus; also called esophagodynia.

esophag'eal. Of or relating to the esophagus.

esophagecta'sia. Esophagectasis; abnormal dilatation of the esophagus.

esophagecta'sis. Esophagectasia.

esophagec'tomy. Surgical removal of a portion of the esophagus.

esophagi'tis. Inflammation of the esophagus.

 peptic e., see reflux esophagitis.

 reflux e., diffuse inflammation of the distal esophagus caused by reflux of gastric or duodenal contents through an incompetent lower esophageal sphincter; frequently associated with a hiatal hernia or a duodenal ulcer; also called peptic esophagitis.

esophagocar'dioplasty. A reparative operation on the esophagus and the cardiac area of the stomach.

esoph'agocele. Protrusion of the mucous membrane of the esophagus through a defect in its muscular layer.

esophagodyn'ia. See esophagalgia.

esophagoenteros'tomy. Surgical connection of the esophagus and intestine after excision of the stomach.

esophagogastrec'tomy. Surgical removal of a portion of the lower esophagus and proximal stomach, usually performed for eradicating neoplasms.

esophagogastros'tomy. The surgical formation of an artificial opening between the esophagus and the stomach.

esophagojejunos'tomy. Surgical union between the esophagus and jejunum.

esophagomala'cia. Softening of the walls of the esophagus.

esophagomyot'omy. Incision through the wall of the esophagus.

 Heller e., a longitudinal extramucosal incision on the esophagus, at the level of its junction with the stomach.

esoph'agoplasty. Surgical repair of a defect of the esophagus.

esophagoplica'tion. Surgical reduction of a pouch or dilatation in the esophagus by making longitudinal folds on its walls.

esoph'agoscope. An instrument for inspecting the interior of the esophagus.

esophagos'copy. Examination of the interior of the esophagus with an esophagoscope.

esophagosteno'sis. Stricture or narrowing of the esophagus.

esophagos'tomy. The surgical formation of an artificial opening into the esophagus.

esophagot'omy. Incision through the esophagus.

esoph'agram. A roentgenogram of the esophagus.

esoph'agus. The musculomembranous tube extending downward from the pharynx to the cardia of the stomach, a distance of about 25 cm (10 inches).

esopho'ria. Condition in which the eyes have a tendency to turn inward, manifested when fusion is prevented by covering one eye.

esophor'ic. Relating to esophoria or the tendency of the eyes to deviate inward.

esotro'pia. Convergent strabismus; see under strabismus.

esotrop'ic. Relating to convergent strabismus or the inward turning of one eye.

ESP. Abbreviation for extrasensory perception.

ESR. Abbreviation for erythrocyte sedimentation rate.

ESRD. Abbreviation for end-stage renal disease.

es'sence. 1. The intrinsic properties or qualities of a thing. **2.** The fluid extract of a substance that retains its fundamental properties, such as the alcoholic solution of a volatile oil.

essen'tial. 1. Necessary. **2.** Having no apparent external cause; said of a disease.

EST. Abbreviation for electroshock therapy.

es'ter. Any of a group of organic compounds formed by the condensation of an alcohol and carboxylic acid.

es'terase. Any enzyme that promotes the hydrolysis of an ester.

esthe'sia. The perception of sense impressions.

esthesiogen'esis. The origin or production of a reaction in a sensory zone.

esthesiog'raphy. 1. Delineating on the skin the areas of tactile and other forms of sensibility. **2.** A description of the mechanism of sensation.

es'tival, aes'tival. Occurring in the summer.

estivoautum'nal. Occurring in summer and autumn.

estradi'ol. An estrogenic hormone obtained commercially from the urine of pregnant mares, hog ovaries, and estrone; also called dihydroxytheelin and dihydroxyestrin.

est'riol. A white, odorless, estrogenic hormone

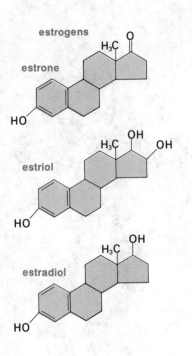

estrogens

estrone

estriol

estradiol

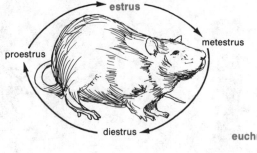

estrus

proestrus

metestrus

diestrus

hetero-chromatin

lymphocyte

euchromatin

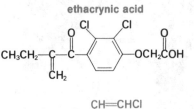

ethacrynic acid

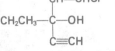

ethchlorvynol (tertiary alcohol)

eversion of upper eyelid

Walker double evertor

present in the urine of pregnant mammals; also called theelol and folliculin hydrate.

es′trogen. General term for the female sex hormones, responsible for stimulating the development and maintenance of female secondary sex characteristics; formed in the ovary, placenta, testis, adrenal cortex, and some plants; therapeutic uses (with natural or synthetic preparations) include the relief of menopausal symptoms and amelioration of cancer of the prostate gland.

es′trone. An estrogenic hormone found in the ovary and in the urine of pregnant mammals.

es′trous. 1. Relating to estrus. 2. In heat.

es′trus. 1. The recurrent period of sexual excitement in the female of animals; also called heat. 2. In mammals, the cycle of changes in the genital tract produced by ovarian hormones.

esu. Abbreviation for electrostatic unit.

ethacrynic acid. An unsaturated ketone derivative of aryloxyacetic acid, a potent diuretic; Edecrin®.

ethambutol hydrochloride. A compound used in the treatment of tuberculosis.

eth′anol. See alcohol (2).

ethchlor′vynol. A hypnotic and anticonvulsant drug, generally used for inducing sleep in simple insomnia and as a daytime sedative; Placidyl®.

e′ther. 1. Any of a group of organic compounds in which two hydrocarbon groups are linked by an oxygen atom. 2. Term used for the anesthetic diethyl ether.

   diethyl e., an inflammable, volatile liquid, $C_4H_{10}O$, obtained from the distillation of ethyl alcohol and sulfuric acid; used as an anesthetic; also called ethyl ether.

   ethyl e., see diethyl ether.

   hydrochloric e., see ethyl chloride.

ethe′real. 1. Relating to, containing, or resembling ether. 2. Evanescent.

etherifica′tion. The conversion of an alcohol into ether.

ether′ify. To convert into ether.

e′therize. To produce anesthesia with ether.

eth′ical. 1. Relating to ethics. 2. Being in accord with professionally accepted codes.

eth′ics. Standards of behavior governing an individual or a profession.

eth′moid. Resembling a sieve.

ethmoidec′tomy. Surgical removal of the ethmoid cells or of part of the ethmoid bone.

ethmoidi′tis. Inflammation of the ethmoid sinus.

ethmosphe′noid. Relating to both the ethmoid and sphenoid bones.

ethnopsychi′atry. The study of varied cultural patterns and their influence on emotional matura-

tion.

eth′yl. The univalent hydrocarbon radical C_2H_5-.

   e. alcohol, see alcohol (2).

   e. chloride, a gas at ordinary temperatures, a volatile liquid when compressed; used to produce local anesthesia by superficial freezing; also called chloroethane and hydrochloric ether.

ethylcel′lulose. An ethyl ether of cellulose, used as a tablet binder; Ethocel®.

eth′ylene. A colorless, flammable gas, CH_2CH_2, somewhat lighter than air; used for inducing general anesthesia; also called ethene.

ethylenediaminetetraacetic acid (EDTA). A chelating agent, or compound used to complex divalent metals.

etio-. Combining form denoting (a) a compound formed by chemical degradation; (b) cause.

etiocholan′olone. A metabolite of adrenocortical and testicular hormones excreted in the urine.

etiolog′ic. Relating to the causes of disease.

etiol′ogy. The study of causes, specifically the cause of a disease.

eu-. Combining form meaning good, well.

Eu. Chemical symbol of the element europium.

Eubacte′rium. A genus of anaerobic bacteria (family Propionibacteriaceae) containing gram-positive rods; some species may be pathogenic.

eubiot′ics. The science of hygienic living.

eucar′yote. See eukaryote.

eucho′lia. The normal state of the bile.

euchro′matin. The lightly stained portion of the cell nucleus containing genetically active DNA: also called true chromatin.

eugen′ics. The branch of science concerned with the study of the hereditary improvement of man by genetic control.

eu′genol. Eugenic acid, a light yellow oily liquid obtained from oil of cloves; used in dentistry as an antiseptic and local anesthetic.

euglob′ulin. A simple protein insoluble in pure water but soluble in saline solutions.

eugon′ic. Growing rapidly on an artificial medium; applied to cultures of the human tubercle bacillus.

eukaryo′sis. The state of having a true nucleus, as in the higher types of cells.

eukar′yote. An organism with cells that have nuclear membranes, membrane-bound organelles, and ribosomes and that exhibit mitosis; also written eucaryote.

eu′nuch. A castrated male, or one whose testes have never developed.

eu′nuchoid. Having the characteristics of a eunuch.

eu′nuchoidism. Condition in which the testes fail to function.

euos′mia. 1. A pleasant odor. 2. A normal state of the sense of smell.

eupep′sia. Good digestion.

eupho′ria. 1. A feeling of well being. 2. In psychiatry, an exaggerated feeling of happiness.

eupla′sia. The normal state of cells or tissues.

euplas′tic. Able to heal readily.

eu′ploidy. In genetics, the condition of having the normal full complement of chromosomes; i.e., the chromosome number of a cell is an exact multiple of the haploid number normal for the species from which it originated.

eupne′a. Normal, easy breathing.

eustachi′tis. Inflammation of the mucous membrane of the auditory (eustachian) tube.

euthana′sia. 1. The act of inducing a painless, easy death, as in persons with a painful terminal illness. 2. Painless death.

euthy′roidism. A normal condition of the thyroid gland.

eutro′phia. A state of normal nourishment and development.

ev. Abbreviation for electron-volt; equal to 1.6×10^{-12} erg.

evac′uant. 1. Promoting a bowel movement. 2. An agent having such an effect.

evac′uate. 1. To empty the bowels. 2. To create a vacuum or very low pressure by removing air or any gas from a closed vessel.

evacua′tion. 1. Emptying of the bowels. 2. The waste material discharged from the bowels. 3. The creation of a vacuum.

evagina′tion. Protrusion of a part or organ.

evanes′cent. Of short life or duration.

evapora′tion. The change of a liquid into a vapor.

eventra′tion. 1. Protrusion of the intestines through an opening in the abdominal wall. 2. Removal of the abdominal organs.

ever′sion. Turning outward, as of a foot, or inside out, as of an eyelid.

evert′. To turn outward.

eviscera′tion. Removal of internal organs.

   e. of the eye, surgical removal of the contents of the eyeball, leaving the sclera intact.

   e. of the orbit, removal of all the contents of the orbit; also called exenteration.

evolu′tion. A continuous and gradual process of change from one state or form to another.

evul′sion. A pulling out or forcible extraction.

Ewart's sign. In large pericardial effusions, bronchial breathing and an area of dullness at the lower angle of the left scapula; also called Pins' sign.

ex-. Prefix meaning out of or away from.

exacerba′tion. Increase in the severity of a disease or any of its symptoms.

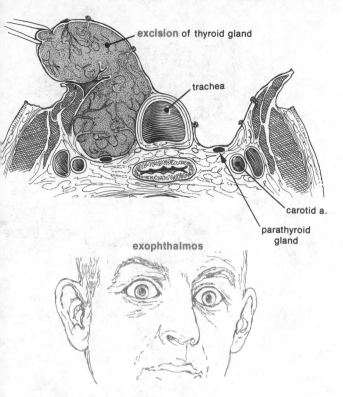

excision of thyroid gland

trachea

carotid a.

parathyroid gland

exophthalmos

exotoxins produced by some bacteria pathogenic to man

TOXIN	DISEASE	SPECIES	ACTION
tetanospasmin	tetanus	*Clostridium tetani*	spastic hemolytic cardiotoxin
diphtheritic toxin	diphtheria	*Corynebacterium diphtheriae*	necrotizing
α-toxin	pyogenic infection	*Staphylococcus aureus*	necrotizing, hemolytic, leucocidic
whooping cough toxin	whooping cough	*Bordetella pertussis*	necrotizing
neurotoxin	dysentry	*Shigella dysenteriae*	hemorrhagic paralytic
neurotoxin	botulism	*Clostridium botulinum*	paralytic

examina′tion. Any inspection or investigation for the purpose of diagnosis.

cytologic e., the microscopic examination of a bodily secretion (especially from the cervix and vagina) for the detection of cancer or for the evaluation of the hormonal condition; also called Papanicolaou examination.

Papanicolaou e., see cytologic examination.

postmortem e., see autopsy.

exam′iner, med′ical. 1. A physician whose function is to ascertain the causes of death of those who die suddenly or as a result of violence. **2.** A physician who examines and reports on the physical condition of applicants for life insurance.

exan′them, exanthe′ma. 1. Any disease accompanied by a skin eruption. **2.** A skin eruption.

e. subitum, an acute febrile disease occurring within the first three years of life, most commonly between six and 18 months; after two to four days of fever the temperature falls by lysis and a macular or maculopapular rash appears; thought to be of viral origin; also called roseola infantum.

exanthem′atous. Relating to any disease accompanied by a rash.

excava′tion. 1. A natural bodily cavity or recess. **2.** A cavity resulting from a pathologic process.

atrophic e., an exaggerated depression of the optic disk caused by atrophy of the optic nerve.

glaucomatous e., glaucomatous cup; see under cup.

physiologic e., physiologic cup; see under cup.

excava′tor. 1. A spoonlike instrument used to scrape out pathologic tissue. **2.** A dental instrument used to remove carious material from a cavity.

excip′ient. A more or less inert substance used as a diluent or vehicle for a drug.

exci′se. To remove surgically.

excis′ion. The surgical removal of a part or organ.

excitabil′ity. The state of being capable of quick response to a stimulus; the property of muscle tissue by virtue of which it reacts to stimulation by propagation of the impulse.

exci′table. Capable of quick response to a stimulus.

excita′tion. 1. Stimulation. **2.** In physics, the increase of energy.

excit′ement. The state of being agitated.

excitoglan′dular. Increasing the activity of a gland.

excitomo′tor. Tending to cause motion.

exci′tor. Tending to produce increased action.

ex′clave. A detached portion of a part.

exclu′sion. Disconnecting from the main part.

excor′iate. To scratch or abrade the skin.

excoria′tion. A scratch mark.

neurotic e., self-inflicted skin lesions by emotionally disturbed persons, usually by the forcible use of fingernails.

ex′crement. Feces.

excres′cence. Any abnormal outgrowth from the surface.

excre′ta. Discharged natural wastes; excreted material, such as sweat, urine, etc.

excrete′. To eliminate waste material from the body.

excre′ter. An individual who is a carrier of disease-causing microorganisms, and who excretes them in the urine or feces.

excre′tion. 1. Process by which the waste products of metabolism, or the undigested food residues, are eliminated from the body. **2.** The product of such a process.

ex′cretory. Relating to or used during excretion.

excur′sion. An oscillating or alternating motion from an axis or a mean position.

exentera′tion. See evisceration of the orbit.

ex′ercise. Physical activity performed to develop or maintain fitness; it may require bodily exertion (active exercise) or effortless motion (passive exercise).

exergon′ic. Indicating a chemical reaction that is accompanied by a release of free energy, regardless of the form of energy involved.

exflagella′tion. The development of microgametes (male gametes) from microgametocytes (mother cells), as in malaria.

exfolia′tion. 1. The shedding, peeling, or scaling of skin; also called desquamation. **2.** In dentistry, the casting off of deciduous teeth.

exhala′tion. 1. The act of breathing out. **2.** Exhaled gas or vapor.

exhale′. 1. To breathe out. **2.** To emit a gas, vapor, etc.

exhaus′tion. 1. Extreme fatigue. **2.** Removal of contents. **3.** Removal of the active ingredients of a drug.

heat e., condition marked by prostration and weakness caused by prolonged exposure to hot temperatures.

nervous e., obsolete term for functional neurosis (neurasthenia) or for a mental disorder.

exhibitionism. A morbid compulsion to expose the genitalia.

exhuma′tion. The process of taking a body out of a place of burial.

ex′itus. 1. Outlet. **2.** Death.

exo-. Prefix meaning external or outward.

exocataphor′ia. A tendency of the eyes to deviate outward and downward.

ex′ocrine. 1. A gland that discharges its secretion

through a duct. **2.** The secretion of such a gland.

exodevia′tion. The outward deviation of one or both eyes in divergent strabismus or in exophoria.

exod′ic. Denoting nerves that convey impulses toward the periphery.

exodon′tics. The branch of dentistry concerned with the extraction of teeth.

exoen′zyme. Any enzyme that performs its functions outside of the cell in which it originates, as a digestive enzyme.

exog′enous. Originating outside the body.

exom′phalos. See omphalocele.

exonu′clease. A nuclease (enzyme) that digests or cleaves DNA from the ends of strands (polynucleotide chains).

exop′athy. Any disease originating from causes outside the body.

exopho′ria. Condition in which an eye has a tendency to turn outward, manifested when fusion is prevented by covering the eye.

exophthal′mic. Relating to or afflicted with exophthalmos.

exophthalmom′eter. An instrument used to measure the degree of protrusion of the eyeball; also called proptometer.

exophthal′mos. Abnormal protrusion of the eyeball.

malignant e., severe, usually bilateral, protrusion of the eyeballs; occurring mostly in middle age; it may be unresponsive to treatment and can lead to blindness.

exoskel′eton. 1. The external, supportive covering of certain invertebrates. **2.** Structures, such as hair, nails, feathers, scales, etc., developed from the ectoderm or mesoderm in vertebrates; also called dermatoskeleton and dermoskeleton.

exosmo′sis. Diffusion from within outward, as from a blood vessel.

ex′ospore. A spore produced by budding, as a fungal spore.

exospo′rium. The outer covering of a spore.

exosto′sis, *pl.* **exosto′ses.** A bony growth on the surface of a bone.

dental e., one projecting from the root of a tooth.

multiple hereditary e., the presence of multiple exostoses in the long bones of children due to a hereditary defect of ossification in cartilage, resulting in severe skeletal deformity and stunting of growth; also called diaphyseal aclasis.

exoter′ic. Belonging to factors outside the organism.

exother′mic, exother′mal. 1. Releasing heat, as certain chemical reactions. **2.** Relating to the external warmth of the body.

exotox′in. A toxin produced and released by bac-

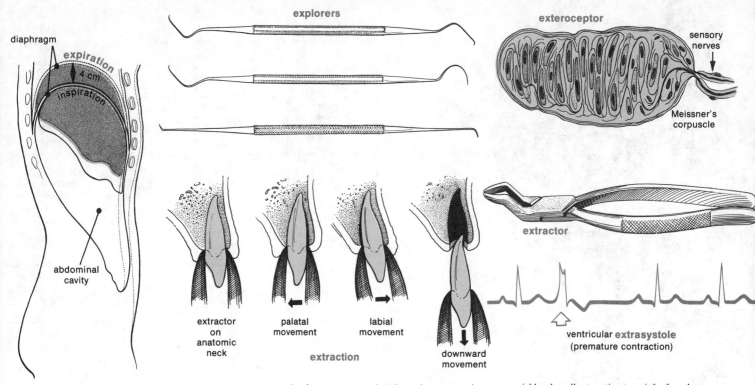

diaphragm

expiration 4 cm **inspiration**

abdominal cavity

explorers

exteroceptor

sensory nerves

Meissner's corpuscle

extractor

extractor on anatomic neck | palatal movement | labial movement | downward movement

extraction

ventricular extrasystole (premature contraction)

---

terial cells as a normal physiologic process; also called extracellular toxin.

exotro'pia. Divergent strabismus; see under strabismus.

expan'siveness. An exaggerated sense of importance.

expec'torant. 1. Promoting the expulsion of mucus or other material from the air passages. **2.** A medicine so acting.

expectora'tion. Sputum; mucus or other secretions coughed up from the air passages.

exper'iment. A test.

   control e., experiment to check the results of other experiments by keeping the same conditions except for one particular factor.

   double blind e., one in which the control is unknown to the experimenter and the subjects.

expira'tion. 1. The act of breathing out. **2.** The act of dying.

expi'ratory. Relating to expiration.

expire'. 1. To exhale; to breathe out. **2.** To die.

explant'. In tissue culture, to transfer living tissue from the body to another medium.

explora'tion. A surgical, digital, or instrumental examination of tissue as an aid in diagnosis; a diagnostic search or investigation.

explor'er. A sharp, curved dental probe used to examine teeth.

explo'sion. 1. A sudden, rapid, violent discharge of force from a confined area. **2.** A sudden outbreak, as an epidemic or population explosion.

expo'nent. 1. A number or symbol written as a superscript, denoting the number of times a factor is to be involved in a repeated multiplication. **2.** One who defines or advocates.

express'. To squeeze out.

expressiv'ity. Strength of the manifestation of a genetic trait in terms of its deviation from the normal.

exsan'guinate. To drain blood; to make bloodless.

exsic'cant. 1. Drying; dehydrating; absorbing. **2.** A dusting or drying powder.

ex'siccate. To dry; to remove moisture.

exsicca'tion. The process of removing moisture.

ex'strophy. Congenital turning inside out of an organ.

   e. of the bladder, malformation in which the interior of the posterior wall of the bladder becomes visible through an opening in the abdominal wall and the anterior bladder wall.

exsuffla'tion. Forcible expiration; forced expulsion of the breath by a mechanical apparatus.

exten'sion. The act of straightening a limb or the condition of being straightened.

exten'sor. A muscle that, by contracting, straightens a limb.

exte'riorize. 1. To expose an organ (temporarily or permanently) as a form of therapy or for the purpose of physiologic experimentation. **2.** In psychiatry, to direct a patient's interests toward others rather than himself.

ex'tern. A nonresident medical student or recent graduate who assists in the care of hospitalized patients.

exter'nal. Situated on the outside; on the surface.

exterocep'tor. A sensory nerve ending in the skin or mucous membrane which is affected primarily by the external environment; e.g., Meissner's corpuscle for touch, Krause's end bulb for cold, Ruffini's corpuscle for warmth, Golgi-Mazzoni corpuscle for pressure, and free nerve endings for pain.

ex'tima. See adventitia.

extinc'tion. 1. In physiology, relating to the point at which a nerve, after responding to a stimulus, becomes completely inexcitable. **2.** In psychology, the process by which a stimulus-response bond is broken.

extirpa'tion. Complete removal of a part or of a pathologic growth.

ex'toplasm. The outer condensation of the cytoplasm of a cell.

extor'sion. The act of rotating outward.

extra-. Prefix meaning outside.

extra-artic'ular. Outside of a joint.

extracap'sular. Located or occurring outside of a capsule, as a fracture occurring outside a joint capsule.

extracel'lular. Occurring outside a cell.

extracorpus'cular. Outside of the blood corpuscles.

extracra'nial. Outside of the skull.

extrac'tion. 1. The act of drawing out or removing. **2.** The process of preparing an extract.

   breech e., the manual removal of an infant from the uterus in breech presentation.

   tooth e., removal of a tooth.

extrac'tor. An instrument used in drawing out a bodily part; especially forceps for extracting teeth.

extradu'ral. Located outside of the dura mater.

extrahepat'ic. Located outside of the liver.

extramed'ullary. Located outside of any medulla.

extra'neous. Originating outside of the organism, or not belonging to it.

extraoc'ular. External to the eye.

extraperitone'al. Located outside of the peritoneal cavity.

extrap'olate. To estimate a value or values beyond the observable range from a known trend of

variables; broadly, to estimate or infer from known values.

extrapul'monary. Located outside of the lungs.

extrapyram'idal. Outside of pyramidal; said of descending nerve tracts that are not part of the pyramids of the medulla.

extrapyramidal disease. Any disease affecting the extrapyramidal areas of the brain.

extrasen'sory. Not perceptible by the senses, as some forms of perception such as telepathy or clairvoyance; also called supernatural.

extrasys'tole. A premature contraction of the heart originating at a site other than the usual (ectopic); it may arise from the atrium, the atrioventricular (A-V) node, or the ventricle; the term is loosely applied to all premature contractions, but more correctly limited to interpolated premature contractions.

   atrial e., one due to an irritability of the atria; the early contractions emanate from an impulse in the atria outside of the sinoatrial (S-A) node.

   atrioventricular nodal e., A-V nodal extrasystole; nodal extrasystole; one emanating from the atrioventricular (A-V) node and leading to a simultaneous or near simultaneous contraction of atria and ventricles.

   A-V nodal e., see atrioventricular nodal extrasystole.

   interpolated e., a ventricular extrasystole which, instead of being followed by a compensatory pause, is sandwiched between two consecutive sinus cycles.

   nodal e., see atrioventricular nodal extrasystole.

   supraventricular e., an extrasystole emanating from a center above the ventricles, i.e., atrium or atrioventricular (A-V) node.

   ventricular e., a premature contraction of the ventricles.

extrau'terine. Located outside of the uterus.

extrav'asate. 1. To escape from a vessel into the tissues. **2.** The material that has escaped.

extravasa'tion. Escape of fluid from a vessel into the surrounding tissues.

extravas'cular. Outside of the blood vessels or lymphatics.

ex'travert. See extrovert.

extraver'sion. See extroversion.

extrem'ity. A limb; an arm or a leg.

extrin'sic. Originating outside of a part where it is found or on which it acts.

extrover'sion, extraver'sion. 1. A turning inside out, as of the uterus. **2.** A personality trait in which a person's interests lie mainly in the environment and others rather than in himself.

ex'trovert, ex'travert. A person whose interests lie outside of himself, or who is outwardly directed.

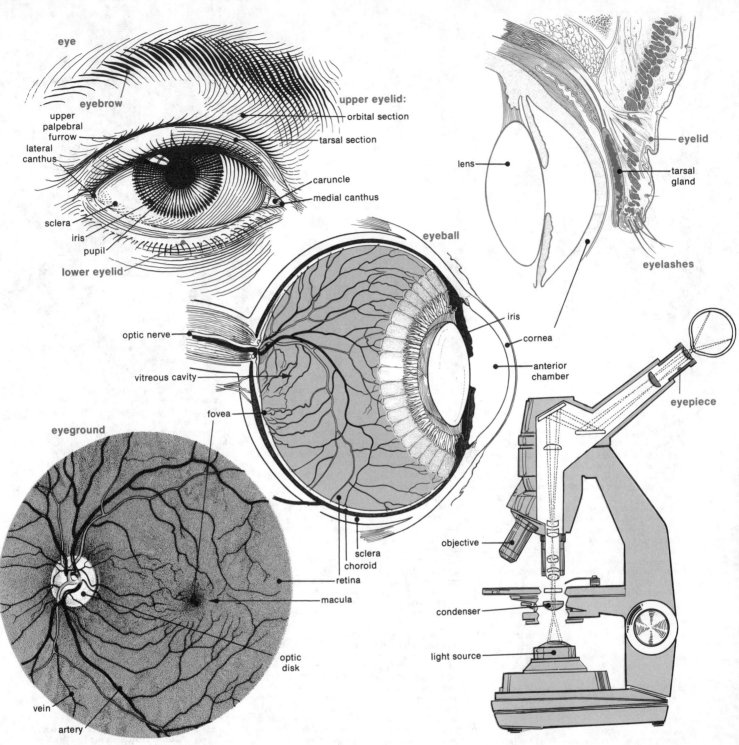

eye

eyebrow

upper palpebral furrow

lateral canthus

sclera

iris

pupil

lower eyelid

upper eyelid:

orbital section

tarsal section

caruncle

medial canthus

eyeball

optic nerve

vitreous cavity

fovea

iris

cornea

anterior chamber

sclera

choroid

retina

macula

optic disk

eyeground

vein

artery

lens

eyelid

tarsal gland

eyelashes

eyepiece

objective

condenser

light source

extrud′e. 1. To push out, or reposition distally. **2.** In dentistry, to move a tooth into a more occlusal position with the teeth of the opposing jaw.

extru′sion. The process of forcing out of a normal position.

extu′bate. To remove a tube, as an intubation tube from the larynx.

extuba′tion. The removal of a tube, specifically, the removal of an intubation tube from the larynx.

ex′udate. Material gradually discharged and deposited in the tissues or a cavity, usually as a result of inflammation.

exuda′tion. The oozing of fluids through the tissues into a cavity or to the surface, usually as a result of inflammation.

exud′ative. Relating to the process of exudation.

exud′e. To ooze; to pass out gradually through the tissues or through an opening.

eye. The organ of vision; in humans, it is a nearly spherical body consisting of three concentric coats: the outermost, fibrous, protective coat, made up of

an opaque, white, posterior portion (five-sixths) called the sclera and an anterior transparent part called the cornea; the middle, vascular, nutritive coat, made up (from behind forward) of choroid, ciliary body, and iris; and the innermost, nervous coat called the retina; within, it contains the anterior and posterior chambers, filled with a clear fluid (aqueous humor), the crystalline lens, and the gelatinous vitreous body.

  fixating e., in strabismus, the eye that is directed toward the object of regard.

  pink e., see pinkeye.

  shipyard e., epidemic keratoconjunctivitis; see under keratoconjunctivitis.

  white of the e., the visible portion of the sclera.

eye′ball. The globe of the eye.

eye′brow. 1. The row of hairs growing between the upper eyelid and the forehead. **2.** The bony ridge over the eye; also called supercilium.

eye′glasses. A pair of ophthalmic lenses mounted on a frame, used as an aid to vision; also

called spectacles and glasses.

eye′ground. The inner surface of the eye seen through the pupil on ophthalmoscopic examination.

eye′lash. One of the short hairs growing on the margin of the eyelid; also called cilium.

eye′lid. One of two folds (upper and lower) which cover and protect the anterior portion of the eyeball.

eye′piece. The lens or system of lenses closest to the eye in an optical instrument such as microscope, that further magnifies the image formed by the objective lens; also called ocular lens.

eye′strain. Fatigue or discomfort associated with the use of the eyes, due to uncorrected errors of refraction, imbalance of the eye muscles, or prolonged use of the eyes.

eye′wash. A medicated irrigating solution used in bathing the eyes, usually containing boric acid, sodium borate, thimerosal, antipyrine, and sodium salicylate; also called collyrium and ophthalmic irrigating solution.

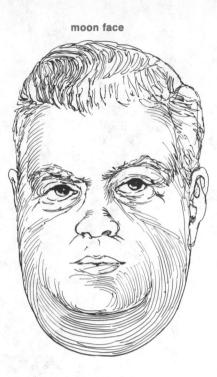

moon face

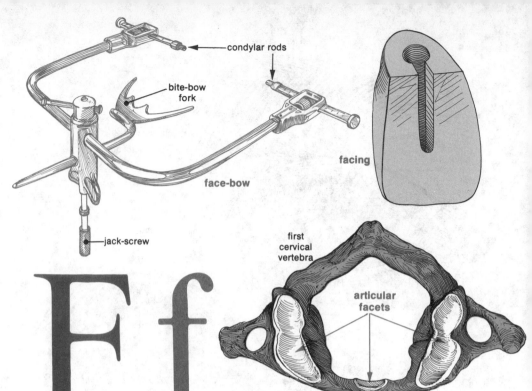

condylar rods

bite-bow fork

face-bow

jack-screw

facing

first cervical vertebra

articular facets

Ff

f. Symbol for focal length.

F₁, F₂, F₃, F₄, etc. Abbreviations for first, second, third, fourth, etc. filial generation; see generation, filial.

Fab. Abbreviation for fragment antigen binding.

F. Symbol for (a) Fahrenheit; (b) farad; (c) visual field; (d) the element fluorine; (d) force; (e) factor.

fabel′la. Latin meaning little bean; in anatomy, the small sesamoid bone sometimes found in the tendon of the lateral head of the gastrocnemius muscle.

fabrica′tion. The feigning of symptoms or illness; the telling of deliberately false statements as if they were true; also called confabulation.

F.A.C.C. Abbreviation for Fellow of the American College of Cardiologists.

F.A.C.D. Abbreviation for Fellow of the American College of Dentists.

face. The front of the head from the forehead to the chin and from ear to ear.

  hippocratic f., hippocratic facies; see under facies.

  masklike f., Parkinson's facies; see under facies.

  moon f., the rounded face observed in individuals with Cushing's disease or in hyperadrenocorticalism.

face-bow. A caliper-like instrument used to record the relationship of the jaws to the temporomandibular joints.

fac′et. An extremely smooth surface on a bone.

  articular f., a small planar or rounded smooth surface on a bone which articulates with another structure.

  costal f., see demifacet.

facetec′tomy. Surgical removal of the facet of a vertebra.

F.A.C.F.P. Abbreviation for Fellow of the American College of Family Physicians.

fa′cial. 1. Of or relating to the face. **2.** The application of cosmetic creams in conjunction with gentle massage of the face.

fa′cies, pl. **fa′cies.** The outward appearance and expression of the face.

  adenoid f., the open-mouthed expression of children with adenoid growths.

  hippocratic f., f. hippocratica, a pinched expression of the face with sunken eyes, hollow cheeks and temples, relaxed lips, and leaden complexion, observed in one dying after an exhausting illness.

  Parkinson's f., one lacking expression due to paralysis agitans.

facilita′tion. The reinforcement of the activity of nervous tissue by the introduction of external impulses; an important protective reflex of the spinal cord; e.g., the reflex withdrawal from pain.

fa′cing. Plastic or porcelain material used to cover the labial or buccal surface of a dental crown.

faciobra′chial. Relating to the face and the arms.

faciocer′vical. Relating to the face and neck.

faciople′gia. Facial palsy; see under palsy.

F.A.C.O.G. Abbreviation for Fellow of the American College of Obstetricians and Gynecologists.

F.A.C.P. Abbreviation for Fellow of the American College of Physicians.

F.A.C.S. Abbreviation for Fellow of the American College of Surgeons.

facti′tious. Artificial; self-induced.

factor. 1. An agent or element that contributes to an action, process, or result. **2.** A gene. **3.** An essential element in a diet, such as a vitamin.

  ABO f.'s, see ABO blood group.

  accelerator f., see factor V.

  antiberiberi f., thiamine.

  antihemolytic f., see factor VIII.

  antihemophilic f. A, see factor VIII.

  antihemophilic f. B, see factor IX.

  antiheparin f., a glycoprotein released from platelets, following platelet aggregation, which shortens the thrombin clotting time in the presence of heparin; also called platelet factor 4.

  antinuclear f., a factor present in serum with strong affinity for nuclei; seen in some collagen disorders including lupus erythematous.

  antipellagra f., nicotinic acid.

  branching f., an enzyme (transglycosylase) in muscle that cleaves α-1,4 linkages in glycogen or starch, transferring the fragments into α-1,6 linkages and creating branches in the polysaccharide molecules; also called α-glucan-branching glycosyltransferase and Q or branching enzyme.

  chemotactic f.'s, soluble substances produced by the reaction of antigen with sensitized leukocytes; they induce migration of neutrophils and monocytes from blood vessels into tissues to ingest and destroy potentially dangerous agents, such as bacteria.

  Christmas f., see factor IX.

  citrovorum f., see folinic acid.

  clotting f.'s, various plasma and tissue components involved in the clotting process.

  corticotropin-releasing f., a substance of hypothalamic origin capable of accelerating pituitary secretion of corticotropin.

  coupling f.'s, proteins that restore phosphorylating ability to mitochondria that have lost it or have become uncoupled.

  erythropoiesis-stimulating f. (ESF), a glycoprotein hormone that stimulates red blood cell production; it acts on the precursor stem cells in the bone marrow, causing them to differentiate into the erythroid cell line; also called erythropoietin.

  extrinsic f., see vitamin B₁₂.

  f. I, fibrinogen, a protein, present in dissolved form in blood plasma; an important factor in the third stage of blood coagulation during which it is converted to fibrin.

  f. II, prothrombin, a stable glycoprotein of plasma which is important in the second stage of blood coagulation where it is converted to thrombin.

  f. III, thromboplastin, a lipoprotein complex liberated from injured tissue.

  f. IV, calcium ions, the presence of which is necessary for many steps of the blood coagulation process.

  f. V, a plasma globulin which acts as an accelerator by speeding the conversion of prothrombin to thrombin in the presence of activated factor X; a congenital deficiency of factor V causes parahemophilia; also known as labile factor or proaccelerin.

  f. VI, no longer considered a coagulation factor; formerly applied to serum accelerator globulin which is activated factor V.

  f. VII, proconvertin, a substance that acts as an accelerator in the extrinsic pathway of prothrombin activation; it is not consumed during the clotting of blood and is, consequently, found in the serum following normal coagulation; congenital or neonatal deficiency of factor VII occurs along with hypoprothrombinemia in hemorrhagic disease of the newborn; it is manifested by purpura and bleeding from the mucous membranes; also called convertin, serum prothrombin conversion accelerator (SPCA), and stable factor.

  f. VIII, the antihemophilic globulin present in plasma, essential in the first phase of clotting; a deficiency of factor VIII causes the hereditary disease, hemophilia A; transmitted by females as a sex-linked characteristic but causes hemorrhagic difficulties almost exclusively in males; also called antihemophilic globulin, antihemophilic factor A, and antihemolytic factor.

  f. IX, a factor essential in the first phase of clotting; a deficiency of factor IX is inherited as a sex-linked recessive trait causing hemophilia B or Christmas disease (after surname of a child in whom this deficiency was first found); also called Christmas factor, plasma thromboplastin component (PTC), and antihemophilic factor B.

  f. X, a procoagulant in normal plasma; a factor required for prothrombin conversion in the presence or absence of tissue extract; a deficiency of factor X may be congenital, but it also occurs in hemorrhagic disease of the newborn, liver disease, and deficiency of vitamin K; also called Stuart-Prower factor.

  f. XI, a factor essential in the first phase of clotting; a deficiency of factor XI is most commonly congeni-

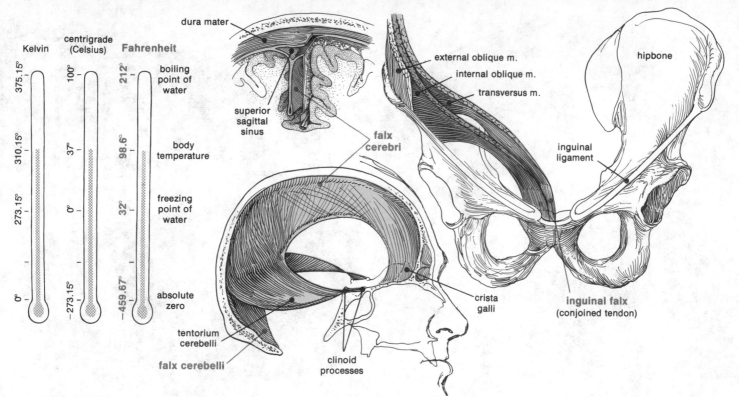

Kelvin — centrigrade (Celsius) — Fahrenheit

- 375.15° / 100° / 212° — boiling point of water
- 310.15° / 37° / 98.6° — body temperature
- 273.15° / 0° / 32° — freezing point of water
- 0° / −273.15° / −459.67° — absolute zero

dura mater

superior sagittal sinus

external oblique m.
internal oblique m.
transversus m.

hipbone

falx cerebri

inguinal ligament

crista galli

inguinal falx (conjoined tendon)

tentorium cerebelli

falx cerebelli

clinoid processes

tal and produces symptoms of mild hemophilia (hemophilia C); also called plasma thromboplastin antecedent (PTA).

f. XII, a stable factor present in normal blood and serum which initiates the process of blood coagulation when the plasma contacts collagen or a foreign surface; it may be bypassed when absent so that hemostasis occurs normally despite a prolonged coagulation time; deficiency of factor XII is caused by an autosomal recessive gene; also called Hageman (after surname of original patient) or contact factor.

f. XIII, a transpeptidase present in normal plasma which cross-links subunits of fibrin monomer to form insoluble fibrin polymer; thrombin catalyzes the conversion of factor XIII into its active form.

follicle-stimulating hormone-releasing f. (FRF), a hypothalamic substance capable of accelerating pituitary secretion of follicle-stimulating hormone; also called FSH-releasing factor.

growth f., any factor capable of promoting growth.

growth hormone-releasing f., (GRF), a substance of hypothalamic origin capable of accelerating pituitary secretion of growth hormone; also called somatotropin-releasing factor.

H f. of Lewis, histamine or histamine-like substance present in the deeper layers of the skin, responsible for inflammatory vascular skin reactions.

Hageman f., see factor XII.

intrinsic f., a mucoprotein produced by the parietal cells of gastric glands essential for absorption of vitamin B_{12} in the ileum; deficiency causes pernicious anemia.

labile f., see factor V.

lipotropic f., choline.

luteinizing hormone-releasing f. (LRF), a substance of hypothalamic origin capable of accelerating pituitary secretion of luteinizing hormone.

pellagra-preventing f. (P-Pf), nicotinic acid.

platelet f. 1 (PF-1), plasma factor V adsorbed on the surface of the platelet.

platelet f. 2 (PF-2), fibrinogen activator on the surface of the platelet.

platelet f. 3, (PF-3), a lipoprotein of the platelet membrane that reacts with factors VIII and IX to activate factor X; it then participates with factor V and with activated factor X to convert prothrombin to thrombin.

platelet f. 4 (PF-4), see antiheparin factor.

prolactin-inhibiting f., a substance of hypothalamic origin capable of inhibiting the synthesis and release of prolactin by the anterior pituitary gland.

releasing f., a substance of hypothalamic origin capable of accelerating the rate of excretion of a given hormone by the anterior pituitary gland.

rheumatoid f., a globulin found in the serum of many individuals with rheumatoid arthritis (70 per cent) and some other conditions; it produces agglutination when added to a suspension of particles coated with pooled human γ-globulin.

secretor f., an inherited factor which permits the secretion of water-soluble forms of A and B-group antigens into saliva and other body fluids.

somatotropin-releasing f., see growth hormone-releasing factor.

somatotropin release-inhibiting f., see somatostatin.

spreading f., hyaluronidase.

stable f., see factor VII.

thyrotropin-releasing f., a substance of hypothalamic origin capable of accelerating pituitary secretion of thyrotropin; thought to be a small basic polypeptide.

tumor-angiogenesis f., a diffusible factor which is mitogenic to capillary endothelium and stimulates rapid formation of new vessels; secreted by malignant tumors and not found in normal tissue with the exception of the placenta; it has a molecular weight of approximately 100,000 and contains 25 per cent ribonucleic acid.

facto'rial. Relating to statistical factors.

fac'ultative. 1. Relating to a mental faculty. **2.** Capable of adapting to varying environmental conditions; e.g., a facultative parasite does not live as a parasite if another food source is available.

fac'ulty. 1. An inherent ability. **2.** Any of the powers of the human mind.

FAD. Abbreviation for flavin adenine dinucleotide.

fagop'yrism, fagopyris'mus. Poisoning by buckwheat, clover, St. John's wort, etc.

Fahr'enheit (F). Denoting a temperature scale that records the freezing point of water at 32° and the boiling point at 212° under normal atmospheric pressure.

fail'ure. 1. The condition of being insufficient. **2.** A cessation of normal functioning.

backward heart f., the theory of backward heart failure maintains that congestive heart failure results from engorgement of the veins causing a "backward" rise in pressure proximal to the failing heart chambers.

cardiac f., heart failure.

congestive heart f., abnormal circulatory congestion resulting from heart failure.

forward heart f., the theory of forward heart failure maintains that congestive heart failure results from inadequate cardiac output, resulting in inadequate kidney blood flow and retention of sodium and water.

heart f., (1) failure of the heart to function effectively as a pump so that it cannot deliver an adequate supply of oxygenated blood to the tissues; also called myocardial failure and cardiac insufficiency or failure; (2) the resulting clinical syndrome.

high output f., condition in which the cardiac output, although at normal levels or higher, is inadequate to meet the demands of the body; seen in states such as marked anemia, Paget's disease, and arteriovenous fistulas.

left ventricular f., heart failure manifested by congestion of the lungs.

low output f., subnormal cardiac output seen in heart failure, usually due to coronary, hypertensive, or valvular disease.

myocardial f., see heart failure. (1).

pacemaker f., failure of an artificial pacemaker to stimulate the heart muscle.

power f., see pump failure.

pump f., failure of the heart as a mechanical pump rather than disturbance of the electrical impulse (arrhythmia); also called power failure.

respiratory f., the failure of the pulmonary system to maintain normal gas tensions of oxygen, carbon dioxide, or both in the arterial circulation.

right ventricular f., heart failure manifested by distention of the neck veins, edema, and enlargement of the liver.

faint. 1. To lose consciousness. **2.** Syncope; generally due to abrupt, usually brief, failure of normal circulation of blood to the brain. **3.** Weak; feeble; lacking strength.

faint'ing. Temporary unconsciousness caused by diminished blood supply to the brain.

fal'ciform, falcat'e. Sickle-shaped.

Falconer-Weddell syndrome. See costoclavicular syndrome.

Fallot's tetralogy. See tetralogy of Fallot.

fall'out. Debris (radioactive material) from the detonation of nuclear weapons that resettles to earth.

local f., dense radioactive particles propelled into the atmosphere by the explosion; they descend to earth within a day or two near the site of the nuclear explosion.

worldwide f., light radioactive particles which ascend into the upper troposphere and stratosphere and are scattered over the earth by atmospheric circulation; they are eventually brought to earth by rain.

falx. A sickle-shaped structure.

f. cerebelli, the fold of cranial dura mater separating the lateral lobes of the cerebellum.

f. cerebri, the fold of cranial dura mater between the cerebral hemispheres.

inguinal f., the united tendons of the transversus

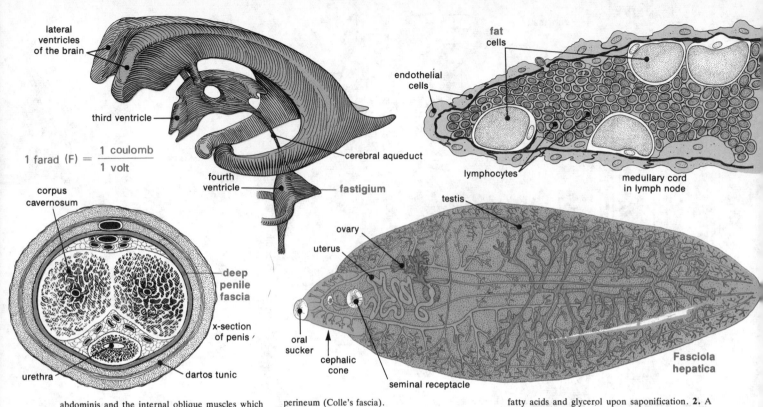

lateral ventricles of the brain

third ventricle

cerebral aqueduct

fourth ventricle

fastigium

$$1 \text{ farad (F)} = \frac{1 \text{ coulomb}}{1 \text{ volt}}$$

corpus cavernosum

deep penile fascia

x-section of penis

urethra

dartos tunic

fat cells

endothelial cells

lymphocytes

medullary cord in lymph node

testis

ovary

uterus

oral sucker

cephalic cone

seminal receptacle

Fasciola hepatica

abdominis and the internal oblique muscles which insert into the crest of the pubic bone and the pectineal line; also called conjoined tendon.

famil'ial. Affecting several individuals in the same family; formerly used to denote disorders caused by a recessive gene; distinguished from hereditary.

fam'ily. In biologic classification, a category ranking above a genus and below an order.

Fanconi's syndrome. A functional disturbance of the proximal kidney tubules resulting in glucosuria, generalized aminoaciduria, phosphaturia, and renal tubular acidosis; it may be inherited, e.g., in cystinosis, or acquired as a consequence of numerous causes including drugs, heavy metals, or disease processes such as amyloidosis and others.

far'ad. A unit of electrical capacity, equal to the capacity of a condenser having a charge of 1 coulomb under an electromotive force of 1 volt.

far'aday. The amount of electricity required to dissolve or deposit 1 gram equivalent weight of a substance in electrolysis, approximately 9.6494×10^4 coulombs.

farad'ic. Relating to induced electricity.

far'cy. A manifestation of glanders; i.e., ulceration of the skin at the site of inoculation of the bacillus followed by involvement of the lymphatic system.

farina'ceous. Of the nature of or containing starch.

farsight'edness. See hyperopia.

fas'cia, *pl.* **fas'ciae.** A sheet of connective tissue that covers the body under the skin, and envelops the muscles and various organs.

  Buck's f., see deep penile fascia.

  bulbar f., connective tissue sheath enveloping the eyeball with the exception of the cornea; attached to the sclera at the sclerocorneal junction; also called Tenon's capsule.

  Camper's f., superficial fatty layer of the superficial fascia of abdomen and perineum.

  Colle's f., the deep membranous layer of the superficial fascia of the perineum.

  deep f., the gray, dense, membranous sheet investing the trunk, neck, limbs, and part of the head; it also covers and holds the muscles and other structures in their proper positions, separating them or joining them for independent or integrated function, respectively.

  deep penile f., a fascial sheath of the penis, derived from the external perineal fascia; also called Buck's fascia.

  f. lata, the broad fascia investing the muscles of the thigh.

  Scarpa's f., the deep membranous layer of the superficial fascia of the abdomen; it is continuous with the deep layer of the superficial fascia of the

perineum (Colle's fascia).

  subcutaneous f., the connective tissue between the skin and the deep fascia, composed of an inner layer and an outer layer that normally contains an accumulation of fat; also called tela subcutanea and superficial fascia.

  subserous f., the layer of connective tissue located beneath the lining of the body cavities and attaching it to the deep fascia; it also covers and supports the viscera; also called tela subserosa.

  transversalis f., the fascial lining of the abdominal cavity between the deep or inner surface of the abdominal musculature and the peritoneum.

  triangular f., reflex inguinal ligament; see under ligament.

fascial. Relating to a fascia.

fasc'icle. A small bundle of fibers, as of nerve or muscle fibers.

fascic'ular. Pertaining to a fascicle or arranged in bundles.

fascicula'tion. 1. The formation of small bundles of fibers (fasciculi). **2.** Involuntary contraction or twitching of a group of muscle fibers; a coarser form of muscular contraction than fibrillation.

fascic'ulus, *pl.* **fascic'uli.** A small bundle of muscle or nerve fibers.

  f. atrioventricularis, atrioventricular bundle; see under bundle.

  inferior longitudinal f., a bundle of association fibers running through the occipital and temporal lobes of the cerebrum.

  medial longitudinal f., a bundle of fibers running under the fourth ventricle from the midbrain to the spinal cord; also called posterior longitudinal bundle.

  proper fasciculi, ascending and descending association fibers surrounding the gray columns of the spinal cord.

Fasci'ola. Liver flukes; a genus of Trematoda.

  F. hepatica, the liver fluke of sheep and cattle; occasionally transmitted to man through the ingestion of uncooked infected liver; formerly called *Distomum hepaticum*.

fascioli'asis. Infection with a species of *Fasciola*.

Fasciolop'sis. A genus of intestinal Trematoda (flukes).

fas'cioplasty. Reparative surgery on a fascia.

fascior'rhaphy. Suture of a fascia or an aponeurosis; also called aponeurorrhaphy.

fasciot'omy. Surgical incision through a fascia.

fast. Resistant to change.

fastig'ium. 1. The peak or highest point of the roof of the fourth ventricle of the brain. **2.** The height of a fever or any acute state; also called maximum.

fat. 1. Any of several organic compounds that yield

fatty acids and glycerol upon saponification. **2.** A mixture of such compounds comprising most of the cell contents of adipose tissue; occurring also in lesser amounts in other animal cells and some plant cells.

  brown f., a lobulated brown mass of tissue composed of cells containing numerous fat globules, found primarily in the interscapular region of the human newborn, hibernating animals, and other mammals; also called interscapular gland.

  saturated f., saturated fatty acid; see under acid.

  unsaturated f., unsaturated fatty acid; see under acid.

fat'al. Causing death.

fatal'ity. Anything resulting in death.

fatigabil'ity. Condition of becoming easily tired.

fatigue. A feeling of exhaustion with decreased efficiency resulting from physical or mental exertion.

  battle f., a severe anxiety state seen in front-line soldiers, characterized by loss of effectiveness, poor judgment, physical complaints, and/or feeling of imminent death.

  flying f., chronic functional disorder occurring to aviators after prolonged piloting of an aircraft; also called aeroasthenia.

fatty acid. See under acid.

fau'ces. The passage from the oral cavity to the oral pharynx, including the lumen and its boundaries; the aperture by which the mouth communicates with the pharynx.

  anterior pillar of the f., palatoglossal fold which rises archlike on each side of the posterior limit of the oral cavity.

  posterior pillar of the f., palatopharyngeal fold just posterior to the palatine tonsil.

fave'olus. A small depression.

fa'vism. Acute hemolytic anemia caused by ingestion of the fava bean or inhalation of the pollen of its flower; seen in individuals of Mediterranean extraction whose red blood cells are deficient in the enzyme glucose 6-phosphate dehydrogenase (not all individuals with this enzyme deficiency are susceptible).

fa'vus. A chronic fungus infection, usually of the scalp, caused by *Trichophyton schoenleini*; also called tinea capitis.

FDA. Abbreviation for Food and Drug Administration.

Fe. Chemical symbol of the element iron, derived from the Latin *ferrum*.

fear. A feeling of apprehension or alarm in response to an external source of danger.

  morbid f., phobia.

features. The outward appearance of the face or

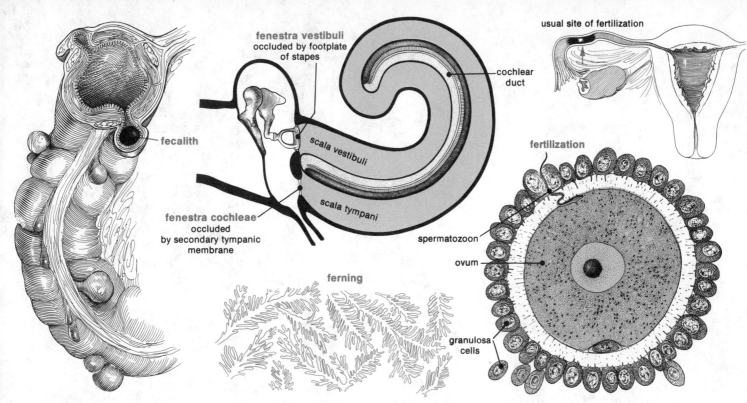

fecalith

fenestra vestibuli
occluded by footplate
of stapes

cochlear duct

scala vestibuli

fenestra cochleae
occluded
by secondary tympanic
membrane

scala tympani

ferning

usual site of fertilization

fertilization

spermatozoon

ovum

granulosa cells

any of its parts.

febrifa′cient. 1. Any substance that produces a fever. **2.** Causing fever.

feb′rile. Having fever.

fe′cal. Relating to feces.

fe′calith. A concretion of feces.

fecalur′ia. The passage of fecal matter with the urine in persons with a connecting channel (fistula) between the rectum and the bladder.

fe′ces. The waste matter discharged from the bowel.

fec′ulent. Fecal; foul.

fe′cundate. To fertilize; to impregnate.

fecunda′tion. Fertilization; impregnation.

fecun′dity. Ability to produce offspring abundantly; pronounced fertility.

fee′ble. Infirm; weak; lacking vitality.

feeblemind′edness. Obsolete term for mental retardation.

feed′back. 1. The process whereby a portion of a system's output, as of an amplifier, is returned to the input; return of information from the output to the control system so as to modify the nature of the control. **2.** The portion of the output so returned. **3.** The feeling created by another person's reactions to oneself.

  negative f., a signal or information returning from the output to the control system which results in reduced output.

  positive f., a signal or information returning to the control system from the output which results in increased output.

feed′ing. Administration of nourishment.

  forced f., the administration of liquid food through a sterile lubricated tube which is passed (nasally or orally) into the stomach.

fee′ling. 1. A sensation perceived by the sense of touch. **2.** Emotional or affective state or process. **3.** A vague belief.

Fehling′s rea′gent. See solution, Fehling's.

fella′tio. Oral penile stimulation.

fel′on. An infection of the distal fat pad at the tip of a finger; manifested by progressive tenderness and throbbing pain.

Felty′s syndrome. Rheumatoid arthritis, leukopenia, and enlargement of the spleen.

fe′male. Relating to or denoting the sex that bears young or produces ova or eggs.

fem′inine. Of or relating to the female sex, or having qualities usually associated with the female.

fem′inism. The possession of feminine characteristics by the male.

feminiza′tion. The development of female characteristics by the male.

fem′oral. Relating to the femur or to the thigh.

femto-. Combining form used in the metric system to indicate one-quadrillionth (10^{-15}) of any unit; e.g., femtoliter.

fe′mur. The thighbone; the longest and strongest bone in the body; see table of bones.

fenes′tra, pl. **fenes′trae.** A window-like opening.

  f. vestibuli, oval window, an oval opening between the middle ear and the vestibule of the internal ear; closed by the footplate of the stapes.

  f. cochleae, round window, a round opening in the medial wall of the middle ear leading into the cochlea.

fen′estrated. Pierced with one or more small window-like openings.

fenestra′tion. 1. The act of perforating. **2.** The surgical creation of an opening in the labyrinth of the internal ear to improve hearing in patients afflicted with otosclerosis.

fer′ment. A substance that causes chemical changes in another substance, without itself changing; formerly used interchangeably with enzyme, now applied to a substance that is not removable from the cell that produces it.

ferment′. To undergo fermentation.

fermen′table. Capable of undergoing fermentation.

fermenta′tion. A chemical decomposition induced in a carbohydrate by a ferment such as yeast, bacterium, or mold.

fermen′tative. Having the ability to cause fermentation.

fer′mium. Radioactive element; symbol Fm, atomic number 100.

fern′ing. The typical palm-leaf pattern formed, upon crystallization, by cervical mucus as a result of electrolyte action on protein; it occurs in the proliferative phase of the menstrual cycle; also called cervical mucus arborization.

ferri-. Combining form denoting iron, especially with a ferric valence.

fer′ric. Relating to or containing iron; especially a salt containing iron in its highest valence (3).

fer′ritin. A protein rich in iron (up to 23 per cent) formed by the union of ferric iron with apoferritin; occurs mainly in the liver, spleen, and intestinal mucosa.

ferro-. Prefix denoting the presence of iron or the divalent ion Fe^{++} in a compound.

ferrocy′anide. A compound containing the negative ion $Fe(CN)_6^{4-}$.

ferropor′phyrin. A derivative of ferrous porphyrin in which a central iron atom is linked to the nitrogen atoms of the porphyrin.

ferropro′tein. A protein containing iron in a pros-

thetic group.

ferroprotopor′phyrin. See heme.

fer′rous. Relating to or containing iron; especially a salt containing iron in its lowest valence (2).

  f. fumarate, a reddish orange compound used as a hematinic; also called iron fumarate.

  f. sulfate, compound widely used in treating uncomplicated iron deficiency anemia; also called iron sulfate and green vitriol.

ferrug′inous. Containing iron; also called chalybeate.

fer′rum. Latin for iron.

fert′ile. Possessing the capacity to reproduce.

fertil′ity. The capacity to initiate or support conception.

fertiliza′tion. The union of a spermatozoon with an ovum.

ferves′cence. An increase of fever.

fes′ter. To form pus.

fes′tinant. Accelerating; rapid.

festina′tion. The involuntary acceleration of walking which occurs when the center of gravity is displaced, as seen in paralysis agitans and some other nervous diseases.

festoon′. A carving in the base material of a denture simulating the contours of the natural tissue that is being replaced by the denture.

  gingival f., swelling or rounding of the marginal gingiva usually due to inflammation.

festoon′ing. The process of cutting, carving, or grinding material to accommodate the contours of natural tissue, as the cutting of a round copper band in order to fit around a prepared tooth and rest snugly on the gingiva prior to taking an impression.

fe′tal. Relating to a fetus.

fe′ticide. The intentional destruction of the embryo or fetus in the uterus; also called induced abortion.

fe′tid. Having a disagreeable odor.

fet′ish. An object to which excessive attention or reverence is attached; often a source of sexual stimulation or gratification.

fet′ishism. Excessive emotional attachment to an inanimate object or body part which serves as a substitute for a human sexual object.

fetog′raphy. Roentgenography of the fetus in utero.

fetol′ogy. The branch of medicine concerned with the fetus and its diseases.

fetom′etry. Estimation of the size of the fetal head prior to delivery.

fetoplacen′tal. Relating to the fetus and placenta.

α-fetoprotein (AFP). A protein substance normally found in the fetus, which also has been found

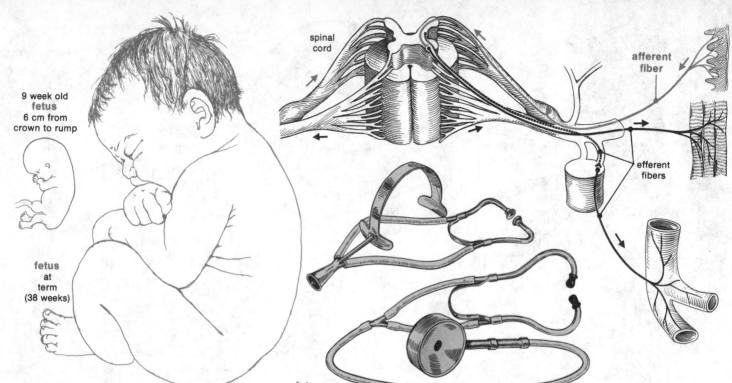

9 week old fetus 6 cm from crown to rump

fetus at term (38 weeks)

spinal cord

afferent fiber

efferent fibers

fetoscopes

in the sera of a large number of individuals with hepatoma.

fe'tor. An offensive odor.

f. ex ore, halitosis.

f. hepaticus, an unpleasant odor of the breath of individuals with severe liver disorders.

f. oris, halitosis.

fet'oscope. Instrument for auscultation of the heart of the fetus; also called fetal stethoscope.

fe'tus. The developing offspring in the uterus, generally from the second month of pregnancy to birth; during the first two months of development, it is called an embryo.

fe'ver. A rise in body temperature above the normal of 98.6°F; usually a temperature of 99.6°F orally or 100°F rectally, or at least 1°F higher than the normal for that individual; also called pyrexia.

blackwater f., malarial hemoglobinuria; see under hemoglobinuria.

canicola f., disease caused by the bacterium *Leptospira canicola;* transmitted to man by contact with infected dog urine.

cat-scratch f., see cat-scratch disease.

Colorado tick f., an acute viral disease (similar to Rocky Mountain spotted fever) transmitted to man by the tick *Dermacentor andersoni;* marked chiefly by fever and leukopenia, but no rash.

desert f., see coccidioidomycosis.

familial Mediterranean f., periodic abdominalgia; see under abdominalgia.

glandular f., infectious mononucleosis; see under mononucleosis.

Haverhill f., disorder caused by infection with *Streptobacillus moniliformis;* marked by fever, rash, and arthritis (usually of the large joints and spine), and lasting from two to three weeks; although the disease is caused by the same organism as that causing rat-bite fever, it is not transmitted by a rat's bite.

hay f., a seasonal irritative inflammation of the mucous membranes of the eye and nose, caused by an allergic reaction to various pollens; not actually associated with a rise in body temperature.

hemorrhagic f., disease of unknown cause marked primarily by fever, capillary hemorrhages, and shock; also called Manchurian or Korean hemorrhagic fever.

icterohemorrhagic f., see Weil's disease.

island f., see tsutsugamushi disease.

jungle yellow f., a form of yellow fever transmitted to man by some forest mosquito in the absence of *Aedes asgipti* (the domestic mosquito).

malignant tertian f., malarial fever usually occurring every other day. See also malaria.

Malta f., see brucellosis.

Mediterranean f., (1) periodic abdominalgia; see under abdominalgia; (2) see brucellosis.

mountain f., altitude sickness; see under sickness.

Oroya f., the acute form and usually the first stage of bartonellosis, endemic disease of the Peruvian Andes; marked by fever, rheumatic pains, anemia, and albuminuria. See also bartonellosis.

paratyphoid f., an infectious disease with symptoms resembling those of typhoid fever, but milder.

pharyngoconjunctival f., fever, pharyngitis, and acute follicular conjunctivitis caused by a virus, usually type 3 adenovirus; conjunctivitis is the chief complaint; it primarily affects children, who acquire it from swimming pools.

pretibial f., a form of leptospirosis first seen at Fort Bragg, North Carolina; marked by mild fever, splenomegaly, and a rash on the anterior surface of the legs; also called Fort Bragg fever.

puerperal f., fever occurring after childbirth.

Q f., a bacterial disease resembling influenza, caused by *Coxiella burneti;* marked by headache, fever, and constitutional symptoms; sometimes associated with inflammation of the lungs; usually acquired by inhalation of the agent.

quartan f., malarial fever in which the paroxysm usually recurs every third day. See also malaria.

quotidian f., daily fever occurring in quotidian malaria. See also malaria.

rat-bite f., disease marked by inflammation of the lymph nodes and lymphatic vessels due to infection with *Spirillum minor* or *Streptobacillus moniliformis;* transmitted by the bite of an infected rat or any rodent; also called headache fever.

recurrent f., relapsing fever.

relapsing f., an acute infectious bacterial disease marked by alternating periods of fever and apyrexia, each lasting about six days; caused by species of the genus *Borrelia;* transmitted to man by either a louse or a soft tick.

rheumatic f., a disease caused by infection with a β-hemolytic streptococcus; it begins with a sore throat and continues with a rapid rise of temperature, prostration, and inflammation of the joints; the heart is often affected.

Rocky Mountain spotted f., an acute infectious bacterial disease marked by fever, bone and muscle pain, headache, and a generalized rash; caused by *Rickettsia rickettsii;* transmitted to man by several varieties of hard ticks; also called spotted or tick fever and tick typhus.

sandfly f., a viral disease transmitted to man by the fly *Phlebotomus papatassi;* marked by fever, ocular pain, and general malaise, followed by complete recovery; also called phlebotomus or pappataci fever.

San Joaquin Valley f., see coccidioidomycosis.

scarlet f., an acute infectious disease marked by high fever, sore throat, and a skin rash; caused by β-hemolytic streptococcus; also called scarlatina.

spotted f., (1) meningococcal meningitis; (2) Rocky Mountain spotted fever.

swamp f., (1) a viral disease of horses marked by fever, staggering gait, and progressive anemia; (2) malaria.

tertian f., malarial fever usually occurring every other day. See also malaria.

tick f., (1) any infectious disease transmitted by the bite of a tick and caused by a protozoan blood parasite; (2) Rocky Mountain spotted fever.

trench f., a relapsing type of fever caused by *Rochalimaea quintana* and transmitted by infected lice; observed in troops during World War I.

tsutsugamushi f., see tsutsugamushi disease.

typhoid f., an acute infectious disease caused by *Salmonella typhi;* marked by a continued fever that has an insidious start, headache, mental depression, prostration, enlargement of the spleen, a maculopapular rash, and sometimes diarrhea.

typhus f., see typhus.

undulant f., see brucellosis.

West Nile f., acute illness marked by fever, headache, a papular rash, lymphadenopathy, and leukopenia; caused by a mosquito-borne virus.

yellow f., an acute infectious disease caused by a specific virus and transmitted by a certain genus of mosquito (*Aedes*); it is characterized by fever, degeneration of the liver (producing jaundice), and intestinal disturbances; also called yellow jack and amarilla.

FF. Abbreviation for filtration fraction.

FHR. Abbreviation for fetal heart rate.

fi'ber. Any slender, threadlike structure.

A f.'s, myelinated fibers of the somatic nervous system having conduction rates from 15 to 100 meters per second.

accelerator f.'s, nerve fibers conveying impulses that increase the force and rapidity of the heartbeat; also called augmentor fibers.

adrenergic f.'s, nerve fibers that release adrenaline-like substances at the synapse.

afferent f.'s, nerve fibers conveying impulses to a nerve center in the brain or spinal cord.

alpha f.'s, somatic motor or proprioceptive fibers having a conduction rate of 100 meters per second.

association f.'s, nerve fibers connecting different areas of the cerebral cortex in the same hemisphere.

augmentor f.'s, see accelerator fibers.

B f.'s, small fibers of the autonomic nervous system having a conduction rate of three to 14 meters per second.

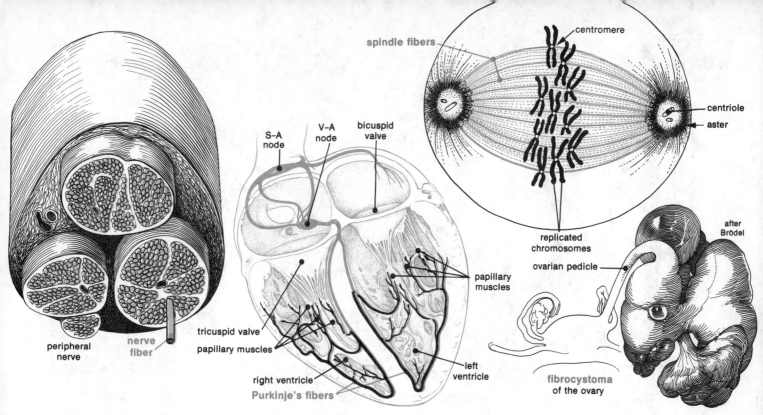

peripheral nerve · **nerve fiber** · **tricuspid valve** · **papillary muscles** · **right ventricle** · **Purkinje's fibers** · **S-A node** · **V-A node** · **bicuspid valve** · **papillary muscles** · **left ventricle** · **spindle fibers** · **centromere** · **centriole** · **aster** · **replicated chromosomes** · **ovarian pedicle** · **fibrocystoma of the ovary** · after Brödel

beta f.'s, somatic nerve fibers having a conduction rate of 40 meters per second.

C f.'s, unmyelinated nerve fibers of the autonomic nervous system having a conduction rate of two meters per second.

cholinergic f.'s, nerve fibers that release acetylcholine at the synapse.

collagen f.'s, collagenous f.'s, the flexible fibers making up the principal constituent of connective tissue; also called white fibers.

depressor f.'s, sensory or afferent nerve fibers which, when stimulated, diminish vascular tone and lower blood pressure.

efferent f., one that conveys impulses from a nerve center in the brain or spinal cord.

elastic f.'s, fibers of elastic properties forming a network in the substance of some connective tissue; also called yellow fibers.

gamma f.'s, somatic nerve fibers having a conduction rate of 20 meters per second.

Golgi's f.'s (types I and II), terms given to the axons of Golgi cells, types I and II.

gray f.'s, see unmyelinated fibers.

inhibitory f.'s, nerve fibers that slow down the action of an organ.

myelinated f.'s, nerve fibers possessing a myelin sheath.

nerve f., one of the slender units of a nerve trunk; the axon of a nerve cell.

nonmyelinated f.'s, unmyelinated fibers.

pressor f.'s, sensory nerve fibers which, upon stimulation, cause narrowing of blood vessels and rise of blood pressure.

projection f.'s, nerve fibers that connect the cerebral cortex with other areas of the brain.

Purkinje's f.'s, specialized fibers formed of modified heart muscle cells located beneath the endocardium; concerned with the conduction of stimuli from the atria to the ventricles.

Sharpey's f.'s, thick perforating collagenous or fibroelastic bundles that attach periosteum to bone; they are continuations of the periosteal fibers and pierce the bone obliquely or at right angles to its long axis.

spindle f., one of several filaments extending between the poles of a dividing cell, forming together a spindle-shaped structure; also called traction fiber.

unmyelinated f.'s, nerve fibers lacking a myelin sheath; also called Remak's or gray fibers.

white f.'s, see collagen fibers.

yellow f.'s, see elastic fibers.

fi′berscope. A viewing instruments with very fine, flexible glass rods for light transmission (fiber optics).

fi′bril. A minute, slender fiber or filament.

Ebner's f.'s, slender collagen fibers in the cementum and dentin of a tooth.

fi′brillar, fi′brillary. 1. Relating to a fibril. **2.** Relating to twitching of small skeletal or smooth muscles.

fi′brillate. 1. To be in a state of fibrillation. **2.** To become fibrillar. **3.** Composed of fibrils.

fibrilla′tion. 1. The rapid contractions or quivering of muscular fibrils. **2.** The formation of fibrils.

atrial f., the replacement of the normal rhythmic contractions of the cardiac atria by rapid irregular quivers.

ventricular f., rapid, irregular twitchings that replace the normal contractions of the muscular walls of the ventricles.

fibril′liform. Having the general configuration of a fibril.

fibrillogen′esis. The normal development of minute fibrils in collagenous fibers of connective tissue.

fi′brin. A fibrous, insoluble protein derived from fibrinogen through the action of thrombin; the basic component of a blood clot.

fi′brination. 1. The formation of a fibrin. **2.** The formation of an abnormally large amount of fibrin; denoting the condition of the blood in certain inflammatory diseases; also called fibrinosis.

fibrin′ogen. Factor I; a protein, present in dissolved form in blood plasma, which is converted into a network of delicate filaments (fibrin) by the action of the enzyme thrombin; the blood cells become entangled in the fibrin network, thus producing coagulation.

fibrin′ogenope′nia. Deficiency in the concentration of fibrinogen in the blood.

fi′brinoid. 1. Resembling fibrin. **2.** An acidophilic, homogeneous, refractile material.

fibrinol′ysin. An enzyme that dissolves fibrin in clotted blood.

fibrinol′ysis. The destruction of fibrin in clotted blood by enzyme action, resulting in the dissolution of a clot.

fibrinopur′ulent. Relating to a discharge that contains pus and a large amount of fibrin.

fibrino′sis. See fibrination (2).

fi′brinous. Relating to or composed of fibrin.

fibro-, fibr-. Combining forms denoting fibrous tissue; e.g., fibroma.

fibroadeno′ma. A benign tumor derived from glandular epithelium.

fibroad′ipose. Containing both fibrous and fatty elements; also called fibrofatty.

fi′broblast. An elongated, flattened, spindle-shaped cell with cytoplasmic processes at each end,

having a flat, oval nucleus showing a finely granular chromatin with one or two nucleoli; one of the most common cell types found in growing connective tissue.

fibrocarcino′ma. See carcinoma, scirrhous.

fibrocar′tilage. A type of cartilage containing collagenic fibers.

fibrochondri′tis. Inflammation of fibrocartilage.

fibrochondro′ma. A benign tumor composed primarily of cartilage and an abundant amount of fibrous tissue.

fi′brocyst. A lesion consisting of a cyst within a fibrous network.

fibrocys′tic. Marked by the presence of fibrocysts.

fibrocystic disease of breast. Benign disease of the female breast marked by one of the three basic morphologic patterns: formation of cysts, overgrowth of stroma and intraductal epithelium, or sclerotic proliferation of gland tissue; there is frequent concurrence of these patterns, with one usually predominating; also called cystic disease of breast, cystic hyperplasia of breast, chronic cystic mastitis, and mammary dysplasia.

fibrocystic disease of pancreas. See cystic fibrosis of pancreas.

fibrocysto′ma. A benign tumor characterized by cysts within a conspicuous fibrous stroma.

fi′brocyte. A resting or quiescent fibroblast.

fibroelas′tic. Made up of collagen and elastic fibers.

fibroelasto′sis. Overgrowth of fibroelastic tissue.

endocardial f., endomyocardial fibroelastosis.

endomyocardial f., congenital heart disease characterized by fibroelastic thickening of the mural endocardium, especially of the left ventricle; the rest of the chambers and the valves may also be involved; also called endocardial sclerosis.

fibroenchondro′ma. A benign tumor located within a bone and composed of mature cartilage and abundant fibrous tissue.

fibroepithelio′ma. A skin tumor composed of fibrous tissue and basal cells of the epidermis; it may be transformed into a basal cell carcinoma; also called premalignant fibroepithelioma and fibroepithelioma of Pinkus.

fibrofat′ty. See fibroadipose.

fi′broid. 1. Resembling or containing fibers. **2.** Colloquial clinical term for certain types of leiomyoma (a benign tumor), especially those occurring in the uterus.

fibrolipo′ma. A tumor composed predominantly of fat cells but containing abundant fibrous tissue; also called lipoma fibrosum.

fibro′ma. A benign tumor derived from fibrous connective tissue; also called fibrocellular tumor.

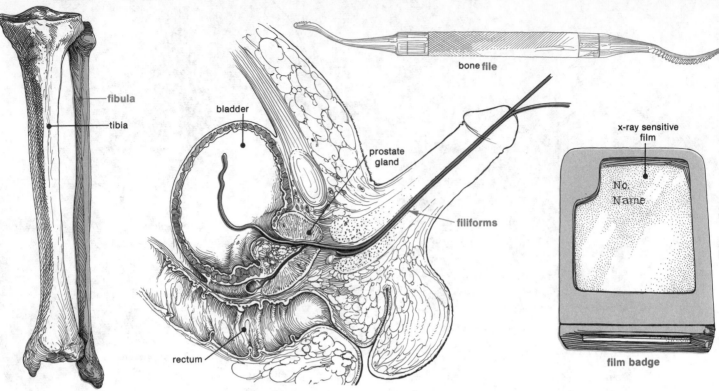

fibula

tibia

bladder

bone file

prostate gland

filiforms

rectum

x-ray sensitive film

No. Name

film badge

concentric f., a benign growth that occupies the entire inner wall of the uterus.

f. molluscum gravidarum, the occurrence of numerous, small fibrous tumors of the skin, colorless or pigmented, appearing during pregnancy and disappearing at its termination.

fibromato'sis. 1. Condition marked by the development of multiple fibromas. **2.** Abnormal overdevelopment of fibrous tissue.

fibromus'cular. Denoting tissues that are both fibrous and muscular.

fibromyo'ma. Leiomyoma; a benign tumor of smooth muscle origin, containing a relatively small amount of fibrous tissue.

fibromyosi'tis. Chronic inflammation of a muscle with overgrowth of its connective tissue.

fibromyxo'ma. Term formerly used to designate connective tissue tumors which are predominantly fibrous but contain abundant acellular elements.

fibropla'sia. Abnormal production of fibrous tissue.

retrolental f., abnormal increase of fibrous tissue behind the lens of the eye, attributed to exposure of newborn infants, usually premature, to 100 per cent oxygen.

fibroplas'tic. Producing fibrous tissue.

fibrosarco'ma. A malignant tumor composed of fibrous connective tissue.

fibro'sis. The formation of fibrous tissue, denoting especially an abnormal degenerative process.

cystic f., see cystic fibrosis of pancreas.

endomyocardial f., thickening of the ventricular myocardium.

hepatic f., a liver disorder marked by an increase in connective tissue without disturbance of the lobular architecture.

perimuscular f., fibrosis involving the renal arteries; also called subadventitial fibrosis.

retroperitoneal f., a disorder, usually of unknown etiology, in which an exaggerated fibrocytic response leads to fibrosis involving retroperitoneal structures, particularly the ureters; rarely are the bile ducts involved; the pharmaceutical preparation methysergide has been implicated in some cases as a cause, although the mechanism remains unclear.

subadventitial f., see perimuscular fibrosis.

fibrosi'tis. Inflammatory hyperplasia of fibrous or connective tissue of the muscles.

fi'brous. Composed of, containing, or resembling fibers of connective tissue.

fib'ula. The lateral and smaller of the two bones of the leg, between the knee and ankle.

fib'ular. Of or relating to the fibula.

fibulocalca'neal. Relating to the fibula and the calcaneus.

Fiedler's myocardi'tis. See myocarditis, acute isolated.

field. A limited area.

auditory f., the area within which a definite sound is heard.

magnetic f., the area of space about a magnet in which its magnetic force is perceptible.

visual f., the area of physical space visible to the eye in a fixed position.

FIGlu. Abbreviation for formiminoglutamic acid.

figure. Shape; form.

mitotic f., the appearance of a cell undergoing mitosis.

fil'ament. A fine threadlike structure.

filament'ous. Threadlike; in bacteriology, denoting a colony made up of long, interwoven, threadlike structures.

Fila'ria. Term formerly used for a genus of parasitic threadworms now given other names.

F. bancrofti, old term for *Wuchereria bancrofti*.

F. malaya, old term for *Brugia malayi*.

F. medinensis, old term for *Dracunculus medinensis*.

F. oculi humani, old term for *Loa Loa*.

fila'ria, *pl.* **fila'rial.** Any nematode worm of the superfamily Filarioidea.

filari'asis. A disease caused by the presence of a parasitic threadworm (filaria) in the body; the best known form of filariasis is elephantiasis.

filar'icide. Any agent that destroys parasitic nematode worms.

filar'iform. Hairlike, as filariae.

Filarioi'dea. A superfamily of true nematode worms that infest man and other vertebrates.

Filaroi'des. A genus of roundworms parasitic in the lungs, bronchi, and trachea of dogs.

file. A device used for cutting, smoothing, or grinding.

fil'ial. Of or relating to a son or daughter.

fili-form. 1. Thread-shaped. **2.** An extremely slender bougie. **3.** In bacteriology, denoting an even, hairlike growth along the line of inoculation in streak or stab cultures.

fil'let. 1. A thin strip of bandage or tape used for making traction. **2.** A band of fibers; also called lemniscus.

filling. Any substance used to fill a space, cavity, or container; e.g., amalgam placed into a tooth cavity to restore the missing portion of the tooth.

acrylic resin f., a material used for restorations in teeth when esthetic properties are needed.

combination f., a tooth restoration composed of two or more layers of different materials.

compound f., a restoration which involves more than one surface of a tooth.

direct f., one that is prepared directly in the tooth cavity.

indirect f., one that is constructed from an accurate impression of the tooth and then cemented into the tooth cavity.

overhanging f., one with excessive material at the junction of the filling and the tooth.

permanent f., one intended to be functional for as long a period as possible.

root canal f., material placed in the root canal of a tooth to eliminate the space once occupied by the dental pulp.

silicate f., a restoration of lost tooth structure made with silicate cement, essentially acid-soluble glass.

temporary f., an interim filling.

treatment f., a temporary filling for allaying the sensitivity of dentin prior to placing the final restorative material.

zinc oxide-eugenol f., a temporary filling material often referred to as ZOE.

film. 1. A thin adherent coating on the surface of teeth consisting chiefly of a mucinous mixture of saliva, microorganisms, and blood and tissue elements. **2.** A thin cellulose sheet coated with a light-sensitive emulsion used in taking photographs.

bite wing f., dental roentgenographic film with an appendage that is held between the occlusal surface of the teeth.

f. badge, a small device containing x-ray sensitive film, worn by individuals who are exposed to ionizing radiation, to record the amount of radiation to which they have been exposed; exposure is determined by measuring the degree of darkening of the film.

f. fault, a defect in an x-ray film due either to physical or chemical causes or to electrical errors in its production.

f. holder, a light-tight film container used in extraoral roentgenography.

fogged f. fault, hazy appearance of a roentgenogram caused by exposure of film to light or stray radiation, subjection to unusual temperatures or chemical actions, or use of outdated film.

filopo'dium, *pl.* **filopo'dia.** A slender process used for locomotion by certain free-living amebae.

fil'ter. 1. A porous substance or screen through which liquids or gases are passed in order to separate any suspended material. **2.** A device or screen that permits the passage of rays of certain wavelengths only. **3.** To pass a substance or rays through such devices.

Berkefeld f., one made of diatomaceous earth through which bacteria do not pass; available in three grades of porosity: W, fine; N, normal; V,

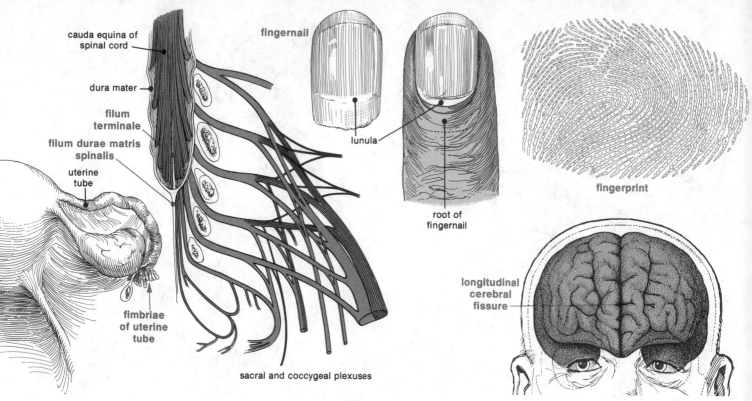

cauda equina of
spinal cord

dura mater

**filum
terminale**

**filum durae matris
spinalis**

uterine
tube

fimbriae
of uterine
tube

fingernail

lunula

root of
fingernail

fingerprint

longitudinal
cerebral
fissure

sacral and coccygeal plexuses

---

coarse.

fil'terable, fil'trable. 1. Capable of passing through a filter. **2.** Applied to viruses, minute enough to be able to pass through a fine filter.

fil'trate. Liquid that has passed through a filter.

filtra'tion. The process of passing a fluid through a filter employing differential pressure.

fi'lum, *pl.* **fi'la.** Latin for thread; a filamentous or threadlike structure or part.

f. durae matris spinalis, filament of the spinal dura mater; the thin sheath covering the filum terminale and attached to the periosteum of the coccyx; it is continuous above with the dura.

f. radicularia nervorum spinalium, root filament of the spinal nerve emerging from the spinal medulla.

f. terminale, the slender fibrous prolongation of the spinal medulla which anchors the spinal cord to the coccyx; it extends from the level of the second lumbar vertebra to the coccyx.

fim'bria, *pl.* **fim'briae. 1.** Any fringelike structure. **2.** See pilus (2).

f. hippocampi, a narrow band of white fibers along the medial border of the hippocampus.

fimbriae of uterine tube, the numerous irregular fringelike processes on the distal part of the uterine tube.

fim'briate, fim'briated. 1. Fringed; having fimbriae. **2.** In bacteriology, denoting a colony with slender fringelike projections.

fim'brioplasty. A corrective operation on the fringed processes of the uterine tube.

fing'er. One of five digits of the hand.

baseball f., see mallet finger.

drop f., see mallet finger.

clubbed f., see digit, clubbed.

drumstick f., clubbed digit; see under digit.

fifth f., the little finger.

first f., the thumb.

fourth f., the ring finger, the thumb being considered the first.

hammer f., see mallet finger.

hippocratic f., clubbed digit; see under digit.

index f., the second digit, the thumb being considered the first; the finger next to the thumb; also called forefinger.

mallet f., a finger marked by constant flexion of the distal phalanx; it cannot be actively extended due to detachment of the extensor tendon; also called baseball finger, drop finger, and hammer finger.

middle f., the third finger.

ring f., the fourth finger.

second f., the index finger.

snapping f., see trigger finger.

third f., the middle finger.

trigger f., one that locks in a flexed position; it can be extended only with difficulty associated with a snapping or clicking noise; it is due to narrowing of the flexor sheath at the level of the metacarpal neck; also called snapping finger.

webbed f.'s, congenital abnormality in which two or more fingers are united in various degrees by a fold of skin.

fingeragno'sia. Loss of ability to recognize the individual fingers of the hand.

fing'er cot. A protective rubber covering for the finger.

fing'ernail. A horny plate on the dorsal surface of the tip of each finger. See also nail.

fing'erprint. An ink impression of the configuration of the ridges on the skin surface of the distal phalanx of a finger; usually used as a means of identification; the patterns are sometimes of clinical significance.

Galton's system of classification of f.'s, the arch-loop-whorl system of classifying variations in the patterns of the ridges.

first aid. Emergency assistance given to the injured or sick before the availability of professional medical care.

fis'sion. 1. Division of a cell; form of asexual reproduction. **2.** The splitting of an atom in two parts.

fissip'arous. Reproducing by fission.

fissu'ra, *pl.* **fissur'ae.** Fissure; cleft.

fissura'tion. 1. The condition of being fissured. **2.** The formation of a fissure.

fissure. A cleft, groove, or slit.

anal f., a painful, difficult to heal slit in the mucous membrane of the anus.

anterior median f., the deep groove in the midline of the anterior aspect of the spinal cord.

auricular f., a groove, between the tympanic and the squamous and mastoid parts of the temporal bone, in which the auricular branch of the vagus nerve is located.

central f., a deep fissure on the lateral surface of each cerebral hemisphere, between the parietal and frontal lobes; also called central sulcus and fissure of Rolando.

dentate f., hippocampal fissure.

enamel f., a deep groove on the surface of a tooth resulting from imperfect fusion of adjoining dental lobes.

f.'s of lungs, those separating the lobes of the lungs.

f. of Rolando, see central fissure.

f. of Sylvius, see lateral cerebral fissure.

hippocampal f., one located between the hippo-

campal convolution and the fascia dentata of the brain.

horizontal f. of cerebellum, a deep cleft encircling the circumference of the cerebellar hemispheres; also called horizontal sulcus of cerebellum.

inferior orbital f., a groove between the greater wing of the sphenoid and the orbital plate of the maxilla.

lateral cerebral f., a deep fissure separating the frontal, temporal, and parietal lobes of each cerebral hemisphere; also called fissure of Sylvius.

longitudinal cerebral f., the deep median groove that divides the cerebrum into right and left hemispheres.

superior orbital f., a cleft between the greater and lesser wings of the sphenoid bone; also called sphenoidal fissure.

transverse cerebral f., a cleft between the corpus callosum and the fornix above and the diencephalon below.

fis'tula. An abnormal passage between two internal organs, or from an organ to the surface of the body; usually designated according to the organs with which it communicates.

anal f., one opening near the anus; it may or may not open into the rectum.

arteriovenous f., an abnormal communication (congenital or traumatic) between an artery and a vein.

branchial f., a congenital defect consisting of a narrow canal on the lateral aspect of the neck in front of the sternocleidomastoid muscle, resulting from incomplete closure of a branchial cleft.

bronchoesophageal f., passage between a bronchus and the esophagus.

bronchopleural f., one connecting a bronchus and a collection of pus in the pleural cavity.

carotid-cavernous f., arteriovenous connection formed by rupture of the intracavernous portion of the carotid artery.

colovesical f., one between the colon and the bladder; also called vesicocolonic fistula.

Eck f., one formed by the experimental anastomosing of the vena cava and portal vein with subsequent ligation of the portal vein, for the purpose of shutting off the liver of an experimental animal from its portal circulation.

enterovaginal f., a fistula between the small intestine and the vagina, usually associated with intestinal disease, especially diverticulitis.

gastrocolic f., one between the stomach and the colon.

internal f., abnormal passage between two internal organs.

pilonidal f., pilonidal sinus; see under sinus.

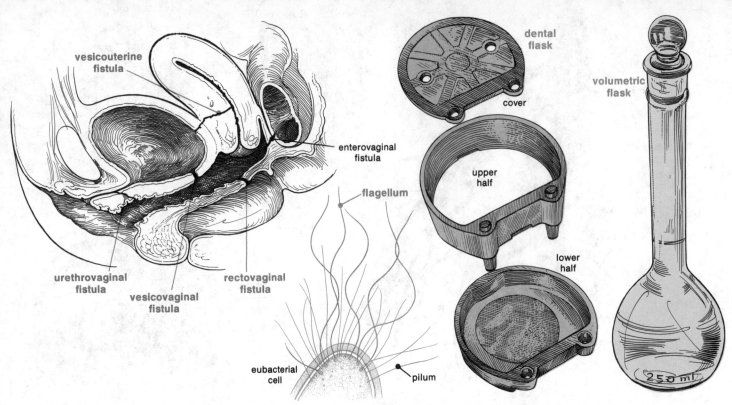

dental flask

cover

volumetric flask

vesicouterine fistula

enterovaginal fistula

flagellum

upper half

lower half

urethrovaginal fistula

vesicovaginal fistula

rectovaginal fistula

eubacterial cell

pilum

250 ml

rectovaginal f., one between the rectum and the vagina, caused by direct surgical damage, disease of the rectum, or obstetrical injury.

Thiry's f., artificial fistula made for collecting the intestinal juice of an experimental animal; consisting of an isolated segment of intestine, having one end closed and the other attached to the skin of the abdomen.

Thiry-Vella f., experimental fistula created by suturing to the skin of the abdomen the two ends of an isolated segment of intestine; also called Vella's fistula.

tracheoesophageal f., congenital fistula between the trachea and esophagus.

urachal f., congenital abnormality which occurs when the lumen of the embryonic allantois (which extends from the navel to the bladder) persists over the entire length, allowing urine to drain from the navel; also called patent urachus.

urethrovaginal f., one between the urethra and the vagina; may be due to obstetrical injury or may be congenital.

Vella's f., see Thiry-Vella fistula.

vesicocolonic f., see colovesical fistula.

vesicouterine f., one between the bladder and the uterus, usually caused by cancer of the cervix or by surgical injury to the bladder.

vesicovaginal f., one between the bladder and the vagina, often the result of traumatic delivery; almost invariably causes urinary incontinence.

fistula'tion, fistuliza'tion. Formation of a fistula.

fis'tulatome. A thin-bladed long knife used for slitting a fistula; also called syringotome.

fistulat'omy. See fistulotomy.

fistulec'tomy. Surgical repair of a fistula by the removal of its walls.

fistuliza'tion. See fistulation.

fistulot'omy. Surgical incision of a fistula; also called fistulatomy and syringotomy.

fis'tulous. Relating to or having fistulas.

fit'ness, phys'ical. A state of well being which enables a person to perform his daily work without undue fatigue.

Fitz-Hugh-Curtis syndrome. Perihepatitis; a complication in women with gonococcal inflammation of the pelvic organs, resulting from the spread of gonoccoci to the upper abdomen.

fixa'tion. 1. The process of making stationary. **2.** In psychiatry, the persistence of immature or earlier patterns of behavior. **3.** In histology, the preservation of tissue elements with minimal alteration of the normal state. **4.** In chemistry, the conversion of a gaseous compound into solid or liquid form. **5.** In ophthalmology, the act of directing the eye toward

an object, causing its image to fall on the fovea.

bifoveal f., fixation in which the images of the object of regard center simultaneously on the foveae of both eyes, as occurs in normal vision.

binocular f., bifoveal fixation.

external f., the holding together of a broken bone by means of a plaster cast encircling the injured part or a plaster splint until successful healing occurs.

f. of the complement, fixation which occurs when an antigen is allowed to combine with its specific antibody in the presence of complement.

f. disparity, condition in which the images of the object of regard do not fall on corresponding retinal points, due to a slight over- or underconvergence of the eyes.

internal f., the use of devices such as metallic pins, screws, wires, or plates, applied directly to the bony fragments to hold them in apposition and alignment.

fix'ative. A substance used to preserve histologic specimens.

flac'cid. Flabby.

flagellant'ism. Erotic stimulation derived from whipping, or being whipped by, a sexual partner.

Flagella'ta. A class of unicellular organisms having one or more whiplike processes (flagella) used for locomotion; also called Mastigophora.

flagellate. A protozoon having one or more flagella.

flagello'sis. Infection with flagellated protozoa.

flagel'lum, *pl.* **flagel'la.** A hairlike protoplasmic structure, present in some microorganisms; it is usually several microns in length and composed of two tightly entwined filaments, each about 100 Å in diameter; it grows out from the basal body in the cytoplasm of the cell and is used for locomotion.

flange. 1. A protruding rim or edge. **2.** In dentistry, the part of the denture base which extends from the cervical ends of the teeth to the border of the denture.

buccal f., the portion of the flange of a denture which occupies the vestibule of the mouth adjoining the cheek.

denture f., the nearly vertical extension from the body of a denture into any of the oral vestibules.

labial f., the portion of the flange of a denture which occupies the vestibule of the mouth adjoining the lips.

lingual f., the portion of the flange of a mandibular denture which occupies the space adjacent to the tongue.

flank. The side of the body between the ribs and the pelvis; also called latus.

flap. 1. A flat piece of tissue cut away from the underlying parts but attached at one end; used to

cover a defect in a neighboring part or the sawn end of a bone after amputation. **2.** A characteristic flapping movement of the hands in certain disorders.

bone f., in neurosurgery, a section of the skull attached to muscles and/or other structures which serve as a hinge.

liver f., see asterixis.

pedicle f., a piece of detached tissue (including skin and subcutaneous tissues) in which the attached end or base contains an adequate blood supply.

sliding f., one used to either lengthen or shorten a localized area of tissue.

flare. Diffuse redness of the skin surrounding an injured point.

flaring of the alae nasi. The enlargement of both nostrils during inspiration, due to contraction of the anterior and posterior dilatores naris muscles; a sign of dyspnea since it implies that greater than normal work is required for breathing.

flash. 1. A sudden, brief, intense burst of light or heat. **2.** In dentistry, excess material squeezed out of the sections of a mold.

hot f., sudden sensation of heat through the whole body; a vasomotor symptom of menopause.

flash'back. The spontaneous and unpredictable reversion of perceptual distortions resulting from having previously taken psychedelic drugs; it can last from several seconds to half an hour.

flash'blindness. Temporary loss of vision caused by exposure to intense light.

flask. 1. A bottle with a narrow neck, used in the laboratory. **2.** A metal case or tube used in investing procedures.

casting f., refractory flask.

crown f., a small dental flask.

dental f., a metal case in which a sectional gypsum mold is made for the purpose of shaping and curing resinous structures, such as dentures or other resinous restorations.

Dewar f., a glass vessel, often silvered, with two walls; used for maintaining materials at constant temperature or, more usually, at low temperature; also called vacuum flask.

Erlenmeyer f., one with a conical body and broad base and a narrow neck.

Florence f., a globular long-necked bottle of thin glass used for holding water or other liquid in laboratory work.

refractory f., a metal tube in which a refractory mold is made for casting metal dental restorations or appliances; more commonly known as a casting ring.

vacuum f., see Dewar flask.

volumetric f., a flask calibrated to contain or to deliver a definite amount of liquid.

fistula | flask

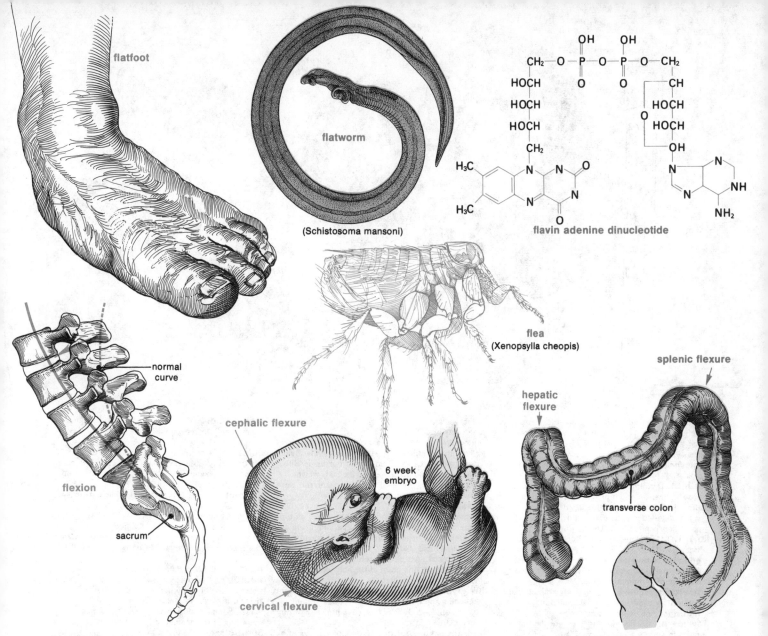

flatfoot

flatworm

(Schistosoma mansoni)

flavin adenine dinucleotide

flea
(Xenopsylla cheopis)

splenic flexure

hepatic flexure

normal curve

cephalic flexure

flexion

6 week embryo

transverse colon

sacrum

cervical flexure

flask'ing. In dentistry, the investing of the cast and a wax denture prior to molding the denture-base material into the form of the denture.

flat'foot. Condition marked by varying degrees of diminution or depression of the longitudinal arch of the foot, resulting in impairment of its weight-bearing capability; it may be congenital or acquired; also called pes planus and weak or splay foot.

flat'ulence. Excessive quantities of gas in the stomach and intestines, causing distention.

flat'ulent. Relating to flatulence.

fla'tus. Intestinal gas expelled through the rectum.

flat'worm. Any member of the phylum Platyhelminthes; e.g., tapeworms and flukes.

fla'vin. Any of various nitrogenous yellow pigments present in numerous plant and animal tissues.

  f. adenine dinucleotide (FDA), a nucleotide containing riboflavin which participates as a coenzyme in oxidation-reduction reactions.

  f. mononucleotide (FMN), a cofactor containing riboflavin in cellular oxidation-reduction systems.

Flavobacte'rium. A genus of bacteria; gram-negative rods which, when motile, move by means of flagella located around the mouth opening; they characteristically produce yellow, orange, red, or yellow-brown pigments; some species are pathogenic.

flavoen'zyme. Any enzyme having a flavin nucleotide as coenzyme.

fla'vor. 1. The distinctive taste of any substance. **2.** Inert substance added to a pharmaceutical preparation to give it a pleasing taste.

flea. A blood-sucking insect of the genus *Pulex.*

  rat f., a general term for *Pulex fasciatus, Pulex*

pallidus, Typhlopsylla musculi, and *Xenopsylla cheopis*; parasitic on the rat and a vector for bubonic plague.

  sand f., see chigoe.

flesh. 1. Muscular tissue and other soft tissues of the body excluding the viscera. **2.** The meat of animals. **3.** Excess tissue; stoutness.

  goose f., temporary rough appearance of the skin caused by contraction of the arrectores pilorum muscles (erectors of the hair) as a reaction to cold, fear, or other stimuli; also called goose pimples or bumps.

  proud f., excessive granulation on the surface of a wound or ulcer.

flex. To bend or approximate two parts which are united by a joint.

flexibilitas cerea. See cerea flexibilitas.

flexim'eter. Instrument used to measure the degree of flexion possible in a joint.

flex'ion. 1. The act of bending a limb at a joint so that its proximal and distal parts are brought together; the bending forward of the spine. **2.** The condition of being bent.

  palmar f., flexion at the wrist, causing the hand to be bent toward the anterior surface of the forearm.

  plantar f., flexion at the ankle joint, causing the foot to be bent downward.

flex'or. A muscle that flexes a joint; see table of muscles.

flexu'ra. Latin for a bend.

flex'ure. A bend.

  caudal f., the bend at the caudal end of the embryo; also called sacral flexure.

  cephalic f., the bend at the cephalic region of the

embryo; also called cranial flexure.

  cervical f., the bend at the junction of the embryonic brain and spinal cord.

  cranial f., see cephalic flexure.

  hepatic f., the bend between the ascending and transverse colon, near the liver.

  pontine f., a concave flexure dividing the rhombencephalon portion of the embryonic brain into anterior and posterior halves.

  sacral f., see caudal flexure.

  splenic f., the bend between the transverse and descending colon, near the spleen.

flick'er. Visual sensation consisting of variations in brightness or hue caused by stimulation by intermittent light flashes.

floater. Opaque deposit in the normally transparent vitreous body; may be congenital or due to degenerative changes of the retina or of the vitreous body.

floating. Unattached; unduly movable.

floating kidney. see kidney, floating.

floating rib. see rib, floating.

floccila'tion. Aimless plucking at the bedclothes, occurring in delirious patients; also called carphologia and crocidismus.

floccula'tion. The formation of flaky masses or precipitation in a solution being tested.

floc'culent. 1. A fluid containing irregularly shaped fluffy particles. **2.** In bacteriology, denoting a liquid culture containing small adherent masses of bacteria.

floc'culus. Latin for small tuft; in anatomy, the small lobule of the posterior lobe of the cerebellum, which adjoins the middle cerebellar peduncle and is continuous with the nodule of the vermis.

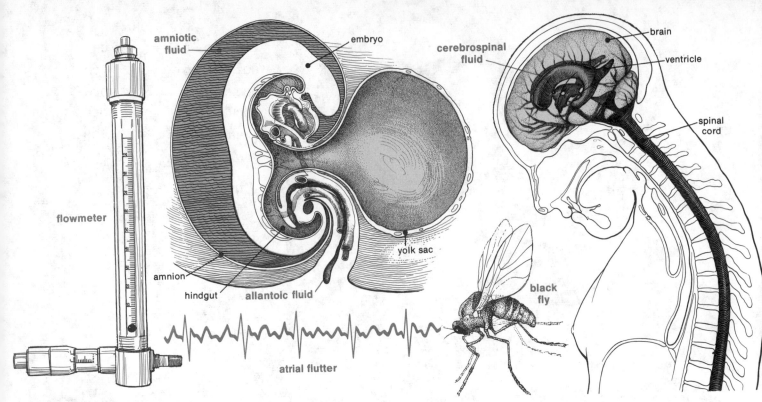

amniotic fluid
embryo
cerebrospinal fluid
brain
ventricle
spinal cord
flowmeter
amnion
hindgut
allantoic fluid
yolk sac
black fly
atrial flutter

flood. 1. To bleed profusely from the uterus, as after childbirth. **2.** Colloquial term for a profuse menstrual flow.

flora. Plant life.

intestinal f., the bacteria in the intestinal contents.

flor'id. 1. Denoting a flushed appearance, as of the skin. **2.** Having a bright red color, as of a lesion.

floss. 1. To use waxed thread (dental floss) or, waxed ribbon (dental tape) to remove particles from spaces between teeth. **2.** Dental floss.

flow. 1. To circulate; to move freely. **2.** Menstrual discharge.

effective renal plasma f. (ERPF), the amount of plasma passing through the kidneys as measured by clearance of *p*-aminohippurate.

flowers. In chemistry, a powdery mineral substance produced by condensation or sublimation.

f. of zinc, zinc oxide.

flow'meter. Device used to measure the flow of liquids in vessels.

floxur'idine (5-FUDR). 5-Fluoro-2'-deoxyuridine; a derivative of fluorouracil; used in the treatment of gastrointestinal cancer.

flu. A general term given to many brief illnesses, presumed to be caused by viruses, mostly the influenza virus; symptoms usually include sudden onset of fever, shivering, headache, muscular aches, and malaise; fever generally lasts three to four days.

fluc'tuant. Having a yielding feel to palpation, suggesting a liquid center.

fluc'tuate. 1. To vary irregularly or change from time to time. **2.** To undulate or move in waves.

fluctua'tion. 1. A variation. **2.** A wavelike motion produced when a body cavity filled with fluid is palpated.

fluid. 1. Any nonsolid substance, either liquid or gas. **2.** Flowing.

allantoic f., the fluid within the allantoic cavity.

amniotic f., the fluid in the amnion in which the fetus floats.

cerebrospinal f., the fluid filling the ventricles of the brain and the subarachnoid spaces of the brain and spinal cord.

extracellular f. (ECF), the body fluid outside of the cells, comprised of interstitial fluid, blood, plasma, and lymph; approximately 20 per cent of body weight.

follicular f., an albuminous fluid secreted by the granulosa (follicle) cells in a developing ovarian follicle; it creates intercellular spaces which eventually give rise to a follicular cavity, the antrum; also called liquor folliculi.

infranatant f., the clear liquid that locates on the bottom of a container after separation from an in-

soluble liquid or solid through the action of gravity or a centrifugal force.

interstitial f., fluid lying in the spaces between cells; comprises the major part of extracellular fluid.

intracellular f., the fluid within the tissue cells, constituting about 40 per cent of the body weight.

intraocular f., the fluid within the anterior and posterior chambers of the eye.

seminal f., see semen.

supernatant f., the clear fluid that settles on top of the contents of a vessel after separating from an insoluble liquid or solid through normal gravity or a centrifugal force.

fluidex'tract. An alcohol solution of a vegetable drug containing one gram of the active principle of the drug in each milliliter.

fluidglycerate. A pharmaceutical preparation containing approximately 50 per cent by volume of glycerin and one gram of the active principle of the specific drug in each milliliter.

fluidram', fluidrachm'. A teaspoonful; 1/8 of a fluid ounce; either of two units of liquid capacity: (1) in the U.S. Customary System, the equivalent of 0.225 cubic inches; (2) in the British Imperial System, the equivalent of 0.2167 cubic inches.

fluke. Common name for species of the class Trematoda (flatworms), especially the parasitic variety.

blood f., fluke of the genus *Schistosoma*, parasitic in the mesenteric-portal blood stream and the vesical and venous plexuses.

Chinese liver f., *Clonorchis sinensis*; a fluke parasitic in the bile ducts.

intestinal f., *Fasciolopsis buski*; large fluke parasitic in the intestines.

liver f., see *Fasciola hepatica*.

lung f., *Paragonimus westermani*; a fluke parasitic the lungs.

flumina pilorum. Hair streams; the lined pattern along which hairs grow on the head and throughout the body.

fluocinolone acetonide. A fluorinated corticosteroid used topically in the treatment of certain dermatoses.

fluores'cein. A material used, because of its fluorescence, as a marker, as in immunofluorescent studies and in circulatory studies, particularly of the eye.

sodium f., an orange-red powder used in solution to detect lesions of the cornea.

fluores'cence. The ability of certain substances to emit light, to become self-luminous, while exposed to direct light rays from another source, especially ultraviolet rays.

fluor'idate. To add fluorine salts to a water supply; also called fluorinate.

fluorida'tion. The addition of fluoride (fluorine compound) to the public water supply to prevent tooth decay.

flu'oride. A compound containing fluorine.

flu'orine. A gaseous chemical element of the halogen group; symbol F, atomic number 9, atomic weight 19.

fluorom'eter. A device for detecting and measuring fluorescence; also called fluorimeter.

fluor'oscope. A type of x-ray apparatus in which x rays going through part of the body strike upon a fluorescent screen of calcium tungstate, rendering an image on the screen of varying densities of the body.

fluoroscop'ic. Relating to fluoroscopy.

fluoros'copy. Direct examination of the inner parts of the body by use of the fluoroscope.

fluoro'sis. Abnormal condition caused by an excessive intake of fluorine, manifested mainly by mottling of the enamel of the teeth.

fluorou'racil (5-FU). 5-Fluorouracil; an antineoplastic drug, $C_4H_3FN_2O_2$, used in the treatment of gastrointestinal cancer and topically for the treatment of multiple premalignant actinic keratoses.

flush. 1. To wash with a brief gush of water. **2.** Sudden redness of the skin, especially of the face and neck.

hot f., sudden redness of the face and neck with a sensation of heat; a vasomotor symptom of menopause.

flut'ter. Rapid vibrations or pulsations.

atrial f., auricular f., extremely rapid but rhythmic contractions of the cardiac atria, usually at a rate of 240 to 300 per min, often producing "sawtooth" waves in the electrocardiogram.

auricular f., see atrial flutter.

diaphragmatic., rapid contractions of all or part of the diaphragm.

ventricular f., rapid contractions of the ventricles producing electrocardiographic complexes that have a regular undulating pattern without distinct QRS and T waves.

flutter-fibrillation. An electrocardiographic pattern of atrial activity showing both flutter and fibrillation.

flux. 1. Excessive discharge of any bodily secretion. **2.** Denoting the movement of ions or molecules through a membrane. **3.** In dentistry, a substance that increases fluidity of molten metal, thereby promoting fusion; also used to remove oxides from metal surfaces during soldering of dental prostheses.

fly. A winged insect of the family Muscidae.

black f., a small, dark, biting fly of the family Simuliidae; vector of onchocerciasis.

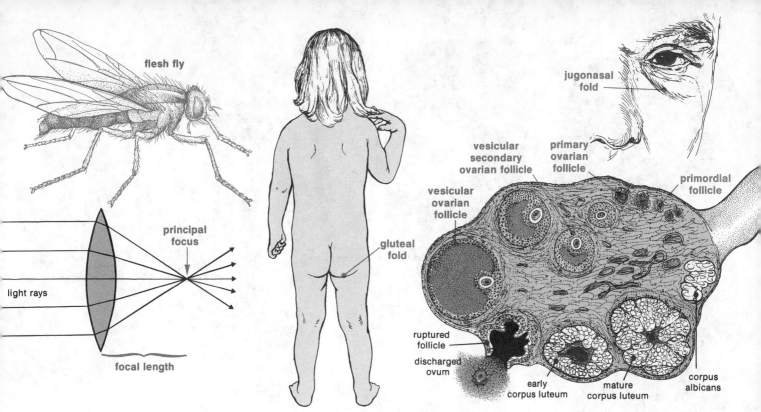

flesh fly

principal focus

light rays

focal length

jugonasal fold

vesicular secondary ovarian follicle

primary ovarian follicle

vesicular ovarian follicle

primordial follicle

gluteal fold

ruptured follicle

discharged ovum

early corpus luteum

mature corpus luteum

corpus albicans

flesh f., a fly whose larvae (maggots) develop in putrifying or living tissues.

fruit f., *Drosophila melanogaster*; a fly used extensively in genetic studies.

mangrove f., species of the genus *Chrysops*; vectors of *Loa loa*.

sand f., a small biting fly of the genus *Phlebotomus*; vectors of leishmaniasis.

Spanish f., see cantharis.

tsetse f., see *Glossina*.

FMN. Abbreviation for flavin mononucleotide.

foam. 1. Collection of numerous small bubbles on the surface of a liquid. **2.** To produce such bubbles.

fo′cal. Relating to a focus; localized.

focal glomerulonephritis. See glomerulonephritis, focal.

focal length. The distance from a point where the image of a distant object is formed (focal point) to a point in or near the lens.

focal plane. The plane at right angles to the optical axis at the focal point.

focal point. The point where the light rays coming from a distant object converge after passing through a lens, coming to a focus and forming an image.

fo′ci. Plural of focus.

focim′eter. Instrument used to determine the vergence power of a lens or system of lenses.

fo′cus, *pl.* **fo′ci. 1.** The point in an optical system where light rays meet. **2.** To adjust a lens system to produce a distinct, clear image. **3.** The principal site of a disease.

conjugate foci, two points in an optical system so interrelated that rays originating at one point are focused at the other, and vice versa.

Ghon′s f., Ghon's primary lesion; see under lesion.

principal f., the real or virtual axial meeting point of rays passing into a lens parallel to its optical axis.

real f., the point at which convergent light rays meet forming a real image.

virtual f., the point at which the backward extensions of diverging light rays intersect, forming a virtual image.

fog. 1. Hazy or dense appearance of a roentgenogram caused by stray radiation, accidental exposure to light, subjection to unusual temperatures or chemical actions, or the use of outdated film. **2.** To subject a film to such conditions.

mental f., a state of bewilderment and confusion.

fogging. In ophthalmology, the deliberate undercorrection of myopia (nearsightedness) or overcorrection of hyperopia (farsightedness); a procedure used to prevent unconscious accommodation of the eye during the testing for astigmatism.

foil. An extremely thin, pliable sheet of metal.

gold f., a foil of pure gold used in dentistry to restore carious or fractured teeth.

platinum f., a foil of pure platinum used in dentistry, because of its high fusing point, as a matrix for soldering procedures and to provide the internal forms of porcelain restorations.

Foix's syndrome. See cavernous sinus syndrome.

fo′late. A salt of folic acid.

fold. The doubling of a part upon itself.

axillary f., one of the musculocutaneous ridges bounding the armpit anteriorly and posteriorly.

glosso-epiglottic fo′s, three folds of mucous membrane reflected from the base of the tongue onto the epiglottis; the fold in the midline is called the median glosso-epiglottic fold and those to the sides are called the lateral glosso-epiglottic folds.

gluteal f., one marking the posterior upper limit of the thigh and the lower limit of the buttock.

jugonasal f., one indicating the confluence of the orbicularis oculi and the quadratus labii muscles.

lacrimal f., a fold of mucous membrane in the nasal cavity at the lower end of the nasolacrimal duct; it keeps air from entering the lacrimal sac when the nose is blown.

medial umbilical f., the fold of peritoneum that covers the obliterated umbilical artery as it ascends from the pelvis toward the umbilicus.

median umbilical f., the fold of peritoneum that covers the median umbilical ligament extending from the apex of the urinary bladder to the umbilicus; also called urachal fold.

neural f., a fold of ectoderm forming the lateral margin of the embryonic neural groove.

rectovesical f., the peritoneal fold that bounds the rectovesical pouch in the male.

salpingopharyngeal f., one of the vertical ridges of mucous membrane extending from the lower portion of the elevation of the auditory tube along the wall of the pharynx on either side.

sublingual f., the fold formed by the mucous membrane of the floor of the mouth, elevated by the sublingual gland and containing its excretory ducts.

transverse f.'s of rectum, rectal valves; the three or four crescentric transverse folds in the rectum.

urachal f., see median umbilical fold.

Vater's f., one located above the greater papilla of the duodenum.

vocal f., the true vocal cord; it contains the vocal ligament.

folia′ceous, fo′liate. Resembling a leaf.

folic acid. A constituent of the vitamin B complex; extracted from liver and green leaves and produced synthetically; deficiency may occur in malnourished individuals, alcoholics, and in malabsorption states

and result in a megaloblastic anemia; also called pteroylglutamic acid.

f. a. antagonist, one of a group of compounds that neutralize the action of folic acid; used in the treatment of neoplastic disorders, especially of the hematopoietic system.

folie′. French for madness; psychosis.

f. à deux, psychosis affecting two closely associated persons in which they share the same delusions; also called communicated or double insanity.

f. gémellaire, psychosis occurring simultaneously in twins who are not necessarily closely associated at the time.

folinic acid. A reduced form of folic acid; also called citrovorum factor and leucovorin.

fo′lium, *pl.* **fo′lia.** A broad thin anatomical structure.

folia of the cerebellum, the numerous long parallel infoldings of the cerebellar cortex.

fol′licle. 1. A somewhat spherical mass of cells usually containing a cavity. **2.** A small crypt, such as the depression in the skin from which the hair emerges. **3.** A small circumscribed body.

atretic ovarian f., one that degenerates before reaching maturity.

graafian f., see vesicular ovarian follicle.

hair f., a saclike invagination of the epidermis from which the root of a hair develops.

lymph f., a small mass of lymphoid tissue as seen in the mucosa of the gut; also called nodulus lymphaticus.

lymphoid f., a collection of proliferating palestaining cells in lymphoid tissue, as in the cortex of lymph nodes.

nabothian f., nabothian cyst; a cyst resulting from obstruction of a mucous gland of the uterine cervix.

ovarian f., the ovum together with its surrounding cells, at any stage of development, located in the cortex of the ovary.

primary ovarian f., a developing follicle in the ovary before the appearance of a fluid-filled antrum; it is composed of a growing primary oocyte and a single or several layers of cuboidal follicular cells surrounded by a sheath of stroma (theca); it usually develops during adolescence.

primordial f., an immature ovarian follicle consisting of the original primordial germ cell, the oogonium, and a thin single layer of squamous (flattened) follicular cells; at birth there are about 400,000 primordial follicles in each ovary; most undergo atresia.

sebaceous f., oil gland of the skin.

solid secondary ovarian f., a follicle in the ovary in which follicular fluid is gradually accumulating between the follicular (granulosa) cells; it first ap-

anterolateral fontanel

anterior fontanel

foramen ovale

base of skull

mastoid fontanel

posterior fontanel

malleus

footplate

stapes

apical dental foramen
(constricting with advancing age)

foramina:
optic
rotundum
ovale
lacerum
jugular
magnum

pears during puberty.

thyroid f., the minute components of the thyroid gland in which the thyroid hormone is stored.

vesicular ovarian f., a large mature follicle in the ovary in which the ovum (oocyte) attains full size (about four times that of the primordial germ cell); at this stage of development, the follicle migrates toward the surface of the ovary, causing a preovulatory swelling; also called graafian follicle.

vesicular secondary ovarian f., one in which the secretion of the follicular fluid gives rise to a cavity (antrum).

follic′ular. 1. Having or resembling a follicle or follicles. **2.** Growing out of follicles.

follicull′tis. Inflammation of hair follicles.

f. barbae, tinea barbae.

folliculo′ma. 1. Granulosal cell tumor; see under tumor. **2.** Cystic enlargement of a vesicular ovarian (graafian) follicle.

folliculo′sis. Abnormally increased development of lymph follicles.

conjunctival f., a chronic condition, frequently found in children, marked by the presence of multiple tiny lymphatic nodules in the conjunctiva of the lower lids.

follic′ulus, *pl.* **follic′uli.** Follicle.

fomenta′tion. The therapeutic application of warmth and moisture.

fo′mes, *pl.* **fo′mites.** Anything (clothing, toys, etc.) capable of transmitting the microorganisms causing a contagious disease.

fontanel′, fontanelle. Any of the membrane-covered spaces between the incompletely ossified cranial bones of an infant; commonly called soft spot.

anterior f., a diamond-shaped fontanel located at the junction of the frontal, sagittal, and coronal sutures; also called frontal or bregmatic fontanel.

anterolateral f., an irregularly shaped fontanel located on either side at the junction of the frontal bone with the sphenoidal angle of the parietal bone, the squamous portion of the temporal bone, and the greater wing of the sphenoid bone; also called sphenoidal fontanel.

bregmatic f., see anterior fontanel.

frontal f., see anterior fontanel.

mastoid f., the fontanel on either side at the junction of the mastoid angle of the parietal bone with the mastoid portion of the temporal bone and the occipital bone; also called posterolateral fontanel.

posterior f., a triangular fontanel at the union of the lambdoid and sagittal sutures; also called occipital fontanel.

posterolateral f., see mastoid fontanel.

sphenoidal f., see anterolateral fontanel.

fontic′ulus. Fontanel.

food. Nourishment, usually of plant or animal origin; also called aliment.

convenience f., food that is partially prepared for cooking so that the time of home preparation is shortened.

conventional f., common food not subjected to unusual processing.

engineered f., food made from vegetable or synthetic substances; also called fabricated food.

enriched f., food to which vitamins (thiamine, niacin, riboflavin) and iron have been added within specified limits; also called fortified food.

fabricated f., see engineered food.

f. analog, engineered food product designed to look like a traditional food item such as chicken or bacon.

formulated f., imitation of common food, such as an imitation dairy product, or new types of food; blended cereal grains, legumes, roots or tubers, and sources of proteins and calories frequently serve as bases.

fortified f., see enriched food.

foot. The termination of the lower extremity.

athlete's f., see tinea pedis.

ball of the f., the anterior padded portion of the sole of the foot.

burning feet, chronic condition marked by pain and burning sensations, especially in the soles of the feet.

cavus f., see clawfoot.

claw f., see clawfoot.

club f., see clubfoot.

drop f., see footdrop.

flat f., see flatfoot.

Friedreich's f., a foreshortened foot with a high arch and clawed toes, occurring in Friedreich's ataxia.

immersion f., a swollen state of the feet after prolonged immersion in cold water, as after shipwreck.

Madura f., see maduromycosis.

march f., painful condition of the feet after prolonged stress; Deutschländer's disease.

splay f., see flatfoot.

trench f., frostbite of the feet after prolonged standing in cold water, snow, or mud; sometimes seen in soldiers on trench duty.

foot and mouth disease. A highly infectious disease of cattle, swine, and sheep; when it occurs in man (rarely), it is characterized by fever and a vesicular eruption of the palms, soles, and the oropharyngeal mucosa.

foot′candle. A unit of illumination on a surface one foot distant from a uniform point source of light of one candela, equal to one lumen per square foot.

foot′drop. Paralysis or weakness of the dorsiflexor muscles of the foot and ankle causing the foot to fall and the toes to drag on the ground during walking; also called toe drop.

foot′plate. The base of the smallest ossicle (stapes) of the middle ear that fits in the oval window.

fora′men, *pl.* **foram′ina.** A natural opening through a bone or a membranous structure; a short passage.

aortic f., see hiatus, aortic.

apical dental f., the opening at the tip of the root of a tooth through which pass the vessels and nerves supplying the pulp.

carotid f., the inferior opening of the carotid canal giving passage to the internal carotid artery.

epiploic f., the opening connecting the two sacs of the peritoneum, namely the greater sac and the lesser sac (omental bursa); also called Winslow's foramen.

ethmoidal f., one of two openings (anterior and posterior) in the orbit, giving passage to vessels and nerves.

external auditory f., see meatus, external auditory.

f. cecum, the pit on the dorsal surface of the tongue representing the remains of the upper portion of the embryonic thyroglossal duct.

f. lacerum, the opening between the apex of the petrous portion of the temporal bone and the body of the sphenoid bone; during life, it is closed with fibrous tissue, giving passage only to the small nerve of the pterygoid canal and a small meningeal branch of the ascending pharyngeal artery; also called lacerated foramen.

f. of Luschka, lateral aperture of the fourth ventricle; see under aperture.

f. of Magendi, median aperture of the fourth ventricle; see under aperture.

f. magnum, the large opening at the base of the skull through which passes the spinal cord; also called great foramen.

f. of Monro, see interventricular foramen.

f. of the vena cava, opening in the diaphragm giving passage to the inferior vena cava; also called foramen quadratum.

f. ovale, (1) the oval opening between the atria of the fetal heart; (2) a large opening in the great wing of the sphenoid bone, through which pass the third portion of the trigeminal nerve and the small meningeal artery.

f. quadratum, see foramen of the vena cava.

f. rotundum, one located in the great wing of the sphenoid bone, through which passes the maxillary nerve; also called round foramen.

follicle | foramen

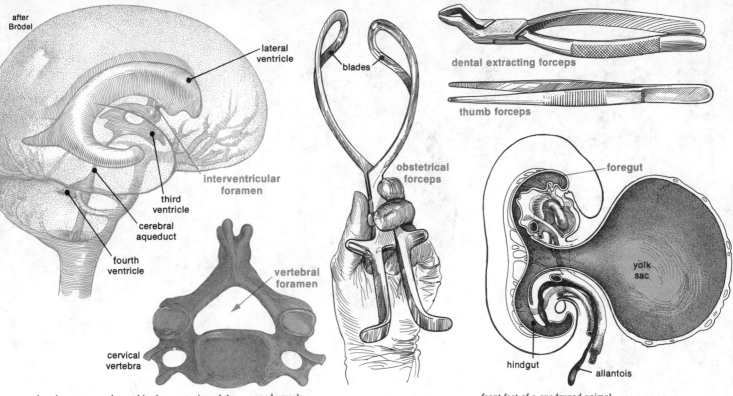

after Brödel

lateral ventricle

blades

dental extracting forceps

thumb forceps

interventricular foramen

third ventricle

cerebral aqueduct

fourth ventricle

vertebral foramen

obstetrical forceps

foregut

yolk sac

cervical vertebra

hindgut

allantois

f. spinosum, one located in the great wing of the sphenoid bone, transmitting the middle meningeal artery.

greater sciatic f., a large opening bounded by the sacrum, the greater sciatic notch of the hipbone, and the sacrotuberous and sacrospinous ligaments.

incisal f., the relatively large opening in the midline of the hard palate just behind the central incisors; the opening of the nasopalatine canal.

inferior dental f., see mandibular foramen.

infraorbital f., the external opening of the infraorbital canal, on the anterior aspect of the maxilla.

interatrial f. primum, (1) the temporary opening of the embryonic heart between the right and left atria; also called ostium primum; (2) the abnormal persistence of such an opening in the adult heart.

interatrial f., secundum, a secondary opening appearing in the embryonic heart between the right and left atria, just prior to the closure of the interatrial foramen primum; also called ostium secundum.

interventricular f., f. of Monro, an oval opening between the third and lateral ventricles of the brain.

intervertebral f., one of several openings into the spinal canal formed by adjoining vertebrae.

jugular f., opening located between the lateral portion of the occipital bone and the petrous portion of the temporal bone.

lesser sciatic f., an opening bounded by the lesser sciatic notch and the sacrotuberous and sacrospinous ligaments.

mandibular f., opening located in the medial aspect of each ramus of the mandible; also called inferior dental foramen.

mental f., one of two lateral openings on the body of the lower jaw, usually beneath the second bicuspid tooth; also called mental canal.

obturator f., the large opening in the hipbone bounded by the pubis and ischium; it is almost completely closed by the obturator membrane except for a small gap (obturator canal) through which the obturator nerve and vessels pass as they leave the pelvis to enter the thigh.

optic f., optic canal, a short canal through the sphenoid bone at the apex of the orbit which transmits the optic nerve and ophthalmic artery into the orbital cavity.

palatine foramina, anterior and posterior openings on either side of the hard palate.

stylomastoid f., opening on the petrous portion of the temporal bone, between the styloid and mastoid processes; it affords passage to the facial nerve and the stylomastoid artery.

supraorbital f., supraorbital notch; a canal or groove in the supraorbital margin of the frontal bone that gives passage to the supraorbital nerve and vessels.

vertebral f., the space between the arch and the body of a vertebra.

Winslow's f., see epiploic foramen.

foram'ina. Plural of foramen.

Forbes-Albright syndrome. Combination of a profuse secretion of milk and absence of the menses, unassociated with recent pregnancy or with acromegaly; believed to be caused by overproduction of prolactin, as in some tumors of the pituitary gland.

force. Strength; capacity to produce work or motion, or cause physical change.

electromotive f. (EMF), force causing the flow of electricity from one point to another, giving rise to an electric current.

f. of mastication, the force applied by the muscles during the act of chewing; also called masticatory force.

masticatory f., see force of mastication.

van der Waals' f.'s, the nondescript, attractive forces between atoms or molecules other than electrostatic (ionic), covalent (sharing of electrons), or hydrogen bending (sharing a proton).

for'ceps. An instrument resembling a pair of tongs, used for grasping, compressing, manipulating, or extracting tissue or specific structures.

bone f., a strong forceps used for grasping and cutting bone.

bulldog f., a forceps for clamping cut blood vessels.

capsule f., one used for extracting the lens in cataract.

chalazion f., a thumb forceps with a flattened plate at the end of one arm and a ring on the other.

dental extracting f., a forceps used for grasping teeth in order to luxate and extract them from the alveolus.

hemostatic f., a forceps with a catch for locking the blades, used for grasping the cut end of a blood vessel to control hemorrhage.

mosquito f., a very small hemostatic forceps.

obstetrical f., a forceps used for grasping and making traction on the fetal head in difficult labor.

rongeur f., a strong biting forceps for gouging away bone.

thumb f., a forceps used by compression with thumb and forefinger for grasping soft tissue; used especially during suturing.

fore'arm. The part of the upper extremity between the elbow and wrist; also called antebrachium.

fore'brain. See prosencephalon.

fore'finger. See finger, index.

fore'foot. 1. The front portion of the foot consisting of the toes and metatarsal bones. **2.** One of the front feet of a quadruped animal.

fore'gut. The cephalic portion of the primitive digestive tract in the embryo; also called headgut.

fore'milk. Colostrum; a thin, sticky secretion of the breasts occurring a few days before and after childbirth.

foren'sic. Relating to or used in legal proceedings.

fore'play. Sexual stimulation leading to sexual intercourse.

fore'pleasure. Pleasurable excitement preceding orgasm.

fore'skin. See prepuce.

fore'waters. In obstetrics, the part of the amniotic sac that pouches into the cervix in front of the fetal head or presenting part.

form. Shape; mold.

accolé f., appliqué form.

appliqué f., a ring of young species of the malarial parasite *Plasmodium falciparum* that parasitize the marginal portion of red blood cells; also called accolé form.

convenience f., in dentistry, a form modified beyond the basic to permit instrumentation for the preparation of a cavity or the insertion of the restorative material.

L-f., L-phase variant; see under variant.

resistance f., in dentistry, the shape given to the prepared cavity of a tooth to enable the restoration to withstand the stress of mastication.

retention f., in dentistry, the provision made in the prepared cavity of a tooth to prevent displacement of the restoration by lateral forces as well as the stress of mastication.

sickle f., see crescent, malarial.

formal'dehyde. A colorless, pungent, gaseous aldehyde, CH_2O, used in solution as a disinfectant and preservative.

for'malin. A 37 per cent aqueous solution of formaldehyde; also called formol.

forma'tio. Any formation or structure of definite shape.

forma'tion. 1. The process of giving form or producing. **2.** Something that is formed.

personality f., the development or structure of the components of the personality.

reaction f., the development of conscious attitudes that are the opposite of certain unconscious components of infantile sexuality; e.g., excessive cleanliness as a reaction to anal interests.

reticular f., a collection of intermingled fibers and gray matter in the pons, the anterolateral portion of the medulla oblongata and the cervical spinal cord; also called reticular substance.

rouleaux f., the arrangement of red blood cells in groups resembling stacks of coins.

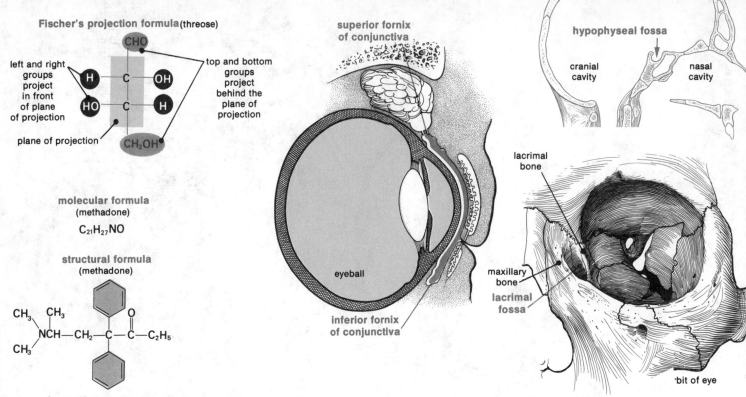

Fischer's projection formula (threose)

left and right groups project in front of plane of projection

top and bottom groups project behind the plane of projection

plane of projection

CHO

H — C — OH

HO — C — H

CH₂OH

molecular formula (methadone)

$C_{21}H_{27}NO$

structural formula (methadone)

superior fornix of conjunctiva

eyeball

inferior fornix of conjunctiva

hypophyseal fossa

cranial cavity

nasal cavity

lacrimal bone

maxillary bone

lacrimal fossa

orbit of eye

---

forme fruste, *pl.* **formes frustes.** French expression for a partial or atypical form of a disease.

for′mic. Relating to ants.

f. acid, a colorless caustic liquid, HCOOH, used in solution as an astringent and counterirritant; it occurs naturally in ants and other insects.

formica′tion. A paresthesia in which there is an abnormal tactile sensation of ants or other small insects crawling over the skin.

formiminoglutamic acid (FIGlu). An intermediate metabolite of histidine which can appear in the urine of folic acid-deficient individuals.

for′mol. See formalin.

for′mula. 1. A symbolic representation of the composition of a chemical substance. 2. An established group of symbols that express a concept. 3. A recipe of ingredients in fixed proportion; e. g., a milk mixture for feeding an infant. 4. A prescription containing directions for the preparation of a medicine.

Arneth f., a formula that expresses the approximate ratio of polymorphonuclear neutrophils in normal individuals, based on the number of lobes in the nuclei, as follows: 1 lobe, 5 per cent; 2 lobes, 35 per cent; 3 lobes, 41 per cent; 4 lobes, 17 per cent; 5 lobes, 2 per cent.

Bazett's f., one for correcting the observed electrocardiogram Q − T interval for cardiac rate: corrected $Q - T = Q - T \sec/\sqrt{R - R}$ sec.

Bernhardt's f., a formula for determining the ideal weight, in kilograms, for an adult; the height in centimeters times the chest circumference in centimeters divided by 240.

empirical f., a chemical formula denoting the proportions of the elements in a substance.

Fischer's projection f., a two-dimensional representation of three-dimensional molecules in which the carbon chain is depicted vertically.

Gorlin f., a formula for calculating the area of the orifices of a cardiac valve, based on the flow across the valve and the mean pressures in the chambers on either side of the valves.

graphic f., see structural formula.

Meeh-Dubois f., a formula for determining the body surface area from the height and weight of an individual: $\mathbf{A} = \mathbf{W} \, 0.425 \times \mathbf{H} \, 0.725 \times$ constant 71.84 (A = surface area in cm², W = weight in kg, and H = height in cm).

molecular f., a chemical formula depicting the number of atoms of each element in the molecules of a substance.

spatial f., see stereochemical formula.

stereochemical f., a formula depicting a spatial representation of the relative positions of the linked atoms, and the numbers of atoms of each element present in a molecule of a substance.

structural f., a graphic chemical formula showing the linkage of the atoms and groups of atoms, as well as their kind and number.

for′mulary. a collection of formulas for the preparation of medicines.

for′myl. The radical −C(H)O of formic acid.

for′nix, *pl.* **for′nices.** Any arched structure, or the space created by such a structure.

f. of the cerebrum, a harp-shaped, bilateral structure in the brain, composed of two posterior pillars (crura of the fornix), the body, and two anterior pillars (columns of the fornix); it is situated under the corpus callosum and is made up of white fibers arising from the hippocampus and terminating mainly in the mammillary bodies.

f. of the conjunctiva, the space formed by the reflection of the conjunctiva from the upper eyelid to the eyeball (superior fornix) and from the eyeball to the lower eyelid (interior fornix).

f. of the vagina, the space between the vaginal wall and the uterine cervix.

fos′sa, *pl.* **fos′sae.** A pit or depression.

acetabular f., a circular, nonarticular depression in the floor of the acetabulum; it lodges a mass of fat.

amygdaloid f., the hollow between the anterior and posterior pillars of the fauces containing the tonsil.

axillary f., the armpit.

coronoid f., the depression on the anterior aspect of the lower end of the humerus where the coronoid process of the ulna rests during full flexion of the forearm.

cranial f., one of three depressions (anterior, middle, and posterior) on the internal aspect of the base of the skull lodging the cerebrum and cerebellum.

cubital f., the depression in front of the elbow; also called bend of the elbow and antecubital space.

glenoid f., the depression in the head of the scapula for articulation with the head of the humerus forming the shoulder joint.

greater supraclavicular f., the triangular depression on each side of the neck above the clavicle, bounded by the lateral border of the sternocleidomastoid muscle, the clavicle, and the omohyoid muscle.

f. ovalis, (1) a depression on the septal wall of the right atrium representing the site of the foramen ovale of the fetal heart; (2) the saphenous opening in the upper thigh, 1½ inches below and lateral to the pubic tubercle, giving passage to the great saphenous vein.

hyaloid f., the concavity on the anterior aspect of the vitreous body in which the crystalline lens lies;

also called lenticular fossa.

hypophyseal f., a pit on the sphenoid bone lodging the pituitary gland; also called pituitary fossa.

lacrimal f., one located in the medial wall of the orbit, formed by the frontal process of the maxilla and the lacrimal bone; it houses the lacrimal gland.

lesser supraclavicular f., the space between the two heads of origin of the sternocleidomastoid muscle; also called Zang's space.

mandibular f., one of two depressions on the temporal bone that receives the condyle of the lower jaw.

olecranon f., a depression on the back of the lower end of the humerus in which the olecranon process of the ulna rests when the elbow is extended.

pituitary f., see hypophyseal fossa.

popliteal f., the diamond-shaped space situated at the back of the knee.

pterygoid f., the fossa between the lateral and medial pterygoid plates of the sphenoid bone.

radial f., a depression on the anterior aspect of the humerus, the site of articulation with the radius.

submandibular f., see fovea, submandibular.

tonsillar f., the depression between the palatoglossal and palatopharyngeal arches occupied by the palatine tonsil.

fossett′e. A small deep ulcer of the cornea.

fos′sula, *pl.* **fos′sulae.** 1. A small depression. 2. One of several small depressions on the surface of the cerebrum.

Foster-Kennedy syndrome. Ipsilateral optic atrophy with contralateral papilledema or choked disk; most commonly caused by a brain tumor at the base of the frontal lobe; also called Kennedy's syndrome.

founda′tion. The basis on which something is supported; a base.

denture f., that portion of the oral structures which supports a denture.

fourchett′e. Tissue connecting posteriorly the labia minora; also called frenulum labiorum pudendi.

fo′vea, *pl.* **fo′veae.** A small depression.

f. centralis, an area approximately 1.5 mm in diameter in the macula lutea of the retina; it is the area of greatest visual acuity.

submandibular f., a pit on the inner surface of the lower jaw on each side which lodges the submandibular gland; also called submandibular fossa.

fo′veate, fovea′ted. Pitted; having small depressions.

fovea′tion. The formation of a pitted scar, as in smallpox.

fove′ola. A minute depression, fovea, or pit.

f. of the coccyx, a small depression or dimple

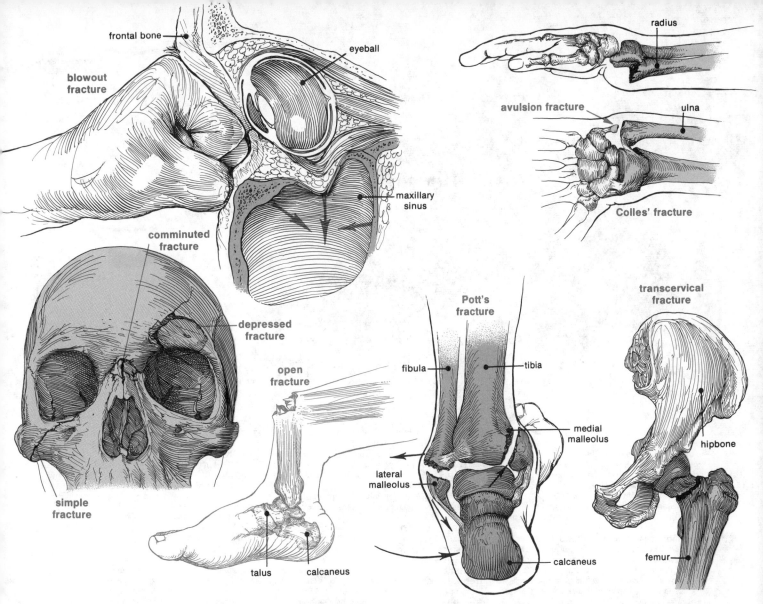

frontal bone

blowout fracture

eyeball

maxillary sinus

comminuted fracture

depressed fracture

simple fracture

open fracture

talus   calcaneus

radius

avulsion fracture

ulna

Colles' fracture

Pott's fracture

fibula   tibia

lateral malleolus

medial malleolus

calcaneus

transcervical fracture

hipbone

femur

often present in the skin over the tip of the coccyx.

gastric f., one of the numerous small pits in the gastric mucosa at the bottom of which open the gastric glands.

granular f. of Pacchioni, one of many depressions in the inner surface of the skull, on either side of the superior sagittal sinus groove, in which are lodged the arachnoid granulations (pacchionian bodies).

fo′veolate. Having minute depressions or pits on the surface.

Fox-Fordyce disease. An uncommon disease of the apocrine glands affecting mainly women from puberty to menopause; characterized by numerous small, follicular, closely aggregated, flesh-colored, intensely pruritic papules in the armpits and on the breasts, pubic area, and perineum; thought to be due to poral closure of the apocrine gland.

fox′glove. Any of various plants of the genus *Digitalis* from which the drug digitalis is prepared.

FPC. Abbreviation for fish protein concentrate.

Fr. Chemical symbol of the element francium.

frac′tion. 1. A quotient of two quantities. **2.** In chemistry, a component of a substance separated by crystallization or distillation.

blood plasma f., the separated components of plasma.

filtration f. (FF), the fraction of plasma entering the kidney that filters into the renal tubules; glomerular filtration rate/renal plasma flow.

fractiona′tion. The breaking up of a total therapeutic dose of radiation into small fractions of low intensity given over a period of time, usually at daily or alternate daily intervals.

frac′ture. The breaking of a bone or cartilage.

articular f., one involving the joint surface of a bone.

avulsion f., a breaking off of a small portion of bone at the site of attachment of a tendon or ligament.

basal skull f., one occurring at the base of the skull.

bimalleolar f., see Pott's fracture.

blow-out f., a fracture of the floor of the orbit caused by a blow to the eye.

Colles' f., a fracture of the lower end of the radius bone.

capillary f., a hairlike fracture.

closed f., a simple fracture; one in which the skin is not broken.

comminuted f., one in which the bone is splintered into several pieces.

compound f., see open fracture.

de Quervain's f., a fracture-dislocation of the wrist; specifically, fracture of the scaphoid (navicular) bone, with dislocation of the lunate bone.

depressed f., a fracture with inward displacement of the skull.

Dupuytren's f., fracture of the lower extremity of the fibula or lateral malleolus, with dislocation of the ankle joint.

extracapsular f., one near but outside of the joint capsule.

fatigue f., see march fracture.

fissured f., see linear fracture.

greenstick f., an incomplete fracture in which one side of the bone is only bent.

impacted f., one in which one fragment is embedded in the substance of the other and fixed in that position.

incomplete f., one in which the line of fracture does not include the whole bone.

intracapsular f., a fracture within a joint capsule.

linear f., one running parallel with the long axis of the bone; also called fissured fracture.

longitudinal f., one in which the direction of the fracture line is along the axis of the bone.

march f., fatigue f., fracture of a metatarsal shaft, usually the second or third, caused by stress associated with prolonged weight bearing, as in walking or marching for long periods of time; seen most commonly in army recruits during basic training.

oblique f., one running obliquely to the axis of the bone.

occult f., condition in which originally there is no evidence of a fracture, but after three or four weeks x ray shows new bone formation.

open f., one that is accompanied by an open wound through which the broken bone may protrude; formerly known as compound fracture.

periosteal f., one occurring beneath the periosteum, without displacement.

Pott's f., a fracture-dislocation of the ankle joint; specifically, fracture of the medial malleolus of the tibia, with fracture of the lower extremity of the fibula (lateral malleolus) and dislocation of the ankle joint; also called bimalleolar fracture.

spiral f., one in which the fracture line runs spirally around the shaft of the bone.

sprain f., avulsion fracture.

stellate f., one with several break lines radiating from a central point.

strain f., the breaking off by sudden force of a piece of bone attached to a tendon or ligament.

stress f., one occurring at the site of a muscle attachment and caused by sudden, violent, endogenous force; e.g., a simple fracture of the fibula in a runner.

supracondylar f., one in the distal end of the humerus.

transcervical f., one through the neck of the

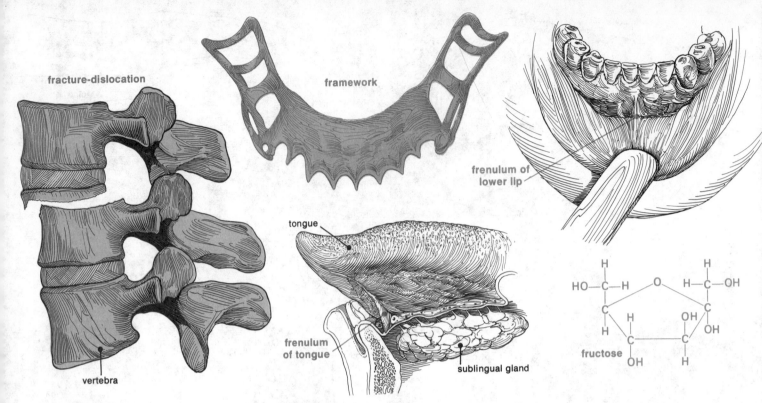

fracture-dislocation

framework

frenulum of lower lip

tongue

frenulum of tongue

sublingual gland

fructose

$$HO-C-H \quad O \quad H-C-OH$$

vertebra

femur.

transcondylar f., one through the condyles of the humerus.

transverse f., one in which the break line runs perpendicular with the axis of the bone.

fracture-dislocation. Dislocation and fracture of a bone near its articulation.

fragil'itas. Latin for brittleness.

f. ossium, brittleness of the bones.

fragil'ity. Brittleness; tendency to break or disintegrate.

erythrocyte f., tendency of the red blood cells to break down due to mechanical or osmotic factors.

mechanical f., tendency of the red blood cells to break down when subjected to mechanical trauma.

osmotic f., tendency of the red blood cells to break down when exposed to increasingly hypotonic saline solutions.

fragment antigen binding. A segment of the IgG-antibody molecule, derived by papain treatment and reduction, containing one antibody reaction site.

frambe'sia. Yaws.

frame. A structure designed to immobilize or give support to a part.

Balkan f., a device used to secure suspension and traction of a fractured limb; it consists of an overhead bar supported from the floor or bed posts; also called Balkan splint.

Foster f., a reversible bed similar to a Stryker frame.

Stryker f., a device that supports the patient and allows turning without individual motion of parts.

frame'work. 1. Stroma. **2.** In dentistry, the skeletal portion of a partial denture around which and to which the remaining portions of the prosthesis are attached.

fran'cium. An unstable radioactive metallic element; symbol Fr, atomic number 87, with mass number 223; the heaviest member of the alkali family of elements; the most stable of its isotopes has a half-life of 21 minutes.

FRC. Abbreviation for functional residual capacity.

freck'le. A brownish spot on the skin; also called ephelis.

freeze-drying. A method of tissue preparation in which the tissue specimen is instantly frozen and then the ice in the specimen is sublimed away in a high vacuum.

freeze-et'ching. A method of tissue preparation in which the tissue specimen is instantly frozen (⁻190°C), fragments are splintered away, and then the ice is sublimed away in a vacuum to a depth of about 100 Å; it produces an etching effect especially suitable for the study of the inner surface of plasma membranes.

freez'ing, gas'tric. Treatment of peptic ulcer by freezing the secretory cells of the stomach for the purpose of reducing or eliminating the production of acid gastric juice.

frem'itus. A vibration usually produced in the chest and felt on palpation.

pleural f., vibration produced by the rubbing together of the roughened surfaces of the pleural membranes, as in pleurisy.

tactile f., vibration felt by the hand when placed on the chest of a person speaking.

vocal f., vibration in the chest produced by the spoken voice.

frenec'tomy. The surgical removal of a frenum.

frenot'omy. The dividing of the frenulum of the tongue for the relief of tongue-tie.

fren'ulum. A small fold of mucous membrane that extends from a fixed to a movable part and limits the motion of the movable part.

f. of the clitoris, a fold connecting the undersurface of the clitoris with the labia minora.

f. of the lips, f. labii, either one of the folds extending from the gums to the midline of the upper or lower lips.

f. of the tongue, f. linguae, one extending from the midline of the undersurface of the tongue to the floor of the mouth.

f. of the prepuce, one that unites the foreskin (prepuce) to the undersurface of the glans penis.

fre'num, *pl.* **fre'na.** A fold of mucous membrane that limits the movement of a part, as the fold passing anteriorly from the gum to the inner surface of the lip.

fre'quency. The number of regular recurrences of a given event.

critical flicker fusion f., critical fusion frequency.

critical fusion f., the minimal number of intermittent or discontinuous visual stimuli per second that gives rise to a continuous visual sensation obliterating the flicker.

dominant f., the particular frequency appearing most frequently in an electroencephalogram (EEG).

FRF. Abbreviation for follicle-stimulating hormone releasing factor.

fri'able. Crumbly; easily torn or damaged.

fric'ative. In phonetics, a sound produced by the forcing of breath through a narrow orifice, as the sounds of the letters f, v, s, z, etc.

Friderichsen's syndrome. Waterhouse-Friderichsen syndrome.

frig'id. 1. Very cold. **2.** Abnormally lacking the desire for sexual intercourse; said chiefly of women. **3.** Unable to achieve orgasm during sexual intercourse.

frigid'ity. A psychologically based inability to respond adequately to a sexual relationship; said chiefly of women.

fringe'. Fimbria.

fringing. Bulbous deformation of the calyx of the kidney and tortuous elongation of the stem sometimes seen in the early stages of tuberculosis of the kidney.

frog in the throat. Accumulation of mucus in the larynx causing hoarseness.

Fröhlich's syndrome. Adiposogenital dystrophy; see under dystrophy.

Froin's syndrome. Clear yellow color of the lumbar spinal fluid with increased protein content and rapid coagulation, indicating that the communication between the lumbar region and the cerebral ventricles has been cut off; seen in certain organic nervous diseases.

Frommel's syndrome. Chiari-Frommel syndrome.

frons. Latin for forehead.

fron'tal. Relating to the forehead.

frost'bite. Local condition of varying degrees of severity caused by freezing of tissues upon exposure to extreme cold temperatures; may lead to gangrene; the fingers, toes, ears, and nose are usually affected. Cf chilblain.

frost, ure'mic. Tiny flakes of urea sometimes seen on the skin of patients with uremia.

fructoki'nase. A liver enzyme that promotes the reaction of ATP (adenosine triphosphate) and D-fructose to form fructose 6-phosphate.

fruc'tosan. A polyfructose, such as inulin, present in certain tubers; also called levan, levulin, and levulan.

fruc'tose. The sweetest of the simple sugars (monosaccharides) present in honey and fruits; in the body it is formed as one of the two products of sucrose hydrolysis; used intravenously as a nutrient replenisher; also called fruit sugar and levulose.

fructose'mia. Hereditary fructose intolerance; a rare genetically determined error of carbohydrate metabolism due to a deficiency of fructose-1-phosphate aldolase.

fructosu'ria. The presence of fructose in the urine; disorder of metabolism in which blood fructose levels are excessive and fructose appears in the urine.

fru'semide. See furosemide.

frustra'tion. In psychology, the denial of gratification by reality.

FSH. Abbreviation for follicle-stimulating hormone.

fuch'sin. Rosaniline monohydrochloride; a bright red dye used in histology and bacteriology.

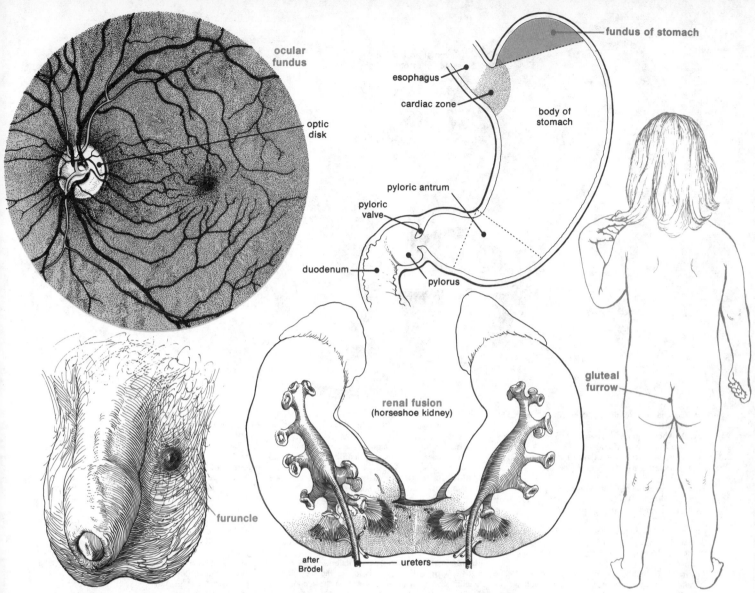

ocular fundus

optic disk

fundus of stomach

esophagus

cardiac zone

body of stomach

pyloric antrum

pyloric valve

duodenum

pylorus

furuncle

renal fusion (horseshoe kidney)

after Brödel

ureters

gluteal furrow

-fuge. Suffix meaning flight or driving away.

fugue. A form of hysterical loss of memory and actual physical flight from a disturbing environment; when the normal mental state returns, the individual has no recollection of his actions during this period.

ful'gurant. Sudden, flashing, like lightning; usually said of pain.

fulgura'tion. Destruction of tissue by means of a high frequency electric current.

ful'minating, ful'minant. Of sudden, violent onset and rapid course.

fumagil'lin. A crystalline antibiotic used as an amebicide.

fumiga'tion. Disinfection by exposure to the fumes of a germicide.

fuming. Releasing a visible vapor.

func'tion. 1. The natural or special type of activity which is proper for an organ or part. **2.** To perform such an action. **3.** The general properties of any substance.

func'tional. 1. Of or relating to a function. **2.** Nonorganic.

fun'dal. Relating to a fundus.

fun'diform. Sling-shaped.

fun'dus. *pl.* **fun'di.** The portion of a hollow organ farthest from, above, or opposite its opening.

  ocular f., the posterior portion of the interior of the eye. See also eyeground.

  f. of the stomach, the dome-shaped part of the stomach above its junction with the esophagus.

  f. of the uterus, the rounded portion of the uterus above the openings of the uterine tubes.

fun'duscope. Ophthalmoscope.

fundus'copy. Ophthalmoscopy.

fun'gal. Of or relating to a fungus.

funge'mia. Fungal disease disseminated through the blood stream.

Fun'gi. A phylum (subkingdom Thallophyta) which includes saprophytic and parasitic plants, those unable to manufacture their own food because they lack photosynthetic pigments.

fun'gi. Plural of fungus.

fun'gicide. Any substance that destroys fungus.

fun'giform. Having the shape of a fungus.

fun'gistat. An agent that inhibits the growth of fungi.

fun'goid. Resembling a fungus.

fungos'ity. A fungus growth.

fun'gous. Of or relating to a fungus.

fun'gus, *pl.* **fun'gi.** A member of the phylum Fungi (subkingdom Thallophyta) characterized by lack of chlorophyll, asexual reproduction, and parasitic qualities.

fu'nic. Of or relating to the umbilical cord.

fu'nicle. A small cordlike structure.

funic'ular. 1. Having a cordlike appearance. **2.** Relating to the umbilical cord.

funiculi'tis. 1. Inflammation of the spermatic cord. **2.** Inflammation of the portion of a spinal nerve located within the intervertebral canal.

funic'ulus, *pl.* **funic'uli. 1.** One of the three main divisions or columns of white matter on either side of the spinal cord, called anterior, lateral, and posterior. **2.** The spermatic cord. **3.** The umbilical cord.

fu'niform. Cordlike.

fu'nis. 1. The umbilical cord. **2.** A cordlike structure.

fun'nel. A conical vessel with a tube extending from its apex; used for pouring liquids, filtering, etc.

  Buchner f., a porcelain funnel consisting of an upper cylindrical portion and a lower conical part, separated by a perforated plate upon which filter paper can be fitted.

FUO. Abbreviation for fever of unknown origin. See also PUE and PUO.

fur'fur, *pl.* **fur'fures.** An epidermal scale.

furfura'ceous. Scaly; denoting a type of desquamation.

furo'semide. A substance used as an oral diuretic; also called frusemide; Lasix®

fur'row. A groove.

  digital f., one of the grooves on the palmar surface of the fingers.

  gluteal f., the groove between the buttocks.

  palpebral f., the groove of the upper eyelid extending from the inner to outer canthi.

fu'runcle. An abscess or pyogenic infection of a sweat gland or hair follicle, usually caused by *Staphylococcus aureus*; also called boil.

furun'cular. Relating to or like a furuncle (boil).

furun'culoid. Like a furuncle (boil).

furunculo'sis. A condition marked by the presence of numerous furuncles (boils).

fusc'in. The brown pigment of the retina.

fu'siform. Tapering at both ends.

fu'sion. 1. The process of melting. **2.** Joining together by surgery, as of a joint. **3.** The integration into one perfect image of the images seen simultaneously by the two eyes. **4.** The abnormal union of two adjacent parts.

  renal f., the abnormal fusion of the kidneys; named according to either the shape or location; e.g., horseshoe kidney, cake or lump kidney, sigmoid kidney, etc.

  spinal f., the fusion of two or more vertebral segments in order to eliminate motion between them.

fusospiroche'tal. Relating to the associated fusiform and spirochetal organisms.

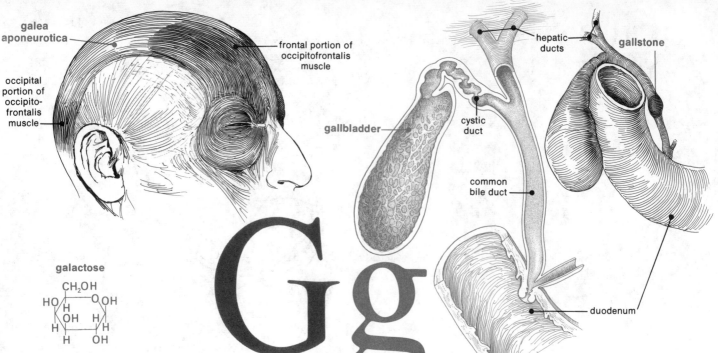

galea aponeurotica

occipital portion of occipitofrontalis muscle

frontal portion of occipitofrontalis muscle

galactose

gallbladder

hepatic ducts

gallstone

cystic duct

common bile duct

duodenum

γ. Gamma. For terms beginning with γ, see under specific term.

G. 1. Abbreviation for gingiva. **2.** Symbol for newtonian constant of gravitation.

g. 1. Abbreviation for (a) gender; (b) gram (also abbreviated gm). **2.** Symbol for acceleration of gravity.

Ga. Chemical symbol of the element gallium.

gadolin'ium. A silvery-white metallic rare-earth element; symbol Gd, atomic number 64, atomic weight 157.25.

gag. 1. To retch; to cause to retch. **2.** An instrument placed between the upper and lower teeth to keep the mouth open during operations on the tongue or throat.

gain. 1. To build up an increase; to acquire. **2.** The ratio of increase of output current, voltage, or power over input; the amplification factor of an electronic circuit.

epinosic g., see secondary gain.

paranosic g., see primary gain.

primary g., the alleviation of anxiety provided by a neurotic illness or symptom; also called paranosic gain.

secondary g., the additional indirect satisfaction or advantage (e.g., manipulating other people or receiving monetary reward) derived from a neurotic illness or symptom; also called epinosic gain.

Gaisböck's syndrome. Hypertension and polycythemia without splenomegaly, occurring in middle aged white males; the polycythemia is relative, with normal red blood cell mass but decreased plasma volume.

gait. A manner of walking or running.

antalgic g., a self-protective limp due to pain.

ataxic g., an unsteady, irregular gait.

cerebellar g., a staggering gait with a tendency to fall, indicative of cerebellar disease.

festinating g., festination.

high steppage g., gait in which the foot is raised high and brought down suddenly, the whole sole striking the ground in a flapping fashion.

tabetic g., a slapping gait characteristic of tabes dorsalis.

galact-, galacto-, galacta-. Combining forms denoting milk or milky; e.g., galactagogue.

galactacra'sia. Abnormal composition of human milk.

galac'tagogue. See galactopoietic. An agent that promotes the flow of milk.

galac'tan. Any of several carbohydrates that yield galactose on hydrolysis.

galac'tic. Relating to milk; inducing the flow of milk.

galac'toblast. Colostrum corpuscle; one of numerous large, round bodies containing fat droplets, present in colostrum; thought to be modified leukocyte.

galac'tocele. A tumor in the breast containing milk; caused by occulsion of a milk duct; also called lactocele.

galactoki'nase. An enzyme that, in the presence of ATP (adenosine triphosphate), promotes the phosphorylation of galactose to galactose 1-phosphate.

galac'tophore. A milk duct.

galactoph'orous. Conveying milk.

galactoph'ygous. Lactifugal; diminishing or arresting the flow of milk.

galactopoi'esis. Milk production.

galactopoiet'ic. 1. Relating to the secretion of milk. **2.** Any agent that promotes the secretion of milk.

galactorrhe'a. Excessive discharge of milk from the breasts after the child has been weaned, or unrelated to a recent pregnancy.

galactosam'ine. A crystalline amino derivative of galactose; also called chondrosamine.

galac'tosan. One of several polysaccharides of galactose; also called polygalactose.

galactosche'sia, galactos'chesis. Suppression of milk secretion; also called galactostasia and galactostasis.

galac'tose. A white crystalline simple sugar, $C_6H_{12}O_6$, not found free in food; it is produced in the body by the digestion of lactose (milk sugar) and then converted into glucose for energy.

galactose'mia. Defect in metabolism of galactose, a nutrient of milk, in which the conversion of galactose to glucose is deficient; the disorder usually becomes evident soon after birth by feeding problems, mental and physical retardation, enlargement of the liver and spleen, and elevated blood and urine galactose levels; can be treated effectively by excluding milk from the diet.

galacto'sis. The formation of milk.

galactosta'sia, galactosta'sis. See galactoschesia.

galactosu'ria. Presence of galactose in the urine.

galactother'apy. Treatment with a milk diet.

galactozy'mase. A starch-hydrolyzing enzyme present in milk.

ga'lea. 1. A helmet-shaped structure. **2.** A form of head bandage.

g. aponeurotica, the aponeurosis of the scalp; it covers the upper part of the skull, connecting the frontal and occipital bellies of the occipitofrontal muscle; also called epicranial aponeurosis.

galeat'omy. Surgical cutting of the epicranial aponeurosis (galea aponeurotica).

gale'na. See lead sulfide.

galeopho'bia. Morbid fear of cats.

gall. 1. Bile. **2.** An erosion.

gallamine triethiodide. A compound used as a skeletal muscle relaxant.

gall'bladder. A pear-shaped sac which stores bile and is situated under the liver.

hourglass g., congenital abnormality of the gallbladder in which a septum divides it into two functioning halves.

strawberry g., gallbladder in which the mucosa is red and congested and dotted with yellowish deposits of cholesterol.

gal'lium. A rare metallic element; symbol Ga, atomic number 31, atomic weight 69.72; liquid near room temperature.

gal'lium-68 (^{68}Ga). A radioactive isotope of gallium, used in bone scanning to detect metastatic bone lesions.

gal'lon. A unit of liquid volume or capacity in the U. S. Customary System, equal to four quarts or 231 cubic inches; it is the equivalent of 3.7853 liters.

gal'lop. A triple or quadruple cadence of heart sounds resembling the canter of a horse, heard on auscultation, due to the addition of a third and/or fourth heart sound; also called cantering or gallop rhythm.

atrial g., presystolic gallop sound related to atrial contraction, occurring in late diastole and designated as a fourth heart sound.

presystolic g., atrial gallop.

protodiastolic g., see ventricular gallop.

summation g., atrial and ventricular gallop sounds occurring simultaneously.

ventricular g., third heart sound occurring in early diastole (0.14 to 0.16 seconds after the second heart sound); also called protodiastolic gallop.

gall'stone. A stone formed in the gallbladder or a bile duct, usually composed of cholesterol crystals; thought to be due to a defect in composition of the bile.

Galton's delta. The middle triangular pattern of the lines of a fingerprint.

galvan'ic. 1. Relating to chemically produced direct current electricity. **2.** Having the effect of an electric shock.

gal'vanism. Direct current electricity, especially when produced by chemical action.

galvaniza'tion. The application of a direct electric current.

gal'vanize. To stimulate with an electric current.

galvano-. Combining form meaning direct electric current.

galvanocau'tery. Cautery with a wire that has

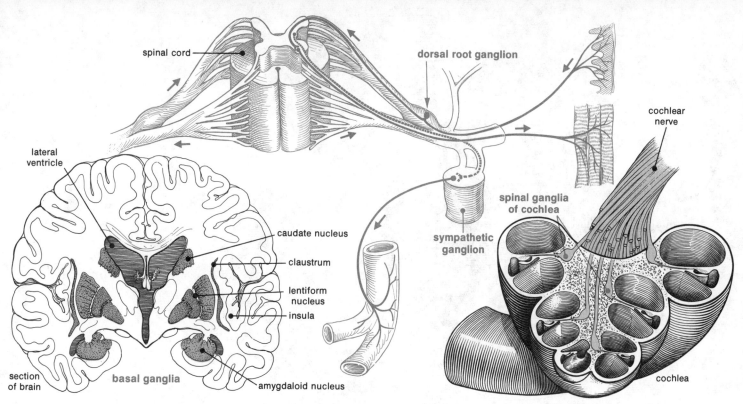

Labels in figure: spinal cord · dorsal root ganglion · cochlear nerve · lateral ventricle · caudate nucleus · claustrum · lentiform nucleus · insula · spinal ganglia of cochlea · sympathetic ganglion · section of brain · basal ganglia · amygdaloid nucleus · cochlea

been heated with a galvanic current.

galvanocontractil'ity. The ability of a muscle to contract under direct current.

galvanofaradiza'tion. The simultaneous application of continuous and interrupted electric currents.

galvanom'eter. Instrument for measuring the strength of a current of electricity.

　Einthoven's string g., see string galvanometer.

　string g., one designed to record the electrical potentials produced in the heart; the forerunner of the electrocardiograph; also called Einthoven's string galvanometer.

galvanopalpa'tion. The testing of cutaneous nerve responses by means of a weak electric current.

gal'vanoscope. Instrument used for detecting the presence and direction of electric currents.

galvanosur'gery. Surgical procedure using a direct electric current.

galvanother'apy. Treatment of disorders by the application of galvanic current; also called galvanotherapeutics.

galvanot'onus. Tonic muscular response to stimulation with an electric current.

gamasoido'sis. Dermatitis resulting from infestation with mites of the family Gamasidae, e.g., the fowl mite, *Dermanyssus gallinae.*

gam'ete. One of two sex cells that combines with another in true conjugation to form a zygote, from which a new organism develops.

gameto-. Combining form denoting gamete; e.g., gametocyte.

gam'etocide. Any agent destructive to gametes.

gam'etocyte. A cell from which gametes are produced by division; a spermatocyte or an oocyte.

gametogen'esis. The production of gametes (ova or spermatozoa).

gametogo'nia. See gametogony.

gametog'ony. Stage in the sexual cycle of protozoa in which gametocytes are formed; also called gametogonia.

gam'ma. 1. The third letter of the Greek alphabet, γ; used to indicate the third in a series. **2.** In chemical nomenclature it indicates (a) the third carbon of an aliphatic chain; (b) the location opposite the alpha position in the benzene ring. **3.** Obsolete term for microgram.

gam'magram. A graphic record of the γ-rays emitted by a substance or tissue.

gamogen'esis. Sexual reproduction.

gamopho'bia. Abnormal fear of marriage.

gang'lia. Plural of ganglion.

gang'liate, gang'liated. Having ganglia.

gangliec'tomy. Surgical removal of a ganglion.

gang'liform. Resembling a ganglion; also called ganglioform.

gang'lioblast. An embryonic cell from which ganglion cells develop.

ganglio'ma. See ganglioneuroma.

gang'lion, *pl.* **gang'lia** or **gang'lions. 1.** A collection of nerve cell bodies located outside of the brain and spinal cord. **2.** A cystic swelling resembling a tumor, occurring on a tendon sheath or joint capsule.

　autonomic g., any ganglion of the sympathetic and parasympathetic nervous systems.

　basal ganglia, ganglia located within the white matter of each cerebral hemisphere; they serve as important links along various motor pathways of the central nervous system; they include the caudate, lentiform, and amygdaloid nuclei and the claustrum.

　cardiac g., one of several ganglia in the cardiac plexus located between the arch of the aorta and the bifurcation of the pulmonary artery.

　celiac g., one of two large sympathetic ganglia in the upper part of the abdomen on either side of the aorta near the origin of the celiac artery; also called solar ganglion.

　cervical g., one of three (superior, middle, and inferior) sympathetic ganglia in the neck.

　ciliary g., a parasympathetic ganglion lying behind the orbit between the optic nerve and the lateral rectus muscle.

　coccygeal g., unpaired ganglion of the sympathetic trunk located on the anterior aspect of the tip of the coccyx; also called ganglion impar.

　dorsal root g., a ganglion located on the dorsal root of each spinal nerve containing the cell bodies of the sensory neurons of the nerve; also called spinal or posterior root ganglion.

　ganglia of glossopharyngeal nerve, the two sensory ganglia (superior and inferior) situated on the glossopharyngeal nerve as it passes through the jugular foramen.

　ganglia of sympathetic trunk, see paravertebral ganglia.

　g. impar, see coccygeal ganglion.

　g. of vagus nerve, inferior, a ganglion situated on the vagus nerve a short distance below the jugular foramen, in front of the transverse processes of the first and second cervical vertebrae.

　g. of vagus nerve, superior, a ganglion situated on the vagus nerve as it passes through the jugular foramen at the base of the skull.

　gasserian g., see trigeminal ganglion.

　geniculate g., a ganglion of the facial nerve.

　otic g., a parasympathetic ganglion located just below the foramen ovale medial to the mandibular

nerve; its preganglionic fibers are derived from the glossopharyngeal nerve and its postganglionic fibers innervate the parotid gland; also called Arnold's ganglion.

　parasympathetic ganglia, aggregations of nerve cell bodies of the parasympathetic nervous system; viz., ciliary, pterygopalatine, otic, and submandibular ganglia of the head and several others located near the organs of the thorax, abdomen, and pelvis.

　paravertebral ganglia, sympathetic ganglia located at intervals on each sympathetic trunk along the side of the vertebral column; generally there are three cervical, 12 thoracic, four lumbar, and four sacral; also called ganglia of sympathetic trunk.

　prevertebral ganglia, the sympathetic ganglia situated in front of the vertebral column and forming the plexuses of the thorax and abdomen; distinguished from the paravertebral ganglia, which lie along each side of the vertebral column.

　posterior root g., see dorsal root ganglion

　pterygopalatine g., the largest of the four parasympathetic ganglia associated with cranial nerves of the head; it is located in the pterygopalatine fossa just posterior to the middle nasal concha; it sends postganglionic parasympathetic fibers to the lacrimal glands, nose, oral cavity, and the uppermost part of the pharynx; also called sphenopalatine ganglion.

　semilunar g., see trigeminal ganglion.

　sphenopalatine g., see pterygopalatine ganglion.

　spinal g., see dorsal root ganglion.

　spiral g. of cochlea, the ganglion of bipolar nerve cell bodies located within the modiolus of the internal ear; it sends fibers peripherally to the spiral organ of Corti and centrally to the cochlear nuclei of the brain stem.

　stellate g., a ganglion of the sympathetic trunk containing two components, the inferior cervical and the first thoracic ganglia, which are often fused.

　submandibular g., one of the four parasympathetic ganglia associated with cranial nerves of the head; it is located just above the deep part of the submandibular gland; its preganglionic fibers are derived from the facial nerve and its postganglionic fibers innervate the submandibular and sublingual glands.

　sympathetic ganglia, those ganglia of the autonomic nervous system that are composed of adrenergic neurons receiving afferent fibers from preganglionic visceral motor neurons located in the lateral horn of the thoracic and upper lumbar segments of the spinal cord; classified according to their location as paravertebral and prevertebral ganglia.

　thoracic g., one on the thoracic portion of the

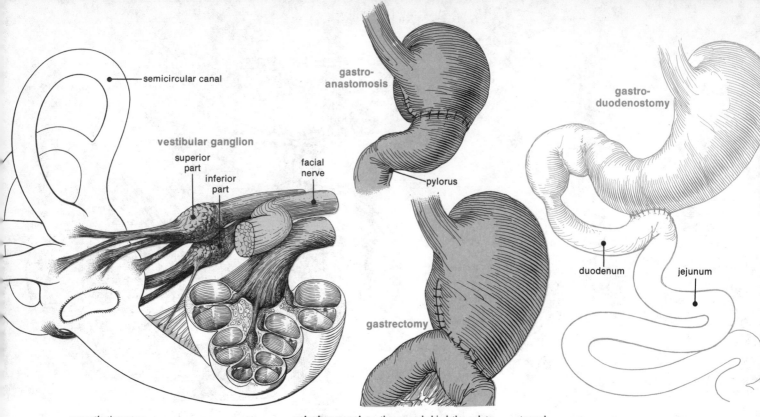

semicircular canal

vestibular ganglion

superior part
inferior part

facial nerve

gastro-anastomosis

pylorus

gastrectomy

gastro-duodenostomy

duodenum

jejunum

sympathetic system.

trigeminal g., the large flattened ganglion on the sensory root of the trigeminal nerve, located on the anterior aspect of the petrous portion of the temporal bone; also called semilunar or gasserian ganglion.

vestibular g., a collection of bipolar nerve cell bodies forming a swelling of the vestibulocochlear nerve in the internal auditory meatus; it is subdivided into superior and inferior parts; also called ganglion of Scarpa.

ganglionec'tomy. Surgical removal of a ganglion.

stellate g., see stellectomy.

ganglioneuro'ma. A small, encapsulated, benign, slow-growing tumor, composed of mature ganglion cells and nerve fibers; also called ganglioma and neurocytoma.

ganglion'ic. Of or relating to a ganglion, generally a nerve ganglion.

ganglioni'tis. Inflammation of any ganglion.

gangliople'gic. Denoting a compound that blocks transmission of impulses (usually for a short period of time) through an autonomic ganglion.

gang'lioside. A class of sphingoglycolipids present in neural tissue containing *N*-acetylneuraminic acid (NANA).

gangliosido'sis. Any disease involving an accumulation of specific gangliosides in the nervous system; also called ganglioside lipidosis.

gango'sa. Ulceration of the soft and hard palate, nasopharynx, and nose; a sequel to yaws; also called rhinopharyngitis mutilans.

gang'rene. Decay of bodily tissue, due to inadequate blood (nutritive) supply; a form of necrosis combined with putrefaction.

cold g., gangrene not preceded by inflammation; also called dry or neurotic gangrene and mummification.

diabetic g., gangrene due to arteriosclerosis accompanying diabetes.

gas g., gangrene occurring in extensively traumatized and soil-contaminated wounds infected with toxigenic anaerobic clostridia, and characterized by the presence of gas in the affected tissue.

moist g., a soft and moist gangrene due to the action of putrefactive bacteria.

gan'grenous. Affected with gangrene.

gap. An interval or an opening.

air-bone g., the lag between hearing acuity by air conduction and by bone conduction.

auscultatory g., a silent interval sometimes noticed during the determination of blood pressure; also called silent gap.

silent g., see auscultatory gap.

velopharyngeal g., the space behind the palate between the nose and throat.

Gardner's syndrome. A hereditary syndrome of polyposis of the rectum and colon, associated with cysts and tumors of skin and bone; transmitted by an autosomal dominant trait; carcinoma of the colon develops in more than 50 per cent of patients by age 40 and colectomy is usually recommended as a prophylactic procedure.

gar'gle. 1. To rinse the throat and mouth by forcing exhaled air through a liquid held in the mouth while the head is tilted back. **2.** A medicated solution used for rinsing the throat and mouth.

gar'goylism. see Hurler's syndrome.

gas, *pl.* **gases, gasses. 1.** An airlike state of matter distinguished from the solid and liquid states by freely moving molecules capable of great expansion and contraction with changes in pressure and temperature; a vapor. **2.** Gaseous anesthesia.

inert g., any of the gases helium, neon, argon, krypton, xenon, and radon (nitron), which are present in the atmosphere and exhibit no chemical affinity; totally unreactive gas, except under extreme conditions.

laughing g., nitrous oxide, a mild anesthetic; so called because its inhalation at times causes a hilarious delirium.

marsh g., see methane.

mustard g., dichlorodiethyl sulfide, an oily, volatile substance used in chemical warfare during World War I as a gaseous blistering agent; inhalation of the poison gas may result in chemical bronchopneumonia; progenitor of the so-called nitrogen mustards used in cancer chemotherapy.

noble g., inert gas.

tear g., any gaseous agent such as chloroacetophenone (CAP) which irritates the eyes, producing blinding tears; usually dispersed through grenades and projectiles.

water g., an industrial fuel gas produced by passing steam over red-hot coal or coke; consists mainly of hydrogen, hydrocarbons, and carbon monoxide.

gas'eous. Relating to or of the nature of a gas.

gash. 1. A flesh wound. **2.** To inflict a wound.

gas'iform. Gaseous.

gasogen'ic. Gas-producing.

gasom'eter. A calibrated apparatus for measuring volume of gases; generally used for measuring respiration gases.

gasom'etry. The scientific measurement of gases; the determination of the relative proportion of gases in a mixture.

gastrec'tomy. Surgical removal of part or all of the stomach; also called gastric resection.

subtotal g., excision of a large portion of the stomach.

gas'tric. Of or relating to the stomach.

gas'trin. One of the gastrointestinal hormones released during digestion; it is secreted by the mucosa of the pyloric region of the stomach upon contact with food; it increases the secretion of hydrochloric acid and, to a lesser degree, of pepsinogen.

gastri'tis. Inflammation of the stomach.

antral g., condition marked by irregular, concentric narrowing of the stomach; also called periantritis.

atrophic g., chronic inflammation of the stomach with degeneration of the mucous membrane.

giant hypertrophic g., see Menétrier's disease.

interstitial g., gastritis involving the submucosa and muscular coat of the stomach.

phlegmonous g., severe inflammation with purulent infiltration of the stomach wall.

pseudomembranous g., inflammation of the stomach marked by the formation of a false membrane.

gastro-, gastr-. Combining forms indicating the stomach; e.g., gastrotomy.

gastroanastomo'sis. Surgical connection of the pyloric and cardiac ends of the stomach; also called gastrogastrostomy.

gastroblenorrhe'a. Excessive secretion of mucus by the stomach.

gastrocam'era. A small camera designed to be swallowed, after which the stomach is inflated and photographs are rapidly taken.

gas'trocele. A hernia of a portion of the stomach.

gastrocne'mius. See table of muscles.

gastrocol'ic. Relating to the stomach and colon.

gastrocoli'tis. Inflammation of the stomach and colon.

gastrocolopto'sis. Downward displacement of the stomach and colon.

gastrocolos'tomy. The surgical construction of a passage between the stomach and colon.

Gastrodiscol'des hom'inis. A species of trematode worms parasitic in the intestines of swine and man.

gastroduode'nal. Relating to both the stomach and the duodenum.

gastroduodenos'copy. The visualization of the interior of the stomach and duodenum with the aid of a gastroscope.

gastroduodenos'tomy. The surgical creation of an artificial passage between the stomach and duodenum.

gastroenter'ic. Gastrointestinal; of or relating to the stomach and intestines.

gastroenteri'tis. Inflammation of the mucous membrane of the stomach and intestines.

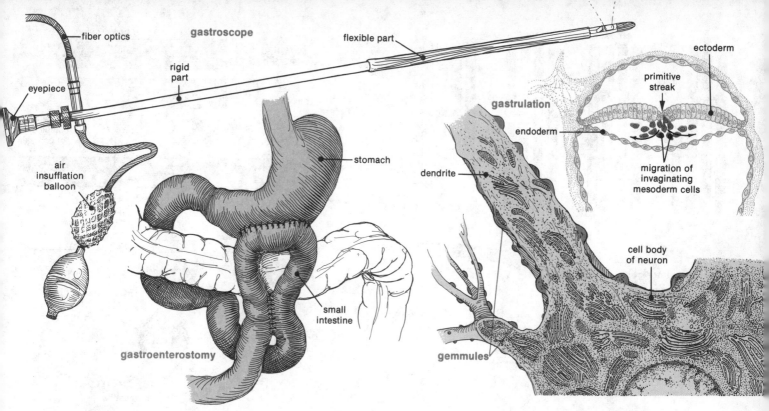

gastroenteroanastomo'sis. A surgical connection between the stomach and any noncontinuous portion of the intestine.

gastroenterol'ogist. A specialist in diseases of the stomach and intestines.

gastroenterol'ogy. The branch of medicine concerned with disorders of the stomach and intestines and also with the esophagus, the liver, and the gallbladder.

gastroenterop'athy. Any disease of the alimentary canal.

gastroenteropto'sis. The downward displacement, or prolapse, of the stomach and a portion of the intestine.

gastroenteros'tomy. The surgical creation of a passage between the stomach and the intestine.

gastroenterot'omy. Surgical incision into the stomach and intestine.

gastroepiplo'ic. Relating to the stomach and greater omentum.

gastroesophage'al. Relating to the stomach and the esophagus.

gastroesophagi'tis. Inflammation of the stomach and esophagus.

gastroesophagos'tomy. The surgical creation of a new opening or connection between the stomach and esophagus.

gastrogastros'tomy. See gastroanastomosis.

gastrogavage'. Feeding by way of a gastrostomy (surgical opening through the stomach wall).

gastrogen'ic. Originating in the stomach.

gas'trograph. Instrument for recording the motions of the stomach.

gastrohepat'ic. Relating to the stomach and the liver.

gastrohydrorrhe'a. Secretion by the stomach of a large quantity of a watery fluid.

gastrointest'inal. Relating to the stomach and intestines; also called gastroenteric.

gastrojejunocol'ic. Relating to the stomach, jejunum, and colon; e.g., a fistula penetrating the three structures.

gastrojejunos'tomy. Surgical creation of an opening or connection between the stomach and jejunum.

gas'trolith. A calculus in the stomach; a gastric calculus.

gastrolithi'asis. The presence of one or more calculi in the stomach.

gastrol'ogy. The scientific study of the stomach and its diseases; the term gastroenterology is more commonly used.

gastromala'cia. Softening of the stomach wall.

gastromeg'aly. Abnormal enlargement of the stomach.

gastrop'athy. Any disease of the stomach.

gas'tropexy. The surgical attachment of the stomach to the abdominal wall.

gastrophren'ic. Relating to the stomach and the diaphragm.

gas'troplasty. Surgical correction of any defect of the stomach.

gastropto'sis, gastropto'sia. Downward displacement of the stomach.

gastropylor'ic. Relating to the stomach as a whole and to the pylorus.

gastror'rhaphy. Suture of the stomach.

gas'troscope. An instrument for viewing the interior of the stomach.

gastros'copy. The examination of the interior of the stomach with the gastroscope.

gastrospas'm. Spasmodic contraction of the stomach.

gastrosteno'sis. Constriction of the stomach.

gastros'tomy. The surgical construction of a passage into the stomach.

gastrot'omy. Surgical incision into the stomach.

gastrotro'pic. Having an effect on the stomach.

gas'trula. An embryo at the stage of development following the blastula when the gastrulation movements occur.

gastrula'tion. The formation of a gastrula; in embryology, the process by which a third germ layer of cells (mesoderm) migrates between the bilaminar disk making it trilaminar (ectoderm, mesoderm, and endoderm); it occurs during the third week of embryonic development.

gath'er. To come to a head; said of a boil when maturing.

gath'ering. 1. The formation of pus in a boil, abscess, etc. **2.** Colloquial term for an abscess, boil, etc.

Gaucher's disease. Disease characterized by the deposit of glucocerebroside, a glycolipid, in reticuloendothelial cells; manifestations include splenomegaly, hepatomegaly, lymph node enlargement, and bone lesions.

gauge. A measuring instrument.

  bite g., gnathodynamometer; a pressure device used in dentistry to determine the biting force.

  Boley g., a caliper-type gauge used in dentistry to obtain measurements necessary for dental prosthesis.

  catheter g., a metal plate with perforations of different sizes used to determine the size of catheters.

Gaulthe'ria. A genus of plants including *Gaultheria procumbens*, commonly known as wintergreen and teaberry; it yields a volatile oil rich in methyl salicylate.

gaunt. 1. Very slim and bony. **2.** Emaciated.

gaunt'let. A glovelike bandage protecting the hand and fingers.

gauze. A thin, open weave surgical dressing or bandage.

  absorbent g., a bleached cotton gauze of varied thread counts and weight.

  petrolatum g., absorbent gauze impregnated with white petrolatum.

gavage'. The passage of nutritive material into the stomach by means of a tube.

g. cal. Abbreviation for gram calorie.

Gd. Chemical symbol of the element gadolinium.

Ge. Chemical symbol of the element germanium.

Geiger-Müller tube. See under tube.

gel. 1. The semisolid state of a coagulated colloid. **2.** To convert a solution into a gel.

gel'ate. To cause the formation of a gel.

gel'atin. A colorless, transparent protein derived from the collagen of tissue by boiling in water; used for nutritional purposes and also as a packaging agent for pharmaceuticals.

  zinc g., jelly containing zinc oxide, gelatin, glycerin, and water; used between layers of bandage as a protective dressing.

gelat'inize. 1. To convert to gelatin. **2.** To become gelatinous.

gelat'inoid. 1. Like gelatin. **2.** Gelatinous.

gelat'inous. 1. Pertaining to or containing gelatin. **2.** Viscous; resembling jelly.

gela'tion. The transformation of a solution to a gel.

gel'ose. In general, any amorphous polysaccharide, such as agar, obtained from red algae and capable of forming a jelly.

gelo'sis. A hard mass in the tissues, especially in a muscle.

gem-. Combining form denoting twin substitutions on a single atom.

gemellol'ogy. The study of twins and twinning.

gem'inate. Occurring in pairs.

gemma'tion. Asexual reproduction in which a new organism develops as an outgrowth of the parent; also called budding.

gem'mule. 1. A bud that develops into a new organism. **2.** One of several spherical enlargements sometimes present on the protoplasmic processes (dendrites) of a nerve cell. **3.** In Darwin's theory of inheritance, particles transferred from body cells to sex cells.

-gen. Combining form meaning producing or precursor of. See also pro-.

gen-, geno-. Combining forms meaning producing.

gen'der. Sex category.

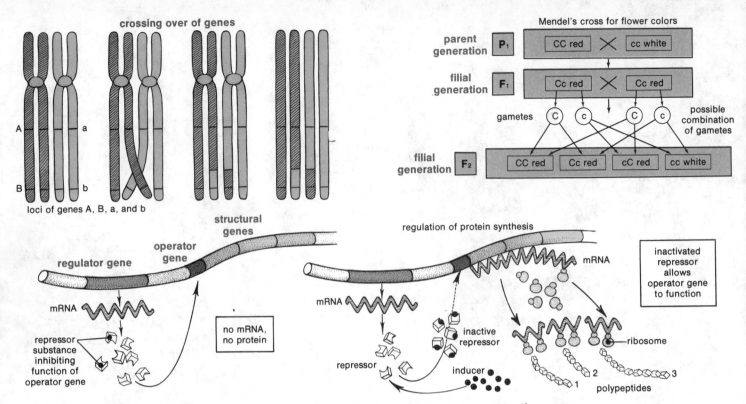

crossing over of genes

loci of genes A, B, a, and b

Mendel's cross for flower colors

parent generation P₁ — CC red × cc white

filial generation F₁ — Cc red × Cc red

gametes C c C c — possible combination of gametes

filial generation F₂ — CC red | Cc red | cC red | cc white

regulator gene — **operator gene** — **structural genes**

mRNA

repressor substance inhibiting function of operator gene

no mRNA, no protein

regulation of protein synthesis

mRNA

inactive repressor

repressor

inducer

inactivated repressor allows operator gene to function

ribosome

polypeptides 1 2 3

---

gene. The hereditary unit occupying a fixed position (locus) in the chromosome, and capable of reproducing itself at each cell division and of managing the formation of protein.

allelic g.'s, different genes located in corresponding positions (loci) in a pair of chromosomes and effecting a similar function.

autosomal g., gene present on any chromosome other than a sex chromosome.

crossing over of g.'s, the exchange of material, including genes, between two paired chromosomes during meiosis.

dominant g., one that produces a recognizable effect in the organism whether paired with an identical or a dissimilar gene.

g. dosage, the number of times a specific gene is present in the nucleus of a cell.

hemizygous g., a gene present in a single dose, or without a partner.

holandric g., Y-linked g., one located on the nonhomologous portion of a Y (male) chromosome.

initiator g., one of the regulator genes that codes for the repressor protein which binds to the DNA.

operator g., one of the regulator genes whose function is to activate messenger-RNA production; it is part of the feedback system for determining the rate of enzyme production.

promotor g., one of the regulator genes on which RNA polymerase attaches and catalyzes the synthesis of messenger-RNA.

recessive g., a gene that does not produce a detectable effect in the organism when combined (heterozygous) with a dominant allele.

regulator g., one which controls the rate of protein synthesis; it controls the production of a repressor protein which acts on the operator gene.

sex-linked g., one located on a sex (X or Y) chromosome.

structural g., one that specifies the formation of a particular polypeptide chain.

X-linked g., one carried on an X (female) chromosome.

Y-linked g., see holandric gene.

gen'era. Plural of genus.

gen'eralist. A physician who treats a broad range of diseases; a family or general physician.

gen'eralize. To become general; said of a primary local lesion that has become widespread or systemic.

genera'tion. A stage in the succession of descent of the offspring of plants or animals.

filial g., offspring resulting from a genetically specified mating: first filial generation (F₁), offspring of the first experimental crossing of animals or plants (parental generation with which the experiment

starts is P₁); second filial generation (F₂), offspring resulting from intercrossing or self-fertilization of F₁ individuals; third, fourth, etc. filial generation (F₃, F₄, etc.), offspring of continued crossing of heterozygotes with continuation of F₂ ratios.

gen'erative. Relating to reproduction.

gen'erator. 1. A machine for producing electrical energy from some other form of energy. **2.** A device that generates vapor, gas, or aerosol from a liquid or solid.

aerosol g., a device for generating airborne suspensions of small particles, usually for inhalation therapy.

asynchronous pulse g., a cardiac pacemaker in which the rate of discharge does not depend on the natural cardiac activity; also called fixed rate pulse generator.

atrial synchronous pulse g., a ventricular stimulating pacemaker whose rate of discharge is determined by the atrial rate; also called atrial triggered pulse generator.

atrial triggered pulse g., see atrial synchronous pulse generator.

demand pulse g., see ventricular inhibited pulse generator.

fixed rate pulse g., see asynchronous pulse generator.

pion g., a device that emits a stream of pions (subatomic particles generated by a high-energy accelerator); used experimentally to kill cancer cells.

pulse g., a generator serving as the source for an artificial pacemaker assembly; it generates and discharges electrical impulses to stimulate the heart.

radionuclide g., a receptacle containing a large quantity of a certain radionuclide which decays down to a secondary radionuclide of shorter half-life; the shorter form affords a continuing supply of relatively short-lived radionuclides for laboratory use; also called "radioactive cow."

standby pulse g., see ventricular inhibited pulse generator.

ventricular inhibited pulse g., a generator which suppresses its electrical output in response to natural ventricular activity but which, in the absence of such cardiac activity, functions as an asynchronous pulse; also called demand pulse or standby pulse generator.

ventricular synchronous pulse g., a pulse generator which delivers its output synchronously with naturally occurring ventricular activity but which, in the absence of such cardiac activity functions as an asynchronous pulse; also called ventricular triggered pulse generator.

ventricular triggered pulse g., see ventricular synchronous pulse generator.

gener'ic. 1. Of or relating to a genus. **2.** General; relating to an entire group.

genesiol'ogy. The study of generation and reproduction.

gen'esis. Creation; origin.

genet'ic. 1. Relating to the study of heredity. **2.** Inherited. **3.** In psychiatry, relating to an earlier period of development in a patient's life in which conflicts or problems originated.

genet'icist. A scientist who specializes in genetics.

genet'ics. The science of heredity; especially the study of the origin of the characteristics of the individual and hereditary transmission.

medical g., the branch of human genetics concerned with the relationship between heredity and disease.

genetotroph'ic. Denoting inherited nutritional factors, applied especially to certain hereditary deficiency disorders.

ge'nial. Of or relating to the chin.

gen'ic. Of or relating to the genes.

-genic. Combining form meaning causing.

genic'ulate, genic'ulated. Shaped like a flexed knee.

genic'ulum pl. **genic'ula.** From Latin, small knee; a sharp kneelike bend in a small structure.

g. of facial canal, the bend in the facial canal which houses the geniculum of the facial nerve.

g. of facial nerve, a kneelike bend of the horizontal portion of the facial nerve at the lateral end of the internal acoustic meatus, above the promontory of the middle ear.

genioglos'sus. See table of muscles.

geniohyoid. See table of muscles.

ge'nioplasty. Reparative or plastic surgery of the chin; also called genyplasty.

gen'ital. Relating to reproduction.

genita'lia. The genitals.

genital'ity. In psychoanalysis, a general term denoting the genital constituents of sexuality.

gen'itals. The organs of reproduction.

genitou'rinary. Urogenital; relating to the organs of reproduction and the urinary tract.

ge'nius. 1. Exceptional intellectual and creative abilities. **2.** One who possesses such abilities.

genodermato'sis. A genetically determined disorder of the skin.

ge'nome. A complete set of chromosomes (with their genes) from one parent; the total genetic endowment.

gen'otype. The genetic or hereditary constitution of an individual.

gentami'cin sul'fate. A broad spectrum antibiotic that inhibits the growth of bacteria; Garamycin®.

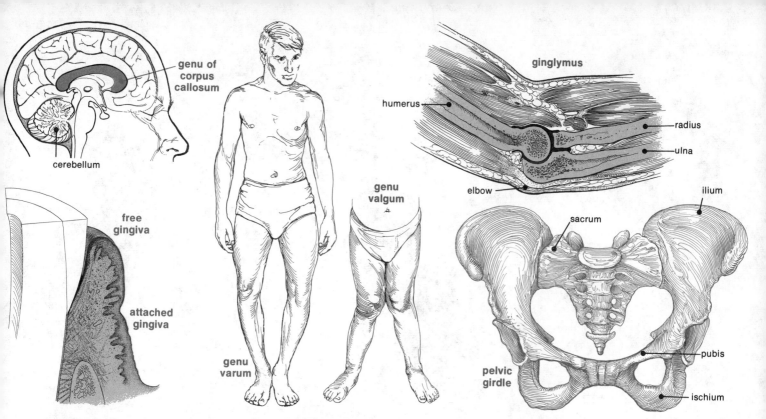

genu of corpus callosum

cerebellum

free gingiva

attached gingiva

genu varum

genu valgum

ginglymus

humerus

elbow

radius

ulna

ilium

sacrum

pelvic girdle

pubis

ischium

gen'tian. Gentian root, the dried roots of the herb *Gentiana lutea*.

g. violet, see under violet.

ge'nu. 1. The knee. **2.** Any structure resembling a flexed knee.

g. of corpus callosum, the anterior extremity of the corpus callosum.

g. recurvatum, the backward bending of the knee joint.

g. valgum, knock knee, a deformity of the leg at the level of the knee, usually bilateral, marked by a lateral angulation of the tibia.

g. varum, bowleg, a deformity, usually bilateral, in which the leg has an outward curvature at the level of the knee.

ge'nus, *pl.* **gen'era.** The biologic classification ranking below a family and above a species; a category denoting resemblances in general features but differences in details.

gen'yplasty. See genioplasty.

geomed'icine. The study of environmental influences on health and disease.

geopathol'ogy. The study of disease as it relates to the environment.

geopha'gia, geoph'agy, geoph'agism. The habit of eating earth, including various forms of clay; a form of pica.

geotricho'sis. Condition caused by infection with the fungus *Geotrichum*.

Geot'richum. A genus of yeastlike fungi, one species of which infects the lungs and bronchi of man.

geriat'ric. Relating to old age.

geriat'rics. The branch of medicine concerned with old age, its physiology and disease.

germ. 1. A pathogenic microbe. **2.** An embryonic structure capable of developing into a new organism; a primordium.

wheat g., the vitamin-rich embryonic or germinating portion of the wheat kernel; used as a cereal or dietary supplement.

germa'nium. A metallic element; symbol Ge, atomic number 32, atomic weight 72.6.

germici'dal. Destructive to disease-causing microorganisms.

ger'micide. An agent that kills germs or microbes.

ger'mifuge. Germicide.

ger'minal. 1. Pertaining to germination. **2.** Pertaining to the nature of a germ.

geroder'ma. Atrophy of the skin.

gerodon'tics, gerodontol'ogy. The diagnosis and treatment of dental disorders of the aged.

geromaras'mus. The atrophy of old age.

geron'tal. Relating to old age; senile.

geronto-, gero-, ger-, gerat-. Combining forms meaning old age.

gerontol'ogy. The study of medical and social problems associated with aging.

geronto'pia. See senopia.

gerontotherapeu'tics. Treatment of diseases of the aged.

gerontox'on. See arcus senilis.

ges'tagen. A general term denoting hormones that produce progestational changes in the uterus.

gestalt'. A unified system of physical, psychological, or symbolic phenomena having properties that cannot be derived solely from its components.

gesta'tion. See pregnancy.

GFR. Abbreviation for glomerular filtration rate.

GH. Abbreviation for growth hormone.

Ghon focus. The primary lesion of pulmonary tuberculosis; that part of the complex which is parenchymal.

Ghon complex. Deposits in the peripheral lung field together with calcified hilar nodes; formerly considered pathognomonic of healed primary tuberculosis but may be mimicked by healed primary lesions of histoplasmosis and coccidioidomycosis; the deposits usually go on to calcification.

ghost, erythrocytic. The remaining membranous sac of a red blood cell after the loss of hemoglobin.

GH-RF. Abbreviation for growth hormone-releasing factor.

GI. Abbreviation for gastrointestinal.

Gianotti-Crosti syndrome. An acute, papular dermatosis of young children, associated with mild fever and malaise; it generally disappears without treatment within 30 to 70 days; also called papulosa infantum and acrodermatitis.

gi'antism. Gigantism.

Giar'dia. A genus of flagellate protozoa some of which are parasitic in the intestinal tract of man and domestic animals.

giardi'asis. Infestation with *Giardia intestinalis*.

gib'berish. Incoherent, rapid talk.

gibbos'ity. 1. A hump or protuberance. **2.** The condition of being humped or protuberant.

gib'bous. Humpbacked.

gib'bus. A hump; a kyphos.

giga-. Combining form used in the metric system meaning one billion (10^9).

gi'gantism. An abnormal condition of excessive growth in height, greatly exceeding the average for the person's race.

giganto-, gigant-. Combining forms meaning exceedingly large or excessive growth.

gi'gavolt. A billion volts.

gil'bert. The electromagnetic unit of electromotive force.

Gilbert's disease. Familial nonhemolytic jaun-

dice; see under jaundice.

Gilles de la Tourette's disease. A rare form of generalized tic usually occurring in childhood; characterized by uncontrolled continuous gestures, facial twitching, foul language, and repetition of sentences spoken by other persons.

gingi'va. The gum; the portion of the oral mucosa which envelops the alveolar process and surrounds the neck of the tooth.

attached g., the portion of the gingiva that extends from the free gingival groove apically and terminates at the mucogingival junction (where alveolar mucosa begins).

free g., the portion of the gingiva that extends from the free gingival groove occlusally, over the free margin of the gingiva, then descends apically into the gingival sulcus and terminates at the epithelial attachment.

gin'gival. Of or pertaining to the gums.

gingivec'tomy. Surgical removal of diseased gingival tissue.

gingivi'tis. Inflammation of the gums.

necrotizing ulcerative g., a bacterial (fusospirochetal) infection, usually of sudden onset, characterized by tender, bleeding gums with ulcer formation (especially between the teeth), a gray exudate, and fetid breath; most commonly occurring in individuals with poor oral hygiene; also called Vincent's disease, infection, or stomatitis, and trench mouth.

gingivo-. Combining form meaning the gums.

gin'givoplasty. Surgical contouring of the gingiva.

gingivo'sis. A noninflammatory desquamative condition of the gums.

gingivostomati'tis. Inflammation of the gums and oral mucosa.

ging'lymus. A hinge joint which has one concave and one convex articulating surface, as the articulation between the ulna and humerus at the elbow; it allows motion in one plane only.

gird'le. 1. An encircling band. **2.** Any encircling structure or region.

pectoral g., see shoulder girdle.

pelvic g., the bony ring formed by the sacrum and the two hipbones.

shoulder g., one formed by the clavicles (collarbones), scapulas (shoulder blades), and the manubrium part of the sternum (breastbone); also called pectoral girdle.

girth. 1. The measure encircling an animal's body slightly behind the forelegs. **2.** Circumference; the distance around anything, particularly the abdomen.

git'alin. Extract of *Digitalis purpurea* used in the treatment of certain heart diseases; also called

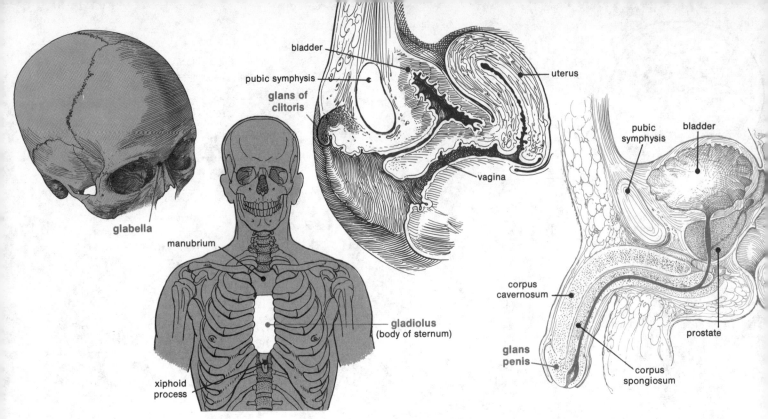

amorphous gitalin; Gitaligin®.

gl. Abbreviation for gland.

glabel′la. The smooth area of the frontal bone located between the eyebrows, immediately above the root of the nose.

gla′brous. Hairless; smooth and bare.

gladi′olus. The body or main portion of the sternum; also called corpus sterni.

gland. A secreting organ.

accessory g., a small detached mass of glandular tissue located near a gland or similar structure.

acinous g., a gland made up of one or several saclike structures.

adrenal g., a flattened, somewhat triangular endocrine gland resting upon the upper end of each kidney; it produces steroid hormones (aldosterone, androgens, glucocorticoids, progestins, and estrogens), epinephrine, and norepinephrine; also called suprarenal gland.

apocrine g., a gland producing a secretion which contains part of the secreting cells.

Bartholin's g., see greater vestibular gland.

Brunner's g.'s, see duodenal glands.

bulbourethral g.'s, two pea-shaped glands situated dorsal and lateral to the membranous portion of the male urethra; during sexual stimulation, the glands secrete a mucus-like substance into the urethra that serves as a lubricant for the epithelium; also called Cowper's glands.

cardiac g.'s, the tubular, branched, slightly coiled, mucus-producing glands located in the transition zone between the esophagus and stomach; they also secrete electrolytes.

compound g., one composed of numerous small sacs (acini) whose excretory ducts combine to form larger ones.

Cowper's g.'s, see bulbourethral glands.

ductless g., one possessing no excretory duct.

duodenal g.'s, small, branched, compound tubular glands in the submucous layer of the first part of the duodenum; they secrete an alkaline mucoid substance into the crypts of Lieberkühn or directly to the surface between the duodenal villi; also called Brunner's glands.

endocrine g., a ductless gland whose secretion (hormone) is absorbed directly into the bloodstream.

endo-exocrine g., one that produces both internal and external secretions, as the pancreas.

excretory g., any gland that separates waste material from the blood.

exocrine g., a gland that discharges its secretion through a duct onto the internal or external surface of the body; it may be simple or compound.

gastric g.'s, numerous, straight, sometimes branched, tubular glands in the mucosa of the fundus and body of the stomach (they are absent in the cardiac and pyloric regions); they contain the cells that produce hydrochloric acid and pepsin; also called fundic glands.

greater vestibular g., one of two small mucoid secreting glands on either side of the vaginal orifice, in the groove between the hymen and the labium minus; its major function is the production of lubrication of the introitus; also called Bartholin's gland.

holocrine g., a gland whose secretion is composed of the disintegrated secreting cell in addition to its accumulated secretion.

interscapular g., brown fat; see under fat.

intestinal g.'s, crypts of Lieberkühn; simple tubular glands in the mucous membrane of the intestines, concerned with the secretion of digestive enzymes and some hormones.

lacrimal g., a gland that secretes tears; located in the upper lateral portion of the orbit.

mammary g., a compound milk-producing gland that forms the major part of the female breast; it consists of 15 to 20 lobes, each of which has a separate duct opening at the apex of the nipple; it reaches functional maturity after pregnancy.

meibomian g., see tarsal gland.

mixed g., a gland in which some secretory units contain both serous and mucous cells; e.g., the submandibular gland.

parathyroid g.'s, the smallest of the endocrine glands, situated between the dorsal borders of the thyroid gland and its capsule; usually four in number, each the approximate size of an apple seed; they produce parathyroid hormone (parathormone) which regulates the calcium and phosphate metabolism of the body.

paraurethral g., one of the larger mucous glands located in the lining of the female urethra, just within the orifice; also called Skene's gland.

parotid g., a salivary gland located below and in front of each ear.

pineal g., see body, pineal.

pituitary g., see hypophysis.

pyloric g., one of the simple, coiled, mucus-producing tubular glands of the pyloric part of the stomach.

racemose g., an acinous gland, like the parotid, whose acini are arranged like grapes on a stem.

sebaceous g., a simple branched holocrine gland in the dermis which usually opens into the distal part of the hair follicle and secretes an oily substance (sebum); some sebaceous glands open directly onto the skin surface, such as on the vermilion border of the lips.

seromucous g., a gland whose secretory cells have histochemical and cytologic characteristics that suggest the elaboration of both serous and mucous secretions.

simple g., a gland consisting of a single system of secretory passages opening into a nonbranching duct; divided into tubular, tubuloalveolar, and alveolar types.

Skene's g., see paraurethral gland.

sublingual g., one of two salivary glands in the floor of the mouth with a series of ducts (10 to 30) opening into the mouth at the side of the tongue's frenulum; most of the secretory units are mucus-secreting with serous demilunes.

submandibular g., one of two predominately serous salivary glands in the upper neck; the main duct opens into the mouth beneath the tongue.

suprarenal g., see adrenal gland.

sweat g.'s, coiled tubular glands, located deep in the skin, that secrete a watery solution rich in sodium and chloride (sweat); also called sudoriferous glands.

tarsal g., one of numerous sebaceous glands in the eyelids; also called meibomian gland.

thymus g., see thymus.

thyroid g., the largest endocrine gland in man, situated in front of the lower part of the neck, and consisting of right and left lobes, on either side of the trachea, joined by a connecting isthmus; it secretes the iodine-rich hormones thyroxin and triiodothyronine which are concerned with regulating the rate of metabolism; also thought to secrete thyrocalcitonin.

tubular g., a gland composed of one or more tubules closed at one end.

urethral g., one of several minute mucous glands located in the lining of the urethra; in the male, also called Littre's glands.

glan′ders. An infectious disease of horses, mules, and donkeys caused by the gram-negative bacillus *Pseudomonas mallei*; marked by fever and ulcers of the respiratory tract or skin; occasionally transmitted to man; also called farcy.

glandilem′ma. The enveloping membrane or capsule of a gland.

glan′dula. A small gland.

glan′dular. Of, relating to, or resembling a gland.

glan′dule. A small gland.

glans, *pl.* **glan′des.** A small glandlike structure.

g. clitoridis, g. of clitoris, a small rounded mass of erectile tissue at the tip of the clitoris.

g. penis, the caplike extension of the corpus spongiosum at the head or tip of the penis.

Glanzmann's disease. See thrombasthenia.

glass. Any of a class of transparent or translucent brittle materials composed of silica with oxides of

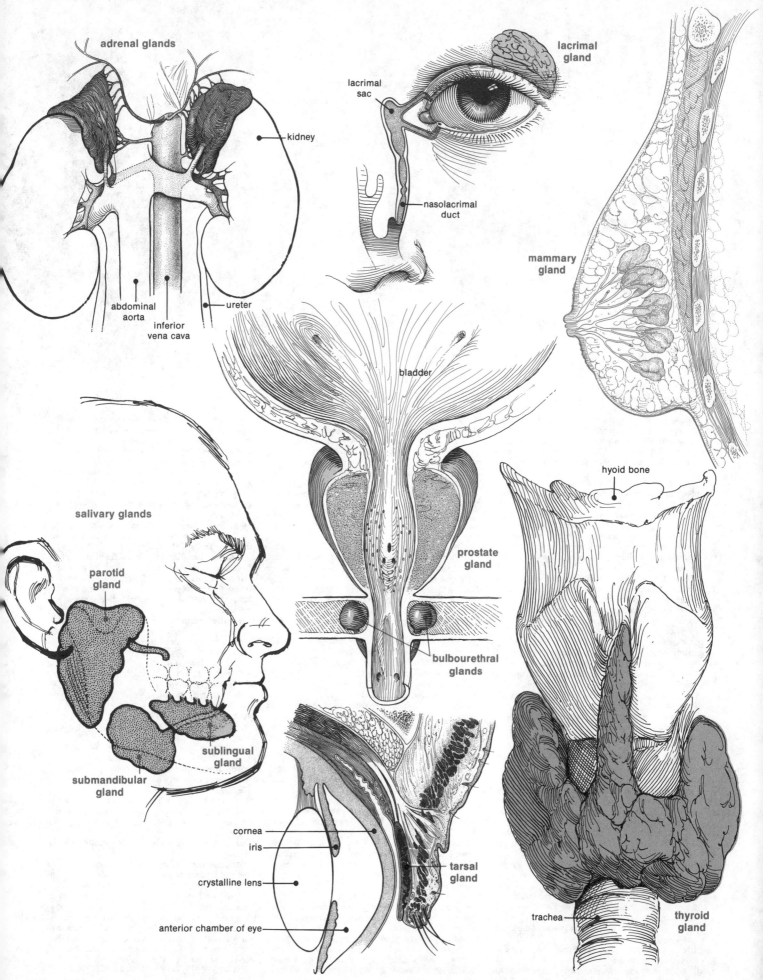

adrenal glands

lacrimal gland

lacrimal sac

kidney

nasolacrimal duct

mammary gland

abdominal aorta

inferior vena cava

ureter

bladder

salivary glands

parotid gland

prostate gland

hyoid bone

sublingual gland

submandibular gland

bulbourethral glands

cornea

iris

crystalline lens

anterior chamber of eye

tarsal gland

trachea

thyroid gland

183

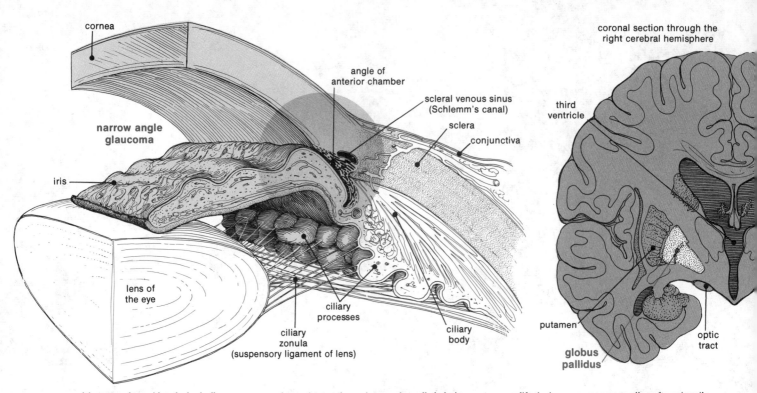

cornea

narrow angle glaucoma

iris

lens of the eye

ciliary zonula (suspensory ligament of lens)

angle of anterior chamber

scleral venous sinus (Schlemm's canal)

sclera

conjunctiva

ciliary processes

ciliary body

coronal section through the right cerebral hemisphere

third ventricle

putamen

globus pallidus

optic tract

several bases, and considered physically as super-cooled liquids instead of true solids.

cover g., a thin piece of glass used to cover an object examined under the microscope.

crown g., glass having a low dispersion and usually a low index of refraction; a compound of lime, potash, alumina, and silica; used in ophthalmic lenses.

flint g., a heavy, brilliant optical glass having a high dispersion and usually a high index of refraction.

optical g., glass carefully manufactured to obtain controlled index of refraction and dispersion, purity, transparency, homogeneity, and workability; the two most common types are crown and flint.

quartz g., crystal made by fusing pure quartz sand; it transmits ultraviolet rays.

Wood's g., a glass containing nickel oxide; used for diagnostic purposes, as in ringworm of the scalp where infected hairs are fluorescent when viewed under light filtered through this glass; also used in conjunction with certain dyes, such as fluorescin, for visualizing abrasions of the cornea.

glas'ses. Eyeglasses. See also spectacles.

glauco'ma. A group of eye diseases characterized by an increase in intraocular pressure, due to restricted outflow of the aqueous humor through the trabecular meshwork and spaces of Fontana in the anterior chamber angle (between the root of the iris and cornea).

acute g., glaucoma due to an acute obstruction of the anterior chamber angle.

congenital g., see buphthalmos.

narrow angle g., a chronic form of glaucoma marked by intermittent attacks during which the space between the base of the iris and the cornea at the trabecular meshwork is narrowed.

open angle g., a chronic, slowly progressive glaucoma due to some defect in the trabecular meshwork of the anterior chamber angle resulting in failure of aqueous humor to drain properly.

GLC. Abbreviation for gas-liquid chromatography.

GLDH. Abbreviation for the enzyme glutamate dehydrogenase.

glenohu'meral. Relating to the glenoid fossa and the humerus.

gle'noid. Resembling a socket; applied to articular depressions forming the shoulder joint (glenoid fossa) and the articulation of the jaw (glenoid or mandibular fossa).

gli'a. Neuroglia; the nonneuronal tissue of the brain and spinal cord.

gli'acyte. A cell of the non-nervous components of nervous tissue (neuroglia).

gli'adin. Any of various simple proteins obtained from wheat and rye glutens; also called glutin.

gli'al. Relating to the non-nervous elements of nervous tissue.

glide, mandib'ular. The side-to-side, protrusive, and intermediate movement of the mandible that occurs when the teeth are in contact.

glioblasto'ma. A general term for malignant forms of neoplasms containing neuroglial cells.

g. multiforme, the most malignant of all gliomas (primary brain tumors); a rapidly growing and fatal tumor of the cerebral hemispheres, composed of undifferentiated cells; the most recent term for this tumor is astrocytoma, grade 3 or 4, grade 4 being the most malignant.

glio'ma. Any tumor derived from the various types of cells that make up brain tissue; e.g. astrocytoma, glioblastoma multiforme, medulloblastoma, ependymoma, oligodendroglioma, etc.

gliomato'sis. Presence within the brain substance of one or several neoplasms originating in the glial cells.

glio'matous. Relating to or of the nature of a glioma.

glio'sis. Tumors of the non-nervous cellular elements of the brain and spinal cord.

gli'osome. One of several granules occurring in the non-nervous cells of nerve tissue.

glo'bi. Brown, granular masses sometimes seen in the granulomatous lesions of leprosy.

glo'bin. A simple protein constituent of hemoglobin.

glob'ule. A minute spherical body, especially a small drop of liquid.

Morgagni's g.'s, minute opaque spheres of fluid beneath the capsule and lens fibers, sometimes seen in cases of cataract; also called Morgagni's spheres.

glob'ulin. Any of a class of simple proteins that are insoluble in water, soluble in saline solutions, and coagulable by heat; found in blood and cerebrospinal fluid; human serum globulin is divided into α, β, and γ fractions on the basis of electrophoretic mobility.

accelerator g. (ac-g), a substance in serum, essential to the clotting process; it accelerates the conversion of prothrombin to thrombin in the presence of thromboplastin and ionized calcium; also called accelerin.

antihemophilic g., (1) see factor VIII; (2) a sterile preparation of normal human plasma which shortens the clotting time of hemophilic blood; used as an antihemophilic.

antilymphocyte g. (ALG), a preparation of purified globulin obtained after injection of human lymphocytes into animals (usually rabbits or horses) containing antibodies against lymphocytes; used to modify the immune response to allografts, primarily by suppressing cell-mediated immunity in the host.

antithymic g. (ATG), a preparation of purified globulin obtained after injection of human thymic cells into animals (usually rabbits or horses) containing antibodies against thymocytes; used to modify the immune response to allografts primarily by suppressing cell-mediated immunity in the host; also called antihuman thymocyte globulin.

α-g., alpha globulin; a plasma globulin that has the greatest electrophoretic mobility in neutral or alkaline solutions.

β-g., beta globulin; a plasma globulin having an electrophoretic mobility intermediate between that of the α- and γ-globulins.

γ-g., gamma globulin; a blood fraction prepared from plasma; composed of a number of molecular classes and subclasses of immunoglobulins and other nonantibody globulins; used in the prophylaxis of numerous diseases, including measles and epidemic hepatitis.

immune serum g., a sterile preparation of globulins containing a number of antibodies normally present in adult human blood; used as an immunizing agent.

thyroxin-binding g., an α-globulin with a strong affinity for thyroxin, thus acting as a carrier of thyroxin in the blood.

globulinu'ria. The presence of globulin in the urine.

glo'bus. A globe or ball.

g. hystericus, a hysterical sensation of having a lump or ball in the throat.

g. pallidus, the inner gray portion of the lentiform nucleus; also called paleostriatum.

glomangio'ma. Painful, small benign tumor of a glomus body, mainly occurring under the nails of the fingers and toes.

glom'erate. Crowded together; a tightly clustered rounded mass; denoting the usual gland structure, consisting of a mass of capillaries surrounding the secretory cells.

glomer'ular. Of, relating to, or resembling a glomerulus.

glomerulonephri'tis (GN). Kidney disease marked by alteration in the structure of the glomeruli; it may be acute, subacute, or chronic.

acute g., disorder occurring primarily in children and sometimes in young adults, most often following streptococcal infections; classical symptoms include fluid retention, periorbital edema, diminished urinary output, dark tea-colored urine, and elevation of the blood pressure; hematuria, red blood cell casts, and proteinuria are characteristic.

chronic g., glomerulonephritis of insidious onset

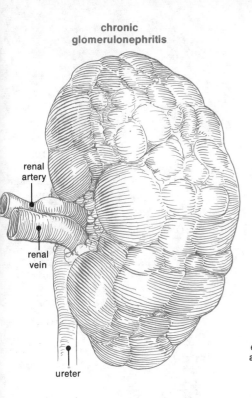

chronic
glomerulonephritis

renal
artery

renal
vein

ureter

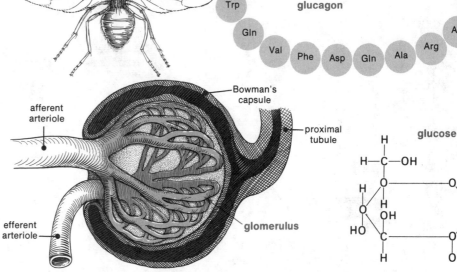

Glossina
palpalis

a tsetse
fly

NH₂ — His — Ser — Glu — Gly — Thr — Phe — Thr — Ser — Asp — Tyr — Ser — Lys — Tyr — Leu — Asp — Ser — Arg — Arg — Ala — Gln — Asp — Phe — Val — Gln — Trp — Leu — Met — Asn — Thr — COOH

glucagon

afferent
arteriole

Bowman's
capsule

proximal
tubule

efferent
arteriole

glomerulus

glucose

or occurring as a sequel to acute glomerulonephritis; marked by kidney failure, hypertension, and proteinuria; the kidneys become symmetrically shrunken and granular.

diffuse g., glomerulonephritis involving most of the renal glomeruli.

Ellis type 1 g., Ellis type 1 nephritis, term formerly used to describe what is now usually called acute glomerulonephritis.

Ellis type 2 g., Ellis type 2 nephritis, term formerly used to describe what is now usually called membranous glomerulonephritis.

focal g., a form of glomerulonephritis in which only some of the glomeruli are affected; may be a benign disease or a manifestation of a more serious, progressive disorder, such as lupus.

focal embolic g., a complication of subacute bacterial endocarditis.

hypocomplementemic persistent g., see membranoproliferative glomerulonephritis.

lobular g., glomerulonephritis marked by separation of the lobules of glomerular tufts and intralobular hyaline deposits, proteinuria, hematuria, and hypertension; often seen in membranoproliferative glomerulonephritis.

membranoproliferative g., mesangiocapillary g., hypocomplementemic persistent g., a form presenting with symptoms suggesting either acute glomerulonephritis or a nephrotic syndrome with microscopic hematuria; the characteristic lesion is an increase in cellularity of the mesangium, increased lobulation of the tufts, and capillary wall thickening commonly associated with hypocomplementemia.

membranous g., a type marked by thickening of the basement membrane in the glomerular capillaries and causing proteinuria and generalized edema; often associated with the nephrotic syndrome; a characteristic spiking appearance is found in the basement membrane on microscopy.

mesangiocapillary g., see membranoproliferative glomerulonephritis.

poststreptococcal g., acute glomerulonephritis.

proliferative g., acute glomerulonephritis.

rapidly progressive g., a form having an insidious beginning, without a previous episode of streptococcal infection, or possibly an unresolved poststreptococcal nephritis with renal insufficiency leading to death within a few months; characterized by marked crescent formation; also called crescent or extracapillary glomerulonephritis.

subacute g., a term used variously to describe rapidly progressive glomerulonephritis or a type of glomerulonephritis with nephrotic syndrome and a prolonged course.

glomer'ulosclero'sis. Fibrosis and degeneration of the structures within the glomeruli of the kidneys.

focal segmental g., a form of progressive renal disease beginning in juxtamedullary capillaries and extending in a centrifugal pattern; usually presents in children or adolescents as a nephrotic syndrome.

intercapillary g., the glomerular lesion present as a complication of diabetes mellitus, associated with albuminuria, edema, and hypertension (Kimmelstiel-Wilson syndrome).

nodular g., a form of diabetic nephropathy in which sclerosis occurs in a peripheral nodular pattern; also called Kimmelstiel-Wilson lesion.

glomer'ulus, *pl.* **glomer'uli. 1.** A small cluster of nerves or capillaries; when used alone the term refers to a tuft of capillaries at the beginning of each uriniferous tubule in the kidney (malpighian tuft). **2.** The coiled secretory portion of a sweat gland.

glo'mus. A minute globular body composed of anastomoses between small arteries and small veins and having a rich nerve supply.

carotid g., carotid body; a small neurovascular structure situated on each side of the neck at the bifurcation of the common cartid artery.

g. intravagale, a collection of chemoreceptor cells on the auricular branch of the vagus nerve; a tumor of this glomus may cause loss of hearing.

g. jugulare, a glomus in the adventitia of the jugular bulb.

glos'sa. Latin for tongue.

glos'sal. Of or relating to the tongue.

glossal'gia. A painful tongue.

glossec'tomy. Amputation of the tongue or of a portion of it.

Glossi'na. A genus of bloodsucking flies, the tsetse flies, which transmit the microorganisms causing African sleeping sickness in humans and domestic animals.

glossi'tis. Inflammation of the tongue.

glosso-, gloss-. Combining forms indicating a relationship to the tongue.

glossodyn'ia. Glossalgia.

glos'sograph. Instrument used to record the movements of the tongue in speaking.

glossola'lia. Meaningless speech; unintelligible and rapid chatter.

glossopharyn'geal. Relating to the tongue and pharynx.

glos'soplasty. Reparative surgery of the tongue.

glossople'gia. Paralysis of the tongue; also called glossolysis.

glossopto'sis, glossopto'sia. Downward displacement of the tongue.

glossor'rhaphy. Suture of the tongue.

glos'sospasm. Spasmodic contraction of the tongue.

glossot'omy. Any surgical incision on the tongue.

glossotrich'ia. Hairy tongue.

glot'tic. Relating to either the tongue or the glottis.

glot'tis. The vocal apparatus located in the larynx, consisting of the vocal cords and the opening between them.

glotti'tis. Glossitis.

glu'cagon. A polypeptide hormone, normally produced by α-cells of the islets of Langerhans in the pancreas when the blood sugar level gets too low; it aids in the breakdown of glycogen in the liver, thus elevating the blood sugar concentration.

glu'can. A polyglucose; e.g., starch amylose, glycogen amylose.

α-glucan-branching glycosyltransferase. Branching factor; see under factor.

α-1,4-glucan 4-glucanohydrolase. Alpha-1,4-glucan 4-glucanohydrolase; an enzyme which, through a reaction with water, breaks down amylose (a straight chain polysaccharide) to form glucose and maltose; present in plants and obtained in crystalline form from pancreatic juice and saliva; formerly known as α-amylase.

α-1,4-glucan maltohydrolase. Alpha-1,4-glucan maltohydrolase; an enzyme which, through a reaction with water, splits amylopectin (a branched polysaccharide) to form maltose; present in soybeans, wheat, barley, and other similar plants; formerly called β-amylase.

glucocor'ticoid. Any steroid hormone of the adrenal cortex (or synthetic steroid) concerned with gluconeogenesis from amino acids and catabolism of protein; this class of compounds has other activities including anti-inflammatory activity and ability to suppress the synthesis of ACTH and MSH; cortisol is the major naturally occurring hormone of this type in humans.

glucogen'ic. Producing glucose.

glucoki'nase. A specific phosphorylation enzyme for glucose present in the liver and muscle; it catalyzes the conversion of glucose to glucose-6-phosphate, in which one molecule of adenosine triphosphate (ATP) is used.

glucokinet'ic. Mobilizing glucose in the body, as in the maintenance of sugar level.

gluconeogen'esis. Formation of glucose from non-carbohydrate sources, such as protein and fat.

gluco'samine. An amino sugar present in mucopolysaccharides; also called chitosamine.

glu'cosan. Any anhydride of glucose; a polysaccharide yielding glucose on hydrolysis; e.g., cellulose, glycogen, starch, and dextrin.

glu'cose. A dextrorotatory monosaccharide or

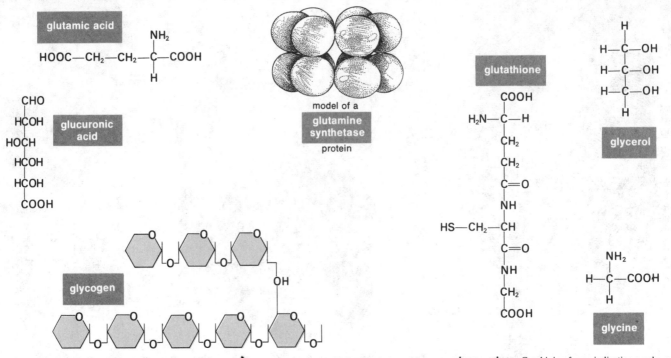

glutamic acid

$$HOOC—CH_2—CH_2—C—COOH$$
with NH_2 and H on the central carbon

glucuronic acid

CHO
HCOH
HOCH
HCOH
HCOH
COOH

glycogen

model of a glutamine synthetase protein

glutathione

COOH
$H_2N—C—H$
CH_2
CH_2
$C=O$
NH
$HS—CH_2—CH$
$C=O$
NH
CH_2
COOH

glycerol

H
H—C—OH
H—C—OH
H—C—OH
H

glycine

NH_2
$H—C—COOH$
H

---

simple sugar, $C_6H_{12}O_6 \cdot H_2O$, occurring as an odorless, sweet, crystalline powder; present in animal and plant tissue and obtained synthetically from starch; used in medicine as an intravenous nutrient; also called blood or grape sugar, dextrose.

glucose-6-phosphatase. A microsomal enzyme catalyzing the hydrolysis of glucose-6-phosphate to glucose and inorganic phosphate; present in liver, kidney, intestinal mucosa, and endometrium; inherited deficiency of this enzyme is thought to be responsible for the glycogen storage disease known as type I glycogenosis or von Gierke's disease.

glucose-6-phosphate dehydrogenase. An enzyme that promotes the oxidation of glucose-6-phosphate to 6-phosphogluconolactone.

glu′coside. One of a variety of substances in nature containing glucose combined by an ether linkage.

glucosu′ria. Presence of glucose in the urine.

glucuronic acid. The curonic acid of glucose, HOOC(CHOH)₄CHO; it inactivates various substances, e.g., benzoic acid, phenol, and the female sex hormones; the glucuronides so formed are excreted in the urine.

β-glucuron′idase. An enzyme catalyzing the hydrolysis of various β-D-glucuronides, liberating free glucuronic acid; active in the liver, spleen, endometrium, breasts, adrenal glands, and testes.

glucuron′ide. A glycoside of glucuronic acid.

glue-sniffing. The intentional inhalation of fumes from plastic cements, resulting in central nervous system stimulation followed by depression.

glutam′ic acid. An amino acid present in protein; involved in ammonia production in the kidney.

glutamic oxaloacetic transaminase (GOT). See under transaminase.

glutamic pyruvic transaminase (GPT). See under transaminase.

glutam′ine. An amino acid found as a constituent of proteins and in free form in blood; it yields glutamic acid and ammonia on hydrolysis.

  g. synthetase, an enzyme that catalyzes the amination of glutamic acid to glutamine which occurs concurrently with the hydrolysis of ATP to ADP and orthophosphate (P₁).

glutaral′dehyde. A tissue fixative which causes a fine precipitation of protein, thus permitting sections to be cut without appreciable distortion of structure; universally used as a prefixer in electron microscopy, generally followed by fixation with osmium tetroxide.

glutathi′one. A crystalline tripeptide of glycine, cystine, and glutamic acid that is present in blood and other tissues; it activates certain proteins and

takes part in oxidation-reduction processes; the reduced form is abbreviated GSH; in the oxidized form two molecules are linked together and abbreviated GSSG.

glu′teal. Of or relating to the buttocks.

glu′telin. One of a number of simple proteins present in the seeds of grain.

glut′en. A mixture of insoluble plant proteins present in grains such as wheat, rye, oats, and barley; used as an adhesive and as a flour substitute.

gluteth′imide. A compound which is a depressant of the central nervous system; used as a hypnotic; Doriden®.

glu′teus, *pl.* **glu′tei.** Any of the three buttock muscles.

  g. maximus, the broad, thick fleshy mass of muscle which forms the prominence of the buttock; it extends and laterally rotates the thigh.

  g. medius, the broad, thick, radiating muscle situated on the outer surface of the pelvis; it abducts the thigh and rotates it medially.

  g. minimus, the smallest of the three glutei; it rotates the thigh medially and abducts it.

glu′tin. See gliadin.

glu′tinous. Sticky.

gluti′tis. Inflammation of the gluteus muscles of the buttock.

glyce′mia. The presence of sugar in the blood.

glyceral′dehyde. Compound formed by the oxidation of glycerol; also called glyceric aldehyde.

glyc′eridase. General term for any of several enzymes that promote the hydrolysis of glycerol esters.

glyc′eride. An ester of glycerol.

glyc′erin. A clear, syrupy, sweet, somewhat colorless liquid, $C_3H_8O_3$, used as a sweetener, a lubricant, and a solvent for drugs. See also glycerol.

gly′cerol. A sweet, syrupy trihydric alcohol, occurring in combinations as glycerides and produced by the fermentation of sugar; pharmaceutical preparations are known as glycerin.

glyc′erose. A sugar resulting from the oxidation of glycerin.

glyc′eryl. Propenyl; the trivalent radical, $C_3H_5O_3$, of glycerol.

  g. guaiacolate, $C_{10}H_{14}O_4$; used to promote the ejection of mucus or exudate from the lungs, bronchi, and trachea.

  g. nitrate, nitroglycerin.

  g. stearate, see stearin.

gly′cine. The principal amino acid present in sugar cane, $C_2H_5NO_2$; the simplest of the amino acids and one of the first to be isolated from proteins; also called aminoacetic acid.

glycinu′ria. The presence of glycine in the urine.

glyco-, glyc-. Combining forms indicating a relationship to sugar.

glycoca′lyx. A carbohydrate-rich outer fuzz coating on the free surface of certain epithelial cells; rich in mucoid components.

glycocholic acid. The principal acid of the bile.

gly′cogen. The form in which carbohydrate is stored in the body, especially in the liver and muscles; a highly branched glucosan of high molecular weight; it is broken down as needed to glucose molecules.

glyco′genase. The enzyme that promotes the breakdown of glycogen to glucose.

glycogen′esis. The formation of glycogen from glucose or other monosaccharides.

glycogenol′ysis. The breakdown of glycogen to simpler products.

glycogeno′sis. Abnormal accumulation of glycogen in the tissues; also called glycogen storage disease.

  type 1 g., disorder thought to be caused by deficiency of the enzyme glucose 6-phosphatase, resulting in excessive accumulation of glycogen in the liver and kidneys; also called von Gierke's disease and glucose 6-phosphatase hepatorenal glycogenosis.

  type 2 g., disease of infancy thought to be caused by deficiency of an enzyme, lysomal α-1,4-glucosidase, resulting in excessive accumulation of glycogen in the heart muscles, liver, and nervous system; associated with marked cardiac enlargement and congestive heart failure usually leading to death within the first year of life; also called generalized glycogenosis and Pompe's disease.

  type 5 g., disorder attributed to deficiency of muscle glycogen phosphorylase (enzyme that catalyzes the splitting of glycogen to glucose), resulting in accumulation of glycogen in the muscles; also called McArdle's syndrome and myophosphorylase deficiency glycogenosis.

glycogen storage disease. See glycogenosis.

glycogeu′sia. A subjective sweet taste in the mouth.

gly′col. One of a group of alcohols containing two hydroxyl groups.

glycol′ysis. The energy-producing process in the body, especially in muscles, in which sugar is broken down into lactic acid; since oxygen is not consumed, it is frequently termed anaerobic glycolysis.

glycolyt′ic. Causing the hydrolysis or digestion of sugar.

glyconeogen′esis. The new formation of sugar; the formation of glucose or glycogen from substances other than carbohydrates, such as protein or fat.

---

glucose-6-phosphatase │ glyconeogenesis

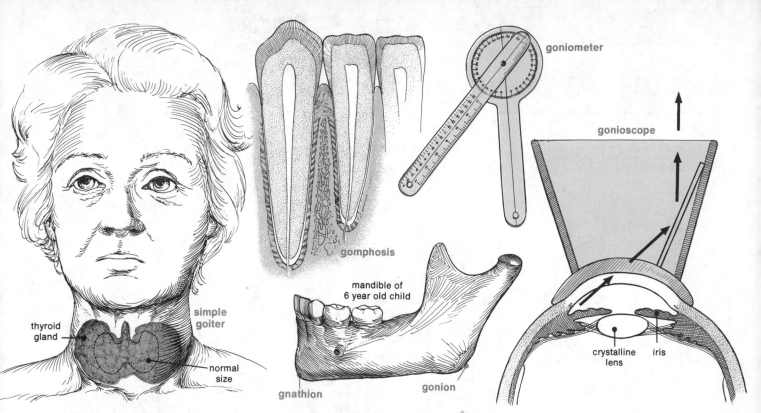

simple goiter
thyroid gland — normal size

goniometer

gonioscope

gomphosis

mandible of 6 year old child

gnathion — gonion

crystalline lens — iris

glycopro'tein. Any of several protein-carbohydrate compounds (conjugated proteins); they include the mucins, the mucoids, and the chondroproteins.

gly'coside. Any of a group of compounds containing a carbohydrate and a noncarbohydrate residue in the same molecule; on hydrolysis they produce sugars and related compounds; found in animal tissues and in many drugs and spices.

glycosphingolip'id. A ceramide linked to one or more sugars by the terminal OH group.

glycostat'ic. Tending to maintain a constant glycogen level in the tissues.

glycosu'ria. Excretion of sugar in the urine in excess of the normal amount; frequently a sign of diabetes mellitus.

renal g., glycosuria occurring with normal blood levels of sugar, due to failure of the renal tubules to reabsorb filtered glucose to the normal degree.

glycyrrhi'za. The dried roots of *Glycyrrhiza glabra;* used in pharmaceutical preparations; also called licorice and licorice root.

glycyrrhizic acid. A glycoside present in glycyrrhiza which in large amounts produces aldosterone-like effects in the kidney, causing retention of sodium and water and excessive excretion of potassium; also called glycyrrhizin.

glyox'aline. See imidazole.

gm. Abbreviation for gram, a unit of weight equivalent to 15.432 grains.

GM counter. Abbreviation for Geiger-Müller counter; see counter, Geiger.

GMP. Abbreviation for guanosine monophosphate (guanosine 5'-phosphoric acid).

GN. Abbreviation for glomerulonephritis.

gnat. One of several minute, winged, biting insects; a midge.

buffalo g., *Simulium pecuarium;* a small, biting, black gnat, vector of onchocerciasis.

gnathal'gia. See gnathodynia.

gnath'ic. Of or pertaining to the jaw.

gnath'ion. The lowest point of the midline of the mandible; a craniometric point.

gnathi'tis. Inflammation of the jaw.

gnatho-, gnath-. Combining forms indicating a relationship to the jaw.

gnathodynamom'eter. Instrument used in dentistry to measure the biting force of the jaws; also called bite gauge and occlusometer.

gnathodyn'ia. Pain in the jaw; also called gnathalgia.

gnath'oplasty. Plastic or reparative surgery of the jaw.

gnathostat'ics. In orthodontic diagnosis, a technique based on relationships between the teeth and certain skull landmarks.

Gnathos'toma. A genus of parasitic, pathogenic, nematode worms (family Gnathostomatidae) formerly called *Chiranthus*.

G. spinigerum, a species frequently transmitted to man by ingestion of the larvae in undercooked fish; it causes migratory swelling of the subcutaneous tissues or abscesses in the intestinal wall; the wandering larvae may also invade the eyes and brain.

gnathostomi'asis. Infection with *Gnathostoma spinigerum*.

-gnosis. Suffix denoting recognition; e.g., diagnosis.

gog'gles. Large, usually tinted, spectacles used as a shield to protect the eyes.

goi'ter. Enlargement of the thyroid gland causing a visible swelling in front of the neck.

adenomatous g., goiter due to the presence of a benign tumor of glandular tissue (adenoma).

colloid g., a soft goiter in which the follicles of the gland are distended and filled with colloid.

cystic g., an enlarged thyroid gland containing one or more cysts.

exophthalmic g., disorder caused by excessive production of thyroid hormone; marked by enlargement of the thyroid gland, bulging eyeballs, muscular tremors, rapid pulse rate, and weight loss; also called Graves' disease.

parenchymatous g., uniform enlargement of the thyroid gland due to excessive proliferation of its follicles and epithelium.

toxic g., one with excessive secretions, causing signs and symptoms of hyperthyroidism.

goi'trogen. Any agent causing goiter.

gold. A soft, deep yellow, corrosion-resistant element; one of the most indestructible, heaviest, and most chemically inert metals known; symbol Au, atomic number 79, atomic weight 196.9.

white g., a gold alloy with a high palladium content.

gold-198 (^{198}Au). A radioactive isotope of gold; used in colloidal suspension for treating some forms of cancer.

gompho'sis. A type of fibrous articulation in which a bony process fits into a socket, as of a tooth and its socket.

gon'ad. A sexual gland.

female g., ovary.

male g., testis.

gonadec'tomy. The surgical removal of an ovary or testis.

gonado-, gonad-. Combining forms relating to a testis or ovary.

gonadoblasto'ma. A benign combined germ-cell and gonadal stromal growth.

gonadogen'esis. The development of the embryonic gonads.

gonadotrop'ic. Influencing the gonads, as the hormones of the anterior pituitary gland which stimulate the ovaries and testes.

gonadotrop'in, gonadotroph'in. A hormone or a substance that stimulates either the ovaries or the testes.

human chorionic g., (HCG), a placental hormone, isolated from the urine of pregnant women.

gonal'gia. Pain in the knee.

gonecys'tolith. A concretion of calculus in a seminal vesicle.

goniom'eter. 1. An instrument for measuring angles. **2.** A device used in testing for labyrinthine disease.

go'nion. The most posterior, inferior, and lateral point of the external mandibular angle.

goniopunc'ture. Operation for congenital glaucoma in which a puncture is made in the trabecular meshwork (at the angle of the anterior chamber) through the corneoscleral junction of the opposite side.

go'nioscope. A combination of a contact lens and mirror which allows the observer to look directly into the angle of the anterior chamber of the eye.

gonios'copy. Examination of the angle of the anterior chamber of the eye by means of a gonioscope.

goniot'omy. Borkan's operation for congenital glaucoma in which abnormal tissue is removed from the filtration angle of the anterior chamber.

gonococ'cal. Relating to gonococci.

gonococce'mia. The presence of gonococci in the blood.

gonococ'cus, *pl.* **gonococ'ci.** The bacterium that causes gonorrhea; an individual organism of the species *Neisseria gonorrhoeae.*

gon'ocyte. A primitive reproductive cell.

gonorrhe'a. A common contagious disease caused by *Neisseria gonorrhoeae* and transmitted chiefly by sexual intercourse; it is marked by inflammation of the mucous membrane of the genital tract, a purulent discharge, and painful, frequent urination; if untreated it may cause complications such as epididymitis, prostatitis, tenosynovitis, arthritis, and endocarditis; in females it may lead to sterility, and in males to urethral stricture.

gonorrhe'al. Relating to gonorrhea.

gonycamp'sis. Any abnormal curvature of the knee.

Goodpasture's syndrome. Glomerulonephritis associated with diffuse pulmonary hemorrhage; caused by an antigen directed against the basement

glycoprotein | **Goodpasture's syndrome**

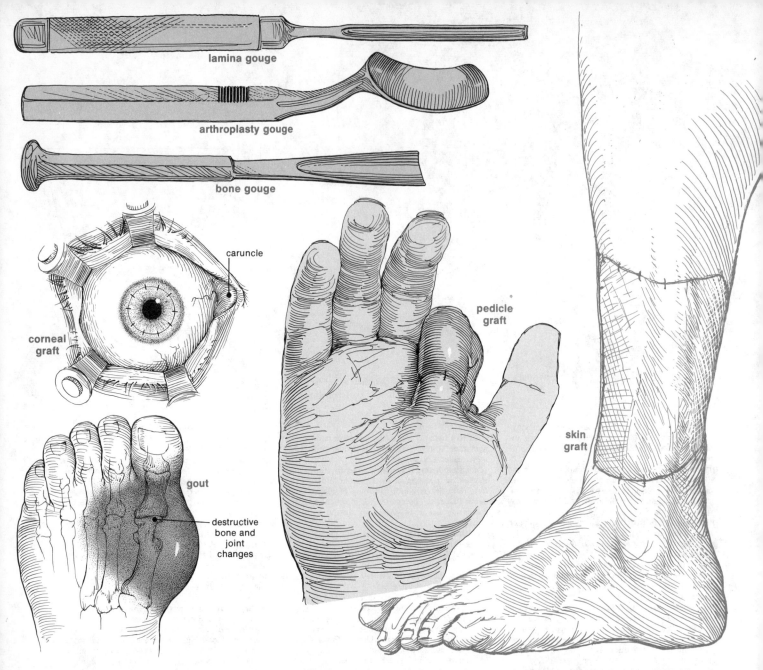

lamina gouge

arthroplasty gouge

bone gouge

corneal graft

caruncle

gout

destructive bone and joint changes

pedicle graft

skin graft

membrane of glomerulus capillaries and pulmonary alveoli; also called hemorrhagic pulmonary-renal syndrome.

gooseflesh. See under flesh.

GOT. Abbreviation for glutamic oxaloacetic transaminase; see under transaminase.

gouge. 1. A strong chisel with a troughlike blade, usually used for cutting and removing bone. **2.** To cut or scoop out in large amounts.

goundou. An endemic disease of West Africa marked by egg-shaped swelling of the maxillary bone, on either side of the nose; associated with yaws.

gout. A metabolic disorder marked by an excess of uric acid in the blood, by painful inflammation of joints, especially of the big toes, and by deposits of sodium biurate in the cartilages of the affected joints and in the kidney.

   saturnine g., gout accompanying lead poisoning.

   secondary g., gout occurring as a result of increased nucleoprotein metabolism and uric acid production.

   tophaceous g., gout marked by the presence of tophi (deposits of sodium urate) about the joints and cartilaginous areas.

gou'ty. Resembling or pertaining to gout.

G.P. Abbreviation for general practitioner (preferred term is family physician).

GPT. Abbreviation for glutamic pyruvic transaminase; see under transaminase.

gr. Abbreviation for grain, a measure of weight.

gra'dient. Rate of change of temperature, pressure, distance, time, or any such variable value.

   concentration g., a solution with a continuous concentration increase of the solute from top to bottom of the container; also called density gradient.

   density g., see concentration gradient.

   mitral g., the difference in diastolic pressure between the left atrium and left ventricle.

   systolic g., the difference in pressure during systole between two communicating chambers of the heart.

   ventricular g., in electrocardiography, the algebraic sum of the areas within the QRS complex and the T wave of the electrocardiogram.

grad'uate. A laboratory vessel, usually of glass, marked with a scale in milliliters or ounces; used to measure liquids.

gradua'ted. Marked by a succession of lines to indicate capacity, degrees, percentages, etc.

Graefe's disease. See ophthalmoplegia progressiva.

Graefe's sign, von Graefe's sign. Immobility or lagging of the upper eyelid on downward movement of the eye; also called lid lag.

graft. 1. A piece of tissue inserted into a bodily part to cover and supply a defect. **2.** To insert such a tissue.

   allogeneic g., allograft; a graft derived from a genetically dissimilar individual of the same species; also called homograft.

   autogenous g., a graft of tissue derived from the same individual or animal to which it is transplanted; also called autograft.

   Blair-Brown g., see split thickness graft.

   Braun g., see full thickness graft.

   checkerboard g., see postage stamp graft.

   corneal g., donor corneal tissue used in keratoplasty to replace diseased corneal tissue; split thickness (lamellar) and full thickness (penetrating) grafts are the most common types used.

   cutis g., a piece of skin from which the epidermis and subcutaneous tissue have been removed.

   delayed g. grafting postponed until infection has been eliminated.

   double end g., see pedicle graft.

   full thickness g., one consisting of skin and subcutaneous tissue; also called Braun graft.

   island g., see pedicle graft.

   isogeneic g., syngeneic graft.

   pedicle g., a stalk of skin and subcutaneous tissue left attached at the donor site until its free end has taken at the recipient site; also called double end or island graft.

   pinch g.'s, circular bits of skin a few millimeters in diameter.

   postage stamp g., multiple, small, thick-split skin graft; also called checkerboard graft.

   skin g., a piece of skin removed from one area of the body, or from another person, to cover a denuded area at another site.

   split thickness g., a graft consisting of a superfi-

gooseflesh | **graft**

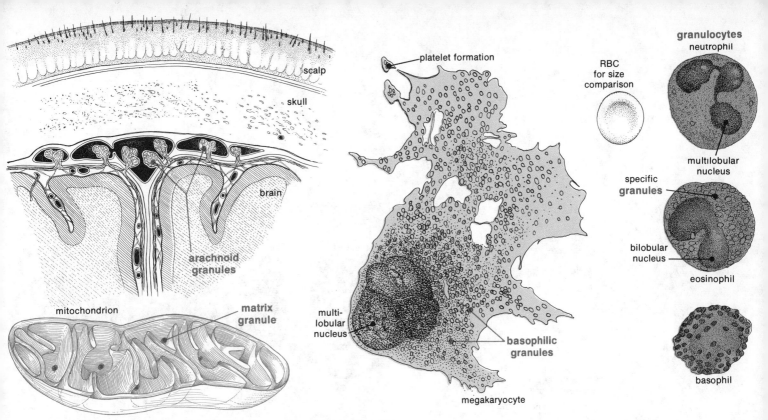

Labels in illustration: scalp; skull; brain; arachnoid granules; mitochondrion; matrix granule; platelet formation; multi-lobular nucleus; basophilic granules; megakaryocyte; RBC for size comparison; granulocytes; neutrophil; multilobular nucleus; specific granules; bilobular nucleus; eosinophil; basophil

cial layer of the dermis; also called Blair-Brown graft.

syngeneic g., see isograft.

tendon g., a piece of tendon used to repair a defect.

thick-split g., one consisting of about three quarters of the skin's thickness.

xenogeneic g., xenograft; a transplant involving two different species, such as the transplantation of a chimpanzee kidney into a human.

graft'ing. Transplantation of tissue from one part of the body to another or from one body to another.

grain. 1. A minute hard particle. **2.** A unit of weight equivalent to 0.0648 gm.

-gram. Combining form denoting something recorded (written or drawn); e.g., electrocardiogram.

gram (gm or g). A metric unit of mass and weight, equal to one-thousandth of a kilogram and approximately one cubic centimeter of water at its maximum density.

gramici'din. A substance produced by the growth of *Bacillus brevis*; used topically to arrest the growth of gram-positive cocci and bacilli.

gram'meter. A unit of energy equal to the force required to raise a weight of one gram to a height of one meter.

gram-mol'ecule. The quantity of a substance that has a weight in grams numerically equal to the molecular weight of the substance; e.g., a gram-molecule of hydrogen weighs two grams; also called mole and mol.

gram-neg'ative. Relating to a microorganism that fails to retain the deep violet dye used in Gram's method of staining bacteria.

gram-pos'itive. Relating to a microorganism that retains the deep violet dye used in Gram's method.

gran'diose. In psychiatry, denoting feeling of great importance; having delusions of grandeur.

grand mal. Generalized epilepsy; see under epilepsy.

gran'ular. 1. Composed of or resembling granules or grains. **2.** Particles with a strong affinity for stains.

gran'ulase. An enzyme capable of splitting starch into dextrins and maltose.

granula'tion. 1. The act or process of dividing substances into small particles or granules; the state of being granular. **2.** The formation of small, rounded, fleshy masses on the surface of a healing wound; also one of these fleshy masses. **3.** A granular mass in or on the surface of an organ or membrane, as a mass of lymphoid tissue on the conjunctiva of the eyelids. **4.** The formation of crystals by prolonged agitation of a supersaturated solution of a salt.

arachnoid g.'s, small masses of arachnoid projecting into the venous sinuses and on the outer surface of the dura mater, causing, through pressure, the pits on the inner surface of the cranium; they usually appear at the age of seven years and increase in size and number as age advances; also called pacchionian bodies or granulations.

pacchionian g.'s, see arachnoid granulations.

gran'ule. 1. A grain or small particle; a minute discrete mass. **2.** A small pill, usually sugar coated.

acidophilic g., one staining readily with acid dyes such as eosin.

basophilic g., one staining readily with basic dyes such as azure A.

chromophobe g., one that does not stain or stains poorly.

Crooke's g.'s, masses of basophilic material in the basophilic cells of the anterior lobe of the pituitary gland; seen in Cushing's disease or after the administration of ACTH.

osmophilic g., one that flourishes in the medium of high osmotic pressure.

Schüffner's g.'s, fine granules present in red blood cells infected with malarial parasites, particularly *Plasmodium vivax*, giving the cells a dotted or stippled appearance.

zymogen g., one of several granules present in enzyme-secreting cells such as those in a salivary gland.

gran'uloblast. Myeloblast; an embryonic blood cell capable of developing into a granulocyte.

gran'ulocyte. A mature granular white blood cell (leukocyte) that develops in the bone marrow from a myeloblast; depending on the specific granules, there are three types: neutrophilic (polymorphonuclear) granulocyte, eosinophilic granulocyte, and basophilic granulocyte.

granulocytope'nia. Deficiency of granular leukocytes (granulocytes) in the blood; also called granulopenia.

granulocytopoie'sis. See granulopoiesis.

granulocyto'sis. The presence of an excessive number of granulocytes in the blood or in the tissues.

granulo'ma. A tumor composed of granulation tissue.

dental g., periapical g., a mass of chronic inflammatory tissue, usually asymptomatic, occurring at the root of a tooth.

eosinophilic g., a relatively benign disorder marked by a simple lesion involving one or several bones, beginning in the marrow and gradually eroding the cortex; occurring predominantly in children and young adults.

g. inguinale, a chronic disease marked by granu-lomatous ulcerations in the inguinal region and the genitalia; caused by *Calymmatum granulomatis*.

periapical g., see dental granuloma.

granulomato'sis. Any disorder marked by the presence of multiple granulomas.

lipoid g., lipid g., see xanthomatosis.

lipophagic intestinal g., see Whipple's disease.

Wegener's g., a rare, often fatal, disease marked by ulceration of the upper respiratory tract progressing to involvement of the lungs, acute necrotizing arteritis, and glomerulonephritis.

granulom'atous. Resembling a granuloma.

granulope'nia. See granulocytopenia.

granuloplas'tic. Capable of forming granules.

granulopoie'sis. The formation of granulocytes; also called granulocytopoeisis.

granulo'sis, granulos'ity. A mass of minute granules.

-graph. A combining form indicating (1) an instrument that makes a recording; e.g., electrocardiograph; (2) something printed; e.g., monograph.

graph. Any pictorial device that displays a relationship of varying values; also called chart.

grapho-, -graphy. Combining forms denoting a relationship to a method of writing or other graphic representation.

graphol'ogy. The study of handwriting as an aid in analyzing the character of the writer.

graph'ospasm. Writer's cramp; see under cramp.

GRAS. Acronym for generally regarded as safe, denoting any safe food additive.

grave. Indicating symptoms of an extremely serious or dangerous character; also called critical.

grav'el. Numerous minute concretions, usually of uric acid, calcium oxalate, or phosphates; formed in the kidney and bladder.

Graves' disease. Exophthalmic goiter; see under goiter.

grav'id. Pregnant.

grav'ida. A woman who is, or has been, pregnant.

gravid'ity. 1. The pregnant state. **2.** The total number of pregnancies a woman has had, including a current pregnancy.

gravim'eter. An instrument used to measure the specific gravity of a liquid; also called hydrometer.

grav'imetric. Of, determined by, or relating to measurement by weight.

grav'ity (G). The gravitational force.

negative g., gravity in a foot-to-head direction in flying, or in standing on one's head.

specific g. (sp gr), the ratio of the mass of any substance (usually liquid) compared to the mass of an equal volume of another substance (usually distilled water at 4°C).

green. A grasslike hue; the color of the spectrum

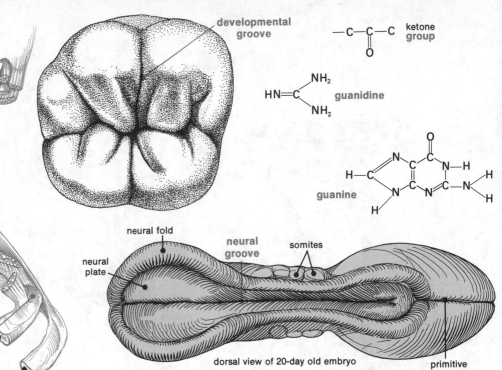

middle and anterior scalene muscles

subclavian grooves

first and second ribs

developmental groove

ketone group

guanidine

guanine

neural fold

neural plate

neural groove

somites

dorsal view of 20-day old embryo

primitive streak

lying between yellow and blue, evoked by radiant energy of wavelengths of approximately 530 nm.

indocyanine g., a dye used in a variety of blood flow, volume, and function studies; most commonly used to measure cardiac output.

Janus g. B, an azo dye used as a supravital stain for the demonstration of mitochondria.

malachite g., green crystalline substance, soluble in water, used as a pH indicator; it changes at pH 1.0 from yellow (acid) to blue-green (alkaline); used also for staining bacteria and as an antiseptic; also called Victoria green.

Paris g., an insecticide composed of copper acetate and copper meta-arsenite.

Victoria g., malachite green.

green vitriol. See ferrous sulfate.

Grey Turner's sign. Areas of discoloration about the navel and the loins occurring in acute hemorrhagic pancreatitis.

GRF. Abbreviation for growth hormone-releasing factor.

grid. A frame of parallel horizontal and vertical lines forming squares of uniform size, used as a reference for plotting curves. 2. In dentistry, an instrument composed of alternate strips of lead and radiolucent material, placed in apposition to a film to absorb secondary or scattered radiation.

Wetzel g., a chart for evaluating the growth and physical fitness of young and adolescent children.

grief. A state of intense mental anguish normally resulting from the loss of a valued object or person.

Griffin claw. See hand, griffin-claw.

grinding, selective. In dentistry, the modification of occlusal surfaces of teeth with the intent of equalizing occlusal stress or of harmonizing cuspal relations, with the aid of articulator paper or equilibration ribbon.

grinding-in. In dentistry, the act of correcting occlusal errors in natural and artificial teeth; also called equilibrating.

grip. 1. Grippe. 2. Grasp.

devil's g., epidemic pleurodynia; see under pleurodynia.

gripe. Colic (2); sharp pain in the intestines.

grippe. From French *gripper*, to seize; flu-like illness; also called influenza and grip.

griseoful'vin. A fungistatic antibiotic derived from a species of *Penicillium*; used systemically in the treatment of superficial fungal infections; Fulvicin-U/F®.

gris'tle. Cartilage.

groin. 1. The inguinal region; the region around the crease formed at the junction of the thigh and trunk. 2. The external genital organs.

Grönblad-Strandberg syndrome. An elastic

tissue degeneration that involves the retina, gastrointestinal tract, and especially the skin.

groove. A narrow, elongated depression.

carotid g., the groove through the sphenoid bone in which the internal carotid artery lies in its course through the cavernous sinus.

costal g., a groove in the lower border of the rib, housing the intercostal vessels and nerve.

developmental g., a groove on the enamel of a tooth, marking the fusion of the lobes of the crown during tooth development.

neural g., the transitory median dorsal groove in the thickened ectoderm (neural plate) of young embryos; the closure of the groove forms a closed tubular structure with a long caudal portion, the future spinal cord, and a broader cephalic portion, which becomes the brain.

subclavian g., a shallow groove on the first rib between the anterior and middle scalene muscles through which the subclavian artery and the inferior trunk of the brachial plexus pass.

group. 1. A collection of related objects. 2. In chemistry, a radical.

characteristic g., a distinctive group of atoms that make one substance different from others.

Lancefield g.'s, Lancefield's classification; see under classification.

symptom g., (1) syndrome; (2) a complex in the electrocardiogram.

growing pains. See under pain.

growth. 1. The progressive development of an organism or any of its parts. 2. A tumor.

appositional g., growth through the addition of layers, typical of rigid structures; also called growth by accretion.

differential g., the various growth rates of related tissues, as in embryonic structures, with resulting change in proportions.

interstitial g., growth through formation of new tissue throughout the structure, as occurs in soft tissues.

psychological g., growth toward self-actualization or personal maturity.

zero population g. (ZPG), the state of a total population that neither increases nor decreases, occurring when the number of births and immigrants equals the number of deaths and emigrants.

grub. The larva of certain insects.

gru'el. Thin porridge; any semifluid food made of cereal boiled in water.

grunt. A deep, guttural sound in the chest; a frequent sign of chest pain implying an acute pneumonic process with pleural involvement; also seen in pulmonary edema and in the respiratory distress syndrome of the neonatal period.

expiratory g., a laryngeal sound sometimes heard during surgical manipulation of the subdiaphragmatic areas.

grypo'sis. Any abnormal curvature.

GSH. Abbreviation for the reduced form of glutathione.

GSSG. Abbreviation for oxidized glutathione.

gt. Abbreviation for Latin *gutta*, drop.

GTT. Abbreviation for glucose tolerance test.

gtt. Abbreviation for Latin *guttae*, drops.

GU. Abbreviation for genitourinary.

guai'acol. A colorless, oily liquid, $C_7H_8O_2$, obtained from creosote or made synthetically from pyrocatechin; used chiefly as an expectorant, intestinal disinfectant, and local anesthetic.

guaneth'idine sul'fate. A potent antihypertensive drug, thought to interfere with the release of norepinephrine at the sympathetic neuroeffector junction; Ismelin Sulfate®.

guan'idine. A strong base obtained from the oxidation of guanine; the amidine of aminocarbamic acid, CH_5N_3, considered by some to be one of the factors responsible for part of the uremic syndrome in renal failure; also called carbotriamine.

guanidine'mia. The presence of guanidine in the blood.

guanidinosuccinic acid. A metabolic by-product found in the body in excessive amounts in renal failure and implicated in the clotting abnormality and the neuropathy of the chronic uremic syndrome.

guan'ine. A crystalline purine base.

guan'osine. 9-β-D-Ribosylguanine; guanine combined with D-ribose.

gubernac'ulum. A guiding cord connecting two structures.

g. dentis, the connective tissue band connecting the permanent tooth follicle to the gingiva.

g. testis, a ligamentous cord extending from the lower end of the fetal testis through the inguinal canal to the floor of the developing scrotum; it guides the descent of the testis from the abdomen into the scrotum.

Guillain-Barré syndrome. Acute segmentally demyelinating polyradiculoneuropathy, a disease complex in which the basic mechanism appears to be an immunizing or allergic reaction commonly occurring after a minor febrile illness; inflammatory changes in the spinal cord produce bilateral weakness or paralysis, most commonly beginning in the lower extremities; recovery is usual if respiratory and vasomotor failure do not occur; the classical findings in the spinal fluid are elevated protein concentration without pleocytosis and under normal pressure; also called infectious polyneuritis and

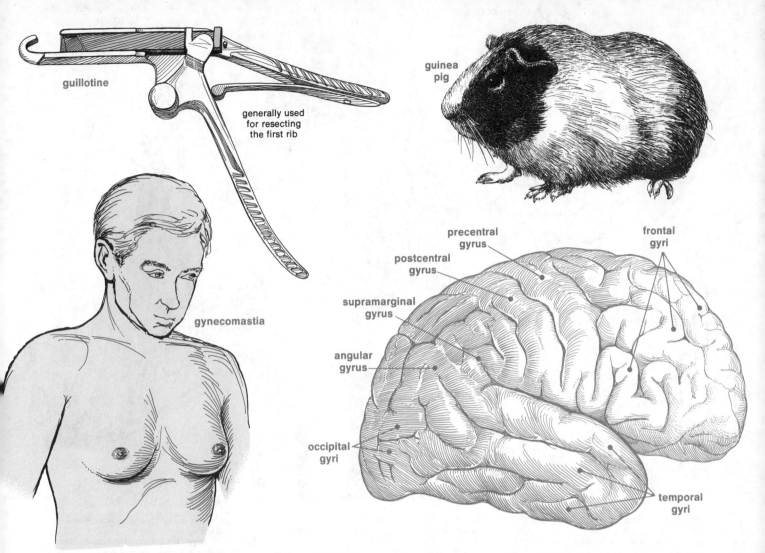

guillotine

generally used
for resecting
the first rib

guinea
pig

gynecomastia

precentral
gyrus

postcentral
gyrus

supramarginal
gyrus

angular
gyrus

occipital
gyri

frontal
gyri

temporal
gyri

acute polyradiculitis.

guil′lotine. A surgical cutting instrument with a knifeblade that slides in the grooves of a guide.

guin′ea pig. Any of several small tropical American burrowing rodents of the genus *Cavia*. used extensively for experimental work.

gul′let. The pharynx and the esophagus; the passage leading from the mouth to the stomach.

gum. 1. The dried viscous sap exuded by certain trees and plants; it is water-soluble, noncrystalline, and brittle. **2.** The gingiva.

  g. arabic, a gummy exudate of various African trees of the genus *Acacia*; used in the preparation of pills.

gum′boil. Colloquial term for a chronic alveolar abscess that drains itself by perforating the gingiva.

gum′ma, *pl.* **gum′mas** or **gum′mata.** A soft, gummy, infectious tumor that occurs, irregularly, during the third stage of syphilis.

gum′matous. Relating to or of the nature of a gumma.

Gunn's sign. Compression of a retinal venule where it is crossed by an overlying arteriole, seen in arteriolar sclerosis.

gusta′tion. 1. The sense of taste. **2.** The act of tasting.

gus′tatory. Of or relating to the sense of taste.

gut. 1. The intestine. **2.** The digestive tube of the embryo.

gut′ta (gt). Latin for a drop; a volume of liquid considered a unit of measure; equivalent to about 1 minim of water.

gut′ta-per′cha. A milky latex sap of several tropical trees (family Sapotaceae); used in the manufacture of splints and as a thin waterproof sheet to protect wounds; in dentistry, used for temporary sealing of dressings in cavities and for filling of root canals.

gut′tate. Resembling a drop; said of certain skin lesions.

gutta′tim. Latin for drop by drop.

gut′tur. Latin for throat.

gut′tural. Relating to the throat.

GVH. Abbreviation for graft vs. host; denoting an immune response of grafted cells against the host cells.

gym′nocyte. A cell without a limiting membrane.

gymnopho′bia. Morbid fear of the sight of the naked body.

GYN. Abbreviation for gynecology or gynecologic.

gy′nandrism. A congenital defect marked by overdevelopment of the clitoris and fusion of the labia majora, having the appearance of a penis and scrotum.

gynan′dromorph. An individual with both male and female characteristics.

gynandromor′phous. Having male and female characteristics.

gynatre′sia. Occlusion of a part of the female genital tract, usually the vagina.

gy′necoid. Resembling a female.

gynecolog′ic. Pertaining to gynecology.

gynecol′ogist. A specialist in gynecology.

gynecol′ogy. The branch of medicine concerned with diseases peculiar to women.

gynecoma′nia. Insatiable sexual desire for women.

gynecomas′tia. Excessive development of the male breast.

gynepho′bia. Morbid fear of or aversion to women.

gyno-, gyn-, gyne-, gyneco-. Combining forms denoting women or female.

gynop′athy. Any disease characteristic of women.

gynoplas′tics. Reparative surgery of the female genitalia.

gyp′sum. The dihydrate of calcium sulfate; $CaSO_4 \cdot 2H_2O$; plaster of Paris and dental stone are derived from it.

gyra′tion. 1. Revolution about a stationary point. **2.** An arrangement or group of gyri in the brain.

gy′ri. Plural of gyrus.

gy′rus. A convolution of the brain.

  angular g., one arching over the upturned end of the superior temporal sulcus.

  cingulate g., a long curved convolution lying above and in front of the corpus callosum; it is continuous posteriorly with the isthmus.

  dentate g., a narrow crenated strip of cortex between the fimbria hippocampi and the hippocampal gyrus; it is continued posteriorly, under the splenium of the corpus callosum, as the delicate fasciolar gyrus.

  fasciolar g., the transitional band between the dentate gyrus and the indusium griseum (supracallosal gyrus); located near the splenium of the corpus callosum.

  frontal g., any of the three (superior, middle, and inferior) gyri of the frontal lobe.

  hippocampal g., one that lies between the collateral sulcus and the hippocampal sulcus, on the inferior surface of each cerebral hemisphere; posteriorly, it is continuous above the cingulate gyrus through the isthmus and below the lingual gyrus; also called parahippocampal gyrus.

  lingual g., a median occipitotemporal gyrus between the calcarine and collateral sulci.

  paraterminal g., a thin sheet of gray matter which covers the undersurface of the rostrum of the corpus callosum.

  postcentral g., the anterior convolution of the parietal lobe, bounded in front by the central sulcus (Rolando) and posteriorly by the interparietal sulcus.

  precentral g., the posterior convolution of the frontal lobe bounded posteriorly by the central sulcus (Rolando) and anteriorly by the precentral sulcus.

  supracallosal g., a thin sheet of gray matter which covers the superior surface of the corpus callosum of the brain; also called indusium griseum.

  supramarginal g., one that arches over the upturned end of the lateral sulcus.

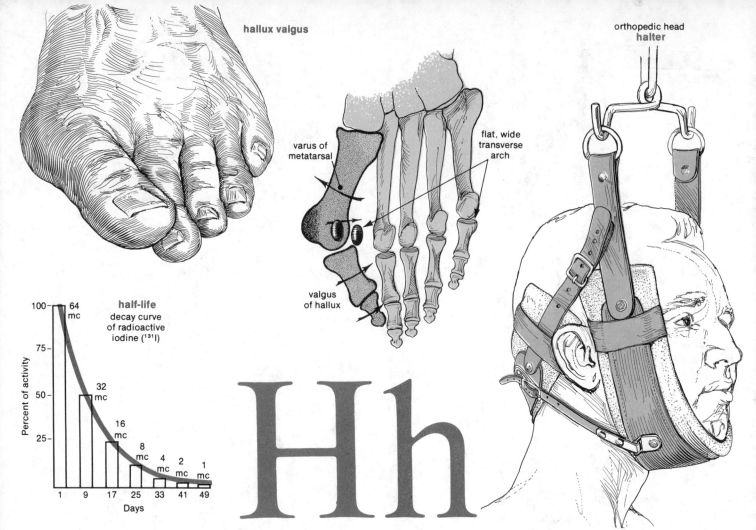

hallux valgus

varus of metatarsal

flat, wide transverse arch

valgus of hallux

orthopedic head
halter

half-life
decay curve
of radioactive
iodine (¹³¹I)

100 — 64 mc
75
50 — 32 mc
25 — 16 mc
8 mc
4 mc
2 mc
1 mc

Percent of activity

Days: 1 9 17 25 33 41 49

Hh

H. 1. Abbreviation for (a) hypermetropia; (b) hyperopia. **2.** Symbol for (a) hydrogen; (b) oersted.

h. Abbreviation for (a) height; (b) horizontal; (c) hundred.

H⁺. Symbol for hydrogen ion.

¹H. Symbol for hydrogen-1.

²H. Symbol for hydrogen-2; also abbreviated D.

³H. Symbol for hydrogen-3.

H disease. See Hartnup disease.

HAA. Abbreviation for hepatitis-associated antigen.

habe′na. 1. A restricting band or frenum. **2.** A restraining bandage.

haben′ula. The dorsal pedicle of the pineal gland.

hab′it. 1. A constant tendency to perform an act, acquired by frequent repetition of the act. **2.** An addiction.

habitua′tion. 1. The process of forming a habit; especially the process of becoming addicted to a drug. **2.** The method by which the nervous system gradually reduces response to a repeated stimulus.

hab′itus. Physical and constitutional characteristics of a person, especially as related to susceptibility to some disease.

Haemaphy′salis. A genus of ticks infesting birds and small mammals; vectors of disease.

  H. leporis palustris, a species that transmits Rocky Mountain spotted fever and tularemia to rabbits but not to humans.

Haemodip′sus ventrico′sus. The rabbit louse; it transmits the causative agent of tularemia in man.

Haemoph′ilus. A genus of bacteria; minute gramnegative, nonmotile, rod-shaped cells, parasitic on media containing blood.

  H. ducreyi, a species that is the causative agent of chancroid (soft chancre); also called Ducrey′s bacillus.

  H. influenzae, the influenza bacillus; a species found in the respiratory tract; causes acute respiratory infections, acute conjunctivitis, and purulent meningitis in children, rarely in adults; also called Pfeiffer′s, Weeks′, or Koch-Weeks bacillus.

  H. parahaemolyticus, a species found in the upper respiratory tract; frequently associated with pharyngitis.

haemorrha′gia. Greek for hemorrhage.

Haemosporid′ia. An order of sporozoa, parasitic in the blood of vertebrates; some of the species cause various diseases.

haf′nium. Chemical element; symbol Hf, atomic number 72, atomic weight 178.50.

Hageman factor. Factor XII.

hagiother′apy. 1. Treatment of disease by placing the patient in contact with religious relics, by visiting shrines, or by participating in religious observances. **2.** Treatment of disease executed by a holy man.

hair. 1. Pilus (1). **2.** A long cylindrical filament.

  embryonic h., see lanugo hair.

  ingrown h., hair that continues to grow but fails to emerge from the pilosebaceous ostium, sometimes causing papules; also called burrowing hair.

  lanugo h., soft, fine hair growing on the body of the newborn; also called embryonic hair.

  tactile h., the whiskers of certain animals.

  taste h., one of the hairlike projections of gustatory cells, formed by the condensation of secretions.

hal′azone. An antibacterial substance used in the sterilization of water supplies.

half-life. The time required for half of the radioactivity originally associated with a radioactive substance to disintegrate (radioactive decay).

  biologic h.-l., (1) the time required for a radioactive isotope within the body to lose half of its activity; this depends both on the natural half-life of the isotope and the rate of excretion from the body; (2) the time it takes for the body to eliminate 50 per cent of a drug; abbreviated $T_{1/2}$.

hal′ide. A salt of a halogen (bromide, chlorine, fluorine, or iodine).

halito′sis. Unpleasant breath; some causes are poor mouth hygiene, infection in the oronasopharyngeal structures, and lung abscess.

hal′itus. 1. Latin for breath. **2.** An exhalation; vapor.

hal′lucal. Of or relating to the big toe.

hallucina′tion. Perception of objects or events which do not exist.

  hypanogogic h., vivid sensory, dreamlike experiences occurring during the period between wakefulness and sleep.

hallu′cinatory. 1. Characterized by hallucination. **2.** Capable of inducing hallucination.

hallu′cinogen. Any agent that induces hallucinations.

hallucino′sis. A psychotic state in which an individual is more or less persistently hallucinated; e.g., chronic alcoholic hallucinosis.

hal′lux, *pl.* **hal′luces.** The big toe; the first digit of the foot.

  h. dolorosa, a painful condition usually associated with flatfoot, in which walking causes severe discomfort in the metatarsophalangeal joint of the big toe.

  h. malleus, hammertoe of the big toe.

  h. rigidus, stiff toe; painful flexion of the big toe due to stiffness in the metatarsophalangeal joint.

  h. valgus, the most common of the painful conditions of the toes, marked by an abnormal angulation of the big toe toward the other toes of the same foot; the condition is generally attributed to narrow or pointed shoes; predisposing congenital and familial factors may exist. Cf bunion.

  h. varus, an abnormal angulation of the big toe away from the other toes of the same foot.

halo, glaucomatous. Colored rings seen around lights by individuals with glaucoma; caused by diffraction of droplets of fluid in the corneal epithelium in the presence of edema of the cornea.

hal′ogen. Any of a group of chemically related nonmetallic elements that form similar saltlike compounds in combination with sodium; they include bromine, chlorine, fluorine, iodine, and the radioactive element astatine.

hal′oid. Resembling a halogen.

hal′ophil, hal′ophile. A microorganism that thrives in a salty environment.

hal′othane. A liquid hydrocarbon used as a general anesthetic; associated with liver damage in susceptible individuals; Fluothane®.

hal′ter. A device for securing the head, particularly for traction.

ham. 1. The buttock and back part of the thigh. **2.**

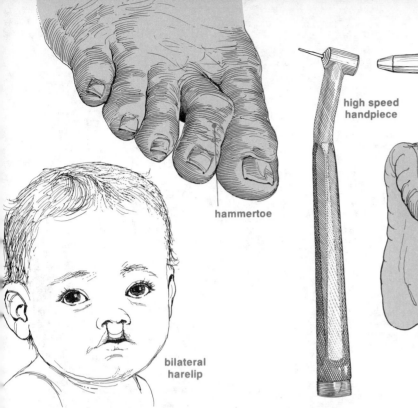

hammertoe

bilateral harelip

high speed handpiece

handpiece

haustra

colon

The popliteal space or poples; the hollow behind the knee.

hamartoblasto'ma. Malignant tumor believed to be derived from a hamartoma.

hamarto'ma. Tumorlike nonmalignant growth composed of cellular elements normally present in that site, but poorly developed.

Hamman-Rich syndrome. Progressive interstitial fibrosis of both lungs leading to pulmonary insufficiency, right-sided heart failure, and death; the cause is unknown.

Hamman's sign. A rasping sound, synchronous with the heart beat, occurring in pneumomediastinum.

ham'mer. See malleus.

ham'mertoe. A deformed toe in which the second and third phalanges are congenitally bent downward.

ham'ster. Any of several ratlike Eurasian rodents (family Cricetidae) extensively used in experimental work.

ham'string. Either of two tendons bounding the popliteal space of the knee; the medial or inner one comprises the tendons of the semimembranosus, semitendinosus, gracilis, and sartorius muscles; the lateral or outer one consists of the tendon of the biceps femoris.

ham'ular. Shaped like a hook.

ham'ulus. Any hook-shaped process, as at the end of a bone.

  h. lacrimalis, the lacrimal hamulus; the hooklike process of the lacrimal bone articulating with the maxilla and forming the upper aperture of the bony nasal duct.

  h. laminae spiralis, the hooklike termination of the spiral lamina bone of the cochlea.

  h. pterygoideus, the hooklike process of the sphenoid bone.

hand. The terminal part of the upper extremity below the forearm.

  accoucheur's h., the characteristic position of the hand produced by spasm in tetany.

  griffin-claw h., permanent extension of the metacarpophalangeal joints; also called griffin claw and main en griffe.

  opera glass h., deformity of the hand marked by shortening of the fingers and transverse folding of the skin caused by absorption of the phalanges, seen in chronic absorptive arthritis; also called main en lorgnette.

  spade h., the characteristic coarse, thick, square hand of acromegaly or myxedema.

H and E stain. Abbreviation for hematoxylin and eosin stain; see under stain.

hand-foot-and-mouth disease. A highly in-

fectious disease of children characterized by painful ulcerative stomatitis of the tongue, soft palate, and oral mucosa, associated with a vesicular eruption on hands and feet; attributed to type A-16 or A-5 Coxsackie virus.

hand'piece. In dentistry, the part of a mechanized, hand-held device that holds rotary instruments such as burs and mandrels during operative procedures; it is connected to a dental engine.

  high-speed h., one that operates at rotational speeds in excess of 12,000 revolutions per minute.

  ultra high-speed h., one that operates at rotational speeds of 100,000 to 300,000 revolutions per minute.

  ultrasonic h., one which vibrates at a frequency of 29,000 cycles per second (above audible range).

  water-turbine h., one with a turbine powered by water under great pressure.

Hand-Schüller-Christian syndrome. Disorder principally of childhood, occasionally of young adulthood, characterized by exophthalmos (unilateral or bilateral), diabetes insipidus, and destruction of bone (especially of the skull), with tumorlike masses of cholesterol-loaded histiocytes; also called Schüller-Christian syndrome and Schüller disease.

hang'nail. A partly detached piece of skin at the base or side of the nail.

Hansen's disease. See leprosy.

hapalonych'ia. A state or condition characterized by soft fingernails or toenails; it can be normal or acquired as a result of malnutrition or debility.

hap'lodont. Having peglike, even-surfaced molar teeth.

hap'loid. Referring to the reduced number of chromosomes in the gametes relative to that in the zygotes or in the body cells (diploid); the haploid number is half the diploid number.

haplo'pia. Single, normal vision, distinguished from double vision or diplopia.

haplo'sis. The meiotic reduction of the diploid number of chromosomes to the haploid number.

hap'ten, hap'tene. Any incomplete antigen which combines specifically with antibody but which does not incite the production of antibody unless attached to a high molecular weight carrier.

haptoglo'bin. A protein present in human blood serum having the ability to combine with hemoglobin; a low level of haptoglobin indicates recent hemolysis.

haptom'eter. Instrument used to determine sensitivity to touch.

hap'tophore. The atom group in the molecule of an antigen or antibody by means of which it becomes attached to a cell or to its corresponding antibody or antigen, respectively.

hard-metal disease. A pneumoconiosis attributed to inhalation of a specific industrial dust, especially of tungsten carbide, silicon carbide, or cobalt.

hardness. The ability of a material to resist scratching, abrasion, or attrition.

harelip. Congenital malformation of the upper lip ranging from a scarlike groove, or a notching of the lip, to a complete cleft extending into the nasal cavity; may be unilateral or bilateral and is frequently accompanied by a cleft palate; also called cleft lip and cheiloschisis.

harmony, occlusal. A contact between upper and lower teeth that is devoid of defects.

harpoon'. An instrument with a barbed head used to remove small pieces of tissue for microscopic examination.

Hartnup disease. A hereditary disorder of amino acid transport, marked by a pellagra-like skin rash upon exposure to sunlight, temporary muscular incoordination, and excretion of excessive amounts of amino acid in the urine; also called H disease and Hartnup syndrome.

Hartnup syndrome. See Hartnup disease.

hasamiyami. A fever occurring in Japan in the autumn, caused by a bacterium (*Leptospira autumnalis*); also called akiyami.

hash'ish. An intoxicating extract made from the dried flowers of the hemp plant, *Cannabis indica*; also written hasheesh.

hat'chet. An angled cutting hand instrument used in dentistry to remove enamel and dentin.

haunch. The region of the upper thigh, buttock, and hip.

hau'stral. Relating to the pouches or sacculations of the colon.

haustra'tion. Increase in size of the sacculations of the large intestine.

hau'strum, *pl.* **hau'stra.** One of the sacculations of the colon.

haver'sian. Term applied to the various osseous structures described by Clopton Havers.

Hb, Hgb. Symbols for hemoglobin.

HBAg. Abbreviation for hepatitis B antigen (hepatitis-associated antigen).

HbCO. Symbol for carboxyhemoglobin.

HbO$_2$. Symbol for oxyhemoglobin.

HbS. Symbol for sickle cell hemoglobin; now called hemoglobin S.

HCG. Abbreviation for human chorionic gonadotropin.

Hct. Abbreviation for hematocrit.

H.d. Abbreviation for Latin *hora decubitus*, at bedtime.

HDC. Abbreviation for human diploid cell.

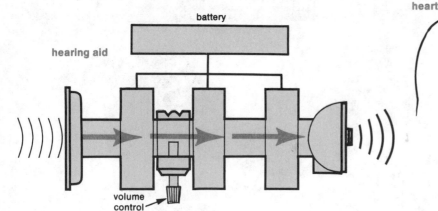

hearing aid

battery

MICROPHONE
microphone collects sounds (just as the ear does) and converts them into electrical impulses

volume control

AMPLIFIER
amplifier, powered by a battery, increases the intensity of the electrical impulses several thousand times; loudness can be adjusted by the volume control

RECEIVER
receiver or speaker changes the amplified electrical impulses back to sound which is delivered many times louder into the ear

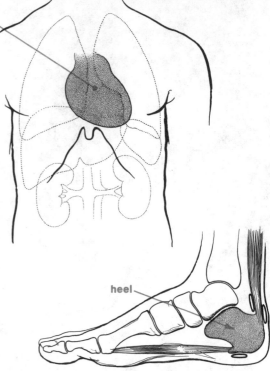

heart

heel

He. Chemical symbol of the element helium.

head. 1. The upper or anterior vertebrate extremity, containing the brain and organs of special senses. **2.** The proximal extremity of a bone; that which is nearer the axial skeleton. **3.** The end of a muscle which is attached to the less movable part of the skeleton. **4.** Slang expression denoting one who frequently uses narcotics.

head′ache. Pain or ache in the head; also called cephalalgia.

  blind h., migraine.

  cluster h., a recurrent unilateral headache in the orbitotemporal area; usually of brief duration, often severe, generally occurring in regular intervals of six-week cycles; usually accompanied by stuffiness of the nose and tearing of the eye on the same side as the pain; can be precipitated by the use of histamine, alcohol, or nitroglycerin; more prevalent among males who smoke heavily; also called histaminic headache or cephalalgia and Horton's headache.

  histaminic h., see cluster headache.

  Horton's h., see cluster headache.

  migraine h., migraine.

  organic h., one caused by disease of the brain or its membranes.

  tension h., one caused by sustained contraction of skeletal muscle about the scalp, face, and especially the neck.

  vascular h., migraine.

head′gear. 1. In orthodontics, an apparatus encircling the head or neck which provides anchorage for the attachment of an intraoral appliance. **2.** In radiology, a protective device to guard the head from injury by radiation.

heal. 1. To close naturally, said of an incision, wound, or ulcer. **2.** To restore to health; to cure.

healer. One who heals or cures, especially a physician.

heal′ing. 1. The process of return to normal health. **2.** Denoting an agent that promotes such a process.

health. 1. The state of an organism with respect to its physical, mental, and social wellbeing. **2.** The state of an organism functioning optimally without disorders of any nature.

heal′thy. Of or pertaining to good health.

hear. To perceive sound.

hearing. The capacity to perceive sound.

  color h., a subjective color sensation produced by certain sound waves; also called pseudochromesthesia.

  conduction h. impairment, reduction of hearing ability caused by interference with the conduction of sound to the end organ.

  h. aid, a small device that amplifies sound; used to compensate for a hearing loss.

  h. impairment, reduction of hearing ability due to either malfunctioning of nerve elements or interference with conduction of sound to the end organ.

  h. level, the measure of hearing ability as read on the hearing loss scale of the audiometer.

  h. loss, reduced auditory sensitivity.

  monaural h., hearing with only one ear.

  sensorineural h. loss, loss of hearing due to dysfunction of the end organ or nerve fibers or both.

heart. The hollow, muscular, four chambered organ that maintains the circulation of the blood by receiving it from the veins and pumping it into the arteries; it lies between the lungs and is enclosed in the pericardium; also called cor.

  dextroposition of h., see under dextroposition.

  h. failure, see under failure.

  left h., the left atrium and left ventricle considered together.

  right h., the right atrium and right ventricle considered together.

heart′burn. Burning sensation in the epigastrium and lower chest caused by irritation of the esophagus; it requires two factors for its genesis; a gastroesophageal sphincter that allows reflux of gastric contents into the esophagus, and an esophagus which is sensitive to that refluxed material; also called pyrosis.

heart′worm. A parasitic nematode worm, *Dirofilaria immitis*, that usually lodges in the right chambers of the heart of dogs and very rarely in man.

heat. 1. A state characterized by elevation of temperature. **2.** A form of energy in transit from a body of higher temperature to another of lower temperature. **3.** Estrus.

  h. of combustion, the quantity of heat released in the complete oxidation of one mole of a substance at constant pressure.

  prickly h., a common, noncontagious skin disorder of hot, humid climates; elevated temperatures cause maceration of the skin, leading to blockage of sweat pores, retention of sweat, and formation of tiny vesicular papules that itch and burn; also called miliaria rubra and heat rash.

heave. Slang term for vomiting.

  dry h., retching without vomiting.

hebephre′nia. A type of schizophrenia, usually developing after the onset of puberty, characterized by shallow, inappropriate emotions, unpredictable childish behavior and mannerisms, and delusions.

hec′tic. 1. Relating to the daily fever characteristic of certain diseases such as tuberculosis. **2.** Feverish; flushed.

hecto-, hect-. Prefixes used in the metric system to indicate one hundred (10^2).

hec′togram (hg). One hundred grams, the equivalent of 1543.7 grains or 3.527 avoirdupois ounces.

hec′toliter. One hundred liters, the equivalent of 105.7 quarts.

hedon′ic. Of, relating to, or characterized by pleasure.

hedon′ics. The study of pleasurable and unpleasurable feelings as they relate to behavior.

hed′onism. A constant pursuit of or devotion to pleasure and avoidance of pain; exhibited in some forms of character disorder.

heel. The rounded posterior portion of the foot.

heel bone. Calcaneus.

Hegar's sign. A compressibility and softening of the lower uterine segment (cervical isthmus) elicited by bimanual examination; a suggestive sign of pregnancy.

hel′icine. Relating to a spiral or helix.

hel′icoid. Spiral.

helicotre′ma. The passage at the apex of the cochlea of the internal ear through which the scala vestibuli and scala tympani communicate with one another.

heliop′athy. Injury from exposure to sunlight.

helio′sis. Sunstroke.

heliotax′is. The tendency of a microorganism to move toward (positive heliotaxis) or away from (negative heliotaxis) a light source.

heliother′apy. A method of treatment by means of direct exposure of the body to the sun's rays.

heliot′ropism. The tendency of plants to turn toward the sunlight.

he′lium. A gaseous element; symbol He, atomic number 2, atomic weight 4.003; present in small amounts in the atmosphere.

he′lix. 1. The folded skin and cartilage forming the margin of the outer ear (auricle). **2.** A coiled curve or structure.

  α-h., the right-handed helical form of many proteins.

  DNA h., see Watson-Crick helix.

  double h., see Watson-Crick helix.

  twin h., see Watson-Crick helix.

  Watson-Crick h., a three-dimensional model of the DNA molecule; it consists of a double helix resembling a ladder that has been twisted into a spiral; the sides of the ladder are formed by the deoxyribose-phosphate units and are held together by rungs composed of pairs of bases (adenine and thymine or cytosine and guanine) joined together by hydrogen bonds; also called DNA, double, or twin helix.

hel′minth. 1. A parasitic intestinal worm, especially the nematode or trematode. **2.** A wormlike

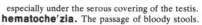

strawberry hemangioma

port-wine hemangioma

parasite.

helminthem'esis. The vomiting of parasitic worms.

helminthi'asis. The condition of having intestinal worms.

helmin'thic. Of, relating to, or caused by worms, especially parasitic intestinal worms.

helmin'thoid. Resembling a worm.

helminthol'ogy. The study of worms, especially the parasitic intestinal worms; also called scolecology.

helo'ma. A corn.

helo'sis. The condition of having horny thickening of the skin, usually on a toe; also called corns.

helot'omy. The surgical removal of corns or of calluses.

hem-, hema-. See hemo-.

hem-. See hemi-.

hemabarom'eter. A device for determining the specific gravity of the blood.

hemacytom'eter. See hemocytometer.

hemacytozo'on. See hemocytozoon.

hemadsorp'tion. Phenomenon in which a substance adheres to the surface of a red blood cell.

hemagglutina'tion. Agglutination (clumping) of red blood cells.

hemagglu'tinin. A protein in blood serum that causes clumping of red blood cells; also present in the surface projections of some viruses.

hem'agogue, hem'agog. Any agent that promotes the flow of blood, particularly during menstruation.

he'mal. 1. Of or relating to the blood or blood vessels. **2.** Relating to or located on the ventral side of the spinal axis where the heart is located; opposed to neural.

hemangiecta'sia, hemangiecta'sis. Dilation of blood vessels.

hemangio-. Combining form indicating a relationship to the blood vessels.

heman'gioblast. An embryonic cell derived from the mesoderm; it develops into cells that give rise to endothelium of blood vessels, to reticuloendothelial elements, and to all types of blood-forming cells.

hemangioblasto'ma. A brain tumor composed of angioblasts; also called angioblastoma.

heman'gioendothe'lioblasto'ma. A tumor of vascular origin in which the endothelial cells seem to be predominantly immature types.

heman'gioendothelio'ma. A tumor derived from blood vessels, composed chiefly of masses of endothelial cells.

hemangio'ma. A benign tumor made up of blood vessels.

capillary h., a congenital tumor composed of mi-

nute, closely packed, thin-walled blood vessels that, for the most part, are of the caliber of capillaries; it varies from bright red to blue and may occur in any tissue or organ; the most common sites are the skin, subcutaneous tissues, and mucous membranes of the oral cavity and lips.

cavernous h., a tumor containing large blood-filled spaces resembling erectile tissue; also called cavernous angioma.

port-wine h., an enlarged red-blue capillary hemangioma that resembles a map, is nonpalpable, and covers large areas of the face and upper trunk; also called port-wine mark, stain, or nevus and nevus flammeus.

senile h., a bright red capillary hemangioma varying in size from pinhead to several centimeters in diameter; may be flat or slightly raised; seen in young adults and, most frequently, in elderly individuals.

spider h., arterial spider; a dilated arteriole of the skin with radiating capillary branches.

strawberry h., a bright red raised tumor; present at birth as a pinhead-sized flat lesion that quickly increases in size and becomes elevated and rough; approximately 90 per cent of these hemangiomas disappear without treatment by the ages of 5 to 7; also called nevus vasculosus.

hemangiomato'sis. The presence of numerous hemangiomas.

hemangiopericyto'ma. A rare tumor believed to be derived from pericytes (connective tissue cells surrounding capillaries).

hemangiosarco'ma. A rare malignant tumor composed chiefly of anaplastic cells derived from blood vessels.

hemarthro'sis. Blood in a joint space, resulting usually in pain, tenderness, and swelling.

hemat-. See hemo-.

hematem'esis. Vomiting of blood.

hem'atherm. Denoting a warm-blooded animal.

hemather'mal. Warm-blooded; said of man and certain animals; also called hemathermous.

hemather'mous. See hemathermal.

hemat'ic. 1. Of, relating to, or contained in blood. **2.** A remedy for blood disorders; hematinic.

hem'atin. 1. The hydroxide of heme. **2.** Heme.

hematin'ic. Any agent that improves the condition of the blood.

hematinu'ria. The presence of heme in the urine.

hemato-. See hemo-.

hem'atoblast. A primitive blood cell from which develop erythroblasts, lymphoblasts, myeloblasts, and other immature blood cells.

hem'atocele. A swelling caused by the effusion and collection of blood into a cavity of the body,

especially under the serous covering of the testis.

hematoche'zia. The passage of bloody stools.

hematocolpome'tra. Accumulation of blood in the uterus and vagina resulting from an imperforate hymen or any other obstruction.

hematocol'pos. Distention of the vagina with accumulated menstrual blood due to an imperforate hymen.

hemat'ocrit (Hct). **1.** The volume percentage of red blood cells in whole blood; in the normal male it constitutes about 45 to 50 per cent of the whole blood volume; in the normal female it constitutes approximately 40 to 45 per cent; also called packed cell volume. **2.** A small centrifuge used to separate the cellular elements of blood from the plasma.

hematocy'anin. See hemocyanin.

hematocys'tis. Effusion of blood into the urinary bladder.

he'matocyte. See hemocyte.

hematocytom'eter. Hemocytometer.

hematocytozo'on. See hemocytozoon.

hematocytu'ria. The presence of red blood cells in the urine; also called true hematuria.

hematogen'esis. See hemopoiesis.

hematogen'ic. Hematogenous.

hematog'enous. 1. Derived from blood. **2.** Relating to anything originating in or circulated by the blood.

hematoid'. 1. Resembling blood. **2.** Bloody.

hematol'din. Pigment derived from the breakdown of hemoglobin; formed in the tissues as a result of hemorrhage.

hematol'ogist. A specialist in the diagnosis and treatment of disorders of blood and blood-forming tissues.

hematol'ogy. The medical specialty which is concerned with blood and blood-forming tissues, and the treatment of blood disorders.

hematol'ysis. See hemolysis.

hemato'ma. A localized mass of blood outside of the blood vessels, usually found in a partly clotted state.

hematomanom'eter. See hemomanometer.

hematome'tra. Distention of the uterus with accumulated blood; also called hemometra.

hematom'etry. Examination of blood to determine (a) the total number, types, and proportions of blood cells; (b) the number or proportion of other formed elements; (c) the percentage of hemoglobin; also called hemometry.

hematomye'lia. Effusion of blood into the spinal cord.

hematopathol'ogy. The branch of medicine concerned with diseases of the blood and blood-forming tissues.

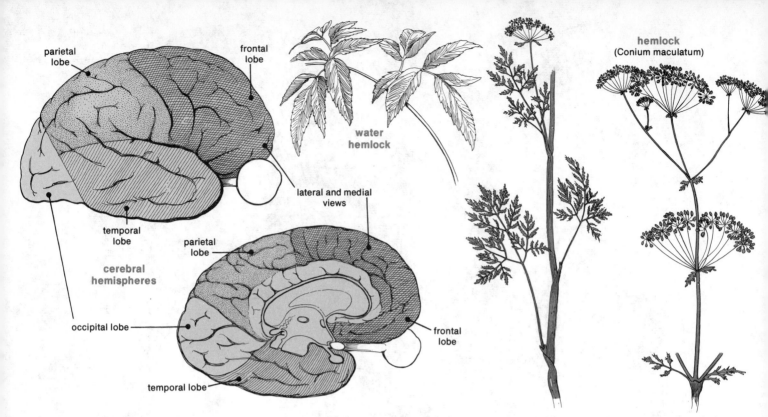

parietal lobe

frontal lobe

temporal lobe

cerebral hemispheres

occipital lobe

parietal lobe

frontal lobe

temporal lobe

lateral and medial views

water hemlock

hemlock (Conium maculatum)

hematop′athy. See hemopathy.

hematope′nia. Blood deficiency.

hematopoietin. See erythropoietin.

hematopor′phyrin. A dark red substance formed by the decomposition of hemoglobin.

hematosal′pinx. Distention of a uterine tube with a collection of blood; also called hemosalpinx.

he′matoscope. 1. Instrument for determining the number of red blood cells suspended in blood by measuring the dispersion of light. **2.** Instrument for determining the percentage of hemoglobin in blood.

hematosep′sis. Septicemia.

hematotax′is. Spontaneous bleeding caused by a blood disease.

hematotrache′los. Distention of the uterine cervix, as with accumulated menstrual blood due to an imperforate hymen.

hematox′ylin. A yellow or orange crystalline compound, extracted from the tropical American tree, logwood; used as a stain in histology and bacteriology.

hematozo′ic. Of, relating to, or caused by hematozoa.

hematozo′on, *pl.* **hematozo′a.** Any parasitic protozoan or microorganism that lives in the circulating blood of its host.

hematu′ria. Discharge of red blood cells in the urine.

heme. The nonprotein, iron-containing porphyrin molecule which forms the oxygen-binding element of hemoglobin; also called ferroprotoporphyrin; formerly known as hematin.

hem′eralo′pia. Defective vision in daylight, with good vision in dim light; also called day blindness and night sight.

hemi-, hem-. Prefixes denoting one-half; e.g., hemianopia.

hemial′gia. Pain on one side of the body only.

hemiamblyo′pia. Reduced vision in one half of the visual field of one or both eyes.

hemianacu′sia. Loss of hearing or deafness in one ear.

hemianalge′sia. Loss of sensibility to pain on one side of the body.

hemianesthe′sia. Loss of sensibility to touch on one side of the body.

  alternate h., hemianesthesia affecting one side of the head and the other side of the body and extremities; also called crossed hemianesthesia.

  crossed h., see alternate hemianesthesia.

hemianop′sia. Loss of vision in one half of the visual field of one or both eyes.

  bilateral h., hemianopsia affecting the visual fields of both eyes.

  binasal h., bilateral hemianopsia affecting the nasal halves of the visual fields of both eyes.

  bitemporal h., bilateral hemianopsia affecting the temporal halves of the visual fields of both eyes.

  congruous h., bilateral hemianopsia affecting the nasal half of one visual field and the temporal half of the other, the defects in the two visual fields being identical in size, shape, and location, resulting in a single defect of the binocular field.

  crossed h., bilateral hemianopsia affecting the upper half of one visual field and the lower half of the other.

  heteronymous h., bilateral hemianopsia affecting either both temporal halves or both nasal halves of the visual fields.

  homonymous h., bilateral hemianopsia affecting the nasal half of one visual field and the temporal half of the other.

  incomplete h., hemianopsia not affecting the entire half of the visual field.

  quadrantic h., see quadrantanopsia.

hemianos′mia. Loss of the sense of smell on one side only.

hemiat′rophy. Atrophy confined to one side of an organ or bodily region, as of the face or tongue.

  facial h., atrophy, usually progressive, affecting the tissues of one side of the face; also called Romberg's disease or syndrome and facial trophoneurosis.

hemibal′lism. Violent, involuntary movements of the extremities involving one side of the body, due to a lesion in the contralateral subthalamic body; also called hemiballismus.

he′mic. Relating to the blood.

hemicel′lulose. Any of a group of polysaccharides whose chemical composition is more complex than sugar and less complex than cellulose.

hemicen′trum. Either lateral half of the body of a vertebra.

hemichore′a. Chorea in which the uncontrollable and irregular movements of the muscles are largely confined to one side of the body.

hemicolec′tomy. Removal of part of the colon.

hemicra′nia. Pain on one side of the head.

hemidiaphore′sis. Sweating on one side of the body.

hemigastrec′tomy. Excision of one half of the stomach, usually the pyloric end.

α-hemihy′drate. Alpha-hemihydrate; $(CaSO_4)_2 \cdot H_2O$; gypsum that has been calcined under steam pressure in an autoclave to 130°C; the resulting crystals are somewhat prismatic; used for making casts and models of the oral cavity; also called dental stone.

β-hemihy′drate. Beta-hemihydrate; $(CaSO_4)_2 \cdot H_2O$; gypsum that has been calcined in the open

air to 110°C; the resulting crystals are irregular in shape; used in the preparation of casts for artificial dentures; also called dental plaster and plaster of Paris.

hemihyper′trophy. Congenital overgrowth of one side of the body.

hemikar′yon. A cell nucleus containing the haploid number of chromosomes.

hemilaminec′tomy. The surgical removal of a portion of the vertebral lamina in order to gain exposure to an underlying nerve root or intervertebral disk; often used to denote unilateral laminectomy.

hemime′lia. A congenital defect marked by absence of all or part of the distal portion of a limb or limbs.

he′min. A crystalline compound, $C_{34}H_{32}N_4O_4FeCl$; the chloride of heme; also called Teichmann's crystals.

heminephrec′tomy. Surgical excision of part of a kidney.

hemipare′sis. Muscular weakness or mild paralysis of one side of the body.

hemiple′gia. Paralysis of one side of the body.

  alternate h., Millard-Gubler syndrome.

hemipleg′ic. One whose body is paralyzed on one side.

Hemip′tera. A large order of insects that includes the common bedbug.

hemisoan′tibody. An antibody that reacts with a surface antigen-determinant or erythrocytes (red blood cells) to cause agglutination of the cells.

hem′isphere. Half of a symmetrical, spherical object.

  cerebral h., the lateral half of the cerebrum.

hemitho′rax. One side of the chest.

hemizygos′ity. The state of having only one of a pair of genes.

hemizy′gote. An individual or cell having only one of a pair of genes.

hemizy′gous, hemizygot′ic. Having unpaired genes; said of the male with respect to the X chromosome.

hem′lock. Any of several poisonous plants (genus *Conium*) capable of producing motor paralysis; more commonly called poison hemlock.

  water h., probably the most poisonous plant in the United States; the poison is found principally in the roots, which are often mistaken for parsnips.

hemo-, hemato-, hemat-, hema-, hem-. Combining forms denoting blood; e.g., hemoglobin.

hemoagglu′tinin. An antibody in serum that causes agglutination of red blood cells (erythrocytes).

hematopathy | **hemoagglutinin**

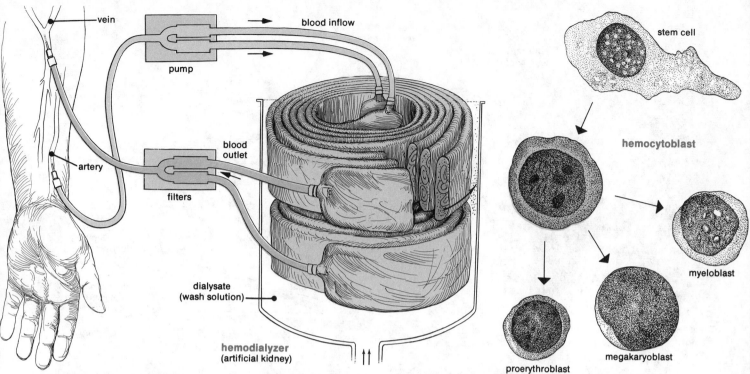

vein — **blood inflow** — **pump** — **blood outlet** — **filters** — **dialysate (wash solution)** — **artery** — **hemodialyzer (artificial kidney)**

stem cell — **hemocytoblast** — **myeloblast** — **megakaryoblast** — **proerythroblast**

---

hemobil′ia. Bleeding into the biliary passages.

hemochromato′sis. A disorder of iron metabolism resulting in accumulation of excess iron in the tissues of many organs, especially the skin, liver, and pancreas, leading to fibrosis and functional insufficiency of those organs which are severely involved; the heart and other muscles and endocrine glands are also affected; deposition of iron in the skin causes a bronzed pigmentation; deposits in the pancreas lead to diabetes; also called iron storage disease and bronze diabetes.

he′mochrome. See hemochromogen.

hemochro′mogen. A substance formed by the union of heme with a nitrogenous compound, as a protein or base; also called hemochrome.

hemochromom′eter. An apparatus for estimating the percentage of hemoglobin in the blood by comparing the solution of bood with a standard solution of an appropriate compound, such as ammonium picrocarminate.

hemocla′sia, hemoc′lasis. Hemolysis or destruction of red blood cells.

hemoconcentra′tion. Increase in the concentration or proportion of formed elements in the circulating blood, usually resulting from the loss of plasma from the blood stream; also called anhydremia.

hemocy′anin. An oxygen-carrying blue respiratory pigment (chromoprotein) occurring in the blood of lower sea animals (e.g., mollusks) in which copper is an essential component; also called hematocyanin.

he′mocyte. Any cell or formed element of the blood; a blood corpuscle; a blood cell; also called hematocyte.

hemocy′toblast. A primitive cell derived from the hemohistioblast; the name given to the cell from which granulocytes, red cell precursors, and megakaryocytes are derived.

hemocytom′eter. An instrument used for estimating the blood cell count in a measured volume of blood; also called hemacytometer, erythrocytometer, and globulimeter.

   Thoma-Zeiss h., an apparatus used to count blood cells; also called Thoma's counting chamber.

hemocytotrip′sis. The destruction of blood cells by mechanical means; e.g., compression between hard surfaces.

hemocytozo′on. An animal parasite of blood cells; also called hemacytozoon and hematocytozoon.

hemodial′ysis. Dialysis accomplished by passing the blood through a semipermeable membrane lying in a bathing solution (artificial kidney), then returning it to the body.

hemodi′alyzer. An apparatus used as a substitute for the kidneys to purify the blood in acute or chronic kidney failure and in certain types of poisoning; toxic elements are removed by passing the blood through a semipermeable membrane lying in a bathing solution, then returning it to the body; commonly called artificial kidney.

   ultrafiltration h., a hemodialyzer that uses fluid pressure differentials to bring about diffusion of protein-free fluid from the blood to the bathing solution.

hemodilu′tion. Increase in the plasma content of the blood with resulting decrease in the concentration of red blood cells.

hemodynam′ic. Of or relating to blood circulation.

hemodynam′ics. The science of the forces connected with the circulation of the blood.

hemoflag′ellates. Flagellated blood parasites.

hemofu′scin. A brown pigment derived from hemoglobin; sometimes found in urine along with hemosiderin; an indication of increased red blood cell destruction.

hemogen′esis. See hemopoiesis.

hemoglo′bin (Hb, Hgb). The oxygen-bearing protein of red blood cells; it is bright red when saturated with oxygen and purple when it is not carrying oxygen.

   fetal h., see hemoglobin F.

   h. A (Hb A), hemoglobin found in normal adults.

   h. A₂ (Hb A₂), hemoglobin which is increased in β-thalassemia; it makes up about 1.5 to 3 per cent of the total hemoglobin concentration in the adult.

   h. C, a slow-moving abnormal hemoglobin characterized by an amino acid substitution (lysine for glutamic acid at position six of the β-chains); it reduces the normal plasticity of red blood cells; associated with chronic hemolytic anemia.

   h. F (Hb F), hemoglobin of a normal fetus; the major hemoglobin component during intrauterine life; also called fetal hemoglobin.

   h. S (Hb S), abnormal hemoglobin characterized by an amino acid substitution (valine for glutamic acid at position six of the β-chain); associated with sickle cell anemia.

   oxygenated h., see oxyhemoglobin.

   reduced h., hemoglobin present in venous blood, after it has released its oxygen in the tissues.

   sickle cell h., hemoglobin S.

hemoglobine′mia. The presence of free hemoglobin in the plasma, resulting from mechanical injury to the red blood cells within the vessels.

hemoglo′binom′eter. An apparatus for estimating the amount of hemoglobin in the blood; also

called hemometer.

hemoglobinop′athy. A hematologic disorder in which the type of hemoglobin within an individual's red blood cells differs qualitatively or quantitatively from that contained in normal red blood cells.

hemoglobinu′ria. The presence of free hemoglobin in the urine, an indication of recent hemolysis of at least moderate severity.

   malarial h., rare condition caused by malignant tertian malaria; also called blackwater or remittent fever.

   paroxysmal nocturnal h., chronic disorder marked primarily by hemolytic anemia, hemoglobinuria (chiefly at night), yellow discoloration of the skin and mucous membranes, and enlargement of the spleen and liver; also called Marchiafava-Micheli syndrome or anemia.

he′mogram. A record of the number, proportion, and morphologic features of the cellular elements of blood.

hemohis′tioblast. An undifferentiated mesenchymal cell of the reticulo-endothelial system from which all blood cells are derived; it is probably similar in morphology to other blood blasts; also called stem cell.

he′molith. A concretion in the wall of a blood vessel.

hemol′ysin. 1. An anti-red blood cell antibody which activates complement (C′) to cause destruction (lysis) of red blood cells; formerly called amboceptor. **2.** Any substance produced by a living agent and capable of destroying red blood cells by liberating their hemoglobin.

   immune h., hemolysin made by injecting an animal with red blood cells or whole blood from another species.

hemolysin′ogen. Antigenic substance in red blood cells that stimulates the formation of hemolysin.

hemol′ysis. Liberation of hemoglobin from the red blood cells; also called erythrocytolysis and hematolysis.

hemolyt′ic. Causing disintegration of red blood cells.

hemolytic disease of the newborn. See erythroblastosis fetalis.

hemolytic-uremic syndrome. A syndrome usually occurring in children, characterized by hemolytic anemia with abnormally shaped erythrocytes, thrombocytopenia, and uremia; minor respiratory or gastrointestinal infection often precedes onset.

he′molyze. To cause the liberation of hemoglobin from red blood cells.

hemomanom′eter. An instrument for determin-

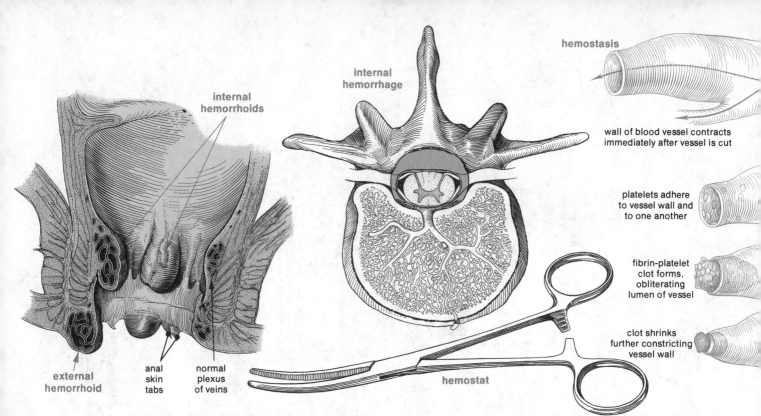

internal hemorrhoids

internal hemorrhage

hemostasis

wall of blood vessel contracts immediately after vessel is cut

platelets adhere to vessel wall and to one another

fibrin-platelet clot forms, obliterating lumen of vessel

clot shrinks further constricting vessel wall

external hemorrhoid

anal skin tabs

normal plexus of veins

hemostat

ing blood pressure; also called hematomanometer.

hemomedias'tinum. Effusion of blood into the mediastinum; also called hematomediastinum.

hemom'eter. 1. See hemoglobinometer. **2.** Term occasionally used for hemocytometer.

hemome'tra. See hematometra.

hemom'etry. See hematometry.

hemop'athy. Any disorder of the blood or blood-forming tissues; also called hematopathy.

hemoperfu'sion. Passage of the blood over a sorbent (e.g., activated charcoal) in order to remove a toxic substance.

hemopericar'dium. Accumulation of blood in the pericardial sac.

hemoperitone'um. Escape of blood into the peritoneal cavity.

hemopex'in. A serum protein in human plasma, containing 20 per cent carbohydrates; important in binding heme and porphyrins.

hemophag'ocyte. A phagocytic cell that engulfs and destroys red blood cells.

hemophagocyto'sis. The process of engulfment of red blood cells by phagocytic cells.

hem'ophil, hem'ophile. Denoting microorganisms that thrive in media containing blood.

hemophil'ia. An inherited hemorrhagic disease characterized by a deficiency of factor VIII (antihemophilic factor), causing excessive and sometimes spontaneous bleeding, and inherited as an X-linked recessive trait; although the heterozygous female is the carrier, she is asymptomatic and the disease is manifested only in the affected sons; also called classic hemophilia and hemophilia A.

h. B., a disorder of the blood clotting process caused by hereditary deficiency of factor IX (plasma thromboplastin component); also called Christmas disease.

hemophil'iac. An individual afflicted with hemophilia; a bleeder.

hemophil'ic. 1. Of or relating to hemophilia. **2.** Thriving in blood, or in culture media containing hemoglobin.

hemopho'bia. An abnormal fear of the sight of blood; also called hematophobia.

hemophthal'mia. Bleeding into the eyeball.

hemopneumopericar'dium. The presence of blood and air in the membrane enveloping the heart; also called pneumohemopericardium.

hemopneumothor'ax. Accumulation of air and blood in the pleural cavity.

hemopoie'sis. The formation of blood cells; also called hematopoiesis; also called hematogenesis and hemogenesis.

hemopoiet'ic. Relating to the formation of blood cells.

hemopor'phyrin. The porphyrin component of heme; $C_{34}H_{38}N_4O_6$; the iron-free heme.

hemoprecip'itin. An antibody that combines with and precipitates soluble antigenic material from erythrocytes; a precipitin specific for blood.

hemopro'tein. A conjugated compound consisting of a protein linked to heme.

hemop'sonin. An antibody that combines with red blood cells and renders them susceptible to phagocytosis.

hemop'tysis. Spitting of blood from lesions in the larynx, trachea, or lower respiratory tract.

hemopyelecta'sia. Dilation of the kidney pelvis with blood and urine.

hemorheol'ogy. The science of the relation of pressures, flow, volumes, and resistances in blood vessels.

hem'orrhage. Bleeding, especially profuse.
accidental h., abruptio placentae.
cerebral h., bleeding from blood vessels within the brain, usually in the area of the internal capsule.
internal h., bleeding into an organ or a body cavity.
secondary h., bleeding that occurs at an interval after an injury or operation.

hemorrhagen'ic. Causing hemorrhage.

hemorrhag'ic. Relating to or characterized by bleeding or hemorrhage.

hemorrhagic disease of the newborn. Disorder occurring during the first few days of life, marked by spontaneous bleeding due to deficiency of procoagulant substances; it is effectively treated with vitamin K.

hemorrhagic pulmonary-renal syndrome. See Goodpasture's syndrome.

hemorrha'gin. Any of a group of toxins that destroy the endothelial cells in capillaries, causing numerous hemorrhages in the tissues; found in certain poisonous substances such as rattlesnake venom, seeds of the castor oil plant, etc.

hem'orrhoid. A dilated (varicose) vein situated at or near the anus; it is present in about 35 per cent of the population, and occurs usually in persons 25 to 55 years old.
external h., varicosities of the inferior hemorrhoidal veins situated external to the rectoanal line and covered by skin.
internal h., varicose enlargement of the superior hemorrhoidal veins situated above the rectoanal line and covered with mucous membrane, causing, at the early stages, intermittent bleeding during or following defecation; the condition may develop in various degrees: (a) the hemorrhoids do not protrude through the anal canal (1st degree); (b) protrusion occurs through the anal canal during defeca-

tion, receding spontaneously afterward (2nd degree); (c) protrusion becomes more pronounced, occurring on any extra exertion and receding only by manual reduction (3rd degree); (d) the hemorrhoids are permanently prolapsed (4th degree).

hemorrhoid'al. 1. Of or relating to hemorrhoids or piles. **2.** Denoting blood vessels supplying the area of the rectum and anus.

hemorrhoidec'tomy. Surgical removal of hemorrhoids.

hemosal'pinx. See hematosalpinx.

he'moscope. Hematoscope.

hemosid'erin. A granular iron-containing yellow pigment formed during decomposition of hemoglobin; deposits are formed in a variety of tissues when there has been red blood cell breakdown.

hemosidero'sis. Deposition of hemosiderin (a yellow substance containing iron) in the tissues.

hemosper'mia. The presence of blood in the seminal fluid.

hemos'tasis. 1. The arrest of bleeding; also called hemostasia. **2.** The arrest of the flow of blood through a part or vessel.

he'mostat. An instrument or an agent that stops bleeding.

hemostat'ic. 1. Arresting hemorrhage. **2.** Any agent that checks bleeding.

hemostyp'tic. A chemical hemostatic; any chemical agent that stops bleeding by astringent properties.

hemotho'rax. Accumulation of blood in the pleural cavity.

hemotox'ic. 1. Causing blood poisoning. **2.** Destructive to blood cells; also called hematotoxic.

hemotox'in. Any toxin that is capable of destroying red blood cells.

hemotym'panum. Collection of blood in the middle ear.

hemozo'on. Hematozoon.

hemp. A herbaceous plant of the genus *Cannabis*.

henry. Unit of electrical induction in which an electromotive force of one volt is induced by a current varying at the rate of one ampere per second.

he'par. Latin for liver.

hep'arin. A mucopolysaccharide acid comprised of D-glucuronic acid and D-glucosamine; found especially in liver and lung tissue; it has the ability to keep blood from clotting and is used chiefly in the prevention and treatment of thrombosis.

hep'arinize. To administer or apply heparin in order to delay the clotting time of blood.

hepatal'gia. Pain in the liver; also called hepatodynia.

hepatec'tomy. Surgical removal of a portion of the liver.

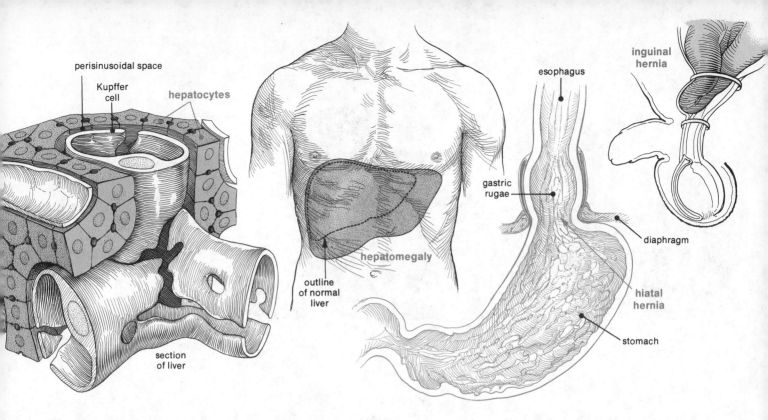

perisinusoidal space

Kupffer cell

hepatocytes

section of liver

esophagus

inguinal hernia

gastric rugae

hepatomegaly

outline of normal liver

diaphragm

hiatal hernia

stomach

hepat'ic. Relating to the liver.

hepati'tis. Inflammation of the liver.

anicteric h., hepatitis in which hyperbilirubinemia is mild, serum transaminase levels are elevated, and liver biopsy resembles icteric forms.

cholestatic h., cholangiolitic h., hepatitis characterized by signs of bile duct obstruction more prominent than the evidence of liver cell necrosis; may be seen occasionally in viral hepatitis or may be drug induced; must be differentiated from extrahepatic obstruction.

chronic aggressive h., progressive destruction of the liver architecture characterized by piecemeal necrosis and formation of intralobular septa leading eventually to cirrhosis and liver failure; often associated with hyperglobulinemia.

chronic persistent h., chronic inflammatory infiltration several months after an episode of acute hepatitis with preservation of lobular architecture and little or no fibrosis; symptoms are usually minor; half of the individuals feel well; mild elevation of transaminase may be seen; up to 80 per cent of individuals have hepatitis B antigen present in the serum.

fulminant h., a rapidly progressive form with necrosis of large areas of the liver; usually fatal within two weeks.

infectious h. (IH) a form of viral hepatitis usually transmitted by the intestinal and oral routes; incubation period is between two and six weeks; may occur sporadically or in epidemics; also called short incubation period, type A, or MS-1 hepatitis.

long incubation period h., see serum hepatitis.

MS-1 h., see infectious hepatitis.

MS-2 h., see serum hepatitis.

serum h. (SH) a form of viral hepatitis formerly thought to be transmitted by injection of infected blood or blood products or by the use of contaminated needles; other forms of transfer are now known to occur commonly; incubation period is between six weeks and six months; associated with an antigen (Australian antigen, hepatitis associated antigen) thought by many to represent the virus; also called long incubation period, type B, or MS-2 hepatitis.

short incubation period h., see infectious hepatitis.

type A h., see infectious hepatitis.

type B h., see serum hepatitis.

viral h., diffuse inflammation of the liver caused by one or more filterable agents.

hepatiza'tion. The conversion of loose tissue into a mass resembling liver, as the consolidation of lung tissue in pneumonia.

hepato-, hepat-. Combining form indicating a relationship to the liver.

hepatocarcino'ma. Malignant tumor of the liver originating in the parenchymal cells; also called hepatoma and primary liver cell carcinoma.

hep'atocyte. A parenchymal liver cell.

hepatoduodenos'tomy. Surgical creation of a passage between the hepatic duct and the duodenum.

hepatodyn'ia. See hepatalgia.

hepatogen'ic. Formed by or originating in the liver; also called hepatogenous.

hep'atogram. A radioisotopic scan of the liver.

hepatog'raphy. 1. The making of a roentgenogram of the liver. **2.** A treatise on the liver.

hepatolienog'raphy. 1. See hepatosplenography. **2.** A treatise on the liver and spleen.

hep'atolith. A calculus in the liver; a biliary calculus.

hepatolithi'asis. Stones in the liver.

hepatol'ogist. A specialist on diseases of the liver.

hepatol'ogy. Study of the liver and its diseases.

hepatol'ysin. An agent destructive to the parenchymal cells of the liver.

hepato'ma. Malignant tumor of the liver originating in the parenchymal cells; also called hepatocarcinoma and primary liver cell carcinoma.

hepatomeg'aly. Enlargement of the liver.

hepatonecro'sis. Death of liver tissue.

hepatop'athy. Any disease of the liver.

hepatore'nal. Relating to the liver and kidney.

hepatorenal syndrome. Renal failure occurring in the presence of severe disease of the liver or biliary tract, characterized initially by oliguria, marked sodium retention, and a rise in blood urea nitrogen usually out of proportion to the increase in serum creatinine.

hepator'rhaphy. The surgical suturing of the liver.

hep'atoscan. The scanning of the liver after intravenous injection of a radioactive substance that is taken up by the hepatic reticuloendothelial system.

hepatosplenog'raphy. Roentgenography of the liver and spleen after introduction of a radiopaque medium.

hepatosplenomeg'aly. Enlargement of the liver and the spleen.

hepatotox'ic. Relating to substances that damage the liver.

hepatotox'in. Any agent that destroys the liver cells.

herbiv'orous. Feeding on plants.

hered'itary. Genetically transmitted from parent to child. Cf heritable.

hered'ity. 1. The genetic transmission of a specific trait from parent to offspring. **2.** The totality of physical and mental traits and potentialities so transmitted to the offspring.

heredo-. Combining form indicating heredity.

heredoatax'ia. Friedreich's ataxia; see under ataxia.

hered'odegenera'tion. Genetic retrogressive change in cells and tissues.

heredopathia atactica polyneuritiformis. See Refsum's syndrome.

her'itable. Capable of being inherited, such as a trait, provided that it is present in the germ cell of a parent. Cf hereditary.

hermaph'rodism. See hermaphroditism.

hermaph'rodite. An individual who has genital tissues of both sexes.

hermaph'roditism, hermaph'rodism. The presence in the same individual of both ovarian and testicular tissues; also called intersexuality.

hermet'ic. Completely sealed against the escape or entry of air.

her'nia. Protrusion of part of an organ through an abnormal opening in the wall that normally contains it.

abdominal h., a hernia protruding through or into any part of the abdominal wall.

concealed h., one not found on inspection or palpation.

Cooper's h., femoral hernia with two sacs, one in the femoral canal and the other passing through a defect in the superficial fascia and appearing immediately beneath the skin.

diaphragmatic h., passage of a loop of intestine through the diaphragm.

epigastric h., one through the linea alba above the navel.

fascial h., see fatty hernia.

fatty h., one in which a mass of adipose tissue escapes through a gap in a fascia or aponeurosis; also called pannicular or fascial hernia.

femoral h., hernia through the femoral canal.

hiatal h., hiatus h., displacement of the upper part of the stomach into the thorax through the esophageal hiatus of the diaphragm.

incarcerated h., one in which the herniated organ (intestine) is tightly constricted and cannot be returned by manipulation; the flow of intestinal contents is arrested but the blood circulation is unaffected.

inguinal h., hernia at the inguinal region; the herniation may pass directly through the abdominal wall (direct inguinal hernia) or through the inguinal canal (indirect inguinal hernia).

irreducible h., one which, as a result of adhesions or for any other reason, cannot be reduced without

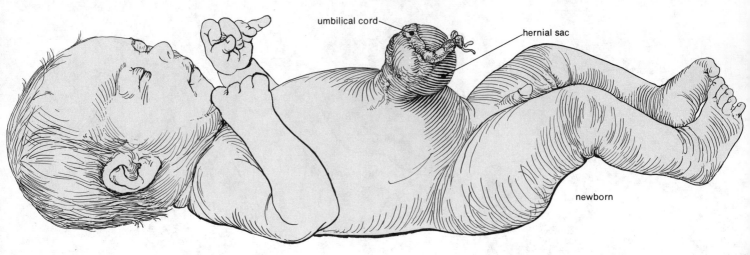

umbilical hernia

umbilical cord

umbilical hernia

hernial sac

newborn

a surgical operation.

pannicular h., see fatty hernia.

reducible h., one whose contents can be returned to their original position by manipulation.

scrotal h., see scrotocele.

sliding hiatal h., sliding esophageal hiatal h., one in which the junction of the stomach and esophagus moves from time to time or permanently into the thorax through the diaphragm.

Spigelian h., an abdominal hernia through the semilunar line.

strangulated h., an incarcerated hernia whose blood supply has been cut off and the herniated intestine has become, or is likely to become, gangrenous.

umbilical h., one in which part of the intestine protrudes through the umbilical ring; it usually results from a fascial and muscular defect with failure of the umbilical ring to close.

ventral h., passage of a loop of intestine through any part of the abdominal wall other than through the inguinal, femoral, or umbilical openings.

her'niated. Pertaining to any structure protruding through a defect or abnormal opening.

hernia'tion. The process of forming an abnormal protrusion.

foraminal h., protrusion of the cerebellar tonsils through the foramen magnum; also called tonsillar herniation.

tonsillar h., see foraminal herniation.

hernior'rhaphy. Surgical repair of a hernia.

her'oin. Diacetylmorphine; a highly addictive narcotic prepared from morphine by acetylization; a white, odorless, bitterish crystalline compound, $C_{17}H_{17}(C_2H_3O_2)_2NO_2$.

herpan'gina. An infection of the throat usually caused by a coxsackie virus (coxsackie A); marked by intense swelling of the area, sudden onset of fever, loss of appetite, difficulty in swallowing (dysphagia), and sometimes abdominal pain, nausea, and vomiting; vesiculopapular lesions about 1 to 2 mm in diameter are present around the tonsillar fauces, and these soon break down to form grayish-yellow ulcers.

her'pes. An inflammatory disease of the skin or mucous membrane marked by eruption of a cluster of vesicles.

h. labialis, herpes simplex of the lips; also called cold sore and fever blister.

h. simplex, a virus infection marked by the appearance of blisters usually on the lips or on the nostrils (cold sores or fever blisters) but may occur also on the conjunctiva, the cornea, or the mucous membrane of the genitalia; also called hydroa febrile.

h. zoster, infection of the ganglia of the posterior roots of the spinal nerves or the fifth cranial nerve by the varicella-zoster virus, which also causes chickenpox; it is marked by a painful eruption of vesicles usually on one side of the body along the course of one or more cutaneous nerves; also called shingles.

her'pesvi'rus. Any of a group of DNA viruses that multiply in the nuclei of cells; members of this group cause herpes simplex, herpes zoster, and varicella; some (such as the Epstein-Barr virus) are believed to cause cancer.

herpet'iform. Resembling herpes.

hetero-, heter-. Combining forms meaning other, another, or different; often denote members of different species.

heterochro'matin. The more darkly stained portion of the cell nucleus containing metabolically inactive DNA.

heterochro'mia. Difference in color of a part or parts that are normally alike in color, as of the two irides.

heteroe'cious. Having more than one host, i.e., spending different stages of its life cycle on two or more unrelated hosts; e.g., tapeworms.

heteroerot'ic. Relating to sexual feelings that are directed toward another person, as opposed to auto-erotic.

heterogamet'ic. Having gametes (sex cells) of different types with respect to the sex chromosomes, as in human males.

heterog'amy. 1. The union of two gametes of different size, structure, and function. 2. Alternation of two kinds of generations, one that reproduces bisexually and another in which the female reproduces without fecundation by the male (parthenogenetic), as in some aphids.

heterogene'ity. The quality of certain genetic disorders which consist of two or more fundamentally distinct entities; formerly thought to represent single entities.

het'erogeneous, het'erogenous. Composed of dissimilar elements or characteristics; not homogeneous.

heterogenet'ic, heterogen'ic. Derived from a different species.

het'erograft. See xenograft.

heterola'lia. Heterophasia; heterophemia; the involuntary uttering of meaningless words instead of those intended.

heterol'ogous. 1. Derived from an individual of a different genetic make-up or species. 2. Relating to tissue not normally located in a designated part or region of the body.

heterol'ysis. Dissolution or digestion of cells of one species by a lytic agent from a different species.

heteromer'ic. 1. Possessing different chemical composition. 2. Denoting spinal nerve cells that have processes crossing the midline to the opposite side of the spinal cord.

heteromorph'ism. In cytogenetics, a difference in shape or size between homologous chromosomes.

heteron'ymous. 1. Relating to different sides of the two visual fields; e.g., the right side of one field and the left side of the other, both nasal fields or both temporal fields. 2. Having different but correlated names.

heteropha'sia. See heterolalia.

heterophe'mia. See heterolalia.

heteropho'nia. 1. The change of voice in the male at puberty. 2. Any abnormality in the voice.

heteropho'ria. The tendency of the optic axes to deviate toward or away from each other.

heterophthal'mia. A difference in appearance of the two eyes, as in the coloration of the irides; also called heterophthalmus.

heterophthal'mus. See heterophthalmia.

Hetero'phyes. A genus of small sized parasitic flukes.

heterophyi'asis. Infection with a heterophyid fluke.

heterophy'id. 1. Relating to flukes of the genus *Heterophyes* (family Heterophilae). 2. A fluke of the genus *Heterophyes*.

heteropla'sia. Alloplasia. 1. The presence of tissue elements in an abnormal location; e.g., the growth of bone where normally there should be fibrous connective tissue. 2. The malposition of a part that is otherwise normal; e.g., the presence of a ureter at the lower pole of a kidney.

het'eroplasty. 1. Surgical grafting of tissue donated from another individual. 2. The replacement of tissue with synthetic material.

het'eroploidy. The state of an individual or cell with a chromosome number other than the normal diploid number.

heterop'sia. Unequal vision in the two eyes.

het'eroscope. Amblyoscope.

heterosexual'ity. The state of having one's sexual interests directed toward a member of the opposite sex, as opposed to homosexuality.

heterospecif'ic. Denoting a graft that is obtained from an individual of a different species; also called heterologous.

heterotax'ia, heterotax'is. Abnormal arrangement of bodily organs or parts; anomalous structural arrangement.

heterotax'ic. Occurring in an abnormal place.

heteroto'pia. The occurrence of a part in an abnormal location.

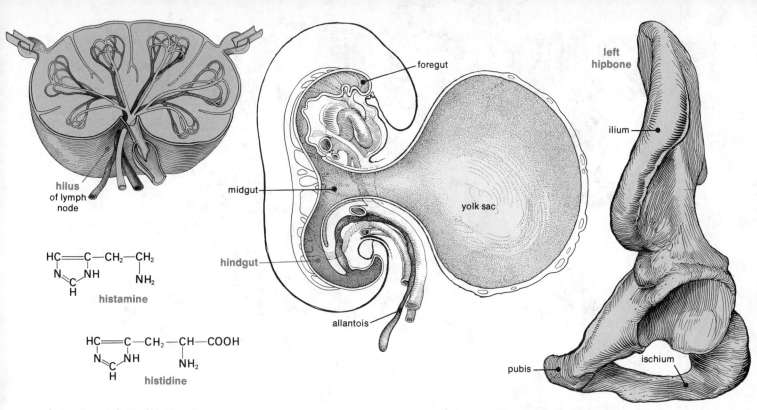

hilus of lymph node

histamine

histidine

foregut

midgut

hindgut

allantois

yolk sac

left hipbone

ilium

pubis

ischium

heterotrans′plant. See xenograft.

heterotro′pia. See strabismus.

heterotyp′ic. Not typical.

heterozygos′ity. The state of having one or more pairs of dissimilar alleles.

heterozy′gote. A zygote produced by the union of two gametes of different genetic composition.

hexa-. Combining form meaning six.

hex′acanth. The motile, six-hooked, first-stage larva of a tapeworm; also called oncosphere.

hex′achlo′rophene. A bactericidal agent, $(C_6HCl_3OH)_2CH_2$, used as a local antiseptic.

hexadecanoic acid. See palmitic acid.

hex′enmilch. German for witch's milk; a milky fluid sometimes secreted by the breasts of newborn infants.

hex′okinase. An enzyme (present in yeast, muscle, and other tissues) that promotes the phosphorylation of glucose and other hexoses to form hexose-6-phosphate.

hexosam′ine. A primary amine derivative of a hexose resulting when NH_2 replaces OH; e.g., glucosamine; also called amino sugar.

hex′osan. Any of several polysaccharides that yield a hexose on hydrolysis.

hex′ose. A monosaccharide having six carbon atoms in the molecule; e.g., glucose and fructose.

hexose-1-phosphate uridylyltransferase. Uridyltransferase; an enzyme system that promotes the interconversion of glucose-1-phosphate and galactose-1-phosphate with simultaneous interconversion of UDP glucose and UDP galactose.

hex′ulose. A ketohexose, as fructose.

hexylresor′cinol. A crystalline phenol used as an anthelminthic.

Hf. Chemical symbol of the element hafnium.

Hfr. Abbreviation for high frequency.

Hg. Chemical symbol of mercury; from Latin *hydrargyrum*.

Hgb. Abbreviation for hemoglobin.

HGH. Abbreviation for human growth hormone.

HHb. Abbreviation for nonionized hemoglobin; also used to denote that hemoglobin acts as an acid.

hia′tus. An opening, aperture, or fissure.

   aortic h., the opening in the diaphragm through which the aorta and thoracic duct pass.

   esophageal h., the opening in the diaphragm through which the esophagus and the two vagus nerves pass.

hiberna′tion. The dormant condition or winter sleep in which certain animals pass the cold months.

hic′cup. A spasm of the diaphragm causing inhalation, followed by sudden closure of the glottis.

hick′ey. 1. Colloquial term for the reddish mark on the skin caused by a playful bite, pinch, or kiss. **2.** A

pimple (papulo-pustule).

hidradeni′tis. Inflammation of a sweat gland.

   h. suppurativa, chronic, relapsing, infectious disease of the apocrine sweat glands; marked by the development of one or more cutaneous pea-sized nodules which undergo softening and suppuration; it occurs most commonly in the genital and perianal regions and in the armpits.

hidradeno′ma. A relatively infrequent benign tumor of sweat gland origin; may be solid or cystic; also written hydradenoma.

hidro′a. Hydroa.

hidrocysto′ma. The cystic deformation of sweat glands.

hidropoie′sis. The formation of sweat.

hidro′sis. 1. Excessive perspiration. **2.** Any sweat gland disorder.

high. A state of drug induced intoxication, as from a narcotic, alcohol, or hallucinogenic agent.

HIID. Abbreviation for hemisoimmune disease, a disorder due to hemisoantibody; e.g., Rh disease.

hi′lar dance. Strong pulsations of the pulmonary arteries seen on fluoroscopic examination in patients with congenital left-to-right shunt.

hi′lus. The point at which nerves and vessels enter and leave an organ.

hind′brain. See rhombencephalon.

hind′foot. 1. The rear portion of the foot consisting of the talus and calcaneus. **2.** One of the back feet of a quadruped animal.

hind′gut. The caudal part of the embryonic alimentary canal.

hip. The lateral area of the body from the waist to the thigh.

   h. pointer, contusion on the iliac crest, or immediately above it.

hip′bone, hip bone. A large, flattened, irregularly shaped bone that forms the anterior and lateral walls of the pelvic cavity; consisting of three parts (ilium, ischium, and pubis); formerly known as the innominate bone.

Hippel-Lindau disease. See von Hippel-Lindau disease.

hippocam′pus. One of two curved bands of a very special type of cortex about 5 cm long, on the floor of the inferior horn of the lateral ventricle on each side of the brain.

Hippoc′rates. A Greek physician known as the "Father of Medicine"; his medical science principles were laid down about 400 years before the birth of Christ.

   aphorisms of H., a collection of observations, rules, and brief statements of clinical wisdom found in Books I to III of the hippocratic writings.

hippocratic facies. See facies, hippocratic.

hippocratic oath. A code of ethical conduct for the medical profession attributed to Hippocrates.

hip′pus. Abnormal, spasmodic, rhythmic contraction and dilation of the pupil.

Hirschsprung's disease. Congenital megacolon; congenital disorder of early infancy characterized by extreme distention of the colon, resulting from absence of ganglion cells of the myenteric plexuses of the rectum and lower colon.

hir′sute. 1. Hairy. **2.** Of or relating to hair.

hir′sutism. Excessive hair on cheek, chin, lip, or chest, especially in women.

hir′udin. An anticoagulant substance secreted by the salivary glands of leeches which prevents coagulation of the blood while the leech is sucking.

His's bundle. See bundle, atrioventricular.

his′tamine. A white crystalline amine, $C_5H_9N_3$, occurring in all animal and plant tissue; formed from histidine by decarboxylation and by the action of putrefactive bacteria; its release within the body causes bronchiolar constriction, arteriolar dilation, increased gastric secretion, and a fall in blood pressure.

his′tidine. α-Amino-β-(4-imidazole) propionic acid; an amino acid.

hist′iocyte. A large mononuclear phagocyte or macrophage; a tissue cell.

histiocyto′sis. A proliferation of histiocytes.

   h. X, the generic name proposed to cover three possibly related entities characterized by histiocytic proliferation of unknown etiology: eosinophilic granuloma, Hand-Schüller-Christian syndrome, and Letterer-Siwe disease.

   nonlipid h., An acute progressive and wasting disease of infants and young children characterized by invasion of the spleen, liver, and bone marrow by proliferating histiocytes, accompanied by generalized involvement of the lymph nodes and enlargement of the spleen and liver; frequently present are a purpuric rash, anemia, and chronic inflammation of the middle ear; also called Letterer-Siwe disease.

histo-, histio-, hist-. Combining forms indicating a relationship to tissue.

histochem′istry. The chemistry of cell components and tissues.

histofluores′cence. Fluorescence of the tissues produced by exposure to ultraviolet rays after injection of a fluorescent substance.

histogen′esis. 1. The origin and development of bodily tissues from undifferentiated cells of the embryonic germ layers. **2.** In myology, the development of muscle fibers from primitive cells.

his′togram. A columnar or bar chart used in descriptive statistics showing the relationship of two factors.

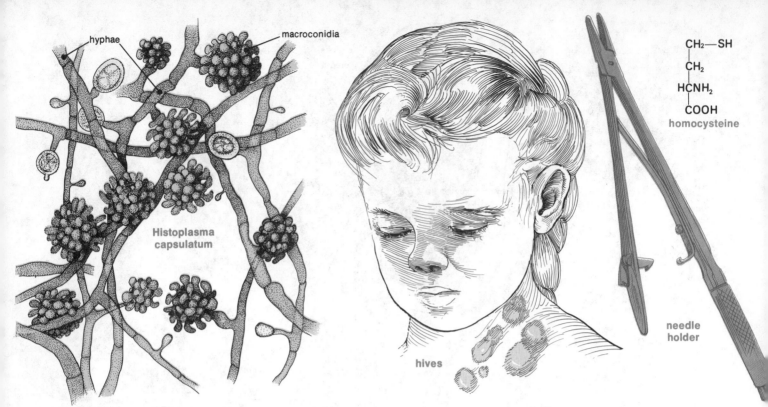

hyphae   macroconidia

Histoplasma
capsulatum

homocysteine

hives

needle
holder

histolog'ic. Pertaining to histology.

histol'ogist. A specialist in histology.

histol'ogy. The branch of anatomy dealing with the microscopic structure of tissues; also called microscopic anatomy and microanatomy.

histol'ysis. The disintegration or breakdown of tissue.

his'tone. Any of several simple water soluble proteins containing a large proportion of basic amino acids; e.g., the globin of hemoglobin.

histopathol'ogy. The pathology of abnormal or diseased tissue; also called pathologic histology.

histophysiol'ogy. The physiology of bodily tissues.

Histoplas'ma. A genus of fungi; some species cause disease in man.

   H. capsulatum, yeastlike fungus occurring in soil; when present in tissue it appears to be encapsulated; the cause of histoplasmosis.

histoplas'min. A concentrate of the growth products of the fungus *Histoplasma capsulatum*; used as a dermal reactivity indicator to detect histoplasmosis.

histoplasmo'sis. A fungal disease caused by *Histoplasma capsulatum*; usually asymptomatic but may produce a benign, mild pulmonary illness; it is a frequent cause of pulmonary nodules; the infection may spread throughout the body, and this disseminated form, though uncommon, is quite serious.

hives. Urticaria; eruption of transitory pruritic wheals, often due to hypersensitivity to foods or drugs or to emotional factors.

HL. Abbreviation for half-life.

Hl. Abbreviation for latent hyperopia.

Hm. Abbreviation for manifest hyperopia.

HMD. Abbreviation for hyaline membrane disease.

HMO. Abbreviation for health maintenance organization.

Ho. Chemical symbol of the element holium.

hoarseness. A harsh, rough, grating quality of the voice.

Hodgkin's disease. A disease of lymphatic tissue characterized by painless enlargement of the lymph nodes with or without systemic symptoms such as fever, sweat, weight loss, and lassitude; if untreated the disease may spread to involve the spleen and other organs; treatment and prognosis depend on the clinical staging.

Hoffmann's sign. Snapping the nail of the middle finger leads to flexion of thumb and fingers; a sign of a pyramidal tract lesion.

holan'dric. Occurring only in males; denoting a character determined by a gene on the Y chromosome.

holarthri'tis. Inflammation of all or most of the joints.

holder, needle. An instrument used for grasping a needle during surgery; also called needle forceps.

ho'lo-, hol-. Combining forms meaning entire or indicating a relationship to the whole.

holoblas'tic. Denoting the complete division of the entire ovum into individual blastomeres.

hol'ocrine. Wholly secretory; relating to a gland whose secretion is composed of the disintegrated secreting cell in addition to its accumulated secretion, e.g., sebaceous glands.

holodias'tolic. Relating to or occupying all of diastole from the second heart sound to the succeeding first heart sound.

holoen'zyme. An enzyme possessing a chemical group that is non-amino acid in nature.

ho'logram. A three-dimensional pattern exposed by holography on a photosensitive surface and then photographically developed.

holog'raphy. The use of lasers to record on a photographic plate the diffraction pattern of an object from which a three-dimensional image can be constructed.

   acoustic h., a technique for detecting breast cancer by transmitting sound waves through breast tissue.

holosys'tolic. Relating to or occupying all of systole; also called pansystolic.

Homans' sign. Pain in the calf or the back of the knee when the foot is dorsiflexed, suggesting the presence of a deep venous thrombosis in the calf.

homeo-, homo-. Combining forms meaning same or similar.

homeomor'phous. Of similar shape.

homeop'athist. One who practices homeopathy.

homeop'athy. A system of therapeutics based on the use of small doses of a drug that in large doses is capable of producing symptoms in healthy individuals which are similar to those of the disease being treated.

homeopla'sia. The formation of new tissue similar to that already existing in, and normal to, the part.

homeosta'sis. A state of physiologic equilibrium in the living body (temperature, blood pressure, chemical content, etc.) under variations in the environment.

homeothera'apy. Treatment or prevention of a disease with a substance similar to, but not identical with, the causative agent of the disease; e.g., vaccination.

homici'dal. Having a tendency to kill.

hom'icide. The killing of a person by another human being.

hom'inid. 1. A member of the family Hominidae. **2.** Relating to the family Hominidae.

Homin'idae. A family of mammals (order Primates) which includes modern and prehistoric man.

Hominoi'dea. 1. In some classifications, a major division of the order Primates which segregates man from the great apes. **2.** A superfamily (suborder Anthropoidea) which includes the great apes and the fossil hominids.

Homo. A genus of Primates consisting of mankind.

   H. sapiens, the present-day human species; modern man.

homo-. See homeo-.

homoblas'tic. Developing from only one type of tissue.

homocen'tric. Having the same center, as rays originating from one source; also called concentric.

homocys'teine. A sulfur-containing amino acid, $HSCH_2CH_2CHNH_2COOH$.

homocys'tine. A sulfur-containing amino acid $(SCH_2CH_2CHNH_2COOH)_2$ formed by oxidation of homocysteine.

homocystinu'ria. A genetically determined disorder of metabolism resulting in a deficiency of activity of the enzyme cystathionine synthase; characterized by an elevation of the concentrations of methionine and of homocystine in the blood, homocystine in the urine (not detectable in normal urine), mental retardation, dislocation of the ocular lenses, skeletal abnormalities (dolichostenomelia, genu valgum, osteoporosis), increased stickiness of platelets in the blood, thromboembolic episodes, and abnormality of the palate with crowding of the teeth.

homoerot'icism. Homosexuality.

homogamet'ic. Producing only one kind of germ cell; especially possessing an X chromosome in cell gametes; also called monogametic.

homog'enate. A substance that has been homogenized; in biochemistry, tissue that has been reduced to a creamy consistency and that has disintegrated cell structure.

homoge'neous. Composed of similar elements throughout; of uniform quality.

homogeniza'tion. The process of making diverse elements homogenous.

homog'enize. To blend diverse elements into a mixture that is uniform in structure or consistency throughout.

homog'enous. 1. In biology, correspondence of parts because of common descent. **2.** Homogeneous.

homogentisate oxygenase. An iron-containing enzyme that promotes the cleavage of the benzene ring in homogentisic acid; congenital absence of this enzyme causes alkaptonuria; also called ho-

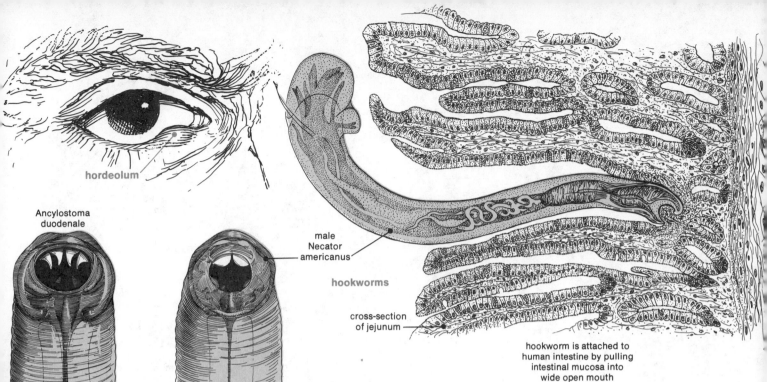

hordeolum

Ancylostoma
duodenale

male
Necator
americanus

hookworms

cross-section
of jejunum

hookworm is attached to
human intestine by pulling
intestinal mucosa into
wide open mouth

mogentisase and homogentisic acid oxidase.

homogentisic acid. An intermediate in the metabolism of the amino acid tyrosine, excreted in the urine of persons afflicted with alkaptonuria; also called alkapton.

h. a. oxidase, see homogentisate oxygenase.

homogentisu'ria. See alkaptonuria.

ho'mograft. See allograft.

homolat'eral. On or relating to the same side; also called ipsilateral.

homol'ogous. Corresponding in structure, position, development, and evolutionary origin, as the wing of a bird, the flipper of a seal, and the arm of man; denoting a homologue.

hom'ologue, hom'olog. Any homologous structure; a part or organ similar in structure, position, and origin to another organ.

homol'ogy. Correspondence in structure, evolutionary origin, or position.

homol'ysin. Isohemolysin.

homomor'phic. Denoting structures of similar size and form.

homon'omous. Denoting parts that are similar in function and structure, as fingers and toes.

homon'ymous. 1. Relating to the same right or left side of the two visual fields; e.g., the nasal half of one visual field and the temporal half of the other. **2.** Having the same name.

ho'moplasty. Repair of a defect with a graft from another member of the same species.

homopol'ymer. A polymer composed of identical units of a single monomer.

homopolypep'tide. A peptide chain containing only one type of amino acid residue, as polyglycine, polyalanine, and polyglutamic acid.

homosex'ual. 1. Relating to or exhibiting homosexuality. **2.** An individual having a sexual interest in or relationship with others of the same sex.

homosexual'ity. Sexual interest or relationship between members of the same sex.

homother'mal. Having a relatively constant body temperature, more or less independent of the environmental temperature; also called warm-blooded, homoiothermal, homothermous, and homothermic.

homotrans'plant. Allograft.

ho'motype. A part or organ having the same structure or function as another.

homozo'ic. Pertaining to the same animal or the same species of animal.

ho'mozygosis. The formation of a zygote by the union of genetically identical gametes.

homozygos'ity. The state of having identical alleles at one or more loci of homologous chromosomes.

homozy'gote. An individual exhibiting homozygosity.

homun'culus. 1. The proportional representation of various parts of the body in the motor or sensory areas of the cerebral cortex. **2.** A minute body imagined by 16th and 17th century biologists to be present in the sperm, from which the human body was supposed to be developed.

motor h., one in which the parts of the figure are roughly proportional to the excitable motor cortex associated with evoking movements of the parts; the figure is generally illustrated upside down on the brain, with the lower extremity on the medial surface of the paracentral lobule and with the head near the lateral cerebral fissure.

sensory h., one in which the parts of the figure are proportional to the amount of cortical area associated with sensory innervation density of the body areas, rather than to the size of the area (e.g., the tongue and thumb have a relatively large representation).

honk, systolic. A loud, vibratory, often musical heart murmur of relatively clear pitch, usually occurring in late systole; believed to originate in the mitral valve; also called systolic whoop.

hook. A metal instrument with a curved or sharply bent tip, used for traction or fixation of a part.

blunt h., one used to make traction upon the groin of a dead infant during a difficult breech presentation.

palate h., one used to pull forward the soft palate to facilitate posterior rhinoscopy.

tracheotomy h., a right-angled hook for holding the trachea steady during tracheotomy.

hook'lets. Small horny residues from *Echinococcus* larval infestation, found in the walls of *Echinococcus* cysts.

hook'worm. Any parasitic roundworm of the genera *Ancylostoma* and *Necator*.

American h., *Necator americanus*.

Old World h., *Ancylostoma duodenale*.

hora decubitus (h.d.), hora somni (h.s.). Latin for at bedtime; used in prescription writing.

horde'olum. A common staphylococcal inflammation of the sebaceous gland of an eyelash, marked by a painful, swollen, erythematous lesion of the external surface of the eyelid; also called stye.

horis'mascope. A U-shaped test tube used to examine the urine for albumin.

hor'monal. Of, relating to, or of the nature of a hormone.

hor'mone. A glandular chemical secretion produced by an organ or part of the body and carried in the bloodstream to another organ or part to stimulate or retard its function; produced by endocrine glands and in the gastrointestinal tract.

adrenocortical h.'s, hormones (steroids) secreted by the human adrenal cortex; the principal ones are cortisol, aldosterone, and corticosterone.

adrenocorticotropic h. (ACTH), a hormone elaborated by the anterior lobe of the pituitary gland which stimulates the adrenal cortex to functional activity; also called adrenocorticotrophin.

adrenomedullary h.'s, any of the hormones formed by the adrenal cortex; e.g., epinephrine, norepinephrine.

androgenic h., any of the masculinizing hormones including testosterone, the most potent one.

antidiuretic h. (ADH), one produced by the posterior lobe of the pituitary gland, having a potent antidiuretic action and some vasoconstrictive action on the visceral circulation; it makes the collecting duct of the kidney tubule permeable to water and allows concentration of urine; also called vasopressin.

chorionic gonadotropic h., chorionic gonadotropin.

erythropoietic h., (1) erythropoietin; (2) any hormone that stimulates the formation of red blood cells; e.g., testosterone.

estrogenic h., estradiol.

female h., estradiol.

follicle-stimulating h. (FSH), a glycoprotein hormone of the anterior lobe of the pituitary gland that stimulates normal cyclic growth of the ovarian follicle in females and stimulates the seminiferous tubules to produce spermatozoa in males.

gastrointestinal h., any secretion of the gastrointestinal mucosa affecting the timing of various digestive secretions; e.g., secretin.

growth h., a hormone secreted by the anterior lobe of the pituitary gland that promotes fat mobilization, inhibits glucose utilization, and affects the rate of skeletal and visceral growth; diabetogenic when present in excess; also called somatotropin.

interstitial cell stimulating h. (ICSH), an anterior pituitary gland secretion which stimulates testicular interstitial cells to produce androgen; ICSH in the male is identical with luteinizing hormone (LH) in the female, which is essential for ovulation and formation of the corpus luteum in the ovary.

luteinizing h. (LH), a glycoprotein hormone of the anterior pituitary gland that promotes maturation of an ovarian follicle, its secretion of progesterone, its rupture to release the egg, and the conversion of the ruptured follicle into the corpus luteum; also called lutein-stimulating hormone (LSH).

lutein-stimulating h. (LSH), see luteinizing hormone.

melanocyte-stimulating h. (MSH), a secretion of the middle lobe of the pituitary gland which in-

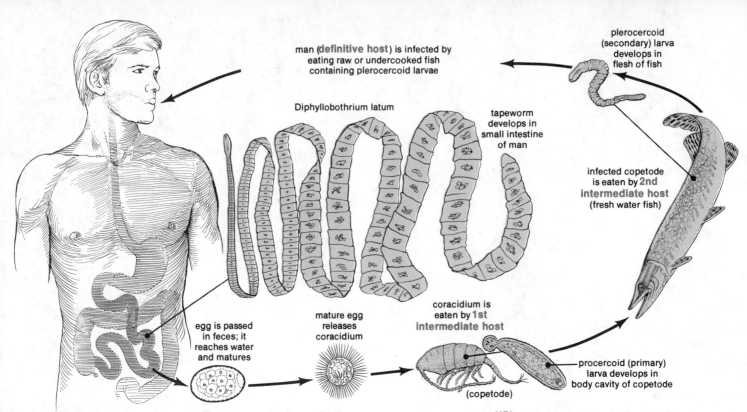

man (definitive host) is infected by
eating raw or undercooked fish
containing plerocercoid larvae

Diphyllobothrium latum

tapeworm
develops in
small intestine
of man

plerocercoid
(secondary) larva
develops in
flesh of fish

infected copetode
is eaten by 2nd
intermediate host
(fresh water fish)

egg is passed
in feces; it
reaches water
and matures

mature egg
releases
coracidium

coracidium is
eaten by 1st
intermediate host

procercoid (primary)
larva develops in
body cavity of copetode

(copetode)

creases deposition of melanin by the melanocytes.

natriuretic h., a postulated hormone which inhibits reabsorption of cations, particularly sodium, from urine; thought to be released by volume expansion.

ovarian h.'s, hormones secreted by the human ovary including estradiol, estrone, estriol, and progesterone.

parathyroid h., (PTH), a protein biosynthesized and secreted into the bloodstream by the four parathyroid glands which are located in the neck behind the thyroid gland; it acts on the cells of bone, kidney, and intestinal tract to maintain a constant concentration of calcium in the blood; also called parathormone.

pituitary growth h. (PGH), the growth hormone of the anterior lobe of the pituitary gland.

placental h., any of the hormones secreted by the placenta, namely, chorionic gonadotrophin, estrogen, progesterone, and human placental lactogen.

progestational h., progesterone.

releasing h., releasing factor; see under factor.

sex h.'s, estrogens (female sex hormones) and androgens (male sex hormones) formed by ovarian, testicular, and adrenocortical tissues.

somatotrophic h., see growth hormone.

testicular h.'s, the hormones elaborated by the human testis, especially testosterone.

thyroid h., a term that commonly refers to thyroxin, but may also include triiodothyronine.

thyrotrophic h., see thyrotropic hormone.

thyrotropic h., a hormone of the anterior pituitary gland that stimulates the growth and function of the thyroid gland; also called thyrotropic hormone, thyrotrophin, and thyrotropin.

hormonogen'ic. Denoting any agent that stimulates the production of a hormone.

hormonother'apy. Medical treatment with hormones.

horn. Any horn-shaped structure or excrescence.

anterior h. of spinal cord, the anterior column of the spinal cord as seen in cross sections.

cutaneous h., a horny growth of the skin; also called warty horn.

posterior h. of spinal cord, the posterior column of the spinal cord as seen in cross sections.

pulp h., a prolongation of vital pulp tissue of a tooth directly under a cusp.

hornet. Any of several stinging wasps, chiefly of the genera *Vespa* and *Vespula*, having a slender, spindle-shaped body with an elongated waist; they usually construct papier-mâché hives; the antigens responsible for hypersensitivity are present in both the venom sac and body of the insect.

horripila'tion. Erection of the fine skin hairs.

hosiery, elastic. Support elastic stockings worn to prevent or alleviate varicose veins.

hos'pital. An institution whose primary aim is caring for or treating patients.

base h., one located in a large military base for the care of patients received from smaller units near the battle front.

closed h., hospital in which only members of the attending and consulting staff may admit and treat patients.

day h., one that provides treatment during the day enabling patients to return home at night; it may be a special facility within a large hospital.

evacuation h., a mobile military hospital where patients are taken and cared for until they can be evacuated to a general hospital.

general h., (1) any large civilian hospital for the care of medical, surgical, and maternity cases; (2) a permanent, large military hospital that receives patients from smaller evacuation hospitals.

mobile Army surgical h. (MASH), see surgical hospital.

proprietary h., a private hospital.

special h., one for the treatment of patients with certain diseases.

surgical h., a mobile military hospital for the immediate care of serious casualties.

voluntary h., one supported by voluntary contributions and controlled by a board of managers, usually self-appointed.

host. 1. An organism that harbors and provides nourishment for another organism (parasite). **2.** The recipient of an organ or tissue transplant from a donor.

alternate h., intermediate host.

definitive h., the organism in which a parasite resides during its adult and sexual phase.

intermediate h., the organism in which a parasite resides during its larval or asexual phase.

primary h., the organism in which the mature parasite resides when it has two or more stages of existence in different organisms.

reservoir h., an animal that serves as a host to species of parasites that are also parasitic for man, and from which man may be infested either directly through ingestion or indirectly through a carrier such as a mosquito.

secondary h., intermediate host.

house'fly. *Musca domestica*; a common, widely distributed member of the insect order Dipter; it breeds in filth and decaying organic waste, and is a transmitter of numerous disease-causing organisms.

Houssay syndrome. Abatement of diabetes mellitus resulting from surgical removal of, or a destructive lesion in, the pituitary gland.

HPL. Abbreviation for human placental lactogen.

h.s. Abbreviation for Latin *hora somni*, at bedtime.

Ht. Abbreviation for total hyperopia.

5-HT. Abbreviation for 5-hydroxytryptamine (serotonin).

hum, venous. A continuous murmur due to altered flow patterns in veins; heard on auscultation over the large veins at the base of the neck when the patient is in a sitting position and looking to the opposite side; commonly heard in association with a goiter.

humec'tant. A substance that helps to retain moisture.

hu'meral. Relating to or located in the proximity of the humerus.

hu'merus. The long bone of the upper arm that extends from the shoulder to the elbow.

humid'ity. Dampness.

absolute h., the amount of water vapor present in the air when saturated at a given temperature, expressed in grains per cubic feet.

relative h., the percentage of water vapor present in the atmosphere, as compared to the amount necessary to cause saturation, regarding saturation at 100.

hu'mor. Any fluid or semifluid occurring normally in the body.

aqueous h., the clear, watery fluid filling the anterior and posterior chambers of the eye.

vitreous h., see body, vitreous.

hu'moral. Relating to or arising from any of the bodily fluids.

hunch'back, hump'back. 1. Kyphosis; an abnormally curved spine. **2.** One afflicted with the deformity.

hunger. 1. A strong craving for nourishment. **2.** A strong desire for anything.

air h., dyspnea characterized by deep, labored respiration, as may occur in acidosis.

Hunter's canal. See canal, adductor.

Hunter's syndrome. A hereditary, X-linked recessive condition characterized by stiff joints, enlargement of the liver and spleen, cardiac involvement, mild retardation, and progressive deafness; also called mucopolysaccharidosis II.

Huntington's chorea. See chorea, hereditary.

Huntington's disease. An inherited disorder of the nervous system transmitted by an autosomal dominant gene and marked by degeneration of the basal ganglia and cerebral cortex; manifestations include choreiform movements, intellectual deterioration, and personality changes; onset is usually insidious and occurs in middle life; the disease is often fatal within five to 15 years after onset.

Hurler's syndrome. An inherited metabolic dis-

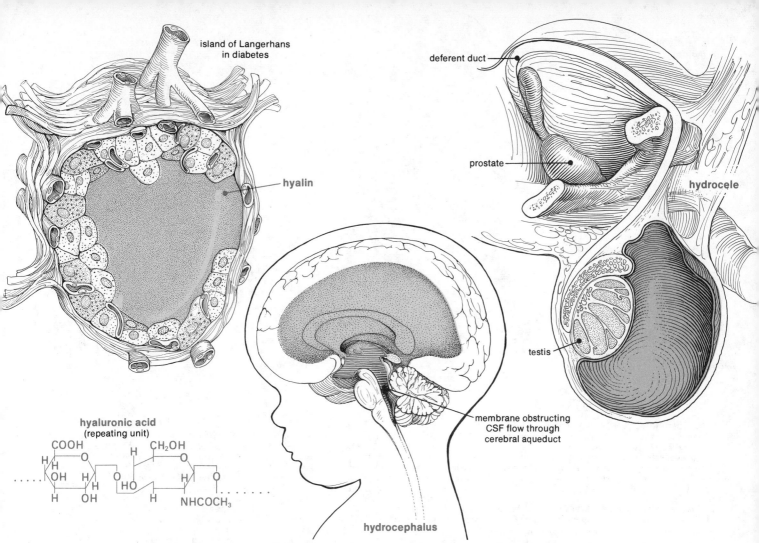

island of Langerhans in diabetes

hyalin

hyaluronic acid (repeating unit)

deferent duct

prostate

hydrocele

testis

membrane obstructing CSF flow through cerebral aqueduct

hydrocephalus

order marked by skeletal deformities, mental retardation, and early death; characterized by an accumulation of an abnormal intracellular material, a deficiency of the enzyme α-L-iduronidase, and excretion of chondroitin sulfate B and heparitin sulfate in the urine; also called mucopolysaccharidosis 1 (MPS 1), gargoylism, dysostosis multiplex, and lipochondrodystrophy.

hy′alin. 1. The homogeneous matrix of hyaline cartilage. **2.** A clear homogeneous substance, occurring in degenerative diseases.

hy′aline. Glassy or translucent in appearance.

hyaline membrane disease of the newborn. Condition, usually fatal, occurring in premature babies with respiratory distress, marked primarily by the lining of the air spaces of the lungs with an eosinophilic membrane; the symptoms usually appear a few hours after the birth of an apparently healthy infant.

hyali′tis. Inflammation of the vitreous body.

hyalo-, hyal-. Combining forms denoting a resemblance to glass.

hy′aloid. Glassy or translucent in appearance.

hy′alomere. The pale, homogeneous, nonrefractile portion of a blood platelet; found in it are elements of chromatomeres, microtubules, mitochondria, microfilaments, and Golgi vesicles.

hyaluronic acid. A mucopolysaccharide present in the form of a gelatinous material in the tissue spaces, thus binding cells together and holding water in the tissues; it has the property of increasing the slipperiness of fluids and of the lubricating and shock absorbing system of joints.

hyaluron′idase. An enzyme, found in sperm, snake and bee venom, and pathogenic bacteria; it causes the breakdown of hyaluronic acid in the tissue spaces, thus enabling the invading agent to enter cells and tissues; also called spreading factor.

hybarox′ia. Oxygen therapy with pressures greater than one atmosphere applied in a room or chamber.

hy′brid. The offspring (plant or animal) of parents who are genetically dissimilar.

hy′datid. 1. A cystic structure containing the embryo of the *Taenia echinococcus*; a hydatid cyst. **2.** Any structure resembling a cyst.

  h. of Morgagni, (1) testicular appendage; (2) vesicular appendage; see under appendage.

hydatid disease. See echinococcosis.

hydatid mole. Hydatidiform mole; see under mole.

hydatid′iform. Resembling a hydatid.

hydr-. See hydro-.

hydralazine hydrochloride. An adrenergic blocking agent that lowers blood pressure by acting directly on arteriolar smooth muscle; it may also increase renal blood flow; Apresoline®.

hydram′nios, hydram′nion. The presence of an excessive quantity of amniotic fluid.

hydrar′gyrism, hydrargyr′ia. Mercury poisoning; see under poisoning.

hydrar′gyrum. Latin for mercury.

hydrarthro′sis. Collection of fluid in a joint.

hy′drase. An enzyme that promotes the addition of water, or its removal from a molecule.

hy′drate. Any compound containing water which is retained in its molecular state.

hy′drated. Combined with water.

hydra′tion. The combination of a substance with water.

hydrenceph′alocele. Hernial protrusion, through a defect in the skull, of brain substance with cerebrospinal fluid; also called hydrocephalocele and hydroencephalocele.

hydrenceph′alomenin′gocele. Hernial protrusion of the meninges, brain substance, and cerebrospinal fluid through a defect in the skull.

hydrenceph′alus. Internal hydrocephalus; see hydrocephalus.

hydriat′ic. Applied to the use of water in treating disease; also called hydrotherapeutic.

hy′dride. A compound of hydrogen with a more positive element or group, thus assuming a formal negative charge.

hydro-, hydr-. Combining forms indicating a relationship to water or to hydrogen.

hydro′a. Any vesicular skin eruption.

  h. aestivale, see hydroa vacciniforme.

  h. febrile, see herpes simplex.

  h. herpetiforme, see dermatitis herpetiformis.

  h. puerorum, see hydroa vacciniforme.

  h. vacciniforme, a recurrent form occurring during the summer months; also called hydroa aestivale or puerorum.

hydroappen′dix. Distention of the vermiform appendix with a serous fluid.

hydrobleph′aron. Edema of the eyelid.

hydrocar′bon. A compound containing hydrogen and carbon only.

hy′drocele. Abnormal collection of fluid in any sacculated cavity in the body, especially under the serous covering of the testis or along the spermatic cord.

  hernia h., one in which the hernial sac is filled with a fluid.

hydrocelec′tomy. Surgical removal of a hydrocele.

hydrocephal′ic. Relating to or afflicted with hydrocephalus.

hydroceph′alocele. See hydrencephalocele.

hydroceph′alus. Excessive accumulation of cerebrospinal fluid in the ventricles of the brain (internal hydrocephalus) or in the subarachnoid spaces (external hydrocephalus), causing enlargement of the head and compression of the brain.

  communicating h., one in which there is no obstruction between the ventricles.

  noncommunicating h., obstructive h., one in which there is an obstruction between the ventricles.

  obstructive h., see noncommunicating hydrocephalus.

hydrochloric acid. A colorless, compound of hydrogen chloride (HCl); the acid secreted by the stomach to facilitate digestion.

hydrochlor′ide. Compound formed by the reaction of hydrochloric acid with an organic base.

hydrochlo′rothi′azide. A thiazide compound used as an oral diuretic.

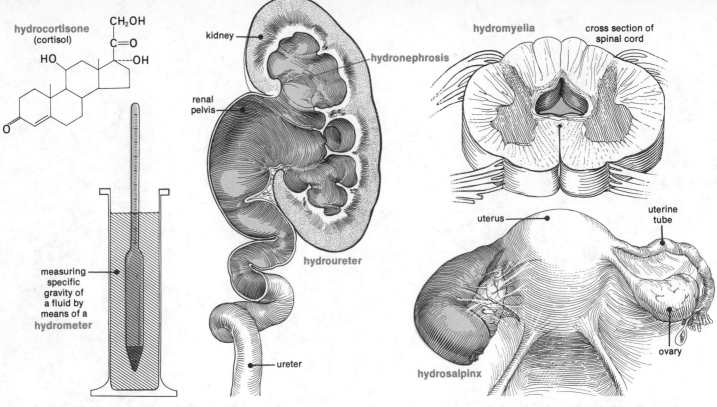

hydrocortisone (cortisol)

CH_2OH
$C=O$
OH
HO
O

measuring specific gravity of a fluid by means of a hydrometer

kidney —
— hydronephrosis
renal pelvis —

hydroureter

— ureter

hydromyelia
cross section of spinal cord

uterus —
— uterine tube

ovary

hydrosalpinx

---

hydrocol′loid. A gelatinous colloid in unstable equilibrium with its contained water, used in dentistry as an elastic impression material.

 irreversible h., a hydrocolloid such as alginate, whose physical condition is changed by an irreversible chemical reaction when mixed with water; used in making diagnostic casts of teeth and partial denture impressions.

 reversible h., a hydrocolloid of agar-agar base whose physical state is altered to a liquid by the application of heat and then changed to that of an elastic gel by cooling.

hydrocol′pocele, hydrocol′pos. An accumulation of fluid in the vagina.

hydrocor′tisone. Cortisol; a steroid hormone isolated from the adrenal cortex or produced synthetically; of the naturally occurring adrenal cortical hormones, hydrocortisone is most capable of correcting by itself the effects of adrenalectomy; provides resistance to stresses and maintains a number of enzyme systems.

hydrocyan′ic acid. A colorless, volatile, poisonous compound with an almond odor, (HCn); used as an insecticide and disinfectant; also called hydrogen cyanide and prussic acid.

hydrodynam′ics. The branch of physics concerned with fluids in motion and the forces affecting the motion.

hydroenceph′alocele. See hydrencephalocele.

hy′drogel. A gel having water as its dispersion medium. Cf hydrosol.

hy′drogen. A colorless, flammable, gaseous element; the lightest of all known chemical elements; symbol H, atomic number 1, atomic weight 1.0080.

 activated h., hydrogen removed from a compound (donor) by a dehydrogenase.

 heavy h., see hydrogen-2.

 h. acceptor, (1) hydrogen carrier; (2) a metabolite that transports hydrogen during metabolism.

 h. carrier, a molecule that carries hydrogen from one substance (oxidant) to another (reductant) or to molecular oxygen to form water (H_2O).

 h. cyanide, see hydrocyanic acid.

 h. donor, substance that gives up hydrogen atoms to another substance.

 h. ion, the positively charged nucleus of the hydrogen atom, $H°$ or H^+, formed by removal of the electron; it exists in aqueous solution as a hydronium ion, OH_3^+.

 h. number, a measure of the amount of unsaturated fatty acids in fat, equal to the quantity of hydrogen that 1 gm of fat will absorb.

 h. sulfide, H_2S; a colorless, flammable, poisonous gas with a rotten egg odor; used as a reagent and in chemical manufacturing; also called sulfuretted hydrogen.

 h. transport, the transfer of hydrogen from one substance to another; the former is thus oxidized and the latter is reduced.

 sulfuretted hydrogen, see hydrogen sulfide.

hydrogen-1 (^1H). The hydrogen isotope that makes up about 99 per cent of the hydrogen atoms occurring in nature; a mass 1 isotope; also called protium.

hydrogen-2 (^2H, D). Deuterium; an isotope of hydrogen having an atomic weight of 2.0141, consisting of one proton and one neutron in the nucleus; a mass 2 isotope; also called heavy hydrogen.

hydrogen-3 (^3H). The heaviest of the three isotopes of hydrogen with an atomic mass of 3; weakly radioactive; half-life 12.4 years; a mass 3 isotope; made artificially by bombardment of other species; also called tritium.

hydrogena′tion. The combination of an unsaturated compound with hydrogen.

hydrokinet′ics. The study of fluids in motion under a force.

hydrolab′yrinth. Abnormal increase in the amount of endolymph in the labyrinth of the inner ear; thought to be the cause of aural vertigo.

hy′drolase. An enzyme that promotes the hydrolysis of a compound.

hydrol′ysate. Any product produced by hydrolysis.

 protein h., a mixture of amino acids produced by splitting the protein molecule with acid, alkali, or enzyme; used in diets of infants allergic to milk or in special diets for individuals unable to eat ordinary food proteins.

hydrol′ysis. The decomposition or splitting of a compound into simpler substances by the addition of the elements of water; a hydrogen is added to one portion and a hydroxyl group to the other.

hydrolyt′ic. Relating to, characterized by, or causing hydrolysis.

hy′drolyze. To subject to hydrolysis.

hydromassag′e. Massage effected with streams of water.

hydrom′eter. An instrument used to measure the specific gravity of a liquid such as urine; also called gravimeter.

hydrome′tra. Accumulation of a watery fluid in the uterus.

hydrome′trocol′pos. Accumulation of fluid in the uterus and vagina.

hydrom′etry. The determination of the specific gravity of a fluid.

hydrom′phalus. A cystlike tumor of the umbilicus.

hydromye′lia. An increase of cerebrospinal fluid in the enlarged central canal of the spinal cord.

hydromy′elocele. A fluid-filled saclike protrusion of the spinal cord through a spina bifida.

hydronephro′sis. Distention of the pelvis and calyces of one or both kidneys with urine as a result of obstruction; also called nephrohydrosis.

hydro′nium. The hydrated hydrogen ion, H_3O^+, as it exists in water; also called hydronium ion.

hydropericar′dium. Abnormal accumulation of serous fluid in the sac around the heart (pericardium).

hydroperitone′um. See ascites.

hydrophil′ia. Affinity for water.

hydrophil′ic, hy′drophile. Readily absorbing water; opposite of hydrophobic.

hydropho′bia. See rabies.

hydropho′bic. 1. Relating to rabies (hydrophobia). **2.** Tending to repel water; opposite of hydrophilic.

hydrophthal′mos. See buphthalmos.

hydropneumo′gony. The injection of air into a joint to determine the amount of effusion in it.

hydropneumopericar′dium. The collection of serous effusion and gas within the pericardial cavity.

hydropneumothor′ax. Pneumohydrothorax; the presence of both gas and serous fluids in the pleural cavity.

hy′drops. Accumulation of clear fluid in bodily tissues or cavities; also called dropsy.

 endolymphatic h., see Ménière's syndrome.

 fetal h., hydrops occurring in the fetus, as in erythroblastosis fetalis.

 h. fetalis, fetal hydrops.

hydropyonephro′sis. The collection of urine and pus in the pelvis and calices of the kidney, usually caused by obstruction of the ureter.

hydror′chis. Collection of fluid within the serous covering of the testis.

hydrorrhe′a. Profuse watery secretion.

 h. gravidarum, profuse secretion of a clear fluid from the uterus during pregnancy.

hydrosal′pinx. Accumulation of serous fluid in the uterine tube.

hy′drosol. A colloid in aqueous solution; a sol in which the dispersing medium is water. Cf hydrogel.

hydrospirom′eter. A spirometer in which the force of the expired air (air pressure) is indicated by the rise and fall of a column of water.

hydrostat′ic. Relating to the pressures exerted by liquids at rest; opposed to hydrokinetic.

hydrotherapeu′tic. See hydriatic.

hydrother′apy. The therapeutic application of water in the treatment of certain diseases.

hydrother′mal. Relating to hot water.

hydrotho′rax. Noninflammatory accumulation of

---

hydrocolloid | **hydrothorax**

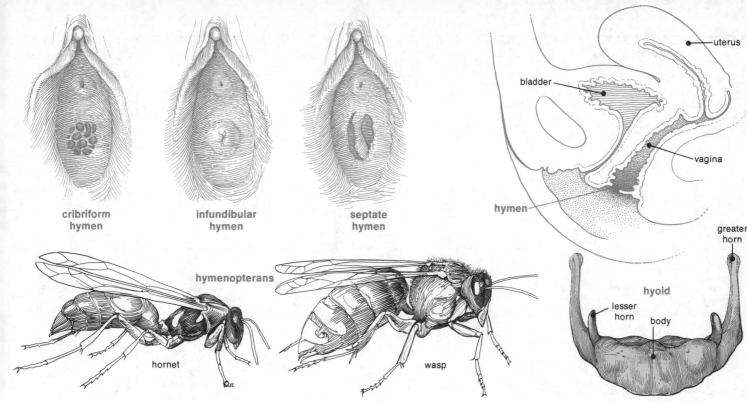

cribriform hymen | infundibular hymen | septate hymen

hymenopterans

hornet

wasp

hyoid

uterus

bladder

vagina

hymen

greater horn

lesser horn

body

serous fluid in the pleural cavity.

hydrot'ropism. Growth or movement of an organism toward a moist surface (positive hydrotropism) or away from a moist surface (negative hydrotropism).

hydroure'ter. Abnormal distention of the ureter with urine due to obstruction.

hy'drous. Containing water.

hydrox'ide. Any chemical compound of hydroxyl (OH) with another element or radical.

hydrox'y-. Prefix indicating the presence of the hydroxyl group, OH.

hydroxyap'atite. A mineral compound used in chromatography of nucleic acids.

25-hydroxycholecalcif'erol. A product of metabolism of cholecalciferol (vitamin D_3), produced mainly in the liver by addition of a hydroxy group on the 1 position by the kidney; converted to 1,25-dihydroxycholecalciferol, thought to be the most active form of vitamin D.

hydroxycor'tisone. Cortisol.

hydrox'yl. The univalent radical or group OH.

hydroxyl'ysine. A basic amino acid found, thus far, only in collagen and gelatin.

hydroxyphenylu'ria. Excretion of tyrosine and phenylalanine in the urine, usually resulting from ascorbic acid deficiency.

hydroxypro'line. 4-hydroxy-2-pyrrolidinecarboxylic acid; $C_5H_9NO_3$; a nutritionally nonessential amino acid found among the hydrolysis products of collagen; not found in proteins other than those of connective tissue.

hydroxyprolinе'mia. An inborn error of metabolism characterized by increased blood levels and urinary excretion of free hydroxyproline; associated with severe mental retardation.

5-hydroxytryp'tamine. See serotonin.

o-**hydroxyty'ramine.** See dopamine.

hy'giene. The science concerned with the methods of achieving or maintaining good health.

oral h., the proper care of the mouth and teeth for the prevention of disease.

hy'gienic. 1. Of or relating to hygiene. **2.** Sanitary; clean.

hygien'ist. One who is skilled in the science of health and the prevention of disease.

dental h., a person trained in the techniques of removing plaques from teeth and other preventive treatments.

hygieol'ogy. 1. The study of hygiene. **2.** The sum of all measures for the dissemination and popularization of public health knowledge.

hygro-. Combining form denoting wet or moist; e.g., hygroma.

hygro'ma. A bursa or cyst containing fluid.

subdural h., a collection of fluid beneath the dura mater (subdural space).

hygrom'eter. Any of several devices for measuring the atmospheric moisture.

hygroscop'ic. Readily absorbing moisture.

hy'men. The membranous fold which partly or completely closes the vaginal orifice in the virgin.

cribriform h., one with a number of small perforations.

denticular h., one in which the opening has serrated edges.

imperforate h., one which completely closes the vaginal orifice.

infundibuliform h., a protruding hymen with a central opening.

septate h., one in which the opening is divided by a narrow band of tissue.

hy'menal. Relating to the hymen.

hymenec'tomy. Excision of the hymen.

Hymenol'epis. A genus of tapeworms of the class Cestoda.

H. nana, a small tapeworm (seven to 10 mm long) parasitic in rats, mice, and children; also called dwarf or dwarf mouse tapeworm.

Hymenop'tera. An order of membrane-winged insects that includes many common stinging members such as the honeybee, yellow jacket, wasp, hornet, and fire ant; the stings are capable of causing severe hypersensitivity reactions and, in some cases, death.

hymenop'teran. Any of the membrane-winged insects of the order Hymenoptera, including the bees, wasps, and ants.

hymenor'rhaphy. 1. The closing of the vagina by suturing of the hymen. **2.** Suture of any membrane.

hymenot'omy. Surgical incision of the hymen, especially an imperforate hymen.

hyoepiglot'tic. Relating to the hyoid bone and the epiglottis.

hyoglos'sal. 1. Relating to the hyoid bone and the tongue. **2.** The twelfth cranial nerve; see table of nerves.

hy'oid. U-shaped; specifically, the horseshoe-shaped bone in the throat between the thyroid cartilage and the root of the tongue.

hyoscy'amine. A poisonous alkaloid, $C_{17}H_{23}NO_3$, occurring in plants such as belladonna, duboisia, hyoscyamus, and stramonium; isometric with atropine; used as an antispasmodic, analgesic, and sedative; also called daturine and *l*-tropine tropate.

hyp-. See hypo-.

hypacu'sis. Impairment of hearing; reduction in ability to perceive sound, usually attributable to conductive or neurosensory deficiency in the pe-

ripheral organs of hearing; also called hypoacusis and hypacusia.

hypalge'sia. Decreased sensitivity to pain.

hypam'nios, hypam'nion. The presence of an abnormally small amount of fluid in the amniotic sac.

hypenceph'alon. The midbrain, pons, and medulla.

hyper-. Prefix indicating excessive or above the normal.

hyperabduction syndrome. Pain and numbness of the arm and hand occurring after prolonged abduction of the arm, as during sleep, which compresses the axillary vessels and brachial plexus.

hyperacid'ity. Superacidity; an excessive degree of acidity.

hyperactiv'ity. Excessively increased activity.

hyperactivity syndrome. See hyperkinetic syndrome.

hyperacu'sia, hyperacu'sis. Exaggerated hearing acuteness; also called auditory hyperesthesia.

hyperadre'nocor'ticism. Excessive secretion of adrenocortical hormones.

hyperaldoster'onism. Aldosteronism; condition caused by excessive secretion of aldosterone by the adrenal cortex.

hyperalge'sia. Excessive sensitiveness to pain.

hyperalimenta'tion. Overfeeding for therapeutic purposes.

parenteral h., the continuous administration of fluids containing nutrients (particularly a solution of amino acids and sugar) into the superior vena cava through a catheter.

hyperbar'ic. Relating to or occurring at pressures greater than atmospheric pressure; e.g., hyperbaric chamber.

hyperbar'ism. Condition resulting from the pressure of ambient gases in excess of that within the body.

hyperbetalipoproteine'mia. Type II familial hyperlipoproteinemia; see under hyperlipoproteinemia.

hyperbilirubine'mia. The presence of an abnormally large amount of bilirubin in the blood.

hypercalce'mia. Abnormally high concentration of calcium in the blood.

idiopathic h. of infants, persistent hypercalcemia affecting infants, associated with osteosclerosis, renal insufficiency, and sometimes hypertension.

hypercalciu'ria. Elevated amounts of calcium in the urine, usually a result of hypercalcemia, as in hyperparathyroidism, bone neoplasm, and vitamin D intoxication; also called hypercalcuria and hypercalcinuria.

Classification of Hyperlipoproteinemia

Type and prevalence	I RARE	II COMMON	III FAIRLY COMMON	IV COMMON	V UNCOMMON
Appearance of plasma	creamy layer over clear infranatant on standing	clear or only slightly turbid	clear, cloudy, or milky	clear to grossly turbid	creamy layer over turbid infranatant on standing
Cholesterol level	↑	↑↑	↑↑	↑	↑↑
TG level	↑↑	↑	↑↑	↑↑	↑↑
Signs and symptoms	abdominal pain hepatosplenomegaly lipemia retinalis eruptive xanthomas	tendon xanthomas tuberous xanthomas corneal arcus accelerated atherosclerosis	tendon, tuboeruptive, and planar xanthomas accelerated atherosclerosis	accelerated coronary atherosclerosis abnormal glucose tolerance	abdominal pain hepatosplenomegaly lipemia retinalis eruptive xanthomas abnormal glucose tolerance

idiopathic h., condition of elevated amounts of calcium in the urine not explained by hypercalcemia.

hypercap′nia, hypercar′bia. The presence of abnormally high concentration of carbon dioxide in the blood.

hypercemento′sis. Overdevelopment of cementum over the root surface of teeth.

hyperchlore′mia. Abnormal increase of chloride in the blood.

hyperchlorhyd′ria. Excessive secretion of gastric juice; may be due to a temporary disturbance of stomach function; chronic hyperchlorhydria may be associated with peptic ulcer.

hypercholesterole′mia, hypercholestere′mia. The presence of an abnormally excessive amount of cholesterol in the blood.

hypercho′lia. A condition in which an excessive amount of bile is secreted by the liver.

hyperchroma′sia. Hyperchromatism.

hyperchromat′ic. Overpigmented; having excessive coloration; said especially of a cell which stains more intensely than normal.

hyperchro′matism. 1. Excessive pigmentation. **2.** Degeneration of a cell nucleus which becomes filled with an excessive amount of pigment particles.

hyperchro′mia. 1. Abnormal increase in the hemoglobin content of red blood cells, usually seen in macrocytic cells where the concentration of hemoglobin is normal but the quantity is increased because the cells are larger than normal. **2.** Hyperchromatism.

hyperchro′mic. 1. Overpigmented. **2.** Relating to an increase in light absorption.

hyperchy′lia. An excessive secretion of gastric juice.

hyperchylomicrone′mia. Type I familial hyperlipoproteinemia; see under hyperlipoproteinemia.

hypercor′ticoidism, hypercor′ticism. Condition caused by an excess of one or more steroids of the adrenal cortex, or by the administration of large quantities of steroids having glucocorticoid qualities.

hypercryalge′sia, hypercryesthe′sia. Excessive sensitivity to cold.

hypercupre′mia. Abnormally high copper content in the blood.

hypercythe′mia. The presence of an abnormally large number of erythrocytes in the circulating blood.

hypercyto′sis. Any condition in which there is an abnormal increase in the number of blood cells, especially of leukocytes.

hyperdip′sia. Intense thirst.

hyperdisten′tion. Extreme distention.

hyperdynam′ia. Extreme muscular activity or restlessness; exaggeration of function.

hyperdynam′ic. Marked by hyperdynamia.

hyperem′esis. Excessive vomiting.

h. gravidarum, pernicious vomiting of pregnancy.

hypere′mia. Excess of blood in an area of the body; congestion.

active h., hyperemia caused by increased inflow of arterial blood resulting in dilatation of arterioles and capillaries, as in inflammation.

collateral h., increased blood flow through collateral vessels due to an arrest of the flow through the main artery.

passive h., hyperemia resulting from an obstruction to the outflow of blood from the affected area.

hyperesthe′sia. Abnormally increased sensitivity to sensory stimuli.

hyperexten′sion. Extension of a part of the body beyond the normal limit; also called superextension.

hyperflex′ion. Flexion of a limb or part beyond the normal limit; also called overflexion and superflexion.

hypergammaglobuline′mia. Excess of γ-globulin in the blood.

hypergen′italism. Overdeveloped genitalia for age of individual.

hyperglobuline′mia. Excess of globulin in the blood.

hyperglyce′mia. Abnormally high concentration of sugar (glucose) in the blood.

hyperglycorrha′chia. An excessive amount of sugar (glucose) in the cerebrospinal fluid (CSF).

hypergo′nadism. Abnormally increased physiologic activity of the gonads (testes or ovaries), with enhanced secretion of gonadal hormones, marked growth, and precocious sexual development.

hyperhidro′sis. Excessive perspiration.

hyperhydra′tion. See overhydration.

hyperin′sulinism. 1. Excessive secretion of insulin by the islets of Langerhans, causing the level of sugar in the blood to fall considerably. **2.** Insulin shock from excess dosage of insulin.

hyperkale′mia. An elevated potassium concentration in the blood; it may cause changes in cardiac function leading to cardiac arrest; also called hyperpotassemia.

hyperkerato′sis. Overgrowth of the horny layer of the skin.

hyperkine′sia, hyperkine′sis. Abnormally increased muscular activity, as seen in some psychiatric disorders, especially in children.

hyperkinet′ic. Of or relating to a state of muscular overactivity.

hyperkinetic syndrome. Condition marked by excessive energy, emotional instability, and short attention span; may be seen in children with minimal brain dysfunction; also called hyperactivity syndrome.

hyperlacta′tion. Excessive or prolonged secretion of milk.

hyperlipe′mia. Excessive amounts of lipids in blood plasma.

hyperlip′oproteine′mia. Disorder of fat metabolism marked by high concentrations of lipoproteins in the blood.

type I familial h., rare disorder characterized by accumulation of chylomicrons in the blood, proportional to intake of dietary fat; inherited as a recessive trait; also called hyperchylomicronemia and exogenous hyperlipemia.

type I h., secondary, a form seen in diseases in which there are abnormal circulating globulins, such as multiple myeloma, macroglobulinemia, etc.

type II familial h., a disorder of autosomal inheritance characterized by increased plasma concentration of low-density (beta) lipoproteins, cholesterol, and phospholipids, with normal levels of triglyceride; associated with xanthomas in the Achilles, patellar, and digital extensor tendons, and susceptibility to atherosclerosis; manifestations are usually detected in infants and young adults; also called familial hypercholesterolemia and hyperbetalipoproteinemia.

type III familial h., a rare form, probably inherited as an autosomal recessive trait, characterized by increased plasma levels of abnormal very low-density (pre-beta) lipoproteins and cholesterol, flat, yellowish-orange xanthomas (usually on the palmar and digital creases), glucose intolerance, and premature atherosclerosis; usually detected in young adults; also called broad-beta disease.

type IV familial h., a common disorder, usually detected in middle life, probably inherited as an autosomal recessive trait; characterized by increased levels of plasma triglyceride of hepatic origin, contained primarily in very low-density (pre-beta) lipoproteins, and by a predisposition to atherosclerosis; also called endogenous hyperlipemia and hyperprebetalipoproteinemia.

type IV h., secondary, a form seen in a variety of metabolic disorders including diabetes mellitus, hypothyroidism, and the nephrotic syndrome.

type V familial h., a rare form with characteristics of both type I and IV, which include increased plasma levels of chylomicrons, very low-density (pre-beta) lipoproteins, and triglycerides while on ordinary diets, with eruptive xanthomas and recurrent acute pancreatitis; occurs chiefly during adolescence and middle life, probably as an autosomal recessive inheritance; also called mixed hyperlipe-

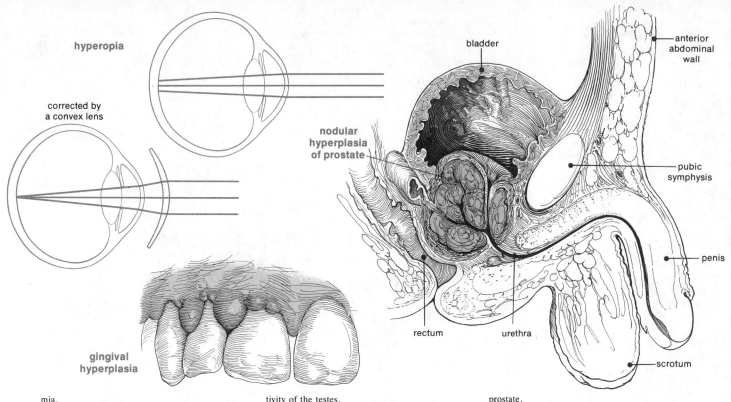

hyperopia

corrected by
a convex lens

gingival
hyperplasia

nodular
hyperplasia
of prostate

bladder

anterior
abdominal
wall

pubic
symphysis

penis

rectum | urethra

scrotum

---

mia.

type V h., secondary, a form seen in association with any of the diseases capable of producing secondary type IV hyperlipoproteinemia.

hyperlysine′mia. A hereditary metabolic disorder in which there is an abnormal increase of lysine in the circulating blood; associated with physical and mental retardation, anemia, hypotonia, convulsions, and impaired sexual development; autosomal recessive inheritance.

hyperlysinu′ria. An abnormally high concentration of lysine in the urine.

hypermas′tia. Overgrowth of the mammary glands.

hypermenorrhe′a. Menorrhagia; prolonged or profuse menses.

hypermetab′olism. An unusually high metabolic rate; heat production by the body above normal, as in thyrotoxicosis.

hyperme′tria. A manifestation of ataxia characterized by voluntary muscular movement overreaching the intended goal.

hypermetro′pia. See hyperopia.

hypermne′sia. Unusually exaggerated activity of memory.

hy′permorph. A tall, usually slender person whose standing height is great in proportion to the sitting height, owing to very long legs.

hypermyoto′nia. Marked development of muscular tonicity.

hypermyot′rophy. Marked development of muscular tissue; also called muscular hypertrophy.

hypernatre′mia. Abnormally high sodium concentration in the blood.

hypernephro′ma. Renal cell carcinoma; see under carcinoma.

hyperoncot′ic. Denoting an oncotic pressure higher than normal.

hyperonych′ia. Hypertrophy of the nails.

hy′perope. One afflicted with hyperopia.

hypero′pia, hypermetro′pia. A condition of the eye in which parallel light rays (rays of light from distant objects) entering the eyeball focus behind the retina, because the eyeball is short or the refractive power of the lens is weak; also called farsightedness and far sight.

latent h., the portion of the total hyperopia that is not revealed because it is compensated for by the tonicity of the ciliary muscle.

manifest h., the portion of the total hyperopia that may be measured by the relaxation of accommodation.

total h., the sum of the latent and the manifest hyperopia.

hyperor′chidism. Increased size of functional ac-

tivity of the testes.

hyperos′mia. An exaggerated sense of smell.

hyperost′osis. 1. Hypertrophy or abnormal growth of bone tissue. **2.** Exostosis.

h. frontalis interna, abnormal deposition of bone on the internal surface of the frontal bone.

hyperova′rianism. Abnormally increased functional activity of the ovaries, usually leading to sexual precocity in young girls.

hyperoxalu′ria. An unusually large amount of oxalic acid or oxalates in the urine; caused by a genetic disorder affecting the metabolism of glyoxylic acid, which forms oxalate rather than glycine; it is one of the common causes of nephrolithiasis and nephrocalcinosis in children.

hyperox′ia. Excessive amount of oxygen in the tissues.

hyperpan′creatism. Abnormally increased functional activity of the pancreas.

hyperparathy′roidism. Excessive secretion of parathyroid hormone.

primary h., excessive secretion of parathyroid hormone resulting from an adenoma or chief cell or clear cell hyperplasia (80 per cent of cases), or carcinoma (20 per cent); the classic laboratory manifestations are high serum calcium and low serum phosphate.

secondary h., hyperplasia of the parathyroid glands and increased secretion of parathyroid hormone secondary to abnormal calcium and phosphorus metabolism in chronic renal disease.

hyperpath′ia. Exaggerated response to pain.

hyperpep′sia. 1. Excessive rapid digestion. **2.** Impaired digestion with hyperchlorhydria.

hyperpepsin′ia. Excessive secretion of pepsin in the stomach.

hyperperistal′sis. Increase in the rate of peristalsis; peristaltic unrest; excessive rapidity of the passage of food through the stomach and intestine.

hyperpha′gia. Overeating.

hyperpho′ria. Tendency of one eye to deviate upward.

hyperphosphatu′ria. Abnormal amount of phosphates in the urine.

hyperpigmenta′tion. Excessive coloration or pigmentation in a tissue or part.

hyperpitu′itarism. Excessive production of growth hormone by the pituitary gland due to a tumor, causing gigantism in children and acromegaly in adults.

hyperpla′sia. The increased size of an organ or part due to the excessive but regulated increase in the number of its cells. Cf neoplasm and hypertrophy.

benign prostatic h., see nodular hyperplasia of

prostate.

congenital adrenal h., adrenal hyperplasia with excessive secretion of androgens resulting from enzymatic defects in the biosynthesis of corticosteroids; there are four major types: (a) simple virilizing form; (b) sodium-losing form; (c) hypertensive form; and (d) 3 β-hydroxysteroid dehydrogenase defect, which may produce feminization of male genitalia.

cystic h. of breast, see fibrocystic disease of breast.

fibromuscular h., fibrosis and hyperplasia of the arterial muscular layer, usually involving the renal arteries.

gingival h., cellular proliferation of the gingiva resulting in swelling.

nodular h. of prostate, a common disorder of men over the age of 50, characterized by the formation of large nodules in the prostate which press against the urethra, thus obstructing the flow of urine; also called benign prostatic hypertrophy or hyperplasia.

hyperplas′tic. Relating to or characterized by hyperplasia.

hyperpne′a. Abnormally rapid and deep breathing.

hyperpolariza′tion. An increase in the positive charges normally present at the surface of a nerve cell membrane.

hyperpotasse′mia. See hyperkalemia.

hyperprebetalipoproteine′mia. Type IV familial hyperlipoproteinemia; see under hyperlipoproteinemia.

hyperproline′mia. An inherited metabolic disorder marked by increased proline in the plasma and excretion of proline, hydroxyproline, and glycine.

hyperproteine′mia. The presence of excessive protein in the blood.

hyperpyret′ic. Relating to high fever; also called hyperpyrexial.

hyperpyrex′ia. Extremely high fever, usually 105.0°F or more.

hyperpyrex′ial. See hyperpyretic.

hyperreflex′ia. Exaggerated deep tendon reflexes.

hyperres′onance. An extreme or exaggerated degree of resonance on percussion as heard in pulmonary emphysema.

hypersecre′tion. Excessive secretion.

hypersen′sitive. Overreactive to a stimulus.

hypersensitiv′ity. 1. Allergy; the altered reactivity to a substance, which can result in pathologic reactions upon subsequent exposure to that particular substance. **2.** Excessive response to a stimulus.

hypersensitiza′tion. The process of creating an

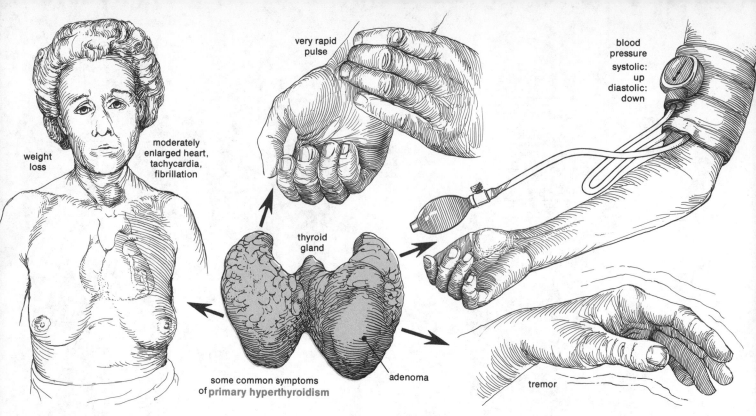

weight loss

moderately enlarged heart, tachycardia, fibrillation

very rapid pulse

blood pressure
systolic: up
diastolic: down

thyroid gland

some common symptoms of **primary hyperthyroidism**

adenoma

tremor

abnormally sensitive state.

hypersialo'sis. Excessive secretion of saliva; also called hypertyalism.

hypersomatotro'pism. Abnormally increased secretion of pituitary growth hormone.

hyperso'mia. Gigantism.

hypersom'nia. Abnormal condition in which the individual sleeps for excessive periods of time.

hyperson'ic. Relating to speeds equal to or exceeding five times the speed of sound (speeds less than hypersonic but greater than the speed of sound are called supersonic).

hypersple'nism. A disorder in which the formed elements of the blood are destroyed by the excessively increased activity of the spleen; it may result in anemic neutropenia, thrombocytopenia, or a combination of these states.

hypersteato'sis. Excessive sebaceous secretion.

hypersthenu'ria. Excretion of urine of abnormally high specific gravity and concentration of solutes, usually resulting from loss or deprivation of water; increased osmolality of the urine.

hypertel'orism. Abnormally increased distance between paired organs or parts.

  ocular h., congenital malformation marked by enlarged sphenoid bone, causing extreme distance between the eyes; also called craniofacial dysostosis.

hyperten'sin. See angiotensin.

hypertensin'ogen. See angiotensinogen.

hyperten'sion. High arterial blood pressure; in adults usually defined as pressures exceeding 140/90 mm Hg.

  essential h., hypertension without a known cause.

  malignant h., severe hypertension that causes degenerative changes in the walls of the blood vessels throughout the body; hemorrhages occur in the retina, the kidney, and other areas; cerebral function is altered.

  portal h., increased pressure in the portal venous system; it may result from: intrahepatic causes, such as cirrhosis of the liver; suprahepatic causes, such as heart failure; infrahepatic causes, such as portal vein thrombosis.

  pulmonary h., hypertension in the pulmonary circulation resulting from primary pulmonary changes such as fibrosis of the lung, or from heart diseases such as mitral stenosis.

  renal h., hypertension secondary to kidney disease.

  renovascular h., hypertension due to obstruction of the renal arteries.

hyperten'sive. Marked by or afflicted with high blood pressure.

hypertheco'sis. Hyperplasia of the theca cells of

the vesicular ovarian (graafian) follicles.

hyperthe'lia. The presence of several nipples but only two breasts.

hyperther'mia. Extremely high body temperature.

hyperthrombine'mia. The presence of excessive thrombin in the blood.

hyperthy'mia. State of increased emotivity or overactivity.

hyperthy'roidism. Condition caused by excessive production or ingestion of thyroid hormone; the most common symptoms include weight loss, increased appetite, rapid heart rate, tremor, and fatigue; when exophthalmos is present, the disease is known as exophthalmic goiter.

  primary h., a form originating within the thyroid gland.

  secondary h., a form caused by abnormal stimulation of the thyroid gland due to a disorder of the pituitary gland.

hyperto'nia. Excessive tension of the muscles or arteries.

hyperton'ic. 1. Having an abnormally increased tension. **2.** Having the greater osmotic pressure of two solutions; frequently, the comparison is to the osmotic concentration of plasma.

hypertonic'ity. The state of being hypertonic.

hypertricho'sis, hypertrichi'asis. A growth of hair in excess of normal for that particular area of the body, e.g., the face in women.

hypertriglyceride'mia. Excessive concentration of triglyceride in the blood.

  familial h., any one of two heritable forms of the disease: (1) exogenous or fat-induced, occurring after meals of normal or high lipid content; (2) endogenous or carbohydrate-induced, occurring after meals rich in carbohydrates.

hyper'trophy. The enlargement of an organ or part due to the increase in size of the cells composing it; the overgrowth meets a demand for increased functional activity. Cf. neoplasm and hyperplasia.

  adaptive h., thickening of the walls of a hollow organ, like the urinary bladder, when the outflow is obstructed.

  compensatory h. of the heart, thickening of the walls of the heart, occurring when a chamber must pump against an increased resistance as in valvular disease or hypertension, thus increasing the power of the heart to maintain the circulation.

  physiologic h., temporary hypertrophy of an organ to meet the demand of a natural increase in functional activity, as in the female breast during pregnancy and lactation.

  vicarious h., hypertrophy of an organ due to dysfunction of another organ of allied activity.

hypertro'pia. Upward deviation of one eye not controllable by fixational efforts; unlike hyperphoria, the condition is continuous.

hyperurice'mia. Excess of uric acid in the blood.

hyperuricosu'ria. Excretion of excessive amounts of uric acid in the urine.

hyperuricu'ria. High level of urinary excretion of uric acid.

hyperventila'tion. A condition marked by fast deep breathing which tends to remove increased amounts of carbon dioxide from the body and lower the partial pressure of the gas, causing buzzing in the ears, tingling of the lips and fingers, and sometimes fainting; also called overventilation.

  central neural h., a pattern of irregular hyperventilation, usually seen in individuals who have a midbrain lesion and who are comatose.

hyperventilation syndrome. A syndrome which is almost always a manifestation of acute anxiety, characterized by difficult, deep, and rapid respiration accompanied by tightness of the chest and a feeling of suffocation; lightheadedness is commonly present and tingling of the hands may appear as a result of marked diminution of carbon dioxide in the blood (hypocapnia), produced by the excessive respiration; it may last half an hour or longer and may recur a few times a day; the attacks may be controlled somewhat by breath-holding or breathing in a paper bag.

hypervitamino'sis. Condition caused by ingestion of excessive amounts of a vitamin preparation.

hypervole'mia. Abnormal increase in the volume of blood, as seen during pregnancy and in some cases of hydatidiform mole.

hypervol'ia. Increased water content or volume of a particular compartment.

hypesthe'sia. See hypoesthesia.

hy'pha, *pl.* **hy'phae.** One of the hairlike structures forming the substance of a fungus.

hyphe'ma, hyphe'mia. Collection of blood in the anterior chamber of the eye.

hyphidro'sis. Diminished or deficient perspiration; abnormally scanty perspiration.

hypnagog'ic. 1. Denoting the transitional state produced by sleep, such as mental images occurring just before sleep. **2.** Inducing sleep; also called hypnotic.

hyp'nagogue. An agent that induces sleep.

hypno-, hypn-. Combining form indicating a relationship to sleep or hypnosis.

hypnoanal'ysis. Psychoanalysis conducted while the patient is under hypnosis.

hypnogen'esis. The process of inducing sleep or a hypnotic state.

hypnol'ogy. The study of sleep or hypnosis.

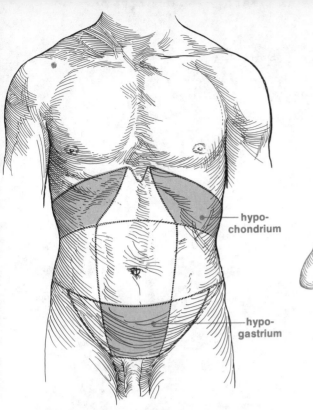

hypo-
chondrium

hypo-
gastrium

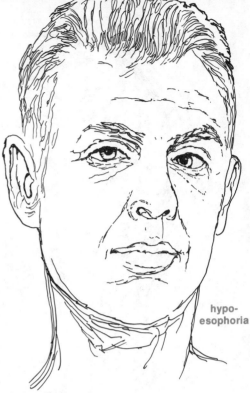

hypodactylia

hypo-
esophoria

hypnopho'bia. Abnormal fear of falling asleep.

hypnopom'pic. Relating to the partially conscious state between the stages of sleep and complete awakening.

hypno'sis. An artificially induced state in which the individual becomes receptive to the hypnotist's suggestions; it may vary in degree from mild suggestibility to a deep sleeplike state with total surgical anesthesia.

hypnother'apy. Treatment using hypnosis.

hypnot'ic. 1. Of, involving, or causing hypnosis. **2.** An individual who is hypnotized. **3.** Any agent that induces sleep.

hyp'notism. 1. The practice of inducing hypnosis. **2.** Hypnosis.

hyp'notist. One who practices hypnotism.

hyp'notize. To put into a hypnotic state.

hypo-, hyp-. Prefixes, equivalent to sub-, indicating beneath, under, deficient, or incomplete.

hy'po. A popular designation for hypodermic injection.

hypoacid'ity. Deficiency of normal acidity; also called subacidity.

hypoadre'nalism. Reduced or deficient adrenocortical function.

hypoadrenocor'ticism. Abnormally low secretion of hormones of the adrenal cortex.

hypoadrenocor'tism. Hypoadrenocorticism.

hypoalbumine'mia. Abnormally low concentration of albumin in the blood.

hypoalimenta'tion. Insufficient nourishment.

hypobar'ic. Relating to or occurring at pressures less than atmospheric pressure.

hypobarop'athy. Condition caused by greatly reduced air pressure and decreased oxygen intake; also called aviator's, altitude, or mountain sickness and Acosta's disease.

hypocalce'mia. A marked reduction of calcium in the blood.

hypocalcifica'tion. Diminished calcification, especially of tooth enamel, producing opaque white spots.

  hereditary enamel h., a hereditary defect of tooth enamel development affecting the primary and secondary teeth; it causes a breaking off of the enamel after tooth eruption, exposing the dentin, which gives the teeth a yellow appearance.

hypocap'nia. Marked diminution in the amount of carbon dioxide in the blood; also called acapnia.

hypochlore'mia. A marked reduction of chloride in the blood.

hypochlorhyd'ria. Abnormally low amount of hydrochloric acid in the gastric juice.

hypochlor'ite. A salt of hypochlorous acid.

hypochlo'rous acid. An unstable acid, HOCl;

used as a bleach and disinfectant.

hypochloru'ria. Abnormally diminished excretion of chloride ions in the urine.

hypocholesterole'mia. Abnormally small amounts of cholesterol in the blood.

hypochon'dria. See hypochondriasis.

hypochon'driac. An individual afflicted with hypochondriasis.

hypochondri'asis. The persistent neurotic preoccupation with one's health and fear of presumed diseases that persist despite reassurances; an exaggerated concern over physical health in absence of organic disease; also called hypochondria.

hypochon'drium. Any of two lateral regions of the upper zone of the abdomen.

hypochromat'ic. Containing a small amount of pigment, or less than the normal amount for the individual tissue; abnormally deficient pigmentation.

hypochrome'mia. Anemia characterized by an abnormally low color index of the blood.

hypochro'mia. 1. Abnormal decrease in the hemoglobin content of the red blood cells. **2.** Hypochromatism.

hypochrom'ic. 1. Having less than the normal amount of pigment. **2.** Relating to a decrease in light absorption.

hypochy'lia. Abnormally low amount of gastric juice.

hypocor'ticoidism. Hypoadrenocorticism.

hypocupre'mia. Abnormally low concentration of copper in the blood.

hypodactyl'ia. The presence of less than the normal number of digits on the hand or foot.

hy'poderm. See hypodermis.

hypoder'mic. Subcutaneous; located in or introduced into the layer beneath the skin; used sometimes to refer not only to the manner of injection, but to the injection per se.

hypoder'mis, hy'poderm. Subcutaneous fascia; see under fascia.

hypodermoc'lysis. The infusion of fluid into the subcutaneous space.

hypodyna'mia. Markedly diminished power.

hypoesopho'ria. Combined downward (hypophoria) and inward (esophoria) deviation of the eyeball.

hypoesthe'sia. Abnormally decreased sensitiveness of the skin; also called hypesthesia.

hypofibrinogene'mia. Deficiency of fibrinogen in the blood, usually below 100 mg per cent; may occur in amniotic fluid embolism, fetal death, abruptio placentae, and occasionally intra-amniotic instillation of hypertonic saline.

hypofunc'tion. Diminished or inadequate func-

tioning of an organ or part.

hypogalac'tia. Insufficient milk production.

hypogam'maglobuline'mia. Lack of γ-globulin in the blood; a deficiency state manifested by recurrent infections; primary forms result from diminished rates of synthesis; secondary forms result from increased catabolism.

hypogas'trium. The middle region of the lower zone of the abdomen.

hypogen'italism. Underdevelopment of the genitalia.

hypoglos'sal. Located beneath the tongue.

hypoglot'tis. The undersurface of the tongue.

hypoglyce'mia. A condition marked by lower than normal level of sugar (glucose) in the blood; characterized clinically by sweating, trembling, palpitation, hunger, weakness, and lightheadedness; the symptoms may vary in duration and often disappear rapidly after eating a snack or a sweet, or drinking a glass of milk; may result from excessive production of insulin by the pancreas or excessive administration of insulin to a diabetic.

hypog'nathous. Having an underdeveloped lower jaw.

hypogo'nadism. A condition resulting from deficient secretion of the gonads.

  hereditary familial h., see Reifenstein's syndrome.

  h. with anosmia, a genetic disorder, usually in males, associated with loss of the sense of smell due to failure of development of olfactory lobes; X-linked inheritance; also called Kallmann's syndrome.

  testicular h., condition caused by a decrease of the internal secretion of the testis and marked by the loss of secondary sexual characteristics.

hypohidro'sis. Abnormally reduced perspiration.

hypokale'mia. Abnormally low level of potassium in the blood; may result in nephropathy, muscle weakness, gastric atony, paralysis of the muscles of respiration, and arrhythmias; also called hypopotassemia.

hypokine'mia. Abnormally reduced cardiac output; reduced circulation rate.

hypomagnese'mia. Abnormally low concentration of magnesium in the blood.

hypoma'nia. A moderate form of manic activity, usually marked by slightly abnormal elation and overactivity.

hypomas'tia. Abnormal smallness of the breasts.

hypomenorrhe'a. Scanty menstrual flow, possibly with shortening of the duration of the menstrual period.

hypometab'olism. Reduced metabolism.

hypome'tria. Loss of power of muscular coordina-

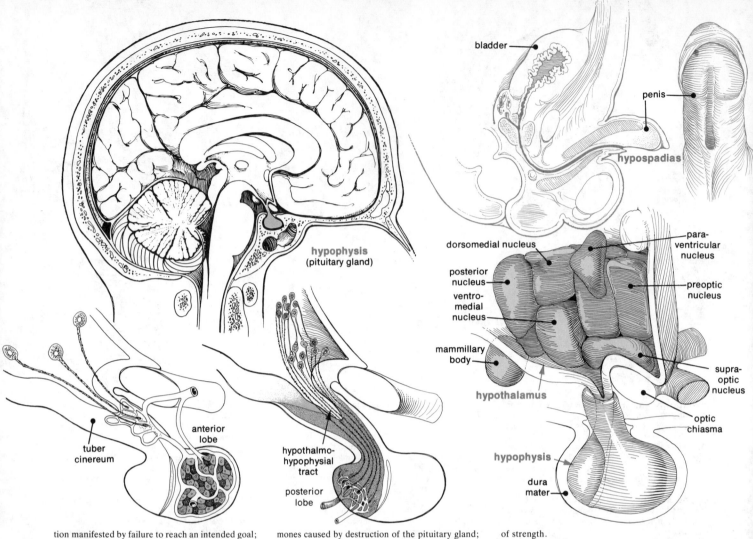

bladder

penis

hypospadias

hypophysis
(pituitary gland)

tuber
cinereum

anterior
lobe

hypothalmo-
hypophysial
tract

posterior
lobe

dorsomedial nucleus

para-
ventricular
nucleus

posterior
nucleus

preoptic
nucleus

ventro-
medial
nucleus

mammillary
body

hypothalamus

supra-
optic
nucleus

optic
chiasma

hypophysis

dura
mater

tion manifested by failure to reach an intended goal; decreased range of voluntary movements.

hy'pomorph. 1. A person who has short legs. **2.** In genetics, a mutant gene that acts in the same direction as the normal allele, but at a lower level of effectiveness.

hyponatre'mia. Low concentration of sodium in the blood.

hyponych'ial. Subungual; beneath a fingernail or toenail.

hyponych'ium. The thickened horny zone of the epidermis beneath the free border of the nail.

hypoova'rianism. Diminished secretion of ovarian hormones.

hypoparathy'roidism. Condition caused by lack of parathyroid secretion, resulting in reduced plasma calcium level and increased plasma phosphate level.

hypophalan'gism. Congenital absence of a phalanx on a finger or toe.

hypopho'ria. Latent condition in which one eye tends to deviate downward.

hypophosphata'sia. Lack of alkaline phosphatase in the blood; a rare inherited disorder characterized by rickets and osteomalacia.

hypophosphate'mia. Deficiency of phosphate in the blood.

hypophys'eal, hypophys'ial. Pertaining to the hypophysis (pituitary gland).

hypophysec'tomize. To remove or destroy the hypophysis (pituitary gland).

hypophysec'tomy. Surgical removal of the hypophysis (pituitary gland).

hypoph'ysis. A gland of internal secretion situated in the hypophysial fossa of the sphenoid bone, attached to the base of the brain by a short stalk; it consists of two main parts, anterior lobe (adenohypophysis) and posterior lobe (neurohypophysis); its secretions are of vital importance to growth, maturation, and reproduction; also called pituitary gland or body.

hypopitu'itarism. A condition due to abnormally diminished production of anterior pituitary hor-

mones caused by destruction of the pituitary gland; it leads to atrophy of the thyroid and adrenal glands and the gonads.

hypopla'sia. Defective or incomplete development of an organ or a part.

  enamel h., failure of the enamel of the teeth to develop completely.

hypoplas'tic. Relating to or characterized by hypoplasia.

hypop'nea. Abnormally shallow breathing.

hypopotasse'mia. See hypokalemia.

hypoproteine'mia. Abnormally small amounts of protein in the blood.

hypoproteino'sis. Dietary deficiency of protein.

hypoprothrombine'mia. Deficiency of prothrombin (blood clotting factor II) in the blood.

hypo'pyon. The presence of pus in the anterior chamber of the eye, secondary to inflammation of the cornea, iris, or ciliary body.

hyporeflex'ia. A condition of weakened reflexes.

hypori'boflavino'sis. Disease caused by insufficient intake of riboflavin; also called ariboflavinosis.

hyposaliva'tion. Diminished flow of saliva.

hyposensitiv'ity. The condition of less than normal sensitivity; one in which the response to a stimulus is unusually delayed or lessened in degree.

hyposensitiza'tion. See immunotherapy (3).

hyposen'sitize. To render insensitive, or less sensitive; to reduce sensitivity, usually with reference to allergy (induced sensitivity); also called desensitize.

hypos'mia. Reduced sense of smell; also called hypospheresia.

hypospa'dia. See hypospadias.

hypospa'dias. A congenital defect in the male in which the urethra opens on the undersurface of the penis; it occurs in approximately 1 in 500 births; there is also a similar defect in the female in which the urethra opens into the vagina; also called hypospadia.

hypos'tasis. 1. A sediment or deposit. **2.** Blood congestion in a part.

hyposthe'nia. A weakened state; decrease or lack

of strength.

hyposthenu'ria. Impairment of ability to concentrate the urine.

hyposto'sis. Inadequate development of bone.

hypotax'ia. Condition marked by imperfect coordination.

hypotel'orism. Abnormally small distance between two organs or parts such as the eyes.

hypoten'sion. Abnormally low blood pressure.

hypoten'sive. Marked by or causing low blood pressure.

hypothal'amus. A deep-lying part of the brain situated just below the thalamus; it forms the floor and part of the lateral walls of the third ventricle; it includes the mammillary bodies, tuber cinereum, infundibulum, and the optic chiasm; the hypothalamic nuclei are concerned with visceral control, e.g., the regulation of water balance and body temperature.

hypoth'enar. The fleshy portion of the palm of the hand, at its medial side.

hypother'mal. Relating to a bodily temperture below normal.

hypother'mia. Abnormally low body temperature, usually below 97°F (36°C).

hypoth'esis. A tentative theory subject to verification.

  Lyon h., the concept that in each somatic cell of normal females only one of the two X-chromosomes is active during interphase; as inactivation of the other X-chromosome takes place randomly, females heterozygous for an X-linked mutant gene may show patches of tissue with the phenotype of the mutant gene while the majority of tissue remains normal.

  Michaelis-Menten h., the assumption that an intermediate complex is formed between an enzyme and its substrate; it is further assumed that the complex decomposes to yield free enzyme and the reaction products, and that the latter rate determines the over-all rate of substrate-product conversion, i.e., enzyme (E) + substrate (S) ⇌ enzyme + substrate complex (ES) → enzyme + products (P).

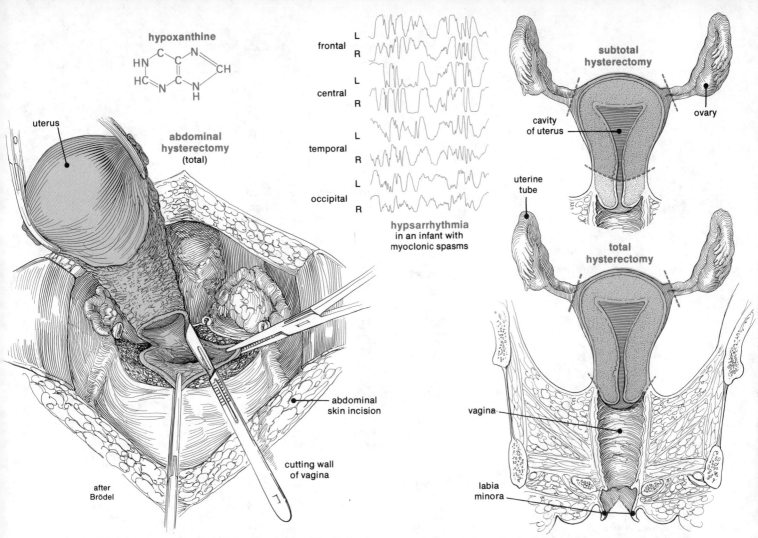

hypoxanthine

abdominal
hysterectomy
(total)

uterus

abdominal
skin incision

cutting wall
of vagina

after
Brödel

frontal L R
central L R
temporal L R
occipital L R

hypsarrhythmia
in an infant with
myoclonic spasms

**subtotal
hysterectomy**

ovary

cavity
of uterus

uterine
tube

**total
hysterectomy**

vagina

labia
minora

---

sequence h., the concept that the amino acid sequence of a protein is determined by a particular sequence of nucleotides in a definite portion of the DNA of the organism producing the protein.

sliding filament h., the assumption that a contracting muscle shortens because two sets of filaments slide past each other.

zwitter h., the supposition that a molecule that behaves as an acid and as a base (ampholytic) yields, in an electrically neutral condition, equal numbers of basic and acid ions, thus becoming an ion (zwitter ion) with an equal number of positive and negative charges.

hypothrombine′mia. Abnormally small amount of thrombin in the blood, resulting in tendency to bleed.

hypothy′roid. 1. Manifested by reduced thyroid function. **2.** A person afflicted with hypothyroidism.

hypothy′roidism. Condition caused by deficient production of thyroid hormone, characterized by a lessened rate of metabolism; clinical features may include cold intolerance, dry skin, hair loss, puffy face, constipation, slow speech, slow heart rate, and retarded mentality; when present at birth it causes cretinism; the severe form is known as myxedema.

hypoto′nia. Lack of muscle tone.

ocular h., abnormally low tension in the eyeball.

hypoton′ic. 1. Having an abnormally reduced tension. **2.** Having the lesser osmotic pressure of two solutions, usually compared to the osmotic concentration of plasma.

hypotoxic′ity. Reduced toxicity.

hypotricho′sis. Scanty hair on the head and body; also called oligotrichosis.

hypotro′pia. Downward deviation of one eye not controllable by fixational efforts; unlike hypophoria, the condition is constant.

hypoventila′tion. Reduced quantity of air entering the lungs.

hypovitamino′sis. Condition marked by deficiency of one or more essential vitamins.

hypovole′mia. Markedly diminished blood volume.

hypovol′ia. Reduced water content of a particular compartment.

hypoxan′thine. A purine present in muscles and other tissues; normally metabolized to uric acid by oxidation, after first being oxidized to xanthine; also called 6-hydroxypurine.

hypoxe′mia. Abnormally low content of oxygen in the arterial blood; also called anoxemia.

hypox′ia. See anoxia.

hypsarrhyth′mia. Abnormal chaotic encephalogram sometimes observed in infants with spasms.

hypsi-, hypso-, Combining form denoting a relationship to height.

hyster-. See hystero-.

hysteral′gia. Pain or discomfort in the uterus.

hysteratre′sia. Pathologic closure of the uterine cavity.

hysterec′tomy. Removal of the uterus.

abdominal h., removal of the uterus through an incision in the abdominal wall.

cesarean h., caesarean h., delivery of a baby through an abdominal and uterine incision, followed by removal of the uterus through the abdominal incision.

subtotal h., removal of the body of the uterus leaving the cervix in place.

total h., removal of the entire uterus.

vaginal h., removal of the uterus through the vagina.

hystere′sis. 1. The failure of coincidence of two associated phenomena, such as the difference between the solidification temperature and the melting temperature of a reversible hydrocolloid. **2.** The lag of a magnetic effect behind its cause.

hyste′ria. An illness resulting from emotional conflict, characterized by lack of control over acts and emotions and other mental and physical symptoms not of organic origin; it is derived from the Greek word for womb, *hystera*, because the illness was originally thought to be caused by disturbances of the uterus.

hyster′ical. Characterized by or pertaining to hysteria.

hyster′ics. Colloquial term for an uncontrollable emotional outburst.

hystero-, hyster-. Combining form indicating the uterus; e.g., hysterotomy.

hysterocol′poscope. Instrument used to inspect the uterine cavity and vagina.

hys′terogram. An x-ray of the uterus utilizing contrast material.

hysterog′raphy. Roentgenography of the uterine cavity after filling it with radiopaque material.

hys′terolith. A calculus of the uterus.

hysterom′eter. A graduated sound for measuring the depth of the uterine cavity.

hysteromyo′ma. A benign tumor of the uterine wall.

hysteromyomec′tomy. Surgical removal of a myoma from the uterus.

hysteromyot′omy. Incision into the muscular wall of the uterus.

hys′tero-oophorec′tomy. Surgical removal of the uterus and ovaries; also called hystero-oothectomy.

hys′teropexy. See ventrofixation of uterus.

hysteror′rhaphy. See ventrofixation of uterus.

hysterosalpingec′tomy. The surgical removal of the uterus and at least one uterine tube.

hysterosalpin′gogram. A roentgenogram detailing the internal structures of the uterus and uterine (fallopian) tubes.

hysterosalpingog′raphy. Roentgenography of the uterus and uterine tubes following the injection of a radiopaque material.

hysterosal′pingo-oophorec′tomy. Surgical removal of the uterus, uterine tubes, and ovaries; also called hysterosalpingo-oothecectomy.

hys′teroscope. A uterine endoscope used for direct visual examination of the cavity of the uterus and cervix.

hysterostomat′omy. An obstetrical surgical procedure; see Dührssen's incisions, under incision.

hysterot′omy. Surgical incision of the uterus.

hysterotrachelec′tomy. Surgical removal of the uterine cervix.

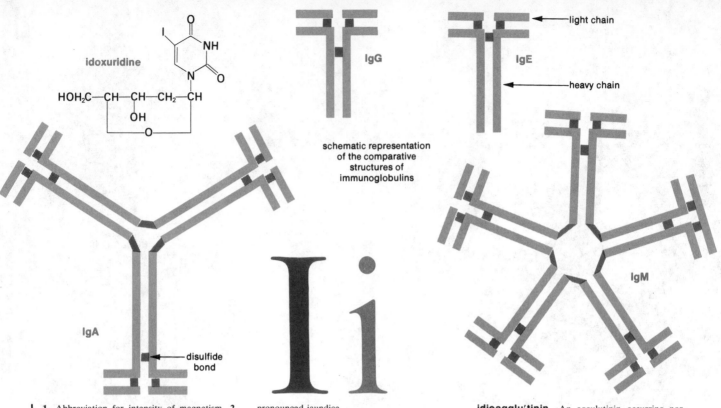

idoxuridine

IgG

IgE

light chain

heavy chain

schematic representation
of the comparative
structures of
immunoglobulins

IgM

IgA

disulfide
bond

I. 1. Abbreviation for intensity of magnetism. **2.** Symbol for (a) electric current; (b) the element iodine; (c) ionic strength; (d) luminous intensity.

^{125}I. Symbol for the radioactive isotope of iodine which has a half-life of 57.4 days.

^{131}I. Symbol for the radioactive isotope of iodine which has a half-life of 8.05 days.

-ia. Suffix signifying a pathologic condition; e.g., hyperplasia, onychia.

IANC. Abbreviation for International Anatomical Nomenclature Committee.

-iasis. Suffix meaning a pathologic condition or state.

-iatrics. Combining form meaning medical treatment; e.g., geriatrics.

iatrogen'ic. Caused by a physician; said of an illness unwittingly induced in a patient by the physician's attitude, treatment, or comments.

iatrog'eny. Abnormal condition caused by a physician.

iat'rotechnique'. Medical and surgical techniques.

-iatry. Combining form meaning medical treatment.

IC. Abbreviation for inspiratory capacity.

-ic. 1. A suffix indicating that the chemical element to which it is added has the higher valence of two possible states. Cf. -ous. **2.** Adjectival ending meaning of, pertaining to, or characteristic of; e.g., dermatologic, psychiatric.

ICD. Abbreviation for International Classification of Diseases of the World Health Organization.

ICDA. Abbreviation for International Classification of Diseases, adapted for use in the United States.

ice. Water in a solid state.

Iceland disease. Epidemic neuromyasthenia; see under neuromyasthenia.

ich'thyoid. Fish-shaped.

ichthyo'siform. Relating to the shape, characteristics, or likeness of ichthyosis.

ichthyo'sis. A disease marked by dry, rough, scaly skin, caused by a congenital defect of the horny layer of the skin; also called fishskin disease and xeroderma.

ichthyotox'in. A toxic substance present in eel serum.

ICP. Abbreviation for intracranial pressure.

-ics. Suffix denoting the science, practice, or treatment of; e.g., genetics.

ICS. Abbreviation for intercostal space.

ICSH. Abbreviation for interstitial cell stimulating hormone.

ic'tal. Relating to a convulsion.

icter'ic. Relating to or having jaundice.

icterogen'ic. Causing jaundice.

icterohepati'tis. Inflammation of the liver with pronounced jaundice.

ic'terus. Jaundice; yellow pigmentation of the skin and/or sclera due to high concentration of bilirubin in the blood.

physiologic i., physiologic jaundice; see under jaundice.

ic'tus, *pl.* **ic'tuses.** A stroke, beat, or sudden convulsion.

i. epilepticus, an epileptic convulsion.

ICU. Abbreviation for intensive care unit.

-id. Suffix indicating (1) a skin rash, e.g., syphilid; (2) a family relationship, e.g., hominid; (3) a small specimen, e.g., spermatid.

id. 1. In Freudian theory, the part of the personality structure associated with the unconscious instinctive impulses and primitive needs of the individual. **2.** A biologic germ structure, supposed to carry the hereditary qualities. **3.** See reaction, id.

-ide. In chemistry, a suffix denoting a binary compound; e.g., hydrogen chloride.

ide'a. A conception existing in the mind as the product of mental activity.

compulsive i., an inappropriate idea that recurs and persists despite reason.

fixed i., a loosely used term to describe a compulsive drive, an obsession, or a delusion; also called idée fixe.

ide'al. A conception regarded as a standard of perfection.

ego i., the part of the personality comprising the goals of the self; it usually refers to the emulation of significant individuals with whom the person has identified.

idea'tion. The formation of ideas or conceptions; indicative of an individual's ability to think.

idée fixe. French for fixed idea.

identifica'tion. A defense mechanism in which a person unconsciously tries to pattern himself after another; distinguished from imitation, which is a conscious process.

iden'tity. The role of a person in society and his perception of it.

ego i., the ego's sense of its own identity.

gender i., the anatomic-sexual identity of an individual.

sense of i., a person's sense of his own selfhood.

ideo-. Combining form relating to ideas.

ideoglan'dular. Eliciting glandular secretions through mental images or thoughts.

ideol'ogy. The intellectual-moral ideas reflecting the needs and aspirations of an individual or group.

ideomo'tion. Muscular movements influenced by a dominant idea.

idio-. Combining form meaning peculiar to; individual.

idioagglu'tinin. An agglutinin occurring normally in the blood of a person or an animal.

id'iocy. Obsolete term for mental retardation; see under retardation.

amaurotic familial i., cerebral sphingolipidosis; see under sphingolipidosis.

idiogen'esis. The origin of an idiopathic disease (one without apparent cause).

id'iogram. A diagrammatic representation of the chromosomal constitution (karyotype) of an organism.

idioheteroagglu'tinin. An agglutinin occurring normally in the blood of one animal (idioagglutinin), but capable of combining with the antigen of another species.

idioisoagglu'tinin. An agglutinin occurring in the blood of an animal (idioagglutinin) of a certain species, capable of agglutinating the cells from animals of the same species.

idiol'ysin. A lysin occurring naturally in the blood of a person or an animal.

idioneuro'sis. A neurosis originating without an apparent cause.

idiono'dal. Arising in the atrioventricular (A-V) node itself.

idiopath'ic. Denoting a disease of unknown cause.

idiophren'ic. Relating to or originating in the mind or brain exclusively, i.e., neither reflex nor secondary.

idiosyn'cracy. 1. A characteristic (physical or behavioral) peculiar to an individual. **2.** A susceptibility, peculiar to an individual, to the action of certain drugs or foods.

idiosyncrat'ic. Of or relating to an idiosyncracy.

id'iot. Obsolete term for retardate.

mongolian i., a person afflicted with Down's syndrome or mongolism.

i.-savant, a mentally retarded individual capable of performing certain remarkable mental tasks, such as solving difficult mathematical problems almost instantly, remembering a variety of facts, etc.

idioventric'ular. Relating to the cardiac ventricles alone, as a cardiac rhythm originating from a ventricular focus.

idoxu'ridine. An antiviral agent used locally for the treatment of herpes simplex infection of the eye.

IDP. Abbreviation for inosine 5'-diphosphate.

Ig. Abbreviation for immunoglobulin.

IgA. Abbreviation for immunoglobulin A (γA globulin); see under immunoglobulin.

IgE. Abbreviation for immunoglobulin E (γE globulin); see under immunoglobulin.

IgG. Abbreviation for immunoglobulin G (γG globulin); see under immunoglobulin.

IgM. Abbreviation for immunoglobulin M (γM

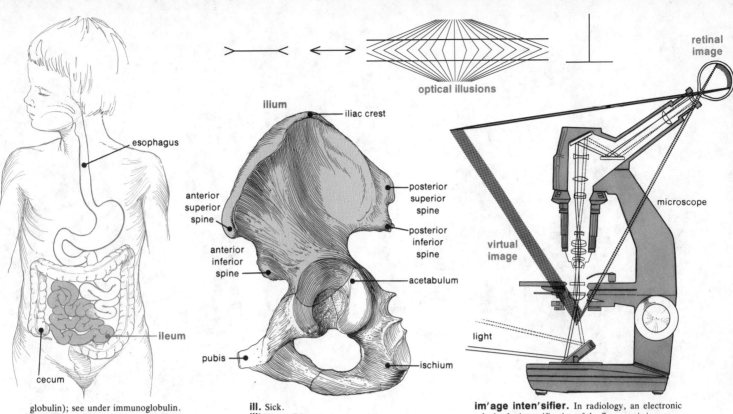

optical illusions

ilium

iliac crest

esophagus

anterior
superior
spine

anterior
inferior
spine

pubis

ileum

cecum

posterior
superior
spine

posterior
inferior
spine

acetabulum

ischium

retinal
image

microscope

virtual
image

light

globulin); see under immunoglobulin.

IH. Abbreviation for infectious hepatitis.

Ile. Symbol for the isoleucine radical.

il'eal. Relating to the ileum.

ilei'tis. Inflammation of the ileum.

  backwash i., inflammation and ulceration of the ileum occurring as an extension of ulcerative colitis.

  regional i., see enteritis, regional.

  terminal i., see enteritis, regional.

ileo-. Combining form indicating a relationship to the ileum.

ileoce'cal. Relating to the ileum and cecum.

ileocecos'tomy. Surgical connection of the ileum and the cecum.

ileoce'cum. The ileum and cecum taken as a whole.

ileocol'ic. Relating to the ileum and the colon.

ileocoli'tis. Inflammation of the ileum and colon.

ileocolos'tomy. Surgical connection of the ileum and colon.

ileoileos'tomy. Surgical connection of two non-continuous portions of the ileum.

ileojejuni'tis. Inflammation of the ileum and jejunum.

ileos'tomy. Surgical establishment of an opening or fistula into the ileum.

ileot'omy. Surgical incision of the ileum.

ileotransversos'tomy. Surgical joining of the ileum and transverse colon.

il'eum. The portion of the small intestine between the jejunum and the cecum; the preferred site for vitamin B_{12} absorption.

il'eus. Obstruction of the intestines accompanied by severe colicky pain, vomiting, and sometimes fever.

  gallstone i., a mechanical intestinal obstruction caused by impaction of one or more gallstones within the bowel lumen.

  meconium i., ileus in the newborn due to obstruction caused by excessively thick meconium; frequently the first evidence of cystic fibrosis.

  paralytic i., ileus resulting from paralysis of the intestinal walls.

il'iac. Relating to the ilium.

ilio-. Combining form meaning ilium.

iliofem'oral. Relating to the ilium and the femur.

ilioing'uinal. Relating to the iliac region and the groin.

iliolum'bar. Relating to the iliac and the lumbar regions.

iliopectin'eal. Relating to the bones ilium and pubis.

il'ium. The superior, broad portion of the hipbone which comprises one of the lateral halves of the pelvis.

ill. Sick.

ill'ness. Disease.

  functional i., see disorder, functional.

  mental i., see disorder, mental.

  terminal i., a sickness that ends in death.

illumina'tion. 1. The process by which light is made to fall on a surface. **2.** In microscopy, the light thrown upon the object to be examined.

  critical i., in microscopy, the focusing of the light source directly on the specimen, creating a narrow, intense light beam.

  dark-field i., illumination of a microscopic specimen by a hollow cone of light; the vertically directed light rays are blocked by a black circular shield and the peripheral rays are directed toward the specimen; the object appears bright on a dark background.

  direct i., one in which the object is illuminated by a beam of light falling almost perpendicular upon it; also called vertical illumination.

  vertical i., see direct illumination.

illumina'tor. In a microscope, the source of light which illuminates the specimen to be viewed.

illu'sion. A false perception of reality.

  optical i., an erroneous interpretation of a visual sensation.

I.M., i.m. Abbreviation for intramuscularly; usually pertaining to an injection.

im'age. 1. A reproduction of the appearance of an object formed by the rays of light emanating from or reflected from it. **2.** A representation or picture of someone or something not present, formed in the mind from memory.

  after-i., afterimage.

  double i., two images of a single object, as formed perceptually in diplopia.

  hypnopompic i., imagery occurring after the sleeping state and before complete awakening, as when a dream figure persists in waking life.

  mental i., image (2).

  mirror i., an image with right and left parts reversed, as the relationship of an object to its image in a mirror.

  real i., an image, formed by converging light rays, which can be seen by inserting a screen, such as a ground glass, into the optical system, or which can be recorded on a photographic plate; the opposite of virtual image.

  retinal i., the image formed on the surface of the retina by the refracting system of the eye.

  virtual i., an image in which light, originating from a point on the object, and having traversed an optical system, appears to be diverging; it cannot be demonstrated on a screen or photographic plate as in the case of a real image.

im'age inten'sifier. In radiology, an electronic device for intensification of the fluoroscopic image.

imbal'ance. Lack of equality or balance.

  autonomic i., imbalance between the sympathetic and parasympathetic nervous systems.

im'becile. Obsolete term for mentally retarded.

imbed'. Variant of embed.

imbibit'ion. The absorption of a fluid, as the taking up of water by a gel.

imbrica'tion. 1. An overlapping of the free edges of tissue in the closure of a wound or the repair of a defect. **2.** A regular overlapping of a surface, as the slight, horizontal, scalelike ridges on the cervical third of the labial surface of some anterior teeth.

imidaz'ole. A heterocyclic compound occurring in histidine; also called glyoxaline.

im'ide. Any compound containing the radical group $=NH$ attached to one bivalent acid radical or two univalent acid radicals.

imido. Relating to the presence of the group $=NH$ attached to acid radicals.

imino. Relating to the presence of the group $=NH$ attached to nonacid radicals.

im'ino acids. Compounds containing both an acid group and an imino group.

imip'ramine hydrochlo'ride. A white crystalline substance, soluble in water; used to treat depression; Tofranil®.

immature'. Not fully developed.

immer'sion. The submerging of an object in a liquid.

  oil i., in microscopy, the use of a layer of oil between the objective and the specimen.

  water i., in microscopy, the use of a layer of water between the objective and the specimen.

immis'cible. Incapable of being mixed; e.g., oil and water.

immobiliza'tion. The act of impeding movement.

immo'bilize. To render incapable of being moved; to fix.

immune'. The state of being secure against harmful effects from pathogenic agents or influences; having immunity.

immune clearance. See clearance, immune.

immune complex disease. A hypersensitivity reaction marked by deposition of antigen-antibody-complement complexes within tissues, especially vascular endothelium.

immune-deficiency syndrome. A group of signs and symptoms indicating impairment of one or more of the major functions of the immune system; i.e., protection against infection (defense), preservation of uniformity of a given cell type (homeostasis), or the removal of malignant cells (surveillance).

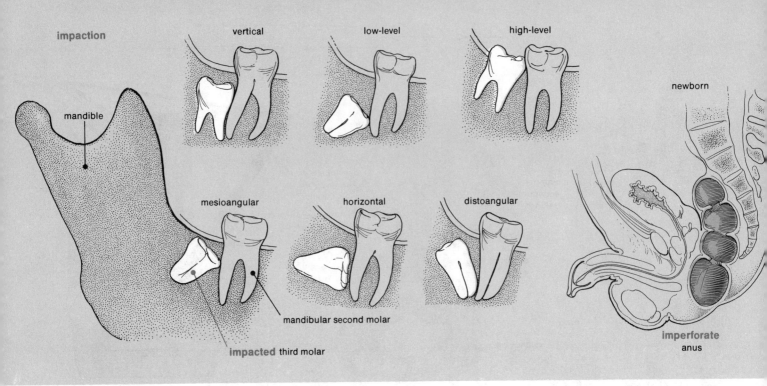

impaction

vertical   low-level   high-level

mandible

mesioangular   horizontal   distoangular

newborn

mandibular second molar

impacted third molar

imperforate
anus

immune response. See response, immune.
immu'nity. 1. The physiologic state which makes the body able to recognize materials as foreign to itself and to neutralize, eliminate, or metabolize them with or without injury to its own tissues. **2.** An inherited, acquired (naturally or artificially), or induced conditioning to a specific pathogen.
  acquired i., immunity acquired after birth.
  active i., immunity acquired as the result of having had a given infectious disease, or by inoculation with a modified form of the causative agent.
  adoptive i., immunity produced by the administration of immune lymphoid cells.
  cell-mediated i., specific immune response conducted by antigen-sensitized lymphocytes; also called cellular immunity.
  congenital i., immunity present at birth.
  local i., immunity manifested by some organs, tissues, or regions of the body.
  passive i., immunity due to receipt of maternal antibody or injection of antibody.
immuniza'tion. The act or process by which a person becomes resistant or immune to a harmful agent.
  active i., the promotion of antibodies when the injected antigen comes in contact with the plasma cells, reticuloendothelial cells, and large lymphoyctes.
  passive i., transient immunization obtained by injection of serum or γ-globulin from an animal or human already rendered immune.
im'munize. The process of making an individual resistant or immune to a harmful agent.
immuno-. Combining form denoting immunity.
immunoagglutina'tion. Agglutination brought about by antibody.
immunochem'istry. The chemistry of immunologic processes.
immunoconglu'tinins. Conglutinins synthesized in response to antigenic stimulation; these antibodies react with certain antigens masked in molecules of native complement and exposed after the components of complement have been fixed on the antigen-antibody complex.
im'munocyte. A lymphoid cell capable of reacting with antigen to produce a specific cell product called antibody.
immunoelectrophore'sis. A form of electrophoresis which in addition employs immune precipitation (antigen-antibody reaction); also called immunophoresis.
immunofluores'cence. The use of fluorescein-labeled antibodies to identify antigenic material specific for the labeled antibody.
immu'nogen. An antigen which stimulates specific immunity.

immunogenet'ics. The study of all the factors controlling immunologic reactions and the transmission of antigenic specificities from generation to generation.
immunogen'ic. 1. Producing immunity. **2.** Relating to an immunogen.
immunoglob'ulin (Ig). A protein molecule functioning as a specific antibody; it brings about the humoral phase of immunity; also called immunoprotein.
  i. A, IgA, the second most abundant class of immunoglobulins; present in secretions and produced especially by lymphoid tissues in the lining of the respiratory, gastrointestinal, and urogenital tracts.
  i. E, IgE, a reaginic antibody that has ability to attach to the skin and initiate immediate hypersensitivity reactions.
  i. G, IgG, the most abundant class of immunoglobulins; present in human serum, they provide immunity to bacteria, viruses, parasites, and fungi which have a blood-borne dissemination.
  i. M, IgM, a class comprised of the largest immunoglobulin molecule (molecular weight 900,000); present in human serum, they agglutinate particulate antigens, such as bacteria and red blood cells.
immunohematol'ogy. The branch of hematology concerned with antigen-antibody reactions and their effect on the blood.
immunologic reaction. The reaction that takes place between an antigen and its antibody; also called immunoreaction.
immunol'ogist. A specialist in immunology.
immunol'ogy. The study of specific processes by which the host maintains constancy of his internal environment when confronted by substances which are recognized as foreign, whether generated from within the host or introduced from the outside.
immunopathol'ogy. The study of disorders caused by antigen-antibody reactions.
immunopharmacol'ogy. The study of drugs and their effects on the immune process and the formation and release of the chemical mediators involved in the genesis of immune injury.
immunoprophylax'is. Prevention of disease through the use of vaccines.
immunopro'tein, immunpro'tein. See immunoglobulin.
immunoreac'tion. See immunologic reaction.
immunoselec'tion. Selective death or survival of fetuses of different genotypes depending on immunologic incompatibility with the mother.
immunosuppres'sion. The modification of the immune response, in a negative way, so it will have a diminished reaction to a foreign substance.

immunosuppres'sive. 1. Modifying the immune response, in a negative way, so it will have a diminished reaction to a foreign substance. **2.** A drug with such a capability.
immunother'apy. 1. Passive immunization through the use of serum or γ-globulin which confers temporary protection to one host by the introduction of antibodies actively produced in another. **2.** The replacement of immunocompetent tissues, e.g., bone marrow, fetal thymus, or other products, in restoring immunocompetence to immune deficient individuals. **3.** The treatment of allergic respiratory disease by injections of extracts of antigens responsible for the illness; formerly known as desensitization or hyposensitization.
immunotol'erance. Immunologic tolerance; see under tolerance.
im'pact. The sudden striking of one body against another.
impact'. To press firmly together.
impac'tion. Tightly wedged together or firmly lodged so as to be immovable.
  ceruminal i., accumulation of earwax in the external auditory canal.
  dental i., condition in which a tooth is so placed in the alveolus as to be incapable of complete eruption.
impair'ment. Damage resulting from injury or disease.
  conduction hearing i., see under hearing.
  hearing i., see under hearing.
  mental i., intellectual defect as manifested by psychologic tests and diminished effectiveness (social and vocational).
impal'pable. Imperceptible to the touch; unable to be grasped or felt.
impa'tent. Closed.
impe'dance. A measure of the total opposition to the flow of electric current in an alternating-current circuit.
imper'forate. Abnormally closed.
imper'meable. Not allowing the entrance of fluids or particular types of ionic or nonionic substances.
impersistence, motor. The loss of ability to sustain a movement.
impeti'go. Contagious skin disease marked by the formation of pustules and caused by staphylococci or streptococci; it occurs mainly in children; the lesions appear as small reddish spots which readily become vesicles and burst, forming a characteristic crust; touching the blisters usually spreads the infection.
im'petus. In psychoanalysis, the motor constituent of an instinct.

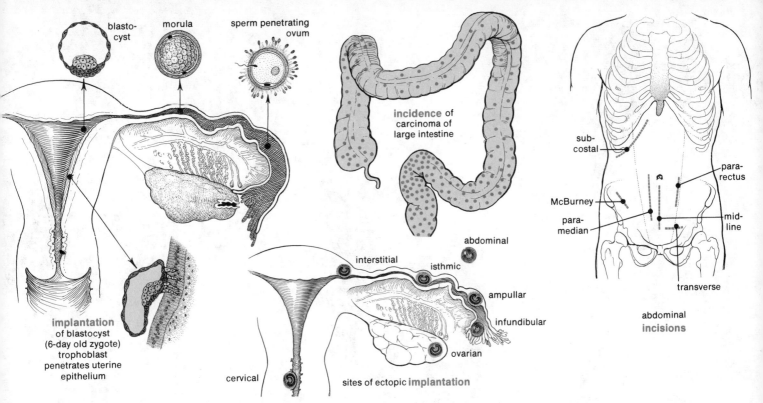

blasto-
cyst

morula

sperm penetrating
ovum

implantation
of blastocyst
(6-day old zygote)
trophoblast
penetrates uterine
epithelium

cervical

incidence of
carcinoma of
large intestine

abdominal

interstitial

isthmic

ampullar

infundibular

ovarian

sites of ectopic implantation

sub-
costal

McBurney

para-
median

para-
rectus

mid-
line

transverse

abdominal
incisions

implant′. 1. To graft. 2. The material grafted.

biocompatible i., an implant of material that permits tissue ingrowth.

dental i., any non-living material placed in a dental socket to substitute for a damaged or missing tooth.

i. denture substructure, a metal framework inserted deeply and in contact with the bone to serve as support for an implant denture superstructure.

i. denture superstructure, a denture placed on, and stabilized by, the implant denture substructure.

implanta′tion. 1. Tissue grafting. 2. The embedding of the fertilized ovum.

im′potence. Lack of power; specifically, lack of copulative power in the male due to failure to achieve adequate erection.

impreg′nate. 1. To render pregnant. 2. To saturate.

impres′sion. An imprint made on a surface by pressure.

complete denture i., an impression of the arch for the purpose of making a complete denture.

dental i., a negative likeness of the teeth or other structures of the oral cavity, made of a setting plastic material which is later filled with plaster of Paris, thus obtaining an exact copy of the structures.

final i., in dentistry, the impression used for making the master cast; also called secondary impression.

secondary i., see final impression.

imprint′ing. A particular way of learning occurring during early life and marked by rapid acquisition and tendency to forget easily.

im′pulse. 1. A sudden urge to act. 2. The transference of energy from one neuron to another; a brief action potential in nerve fibers.

cardiac i., the movement of the chest wall produced by cardiac contraction; the point of maximal impulse (PMI) is normally in the fifth intercostal space, on the midclavicular line or somewhat medial.

in-. Prefix denoting (a) not or without, e.g., inaction; (b) in or within, e.g., intubation; (c) intensive action, e.g., impress; (d) a causative function, e.g., imperil; it becomes im- before b, p, or m.

In. Chemical symbol of the element indium.

inac′tivate. To render anything inactive or inert; may be done by using heat or other methods.

inad′equacy. 1. A state of being deficient. 2. A failing.

sexual i., insufficient sexual response (constant or transitory).

inan′imate. Without life.

inani′tion. Debility resulting from lack of food or defect in assimilation.

inappar′ent. Not apparent; said of certain infections.

inartic′ulate. 1. Not articulate; speechless. 2. Not joined; not having functional joints.

inattention, selective. In psychiatry, failure to pay attention to a part of the perceived situation.

in′born. An ambiguous term generally meaning acquired genetically; distinguished from congenital, meaning present at birth.

in′breeding. The mating of closely related individuals, occurring naturally or as a deliberate process for the purpose of preserving desirable characters.

incapari′na. Generic name for a mixture of cereal grains and oilseed meals of a given general range of protein quality, fortified with vitamins and minerals.

incar′cerated. Confined; held fast, as an irreducible hernia.

in′cest. Sexual intercourse between male and female who are blood-related.

inces′tuous. Relating to or involving incest.

in′cidence. The frequency at which an event occurs, such as the number of cases of a disease.

in′cident. 1. A distinct occurrence or event. 2. Falling upon, as incident rays.

incip′ient. Beginning to appear; in an initial stage.

inci′sal. Cutting; pertaining to the cutting edges of the anterior teeth.

incise′. To cut with a knife.

inci′sion. A surgical cut into soft tissue.

Dührssen's i.'s, two or three incisions made on the partially dilated uterine cervix to facilitate delivery of the child.

Halsted's i., see operation, Halsted's.

McBurney's i., an oblique abdominal incision parallel to the fibers of the external oblique muscle, approximately one inch from the anterior superior iliac spine; used in the operation for appendicitis.

inci′sor. Any of the eight front cutting teeth, four in each jaw.

central i., the tooth closest to and on either side of the midsagittal plane of the head, on either jaw.

lateral i., the second tooth, mandibular or maxillary, on either side of the midsagittal plane of the head.

incisu′ra, *pl.* **incisu′rae.** A notch or indentation on any structure; also called incisure.

inci′sure. See incisura.

inclina′tion. 1. A trend or disposition toward a particular condition. 2. The state of being inclined; a leaning or sloping. 3. In dentistry, the angle of the long axis of a tooth from the perpendicular.

inclu′sion. The act of enclosing or the state of being enclosed.

cell i., transient substance in a cell that does not participate in the cell's function; e.g., pigmented granules, crystals, lipids, etc.

dental i., a tooth enclosed in bone and unable to erupt.

fetal i., unequal conjoined twins in which the less developed one is enclosed within the body of the other.

lipid i., see droplet, lipid.

incoher′ent. Disoriented; confused.

incompat′ible. Incapable of being mixed or used simultaneously without undergoing chemical changes or producing undesirable effects, as two types of blood or certain drugs; also called antagonistic.

incom′petence, incom′petency. The state of lacking functional ability.

aortic i. failure of the aortic valve to close tightly, allowing regurgitation of blood into the left ventricle during diastole.

mitral i., defective closure of a mitral valve, allowing regurgitation of blood into the left atrium during systole.

muscular i., defective action of the papillary muscles of the heart, resulting in imperfect closure of a normal valve.

pulmonary i., pulmonic i., imperfect closure of a pulmonic valve, allowing regurgitation of blood into the right ventricle during diastole.

pyloric i., a relaxed state of the pylorus, allowing food to pass from the stomach into the intestine before gastric digestion is completed.

tricuspid i., imperfect closure of a tricuspid valve, allowing regurgitation of blood into the right atrium during systole.

valvular i., failure of one or more heart valves to close completely.

incon′stant. 1. Variable; irregular. 2. In anatomy, denoting a structure that may or may not be present; suggesting a tendency to change; or is given to change of location.

incon′tinence. 1. Inability to control the passage of urine or feces. 2. Lack of sexual self-control.

stress i., involuntary urination occurring during straining, coughing, or sneezing.

incoordina′tion. Inability to produce harmonious voluntary muscular movements.

incorpora′tion. The act of making something part of oneself, either by eating and digesting food or by taking in and adopting knowledge or the attitudes of another person (especially in psychoanalysis).

in′crement. 1. The process of augmenting or increasing. 2. An addition.

incrusta′tion. 1. The formation of a scab. 2. A scab.

incuba′tion. 1. The maintenance of optimal condi-

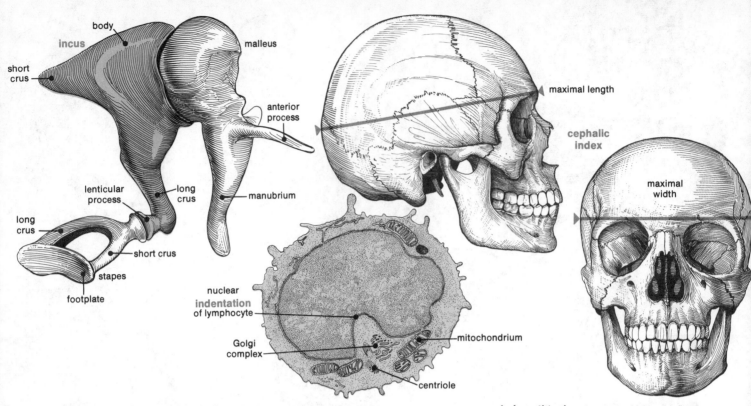

tions of the environment, such as the proper temperature and gas content, for bacterial growth or the development of a premature newborn. **2.** The phase of an infectious disease from the time of introduction to the appearance of the first symptoms.

incuba′tor. One of a variety of apparatuses designed to maintain a constant temperature; used to preserve the life of a premature baby, to grow bacterial cultures, etc.

incu′rable. Not curable.

in′cus. The middle of the three auditory ossicles in the middle ear, situated between the malleus and the stapes; also called anvil.

indenta′tion. 1. A deep recess in a boundary; a notch, dent, or impression. **2.** The act of indenting or notching.

in′dex, *pl.* **in′dexes** or **in′dices. 1.** The forefinger or second digit. **2.** A value expressing the ratio of one measurement to another. **3.** A mold used to record or maintain the relative position of teeth to one another and/or to a cast. **4.** A guide used to reposition teeth, casts, or parts.

  Arneth i., a value obtained by adding the percentages of polymorphonuclear neutrophils with one or two lobes in their nuclei plus one half the percentage of those with three lobes; the normal value is 60 per cent.

  cardiac i., the cardiac output per minute per square meter of body surface.

  cardiothoracic i., the ratio of the maximal transverse diameter of the heart shadow on an x-ray to the maximal transverse diameter of the chest, normally less than one half.

  cephalic i., the ratio of the maximal breadth to the maximal length of the head.

  chemotherapeutic i., the ratio of the minimal effective dose of a drug to the maximal tolerated dose.

  color i. (CI), the ratio of the amount of hemoglobin to the number of red blood cells; also called blood quotient and globular value.

  icterus i., one indicating the amount of bilirubin in the blood.

  maturation i., one used to detect estrogenic activity; it indicates the percentage of mature cells exfoliated from the vagina; the action of an estrogen matures vaginal epithelium; therefore, the higher percentage of mature cells exfoliated suggests increased estrogenic activity.

  nasal i., the ratio of the greatest width of the nose to its length.

  orbital i., the ratio of the height of the orbit to its width.

  pelvic-outlet i., relation of the anteroposterior diameter of the pelvis to the greatest transverse

width across the inlet.

  refractive i. (n), the ratio of the speed of light in a medium of reference (vacuum, air, etc.) to the speed of light in a given medium.

  therapeutic i., the ratio of the dose that is fatal to 50 per cent of test animals (LD_{50}) to the dose that produces the desired effect in 50 per cent of test animals (ED_{50}); used in quantitative comparison of drugs.

  thoracic i., the ratio of the anteroposterior to the transverse diameter of the chest.

  vital i., the ratio of births to deaths in a given population during a given time.

in′dican. 1. A water-soluble glucoside that hydrolyzes to glucose and indoxyl, present in plants yielding the blue dye indigo. **2.** Potassium indoxyl sulfate, a product of decomposition of the amino acid trytophan; formed in the intestines and excreted in the urine.

in′dicant. Serving to indicate, as a symptom that indicates a mode of treatment.

indicanu′ria. The presence of increased indican in the urine; a sign of protein putrefaction mainly in the intestines.

indica′tion. Anything that suggests the proper treatment of a disease.

indica′tor. In chemistry, any of various substances (e.g., litmus) that, by means of changing color, indicate the presence, absence, or concentration of a substance, or the degree of completion of a chemical reaction between two or more substances.

indig′enous. Occurring naturally in an area; also called native.

indiges′tible. 1. Not capable of being digested. **2.** Difficult to digest.

indiges′tion. 1. Discomfort caused by a temporary inability to digest food properly. **2.** Failure of digestion.

  nervous i., indigestion caused by emotional disturbances.

in′digo. A blue dye obtained from plants of the genus *Indigofera* or produced synthetically.

  i. carmine, a blue dye, sodium indigotindisulfonate.

indisposition. Malaise.

in′dium. A soft, silvery-white metallic element; symbol In, atomic number 49, atomic weight 114.82.

in′dium-111 (^{111}In.) A gamma-emitting radionuclide used as a tracer, as in tumor localization.

in′dole. A normal product of protein decomposition in the large intestine; also called ketol.

in′dolent. 1. Sluggish. **2.** Causing little or no pain.

indolic acids. Products of metabolism of the amino acid tryptophan.

indometh′acin. A nonsteroidal anti-inflammatory compound; an inhibitor of prostaglandin synthetase; used in the treatment of rheumatoid arthritis, osteoarthritis, acute gout, and other musculoskeletal disorders; Indocin ®.

induce′. 1. To bring on or about by stimulation; to cause; to effect. **2.** In psychology, to arouse by indirect influence.

indu′cer. A small molecule, usually a substrate of a specific enzyme pathway, capable of combining with the repressor to form an inactive complex that cannot combine with the operator, and as a result permits mRNA synthesis.

induc′tance. A circuit element, typically a conducting coil in which a magnetic field is associated with the circuit when the circuit is carrying current; the unit of induction is the henry (H).

induc′tion. Stimulation of the synthesis of an enzyme from amino acids programmed by a structural gene in the presence of a small inducer molecule.

induc′tor. An agent that brings about induction.

inducto′rium. Instrument designed to generate currents of electricity for stimulation of a nerve or a muscle.

in′durated. Hardened; denoting normally soft tissues that have become abnormally firm.

indura′tion. 1. The hardening of a tissue. **2.** An abnormally hard spot or area.

  black i., pigmentation and hardening of lung tissue, as in pneumonia.

  cyanotic i., one caused by chronic venous congestion of an organ.

indusium griseum. Supracallosal gyrus; see under gyrus.

indwel′ling. Denoting a catheter or drainage tube which is fixed and held in position for a period of time.

ine′briant. Any intoxicating agent; an intoxicant.

inebria′tion. The condition of being intoxicated.

inert′. 1. Slow to move or act; sluggish. **2.** Resisting action. **3.** Devoid of chemical activity, as the inert gases. **4.** Denoting a compound or drug having no therapeutic action.

iner′tia. 1. Resistance offered by a mass to a change in its position of rest or motion. **2.** Denoting inability to move unless stimulated by an external force.

  colonic i., sluggish muscular activity of the colon.

  uterine i., absence of effective uterine contractions during labor.

in extre′mis. Latin for at the point of death.

in′fancy. Babyhood; approximately the first two years of life.

in′fant. A child under the age of two years.

  LBW i., one with a low birth weight.

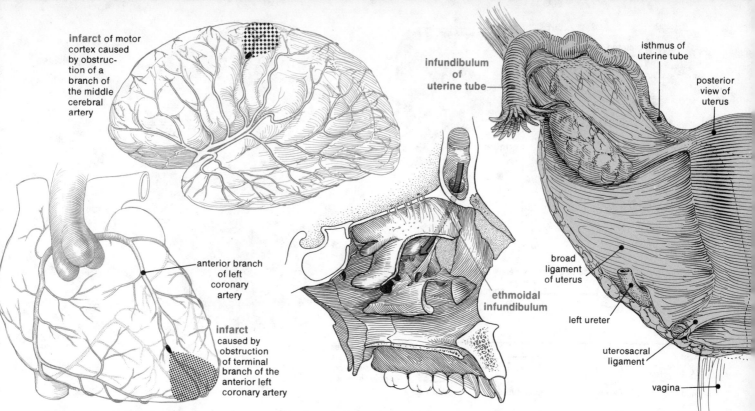

infarct of motor cortex caused by obstruction of a branch of the middle cerebral artery

anterior branch of left coronary artery

infarct caused by obstruction of terminal branch of the anterior left coronary artery

infundibulum of uterine tube

ethmoidal infundibulum

isthmus of uterine tube

posterior view of uterus

broad ligament of uterus

left ureter

uterosacral ligament

vagina

premature i., an infant born after a gestation period of less than the normal length of time; one born before term.

infan'ticide. The killing of an infant.

in'fantile. Relating to an infant.

infantile polycystic disease of kidneys. See polycystic disease of kidney.

infan'tilism. Extremely slow development of mind or body, or both.

in'farct. An area of necrosis in a tissue caused by obstruction in the artery supplying the area.

anemic i., one caused by the sudden interruption of circulation in the terminal artery; also called pale infarct.

hemorrhagic i., an infarct which is red and swollen due to infiltration of blood into the dead area; also called red infarct.

pale i., see anemic infarct.

red i., see hemorrhagic infarct.

infarc'tion. 1. The formation of an infarct. **2.** Infarct.

myocardial i., deterioration and/or death of a portion of the heart muscle as a result of deprivation of its blood supply, usually due to occlusion of the artery supplying blood to the area; the occlusion may or may not be due to a thrombus (blood clot).

pulmonary i., an airless area of lung tissue filled with blood cells as a result of the interruption of the blood supply to the tissues by a clot.

subendocardial myocardial i., one involving the layer of muscle adjacent to the lining of the heart chambers.

transmural i., a myocardial infarction thought to involve the whole thickness of the heart muscle, extending through all layers of the myocardium rather than being restricted to the subendocardial region.

infect'. To contaminate with harmful agents.

infec'tion. Invasion of the body by living microorganisms; it may or may not result in an illness.

clinical i., one that has become sufficiently active to give rise to signs and symptoms of a disease (infectious disease).

focal i., one in which the microorganisms remain in a limited area.

inapparent i., subclinical i., one which is not sufficiently active to give rise to recognizable signs and symptoms of disease.

latent i., a persistent inapparent infection in which the presence of the organism cannot be detected by currently available methods; it flares up from time to time under certain conditions; e.g., a herpes simplex infection (cold sore).

secondary i., one occurring in an individual who is already suffering from a previous infection by another microorganism.

subclinical i., see inapparent infection.

terminal i., an acute infection taking place toward the end of another disease (usually chronic) and generally causing death.

infec'tious. Capable of being transmitted or capable of causing infection.

infecun'dity. Inability of a woman to bear children.

inference, statistical. In biostatistics, the procedure in which a conclusion is made on the basis of a drawn sample; usually a statistic is computed and, from that, a conclusion is formed about the corresponding parameters.

infe'rior. Located in a lower position in relation to another structure.

inferti'lity. The failure to conceive or induce conception, although the potential for reproduction is present.

infest'. To attack or live on a host as a parasite.

infesta'tion. Presence of parasites on the body (e.g., ticks, mites, lice, etc.), or in the organs (e.g., worms).

infil'trate. 1. To pass into the interstices of a tissue or substance, as a cancer. **2.** The material that has infiltrated into the tissue; e.g., a pulmonary infiltrate noted on chest x-ray.

infiltra'tion. The process of seepage or diffusion into tissue of substances that are not ordinarily present; invasion by cells that are not normal to the location.

fatty i., accumulation of fat globules in the cells.

infirm'. Weak in body due to disease or old age.

infir'mary. A dispensary for the care of the sick or injured, especially in a school or camp.

infir'mity. 1. A disabling state of the mind or body. **2.** A disease or condition causing bodily debilitation.

inflamma'tion. A tissue reaction to irritation, infection, or injury, marked by localized heat, swelling, redness, pain, and sometimes loss of function.

inflam'matory. Relating to, marked by, resulting from, or causing inflammation.

infla'tion. The act of distending or the state of being distended by gas or liquid.

inflec'tion, inflex'ion. The act of turning inward, or a state of being turned inward.

influen'za. A contagious infectious disease attributed to a filtrable virus and causing fever, headache, pain in the back and limbs, and inflammation of the respiratory tract; it occurs in epidemics and sometimes pandemics (world epidemics); also called flu and grippe.

infold'. To fold inward.

infra-. A prefix meaning below or beneath; denot-

ing a position below the element indicated by the word to which it is joined; e.g., infrascapular.

infraclavic'ular. Situated below a clavicle (collarbone).

infraclu'sion. Condition in which a tooth fails to erupt; also called infraocclusion.

infrahy'oid. Located below the hyoid bone.

inframandib'ular. Below the lower jaw.

infrana'tant. The clear fluid seen after the flotation of particulate matter in a suspension.

infraocclu'sion. See infraclusion.

infraor'bital. Located beneath or in the floor of the orbit of the eye.

infrapatel'lar. Located below the kneecap (patella), such as a bursa.

infrared'. The electromagnetic radiation beyond the red end of the spectrum, with wavelengths that are too long (greater than 7700 Å) to be seen by the human eye.

infrascap'ular. Located below the scapula (shoulder blade).

infraspi'nous. Located below a spinous process.

infrasplen'ic. Located below or beneath the spleen.

infraster'nal. Below the sternum (breastbone).

infratroch'lear. Located below the pulley (trochlea) of the superior oblique muscle of the eye.

infraumbil'ical. Under the navel.

infundib'uliform. Shaped like a funnel.

infundib'ulum. Latin for funnel; most commonly refers to the funnel-shaped stalk of the pituitary gland.

ethmoidal i., the long, curved, funnel-shaped passage connecting the anterior ethmoid cells and the frontal sinus with the nasal cavity.

i. of uterine tube, the lateral, funnel-shaped extremity of the uterine (fallopian) tube.

infu'sible. 1. Resistant to heat. **2.** Capable of being infused.

infu'sion. 1. The introduction of a fluid into a vessel. **2.** The soaking or steeping of a substance in water in order to extract its soluble parts. **3.** The resulting liquid.

Infuso'ria. Former term for the protozoan class Ciliata.

inges'ta. Food taken into the body.

inges'tion. 1. The introduction of food, drink, or medicines into the stomach. **2.** Process by which a cell or a unicellular organism takes in foreign material.

in'guinal. Pertaining to the groin.

INH. Abbreviation for isonicotinic acid hydrazide; see isoniazid.

inha'lant. A remedy taken by inhalation.

inhala'tion. The act of breathing in; breathing in

infant | inhalation

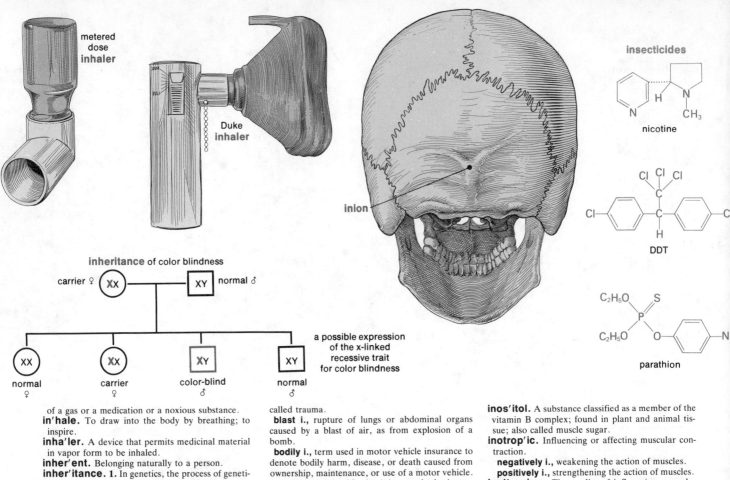

metered
dose
inhaler

Duke
inhaler

inion

insecticides

nicotine

DDT

parathion

inheritance of color blindness

carrier ♀ (XX) ──── (XY) normal ♂

XX normal ♀

XX carrier ♀

XY color-blind ♂

XY normal ♂

a possible expression
of the x-linked
recessive trait
for color blindness

of a gas or a medication or a noxious substance.

in'hale. To draw into the body by breathing; to inspire.

inha'ler. A device that permits medicinal material in vapor form to be inhaled.

inher'ent. Belonging naturally to a person.

inher'itance. 1. In genetics, the process of genetically transmitting characters from parent to offspring. **2.** The characters so transmitted.

dominant i., see gene, dominant.

holandric i., transmission of a character determined by a gene on the Y chromosome, i.e., occurring only in males.

hologynic i., transmission of a trait from mother to all daughters but to no sons, i.e., occurring only in females.

Mendelian i., Mendel's laws; see under law.

mosaic i., inheritance characterized by the dominance of paternal influence in one group of cells and the dominance of the maternal in another.

recessive i., see gene, recessive.

sex-linked i., sex linkage; see under linkage.

inhibition. The restriction or arrest of a function or specific activity.

inhib'itor. An agent or nerve that represses physiologic activity.

allosteric i., a substance that decreases enzymatic activity through noncompetitive binding to the enzyme molecule at a site (allosteric site) other than the active site of the enzyme.

in'ion. The most prominent point of the external occipital protuberance to the skull; used as a fixed craniometric point.

initiator. A substance, necessary to the process of building certain giant molecules, which helps bring about such reactions and, unlike a catalyst, is altered and may appear in the final product.

inject'. To drive a fluid into a part.

inject'able. Any substance that may be injected.

injec'tion. 1. The act of forcing or driving a fluid into a part, such as the subcutaneous tissue or a bodily cavity. **2.** The fluid injected. **3.** The state of being injected; also called congestion and hyperemia.

retrograde i., introduction of a solution into an organ against the normal direction of flow, as injection of a radiopaque solution into the kidney via the ureter.

injec'tor. A device for administering injections.

jet i., a machine that, through high pressure, forces a liquid through a small orifice at high velocity; the liquid is thus able to penetrate the unbroken skin without causing pain.

in'jure. To wound or hurt.

in'jury. A specific bodily damage or wound; also

called trauma.

blast i., rupture of lungs or abdominal organs caused by a blast of air, as from explosion of a bomb.

bodily i., term used in motor vehicle insurance to denote bodily harm, disease, or death caused from ownership, maintenance, or use of a motor vehicle.

countercoup i. of brain, injury to the brain at a site opposite to the point of impact.

whiplash i., a nonspecific term applied to an injury of the spine, usually at the junction of the fourth and fifth cervical vertebrae, caused by an abrupt jerking motion of the head; also called hyperextension-hyperflexion injury.

in'lay. A solid restorative material (gold, fired porcelain, plastic) that is fitted and cemented to a tapered cavity preparation in a tooth.

in'let. A passage that leads to a cavity.

in'nate. Present at birth.

innerva'tion. The nerve supply of a given area or structure.

innidia'tion. The multiplication of cells in a location where they have been carried by lymph or the blood stream.

in'nocent. Benign; said of a tumor.

innoc'uous. Harmless.

innom'inate. Unnamed.

innominate artery. Brachiocephalic trunk; see under trunk.

innominate bone. See hipbone.

innnominate vein. See table of veins.

innox'ious. Harmless; not injurious.

inoc'ulable. 1. Transmissible by inoculation. **2.** Susceptible to a disease which is transmissible by inoculation.

inoc'ulate. To introduce a virus into the body; to introduce vaccines, immune sera, or other antigenic material into the body in order to prevent, cure, or experiment.

inocula'tion. The introduction into the body of disease-causing microorganisms.

therapeutic i., the introduction of an antiserum for curative purposes.

inoc'ulum. Material containing microorganisms introduced by inoculation.

inop'erable. That which cannot be operated upon or which cannot be removed by surgery.

inorgan'ic. Neither composed of nor derived from organic matter (animal or vegetable); designating compounds that do not contain carbon.

inos'culate. To make continuous or unite by small openings or anastomoses.

in'osine 5'-diphos'phate (IDP). A nucleotide which participates in high-energy phosphate transfer.

inos'itol. A substance classified as a member of the vitamin B complex; found in plant and animal tissue; also called muscle sugar.

inotrop'ic. Influencing or affecting muscular contraction.

negatively i., weakening the action of muscles.

positively i., strengthening the action of muscles.

inot'ropism. The quality of influencing muscular contraction.

in'patient. A patient staying overnight in a hospital.

insaliva'tion. The mixing of food with saliva in chewing.

insane. Relating to insanity, or to one who is of unsound mind.

insan'ity. In law, a mental state in which one is legally nonresponsible or incompetent for some or all purposes. Originally a medical term referring to loss of reason, by the end of the 19th century it came to include diseases of the intellect, the will, or the emotions; since the 1920s, the term has not been used in the United States for medical purposes, but continues to have multiple legal meanings, all of which involve some degree of nonresponsibility or incompetence for legal purposes. The law defines different kinds or degrees of insanity (e.g., for making a will, making a business contract, committing criminal acts, or reasonable likelihood of imminent danger to oneself or others); insanity for one act may not necessarily mean insanity for other kinds of acts.

inscrip'tion. The part of a prescription that stipulates the names and amounts of ingredients to be used by the pharmacist. See also superscription, subscription, and signature.

insecta'rium. A place in which living insects are kept and bred for scientific purposes.

insec'ticide. Any agent that kills insects.

insec'tifuge. Any substance that drives away insects.

insemina'tion. 1. Introduction of seminal fluid into the vagina. **2.** Fertilization of an ovum.

artificial i., deposit of seminal fluid in the vagina by means other than sexual intercourse.

insen'sible. 1. Imperceptible by the senses. **2.** Unconscious.

inser'tion. 1. The site of attachment of a muscle to a bone which is more movable than the one from which it originated. **2.** The act of introducing or implanting.

insid'ious. Spreading or developing harmfully in a subtle or imperceptible way; applied to certain diseases.

in'sight. 1. The ability to understand the real nature of a situation. **2.** Self-understanding.

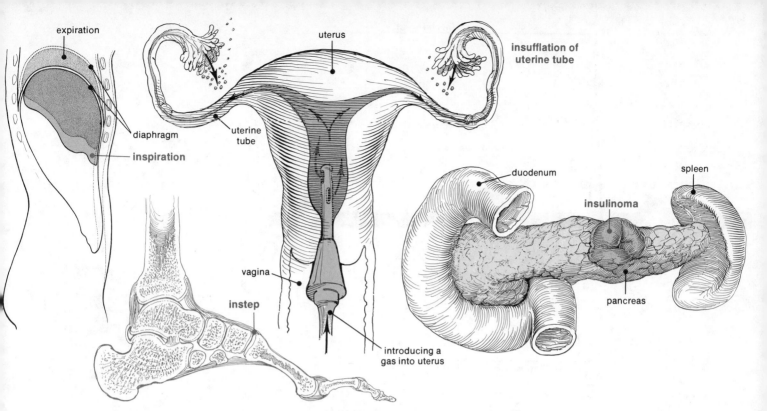

expiration

diaphragm

inspiration

uterus

uterine tube

insufflation of uterine tube

duodenum

insulinoma

spleen

pancreas

vagina

instep

introducing a gas into uterus

in si′tu. Latin for in place.

insol′uble. Not capable of entering into solution.

insom′nia. Inability to sleep under normal conditions; three varieties are recognized: inability to fall asleep upon retiring; intermittent waking after falling asleep; early awakening.

insom′niac. A person suffering from insomnia.

inspira′tion. Breathing in.

inspi′ratory. Relating to inhalation.

inspire′. To inhale; to breathe in.

inspissa′tion. The process of thickening as by evaporation of fluid.

inspis′sator. A device used to air-dry fluids.

in′step. The arched middle part of the dorsum of the human foot.

instilla′tion. The gradual, drop by drop, pouring of a liquid.

in′stinct. An inherent drive or tendency to act in a certain way without the aid of reason.

instrumenta′tion. The utilization of instruments in the treatment of a patient.

in′sudate. The material passed into vessel walls; from Latin, sweating inward.

insuffic′iency. Inability to perform a normal function; said of an organ or structure.

  adrenal i., see Addison's disease.

  aortic i., insufficiency of the aortic valve.

  cardiac i., heart failure; see under failure.

  coronary i., insufficient blood flow to the cardiac muscle, leading to prolonged pain or discomfort (angina).

  mitral i., insufficiency of the mitral valve.

  pulmonary i., insufficiency of the pulmonary valve.

  renal i., defective kidney function, especially a decrease in glomerular filtration manifested by a consequent increase in blood levels of urea and creatinine.

  tricuspid i., insufficiency of the tricuspid valve.

  valvular i., failure of a heart valve to close tightly, thus allowing regurgitation of blood; named according to the valve involved, aortic, mitral, pulmonary, or tricuspid.

  venous i., inadequate drainage of blood from a part, resulting in edema.

insufficiency disease. See disease, deficiency.

insuf′flate. 1. To blow into, as in artificial respiration. **2.** To blow medicated vapor, powder, etc. into a bodily cavity.

insuffla′tion. The act of blowing air, medicated vapor, powder, or anesthetic into a body cavity.

  cranial i., the forcing of air into the ventricles of the brain.

  perirenal i., injection of air or carbon dioxide in the area around the kidneys for roentgen visualiza-

tion of the adrenal glands.

  tubal i., uterotubal i., the passage of a gas, usually carbon dioxide, into the uterus to determine the patency of the uterine (fallopian) tubes.

  uterotubal i., see tubal insufflation.

in′sufflator. Instrument used in insufflation.

in′sula. The central lobe of the cerebrum, lying deeply in the lateral cerebral fissure (fissure of Sylvius); also called island of Reil and central lobe.

in′sular. Relating to an insula, especially the central lobe of the cerebrum (island of Reil).

in′sulate. To prevent the passage of heat, sound, or electricity from one body or region to another by interposing material with nonconductive properties.

insula′tion. 1. The act of insulating. **2.** The material used to insulate. **3.** The state of being insulated.

insula′tor. Any nonconductive material used to effect insulation.

in′sulin. A hormone produced in the islets of Langerhans in the pancreas, concerned with the regulation of carbohydrate metabolism by controlling glucose levels in the blood; it is extracted from the pancreas of beef or pork for use in the treatment of diabetes.

in′sulinase. Enzyme capable of destroying or inactivating insulin.

insulino′ma, insulo′ma. An insulin-producing islet cell adenoma of the pancreas.

in′sult. An injury or irritation.

integra′tion. 1. The condition of being combined. **2.** The process of bringing all parts together to form a whole, as the building up of living substance by assimilation of nutritive material.

integ′ument. A covering or coat, as the skin or the membrane covering an organ; also called tegument.

intel′ligence. 1. The faculty of thought, reason, and understanding. **2.** The ability to acquire and apply knowledge.

  abstract i., the ability to acquire and understand abstract ideas and symbols.

  i. quotient (IQ), see under quotient.

  mechanical i., the ability to acquire knowledge and understanding of technical mechanisms.

  social i., ability to understand and manage social relationships.

intem′perance. Lack of self-restraint, as in the indulgence of alcoholic beverages.

inten′sity. Degree of activity, tension, strength, etc., usually implying a large measure.

inten′sive. Of or characterized by intensity; applied to an exhaustive and concentrated form of treatment.

inten′tion. 1. A process. **2.** Objective.

  healing by first i., the immediate healing of a wound without suppuration or granulation.

  healing by second i., healing by the union of two granulating surfaces after some suppuration has taken place.

  healing by third i., filling of a wound with granulations followed by the formation of scar tissue.

inter-. Prefix meaning between, among.

interac′inous. Between the acini of a gland.

interalve′olar. Between alveoli.

interan′nular. Located between two ringlike structures.

interartic′ular. Located between two joints or joint surfaces.

intera′trial. Situated between the atria of the heart.

interca′dence. The occurrence of an extra pulse beat, between two regular beats.

inter′calary. Occurring between parts; also called interpolated and interposed.

inter′calate. To interpose or insert between others; to interpolate.

interclavic′ular. Located or occurring between the clavicles (collarbones).

intercon′dylar, intercondyl′ic, intercon′-dyloid. Located between two condyles.

intercos′tal. Located or occurring between successive ribs.

in′tercourse. 1. Interchange between individuals. **2.** Coitus.

intercris′tal. Located between two crests.

intercur′rent. Occurring during the course of an already existing disease.

intercuspa′tion. The fitting together or interlocking of the cusps of opposing teeth.

interden′tal. Between the teeth.

interden′tium. The space between two adjacent teeth.

interdig′ital. Between the fingers or toes.

interdigita′tion. 1. Interlocking of structures by means of finger-like processes. **2.** The processes so interlocked.

interepithe′lial. Situated or passing between epithelial cells.

in′terface. A surface forming a common boundary between two bodies.

interfa′cial. Relating to an interface.

interfe′rence. 1. The coming together of waves in various media in such a way that the crests of one series correspond to the hollows of the other; when they cross, they reinforce each other at certain points and neutralize each other at other points. **2.** The collision of two waves of excitation in the myocardium, seen in fusion beats. **3.** In A-V (atrioventricular) dissociation, the disturbance of the rhythm of the heart ventricles by a conducted impulse from the atria. **4.** Superinfection, as occurs when cells are

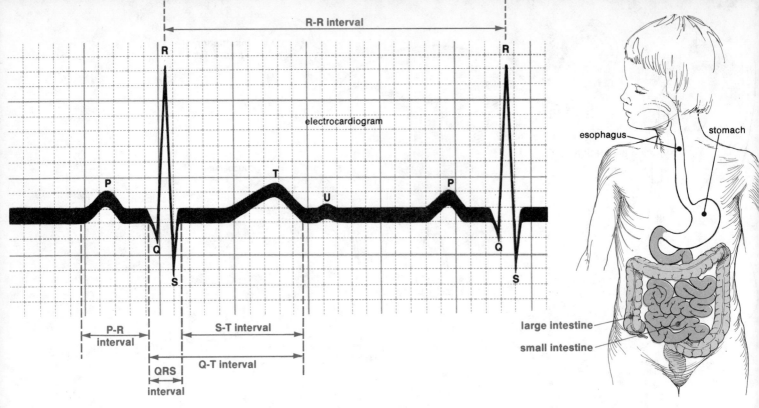

electrocardiogram

R-R interval

P-R interval

S-T interval

QRS interval

Q-T interval

esophagus

stomach

large intestine

small intestine

exposed to two viruses.

interfer′on. A protein substance produced by body cells in response to invasion by viruses and other intracellular parasites; it interferes with the synthesis of new virus and is effective against certain protozoal parasitic infections, such as malaria.

interic′tal. Denoting the interval between convulsions.

interlo′bar. Located between lobes.

interlob′ular. Located between lobules.

interme′diate. 1. Occurring between two extremes. **2.** A substance formed in the course of chemical reactions, which then proceeds to participate rapidly in further reactions, so that at any given moment it is present in minute concentrations only.

metabolic i.'s, substances which appear in the course of the reactions involved in metabolism.

intermediate coronary syndrome. Episodes of precordial pain which are too severe or protracted to be called angina, yet are not accompanied by the symptoms of a myocardial infarction; also called acute coronary insufficiency.

intermens′trual. Denoting the interval between two consecutive menstrual periods.

intermit′tency, intermit′tence. The quality of being recurrent (often at regular intervals); not continuous.

intermus′cular. Located between muscles.

in′tern. A recent medical school graduate who receives supervised practical training by assisting in the medical and surgical care of patients at a hospital.

inter′nal. Located within or on the inside; away from the surface.

International Systems of Units (SI). A complete system of units for international scientific and technologic work; based on the metric system to which are added units of time, electric current, temperature, and luminous intensity; the abbreviation is from the French equivalent, Système International.

interneu′ron. Excitatory or inhibitory neuron in the central nervous system which is situated between the primary afferent neuron and the final motor neuron; it usually has a short range of action.

inter′nist. A specialist in internal medicine.

interno′dal. Between two nodes; applied to the segment of a nerve fiber between two successive nodes.

internu′clear. Between two nuclei.

internun′cial. Denoting a connecting agent or part, as a nerve cell connecting two other nerve cells.

interocep′tor. Any one of the sensory nerve endings which are located in, and receive stimuli from,

visceral tissues and blood vessels.

interos′seous. Connecting or lying between bones.

interphalan′geal. Positioned between two contiguous phalanges of either the fingers or the toes.

in′terphase. The interval between two successive mitotic divisions; the phase when the cell is not dividing; improperly called "resting stage."

in′terplanting. In experimental embryology, the transferring of an embryonic part from one embryo to an indifferent environment in another embryo.

interpreta′tion. In psychoanalysis, the process by which the therapist explains to the patient the meaning of a particular aspect of his problems.

interprox′imal. Between adjacent surfaces, as the space between adjacent teeth in the same dental arch.

interradic′ular. Situated between the roots of a tooth.

interscap′ular. Positioned between the scapulae.

intersep′tal. Situated between two septa.

in′tersex. See hermaphrodite.

intersexual′ity. See hermaphroditism.

in′terspace. Space between two similar structures.

interspi′nal. Between the spinous processes of the vertebrae; also called interspinous.

inter′stice. A minute space in the substances of an organ or tissue.

intersti′tial. Pertaining to or situated in the spaces within a tissue.

intersti′tium. Structures such as fibers, located between bodily parts, that form a supporting framework of tissue which binds organs together.

intertrig′inous. Characterized by or related to intertrigo.

intertri′go. Skin eruption occurring between two adjacent surfaces, as between the scrotum and the thigh.

intertrochanter′ic. Located between the two trochanters of the femur.

in′terval. 1. The lapse of time between two events or between the recurrence of similar episodes of a disease. **2.** A distance between two objects. **3.** A gap in a continuous process.

coupling i., the interval between a premature heart beat and the normal beat preceding it.

lucid i., a period of mental clarity occurring in the course of a mental disorder.

P-P i., the distance between the same points on two consecutive P waves of the electrocardiogram.

P-R i., the atrioventricular conduction time, measured from the beginning of the P wave to the beginning of the QRS complex of the electrocardiogram; it includes the time required for atrial depo-

larization and repolarization plus the normal delay of excitation in the atrioventricular node.

Q-R i., the interval from the beginning of the QRS complex to the peak of the R wave in the electrocardiogram.

QRS i., the duration of the QRS complex, representing the measurement of total ventricular depolarization.

Q-T i., the interval between the onset of the Q wave and the end of the T wave of the electrocardiogram; it measures the duration of electrical systole.

R-R i., the interval between two consecutive QRS complexes of the electrocardiogram.

interver′tebral. Between two vertebrae.

intervil′lous. Located among villi.

intes′tinal. Relating to the intestine or bowel.

intes′tine. The portion of the alimentary canal from the stomach to the anus.

large i., the sacculated portion of the intestine, extending from the ileum to the anus and forming an arch over the convolutions of the small intestines; composed of three parts: cecum, colon, and rectum.

small i., the convoluted portion of the intestine extending from the stomach to the cecum; divisible into three portions: duodenum, jejunum, and ileum.

in′tima. The inner layer of a blood vessel.

in′toed. See pigeon-toe.

intol′erance. Unfavorable reaction to a substance.

hereditary fructose i., metabolic defect due to an autosomal recessive inheritance; marked by a deficiency of fructose 1-phosphate aldolase, causing vomiting and hypoglycemia upon ingestion of fructose; repeated ingestion of fructose by infants with this disorder may result in severe disease; also called fructosemia.

lactose i., intolerance to lactose due to presence of less than the normal amount of the enzyme lactase; manifested by abdominal cramps and diarrhea upon ingestion of milk and milk products.

intor′sion, intor′tion. The real or apparent inward turning of one or both eyes.

intor′tor. A muscle, as an extraocular muscle, that turns a part inward.

intox′icant. An intoxicating agent, especially alcohol.

intoxica′tion. 1. Poisoning. **2.** Acute alcoholism; see under alcoholism.

intra-. Prefix meaning within.

intra-abdom′inal. Situated within the abdomen.

intra-artic′ular. Located within a joint's cavity.

intracap′sular. Within a capsule, especially the capsule of a joint.

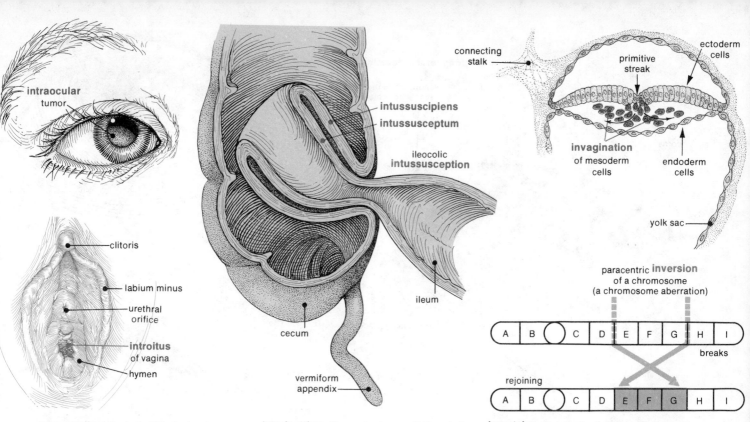

intraocular
tumor

clitoris
labium minus
urethral
orifice
introitus
of vagina
hymen

intussuscipiens
intussusceptum
ileocolic
intussusception

ileum
cecum
vermiform
appendix

connecting
stalk
primitive
streak
ectoderm
cells
invagination
of mesoderm
cells
endoderm
cells
yolk sac

paracentric **inversion**
of a chromosome
(a chromosome aberration)

| A | B | | C | D | E | F | G | H | I |

breaks

rejoining

| A | B | | C | D | E | F | G | H | I |

intracar′diac. Located within the heart.
intracath′eter. A slender plastic tube inserted into a vein for injection, infusion, or venous pressure monitoring.
intracel′lular. Located or occurring within a cell or cells.
intracer′ebral. Within the cerebrum.
intracos′tal. Situated on the inner surface of a rib or ribs.
intracra′nial. Within the skull.
intracuta′neous. Within the layers of the skin.
intrader′mal. Within the dermis (layer of skin also called true skin).
intradu′ral. Situated within the dura mater, the outermost membrane surrounding the brain and spinal cord.
intraepithe′lial. Situated within, or passing through, the epithelial cells.
intrahepat′ic. Located within the liver.
intralu′minal. Within the lumen of a tubule or tubular structure.
intramed′ullary. Within the bone marrow, the spinal cord, or the medulla oblongata.
intramem′branous. Between layers of a membrane.
intramolec′ular. Occurring or located within the molecule.
intramu′ral. Situated within the wall of an organ or cavity.
intramus′cular. Within the substance of a muscle.
intrana′sal. Located or occurring within the nasal cavity.
intraneu′ral. Within a nerve.
intraoc′ular. Within the eyeball.
intrao′ral. Within the mouth.
intraor′bital. Within the orbit.
intraos′seous. Within bone tissue.
intraperitone′al. Within the peritoneal cavity.
intrapsy′chic. Taking place within the mind.
intrapul′monary. Within the lungs.
intrare′nal. Located within the kidney.
intrathe′cal. Within a sheath.
intrathoracic. Within the chest cavity.
intrau′terine. Within the uterus.
intravas′cular. Within the blood or lymphatic vessels.
intrave′nous. Within a vein.
intraventric′ular. Within a ventricle of the heart or brain.
intrin′sic. Belonging or situated entirely within a part.
intro-. Prefix meaning in or into.
introdu′cer. Instrument used to introduce a tube into the trachea; also called intubator.
intro′itus. Entrance into a cavity or hollow organ.

introjec′tion. The unconscious symbolic assimilation of a loved or hated object, making it a part of the self.
intromis′sion. Insertion; introduction.
introspec′tion. Examination of one's own mental processes.
introver′sion. 1. Preoccupation with one's own interests and experiences. **2.** The process of turning an organ or part inward.
in′trovert. One whose thoughts are predominantly about himself.
introvert′. To turn inward.
in′tubate. To introduce a tube into the trachea or the larynx.
intuba′tion. 1. Introduction of a tube into any canal. **2.** Insertion of a tube into the trachea to allow air to enter the lungs.
in′tubator. See introducer.
intumesce′. To swell.
intumes′cence. A swelling.
intumes′cent. Enlarging; swelling.
intussuscept′. To turn inward.
intussuscep′tion. Condition in which one part of the intestine becomes pushed into the lumen of an adjoining segment; it occurs chiefly at the iliocecal junction, causing acute abdominal symptoms; seen most commonly among children.
intussuscep′tum. The inner or ensheathed segment of intestine in an intussusception.
intussuscip′iens. The outer portion of intestine surrounding the inner segment in an intussusception.
in′ulin. A fructose polysaccharide found in the roots and underground stems of several plants; used in kidney function tests as a measure of glomerular filtration rate, since it is filtered at the glomerulus, and neither secreted nor reabsorbed by the tubules.
inunc′tion. 1. The rubbing or smearing of a drug, in ointment form, into the skin. **2.** Ointment.
in u′tero. Latin for within the uterus.
in vac′uo. Latin for in a vacuum.
invag′inate. To turn within or enclose; to ensheathe; to infold one part within another part of the same structure.
invagina′tion. Ensheathing or infolding of a part within itself.
in′valid. A person disabled by a chronic illness or infirmity.
inva′sion. 1. The spread of a malignant tumor to adjacent tissues. **2.** The beginning of a disease.
inva′sive. Having a tendency to spread or to invade healthy tissue.
inventory, personality. A psychological test for evaluation of personal characteristics; usually a checklist answered by the person about himself.

inver′sion. 1. A turning inside out. **2.** Any reversal of the normal relation with other organs. **3.** In psychiatry, homosexuality. **4.** In genetics, a chromosome aberration resulting from fragmentation of a chromosome by two breaks, followed by a turning end for end of the fragment and refusion.
i. of the uterus, a turning of the uterus inside out, exposing the lining membrane (endometrium).
invert′. To turn upside down.
in′vertase. An enzyme that converts sucrose into glucose and fructose; found in the small intestine; also called sucrase.
Invertebra′ta. A division of the animal kingdom comprised of animals without spinal columns.
inver′tebrate. An animal that does not have a spinal column.
inver′tor. A muscle that turns a part inward.
in′vertose. Invert sugar; a mixture of equal parts of glucose and fructose.
invest′. To envelop; to cover completely.
invest′ing. 1. In dentistry, the process of covering an object, such as a wax pattern of a tooth restoration or a denture, with a refractory investment material before casting or curing. **2.** In psychoanalysis, affecting an object with psychic energy or cathexis.
vacuum i., forming a mold around a pattern in a vacuum in order to avoid trapping air in the investment material.
invest′ment. 1. Any material used to invest an object. **2.** In psychoanalysis, the affective charge invested in or given to an idea or object.
casting i., the material from which the mold is made in fabrication of a metal cast.
refractory i., any material which can withstand the high temperatures used in soldering or casting.
in vitro. In an environment outside of the body, usually in a test tube or similar artificial environment.
in vivo. Within the living body.
involu′crum. An enveloping sheath of new bone, such as that developed around a necrosed bone as a response to infection.
invol′untary. 1. Performed independently of one's own free will. **2.** Not performed willingly.
involu′tion. A retrograde process resulting in lessening in the size of a tissue, as the return to normal size of the uterus after childbirth, or the shrinking of organs and tissues in old age.
involu′tional. Relating to involution.
i′odate. 1. A salt of iodic acid. **2.** To iodize.
io′derma. Any cutaneous reaction caused by iodine and compounds thereof; lesions may vary from mild acneform to granulomatous.
iod′ic acid. A white or colorless crystalline powder, HIO_3; used as an antiseptic and deodorant.

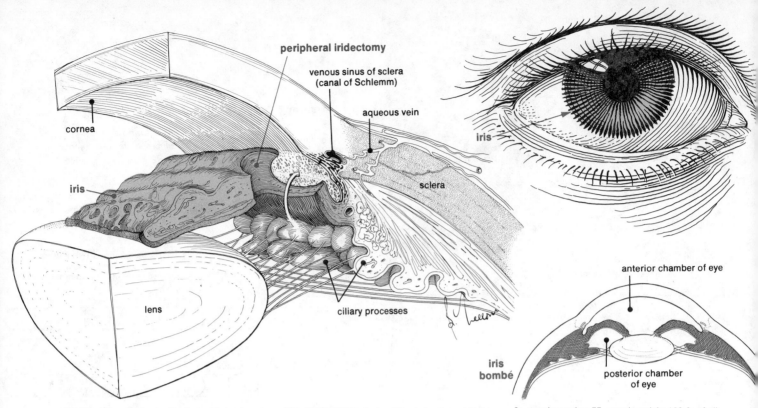

peripheral iridectomy

venous sinus of sclera (canal of Schlemm)

aqueous vein

cornea

iris

iris

sclera

lens

ciliary processes

anterior chamber of eye

iris bombé

posterior chamber of eye

---

i'odide. A compound of iodine with another element, especially with potassium or sodium.

iodim'etry. See iodometry.

i'odine. A lustrous, grayish-black, corrosive, nonmetallic element; symbol I, atomic number 53, atomic weight 126.91; used as an antiseptic and in the diagnosis and treatment of thyroid disease; it has no natural isotopes; its most widely used artificial isotopes are ^{131}I and [125]I.

   protein-bound i. (PBI), thyroid hormone in its circulating form, consisting of one or more of the iodothyronines bound to one or more of the serum proteins; also called serum protein-bound iodine.

i'odine-125 (^{125}I). One of the lower energy isotope-labeled agents used as a tracer in thyroid studies and as therapy in hyperthyroidism; has a half-life of 57.4 days.

i'odine-131 (^{131}I). A beta-emitting radioactive iodine isotope used as a tracer, as in thyroid studies and in brain tumor localization; has a half-life of 8.05 days.

i'odism. Poisoning from the prolonged use of iodine or an iodide.

i'odize. To treat or combine with iodine.

iodochlor'hydrox'yquin. Compound used topically for a variety of skin disorders; also used as an amebicide; Vioform®.

io'doform. A lemon-yellow iodine compound used as an antiseptic.

iodohippurate sodium. A radiopaque compound used in radiography of the urinary tract.

iodom'etry. The volumetric determination of the amount of iodine in a compound; also called iodimetry.

iodophil'ia. Affinity for iodine; said of certain cells.

iodop'sin. A color-sensitive violet pigment composed of a vitamin A derivative and a protein; present in the cones of the retina and important in color vision; also called visual violet.

i'on. An atom or group of atoms or molecules having acquired an electric charge by gaining (cations) or losing (anions) electrons.

   dipolar i., an ion that carries both a positive and a negative charge; amino acids are the most notable dipolar ions, containing the positively charged NH_3 group and the negatively charged COO group; also called zwitterion.

   i. pair, two particles of opposite charge formed during the interaction of radiation and matter.

ion exchange. Chemical reaction between an insoluble solid and a solution surrounding the solid through which ions of like charge are interchanged; used in the separation of radioactive isotopes and in water softening.

ion exchanger. 1. A solid substance used in ion exchange. **2.** Apparatus used to effect ion exchange.

ion'ic. Of, containing, or relating to an ion or ions.

ioniza'tion. Production of ions (electrically charged atoms or molecules) from neutral atoms or molecules; radiation creates ions by dislocating negatively charged electrons from the atoms they impinge upon.

i'onize. To separate into ions, totally or partially.

iontophore'sis. 1. Term suggested to denote the movement of ions through an electric field. **2.** Introduction of the ions of a medication through intact skin by means of an electric current; also called ion transfer, ionization, and ionic medication.

IOP. Abbreviation for intraocular pressure.

iopanoic acid. A radiopaque iodine compound used in x-ray examination of the gallbladder and ducts.

I.P., i.p. Abbreviation for intraperitoneal.

ip'ecac, ipecacuan'ha. The dried root of *Cephaelis ipecacuanha* or *Cephaelis acuminata,* a shrub of South America; used as an emetic, as an expectorant, and in the treatment of amebic dysentery.

   i. syrup, a suspension of ipecac alkaloids that induces vomiting; available without prescription.

IPPB. Abbreviation for intermittent positive-pressure breathing.

ipsilat'eral. On the same side; describing symptoms occurring on the same side as a lesion, such as a brain lesion.

IPSP. Abbreviation for inhibitory postsynaptic potential (a hyperpolarizing response).

IQ. Abbreviation for intelligence quotient; see under quotient.

Ir. Chemical symbol of the element iridium.

iridec'tomy. Surgical removal of a portion of the iris.

   peripheral i., surgical removal of a minute portion of the periphery of the iris, as in the treatment of narrow angle glaucoma.

iride'mia. Bleeding from the iris.

iridenclei'sis. One of the filtering operations for glaucoma in which a portion of the iris is cut and incarcerated in an incision on the border of the cornea for the purpose of draining the fluid from the anterior and posterior chambers of the eye.

ir'ides. Plural of iris.

irides'cent. Displaying a changeable, colorful, metallic luster.

irid'esis. Surgical procedure in which a portion of the iris is brought out through an incision in the cornea and fixed with a suture.

irid'ic. Relating to the iris.

irid'ium. A whitish-yellow metallic element, symbol

Ir, atomic number 77, atomic weight 192.2; of all chemical elements, it has the greatest resistance to corrosion.

iridiza'tion. The multicolor halo around a bright light observed by persons afflicted with glaucoma.

irido-. Combining form denoting the iris.

iridocapsuli'tis. Inflammation of the iris and the capsule of the lens of the eye.

irid'ocele. Protrusion of a portion of the iris through a defect or wound in the cornea.

iridochoroidi'tis. Inflammation of both the iris and the vascular coat of the eyeball.

iridocolobo'ma. Congenital absence of a portion of the iris.

iridoconstric'tor. 1. Anything that causes contraction of the pupil, as a nerve or a chemical. **2.** The circular muscle fibers of the iris.

iridocyclec'tomy. Surgical removal of the iris and ciliary body.

iridocycli'tis. Inflammation of the iris and the ciliary body; also called anterior uveitis.

iridodial'ysis. Separation of a portion of the iris from its attachment to the ciliary body.

iridodila'tor. Something causing dilation of the pupil; denoting the sympathetic ciliary nerve fibers that innervate the pupillary dilator muscle or any chemical that causes constriction of that muscle.

iridodone'sis. Abnormal trembling of the iris upon movement of the eye, as may occur in partial dislocation (subluxation) of the lens.

iridokerati'tis. Inflammation of the iris and cornea.

iridokine'sia, iridokine'sis. The movement of the iris resulting in dilation and contraction of the pupil.

iridomala'cia. Degenerative softening of the iris as a result of disease.

iridople'gia. Paralysis of the iris.

iridosclerot'omy. Incision into the sclera and the margin of the iris.

iridot'omy. Incision into the iris.

i'ris, *pl.* **ir'ides.** The doughnut-shaped part of the eye, situated between the cornea and the crystalline lens and separating the anterior and posterior chambers; the contraction of the iris alters the size of the pupil; the amount of pigment in it determines the color of the eye.

   i. bombé, a bulging forward of the iris caused by pressure from the aqueous humor in the posterior chamber, which cannot pass to the anterior chamber because of adhesion of the pupillary border of the iris to the anterior surface of the lens.

irit'ic. Relating to iritis.

iri'tis. Inflammation of the iris.

i'ron. A metallic element, symbol Fe, atomic num-

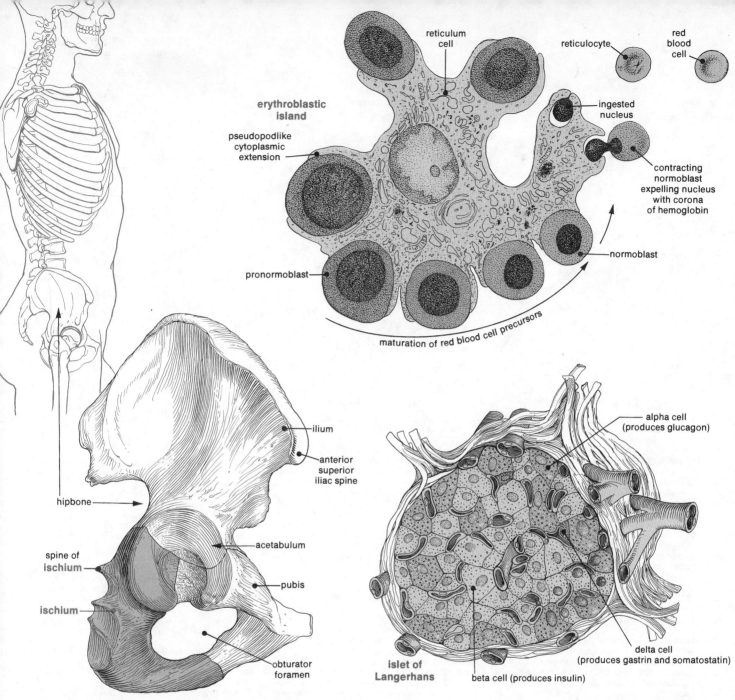

erythroblastic island

reticulum cell

pseudopodlike cytoplasmic extension

pronormoblast

reticulocyte

red blood cell

ingested nucleus

contracting normoblast expelling nucleus with corona of hemoglobin

normoblast

maturation of red blood cell precursors

ilium

anterior superior iliac spine

hipbone

acetabulum

spine of ischium

pubis

ischium

obturator foramen

alpha cell (produces glucagon)

islet of Langerhans

delta cell (produces gastrin and somatostatin)

beta cell (produces insulin)

ber 26, atomic weight 55.85; present in the body as a component of hemoglobin, myoglobin, cytochrome, and the proteins catalase and peroxidase; its role in the body is predominantly concerned with cellular respiration.

i′ron-59 (^{59}Fe). A radioactive beta-emitter iron isotope with a half-life of 45.1 days; used as a tracer for erythrocyte studies and ferrokinetics.

iron storage disease. Hemochromatosis; accumulation of excess iron in the tissues of many organs, especially the liver and pancreas, leading to fibrosis and functional insufficiency.

irra′diate. To treat with or expose to radiation.

irradia′tion. 1. Exposure to the action of rays. **2.** The condition of having been subjected to radiation. **3.** Therapy by exposure to radiation.

irrational. Contrary to reason or to the principles of logic.

irredu′cible. Incapable of being reduced in size or made simpler.

ir′responsibil′ity. The state of not being responsible.

  criminal i., the state of not being responsible for one's own criminal acts, due to a mental defect or disorder.

ir′rigate. To wash out a wound or bodily cavity with water or a medicated liquid.

ir′riga′tion. The washing out of a wound or a bodily cavity with a stream of fluid.

ir′ritabil′ity. 1. Responsiveness to stimuli. **2.** Exaggerated responsiveness to a stimulus.

ir′ritable. Capable of reacting, or tending to overreact, to a stimulus.

ir′ritant. 1. Causing irritation. **2.** A stimulus.

ir′rita′tion. 1. Incipient inflammation of a bodily part. **2.** The act of eliciting a reaction (normal or exaggerated) in the tissues.

IRV. Abbreviation for inspiratory reserve volume.

ische′mia. Lack of blood in an area of the body due to mechanical obstruction or functional constriction of a blood vessel.

  myocardial i., ischemia of the heart muscle, usually due to coronary heart disease.

ische′mic. Relating to local deficiency of blood.

is′chia. Plural of ischium.

is′chial. Relating to the ischium.

ischio-. Combining form referring to the ischium (one of the bones forming the hipbone).

ischiodyn′ia. Pain in the hip.

is′chium. The lowest of three bones comprising each half of the hipbone; the bone on which the body rests when sitting.

ischu′ria. Suppression or retention of the urine.

i′sland. An isolated structure or cluster of cells.

  erythroblastic i., one or two central reticulum cells of the bone marrow surrounded by normoblasts at various stages of development; the reticulum cells phagocytize the ejected nuclei of the developing normoblasts just prior to their release into the marrow capillaries as erythrocytes; they also ingest worn out or damaged red blood cells, conserving their iron as ferritin.

  i. of Langerhans, islet of Langerhans; see under islet.

  Reil's i., see insula.

i′slet. Small island.

  i. of Langerhans, cluster of cells in the pancreas that produce insulin; also called island of Langerhans and pancreatic islet.

-ism. Suffix indicating (a) an abnormal condition; (b) a characteristic quality; (c) a process or action.

iso-, is-. Prefix indicating identical, equal, or similar.

isoagglu′tinin. An antibody directed against antigenic sites on the red blood cells of individuals of the same species and causing agglutination of the cells.

isoallel′e. A normal allelic gene which can be distinguished from other normal ones only by the differences in the expression of a dominant trait when paired with another gene in a heterozygous

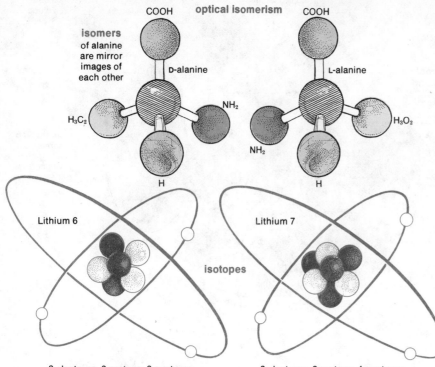

isomers of alanine are mirror images of each other

optical isomerism

COOH
D-alanine
H₃C₂
NH₂
H

COOH
L-alanine
H₃O₂
NH₂
H

Lithium 6

Lithium 7

isotopes

3 electrons, 3 protons, 3 neutrons

3 electrons, 3 protons, 4 neutrons

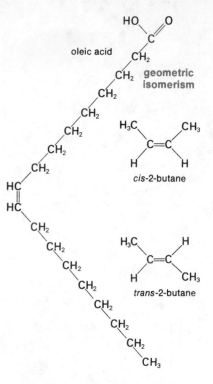

oleic acid

geometric isomerism

H₃C   CH₃
   C=C
H   H

cis-2-butane

H₃C   H
    C=C
H   CH₃

trans-2-butane

person.

isoan'tibody. An antibody produced by one individual which reacts with antigens of another individual of the same species.

isoan'tigen. Homologous antigen; an antigen produced by one individual which incites the formation of antibodies in another individual of the same species; also called alloantigen.

i'sobar. 1. Any one of two or more atomic species that have the same atomic weight but not necessarily the same atomic number. **2.** A line on a chart connecting two points of equal barometric pressure at a given time.

isobar'ic. Denoting atoms having the same weight.

isocel'lular. Composed of cells similar in size and character.

isochromat'ic. Of uniform or equal color.

isochro'mosome. A chromosome with two identical arms, resulting from transverse rather than longitudinal division of the centromere during meiosis.

isoco'ria. Equal size of the two pupils.

isocor'tex. The non-olfactory, phylogenetically younger part of the cerebral cortex; so called because its cellular and fibrous layers are distributed in a uniform pattern; also called neocortex and neopallium.

isodynam'ic. Of equal strength.

isoelec'tric. Having an equal number of positive and negative charges; electrically neutral; said of certain molecules.

isoen'zyme. See isozyme.

isogam'ete. A gamete that has the same size as the one with which it unites.

isog'amy. Conjugation or fusion of morphologically identical gametes.

isogene'ic. See isogenic.

isogen'ic. Isogeneic; genetically alike.

i'sograft. A tissue transplant involving two genetically identical or near-identical individuals, such as identical twins or highly inbred animals; also called syngeneic or isogeneic graft and isotransplant.

isohemagglu'tinin. An antibody that agglutinates blood cells of another individual of the same species; the antibody of blood groups.

isohemol'ysin. Homolysin; a specific antibody from one individual that reacts with antigen in red blood cells of another individual of the same species, resulting in cell destruction.

isohemol'ysis. Dissolution of red blood cells caused by reaction between specific antigens present in the cells and antibodies (isohemolysins) from another individual of the same species.

isoimmuniza'tion. The development of a significant concentration of specific antibody stimulated by the presence of antigens from another individual of the same species, as when fetal cells or other proteins gain access to the maternal circulation, with resulting maternal immunization to the paternal antigens present in the fetal material.

i'solate. 1. To separate from a group; to set apart by oneself, as to place an individual in quarantine. **2.** To free or separate (a substance) from a combined form. **3.** In psychoanalysis, to dissociate experiences or memories from the effects pertaining to them, so as to render them a matter of indifference; a defense mechanism against anxiety.

isoleu'cine. An essential amino acid.

isol'ogous. Marked by an identical genotype; also called isoplastic.

i'somer. One of two or more compounds that have the same percentage composition and molecular weight but different physical or chemical properties due to a different arrangement of the atoms in the molecule.

isom'erase. An enzyme that catalyzes the conversion of a substance to an isomeric form; e.g., glucosephosphate isomerase.

isomer'ic. Relating to or displaying isomerism.

isom'erism. The existence of a compound in two or more forms having the same percentage composition and molecular weight but differing in chemical and physical properties, and also in the arrangement of the atoms within the molecule.

   chain i., a form of structural isomerism in which the linkages in the basic chain of carbon atoms vary.

   geometric i., one in which free rotation about a carbon bond is restricted.

   optical i., stereoisomerism involving the arrangement of substituents about asymmetric carbon atoms which can rotate the plane of polarized light passing through the substance.

   structural i., isomerism involving the same atoms in different structural formulas.

isomeriza'tion. The process in which an isomer is converted into another, as in the action of isomerases.

isomet'ric. 1. Denoting the contraction of a muscle in which its tension is increased without shortening its length; opposed to isotonic. **2.** Of equal dimensions.

isomor'phism. Similarity of shape or structure.

isoni'azid. Isonicotinic acid hydrazide (INH); used in the treatment of tuberculosis.

isoplas'tic. See isologous.

isopropamide iodide. Compound used as an antispasmodic and antisecretory agent.

isopropyl alcohol. A secondary toxic alcohol, (CH₃)₂CHOH; used in the preparation of cosmetics and medicines for external use.

isoproterenol hydrochloride. A crystalline compound used as a cardiac stimulant and in the treatment of bronchial asthma; a β-adrenergic stimulant; Isuprel®.

isoproterenol sulfate. Compound used as an inhalation in the treatment of asthma and emphysema.

isop'ter. A contour line in a visual field representing the area in which the visual acuity is the same as that measured with a specific test target.

isosex'ual. 1. Relating to characteristics of both sexes in one person. **2.** Denoting the traits of an individual which are characteristic of the sex to which the individual belongs.

Isos'pora. A genus of coccidia; some species are parasitic in man's intestines and pathogenic.

i'sosthenu'ria. Lack of variation in the specific gravity of urine, regardless of amount of fluid intake; inability to concentrate or dilute the urine above or below, respectively, the osmolality of plasma, generally corresponding to a specific gravity of 1.010.

isother'apy. Prevention of disease by using the agent that causes the disease, i.e., vaccines.

isother'mal. Relating to or of the same temperature.

isoton'ic. Of equal tension or osmotic pressure, usually referring to the osmotic concentration of blood plasma.

isotonicity. 1. Equality of tension, as between two muscles. **2.** Equality of osmotic pressure, as between two solutions.

i'sotope. One of two or more chemical elements in which all atoms have the same atomic number but varying atomic weights, due to unequal numbers of neutrons in their nuclei; many are radioactive; designated by the chemical symbol and a superscript number representing the atomic weight, as ¹²C (isotope of carbon with atomic weight of 12).

   radioactive i., one with an unstable nucleus that emits ionizing radiation in stabilizing itself.

   stable i., an isotope of a chemical element that shows no inclination to undergo radioactive breakdown; a nonradioactive nuclide.

isotox'in. A poison in the blood or tissues of an animal that only has toxic effects on other animals of the same species, not on that animal itself.

isotrans'plant. See isograft.

isotrop'ic, isot'ropous. Equal in all directions.

isovalericacide'mia. A disorder of leucine metabolism characterized by elevated serum isovaleric acid upon protein ingestion or during infectious episodes; associated with recurrent episodes of coma, acidosis, and malodorous sweat; autosomal recessive inheritance.

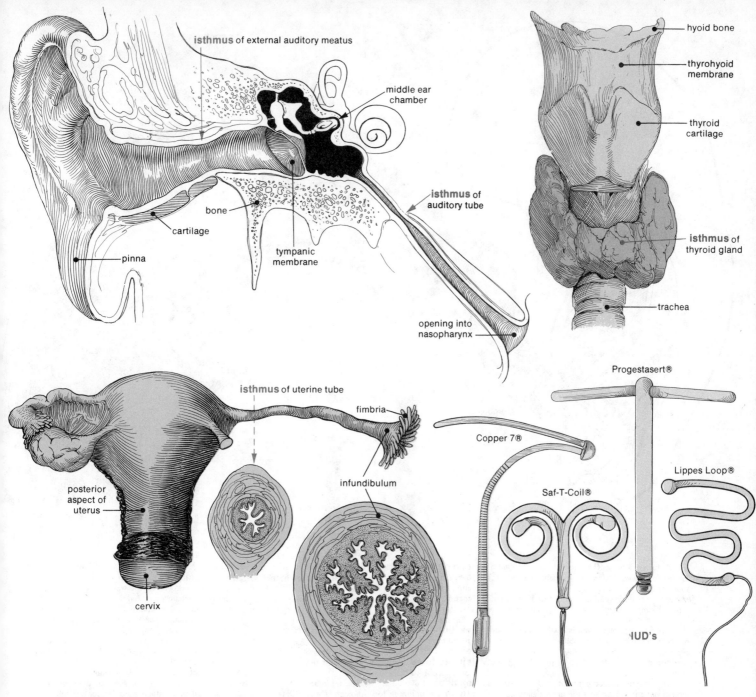

isthmus of external auditory meatus

middle ear chamber

isthmus of auditory tube

bone

cartilage

tympanic membrane

pinna

opening into nasopharynx

hyoid bone

thyrohyoid membrane

thyroid cartilage

isthmus of thyroid gland

trachea

isthmus of uterine tube

fimbria

infundibulum

posterior aspect of uterus

cervix

Progestasert®

Copper 7®

Saf-T-Coil®

Lippes Loop®

IUD's

isovolu'mic, isovolumet'ric. Equal or unchanged volume; occurring without an associated alteration in volume, as when, in early ventricular systole, the muscle fibers initially increase their tension without shortening so that ventricular volume remains unchanged.

i'sozyme, isoen'zyme. One of a group of enzymes that catalyze the same chemical reaction but have different physical properties.

is'thmus. 1. A narrow section of tissue connecting two larger parts. **2.** A narrow passage connecting two larger cavities.

i. of aorta, a slight constriction of the aorta between the left subclavian artery and the ligamentum arteriosum.

i. of auditory tube, the narrowest part of the auditory (eustachian) tube, at the junction of the bony and cartilaginous portions.

i. of cingular lobe, the narrow posterior portion of the cingulate gyrus which joins the hippocampal gyrus; also called isthmus of the limbic lobe.

i. of external auditory meatus, the narrowest portion of the auditory tube near the junction of the bony and cartilaginous parts.

i. of limbic lobe, see isthmus of the cingular lobe.

i. of nasopharynx, the opening between the free edges of the soft palate and the posterior pharyngeal wall.

i. of oropharynx, the constricted aperture by which the mouth is connected with the pharynx; located at the interval between the two palatoglossal arches.

i. of prostate, the anterior portion of the base of the prostate gland.

i. of rhombencephalon, a marked constriction of the brain in the fetus connecting the rhombencephalon with the mesencephalon, from which the anterior medullary velum is formed.

i. of thyroid, the narrow, central portion connecting the two lateral lobes of the thyroid gland.

i. of urethra, the slightly constricted junction of the urethra between the cavernous and membranous portions.

i. of uterine tube, the narrow, medial portion of the uterine tube at its junction with the uterus.

i. of uterus, the elongated constricted part of the uterus between the cervix and the uterine body; it is about 1 cm in length.

i. Vieussensi, the ring or margin of the fossa ovalis.

itch. 1. A skin sensation and/or irritation causing a desire to scratch. **2.** Common name for scabies.

barber's i., see tinea barbae.

swimmer's i., an itchy rash caused by penetration of the skin by the larvae of the worm *Schistosoma mansoni* during immersion in contaminated fresh water.

-ite. Suffix meaning (1) resembling or of the nature of; (2) in chemistry, a salt; (3) in biology, an essential portion of a structure.

i'ter. A passageway leading from one anatomic part to another.

-itis. Suffix meaning inflammation.

ITP. Abbreviation for idiopathic thrombocytopenic purpura.

IU. Abbreviation for International Unit.

IUCD. Abbreviation for intrauterine contraceptive device.

IUD. Abbreviation for intrauterine device.

I.V., i.v. Abbreviation for intravenously.

IVP. Abbreviation for intravenous pyelogram (urogram).

Ixo'des. A genus of parasitic ticks of the family Ixodidae.

ixodi'asis. A condition marked by skin lesions and fever caused by ticks, particularly those of the family Ixodidae (hard-bodied ticks).

ixod'ic. Relating to or caused by ticks.

Ixod'idae. A family of ticks of the order Acarina; the transmitters of several diseases including tick paralysis; also called hard ticks.

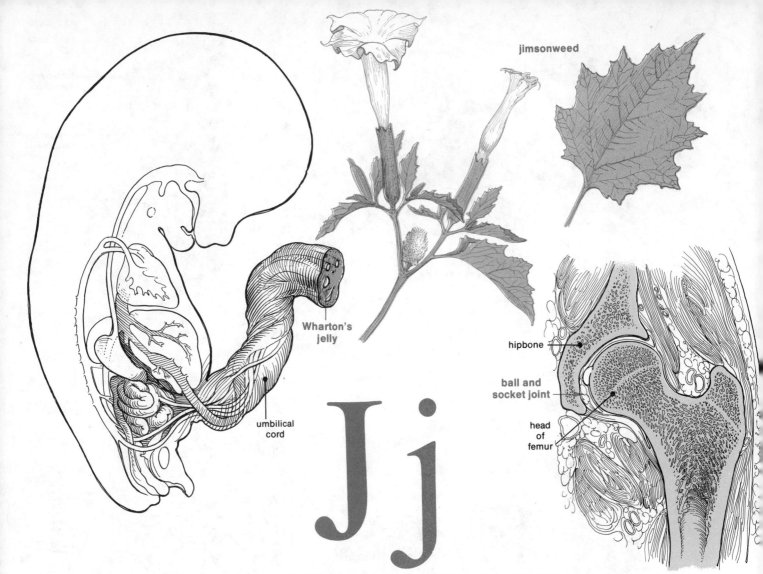

jimsonweed

Wharton's jelly

umbilical cord

hipbone

ball and socket joint

head of femur

J j

J. 1. Abbreviation for Kidd blood factor. **2.** Symbol for (a) Joule's equivalent; (b) radiant intensity; (c) sound intensity.

jack'et. An outer casing, bandage, or garment, especially one extending from the shoulders to the hips.

 Minerva j., a plaster of Paris cast extending from the chin to the hips for immobilization of the lower cervical or upper thoracic spine.

 porcelain j., in dentistry, a porcelain jacket crown.

 strait j., a long-sleeved garment used to restrain a violent patient by securing the arms tightly against the body.

jack'screw. A device used to approximate or separate teeth or jaw segments.

Jackson's syndrome. Paralysis of one side of the tongue, palate, and larynx; also called syndrome of vago-accessory-hypoglossal paralysis.

jactita'tion. The tossing to and fro of a distressed patient in bed; extreme restlessness.

Jakob-Creutzfeldt disease. See Creutzfeldt-Jakob disease.

Jansky-Bielschowsky disease. Cerebral sphingolipidosis; see under sphingolipidosis.

jar'gon. 1. Language peculiar to a trade, profession, class, etc. **2.** Incoherent, meaningless utterance. See also paraphasia.

jaun'dice. Yellow pigmentation of the skin and/or sclera caused by high levels of bilirubin in the blood; also called icterus.

 familial nonhemolytic j., jaundice in the absence of liver damage, biliary obstruction, or hemolysis; the unconjugated bilirubin is elevated; believed to be due to an inborn error of metabolism; also called Gilbert's disease.

 hemolytic j., jaundice resulting from hemolysis.

 physiologic j., mild jaundice of the newborn, primarily due to immaturity of the liver; also called physiologic icterus.

jaun'diced. 1. Marked by jaundice. **2.** Yellowish.

jaw. One of the two bones supporting the teeth; the upper one is the maxilla and the lower one is the mandible.

 lock-j., see trismus.

 lumpy j., see actinomycosis.

jaw'bone. Any bone of the two jaws, especially the mandible.

jeju'nal. Of or relating to the jejunum.

jejunec'tomy. Surgical removal of the jejunum, or a portion of it.

jejuni'tis. Inflammation of the jejunum.

jejuno-. Combining form indicating a relationship to the jejunum.

jejunocolos'tomy. Operation in which a communication between the jejunum and the colon is established.

jejunoilei'tis. Inflammation of the jejunum and ileum.

jejunoileos'tomy. Surgical connection between the jejunum and a noncontinuous segment of the ileum.

jejunojejunos'tomy. Surgical joining of two noncontinuous segments of the jejunum.

jejuno'plasty. Corrective surgery on the jejunum.

jejunos'tomy. The formation of a permanent opening through the abdominal wall into the jejunal part of the small intestine.

jejunot'omy. Cutting into the jejunum.

jeju'num. The portion of the small intestine between the duodenum and the ileum; in the adult it is about eight feet in length, with a diameter of approximately four cm.

Jellinek's sign. Brownish pigmentation of the eyelids, seen in cases of exophthalmic goiter.

jel'ly. A semisolid substance having resilient consistency.

 Wharton's j., the soft, homogenous connective tissue comprising the matrix of the umbilical cord and supporting the umbilical vessels.

jel'lyfish. A free-swimming marine coelenterate having a gelatinous, umbrella-shaped body and tentacles hanging down into the water; in the tentacles are hairlike structures, called nematocysts, that can be forcibly ejected in order to deposit toxins into the victim's skin; human reaction to stings ranges from skin rashes to death, depending on the species of jellyfish and the sensitivity of the individual; the more sensitive persons experience the symptoms of anaphylactic shock.

Jensen's disease. See chorioretinitis.

jerk. 1. A sudden abrupt or spasmodic movement. **2.** A sudden involuntary muscular contraction following a tap on the muscle or its tendon; also called muscular reflex.

 ankle j., calcaneal tendon reflex; see under reflex.

 crossed j., a muscular contraction on one side following a tap on the other side.

 crossed knee j., movement of one leg when the patellar tendon of the other leg is tapped.

 elbow j., triceps reflex; see under reflex.

 knee j., patellar reflex; see under reflex.

JG. Abbreviation for juxtaglomerular.

JGA. Abbreviation for juxtaglomerular apparatus.

jig'ger. Sand flea.

jim'sonweed. A poisonous plant, *Datura stramonium*, having large funnel-shaped white or purple flowers and prickly fruit; also called stramonium and thorn apple.

jit'ters. Extreme nervousness.

joint. The point of connection between two or more bones; an articulation.

 amphiarthrodial j., one in which the articulating surfaces are united by an articulating disk of fibrocartilage, allowing only slight motion, as between the bodies of the vertebrae; also called cartilaginous joint and amphiarthrosis.

 ball and socket j., spheroidal j., a type of diarthrodial joint in which the globular end of one bone fits into the cuplike cavity of the other, permitting

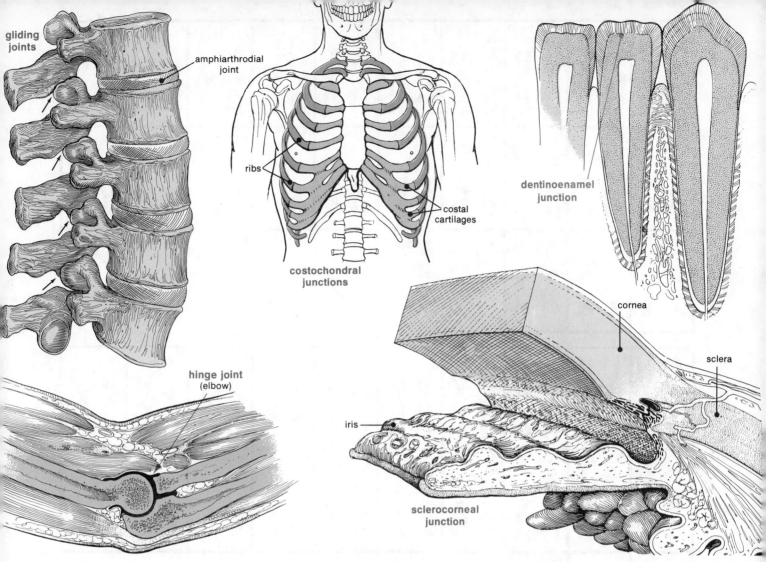

gliding joints

amphiarthrodial joint

ribs

costal cartilages

costochondral junctions

dentinoenamel junction

cornea

sclera

hinge joint (elbow)

iris

sclerocorneal junction

extensive movement in any direction, as seen in the hip and shoulder; also called enarthrosis.

condyloid j., a type of diarthrodial joint in which the ovoid articular surface of one bone fits into the elliptical cavity of another, allowing all movements except axial rotation.

diarthrodial j., synovial j., a joint that permits relatively free movement, characterized by the presence of (a) a layer of cartilage covering the articular surfaces of the bones (b) a cavity between the bones, the whole being surrounded by a capsule which is lined by synovial membrane; also called synovial or movable joint and diarthrosis.

gliding j., a type of diarthrodial joint in which the apposed surfaces are more or less flat, permitting a gliding motion, as between the articular processes of the vertebrae; also called plane joint and arthrodia.

hinge j., a variety of diarthrodial joint which permits only a forward and backward movement, as the hinge of a door; e.g., the interphalangeal joints.

rotary j., a type of diarthrodial joint in which a pivot-like process fits and rotates within a ring which is formed partly of bone and partly of ligaments, as the proximal radioulnar articulation; also called pivot or trochial joint.

saddle j., a type of synovial joint in which the articlar surface of one bone is concave in one direction and convex in a direction at right angles to the first, with the articular surface of the other bone reciprocally convex and concave, as the carpometacarpal joint of the thumb.

spheroidal j., see ball and socket joint.

synarthrodial j., one in which two bones are united by fibrous tissue permitting little or no movement between the bones, as the joints between the bones of the skull; also called fibrous or immovable joint and synarthrosis.

synovial j., see diarthrodial joint.

joule. 1. A unit of energy equivalent to that expended when a current of one ampere is passed

through a resistance of one ohm for one second. **2.** A unit of energy equivalent to the work done in moving a body one meter against a force of one newton.

JRA. Abbreviation for juvenile rheumatoid arthritis.

ju′gal. 1. Connecting. **2.** Relating to the cheek.

ju′gular. 1. Relating to the neck. **2.** Denoting certain structures in the neck, as a vein.

ju′gulum. The neck or throat.

ju′gum, *pl.* **ju′ga.** A ridge connecting two structures.

juga alveolaria, eminences on the anterior surface of the alveolar processes of the maxilla and mandible, caused by the roots of the incisors and cuspids.

juga cerebralia, the cerebral ridges on the internal surface of the cranial bones corresponding to the sulci of the brain; also called cerebral ridges of cranium.

j. petrosum, the eminence of the petrous part of the temporal bone formed by the superior semicircular canal; also called petrosal ridge.

j. sphenoidale, the elevated smooth anterior surface of the body of the sphenoid bone that connects the lesser wings; it forms part of the anterior cranial fossa.

juice. A digestive secretion; e.g., gastric juice, pancreatic juice, etc.

junc′tion. 1. A joint or articulation. **2.** The line of union of two parts or surfaces.

cementodentinal j., the surface at which the cementum and dentin of a root of a tooth meet.

cementoenamel j., the line around a tooth where the enamel of its crown and the cementum of its root meet; also called cervical line.

conjunctivocorneal j., the area of the eye, at the limbus, where the fibrous membrane of the conjunctiva ends and only the epithelium continues centrally to cover the cornea.

costochondral j., the point of articulation between the sternal end of a rib and the lateral end of its cartilage.

dentinoenamel j., the surface at which the dentin and the enamel of the crown of a tooth meet.

esophagogastric j., the junction of the esophagus and the stomach.

J j., J point, the point at the end of the QRS complex of the electrocardiogram (principal deflection) and the beginning of the ST segment (segment immediately following the QRS complex).

mucocutaneous j., the area of transition from a mucous membrane to the epidermis.

myoneural j., neuromuscular junction.

neuromuscular j., the area of contact between the motor nerve and the muscle; the end of the nerve broadens into an endplate that fits into a depression in the muscle fiber.

sclerocorneal j., the area of the eye, at the limbus, where the sclera and cornea join.

junctu′ra, *pl.* **junctu′rae.** Latin for a joining; also called articulation.

jurisprudence, medical. The application of medical knowledge to legal questions; e.g., in cases of death by poisoning; also called forensic or legal medicine.

jur′y-mast. An upright bar used in conjunction with a plaster of Paris jacket; used as a head support in cases of diseases of the spine, as in Pott's disease.

jux′ta-. Prefix denoting near.

juxtamed′ullary. Referring to that portion of the inner cortex of the kidney adjacent to the medulla, e.g., juxtamedullary glomeruli.

juxtamed′ullary. Referring to that portion of the inner cortex of the kidney adjacent to the medulla, e. g., juxtamedullary glomeruli.

juxtapose′. To position side by side.

juxtaposi′tion. The state of being side by side; the act of placing side by side.

juxtapylor′ic. Located near the pylorus.

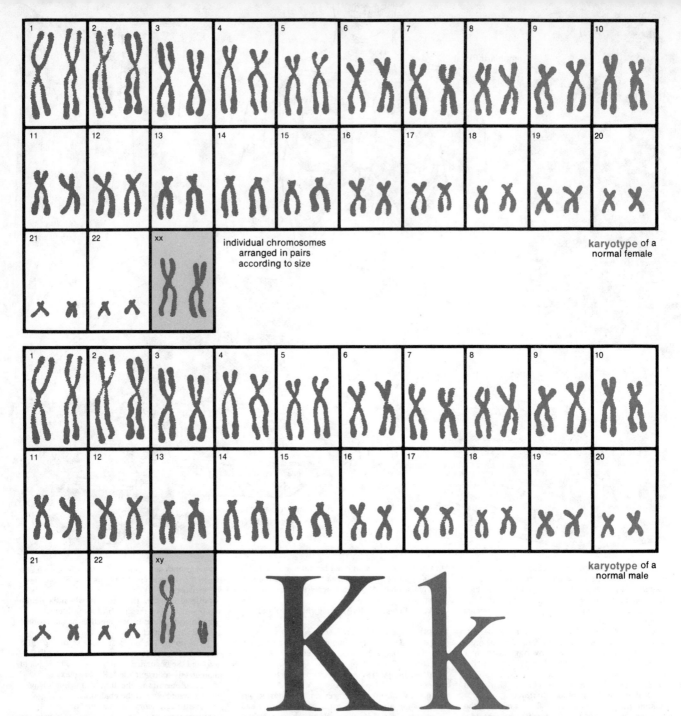

individual chromosomes
arranged in pairs
according to size

karyotype of a
normal female

karyotype of a
normal male

K k

K. Symbol for (a) dissociation constant; (b) Kelvin (temperature scale); (c) the element potassium.

k. **1.** Abbreviation for (a) cathode; (b) kilo-. **2.** Symbol for (a) constant; (b) kelvin (unit of temperature).

Ka. Abbreviation for cathode.

kal-, kali-. Combining forms meaning potassium.

kala azar. Visceral leishmaniasis; see under leishmaniasis.

kaliope′nia. Potassium deficiency in the body.

ka′lium. Latin for potassium.

kaliure′sis. Increased excretion of potassium in the urine; also called kaluresis.

kaliuret′ic. **1.** Relating to kaliuresis. **2.** An agent which induces kaliuresis.

Kallmann′s syndrome. Hypogonadism with anosmia; see under hypogonadism.

kalure′sis. See kaliuresis.

K and k blood groups. See Kell blood group.

ka′olin. A fine, whitish clay used in ceramics and as a demulcent and absorbent; also called Fuller′s earth and terra alba.

kap′pa. 1. The tenth letter of the Greek alphabet, κ; used to denote the tenth in order of importance. **2.** Symbol for the tenth carbon atom.

Kartagener′s syndrome. Displacement of the viscera to the opposite side of the body (situs inversus) associated with dilation of the bronchial tubes (bronchiectasis) and chronic sinusitis.

karyo-, kary-, caryo-. Combining forms denoting a relationship to the nucleus of a living cell; e.g., karyoplasm.

kar′yochrome. A nerve cell having a nucleus that stains deeply.

kar′yocyte. A nucleated cell; usually referring to a young nucleated red blood cell (normoblast).

karyog′amy. Fusion of the nuclei of two cells during cell conjugation.

karyogen′esis. The formation of a cell nucleus.

kar′yogram. See karyotype.

karyokine′sis. See mitosis.

karyolob′ic. Having a lobulated nucleus.

kar′yolymph. The clear homogeneous liquid part of a cell nucleus.

karyoly′sis. The destruction or dissolution of the nucleus of a cell.

karyomor′phism. 1. Development of a cell nucleus. **2.** Referring to the nuclear shapes of cells.

kar′yon. The cell nucleus.

karyoplas′m. Nucleoplasm; the protoplasm of the cell nucleus.

karyopykno′sis. Shrinkage of cell nuclei and con-

densation of the chromatin.

karyorrhex′is. Fragmentation of the cell nucleus.

kar′yosome. One of the spherical masses of chromatin resembling a knot in the chromatin network of a resting nucleus during mitosis; also called net knot and chromatin or false nucleolus.

kar′yotype. 1. The chromosome characteristics of an individual or a species. **2.** A systematized presentation of individual chromosomes of a single cell, photographed during the metaphase stage of mitosis and arranged in pairs according to size.

kar′yoty′ping. Analysis of chromosomes.

Kell blood group. K and k blood groups; red blood cell antigens, specified by the K gene; antibody to the K antigen (anti-K) is the cause of hemolytic disease of the newborn; named after a Mrs. Kell, in whose blood the antibodies were discovered.

ke′loid. A nodular, nonencapsulated, highly hyperplastic mass of scar tissue.

keloido′sis. The presence of multiple keloids.

ke′loplasty. Surgical removal of a scar or keloid.

Kel′vin. Relating to the absolute scale of temperature; see scale, absolute.

Kennedy′s syndrome. See Foster-Kennedy syndrome.

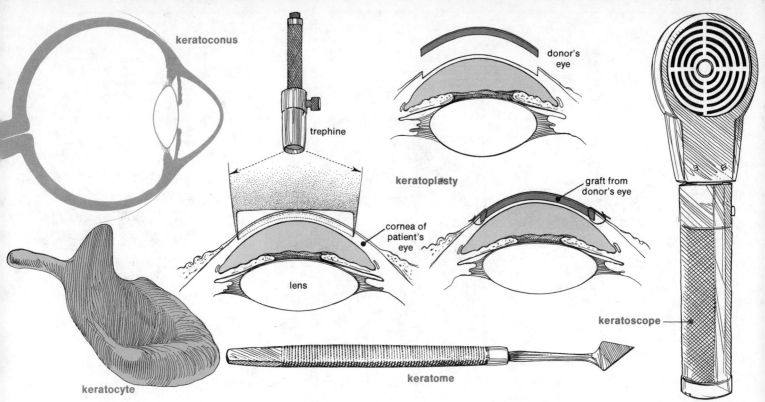

keratoconus

trephine

keratoplasty

donor's eye

graft from donor's eye

cornea of patient's eye

lens

keratocyte

keratome

keratoscope

Kent's bundle. Atrioventricular bundle; see under bundle.

keratal'gia. Pain in the cornea.

keratecta'sia. Protrusion or bulging of the cornea due to a thinning or weakening of the corneal tissue; also called kerectasis.

keratec'tomy. Surgical removal of the superficial layers of the cornea affected by scarring or degeneration, without replacing the excised tissue with a graft.

kerat'ic. 1. Horny. **2.** Relating to the cornea.

ker'atin. The protein present largely in, and forming the main components of, epidermal structures such as hair, nails, horns, feathers, etc.

α-ker'atin. Keratin in its folded form (as in normal hair).

β-ker'atin. Keratin in its extended form (as in stretched hair).

keratiniza'tion. The formation of keratin or a horny layer.

ker'atinize. To become horny.

kerat'inosome. An intracytoplasmic granule unique to mammalian keratinized epithelial cells, that is about 300 nm in diameter, is bound by a membrane, and contains lamellae; considered by some to be a specialized epidermal lysosome.

kerat'inous. Relating to or consisting of keratin.

kerati'tis. Inflammation of the cornea; also called corneitis.

band k., a grayish opacity extending across the cornea under the eyelid.

fascicular k., superficial corneal ulcer that moves from the periphery to the center of the cornea, carrying with it a narrow band of blood vessels from the conjunctiva; it remains superficial and terminates in a linear opacity; secondary to phlyctenular keratitis.

herpes simplex k., herpes simplex infection of the cornea.

interstitial k., deep inflammation and vascularization of the cornea involving primarily the middle layer; found chiefly in children and young adults as a late manifestation of congenital syphilis.

phlyctenular k., small gray nodules that break down forming a shallow ulcer; usually spreading from the conjunctiva; seen most commonly in the corneal periphery.

kerato-. Combining form meaning cornea or horny tissue.

keratocantho'ma. A rapidly growing benign skin nodule, usually with a central depression, histologically resembling squamous cell carcinoma and occurring chiefly on the face.

ker'atocele. Hernia of the posterior limiting (Descemet's) membrane of the cornea.

keratochromato'sis. Discoloration of the cornea.

keratoconjunctivi'tis. Inflammation of the cornea and conjunctiva.

epidemic k., a contagious form caused by a type 8 adenovirus, occurring mainly in persons exposed to dust and trauma in industry; also called shipyard eye.

keratoconom'eter. An instrument for determining the degree of keratoconus.

keratoco'nus. A degenerative, noninflammatory, central, conical protrusion of the cornea; usually bilateral; inherited as an autosomal recessive trait; also called conical cornea.

ker'atocyte. 1. A ruptured or mutilated red blood cell (erythrocyte). **2.** One of the flattened cells between the lamellae of the cornea; also called corneal corpuscle.

keratoder'mia. Thickening of the horny layer of the skin.

k. blennorrhagica, see keratosis blennorrhagica.

k. palmaris et plantaris, thickening of the skin occurring in symmetrical patches on the palms and soles; also called keratodermia symmetrica.

k. symmetrica, see keratodermia palmaris et plantaris.

keratogen'esis. The formation of horny tissue.

keratog'enous. Causing the production of horny tissue such as nails, feathers, etc.

keratohelco'sis. Ulceration of the cornea.

keratohe'mia. The presence of blood deposits in the cornea.

ker'atoid. Horny.

keratoirid'oscope. Instrument used to examine the cornea and the iris.

keratoiri'tis. Inflammation of the cornea and iris.

keratoleptyn'sis. Plastic surgery of the eye; removal of the anterior surface of the cornea and replacement by bulbar conjunctiva.

keratol'ysis. The peeling and shedding of the epidermis.

keratolyt'ic. Causing scaling of the epidermis; also called desquamative.

keratomala'cia. Dryness, softening, and dissolution of the cornea caused by severe deficiency of vitamin A.

ker'atome. A surgical knife for incising the cornea; also called keratotome.

keratom'eter. An instrument for measuring the curvature of the cornea.

keratom'etry. The measuring of the anterior curvature of the cornea with a keratometer.

keratomyco'sis. Fungus infection of the cornea.

keraton'osus. Any disease of the cornea.

keratonyx'is. Surgical puncture of the cornea, as

for needling the lens for soft cataract.

keratop'athy. A noninflammatory disease of the cornea, distinguished from keratitis.

ker'atoplasty. Operation in which the cornea or a portion of it is removed and replaced by healthy corneal tissue (graft); also called corneal transplantation.

lamellar k., procedure in which only the superficial layer of the cornea is removed for the treatment of superficial corneal opacities or recurrent superficial lesions.

penetrating k., one in which the entire corneal thickness is removed.

keratopros'thesis. Plastic corneal implant.

keratorhex'is. Rupture of the cornea due to a perforating ulcer or to injury; also written keratorrhexis.

keratoscleri'tis. Inflammation of the cornea and the sclera.

ker'atoscope. Instrument containing a disc of concentric rings used to examine the curvature of the cornea.

keratos'copy. Inspection of the anterior surface of the cornea with a keratoscope.

ker'atose. 1. Relating to or marked by keratosis. **2.** Horny.

kerato'sis. A circumscribed overgrowth of the horny layer of the epidermis.

actinic k., see senile keratosis.

arsenical k., keratosis resulting from chronic arsenic poisoning.

k. blennorrhagica, pustules and crusts associated with Reiter's disease; also called keratodermia blennorrhagica.

seborrheic k., flat, warty, benign lesions seen in persons after the third decade of life.

senile k., premalignant warty lesions occurring on the sun-exposed parts of the aged; also called actinic keratosis.

kerat'otome. See keratome.

keratot'omy. Surgical incision through the cornea.

keraunopho'bia. Abnormal fear of thunder and lightning.

kerec'tomy. Keratectomy.

ke'rion. Suppurative inflammation of the scalp, a complication of ringworm; it may simulate a carbuncle, with follicular pustules, exudate, and crusting.

Kerley lines. B lines of Kerley; see under line.

kernic'terus. The neurologic complication of unconjugated hyperbilirubinemia in the infant, causing staining of nuclear masses in the brain and spinal cord by bile pigment, with associated degenerative changes; the clinical signs include spasticity, opisthotonos, twitching, and convulsions.

Kernig's sign. Patient's inability to extend his leg

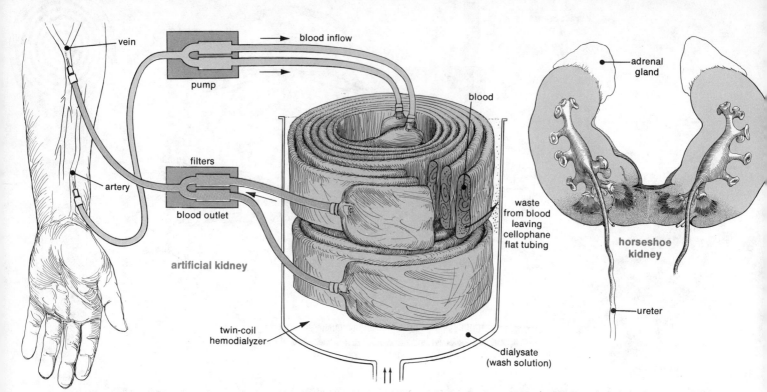

labels on figure:
vein — blood inflow — pump — blood — filters — artery — blood outlet — artificial kidney — waste from blood leaving cellophane flat tubing — adrenal gland — horseshoe kidney — twin-coil hemodialyzer — dialysate (wash solution) — ureter

completely when lying on his back with his thigh flexed at right angles with his trunk; seen in meningitis.

ker'oid. 1. Resembling the cornea. **2.** Horny.

keto-, ket-. Prefixes indicating any compound containing a ketone group (=CO) or ketonic properties.

ke'to acid. An acid having the general formula R—CO—COOH.

ketoacido'sis. Acidosis (diabetic) produced by the presence of an excessive amount of ketone acids in the body.

ketoacidu'ria. Excessive ketonic acids in the urine.

  branched-chain k., see maple syrup urine disease.

ketogen'esis. The production of ketone bodies (acetone substances).

ke'tol. See indole.

ke'tone. Any of a group of compounds having a carbonyl group (CO) linking to hydrocarbon groups.

ketone'mia. The presence of ketone bodies in the blood.

ke'tones. Ketone bodies; see under body.

ketoniza'tion. Conversion into a ketone.

ketonu'ria. The presence of ketone bodies in the urine.

ke'tose. A carbohydrate containing a ketone group in its molecule.

keto'sis. Abnormally large amounts of ketone (acetone) bodies in the tissues and fluids.

17-ketoster'oid. A steroid compound with a ketone radical on the seventeenth carbon; a steroid hormone derived from the adrenal gland or gonads; present in excess in the urine in certain tumors of the adrenal cortex; the metabolites of dehydroisoandrosterone are 17-ketosteroids and the metabolites of other steroids, including cortisol and 17-α-OH progesterone, may be oxidized to 17-ketosteroids; normal values in the urine are 6–18 mg/24 hours in the male and 4–13 mg/24 hours in the female.

ketosuccinic acid. See oxaloacetic acid.

kev. Abbreviation for kilo-electron volt or 1000 electron volts.

kg. Abbreviation for kilogram.

17-KGS. Abbreviation for 17-ketogenic steroids.

kick. A forceful thrust.

  atrial k., a forceful atrial contraction that tends to improve the performance of the ventricle; usually occurring in aortic stenosis or ischemic heart disease.

Kidd blood group. The red blood cell antigens, specified by the Jk gene, that react with the antibodies designated anti-Jk[a] and anti-Jk[b]; Named after a Mrs. Kidd, in whose blood the antibodies were discovered.

kid'ney. One of two bean-shaped organs, approximately four and one-half inches long, located in the posterior part of the abdomen, behind the peritoneum, on either side of the spine; it serves to regulate acid-base concentration and water balance in the tissues and to discharge metabolic wastes as urine.

  artificial k., popular name for hemodialyzer, an apparatus used as a substitute for the kidneys to purify the blood in acute or chronic kidney failure; toxic elements are removed by passing the blood through a semipermeable membrane lying in a bathing solution, then returning it to the body.

  contracted k., a small scarred kidney due to abnormally large amounts of fibrous tissue.

  crush k., degeneration of renal tubule epithelium following crushing injuries of muscle.

  ectopic k., a permanently abnormally placed kidney; distinguished from a floating kidney.

  floating k., the excessively mobile kidney in nephroptosia; distinguished from ectopic kidney; also called wandering kidney.

  Goldblatt k., one with impaired arterial blood supply, causing arterial hypertension.

  horseshoe k., one resulting from the fusion of the lower extremities of the two kidneys across the body midline.

  medullary sponge k., congenital defect marked by cyst formation of the pyramids of the kidney, occasionally associated with dilation of the collecting tubules and formation of stones; often asymptomatic and not generally a cause of renal failure. See also cystic disease of renal medulla.

  movable k., floating kidney.

  polycystic k., a kidney whose substance has been largely replaced by tightly packed cysts of varying sizes resembling a bunch of grapes. See also polycystic disease of kidney.

  sponge k., medullary sponge kidney.

  wandering k., see floating kidney.

kilo-. A prefix used in the metric system signifying one thousand (10^3); thus, a kilogram is 1000 grams.

kil'ocalorie. Large calorie; see under calorie.

kil'ogram (kg). One thousand grams or 2.2046 pounds.

kil'ogram-me'ter. The meter-kilogram-second (mks) gravitational unit of work, equal to the work performed by a kilogram force through a distance of one meter.

kil'oliter (kl). One thousand liters, about 1057 quarts.

kil'ovolt (kv). A thousand volts.

Kimmelstiel-Wilson disease. See Kimmelstiel-Wilson syndrome.

Kimmelstiel-Wilson nodular lesion. Nodular glomerulosclerosis; see under glomerulosclerosis.

Kimmelstiel-Wilson syndrome. Disorder occurring in patients with diabetes mellitus of several years' duration, marked by hypertension, edema, and proteinuria associated with intercapillary glomerulosclerosis; also called Kimmelstiel-Wilson disease.

kin-, kine-. Combining forms meaning motion.

kinanesthe'sia. Loss of ability to perceive sensation of movement.

ki'nase. An enzyme that activates proenzymes or zymogens (inactive enzymes).

kin'dred. An extended group of related persons; also called family group, clan, and tribe.

kinemat'ics. The science of motion, particularly of the bodily parts.

kinesal'gia. Pain occurring during muscular movement.

kin'escope. Instrument for testing the refraction of the eye; consisting of a disc with a slit, moved across the front of the eye, through which the patient observes a fixed object.

kine'sia. Motion sickness.

kine'sics. The study of nonverbal body motion as it relates to communication, as shrugs, waves, etc.

kinesiol'ogy. The study of muscular movement as it applies to treatment.

kinesither'apy. Treatment employing movement; also called kinetotherapy.

kinesthe'sia. The sense perception of muscular movement by which the individual can estimate the position of his body members.

kinet'ic. Relating to or produced by motion.

kinet'ics. The study of all aspects of motion and forces affecting motion.

  chemical k., the study of the velocities of chemical reactions.

  first-order k., the kinetics characteristic of a reaction whose rate of movement is proportional to the concentration of a single substance.

  zero-order k., the kinetics characteristic of a reaction that proceeds at a constant rate regardless of the concentrations of reactants.

kineto-. Combining form meaning motion.

kinetocar'diogram. Graphic representation of chest wall vibrations caused by heart activity.

kinetocar'diograph. Apparatus used to make graphic representations of low-frequency movements of the chest wall over the heart area.

kine'tochore. See centromere.

kine'toplasm. 1. The chromophil substance of nerve cells. **2.** The most contractile portion of a cell.

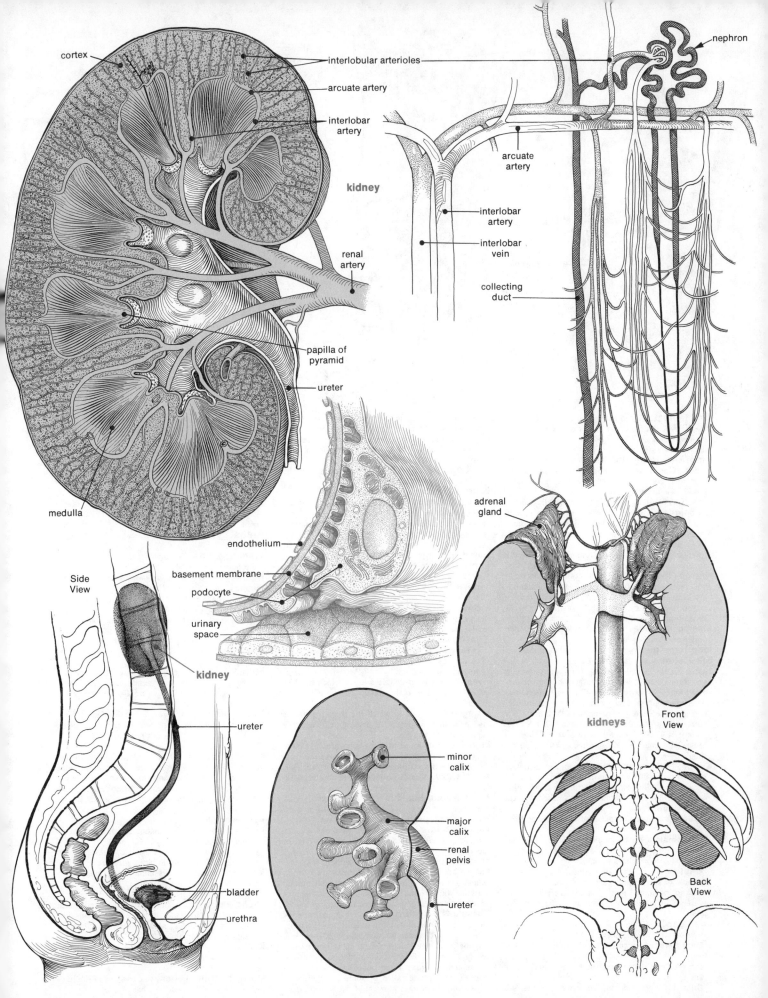

cortex

interlobular arterioles

arcuate artery

interlobar artery

kidney

renal artery

papilla of pyramid

ureter

medulla

nephron

arcuate artery

interlobar artery

interlobar vein

collecting duct

endothelium

basement membrane

podocyte

urinary space

kidney

Side View

ureter

bladder

urethra

adrenal gland

kidneys Front View

minor calix

major calix

renal pelvis

ureter

Back View

233

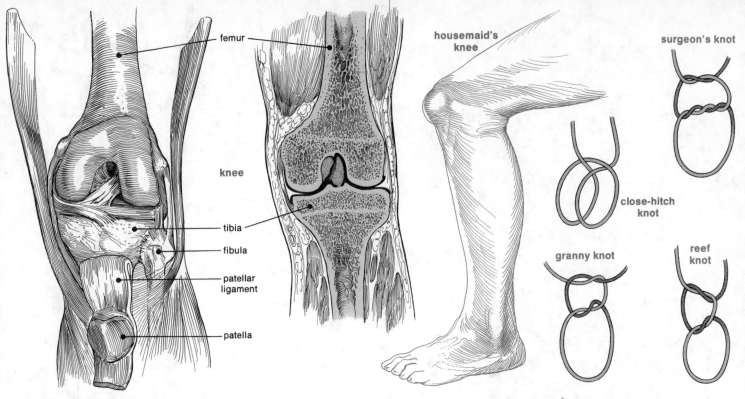

femur

housemaid's knee

surgeon's knot

knee

tibia

fibula

patellar ligament

patella

close-hitch knot

granny knot

reef knot

kine toplast. A rod-shaped structure, located at the base of the flagellum of parasitic flagellates; it divides independently prior to the division of the nucleus.

King-Armstrong unit. King unit; see under unit.

ki′nin. One of several substances, as bradykinin, that cause contraction of smooth muscle and other physiologic effects.

kink. 1. A bend. 2. A muscle spasm, usually painful.

Klebsiella. A genus of coliform bacteria (family Enterobacteriaceae), composed of motile and nonmotile gram-negative microorganisms.

K. pneumoniae, the causative agent of Friedländer's pneumonia; normally found in the nose, mouth, and intestinal tract of healthy persons; it causes less than 10 per cent of all acute bacterial pneumonias and is frequently present as a secondary invader in the lungs of individuals with chronic pulmonary diseases; also called Friedländer's bacillus and pneumobacillus.

kissing disease. Infectious mononucleosis; see under mononucleosis.

klep′toma′nia. A morbid compulsion to steal.

Klinefelter's syndrome. Common form of genetic disease in males arising from aberrations in sex chromosomes; usually characterized by abnormally long legs, extremely small testes, gynecomastia, eunuchoidism, azoospermia, and a general deficiency of secondary male features such as a deep voice and a beard; syndrome exhibits a classic pattern of 47 XXY karyotype (an extra X chromosome); also called XXY syndrome and seminiferous tubule dysgenesis.

Klippel-Feil syndrome. Congenital defect marked primarily by fusion of one or more cervical vertebrae, resulting in a characteristic short, thick neck with limited movements; also called cervical fusion syndrome.

knee. The articulation between the femur and the tibia.

housemaid's k., prepatellar bursitis; inflammation of the bursa in front of the patella (kneecap), usually due to repeated trauma.

k. reflex, see reflex, patellar.

knock k., see genu valgum.

locked k., limited motion of the knee due to the presence of loose tissue, such as cartilage, in the joint.

knee′cap. See patella.

knife. A cutting instrument with a sharp blade.

Bard-Parker k., a surgical knife with a disposable blade.

Blair k., one with a long sharp blade used to cut skin grafts.

Buck k., a periodontal knife with a spearlike

point, used for incising the gums between the teeth.

cautery k., a knife connected to an electric battery that sears tissue while cutting, to control bleeding.

Merrifield k., a gingivectomy knife with a long, narrow, triangular blade.

knit′ting. The union or growing together of the fragments of a broken bone.

knob. A protuberance; a nodule.

knock, pericardial. Heart sound occurring early during diastole, after the second heart sound but earlier than the normal physiologic third sound; common in patients with constrictive pericarditis; also called early diastolic sound and the third heart sound of constrictive pericarditis.

knot. 1. An intertwining of the ends of one or two cords, tapes, sutures, etc., so that they cannot be separated. 2. A node or circumscribed swelling. 3. To join the ends.

clove-hitch k., a knot made with two continuous loops around a part; used for making traction in the reduction of dislocations.

flat k., see reef knot.

granny k., an insecure double knot in which the two stretches of cord do not pass together under the loop but are separated by it.

reef k., flat k., a double knot in which the free ends are parallel to the standing ends of the first knot.

surgeon's k., one in which the thread is passed twice through the loop of the first knot with a simple knot tied over the first.

knuck′le. The dorsal part or region around a joint of the finger, especially of the metacarpophalangeal joints of the flexed fingers.

Koch's law. Koch's postulates; see under postulate.

Koch-Weeks bacillus. See *Haemophilus influenzae*.

koilo-. Combining form meaning concave.

koilonych′ia. A rarely seen symptom of iron deficiency anemia in which the nails are concave or spoon-shaped.

koiloster′nia. Funnel chest; see under chest.

ko′la, co′la. Either of two African trees, *Cola nitida* or *Cola acuminata*, bearing nuts that contain caffeine, theobromine, and colatin; used in the production of beverages and pharmaceutical products.

Korsakoff's syndrome. Severe impairment of recent memory and inability to learn new information, seen in disorders predominantly affecting the hippocampal-mammillary system in the brain, especially thiamine deficiency; confabulation is usually a prominent feature; often associated with Wernicke's disease and called by some the Wernicke-Korsakoff syndrome; also called Korsakoff's psy-

chosis.

Kr. Chemical symbol for the element krypton.

Krabbe's disease. A disease of late infancy marked by progressive cerebral demyelination and large globoid phagocytic cells in the white matter of the brain and spinal cord; the development of the infant usually ceases; also called globoid cell leukodystrophy.

kraurosis vulvae. Drying and shriveling of the vagina and vulva accompanied by itchiness and pain.

Krebs' cycle. Tricarboxylic acid cycle; see under cycle.

krymo-, kryo-. Combining forms meaning cold; alternate form, cryo.

kryp′ton. One of the inert gaseous elements found in the atmosphere; symbol Kr, atomic number 36, atomic weight 83.80.

kryp′ton-85 (^{85}Kr). A radioactive form of krypton, used as a tracer, as in studying regional blood flow.

17-KS. Abbreviation for 17-ketosteroids.

Kufs' disease. Cerebral sphingolipidosis; see under sphingolipidosis.

ku′ru. A progressive fatal disease of the central nervous system seen in certain natives of New Guinea; caused by a slow virus; also called laughing sickness.

Kussmaul's sign. Great increase in jugular venous distention and pressure during inspiration; seen in patients with cardiac tamponade.

kv. Abbreviation for kilovolt.

kwashior′kor. A nutritional deficiency syndrome of children due to inadequate intake of proteins relative to the caloric intake; marked by edema, apathy, anorexia, diarrhea, and skin lesions, with characteristically low serum protein, especially albumin.

kyllo′sis. Clubfoot.

ky′mograph. An instrument for graphically recording pressure variations.

ky′moscope. Apparatus used to measure pulse waves or the variations in blood pressure.

kynuren′ic acid. A crystalline compound; product of trypotophan metabolism.

ky′phos. Greek for hump.

kyphoscolio′sis. Abnormal backward and lateral curvature of the spine; it not only deforms but progressively disables, impairing first lung function and then heart function.

kypho′sis. Abnormal, rearward increase in the curvature of the thoracic spine; also called hunchback and humpback.

kyrtorrhach′ic. Relating to curvature of the lumbar spine with the concavity backward.

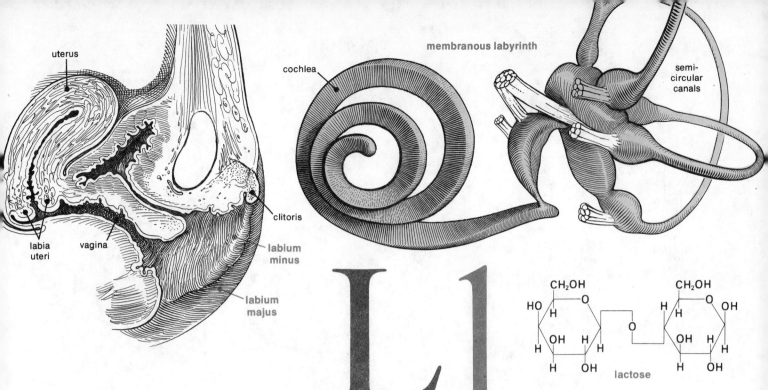

uterus · cochlea · membranous labyrinth · semi-circular canals · clitoris · labium minus · labium majus · labia uteri · vagina · lactose

L l

λ. 1. The eleventh letter of the Greek alphabet, lambda. **2.** Symbol for wavelength.

L. 1. Abbreviation for *Lactobacillus*. **2.** Symbol for (a) inductance; (b) lambert; (c) lethal.

l. 1. Abbreviation for (a) left; (b) length; (c) lumbar. **2.** Symbol for liter.

L-. In chemistry, a prefix printed as a small capital letter, indicating a substance to be structurally related to L-glyceraldehyde (a standard compound).

L+. The lethal plus dose; symbol for a toxin-antitoxin mixture of diphtheria containing a fatal dose in excess, which will kill an experimental animal in four days.

l-. In chemistry, a prefix (abbreviation for levo-, i.e., counterclockwise) indicating the direction in which the plane of polarized light is rotated when passed through a substance; the substance is said to be levorotatory. Opposed to *d-*.

Lo. Symbol for a toxin-antitoxin mixture whic h will produce no reaction in an experimental animal.

La. Chemical symbol for the element lanthanum.

la belle indifference. Belle indifference.

la'bia. Plural of labium.

la'bial. Relating to lips.

la'bile. 1. Unstable or easily changed, as drugs or preparations that are readily altered when exposed to heat. **2.** In psychiatry, emotionally unstable.

labil'ity. Instability or the condition of being changeable.

labio-. Combining form indicating a relationship with the lips.

labiochore'a. Spasm and stiffening of the lips during speech.

labiogin'gival. Relating to the area of junction of the lips and the gums.

la'biograph. Device used to record the movements of the lips in speaking.

labiomen'tal. Relating to the lower lip and the chin.

labiona'sal. Relating to the lips and nose.

la'bioplacement. The abnormal position of a tooth toward the lips.

labioplas'ty. Cheiloplasty; plastic surgery of the lips.

labiover'sion. Deviation of teeth toward the lips.

la'bium, *pl.* **la'bia.** A lip or liplike structure.

 labia majora, the two large folds of tissue surrounding the vulva; commonly called major lips.

 labia minora, the two narrow folds within the labia majora; commonly called minor lips.

 l. uteri, the margin of the vaginal portion of the cervix bounding the opening of the uterus (external os); designated as anterior and posterior labia or lips.

la'bor. Childbirth.

 first stage of l., dilation of the uterine cervix.

 induced l., labor brought on by artificial means.

 premature l., labor occurring before term.

 second stage of l., stage of childbirth beginning with complete dilation of the cervix and ending with delivery of the baby.

 third stage of l., expulsion of the placenta.

lab'oratory. 1. A room or building equipped with scientific equipment for the conduction of experiments, tests, etc. **2.** A place used for the manufacture of drugs and chemicals.

la'brum, *pl.* **la'bra.** A lip, edge, or liplike structure.

lab'yrinth. 1. A group of intercommunicating canals. **2.** Internal ear.

 bony l., a series of cavities in the petrous portion of the temporal bone which houses the membranous labyrinth.

 membranous l., a system of communicating membranous canals, lying within the bony labyrinth.

 ethmoid l., the labyrinth in the lateral part of the ethmoid bone consisting of thin walled cavities or cells; also called ectethmoid.

labyrin'thine. Relating to the labyrinth of the internal ear.

labyrinthi'tis. Inflammation of the labyrinth of the internal ear; also called otitis interna.

labyrinthot'omy. Incision into the labyrinth of the internal ear.

lac, *pl.* **lac'ta.** Latin for milk; any whitish, milky-looking fluid.

lacera'tion. A wound made by tearing of the tissue.

lacin'ia. Fringe; fimbria.

lac'rimal. Relating to tears.

lacrima'tion. The secretion, especially excessive, of tears.

lacrima'tory. Causing discharge of tears.

lacrimot'omy. The operation of incising the lacrimal sac or duct.

lactacide'mia. The presence of lactic acid in the circulating blood; also called lacticacidemia.

lac'tagogue. 1. Any agent that promotes the flow of milk. **2.** Increasing the secretion of milk.

lactal'bumin. An albumin of milk.

lac'tase. An intestinal enzyme that catalyzes the conversion of lactose into glucose and galactose; a sugar splitting enzyme; a deficiency of lactase may lead to gastrointestinal symptoms such as bloating, flatulence, and diarrhea following ingestion of milk and milk products.

lac'tate. 1. To secrete milk. **2.** Any salt or ester of lactic acid.

 l. dehydrogenase, see lactic acid dehydrogenase.

lacta'tion. The production of milk.

lac'teal. 1. A lymph vessel that conveys chyle from the small intestine. **2.** Relating to milk.

lactes'cent. 1. Milky. **2.** Producing a milky fluid, as certain plants and insects.

lac'tic. Relating to milk.

lac'tic acid. A colorless syrupy substance formed by the fermentation of milk sugar (lactose); an end product of anaerobic glycolysis in the body.

 l. a. dehydrogenase, an enzyme that may be measured in serum for diagnosis of some diseases, e.g., acute myocardial infarction and liver disease; also called lactate dehydrogenase.

lacticacide'mia. See lactacidemia.

lactif'erous. Secreting or conveying milk.

lactif'ugal. See galactophygous.

lac'tifuge. An agent that arrests the secretion of milk.

lactig'enous. Producing milk.

lac'tin. Lactose.

lac'tinated. Containing lactose.

lacto-, lact-. Combining forms meaning milk.

Lactobacil'lus. A genus of rod-shaped, nonmotile microorganisms (family Lactobacillacea) that produce lactic acid in the fermentation of carbohydrates, especially in milk.

 L. acidophilus, a species found in the feces of milk-fed infants and individuals on a diet with a high content of milk, lactose, or dextrin.

lac'tobezoar. A coagulum in the stomach formed by the prolonged ingestion of powdered milk which is mixed with an insufficient amount of water.

lac'tocele. See galactocele.

lac'toflavin. 1. Riboflavin. **2.** Flavin in milk.

lac'togen. Any agent that stimulates the production of milk.

human placental l. (HPL, hPL), a polypeptide hormone appearing in the serum of pregnant women at about the sixth week of gestation and rising steadily thereafter; it disappears from the blood immediately after delivery; it is produced by the syncytiotrophoblast (in placenta) and is intimately involved in carbohydrate metabolism of both mother and fetus; also called chorionic somatomammotropin and chorionic growth hormone.

lactogen'ic. Inducing milk production.

lactoglob'ulin. A simple protein found in milk.

lac'tone. A salt of a hydroxyl acid, formed by the removal of water from the acid.

lactopro'tein. Protein normally present in milk.

lactorrhe'a. Galactorrhea.

lac'tose. A sugar formed by the mammary glands and constituting about five per cent of cow's milk; it yields glucose and galactose on hydrolysis; also called milk sugar.

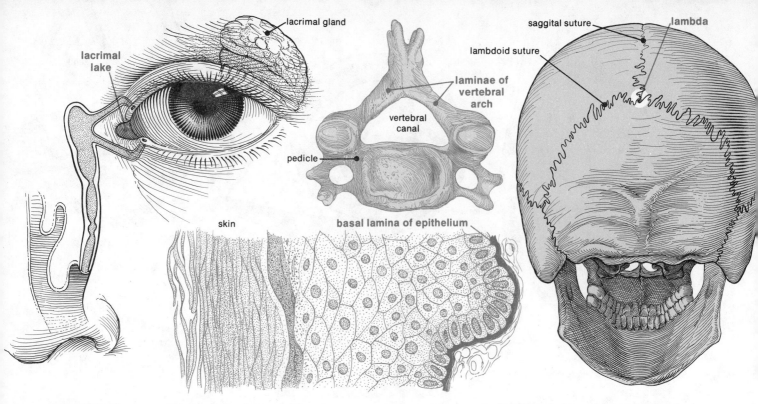

lacrimal lake

lacrimal gland

laminae of vertebral arch

vertebral canal

pedicle

skin

basal lamina of epithelium

saggital suture

lambdoid suture

lambda

lactosu'ria. The presence of lactose in the urine; occurring sometimes in premature newborn infants.

lactovegeta'rian. One who lives on a diet of vegetables, milk, and milk products.

lacu'na, *pl.* **lacu'nae. 1.** A small cavity. **2.** A defect or gap.

   erosion l., a depression in bone caused by resorption of bone tissue by osteocytes; also called Howship's lacuna.

   Howship's l., see erosion lacuna.

la'cus. Latin for lake; a small collection of fluid.

   l. lacrimalis, lacrimal lake; see under lake.

Laënnec's cirrhosis. See cirrhosis, alcoholic.

lag. Lag phase; see under phase.

lagophal'mos, lagophal'mia. Condition in which the eyelids cannot be closed completely; also called hare's eye.

lake. 1. A small accumulation of fluid. **2.** To cause blood plasma to become red as a result of the release of hemoglobin from the erythrocytes.

   lacrimal l., the area of the conjunctiva, between the medial margins of the eyelids at the inner angle, in which the tears collect after bathing the anterior surface of the eyeball; the caruncle lies in its floor; also called lacus lacrimalis.

lalla'tion. 1. Poor articulation, especially speech sounding like the prattling of a baby; babbling. **2.** Defective enunciation of words in which the phoneme (l) is substituted for (r).

lalopathol'ogy. The study of speech disorders.

lalop'athy. Any speech defect.

lalopla'gia. Paralysis of muscles involved in the production of speech.

lam'bda. 1. A craniometric point at the junction of the sagittal and lambdoid sutures. **2.** The Greek letter λ, used as a symbol for wavelength.

lamb'doid. Resembling the shape of the Greek letter lambda (λ); denoting the deeply serrated suture in the skull between the occipital bone and the two parietal bones.

lam'bert. Unit of brightness, equal to the uniform brightness of a perfectly diffusing surface emitting or reflecting light at the rate of one lumen per square centimeter.

lamel'la, *pl.* **lamel'lae. 1.** A thin layer or plate, as of bone. **2.** A medicated gelatin disc, used under the eyelid in place of solutions.

lam'ellar. 1. Scaly. **2.** Relating to lamellae.

lam'ina, *pl.* **lam'inae.** A thin layer or flat plate, as of muscle or bone.

   anterior elastic l. of cornea, Bowman's membrane; see under membrane.

   basal l. of choroid, the transparent, inner layer of the choroid in contact with the pigmented layer of the retina; also called Bruch's membrane and lam-

ina vitrea.

   basal l. of epithelium, a relatively thin layer, about 300 to 1200 Å in thickness, composed of slender filamentous material enmeshed in a mucopolysaccharide matrix; it occurs at the base of epithelial cells where it blends with the reticular lamina to form the basement membrane; also called boundary membrane and basement lamina.

   basement l., see basal lamina of epithelium.

   choroidocapillary l., the layer of the choroid between the basal lamina and the vascular lamina.

   cribriform l., of ethmoid bone, the bony plate which forms part of the roof of the nasal cavity and is transversed by the filaments of the olfactory nerve.

   external cranial l., the outer plate of a cranial bone.

   internal cranial l., the inner plate of a cranial bone.

   interpubic fibrocartilaginous l., the fibrocartilaginous disk uniting the articular surfaces of the pubic bones at the symphysis.

   l. cribrosa sclerae, the sievelike portion of the sclera through the holes of which pass the fibers of the optic nerve.

   l. fusca sclerae, a layer consisting of a delicate mesh of elastic fibers connecting the sclera and choroid.

   l. vitrea, see basal lamina of choroid.

   laminae of vertebral arch, two broad plates directed dorsally and medially from the pedicles of a vertebra; their posterior midline fusion forms the vertebral arch.

   lateral l. of pterygoid process, a broad, thin, and everted plate of the pterygoid process of the sphenoid bone; its lateral surface forms part of the medial wall of the infratemporal fossa; its medial surface forms part of the pterygoid fossa.

   medial l. of pterygoid process, a narrow, long plate of the pterygoid process of the sphenoid bone that curves laterally at its inferior extremity into a hooklike process, the pterygoid hamulus.

   posterior elastic l. of cornea, Descemet's membrane; see under membrane.

   reticular l., a relatively thin layer of reticular and collagenous fibers embedded in a mucopolysaccharide matrix; together with the basal lamina it makes up the basement membrane which holds the basal cells of the epithelium firmly to the underlying connective tissue; it also encloses fat cells, muscle cells, and Schwann cells of peripheral nerves.

   suprachoroidal l., a layer of loose connective tissue forming the external layer of the choroid.

   vascular choroidal l., the layer of the choroid containing the larger blood vessels.

lam'inar. 1. Arranged in layers. **2.** Relating to a bony plate.

lamina'tion. An arrangement in layers.

laminec'tomy. Surgical removal of the posterior arch of a vertebra.

laminot'omy. The surgical division of the lamina of a vertebra.

lamp. Any device for producing light, heat, or therapeutic radiation.

   annealing l., an alcohol lamp with a soot-free flame used for heating and purifying gold leaf intended as a filling for tooth cavities.

   argon l., a lamp radiating chiefly in the near ultraviolet area around 360 nm; used chiefly in conjunction with fluorescein in fitting of contact lenses.

   Eldridge-Green l., a color perception test lamp containing a single light with color filters mounted in rotating disks.

   Kromayer's l., a U-shaped quartz lamp of mercury vapor that generates ultraviolet rays.

   mignon l., a small electric lamp used in the cystoscope.

   slit-l., see slitlamp.

   ultraviolet l., one that emits rays in the ultraviolet band of the spectrum.

   uviol l., an electric lamp with a globe of uviol glass producing light with a high content of ultraviolet rays; used in phototherapy.

lanat'oside A, B, C. Digilanid A, B, and C, the three natural glycosides of *Digitalis lanata*.

lance. To cut into a part, as into a boil.

lan'cet. A small, pointed, double-edged surgical knife.

lan'cinating. Denoting a piercing or cutting pain.

Landry's paralysis. See paralysis, acute ascending.

language. The use of vocal sounds in articulate, meaningful patterns, as a form of communication.

   body l., expression of thoughts and feelings by means of bodily movements.

lan'olin. Fat obtained from sheep's wool; used in the preparation of ointments.

   anhydrous l., see wool fat.

lan'thanum. Metallic rare earth element; symbol La, atomic number 57, atomic weight 138.92.

lanu'ginous. Covered with fine, soft, downlike hair (lanugo).

lanu'go. The fine soft hair covering the body of the newborn.

LAO. In radiology, the abbreviation for left anterior-oblique projection.

laparo-. Combining form denoting the abdomen.

laparohysterec'tomy. Removal of the uterus through an incision of the abdominal wall.

laparohysterot'omy. Incision of the uterus

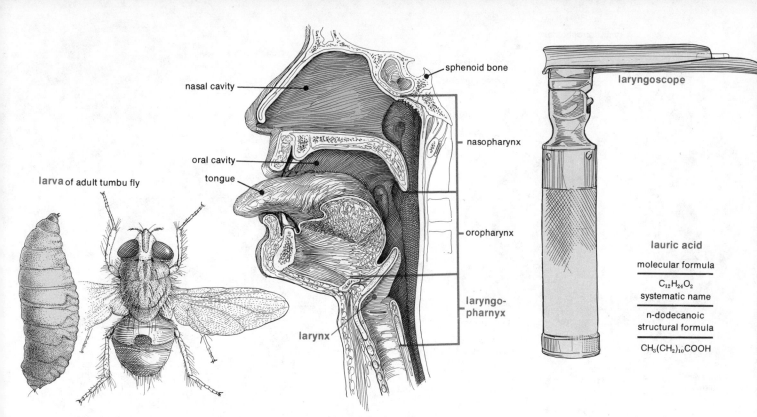

nasal cavity

sphenoid bone

nasopharynx

oral cavity

tongue

oropharynx

larynx

laryngo-pharnyx

larva of adult tumbu fly

laryngoscope

lauric acid

molecular formula

$C_{12}H_{24}O_2$

systematic name

n-dodecanoic

structural formula

$CH_3(CH_2)_{10}COOH$

---

through an incision of the abdominal wall.

lap'aroscope. Instrument for visualizing the peritoneal cavity.

laparos'copy. Visualization of the contents of the abdominal cavity by means of an endoscope; also called celioscopy.

laparot'omy. Surgical incision into the flank or through any part of the abdominal wall; also called celiotomy.

lapsus linguae. Latin for a slip of the tongue; usually due to unconscious factors.

lar'va, *pl.* **lar'vae.** The wormlike early stage in the development of certain animals, bearing little or no resemblance to the adult form.

lar'va mi'grans. Larval worms existing for a period of time in the tissues of a host other than the one to which they are adapted.

cutaneous l. m., a subcutaneous creeping eruption of the skin caused by wandering larvae of *Ancylostoma brazilience* and other domestic animal hookworms; acquired through contact with soil containing contaminated dog or cat feces; also called creeping eruption.

visceral l. m., disease caused by the presence of larvae of *Toxocara canis* (intestinal parasite of dogs) that penetrate the intestinal wall and wander through organs, especially the liver; acquired through consumption of raw vegetables contaminated with eggs of the parasite.

lar'vicide. An agent destructive to larvae.

laryn'geal. Relating to the larynx.

laryngec'tome. A person who has had his larynx removed.

laryngec'tomy. Removal of the larynx.

laryngis'mus. Spasmodic contraction of the larynx.

l. stridulus, a disease of children marked by sudden attacks of spasm of the larynx, lasting a few seconds, with a crowing noise on inspiration and cyanosis; also called crowing convulsions, Kopp's asthma, and pseudocroup.

laryngi'tis. Inflammation of the larynx.

acute l., laryngitis caused by infection or by mechanical irritation; infectious forms are frequently associated with sore throat and cough; characterized by hoarseness which may progress to complete loss of voice.

atrophic l., a chronic form leading to atrophy of the glands of the mucous membrane, diminished secretions, and formation of crusts.

laryngo-, laryng-. Combining forms denoting or relating to the larynx.

laryng'ocele. A congenital anomaly of the larynx; a sac formed by the outpocketing of the laryngeal mucosa reaching upward and outward between the

true and false vocal cords.

laryngocente'sis. A small surgical incision or puncture of the larynx.

laryngofis'sure. Surgical incision of the larynx, usually through the midline, for the removal of a tumor; also called median laryngotomy.

laryn'gograph. Instrument used to make tracings of the movements of the larynx.

laryngol'ogy. The study of the larynx and treatment of its diseases.

laryngoparal'ysis. Paralysis of the larynx.

laryngopharyn'geal. Relating to both the larynx and pharynx.

laryngopharyngec'tomy. Removal of both larynx and pharynx.

laryngophar'ynx. The lower portion of the pharynx from the hyoid bone to the esophagus, with which it is continuous; also called pars laryngea pharyngis. See also pharynx.

laryn'goplasty. Reparative surgery of the larynx.

laryn'goscope. Any tubular instrument used in examining the interior of the larynx.

laryngos'copy. Examination of the larynx with a laryngoscope.

indirect l., examination of the larynx by an instrument giving a reflected view.

laryn'gospasm. A reflex contraction of the laryngeal muscles.

laryngosteno'sis. Stricture or narrowing of the larynx.

laryngos'tomy. Creation of a permanent opening into the larynx.

laryn'gotome. Instrument used to make an incision into the larynx.

laryngot'omy. Surgical incision into the larynx.

laryngotracheobronchi'tis. Acute inflammation of the upper respiratory passages, occurring as a primary infection or attending a systemic disease such as diphtheria, whooping cough, etc.

lar'ynx. The organ of voice production, located at the upper end of the trachea; it is composed of a cartilaginous and muscular frame, lined with mucous membrane, and contains the vocal cords.

lasci'via. Excessive sexual desire; also called nymphomania.

Lasègue's sign. Pain along the course of the sciatic nerve when the patient, lying on his back, flexes his thigh on his abdomen and then extends his leg at the knee; it indicates disease of the sciatic nerve.

la'ser. Any of several devices that convert light of mixed frequencies into coherent, highly amplified visible radiation; used in surgical and physiological procedures; the term is an acronym for light amplification by stimulated emission of radiation; also

called optical maser.

l. beam, the concentrated, nonspreading (coherent) beam of monochromatic visible light emitted by a laser.

l. photocoagulator, a laser combined with an ophthalmoscope; used in the treatment of retinal detachment to direct laser beams into selected areas of the detached retina.

las'situde. Weakness or weariness.

la'tah. Nervous disorder marked by imitative behavior and extreme response to suggestion; observed in natives of Malay.

la'tent. Present but not manifest; concealed.

lat'eral. Located on the side; farther from the middle.

lateral'ity. A tendency to use either the right or the left parts of the body; right or left dominance of the cerebral cortex.

laterodevia'tion. Displacement to one side.

lateroduc'tion. Movement to one side, as of a limb.

lateroflex'ion. Bending to one side.

lateropul'sion. Involuntary movement toward one side, occurring in certain nervous disorders.

laterotor'sion. Rotation of the eye around its anteroposterior axis.

laterover'sion. The displacement of an organ to one side.

lath'yrism. Disease due to poisoning with some species of peas of the genus *Lathyrus*; neurologic symptoms predominate.

latis'simus. Broadest; widest.

Latrodec'tus. A genus of highly poisonous spiders.

L. mactans, see black widow.

LATS. Abbreviation for long-acting thyroid stimulator; see under stimulator.

lat'tice. A regular configuration of ions or molecules in a definite geometric arrangement.

la'tus, *pl.* **lat'era.** The flank; the side of the body between the ribs and the pelvis.

laud'able. Term formerly given to abundant thick pus, thought to indicate the healing of a wound.

lau'danum. A tincture of opium.

Laurence-Biedl syndrome. A recessive hereditary disorder marked by some or all of the following: mental retardation, obesity, polydactyly, hypogonadism, and visual disturbances (retinitis pigmentosa); also called Laurence-Moon-Biedl or Laurence-Moon-Biedl-Bardet syndrome.

lauric acid. A fatty acid present in milk and especially in coconut oil; also called dodecanoic acid.

lavag'e. The washing out of a cavity or a hollow organ.

law. 1. A principle, rule, or formula expressing a

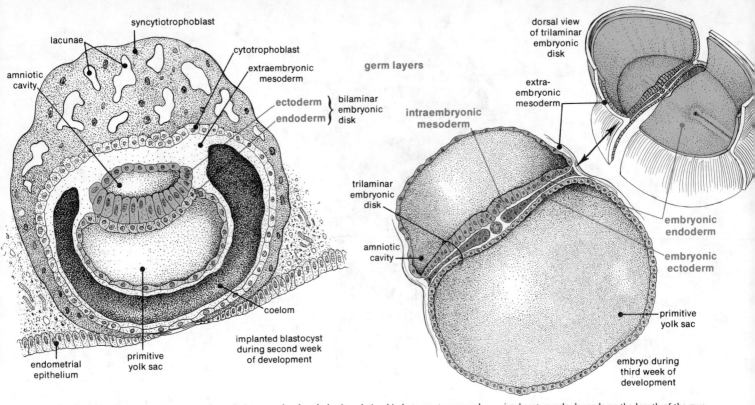

germ layers

lacunae · syncytiotrophoblast · cytotrophoblast · extraembryonic mesoderm · amniotic cavity · ectoderm endoderm } bilaminar embryonic disk · intraembryonic mesoderm · trilaminar embryonic disk · amniotic cavity · coelom · implanted blastocyst during second week of development · endometrial epithelium · primitive yolk sac

dorsal view of trilaminar embryonic disk · extra-embryonic mesoderm · embryonic endoderm · embryonic ectoderm · primitive yolk sac · embryo during third week of development

fact based on observed recurrence, order, relationship, or interactions of natural processes or actions. **2.** A generalization based on the repetition of events.

Arrhenius' l., only those solutions which have high osmotic pressures are electrically conductive.

Avogadro's l., equal volumes of gases contain equal numbers of molecules (pressure and temperature being the same).

Beer's l., the intensity of a light ray is inversely proportional to the depth of liquid through which it is transmitted (the absorption is dependent upon the number of molecules in the ray's path).

Boyle's l., at a fixed temperature, the volume of confined gas varies inversely with the pressure upon it.

Charles' l., all gases expand and contract equally on heating and cooling; also called Gay-Lussac law.

Courvoisier's l., obstruction of the common bile duct is more likely to be caused by gallstones when the gallbladder is contracted due to scarring and inflammation; if the gallbladder is enlarged, obstruction is usually due to other causes, such as carcinoma of the head of the pancreas; also called Courvoisier's sign.

Dalton's l., each gas in a mixture of gases exerts a pressure proportionate to the percentage of its volume in the mixture as if that were the only gas dissolved; also called law of partial pressure.

Dalton-Henry l., in dissolving a mixture of gases, a fluid will absorb as much of each gas in the mixture as if that were the only gas dissolved.

Einthoven's l., Einthoven's equation, in electrocardiography, the potential difference in lead II is equal to the sum of the potential differences of leads I and III.

Faraday's l.'s, (1) in electrolysis, the amount of an ion liberated by an electric current is proportional to the strength of the current; (2) when the same current is passed through several electrolytes, the amounts of different substances decomposed are proportioned to their chemical equivalents.

Galton's l., while offspring generally tend to resemble their parents, the offspring of parents of extreme types tend to regress toward the mean of the population; also called law of partial pressure.

Gay-Lussac l., see Charles' law.

Henry's l., the amount of gas which can be dissolved in a liquid solution is proportional to the partial pressure of the gas; when the pressure is doubled, twice as much gas passes into solution.

inverse square l., one which is especially applied to all point sources of radiation; the intensity of radiation is inversely proportional to the square of the distance.

Laplace's l., the relationship between transmural pressure difference (ΔP), wall tension (T), and diameter (D) related to surface tension in a concave surface: $\Delta P = (4 \, T/D)$.

l. of heart, see Starling's law.

l. of independent assortment, Mendel's second law.

l. of mass action, the speed of a chemical reaction is proportional to the active masses (molar concentration) of the reacting material.

l. of partial pressure, see Dalton's law.

l. of refraction, for two given media, the sine of the angle of incidence is constantly related to the sine of the angle of refraction.

l. of regression, see Galton's law.

l. of segregation, Mendel's first law.

l. of universal gravitation, see Newton's law.

Mendel's l.'s, the principles of heredity summarized in two laws and expressed in modern times as: (1) first law or law of segregation; paired hereditary units (genes) in the offspring (one from each parent) do not mix or alter one another, therefore they are able to separate during the formation of sex cells (gametes) in meiosis and are transmitted independently from generation to generation; (2) second law or law of independent assortment; the corresponding hereditary units in a pair of gametes unite in the offspring to form new combinations and recombinations according to the laws of chance, provided that the two pairs of genes do not lie on the same chromosome; also called mendelian laws.

Mendeleeff's l., see periodic law.

mendelian l.'s, see Mendel's laws.

Newton's l., l. of universal gravitation, all bodies attract each other with a force directly proportional to their masses and inversely proportional to the square of the distance between them.

Ohm's l., the electric current in a circuit is equal to the electromotive force divided by the resistance: amperes = volts/ohms.

Pascal's l., fluids at rest transmit pressure equally in every direction.

periodic l., the elements when arranged in the order of their atomic weights display a periodic variation of their properties; every element of the series is related in its properties to the eighth element before and after it; also called Mendeleef's law.

Poiseuille's l., speed of fluid flowing in a tube is proportional to the cross-sectional area of the tube.

Sherrington's l., every dorsal spinal nerve root supplies a special area of the skin (dermatome), although the area may be overlapped by fibers from adjacent spinal segments.

Starling's l., the energy liberated by the contracting heart muscle depends on the length of the muscle fibers at the end of diastole; within limits, the stroke volume of the heart is determined by the change in myocardial fiber length associated with ventricular filling in diastole; also called law of heart.

van't Hoff's l.'s, (1) in stereochemistry, all optically active substances form an unsymmetrical arrangement in space, owing to their having multivalent atoms united to four different atoms or radicals; (2) the osmotic pressure of a substance in a dilute solution is the same that the same substance would exert if present in the state of an ideal gas occupying the same volume as the solution; (3) the velocity of chemical reactions increases between two- and three-fold each 10°C rise in temperature.

wallerian l., Waller's l., a nerve fiber loses its normal structure and function when continuity with its cell of origin is interrupted.

lawren′cium. Synthetic transuranic element; symbol Lw, atomic number 103, atomic weight 257.

lax′ative. An agent that stimulates evacuation of a soft formed stool by increasing peristalsis or simply through hydration of the stool; distinguished from a cathartic, which produces a stronger effect.

layer. A sheetlike coating, or stratum, covering a surface; also called stratum and lamina.

bacillary l., the layer of rods and cones of the retina.

choriocapillary l., choroidocapillary lamina; see under lamina.

conjunctival l. of bulb, the mucous membrane investing the anterior surface of the sclera, terminating at the margin of the cornea.

conjunctival l. of eyelids, the mucous membrane that lines the posterior surface of the eyelids; it is continuous with the bulbar conjunctiva.

corneal l., the outer layer of the epidermis consisting of several layers of flat keratinized nonnucleated cells.

germ l., any of three primary layers formed in the early development of the embryo, the ectoderm, endoderm, or mesoderm, which give rise to specific tissues of the body.

l.'s of cerebellar cortex, three distinct layers of the cerebellar cortex which, from the surface inward, are: molecular layer, Purkinje cell layer, and granular layer; the granular layer is adjacent to the cerebellar white matter.

l.'s of cerebral cortex, six not too obvious layers of the cerebral cortex that tend to blend into each other; from the surface inward, they are: molecular layer, outer granular layer, pyramidal cell layer, inner granular layer, ganglionic layer, and the fusiform layer.

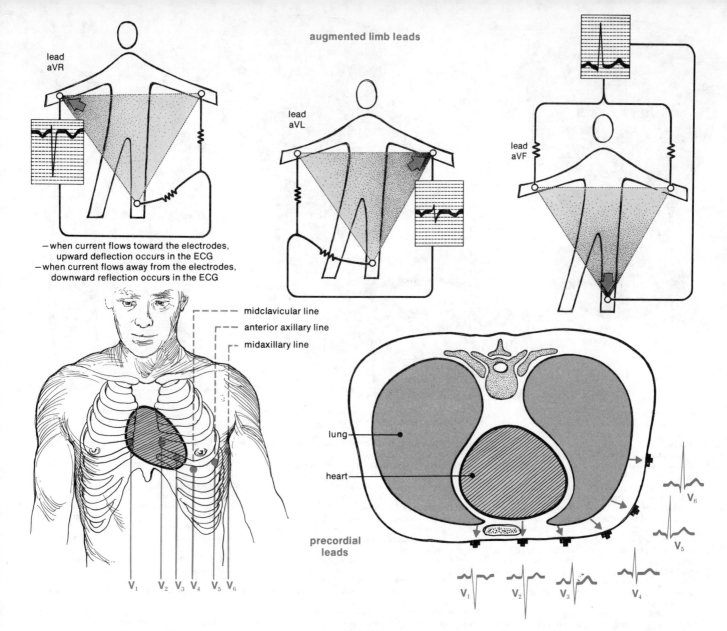

augmented limb leads

lead aVR

—when current flows toward the electrodes, upward deflection occurs in the ECG
—when current flows away from the electrodes, downward reflection occurs in the ECG

lead aVL

lead aVF

midclavicular line
anterior axillary line
midaxillary line

V₁ V₂ V₃ V₄ V₅ V₆

lung

heart

precordial leads

V₆

V₅

V₁ V₂ V₃ V₄

---

l. of rods and cones, a layer of the retina between the pigment epithelium and the external limiting membrane, containing the visual receptors (rod and cone cells).

malpighian l., stratum germinativum; see under stratum.

odontoblastic l., the layer of odontoblast cells lining the pulpal surface of the dentin of teeth.

prickle-cell l., stratum spinosum; see under stratum.

Purkinje's l., the middle of three layers of the cerebellar cortex consisting of large neuron cell bodies.

subendothelial l., the thin layer of connective tissue situated between the endothelium and elastic lamina in the intima of blood vessels.

lay′ering. An arrangement in layers.

LBBB. Abbreviation for left bundle-branch block.

LD. Abbreviation for (a) lethal dose; (b) learning disability.

LD₅₀. Abbreviation for the median dose that will kill within a stated period of time 50 per cent of the animals inoculated.

LDH. Abbreviation for lactic acid dehydrogenase.

LE. Abbreviation for lupus erythematosus.

Le. Abbreviation for Lewis blood group.

leach′ing. Lixiviation; the process of washing out soluble matter from a substance by a percolating liquid.

lead. A specific array of electric connections (electrodes) used for recording the electric potential created by a functioning organ, as the heart (electrocardiography) or brain (electroencephalography).

augmented limb l., one of three unipolar leads

for registering the variations in electric potentials at one point (right arm, aVR; left arm, aVL; or left leg, aVF) with respect to a point which does not vary significantly in electric activity during contraction of the heart; the lead is augmented (increased) by virtue of an electric connection which increases the amplitude; lead aVR records the electric potentials of the right arm with reference to a junction made by connecting the wires from the left arm and the left leg; lead aVL records the potentials at the left arm in reference to a junction made by connecting the wires from the right arm and the left foot; lead aVF records the potentials at the left foot in reference to a junction made by connecting the wire from the left and right arms.

bipolar l., one in which the electrodes detect electric variations at two points and record the difference.

chest l., precordial lead.

direct l., a lead recorded with the exploring electrode placed directly on the surface of the exposed heart.

esophageal l., a record obtained with the exploring electrode lying within the lumen of the esophagus; of particular value in obtaining sizable atrial deflections and therefore useful in the recognition of arrhythmias.

indirect l., standard lead.

intracardiac l., a lead recorded with the exploring electrode placed in one of the heart's chambers, usually by means of cardiac catheterization.

limb l., one of the three bipolar standard leads or one of the three unipolar augmented limb leads (aVR, aVL, aVF).

precordial l., one in which the exploring electrode is on the chest overlying the heart or its vicinity; unipolar chest lead recorded in positions V₁ through V₆ (the V designation denotes that the movable electrode registers the electric potential under the electrode with respect to a V or central terminal connection, which is made by connecting wires from the right arm, left arm, and left leg; the electric potential of the central terminal connection does not vary significantly throughout the cardiac cycle; as a result, the recordings made with the V connection show the electric variations that are taking place under the movable precordial electrode); position V₁ is at the fourth intercostal space at the right sternal border; V₂ is at the fourth intercostal space at the left sternal border; V₄ is at the left midclavicular line in the fifth intercostal space; V₃ is equidistant between V₂ and V₄; V₅ is in the fifth intercostal space in the anterior axillary line; V₆ is at the fifth intercostal space in the left midaxillary line.

standard l., one of the original bipolar limb leads designated I, II, and III; it detects the electric variations at two points and displays the difference; lead I records the potential difference between the right and left arms; lead II records the difference between right arm and left leg; lead III records the difference between left arm and left leg.

unipolar l.'s, those in which the exploring electrode records the variations in electric potential at one point with reference to a point that does not vary significantly in electric activity during cardiac contraction.

V l., a chest lead with the central terminal as the indifferent electrode.

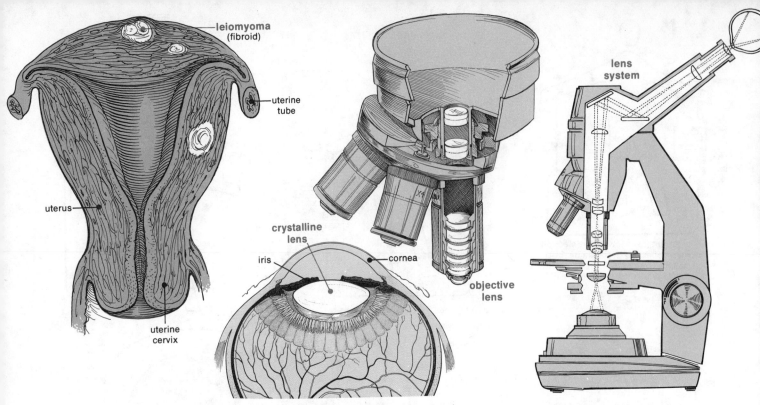

leiomyoma (fibroid) — **uterine tube** — **uterus** — **uterine cervix**

crystalline lens — **iris** — **cornea**

lens system — **objective lens**

lead. A malleable, bluish-gray, dense metallic element, extracted chiefly from lead sulfide; symbol Pb (plumbum), atomic number 82, atomic weight 207.19.

  l. arsenate, a poisonous mixture of arsenate of soda and acetate of lead, $Pb_3(AsO_4)_2$, used as an insecticide.

  l. carbonate, a poisonous white powder, $PbCO_3$, used largely in the manufacture of paint.

  l. chromate, a poisonous lemon-yellow powder, $PbCrO_4$, used as a paint pigment.

  l. sulfide (PbS), the natural form in which lead is usually found; also called galena.

Leber's disease. Leber's hereditary optic atrophy; see under atrophy.

lecithin. One of a group of phospholipids having a yellowish or brown waxy appearance; found in nerve tissue, egg yolks, and cells (both animal and vegetable).

lec'ithinase. See phospholipase.

lec'tin. A protein found predominantly in seeds, particularly those of the legumes; it binds to specific carbohydrate-containing receptor sites on the red blood cell surface, and can cause the cells to agglutinate; also called plant agglutinin, and phytoagglutinin.

leech. Any of various annelid worms (class Hirudinea) of which one blood sucking species, *Hirudo medicinalis* (German leech), was used for bleeding patients.

leg. The lower limb, especially between the knee and the ankle.

Legg-Calvé-Perthes disease. Epiphysial aseptic necrosis; see under necrosis.

Legg-Perthes disease. Epiphysial aseptic necrosis; see under necrosis.

leg'umin. A protein found in peas and beans.

leio-. Combining form meaning smooth.

leiomyofibro'ma. See leiomyoma.

leiomyo'ma. A benign tumor derived from smooth muscle and containing a relatively small amount of fibrous tissue; may occur anywhere in the body but is most frequently seen in the uterus; also called fibromyoma, leiomyofibroma, and fibroid.

leiomyomato'sis. The state of having multiple benign tumors of smooth muscle (leiomyomas).

leiomyosarco'ma. A malignant neoplasm in which smooth (nonstriated) muscle cells proliferate into a fleshy mass.

Leishman'ia. A genus of flagellated parasitic protozoa (family Trypanosomidae) transmitted to humans by the sandfly.

  L. braziliensis, a species that is the causative agent of mucocutaneous leishmaniasis.

  L. donovani, a species of intracellular parasite causing visceral leishmaniasis (kala azar).

  L. tropica, a species that is the cause of cutaneous leishmaniasis.

leishmani'asis, leishmanio'sis. Infection with a species of *Leishmania*.

  cutaneous l., chronic skin lesions with a tendency to ulcerate produced by *Leishmania tropica*; prevalent in tropical and subtropical areas; also called oriental sore and Old World leishmaniasis.

  mucocutaneous l., skin lesions often associated with ulcerative lesions of the mucous membranes of the nose, mouth, and pharynx; caused by *Leishmania braziliensis*; also called American or New World leishmaniasis.

  visceral l., a disease characterized by chronic fever, splenomegaly, anemia, leukopenia, and hyperglobulinemia; caused by *Leishmania donovani*; transmitted by the bite of a sandfly; also called kala azar and tropical splenomegaly.

leish'manid. Any lesion that may be infected with a species of the genus *Leishmania*.

lemnis'cus, *pl.* **lemnis'ci.** A band or bundle of nerve fibers in the central nervous system.

  lateral l., the major auditory pathway to the brain stem; it consists of a band of longitudinal ascending fibers which pass through the pons (in the lateral tegmentum) to the level of the midbrain, where most of the fibers terminate in the inferior colliculus with a few projecting directly to the medial geniculate body.

  medial l., a bundle of ascending fibers which originates in the nuclei of the lower brain stem and terminates in the ventral posterolateral (VPL) nucleus of the thalamus.

  trigeminal l., a band of fibers in the brain stem passing from the sensory nuclei of the trigeminal nerve to the posterior part of the ventral nucleus of the thalamus.

length. Distance between two points.

  bond l., the average distance between the nuclei of two atoms linked by a bond.

  crown-heel l. (C-H length), the length of an embryo from the top of the head to the heel.

  crown-rump l. (C-R length), the length of an embryo from the top of the head to the bottom of the buttocks.

len'itive. 1. A soothing agent. **2.** Soothing.

lens. 1. A transparent object (made of glass, plastic, quartz, etc.) having two polished surfaces of which at least one is curved, usually with a spherical curvature, shaped so that light rays on passing through it are made to diverge or converge. **2.** The crystalline lens, the biconvex transparent structure of the eye located between the iris and the vitreous body.

achromatic l., a compound lens that eliminates or reduces chromatic aberration; made of two kinds of glass with different dispersive powers.

acrylic l., one made of acrylic material; used to replace a cataractous lens.

aplanatic l., one that corrects spherical aberration.

apochromatic l., one that corrects both spherical and chromatic aberrations.

bifocal l., lens having one portion (usually the upper and larger portion) suited for distant vision and the other suited for near vision.

compound l., optical system having two or more lenses.

concave l., one that disperses light rays; also called minus, diverging, myopic, negative, or reducing lens.

concavoconvex l., lens having one concave and one convex surface; also called positive meniscus lens.

contact l., a molded plastic lens that rests directly on the eye in contact with the cornea; used to correct refractive errors.

convex l., one that converges or focuses light rays; also called plus, converging, hyperopic, or magnifying lens.

convexoconcave l., lens having one convex and one concave surface; also called negative meniscus lens.

crystalline l., see lens (2).

cylindrical l., one in which one or both surfaces have the curve of a cylinder, either concave or convex; used to correct astigmatism.

eye l., the lens in an eyepiece which is nearest the eye; it renders light rays from the objective lens parallel prior to entrance into the eye; also called ocular lens.

field l., the lens nearest the objective lens in an eyepiece; it increases the field of view in a microscopic or telescopic system.

immersion l., the lens in a microscope nearest the object, designed so that it can be lowered into contact with a fluid which is placed on the cover glass.

l. system, two or more lenses arranged to work in conjunction with one another in order to accomplish a required function; e.g., microscope, projection lens system, etc.

meniscus l., a crescent-shaped lens; one which is concave on one surface and convex on the other.

minus l., see concave lens.

objective l., the lens in a microscope or telescope nearest the object; it converges light rays from the field of view.

planoconcave l., one that is flat on one surface and concave on the other.

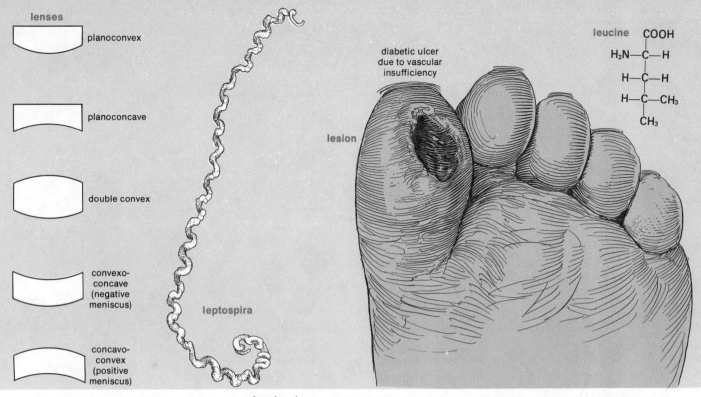

lenses

planoconvex

planoconcave

double convex

convexo-
concave
(negative
meniscus)

concavo-
convex
(positive
meniscus)

leptospira

diabetic ulcer
due to vascular
insufficiency

lesion

leucine

$$COOH$$
$$H_2N-C-H$$
$$H-C-H$$
$$H-C-CH_3$$
$$CH_3$$

planoconvex l., one that is flat on one surface and convex on the other.

plus l., see convex lens.

spherical l., one in which all refractive surfaces are spherical.

sphericocylindrical l., one in which one surface is spherical and the other is cylindrical.

trifocal l., one having three portions with different focal powers; serving for distant, intermediate, and near vision.

lensom′eter. An optical instrument used to determine the refractive power, optical center, cylinder axis, and prismatic effect of ophthalmic lenses.

lentico′nus. A conical protrusion on either the anterior or posterior surface of the lens of the eye, usually affecting only one eye.

lentic′ular. 1. Relating to a lens. **2.** Shaped like a lentil; also called lentiform.

lentic′ulostri′ate. Relating to the lentiform nucleus and the corpus striatum of the brain.

len′tiform. Lenticular (2); shaped like a lentil.

lenti′go, *pl.* **lenti′gines.** A flat, tan or brown spot on the skin which is to be differentiated from a freckle; an early junction nevus.

leonti′asis. The lion-like appearance of the face in some cases of advanced leprosy; i.e., ridges and furrows on the forehead and cheeks.

lep′er. An individual afflicted with leprosy.

lepiodo′sis. Any scaly eruption of the skin.

lep′othrix. See trichomycosis axillaris.

lep′ra. Leprosy.

lep′rid. The early skin lesion of leprosy.

leprol′ogy. The study of leprosy.

lepro′ma. The characteristic lesion of the focus of infection with *Microbacterium leprae*.

lepro′matous. Relating to a leproma.

lep′romin. Extract made from tissue containing the leprosy bacillus *Mycobacterium leprae*, used in skin tests to determine resistance to leprosy.

leprosa′rium. A special hospital for the care and treatment of those afflicted with leprosy.

lepro′sery. A leper colony.

leprostat′ic. An agent that inhibits the growth of the leprosy bacillus (*Mycobacterium leprae*).

lep′rosy. A chronic infectious disease caused by the bacillus *Mycobacterium leprae* (Hansen's bacillus), which produces granulomatous lesions of the skin, mucous membranes, peripheral nervous system, and bones; it occurs almost exclusively in tropical and subtropical regions and its severity can range from noncontagious and remitting forms to highly contagious malignant forms marked by mutilation; also called Hansen's disease and elephantiasis graecorum.

lep′rous. Relating to leprosy.

-lepsis, -lepsy. Combining forms meaning seizure.

lep′to-, lept-. Combining forms denoting slender, thin, or light.

lep′tocyte. A thin red blood cell having a pigmented border surrounding a clear area with a pigmented center.

leptocyto′sis. The presence of leptocytes in the blood, occurring in certain disorders, including thalassemia.

leptoder′mic. Thin-skinned.

leptomenin′geal. Relating to the pia mater and arachnoid collectively (leptomeninges).

leptomen′inx, *pl.* **leptomenin′ges.** The pia-arachnoid.

leptomo′nad. 1. A member of the genus *Leptomonas*. **2.** Former term for promastigote.

Leptospi′ra. A genus of spiral, hook-ended spirochetes, bacteria of the order Spirochaetales.

leptospi′ra. Any organism belonging to the genus *Leptospira*.

leptospiro′sis. Infection with bacteria of the genus *Leptospira*; the clinical picture may vary from a mild fever to a fulminating, toxic illness with jaundice and renal failure; specific syndromes include aseptic meningitis and pretibial fever, the latter associated with a pretibial eruption and splenomegaly.

l. icterohemorrhagia, see Weil's disease.

lep′totene. In meiosis, the first stage of prophase in which the chromosomes appear as individual, slender threads, well separated from each other.

Leptotrich′ia. A genus of anerobic, nonmotile bacteria indigenous to the oral cavity of man.

Leriche's syndrome. See aortoiliac occlusive disease.

LES. Abbreviation for lower esophageal sphincter.

les′bian. 1. A homosexual female. **2.** Relating to lesbianism. **3.** With a capital L, relating to the Island of Lesbos.

les′bianism. Female homosexuality.

Lesch-Nyhan syndrome. A disorder of purine metabolism and excess uric acid; clinical features include severe mental retardation and compulsive, self-mutilating behavior; death usually occurs during childhood due to kidney damage.

le′sion. Any morbid change in the structure or function of tissues due to injury or disease.

Ghon's primary l., the primary lesion of pulmonary tuberculosis, appearing in the roentgenogram as a small sharply defined shadow; also called Ghon's focus.

Janeway l., a small hemorrhagic lesion on the palm or sole, occurring in some cases of bacterial endocarditis.

Kimmelstiel Wilson nodular l., nodular glomerulosclerosis; see under glomerulosclerosis.

le′thal. Deadly.

le′thal blood lev′el. See under level.

leth′argy. A state of drowsiness and sluggishness.

Letterer-Siwe disease. Nonlipid histiocytosis; see under histiocytosis.

Leu. Symbol for leucine radical.

leuc-, leuco-. Combining forms meaning white or colorless. For terms beginning thus and not found here, see leuk-, leuko-.

leu′cine. An essential amino acid formed by the hydrolysis of protein; found in many tissues, especially the pancreas and spleen.

leucovo′rin. See folinic acid.

leuk-. see leuko-.

leukapher′esis. Procedure in which white blood cells are removed from withdrawn blood which is then retransfused into the patient.

leuke′mia. Disease characterized by the appearance of great numbers of immature and abnormal white blood cells in the bone marrow and often in the spleen and liver; usually these cells appear in the peripheral blood and may also invade other tissues; classified acute or chronic and also on the basis of the dominant type of cell involved (granulocytic, lymphocytic and monocytic); determination of acute or chronic refers in part to the rapidity of its course but more to the degree of immaturity of the predominant cells.

aleukemic l., a form in which the abnormal cells are present in the blood-forming tissues but not in the circulating blood; usually associated with decreased total number of normal white blood cells.

basophilic l., a type marked by the presence of great numbers of basophilic leukocytes in the blood and tissues; also called mast cell leukemia.

embryonal l., see stem cell leukemia.

eosinophilic l., a form in which eosinophilic white cells are present in great numbers in the blood and/or bone marrow.

granulocytic l., a type characterized by (a) massive proliferation of myelopoietic cells, chiefly in the bone marrow, and (b) the presence of large numbers of mature and immature granulocytes (especially neutrophils) in the tissues and circulating blood; also called myelocytic, myelogenic, or myelogenous leukemia.

l. cutis, massive accumulation of leukemic cells in the skin, forming red, brown, or purple nodules which may be localized (usually on the face and neck) throughout the body; also called lymphoderma perniciosa.

lymphatic l., see lymphocytic leukemia.

lymphoblastic l., acute lymphocytic leukemia in which the abnormal cells are the large immature

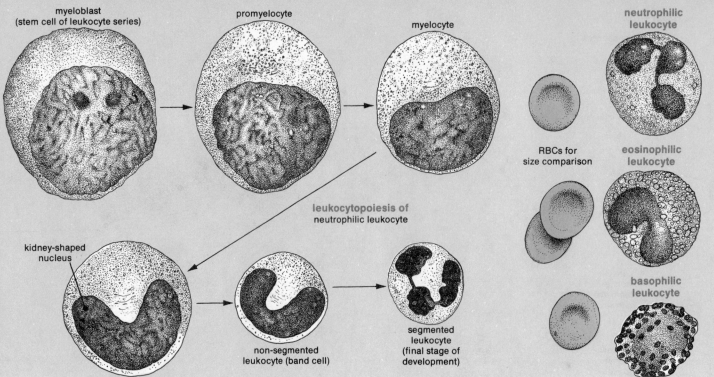

myeloblast
(stem cell of leukocyte series)

promyelocyte

myelocyte

neutrophilic
leukocyte

RBCs for
size comparison

eosinophilic
leukocyte

leukocytopoiesis of
neutrophilic leukocyte

kidney-shaped
nucleus

basophilic
leukocyte

non-segmented
leukocyte (band cell)

segmented
leukocyte
(final stage of
development)

metamyelocyte

forms of cells (lymphoblasts), which make up 50 to 90 per cent of the total, with most of the remainder made up of mature lymphocytes.

lymphocytic l., lymphatic l., an acute form occurring predominantly in children, characterized by the occurrence of lymphoblasts in the blood-forming tissues (particularly bone marrow, spleen, and lymph nodes); normal bone marrow elements may be replaced by the abnormal cells; a chronic form is usually seen in older people, with rather mature lymphocytes abundantly present in the blood; also called lymphoid leukemia.

lymphoid l., see lymphocytic leukemia.

mast cell l., see basophilic leukemia.

megakaryocytic l., a rare form characterized by uncontrolled proliferation of megakaryocytes in the bone marrow and the presence of a considerable number in the circulating blood.

monocytic l., a variety in which the predominant abnormal cells are monocytes; in the Naegeli type of monocytic leukemia the cells are thought to arise from myeloblasts, and are associated with neutrophils; in the Schilling type, the latter are not very evident.

myeloblastic l., leukemia characterized by an increase in myeloblasts which fail to mature (constituting approximately 30 to 60 per cent of increased total of white blood cells) and a reduction of the mature forms.

myelocytic l., see granulocytic leukemia.

myelogenic l., see granulocytic leukemia.

myelogenous l., see granulocytic leukemia.

myelomonocytic l., a form of monocytic leukemia in which a moderately large number of monocytes is formed; considered by Naegeli to be a variant of granulocytic leukemia because he believed monocytes to be derived from myeloblasts in bone marrow; also called Naegeli type of monocytic leukemia.

Naegeli type of monocytic l., myelomonocytic leukemia.

plasma cell l., an unusual type of leukemia marked by increase of plasma cells and occurring in association with uncontrolled proliferation of plasma cells in bone (multiple myeloma) and in soft tissues (plasmacytoma).

Schilling type of monocytic l., monocytic leukemia.

stem cell l., an extremely acute and uncommon type in which the abnormal cells are so primitive and immature that it is impossible to differentiate them, but they are thought to be the precursors of lymphocytes, myeloblasts, and monoblasts; also called embryonal leukemia.

subleukemic l., condition marked by the presence of small numbers of immature cells in the circulating blood; the total count of white blood cells is normal or subnormal.

leukem'ic. Relating to or suffering from leukemia.

leukemogen'esis. The cause and development of a leukemic disease.

leuke'moid. Resembling the blood changes of leukemia.

leuko-, leuk. Combining forms meaning white or colorless.

leukoagglu'tinin. Antibody that agglutinates white blood cells.

leu'koblast. An immature white blood cell.

leukocytac'tic. See leukocytotactic.

leukocytax'ia. See leukocytotaxia.

leu'kocyte. A white blood cell; any of the colorless cells of the blood; divided into two main groups according to their staining reactions: (1) granular or polymorphonuclear leukocytes, which have readily stainable cytoplasmic granules and lobulated nuclei; they include the neutrophils, eosinophils, and basophils; (2) nongranular leukocytes, which have minute cytoplasmic granules, not detectable with ordinary methods; they include lymphocytes and monocytes.

agranular l.'s, see agranulocytes.

basophilic l., a white blood cell containing large coarse granules that stain readily with basic dyes (e.g., methylene blue); it constitutes about 0.5 per cent of the total white blood cell count; also called basophil and mast leukocyte.

eosinophilic l., a granular white blood cell with a bilobed nucleus and numerous, large cytoplasmic granules that stain intensely with acid dyes (e.g., eosin); it constitutes two to five per cent of the total white blood cell count and increases in number during parasitic infestations and allergic states; also called eosinophil, acidophil and oxyphil.

filamentous polymorphonuclear l., a polymorphonuclear leukocyte whose nuclear segments are united by threadlike filaments of chromatin.

neutrophilic l., a mature granular white blood cell having a nucleus of three to five distinct lobes joined by thin strands of chromatin and having granules that stain with a mixture of acid and basic dyes; it constitutes about 50 to 75 per cent of the total white blood cell count; its primary function is ingestion and digestion of particulate matter, especially virulent bacteria; also called neutrophil and neutrophilic granulocyte.

nonfilamentous polymorphonuclear l., a polymorphonuclear leukocyte whose nuclear segments are united by wide bands of chromatin.

polymorphonuclear l., common term for any granular leukocyte, especially a neutrophilic leukocyte.

leukocy'toblast. General term denoting any immature white blood cell.

leukocytogen'esis. The formation of white blood cells.

leukocytol'ysin. Any agent causing dissolution of white blood cells.

leukocytol'ysis. The dissolution of white blood cells; also called leukolysis.

leukocytom'eter. A standarized glass slide used to count leukocytes.

leukocytope'nia. See leukopenia.

leukocytopoie'sis. The formation of white blood cells.

leukocyto'sis. Abnormal increase in the number of white corpuscles in the blood.

leukocytotac'tic. Relating to leukocytotaxia; also called leukocytactic and leukotactic.

leukocytotax'ia. The tendency of white blood cells to move either toward (positive leukocytotaxia) or away from (negative leukocytotaxia) certain microorganisms and substances formed in inflamed tissue; also called leukocytaxia and leukotaxis.

leukocytox'in. Any agent that causes degeneration of leukocytes.

leukoder'ma. Absence of pigment in the skin; also called achromia.

acquired l., see vitiligo.

congenital l., see albinism.

leukodys'trophy. Disease occurring early in life and affecting primarily the white matter of the brain, especially the cerebral hemispheres; thought to be a congenital defect in the formation or maintenance of myelin.

globoid cell l., see Krabbe's disease.

metachromatic l., a progressive disorder of sphingolipid metabolism in which sulfatide accumulates in the tissues; it affects both the central and peripheral nervous systems, causing blindness, deafness, muteness, and quadriplegia; death usually follows a few years from onset; most commonly seen in infants and young children; also called sulfatide lipidosis.

leukoerythroblasto'sis. Any anemic condition resulting from lesions in the bone marrow.

leukoencephalop'athy. Leukodystrophy.

leukoko'ria. Any eye condition that causes a white reflection from behind the clear crystalline lens, giving the appearance of a white pupil.

leukol'ysis. See leukocytolysis.

leuko'ma. An opaque white spot on the cornea.

leukomyeli'tis. Inflammation of the white tracts of the spinal cord.

leukomyelop'athy. Any disease that involves the

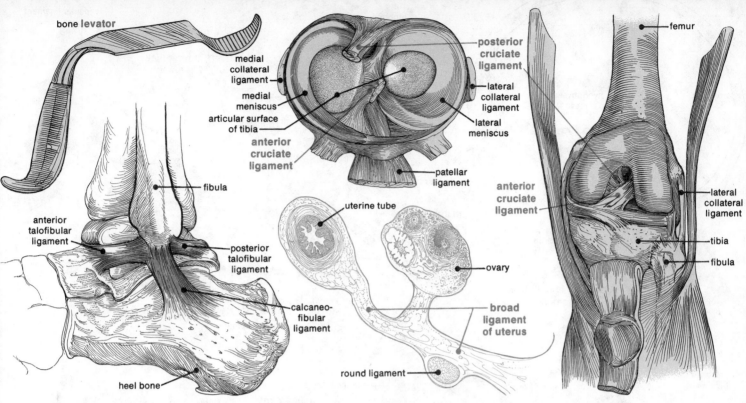

Labels on figure (left to right, top to bottom): bone **levator**, medial collateral ligament, medial meniscus, articular surface of tibia, **anterior cruciate ligament**, **posterior cruciate ligament**, lateral collateral ligament, lateral meniscus, patellar ligament, femur, **anterior cruciate ligament**, lateral collateral ligament, tibia, fibula, fibula, anterior talofibular ligament, posterior talofibular ligament, calcaneofibular ligament, heel bone, uterine tube, ovary, **broad ligament of uterus**, round ligament

white tracts of the spinal cord.

leukonych'ia. Unduly white nails; especially white spots or patches under the nails.

l. totalis, leukonychia in which the entire nail is white.

l. striata, leukonychia in which the nail plate is marked by horizontal streaks of whiteness.

leukopath'ia, leukop'athy. Leukoderma.

leukopede'sis. Movement of white blood cells through the capillary walls into the tissues.

leukope'nia. Abnormal reduction in the number of white corpuscles in the blood; also called leukocytopenia.

leukopla'kia. A disease affecting the mucous membrane of the cheeks, tongue, gums, penis, or vulva, manifested by the formation of white, irregular thickened patches; a chronic inflammatory process, which may ultimately become a squamous cell carcinoma; continued mechanical and chemical irritation is considered the most frequent direct cause; when the lesion is in the oral cavity it is also called smoker's patch.

leukopoie'sis. The production of white blood cells.

leukopro'tease. An enzyme, the product of polynuclear leukocytes, formed in an area of inflammation and causing liquefaction of dead tissue.

leukorrhe'a. An abnormal, white or yellowish discharge from the vagina, containing mucus and pus cells.

leuko'sis. Abnormal proliferation of tissues that form white blood cells.

leukotac'tic. See leukocytotactic.

leukotax'ine. A crystalline nitrogenous substance prepared from inflammatory exudates and injured degenerating tissue.

leukotax'is. See leukocytotaxia.

leukot'omy. Surgical incision into the white matter of the frontal lobe of the brain.

prefrontal l., see lobotomy, prefrontal.

transorbital l., see lobotomy, transorbital.

leukovi'rus. Any of a group of RNA viruses known to cause cancer, under natural conditions, in chickens; they affect the lymphoid and blood forming tissues; also produce solid tumors; e.g., Rous sarcoma.

levallorphan tartrate. White, bitter, crystalline, antianalgesic substance; used in the treatment of narcotics overdose.

levarterenol bitartrate. A white, crystalline, sympathomimetic substance that is soluble in water.

leva'tor. 1. A muscle that raises a part. **2.** Surgical instrument used to lift a structure or a depressed part such as that of a fractured skull.

lev'el. A standard.

lethal blood l., level of concentration of a drug in the blood at which death has been reported to ensue, or which is so far above therapeutic or toxic concentrations that it might cause death.

l. of significance, the probability that an observed difference is due to some factor or factors other than chance.

therapeutic blood l., level of concentration of a drug in the blood at which therapeutic effects are attained.

toxic blood l., level of concentration of a drug in the blood at which toxic symptoms are seen.

levo-. Combining form denoting the left side.

levoro'tatory. Denoting the property of certain substances, as levulose, that turn the plane of polarized light counterclockwise.

lev'ulose. See fructose.

levulosu'ria. Hereditary fructose intolerance; see fructose intolerance.

Lewis blood group. Antigens of red blood cells, saliva, and other body fluids, specified by the Le gene, that react with the antibodies designated anti-Le[a] and anti-Le[b]; named after a Mrs. Lewis in whose blood the antibodies were discovered.

lew'isite. An oily liquid $C_2H_2AsCl_3$, used to make a highly poisonous war gas.

-lexis, -lexy. Combining forms relating to speech.

LGV. Abbreviation for lymphogranuloma venereum.

LH. Abbreviation for luteinizing hormone.

LH-RF. Abbreviation for luteinizing hormone-releasing factor.

Li. Chemical symbol of the element lithium.

libid'inous. Erotic.

libi'do. 1. The emotional energy associated with primitive biologic impulses. **2.** In psychoanalysis, the term is applied to the motive force of the sexual instinct.

Libman-Sacks syndrome. Nonbacterial verrucous endocarditis associated with lupus erythematosus; also called atypical verrucous endocarditis.

lice. Plural of louse.

li'chen. Any eruption of the skin.

l. planus, an eruption of flat, glistening papules with depressed purplish centers.

lichenifica'tion. Hardening and thickening of the skin resulting from long-continued irritation.

lic'orice. See glycyrrhiza.

lidocaine hydrochloride. A widely used local anesthetic; also used in the treatment of cardiac arrhythmias; Xylocaine Hydrochloride®.

lie of the fetus. The relation that the long axis of the fetus bears to that of the mother.

longitudinal l., relationship in which the long axis of the fetus is roughly parallel to the long axis of the

mother; noted in about 99 per cent of all labors at term.

transverse l., relationship in which the long axis of the fetus is at right angles to that of the mother.

li'en. Latin for spleen.

lieno-, lien-. Obsolete prefixes indicating a relationship to the spleen; preferred prefixes are spleno- and splen-.

lienore'nal. Splenorenal.

life. The state or quality manifested by active metabolism; also called vitality.

lig'ament. 1. Any band of fibrous tissue connecting bones. **2.** Any membranous fold, sheet, or cordlike structure that holds an organ in position.

acromioclavicular l., one extending from the acromion process of the scapula to the clavicle.

alar l., one of two short, rounded cords connecting the second vertebra (axis) to the skull; also called odontoid or check ligament.

alveolodental l., periodontal ligament.

annular l., any ligament encircling a structure.

apical odontoid l., one that extends from the apex of the odontoid process of the axis (second vertebra) to the anterior margin of the foramen magnum.

arcuate l.'s, two ligaments (lateral and medial) that attach the diaphragm to the first lumbar vertebra and the twelfth rib on either side.

arcuate l., median, one between the crura of the diaphragm.

broad l. of uterus, one of two fibrous sheets covered on both sides with peritoneum, extending from the uterus to the lateral pelvic wall, on both sides.

capsular l., the fibrous membrane of a joint capsule.

crural l., inguinal ligament.

cardinal l., a sheet of subserous fascia embedded in the adipose tissue of the lower uterine cervix and vagina, on either side, extending in close association with the vaginal arteries.

Cooper's l., (1) see pectineal ligament; (2) see suspensory ligament of breast.

cricothyroid l., a well defined band of elastic tissue extending from the superior border (midline) of the cricoid cartilage to the inferior border of the thyroid cartilage.

cruciate l.'s of knee, two ligaments (anterior and posterior) of considerable strength situated in the middle of the knee joint; they cross each other somewhat like the letter X.

cruciform l. of atlas, a cross-shaped ligament consisting of two parts: (1) a thick strong transverse band which arches across the ring of the first vertebra (it retains the dens of the second vertebra in

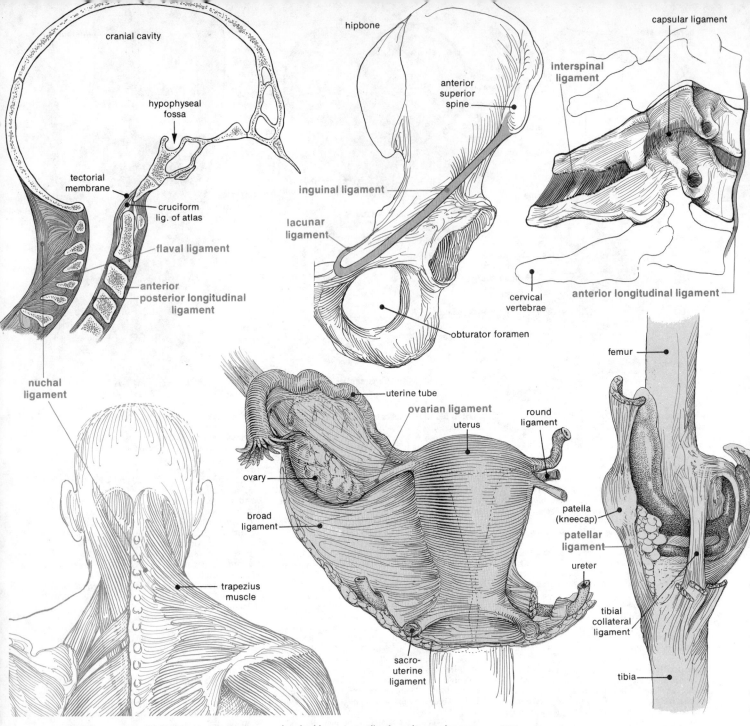

place); (2) a small longitudinal band which divides the ring of the first vertebra into anterior and posterior parts.

deltoid l., the medial reinforcing ligament of the ankle joint.

falciform l. of liver, a sickle-shaped ligament composed of two layers of peritoneum that ascends from the navel to the liver; it attaches the liver to the abdominal wall.

fibular collateral l., a strong, round, fibrous cord, situated on the lateral side of the knee joint; it is attached from the lateral condyle of the femur to the lateral side of the head of the fibula; also called lateral collateral ligament.

flaval l.'s, a series of yellow elastic bands which bind together the laminae of adjacent vertebrae from the axis to the first segment of the sacrum; they serve to maintain the upright position.

fundiform l. of penis, a fibroelastic tissue that is intimately adherent to the linea alba and the pubic symphysis and is extended on to the dorsum of the penis.

hypoepiglottic l., a short triangular elastic band that unites the epiglottis to the upper part of the hyoid bone.

inguinal l., one extending from the anterior superior spine of the ilium to the tubercle of the pubic bone; it is actually the rolled inferior margin of the aponeurosis of the external oblique muscle; also called Poupart's or crural ligament.

interfoveolar l., the thickened portion of the transverse fascia that lies medial to the deep inguinal ring, connecting the transverse muscle of the abdomen to the inguinal ligament and pectineal fascia; also called Hesselbach's ligament.

interspinal l., short bands of fibrous tissue that interconnect the spinous processes of adjacent vertebrae.

lacunar l.'s, a triangular band extending horizontally from the inguinal ligament to the iliopectineal line of the pubis.

longitudinal l., anterior, a broad, flat, strong band of fibers which extends along the anterior surface of the vertebral bodies from the axis (second vertebra) to the sacrum; it is thickest in the thoracic area.

longitudinal l., posterior, a broad, flat, strong band of fibers in the vertebral canal, extending along the posterior surface from the axis (second vertebra) to the sacrum; it is thickest in the thoracic

area.

nuchal l., a broad, somewhat triangular membranous septum in the back of the neck extending from the tips of the cervical spinous processes to the external occipital crest; it forms a septum for attachment of muscles on either side of the neck.

ovarian l., a cordlike bundle of fibers between the folds of the broad ligament, joining the uterine end of the ovary to the lateral margin of the uterus, immediately behind the attachment of the uterine tube.

palpebral l., medial, fibrous bands about four mm in length that connect the medial ends of the tarsi to the frontal process of the maxilla in front of the nasolacrimal groove.

patellar l., the continuation of the central part of the common tendon of the quadriceps muscle of the thigh (quadriceps femoris) from the patella to the tuberosity of the tibia; it is about eight centimeters in length.

pectineal l., a strong aponeurotic band extending from the pectineal line of the pubis to the lacunar ligament with which it is continuous; also called Cooper's ligament.

periodontal l., connective tissue fibers that attach

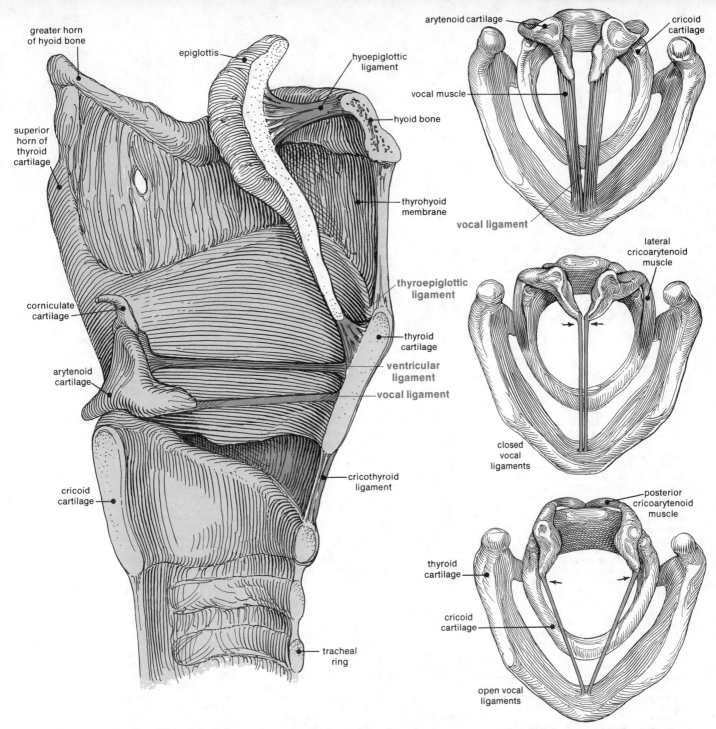

greater horn
of hyoid bone

epiglottis

hyoepiglottic
ligament

superior
horn of
thyroid
cartilage

hyoid bone

thyrohyoid
membrane

cornuculate
cartilage

thyroepiglottic
ligament

arytenoid
cartilage

thyroid
cartilage

ventricular
ligament

vocal ligament

cricoid
cartilage

cricothyroid
ligament

tracheal
ring

arytenoid cartilage

cricoid
cartilage

vocal muscle

hyoid bone

vocal ligament

lateral
cricoarytenoid
muscle

closed
vocal
ligaments

posterior
cricoarytenoid
muscle

thyroid
cartilage

cricoid
cartilage

open vocal
ligaments

a tooth to the bone; also called periodontal membrane.

Poupart's l., see inguinal ligament.

radial collateral l., a large bundle of fibers that crosses the lateral side of the elbow joint; it is attached above to the lateral epicondyle of the humerus, and below to the annular ligament and neck of the radius.

reflected inguinal l., a small, frequently absent, triangular sheet extending from the medial part of the inguinal ring to the linea alba.

round l. of liver, a fibrous cord (the remains of the umbilical vein) extending from the navel to the anterior border of the liver; also called ligamentum teres hepatis.

round l. of uterus, a fibromuscular cord extending from the uterus, on either side, in front and below the uterine tube to the labium major (usually passing through the inguinal canal).

sacrospinous l., a strong triangular ligament attached by its apex to the spine of the ischium and by its base to the lateral part of the sacrum and the coccyx.

sacrotuberous l., a strong ligament extending from the tuberosity of the ischium to the lateral part

of the sacrum and coccyx and to the posterior inferior iliac spine.

sphenomandibular l., a flat, thin band which extends from the spine of the sphenoid bone to the lingula of the lower jaw.

stylomandibular l., a condensed band of cervical fascia which extends from the apex of the styloid process to the posterior border of the angle of the lower jaw.

suspensory l. of breast, one of numerous fibrous bands distributed between the lobes of the mammary glands, extending from the skin to the deep layer of the superficial fascia; also called Cooper's ligament.

suspensory l. of crystalline lens, ciliary zonula; see under zonula.

suspensory l. of ovary, a band of peritoneum arising from the ovary and extending upward over the iliac vessels to become continuous with the peritoneum on the psoas major muscle; it contains the ovarian vessels and nerves.

thyroepiglottic l., an elastic ligament that attaches the petiole of the epiglottis to the thyroid cartilage.

tibial collateral l., a broad, flat, membranous band, situated toward the medial and posterior part

of the knee joint; it is attached from the medial condyle of the femur to the medial condyle and medial surface of the tibia; also called medial collateral ligament.

ulnar collateral l., a thick triangular band of fibers that crosses the medial side of the elbow joint; it is attached above to the medial epicondyle of the humerus, and below to the coronoid process of the ulna (anterior portion) and to the medial margin of the olecranon (posterior portion).

uterosacral l., a fibrous band of subserous fascia extending from the uterine cervix, along the lateral wall of the pelvis, to the sacrum.

ventricular l. of larynx, a thin fibrous membrane in the ventricular fold of the larynx that extends from the thyroid cartilage to the arytenoid cartilage; also called vestibular ligament.

vocal l., the band that extends on either side from the thyroid cartilage to the vocal process of the arytenoid cartilage; it represents the upper border of the conus elasticus of the larynx.

ligamen′tous. Of the nature of a ligament.

li′gand. An organic molecule attached to a central metal ion by multiple coordination bonds, as oxygen is bound to the central iron atom of hemoglobin.

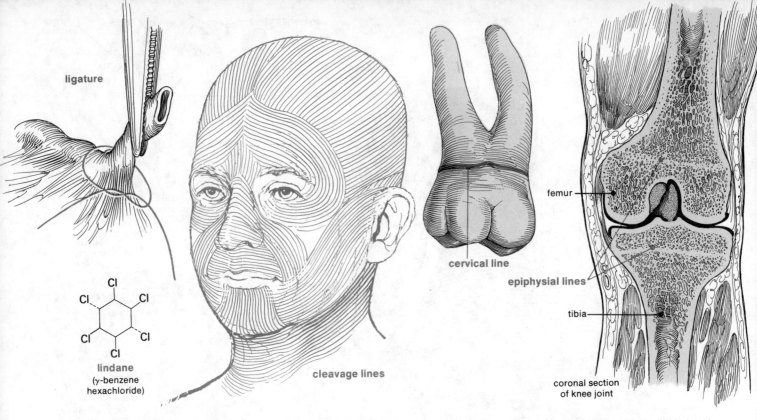

ligature

lindane
(γ-benzene
hexachloride)

cleavage lines

cervical line

epiphysial lines

femur

tibia

coronal section
of knee joint

li′gase. Enzyme that catalyzes the joining of two molecules coupled with the breakdown of ATP or some other nucleoside triphosphate.

li′gate. To constrict a blood vessel, a duct, or the pedicle of a tumor by means of a tightly tied thread (ligature).

liga′tion. The tying of a blood vessel.

li′gator. An instrument used for ligating blood vessels which are generally deep or nearly inaccessible.

lig′ature. A thread used for tying vessels.

light. An electromagnetic radiation capable of inducing visual sensation through the eye; radiant energy, approximately between 380 and 760 nm.

axial l., rays of light parallel to each other and to the axis of an optical system.

cold l., (1) light producing little or no heat, as that by certain luminous insects; (2) any visible light essentially devoid of infrared radiation.

diffused l., light whose rays have no predominant directional component.

coherent l., electromagnetic radiation in which waves have a continuous relationship among phases.

infrared l., infrared rays; see under ray.

Minin l., a lamp that generates violet and ultraviolet light for therapeutic radiation.

polarized l., light of which the vibrations are all in one plane, transverse to the ray, instead of in all planes.

reflected l., light whose rays have been bent by a mirror-like surface and which continues to travel in the altered direction.

refracted l., light whose pathway is altered from its original direction as a result of passing from one transparent medium to another of different density.

transmitted l., light which passes or has passed through a transparent medium.

ultraviolet l., ultraviolet rays; see under ray.

Wood's l., a lamp that generates ultraviolet radiation in the region near the visible spectrum; used in diagnosis and treatment of skin diseases, detection of corneal abrasions, and the evaluation of the fit of contact lenses.

light′ening. The sinking of the fetal head into the pelvic inlet causing the uterus to descend to a lower level and fall forward, thus relieving pressure on the diaphragm and making breathing easier.

Lignac-De Toni-Fanconi syndrome. A childhood form of cystinosis; a rare genetic disorder marked by widespread deposits of cystine throughout the body and dysfunction of the renal tubules, associated with vitamin D-resistant rickets, acidosis, dwarfism, glycosuria, and albuminuria.

limb. An extremity; an arm or leg.

lower l., the lower extremity that includes the hip, buttock, thigh, leg, and foot.

phantom l., a phenomenon often experienced by amputees in which sensations, sometimes painful, seem to originate in the amputated limb.

upper l., the upper extremity that includes the shoulder, arm, forearm, and hand.

lim′bic. 1. Relating to a limbus or border. **2.** Relating to the limbic system of the brain, comprising the cortex and related nuclei; thought to control emotional and behavioral patterns.

lim′bus, *pl.* **lim′bi.** A border.

l. of cornea, the highly vascular band at the junction of the cornea and sclera.

lime. Calcium oxide, CaO; a white caustic powder used in waste treatment, insecticides, and in several industries; also called quicklime, unslaked lime, and calx.

li′men, *pl.* **li′mina.** A threshold; a border; the beginning point; the entrance to a structure.

l. insulae, threshold of the insula (island of Reil) of the brain; a narrow tongue of insular cortex extending ventromedially toward the anterior perforated substance; it receives fibers from the lateral olfactory stria.

l. nasi, the threshold of the nose; the curved ridge which forms the superior and posterior boundary between the nasal cavity proper and the vestibule, where the skin is replaced by mucous membrane.

li′minal. Having the lowest amount of strength necessary to elicit a response; said of a stimulus.

liminom′eter. Instrument to measure a stimulus that has the lowest amount of strength necessary to produce a reflex response.

limp. 1. To walk lamely, with a yielding step. **2.** An uneven gait, favoring one leg. **3.** Flaccid.

lincomy′cin. Substance produced by *Streptomyces lincolnensis*; it has antibacterial action against gram-positive organisms.

lin′dane. γ-Benzene hexachloride; a drug that repels ticks and kills lice.

Lindau's disease. See von Hippel-Lindau disease.

line. 1. A thin, continuous strip, mark, or ridge. **2.** A skin crease; a wrinkle. **3.** An imaginary mark connecting landmarks on the body or passing through them. **4.** A boundary or limit.

absorption l.'s, numerous dark lines in a spectrum due to absorption of specific wavelengths of light by the substance through which it passes.

axillary l., one of three imaginary vertical lines associated with the axilla: the anterior axillary line passes through the anterior fold of the axilla; the posterior passes through the posterior fold; the midaxillary passes through the center of the axilla.

B l.'s of Kerley, horizontal lines in the chest x-ray (above the costophrenic angle) of individuals with pulmonary hypertension secondary to mitral stenosis.

blue l., see lead line.

cervical l., the line around a tooth marking the junction of the enamel of its crown and the cementum of its root.

cleavage l.'s, definite linear clefts in the skin indicative of the direction of the underlying subcutaneous fibrous connective tissue bundles; also called Langer's lines.

dentate l., see pectinate line.

epiphysial l., the line of junction of the epiphysis and diaphysis of an adult long bone.

finish l., in the preparation of a dental cavity, the minimal line of demarcation of the wall of the preparation at the cavosurface.

Fleischner l.'s, linear shadows on a chest x-ray, indicating foci of atelectasis.

fulcrum l., an imaginary line of dental appliance rotation; also called rotational axis.

gingival l., the position of the margin of the gingiva as it extends onto a tooth; also called gum line.

gluteal l., one of three rough curved lines on the outer surface of the iliac part of the hipbone, named anterior, posterior, and inferior.

gum l., see gingival line.

Hampton l., in radiography, a line of decreased density surrounding a benign stomach ulcer.

iliopectineal l., an oblique ridge on the surface of the ilium and continued on the pelvis, which forms the lower boundary of the iliac fossa; it separates the true from the false pelvis; also called linea terminalis.

Langer's l., see cleavage lines.

lead l., a dark bluish area of abnormal pigmentation of the gingival tissues, usually 1 mm from the gingival crest, associated with lead poisoning; also called blue line.

l. of occlusion, the alignment of the occluding surface of the teeth in the horizontal plane.

l. of accomodation, the linear extent to which an object can be moved closer to or away from the eye in a given state of refraction without causing noticeable blurriness.

M l., a line formed by the nodular thickenings of the myofilament (myosin) bisecting the H zone of striated muscle myofibrils.

median l., a vertical center line dividing the body surface into right and left parts.

mercurial l., a linear discoloration of the gingival tissues associated with mercury poisoning; seen along the gingival margin, it can be bluish, purplish, or muddy red in coloration.

midaxillary l., an imaginary vertical line passing

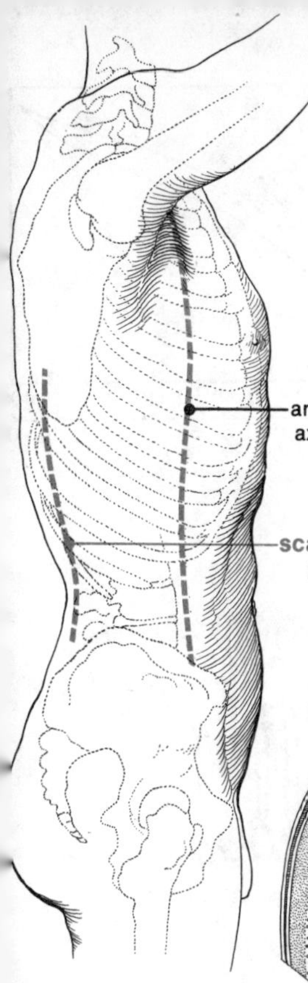
anterior
axillary
line
scapular
line

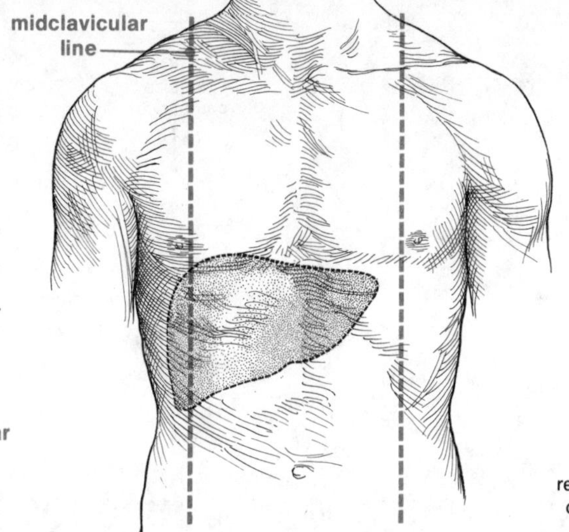
midclavicular
line

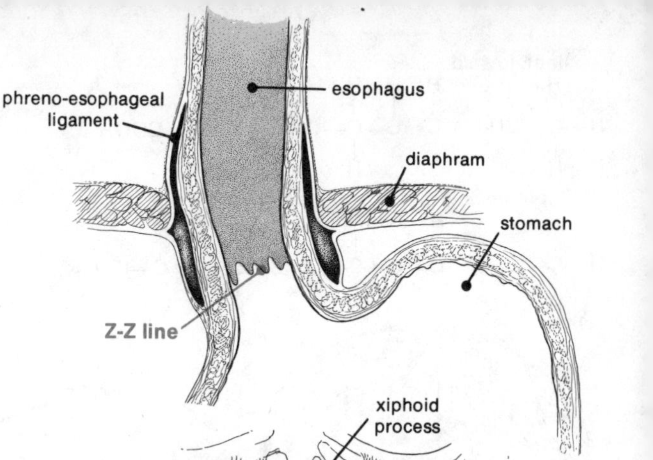
phreno-esophageal
ligament
esophagus
diaphram
stomach
Z-Z line

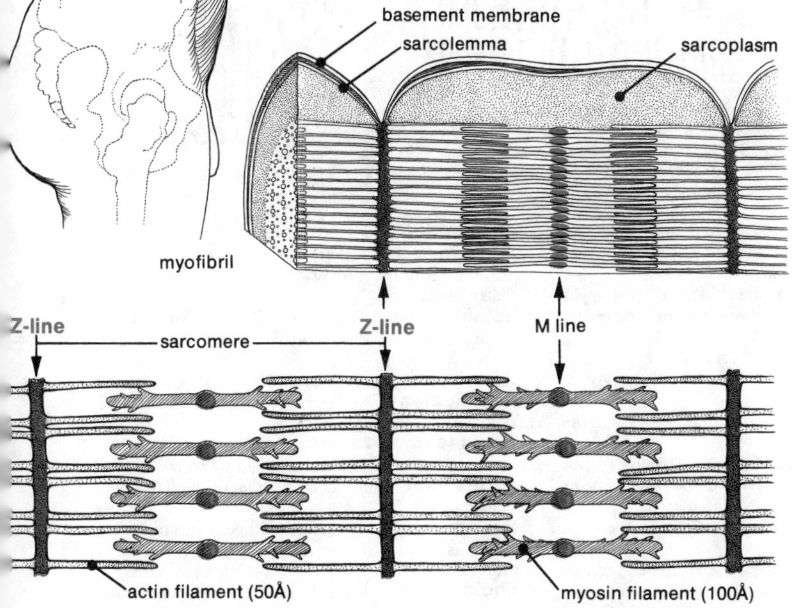
basement membrane
sarcolemma
sarcoplasm
myofibril
Z-line
sarcomere
Z-line
M line
actin filament (50Å)
myosin filament (100Å)

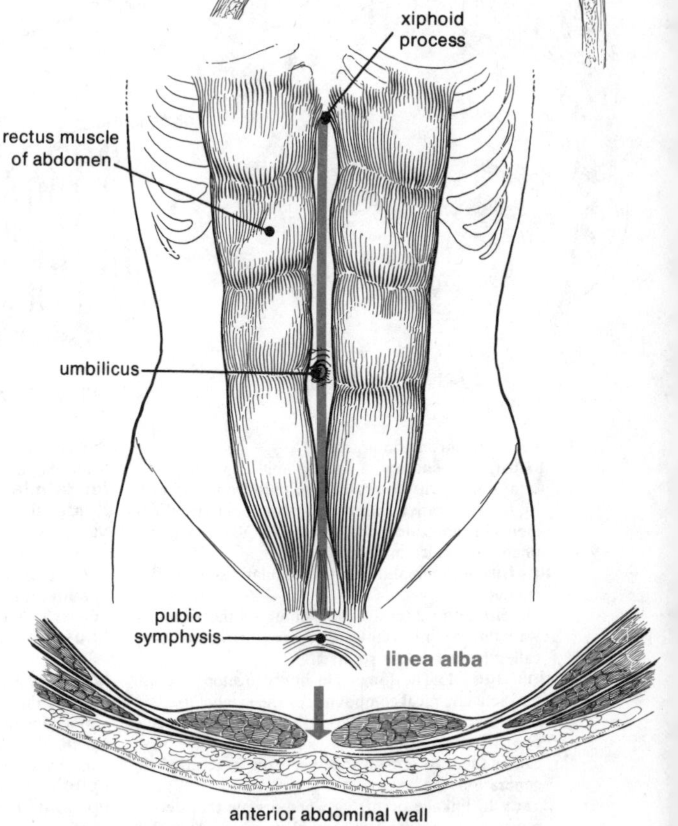
xiphoid
process
rectus muscle
of abdomen
umbilicus
pubic
symphysis
linea alba
anterior abdominal wall

through the middle of the axilla.

midclavicular l., a vertical line passing through the midpoint of the clavicle on either side; it corresponds closely to a perpendicular line passing through the nipple.

milk l., the line or ridge of thickened epithelium in the embryo, extending from the axillary to the inguinal region, along which the mammary glands are developed.

nipple l., a vertical line passing through the nipple on either side.

nuchal l.'s, three lines or ridges (inferior, superior, and highest) on the exterior surface of the occipital bone of the skull.

pectinate l., the line between the rectal mucosa and the skin lining the anus; also called dentate line.

pectineal l., the line on the superior ramus of the pubic bone from the pubic tubercle to the iliopubic eminence; also called pecten pubis.

pure l., a strain of animals inbred for many generations, homozygous for certain specific genes; also called isogenic strain.

scapular l., an imaginary vertical line passing through the lower angle of the scapula on either side.

Schwalbe's annular l., one formed by the peripheral limit of Descemet's membrane of the cornea, indicating the anterior edge of the trabeculae and spaces of Fontana.

survey l., (1) a line inscribed on a cast of a tooth by a surveyor scriber; it marks the greatest height of contour in relation to the chosen path of insertion of the restoration; (2) the line denoting the height of contour of a tooth after the cast has been positioned according to the chosen path of insertion; also called clasp guideline.

temporal l.'s, the two curved lines (inferior and superior) on the outer surface of the parietal bones of the skull.

visual l., an imaginary straight line extending from the object seen to the fovea centralis of the retina; also called visual axis.

Wagner's l., a narrow line representing the area of preliminary calcification, at the junction of the epiphysis and diaphysis of a long bone.

Z l., one of the transverse septa dividing the myofibrils of skeletal muscle into longitudinally arranged sarcomeres; the region between two Z lines consists of overlapping thick and thin myofilaments; also called Z band.

zigzag l., see Z-Z line.

Z-Z l., the transition line from esophageal to gastric mucosa; it appears as an irregular dentate or zigzag line; also called zigzag line.

lin'ea, *pl.* **lin'eae.** A line.

l. alba, the narrow portion of the anterior aponeurosis running down the midline of the abdominal wall from the pubic symphysis to the xiphoid process; also called white line.

l. aspera, a longitudinal ridge with two prominent lips, on the posterior surface of the femur; also called rough line.

l. nigra, the dark streak on the abdomen of pregnant women, between the umbilicus and the pubic symphysis.

l. semilunaris, the lateral edge of the abdominal rectus muscle; it crosses the costal margin at the tip of the ninth costal cartilage.

l. terminalis, iliopectineal line; see under line.

line'breeding. A method of breeding designed to perpetuate the desirable traits of an animal by crossbreeding its descendants.

liner. A layer of asbestos applied to the inside of a dental casting ring in order to free the investment from the restraint of the ring during heating.

lin'gua. Latin for tongue; denotes any tongue-like anatomic structure.

ling'ual. Pertaining to the tongue.

ling'ually. Toward the tongue.

lin'gula. Any tongue-shaped process.

l. of cerebellum, the most anterior tongue-shaped lobule of the superior vermis of the cerebellum.

l. of lung, a projection from the upper lobe of the left lung just beneath the cardiac notch.

l. of mandible, a projection of bone overlapping the mandibular foramen on the inner surface of the ramus of the mandible; it serves for the attachment of the sphenomandibular ligament.

lingulec'tomy. Surgical removal of the lingular portion of the upper lobe of the left lung.

linguo-. Combining form denoting a relationship to the tongue.

linguoclu'sion. The displacement of a tooth or group of teeth toward the tongue; also called lingual occlusion.

lin'guo-occlu'sal. Relating to the lingual and occlusal surfaces of a posterior tooth; usually denoting the line angle formed by the junction of the two surfaces.

linguopapilli'tis. Small painful ulcers around the papillae on the tongue margins.

linguover'sion. Malposition of a tooth toward the tongue.

lin'iment. An oily medicinal liquid applied to the skin by friction as a counterirritant.

li'nin. The fine, threadlike, nonstaining (achromatic) substance of the cell nucleus that intercon-

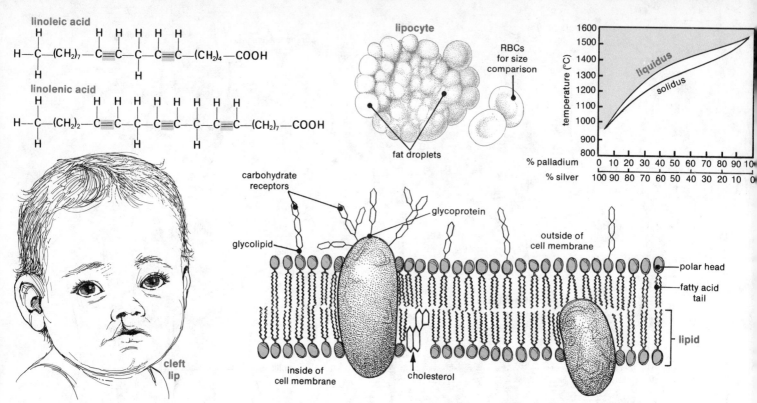

linoleic acid

linolenic acid

lipocyte

RBCs for size comparison

fat droplets

carbohydrate receptors

glycoprotein

glycolipid

outside of cell membrane

polar head

fatty acid tail

lipid

inside of cell membrane

cholesterol

cleft lip

% palladium

% silver

liquidus

solidus

nects the chromatin granules.

li'ning. In dentistry, a coating applied to the walls of a tooth cavity to protect the pulp from irritation by the restorative filling; most commonly used cements include zinc-oxide eugenol (ZOE), zinc phosphate, and calcium hydroxide.

lini'tis. Inflammation of the cellular tissue of the stomach.

l. plastica, extensive thickening of the stomach wall due to infiltrating scirrhous carcinoma; also called leather-bottle stomach.

link'age. 1. The force that holds together the atoms in a chemical compound, or the symbol used to represent it. **2.** The relationship existing between two or more genes in the same chromosome that causes them to remain together from generation to generation.

sex l., linkage occurring when a gene that determines a certain trait is carried in a sex (X or Y) chromosome. See also X linkage.

X l., sex linkage occurring when a gene that determines a trait is located on the X chromosome; the term sex linkage is often used synonymously with X linkage, but since a Y-linked trait is also sex-linked, the preferred term is X linkage.

linoleic acid. A light straw-colored polyunsaturated fatty acid, $C_{18}H_{32}O_2$, that is essential in the human diet; it strengthens capillary walls, lowers serum cholesterol, and prolongs blood clotting time.

linolenic acid. A colorless polyunsaturated fatty acid, $C_{18}H_{30}O_2$, that is essential in the human diet.

liothy'ronine. 3,5,3'-Triiodothyronine.

lip. 1. One of the two fleshy folds forming the anterior boundary of the mouth. **2.** Any liplike structure.

cleft l., harelip; congenital malformation of the upper lip ranging from a scarlike groove, or a notching of the lip, to a complete cleft extending into the nasal cavity.

double l., an oral anomaly consisting of a fold of excess or redundant tissue on the mucosal side of the lip; the upper lip is involved more than the lower one.

lip'ase. A fat-splitting enzyme present in pancreatic juice, blood, and many tissues.

lipec'tomy. Surgical removal of adipose tissue, as for certain cases of obesity; also called adipectomy.

lipede'ma. Chronic swelling of the legs, seen most frequently in middle-aged women.

lipe'mia. The presence of an abnormally large amount of fat in the blood; also called lipidemia.

lip'id. 1. Generally any fat, oil, or wax, or any derivative of these materials; soluble in organic compounds like alcohol and insoluble in water. **2.** Specifically, the fats and fat-like materials which,

together with carbohydrates and proteins, constitute the main structural substance in the living cell.

lipide'mia. See lipemia.

lipido'sis, pl. **lipido'ses.** General term applied to disorders marked by abnormal concentration of lipids in the tissues.

ganglioside l., see gangliosidosis.

sulfatide l., metachromatic leukodystrophy; see under leukodystrophy.

lipo-, lip-. Combining forms indicating a relationship to lipids.

lipoat'rophy, lipoatro'phia. Atrophy of body fat, as the loss of subcutaneous fat after repeated injections of insulin into the same area.

lip'ocele. A hernial sac containing adipose tissue; also called adipocele.

lipochondrodys'trophy. See Hurler's syndrome.

lip'ochrome. Any of various naturally occurring fatty pigments such as carotene and lipofuscin.

lip'ocyte. Fat cell; see under cell.

lipodys'trophy. Defective or faulty metabolism of fat.

lipofibro'ma. A benign tumor composed of fibrous connective tissue and fatty tissue.

lipofus'cin. A golden brown lipid-containing pigment that represents the indigestible residue of cellular lysosomal activity, associated with normal wear and tear; sometimes called old age pigment.

lipogen'esis. The formation of fat.

lipogen'ic. Fat-producing; also called adipogenic.

lip'oid. Resembling fat.

lipoido'sis. The presence of lipid material deposited in various organs.

lipolipoido'sis. Fatty infiltration of the cells.

lipol'ysis. The splitting up or chemical decomposition of fat.

lipo'ma. A benign tumor composed of mature fat cells; also called adipose tumor.

l. fibrosum, see fibrolipoma.

lipo'matoid. Resembling a tumor of fatty tissue.

lipomato'sis. Deposition of fat, either local or general; also called liposis.

lipo'matous. 1. Of the nature of lipoma. **2.** Marked by the presence of a lipoma.

lipope'nia. An abnormally small amount of lipids in the body.

lip'ophage. A fat-absorbing cell.

lipophag'ic. Ingesting or absorbing fat.

lip'ophil. Having affinity for lipids.

lipopro'tein. A conjugated protein containing fat as the nonprotein substance.

liposarco'ma. A rare malignant tumor usually found in the retroperitoneal and mediastinal fat deposits of elderly individuals.

lipo'sis. See lipomatosis.

lipotrop'ic. Relating to lipotropy.

lipot'ropy. 1. Prevention of excessive accumulation of fat in the liver. **2.** Affinity of basic dyes for fatty tissue.

lip'ping. The formation of a liplike border at the articular end of a bone in degenerative bone disease.

lipu'ria. The presence of fat in the urine.

liquefa'cient. An agent that causes a solid to dissolve or become liquid.

liquefac'tion. 1. The act of liquefying. **2.** The state of being converted into a liquid form.

liques'cent. Entering or tending to enter the liquid state.

liq'uid. A substance, neither solid nor gaseous, that exhibits a characteristic readiness to flow, like water.

liquid air. Air in the liquid state; air which has been made liquid by means of intense cold and pressure; used as a source of oxygen and nitrogen, and as a refrigerant.

liq'uidus. The temperature line on a constitution diagram above which the indicated metal element or alloy turns to liquid.

liq'uor, pl. **liquo'res. 1.** A liquid substance. **2.** A solution of a nonvolatile substance in water.

Lister'ia. A genus of bacteria (family Corynebacteriaceae) containing small, gram-positive, aerobic rods; found in feces, sewage, and vegetation.

L. monocytogenes, a species causing meningitis, septicemia, abscesses, and local purulent lesions.

listerio'sis. Infection with bacteria of the genus *Listeria;* commonly occurring in animals but occasionally transmitted to man, where it may produce a clinical picture resembling infectious mononucleosis or an acute meningitis.

li'ter. A metric unit of capacity equal to a cubic decimeter, or 1000 cubic centimeters; approximately 1.056 liquid quarts.

lith-. See litho-.

lith'agogue. An agent that causes the dislodging or expulsion of a calculus, especially of a urinary calculus.

lithec'tasy. The extraction of a bladder stone through the previously dilated urethra.

lithe'mia. See uricemia.

lithi'asis. The formation of stones, especially biliary or urinary stones.

lith'ium. A silvery, soft, highly reactive metallic element; symbol Li, atomic number 3, atomic weight 6.939; used in the treatment of mental illness, particularly in manic disorders.

litho-, lith-. Combining forms meaning stone.

lithocystot'omy. Removal of stones from the bladder.

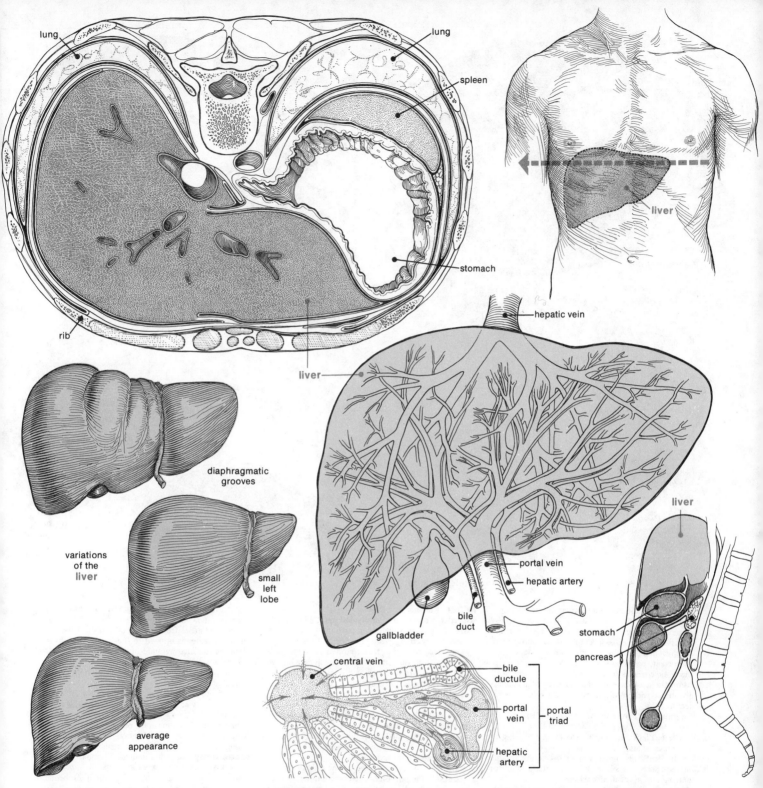

lithodial′ysis. The crushing or dissolving of a stone in the bladder.

lithogen′esis, lithog′eny. The formation of stones within the body.

lithog′enous. Causing the formation of stones.

lithol′apaxy. The operation of crushing a stone in the urinary bladder by means of the lithotrite, and then washing out the fragments through a wide transurethral catheter.

lithol′ogy. The study of pathologic stone formation.

lithol′ysis. Dissolution of stones.

lithome′tra. Calcification of the tissue of the uterus.

lithoneph′ria. Stone in the kidney.

lithonephrot′omy. Incision into the kidney parenchyma or pelvis for removal of a stone; also called renal lithotomy.

lithope′dion. A retained calcified fetus.

lithot′omy. Operation for the removal of a stone, especially from the bladder.

lithotre′sis. The boring of holes in a calculus to facilitate its crushing and removal.

lith′otripsy. The operation of crushing a stone (calculus) in the urinary bladder.

lith′otrite. Instrument for crushing stones in the bladder.

lith′ous. Relating to a calculus or stone.

lithure′sis. The passage of minute stones or gravel in the urine.

lithu′ria. A condition marked by excess uric (lithic) acid or urates in the urine.

lit′mus. A blue pigment, obtained from *Roccella tinctoria* and other lichens, that turns red with increasing acidity and blue with increasing alkalinity.

  l. paper, white paper impregnated with litmus powder and used as a test for acidity and alkalinity; the acid-base pH range is from 4.5 to 8.3.

lit′ter. 1. A stretcher for transporting the disabled. 2. A group of animals produced at one birth by a multiparous mammal; also called brood.

live′do reticula′ris. Circulatory disorder of unknown origin causing constant bluish discoloration on large areas of the extremities.

liv′er. A large, dark red gland that produces and secretes bile, and plays an important role in the metabolism of carbohydrates, fats, protein, minerals, and vitamins; located beneath the entire right dome of the diaphragm and approximately one-third of the left dome; it is the largest glandular organ in the body, weighing from 1200 to 1600 g in the adult (about 1/40 the weight of the body); on the basis of the internal distribution of the blood veesels and bile ducts, the liver may be divided into nearly equal right and left lobes; also called hepar.

  cirrhotic l., a fibrotic liver associated with alterations of the lobular structure and the presence of

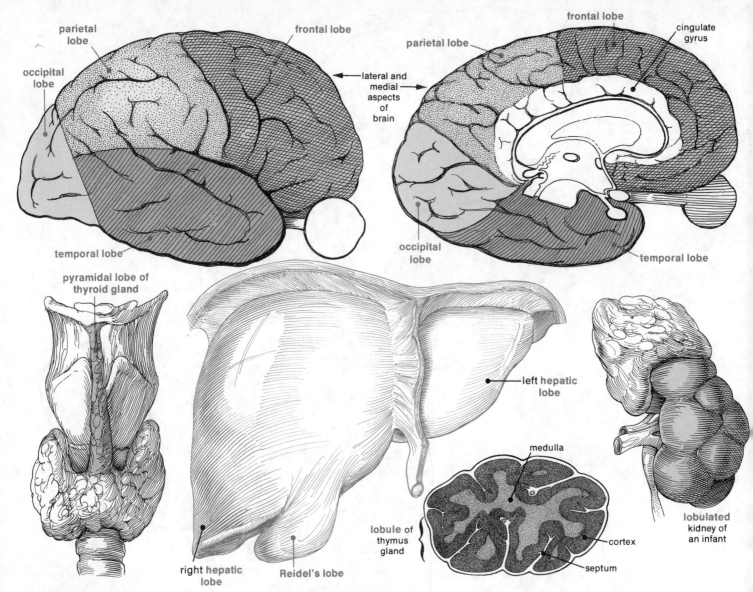

parietal lobe

frontal lobe

frontal lobe

cingulate gyrus

parietal lobe

occipital lobe

lateral and medial aspects of brain

occipital lobe

temporal lobe

temporal lobe

pyramidal lobe of thyroid gland

left hepatic lobe

medulla

lobulated kidney of an infant

lobule of thymus gland

cortex

septum

right hepatic lobe

Reidel's lobe

---

regenerative nodules and vascular anastomoses.

fatty l., an enlarged, doughy liver due to fatty degeneration and infiltration (fatty metamorphosis); it may develop as a complication of any disease in which malnutrition, especially protein deficiency, is present; commonly seen in the early stages of alcoholic cirrhosis or in diabetes.

fibrotic l., a liver marked by an increase in connective tissue without disturbance of the lobular architecture.

nutmeg l., a liver presenting a mottled or polymorphic appearance when sectioned.

liv′id. 1. Black and blue. **2.** Denoting a bluish-gray complexion; also called cyanotic.

lixivia′tion. The process of removing the soluble ingredients from a substance by repeated washing or percolating; also called leaching.

lixiv′ium. The soluble ingredients removed from any substance by leaching; also called lye.

L.M. Abbreviation for licentiate in midwifery.

Lo′a. Congolese for eyeworm; a genus of filarial roundworms.

L. loa, the so-called eyeworm, a threadlike roundworm that infests the subcutaneous tissues, causing tumefactions; the worms migrate rapidly and are usually noticed when passing through the conjunctiva across the eyeball or over the bridge of the nose; indigenous to the western part of equatorial Africa.

load. 1. The quantity borne or sustained by an organism or a part. **2.** A deviation from normal of any body contents (water, salt, etc.); positive load is more than normal and negative load is less than normal.

loai′asis, lo′asis. Condition of infestation with worms of the genus *Loa*.

lo′bar. Relating to a lobe.

lob′ate. Composed of or divided into lobes; lobed.

lobe. 1. A fairly well defined portion of an organ or gland bounded by structural borders such as fissures, sulci, or septa. **2.** A rounded anatomic projecting part, as the fatty lobule of the human ear. **3.** One of the main divisions of the crown of a tooth, formed from a distinct point of calcification.

azygos l., an occasional small triangular lobe on the mediastinal surface at the apex of the right lung, which is delimited by the arch of the azygos vein embedded in the lung substance.

caudate l., a small lobe of the liver situated posteriorly between the inferior vena cava and the fissure for the ligamentum venosum.

ear l., the lower fleshy part of the auricle.

frontal l., the portion of each cerebral hemisphere bounded behind by the central and below by the lateral sulci.

hepatic l., any of the liver lobes, designated right, left, caudate, and quadrate.

limbic l., a general term which usually denotes the cingulate and parahippocampal gyri along with the olfactory bulb and stalk and the parolfactory and olfactory gyri.

occipital l., the most posterior portion of each cerebral hemisphere, bounded anteriorly by the parieto-occipital sulcus and the line joining it to the preoccipital notch.

olfactory l., a general term which usually denotes the olfactory bulb, tract, and trigone plus the anterior perforated substance.

parietal l., the upper central portion of each cerebral hemisphere between the frontal and occipital lobes, and above the temporal lobe; it is separated from the frontal lobe by the central sulcus.

pyramidal l. of thyroid gland, an inconstant, narrow, somewhat cone-shaped lobe of the thyroid gland that arises from the upper border of the isthmus and extends upward to the level of the hyoid bone; also called pyramid of thyroid gland.

Riedel's l., a tongue-shaped mass of tissue occasionally extending downward from the right lobe of the liver.

quadrate l., a small lobe on the inferior surface of the liver between the gallbladder and the ligamentum teres.

temporal l., a long lobe on the outer side and under surface of each cerebral hemisphere; it is bounded above by the lateral sulcus.

lobec′tomy. Surgical removal of a lobe.

lobe′lia. The dried leaves and tops of *Lobelia inflata;* contains several alkaloids including lobeline, norlobelanine, and isolobelanine.

lob′eline. A mixture of alkaloids derived from plants of the genus *Lobelia;* it has actions similar to those of nicotine, but less potent.

lobot′omy. Surgical incision into a lobe.

prefrontal l., a psychosurgical procedure consisting of division of the fibers in the brain connecting the prefrontal and frontal lobes with the thalamus; also called prefrontal leukotomy.

transorbital l., lobotomy through the roof of the orbit; also called transorbital leukotomy.

lob′ulated. Consisting of or divided into lobules.

lob′ule. A small lobe.

lob′ulet, lobulette′. A very small lobule or a section or subdivision of a lobule.

lob′ulus, *pl.* **lob′uli.** Latin for lobule.

lo′bus, *pl.* **lo′bi.** Latin for lobe.

lo′cal. Confined to a limited area.

localiza′tion. 1. Restriction of a process to an

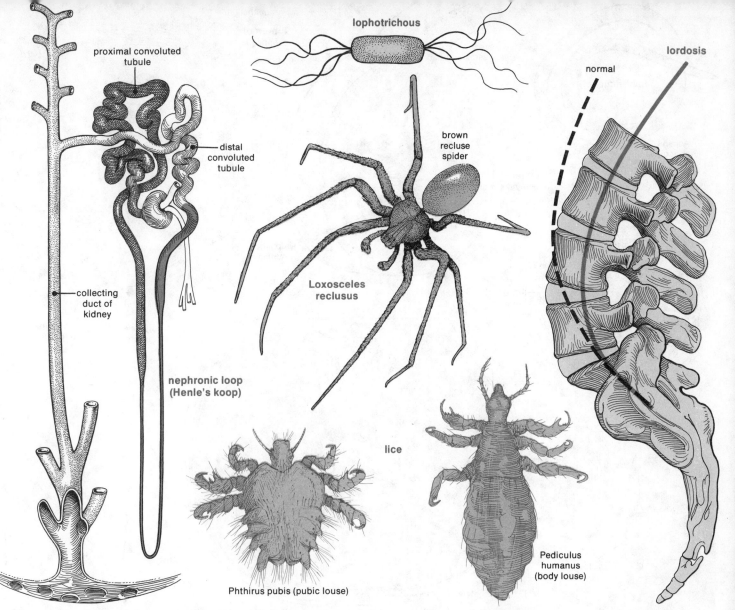

lophotrichous

proximal convoluted tubule

distal convoluted tubule

collecting duct of kidney

nephronic loop (Henle's koop)

brown recluse spider

Loxosceles reclusus

lice

normal

lordosis

Pediculus humanus (body louse)

Phthirus pubis (pubic louse)

area. **2.** The determination of the site of a morbid process.

lo′calized. Limited to a definite part; generally applied to changes that are restricted or confined to a particular area or part.

lo′calizer. A visual training instrument used in the treatment of amblyopia or anopsia.

lo′chia. The bloody discharge from the uterus following childbirth.

lochiome′tra. Retention of blood and mucus (lochia) in the uterus following childbirth.

lochiometri′tis. Inflammation of the uterus following childbirth.

lochiorrhe′a. Excessive flow of discharges after childbirth.

lochios′chesis. Retention in the vagina of the post-delivery discharges (lochia).

lo′ci. Plural of locus.

lock′jaw. 1. See tetanus. **2.** A symptom of tetanus; see trismus.

lo′co. A condition affecting cattle who eat loco weed; marked primarily by incoordination and dullness; also called loco-weed disease.

locomo′tor. Relating to motion.

loco-weed disease. See loco.

loc′ular. Of or relating to a loculus.

loc′ulate, loc′ulated. Divided into or containing numerous loculi.

locula′tion. 1. A structure or tissue having numerous small cavities. **2.** The formation of small cavities or loculi.

loc′ulus, *pl.* **loc′uli.** A small cavity.

lo′cum te′nens. A physician who substitutes for another professionally.

lo′cus, *pl.* **lo′ci.** A place or spot, as the specific site occupied by a gene in a chromosome.

l. ceruleus, a bluish gray area in the floor of the fourth ventricle.

Löffler's disease. An uncommon but distinctive form of disease in which the heart is the organ mainly affected by an eosinophilic arteritis, probably of an allergic type; characterized by progressive congestive heart failure, multiple systemic emboli, and eosinophilia; also called eosinophilic endomyocardial disease and Loffler's endocarditis.

Löffler's syndrome. Disorder, usually lasting less than a month, marked by transient infiltrates of the lungs, low fever, and increased number of eosinophils in the peripheral blood.

logop′athy. Any disorder of speech.

logople′gia. Paralysis of the speech organs.

logorrhe′a. Excessive, uncontrollable talking.

-logy. Combining form meaning the study or science of a subject.

loin. The part of back and sides of the body between the ribs and the pelvis.

loop. 1. A bend in a cord or cordlike structure. **2.** A platinum wire attached to a handle at one end and bent into a circle at the other; used to transfer bacterial cultures.

Henle's l., see nephronic loop.

nephronic l., the U-shaped portion of the nephronic tubule, between the proximal and distal convoluted portions; also called Henle's loop or ansa.

lophot′richous. Referring to a bacterial cell with two or more flagella or cilia at one or both poles.

lordoscolio′sis. An abnormal backward and lateral curvature of the spine.

lordo′sis. Abnormally increased forward curvature of the lumbar spine; also called sway-back.

lordot′ic. Of, relating to, or characterized by lordosis.

lo′tion. 1. Any of various medicated liquids for external application, especially those containing one or more insoluble substances in suspension. **2.** Any of various liquid cosmetic preparations, usually applied to the face and hands.

calamine l., a preparation of mineral oil with zinc oxide, ferric oxide, glycerin, bentonite magma, and calcium hydroxide solution.

loupe. A small magnifying lens, usually set in an eyepiece.

louse, *pl.* **lice. 1.** Any of various small, wingless, flat-bodied, parasitic insects of the orders Anoplura and Mallophaga. **2.** Common name for *Pediculus humanus capitis*.

body l., see *Pediculus humanus corporis*.

crab l., see *Phthirus pubis*.

head l., see *Pediculus humanus capitis*.

pubic l., see *Phthirus pubis*.

Lowe's syndrome. See oculocerebrorenal syndrome.

Loxos′celes reclu′sus. North American brown recluse spider; volume for volume its venom is more potent than a rattlesnake's; its bite is potentially about as lethal as that of the black widow spider.

loxos′celism. A condition resulting from the bite of the North American brown recluse spider, *Loxosceles reclusus*; characterized by gangrenous slough at the affected area, nausea, malaise, fever, hemolysis, and thrombocytopenia.

loxot′omy. Surgical amputation by means of an oblique incision through the soft tissue; distinguished from a circular amputation.

loz′enge. A medicated disk-shaped tablet for local treatment of the mouth or throat; also called troche.

L.P. Abbreviation for light perception.

LPN. Abbreviation for licensed practical nurse.

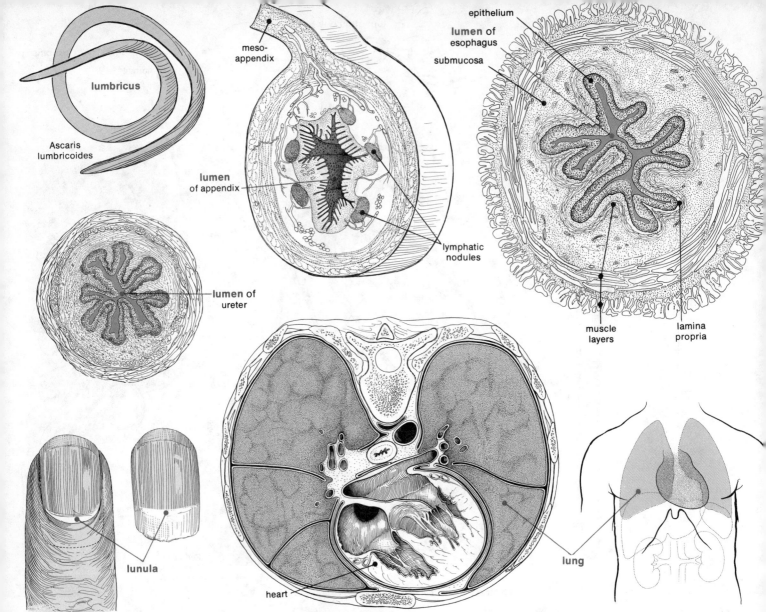

Lr. Symbol for a toxin-antitoxin mixture which will produce a minimal, positive reaction at the site of injection in an experimental animal

LRF. Abbreviation for luteinizing hormone-releasing factor.

LSD. Abbreviation for lysergic acid diethylamide.

LSH. Abbreviation for lutein-stimulating hormone.

Lu. Chemical symbol of the element lutetium.

lu'bricant. Any substance or secretion acting as a surface coating that reduces friction, heat, and wear.

   vaginal l., the transudate-like secretion which appears on the walls of the vagina shortly after the onset of effective sexual stimulation.

lubrica'tion. The process of lubricating or making slippery.

lucif'ugal. Avoiding light.

lues. Syphilis.

luet'ic. Syphilitic.

lumba'go. Backache in the lumbar region.

lum'bar. Relating to the loins.

lumbariza'tion. Fusion between the transverse processes of the lowest lumbar and the adjacent sacral vertebrae.

lumbosa'cral. Relating to the lumbar portion of the spine and the sacrum.

lum'brical. 1. Pertaining to or resembling an earthworm. **2.** See table of muscles.

lum'bricoid. Resembling an earthworm.

lum'bricus. A worm parasitic in the intestine, *Ascaris lumbricoides.*

lu'men. 1. The interior space of a tubular structure, as a blood vessel or the esophagus. **2.** A unit of emitted light; one lumen equals 0.001946 watt.

lu'mina. One of the plural forms of lumen.

lu'minal. Relating to the lumen of a blood vessel, intestine, or other tubular structure.

lumines'cence. The property of giving off light by processes that derive energy from essentially nonthermal sources.

luminif'erous. Producing, conveying, or transmitting light.

lu'minophore. 1. Any substance that emits light at room temperature. **2.** An organic radical that produces or increases the property of luminescence of certain organic compounds.

lu'minous. Emitting or reflecting light.

lumirhodop'sin. An intermediate product in the bleaching process of rhodopsin by the action of light prior to the formation of metarhodopsin and the retinene.

lumpec'tomy. Surgical removal of a hard mass of tissue, especially from the breast.

lu'nacy. Obsolete word for a major mental illness.

lung. The paired organ of respiration occupying the chest cavity (together with the heart) and enveloped by the pleura; generally the right lung is slightly larger than the left and is divided into three lobes, while the left has but two; the primary purpose of the lung is the uptake of oxygen and the elimination of carbon dioxide; it is accomplished by the following processes: (a) ventilation (inspired air reaches the alveoli and is distributed evenly to the millions of alveoli in the lungs); (b) diffusion (oxygen and carbon dioxide pass across the alveolar capillary membranes); (c) pulmonary capillary blood flow (flow is distributed evenly to all the ventilated alveoli).

   black l., a form of pneumoconiosis common in coal miners, characterized by heavy deposit of coal dust in the lung; chronic bronchitis and emphysema may be associated with the condition.

   coal miners' l., black lung.

   farmer's l., an acute reaction or condition due to inhalation of moldy hay dust, usually from handling grains particularly in threshing; thought to be of allergic origin; the symptoms are distressing dyspnea, cyanosis, and a dry cough; also called thresher's lung.

   honeycomb l., a lung marked by a spongy or honeycomb appearance from numerous small cysts resulting from diffuse fibrosis and cystic dilation of bronchioles.

   iron l., a popular name for the Drinker respirator; see under respirator.

   miners' l., black lung.

   rheumatoid l., infiltrates in the lung associated with rheumatoid arthritis.

   thresher's l., see farmer's lung.

   welder's l., relatively benign form of pneumoconiosis due to deposition of fine metallic particles in the lung; occupational hazard among welders.

   wet l., accumulation of fluid in the lung as in pulmonary edema.

lung'worm. Any of various nematode worms parasitic in the air passages of animals.

lu'nula. The pale semicircle at the root of each nail; also called half moon.

lu'poid. Resembling lupus.

lu'pus. A general term denoting any of several diseases manifested by characteristic skin lesions; used with a qualifying adjective.

   discoid l. erythematosus, a disease confined to the skin, marked by a scaly rash, usually in a butterfly pattern over the nose and cheeks, sometimes extending to the scalp and causing baldness.

   l. pernio, sarcoid lesions of the hands and face, especially the ears and nose, resembling frostbite.

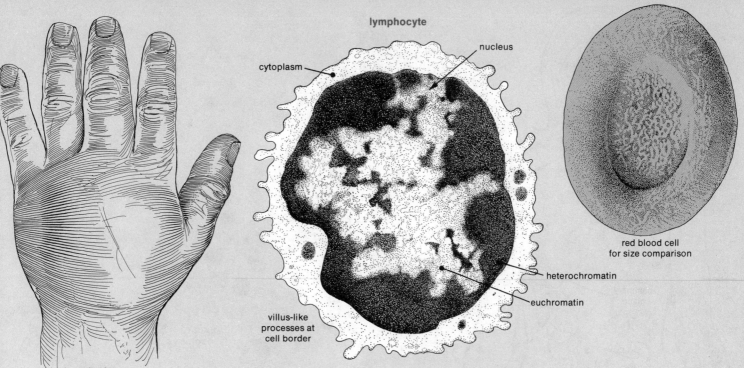

lymphedema

lymphocyte

cytoplasm — nucleus

villus-like processes at cell border

heterochromatin

euchromatin

red blood cell for size comparison

---

l. vulgaris, infection of the skin with the bacillus of tuberculosis, causing red-brown nodular lesions most frequently on the face.

systemic l. erythematosus (SLE), a chronic disease of unknown origin commonly marked by an erythematous rash on the face and other areas exposed to sunlight; it is much more common in women than men and occurs most often in the third and fourth decades; it involves the vascular and connective tissues of many organs, resulting in a multiplicity of local and systemic manifestations; serlogic abnormalities including false positive VDRL and antinuclear antibodies are manifestations, as well as a positive LE cell test; anti-DNA antibodies appear to be specific for SLE.

lu'teal. Relating to the corpus luteum of the ovary.

lu'tein. The yellow pigment of egg yolks, corpus luteum, and fat cells.

luteiniza'tion. The formation of luteal tissue; process in which the mature ovarian follicle after discharging the egg, becomes hypertrophied and yellow, thus forming the corpus luteum.

lu'teinizing. See luteogenic.

Lutembacher's syndrome. Congenital abnormality of the heart marked by an interatrial defect and mitral stenosis.

lu'teogenic. Luteinizing; inducing the development of corpora lutea.

luteo'ma. An uncommon ovarian tumor believed to be formed in the same way that the lutein cells of the corpus luteum are produced.

lu'teotrophic, lu'teotropic. Having a stimulating action on the development and function of the corpus luteum.

lute'tium. A silvery-white rare earth element, symbol Lu, atomic number 71, atomic weight 174.97; the final member of the lanthanide rare earth series; used in nuclear technology.

Lutheran blood group. Antigens of red blood cells, specified by the Lu gene, that react with antibodies designated anti-Lu^a and anti-Lu^b; first detected in the serum of an individual who had received many transfusions and who developed antibodies against the erythrocytes of a donor named Lutheran.

lux. A unit of illumination, equal to one lumen per square meter.

luxa'tion. Dislocation.

LV. Abbreviation for left ventricle.

LVH. Abbreviation for left ventricular hypertrophy.

Lw. Chemical symbol of the element lawrencium.

lye. 1. Sodium or potassium hydroxide. **2.** Lixivium.

lying-in. Confinement of a woman during childbirth.

lymph. A transparent or slightly opalescent fluid containing a clear liquid portion, a varying number of white blood cells, chiefly lymphocytes, and a few red blood cells; it is absorbed from the tissue spaces by the lymphatic capillaries (a system of closed tubes), conveyed, and eventually returned to the bloodstream by the lymphatic vessels, after it flows through a filtering system (lymph nodes).

lymph'aden. Lymph node.

lymphadenecta'sia. Enlargement of lymph nodes with excessive lymph.

lymphadenec'tomy. Surgical removal of lymph nodes.

lymphade'nia. Chronic overgrowth of lymphoid tissue.

lymphadeni'tis. Inflammation of the lymph nodes.

lymphadenog'raphy. Roentgenographic examination of a lymph node.

lymphadeno'ma. See lymphoma. Any tumor made up of lymphoid tissue.

lymphadenomato'sis. A condition marked by the presence of numerous enlarged lymph nodes, as in malignant lymphoma.

lymphadenop'athy. Any disorder of the lymph nodes or lymph vessels.

lymphadeno'sis. Generalized enlargement of the lymph glands and lymphatic tissue of the organs; proliferation of lymphoid tissues.

benign l., infectious mononucleosis.

malignant l., lymphoma.

lymph'agogue. An agent that increases the formation and flow of lymph.

lymphangiecta'sia, lymphangiec'tasis. Abnormal dilatation of lymphatic vessels; also called telangiectasia lymphatica.

lymphangiec'tomy. Surgical excision of a lymphatic vessel.

lymphan'gioendothelio'ma. A tumor composed of small masses of endothelial cells and aggregations of tubular structures thought to be lymphatic vessels.

lymphangiog'raphy, lymphog'raphy. Roentgenographic visualization of lymphatic vessels after injection of a contrast medium.

lymphangiol'ogy. See lymphology.

lymphangio'ma. A tumor-like mass of dilated lymphatic vessels.

lymphangi'tis. Inflammation of the lymphatic vessels; a common manifestation of a bacterial infection, usually caused by the hemolytic streptococcus.

lymphat'ic. Relating to lymph, lymph nodes, or lymph vessels.

lymphecta'sia. Dilatation of the lymphatic vessels.

lymphede'ma. Chronic unilateral or bilateral swelling of the extremities caused by obstruction of the lymphatic vessels or disease of the lymph nodes.

lympho-, lymph-. Combining forms indicating a relationship to lymph.

lymph'oblast. An immature cell that is the precursor of the lymphocyte; also called lymphocytoblast and immunoblast.

lymphoblas'tic. Relating to lymphoblasts or the production of lymphocytes.

lymphoblasto'ma. A tumor arising in a lymph node or group of nodes, composed mainly of lymphoblasts; a form of malignant lymphoma.

lymphoblasto'sis. Excess of lymphoblasts in the blood.

lym'phocele. A cystic mass that contains lymph; also called lymphocyst.

lymph'ocyte. A white blood cell formed in lymphoid tissue and constituting normally from 25 to 33 per cent of all white blood cells in adult peripheral blood.

B l.'s, lymphocytes derived from bone marrow; they interact chiefly with the humoral immune system which involves substances such as antibodies, antigens, and serum complement enzymes in the blood.

T l.'s, lymphocytes derived from the thymus gland; they play a large role in the cellular immune system by responding to antigens and triggering reactions in other cells such as macrophages.

virgin l., inducible cell; see under cell.

lymphocyt'ic. Relating to lymphocytes.

lymphocy'toblast. See lymphoblast.

lymphocyto'ma. A tumor of low grade malignancy, arising in a lymph node or group of nodes; made up chiefly of adult lymphocytes.

lymphocytope'nia. Marked reduction in the number of lymphocytes in the blood.

lymphocytopoie'sis. The formation of lymphocytes.

lymphocyto'sis. Excessive number of lymphocytes in the blood.

lymphoder'ma pernicio'sa. See leukemia cutis.

lymphoepithelio'ma. A malignant tumor derived from the epithelium of the area around the tonsils and nasopharynx, and containing abundant lymphoid tissue.

lymphogen'esis. The production of lymph.

lymphog'enous. 1. Originating from lymph. **2.** Producing lymph.

lymphogranulo'ma vene'reum. (LGV). A viral infection marked by the appearance of a transient ulcer on the genitalia and enlargement of the lymph nodes of the groin in the male and the

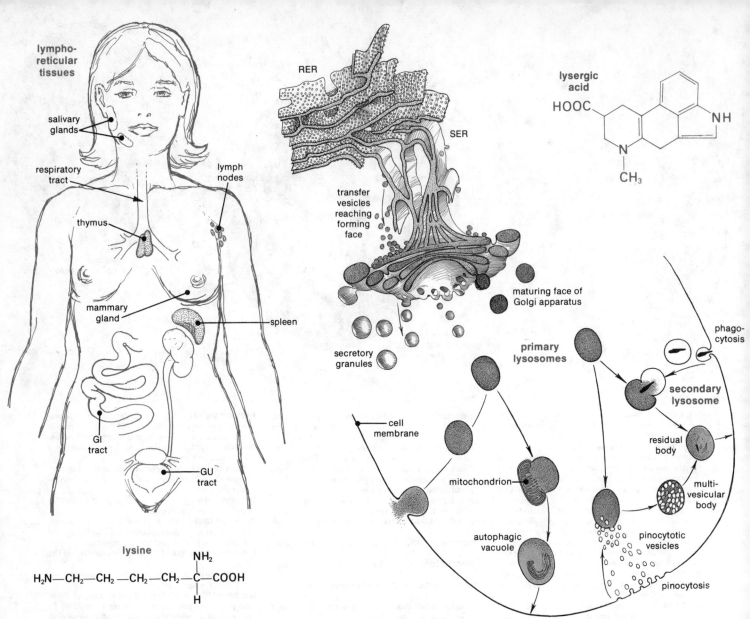

lympho-reticular tissues

salivary glands

respiratory tract

thymus

mammary gland

lymph nodes

spleen

GI tract

GU tract

RER

SER

transfer vesicles reaching forming face

maturing face of Golgi apparatus

secretory granules

primary lysosomes

phago-cytosis

secondary lysosome

residual body

multi-vesicular body

cell membrane

mitochondrion

autophagic vacuole

pinocytotic vesicles

pinocytosis

lysergic acid

HOOC

NH

N

CH₃

lysine

$H_2N-CH_2-CH_2-CH_2-CH_2-\overset{\overset{\displaystyle NH_2}{|}}{\underset{\underset{\displaystyle H}{|}}{C}}-COOH$

---

pararectal nodes in the female, with attending stricture of the rectum; also called tropical bubo and lymphogranuloma inguinale; formerly called lymphopathia venereum..

lymphog'raphy. See lymphangiography.

lym'phoid. Pertaining to or resembling lymph or lymphatic tissue.

lymphoidec'tomy. Surgical excision of lymphoid tissue, such as adenoids.

lymphokine'sis. 1. Circulation of lymph through the lymphatic vessels and nodes. **2.** The movement of endolymph in the membranous labyrinth of the internal ear.

lymphol'ogy. The science of the lymphatic system comprising lymph, lymphocytes, lymph nodes, and lymph vessels; also called lymphangiology.

lympho'ma. Any of a group of malignant diseases originating in the lymphoreticular system, usually in the lymph nodes.

   Burkitt's l., a malignant tumor affecting children of the middle African regions; it involves primarily the jaw and abdominal area; also called African lymphoma.

   giant follicular l., a malignant tumor of lymphoid tissue characterized by multiple proliferative, follicle-like nodules.

lymphomato'sis. Any condition characterized by the presence of multiple lymphoid tissue tumors (lymphomas).

lymphopath'ia vene'reum. Old term for lymphogranuloma venereum.

lymphop'athy. Any disease of the lymphatic system.

lymphope'nia. Reduction in the number of lymphocytes in the blood.

lymphopoie'sis. The formation of lymphocytes.

lymphoretic'ular. Relating to a tissue containing a variety of cell types involved in the elaboration of a cell product when confronted with a substance which is recognized as foreign; the tissue is located within the thymus gland, lymph nodes, spleen, and the lining of the lymphatic and vascular channels, as well as in bodily tracts exposed to the outside.

lymphosarco'ma. A malignant tumor of lymph nodes composed of lymphoblasts and lymphocytes which enlarges and invades adjacent tissues.

lymphos'tasis. Obstruction of the normal flow of lymph.

ly'ophil. Any substance that easily goes into solution; lyophilic material.

lyophil'ic. Denoting a pronounced affinity between the dispersed particles and the solvent (dispersing medium) of a colloid.

lyoph'ilization. 1. The process of freeze-drying; the act of separating a solid substance from solution by freezing the solution and evaporating the ice under vacuum. **2.** Process used for preservation of a variety of tissues and bacteria.

lyophil'ize. To separate a solid from solution by rapid freezing and dehydration under vacuum; to freeze-dry.

lyopho'bic. Denoting a lack of affinity between the dispersed particles and the solvent of a colloid.

lyotrop'ic. Readily soluble.

lyse. To effect lysis (disintegration of cells).

lysergic acid. A crystalline compound derived from ergot.

   l. a. diethylamide (LSD), a hallucinogenic drug derived from lysergic acid.

ly'sin. An antibody that destroys cells by dissolving them, as hemolysin and bacteriolysin which destroy blood cells and bacteria, respectively.

ly'sine. One of the essential amino acids; produced by the hydrolysis of casein and other proteins.

-lysis. Combining form meaning dissolution, separation, loosening, or rupture.

ly'sis. 1. Destruction of cells by a specific lysin. **2.** The gradual recovery from an acute disease.

ly'sogen. An antigen that stimulates the formation of a specific lysin.

lysogen'esis. The production of antibodies that cause dissolution of cells and tissues.

ly'sokinase. An activator agent of the fibrinolytic system, such as streptokinase or staphylokinase, that produces plasma by indirect or multiple-stage action on plasminogen.

lysolecithin. A lecithin (phosphatidyl choline) from which the unsaturated fatty acid residue has been removed by partial hydrolysis; it has strong hemolytic properties and is a good detergent and emulsifier of dietary lipid.

ly'sosome. One of the large cytoplasmic particles in a cell containing a powerful digestive juice (hydrolyzing enzyme or lysozyme) capable of breaking down most of the constituents of living matter; it is present in all animal cells, being particularly large and abundant in white blood cells.

   primary l., a lysosome that has not engaged in any digestive activity.

   secondary l., a vacuolated lysosome that is the site of current or previous digestive activity.

ly'sozyme. An antibacterial enzyme naturally present in tear fluid, sweat, saliva, and nasal secretions; also called mucopeptide glucohydrolase.

lyt'ic. Relating to or causing disintegration of cells.

colony

macrodactylia

macrophage

macroconidium

Microsporum canis

nucleus

Mm

μ. The Greek letter mu; symbol for micron.

μCi. Abbreviation for microcurie; formerly μc.

μg. See mcg.

μμ. Symbol for micromicron.

M. 1. Abbreviation for (a) metal; (b) *Micrococcus;* (c) *misce* (in prescriptions, mix); (d) molar; (e) muscle; (f) myopia. **2.** Symbol for (a) a blood factor; (b) molecular weight.

M. Abbreviation for molar concentration.

m. Abbreviation for (a) meter; (b) a unit of fluid measure.

mμ. Symbol for millimicron.

ma. Abbreviation for milliampere.

Macaca. A genus of monkeys of the family Cercopithecidae.

M. mulatta, the rhesus monkey from which the Rh antigen was originated.

Mace. Proprietary name for the lacrimator chloracetophenone, combined with a light petroleum dispersant and a Freon-like propellant; used in aerosol form as a defensive weapon to disable with intense burning eye pain and respiratory distress.

macerate. To soften a solid or a tissue by soaking in a fluid.

macera'tion. 1. The softening of a solid or the separation of its constituents by soaking it in a liquid. **2.** In obstetrics, the softening and disintegration of a fetus remaining in the uterus after its death.

machine. A device that accomplishes a specific objective.

heart-lung m., any of various machines that make it possible to support the circulation with oxygenated blood while keeping the heart essentially free of blood and permitting surgery within the heart, coronary arteries, and ascending arch of the aorta under direct vision; venous blood ordinarily returning to the right atrium is diverted to an oxygenator (artificial lung) where it takes up oxygen and gives off carbon dioxide; the refreshed blood is pumped into the individual's arterial system.

Holtz m., a device for developing high-voltage static electricity by multiplication of an induced charge.

kidney m., artificial kidney; see under kidney.

panoramic rotating m., an x-ray machine capable of radiographing all the teeth and surrounding structures by using a reciprocating motion of the tube and extraoral film.

Van de Graaf m., an electrostatic machine that produces high potential; used for generating high-voltage x rays.

Wimshurst's m., a machine capable of converting mechanical energy into electrical energy by electrostatic action.

macrenceph'aly, macrencepha'lia. Macroencephaly.

macro-, macr-. Combining forms denoting (1) large or long; e.g., macronucleus; (2) abnormal enlargement; e.g., macroencephaly.

macroam'ylase. A form of serum amylase in which the enzyme occurs as a complex joined to a globulin.

macrobra'chia. Condition of having abnormally long arms.

macroceph'alous. Having an abnormally large head.

macrochi'lia. 1. Unusually large lips. **2.** A condition of permanently enlarged oral lips, usually due to the presence of distended lymph spaces.

macrochi'ria. Megalochiria; a condition of unduly enlarged hands.

macroconid'ium. A large exospore or conidium.

macrocor'nea. See megalocornea.

macrocra'nia. Abnormal general enlargement of the head; distinguished from enlargement of the head in one direction only.

macrocryoglobuline'mia. The presence of cold precipitating macroglobulins (cold hemagglutinins) in the peripheral blood.

mac'rocyte. A large red blood cell at least two microns larger than normal; can be seen in the blood of individuals with pernicious anemia, folic acid deficiency, and other anemias; also called megalocyte.

macrocythe'mia. See macrocytosis.

macrocyto'sis. A condition in which the red blood cells are larger than normal; also called macrocythemia.

macrodactyl'ia, macrodac'tyly. A condition in which fingers or toes are abnormally large; also called dactylomegaly and megalodactylism.

mac'rodont. 1. An abnormally large tooth. **2.** Denoting a skull with a dental index over 44.

macrodon'tia. The condition of having abnormally large teeth.

macroenceph'aly. Malformation and great increase in size and weight of the brain due partly to proliferation of the glia (nonneuronal tissue); associated with small ventricles, enlargement of the head, and mental retardation.

macrogam'ete. The female of certain unicellular organisms.

macrogame'tocyte. A mother cell producing the females or macrogametes of certain protozoa.

macrogenitoso'mia. Disorder of the adrenal cortex affecting male children, believed by some to originate during prenatal life; characterized by early enlargement of the penis with frequent erections, associated with rapid growth of the skeleton, mus-

cles, body hair, and larynx; ossification of the skeleton occurs prematurely, resulting in abnormally short stature.

macrogin'givae. Abnormal enlargement of the gums.

macrog'lia. The astrocyte and oligodendrocyte, the two neuroglial elements of ectodermal origin.

macroglob'ulin. Unusually large plasma globulin (protein); molecular weight is often about 1,000,000.

macroglobuline'mia. A plasma cell dyscrasia; a disorder marked by excessive production of gamma M globulin; common findings include anemia and bleeding manifestations; also called primary macroglobulinemia and Waldenström's syndrome.

macroglos'sia. Enlargement of the tongue; also called megaloglossia.

macrogna'thia. Abnormal largeness of the jaw.

macrogy'ria. A congenital malformation in which the convolutions of the cerebral cortex are larger than normal due to a reduction in the number of sulci.

mac'rolides. A group of antibiotics having molecules made up of large-ring lactones; e.g., erythromycin.

macromas'tia, macroma'zia. Abnormally large breasts.

macrome'lia. A condition of unduly enlarged limbs; abnormal size of one or more of the extremities; also called megalomelia.

mac'romethod. A chemical test using ordinary (not minute) quantities.

macromol'ecule. Any molecule composed of several monomers, notably proteins, nucleic acids, polysaccharides, glycoproteins, and glycolipids.

macronu'cleus. 1. A nucleus that occupies a large area of the cell. **2.** The larger, nonreproductive nucleus in ciliated protozoa.

macropar'asite. A parasite that is visible to the unaided eye; e.g., a louse.

macropath'ology. Gross anatomic changes caused by disease.

mac'rophage. A large mononuclear cell which ingests degenerated cells and blood tissue; found in large numbers throughout the body, with the greatest accumulation in the spleen, where they remove damaged or aging red blood cells from the circulation; in the brain and spinal cord they are known as microglia; in the blood they are called monocytes.

alveolar m., a cell that moves about on the alveolar surface of the lung engulfing airborne particles that reach the alveolus; derived from the hematogenous monocyte; also called dust cell and alveolar phagocyte.

macrophthal'mia. Abnormal enlargement of the

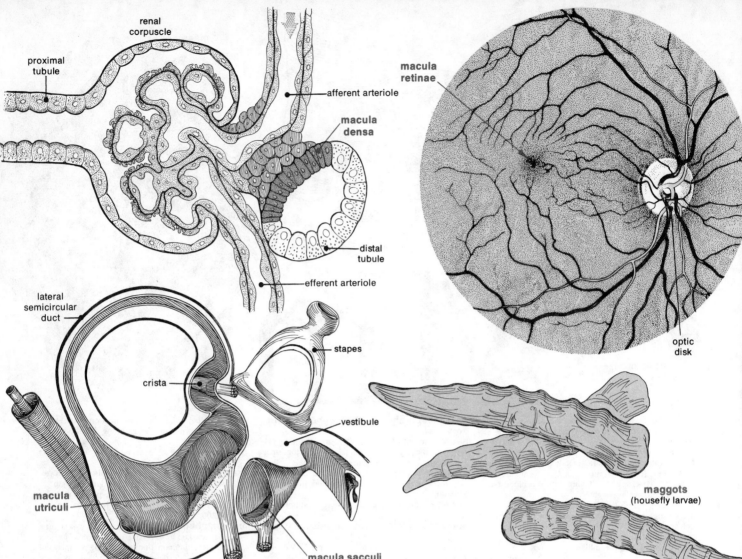

renal corpuscle

proximal tubule

afferent arteriole

macula retinae

macula densa

distal tubule

efferent arteriole

optic disk

lateral semicircular duct

crista

stapes

vestibule

macula utriculi

macula sacculi

maggots (housefly larvae)

eyeballs.

macropla′sia. Gigantism.

macropol′ycyte. An extremely large polymorphonuclear neutrophilic leukocyte having a nucleus with numerous segments.

macrop′sia. The condition of seeing objects as larger than their actual sizes; also called megalopsia.

macrorrhin′ia. The condition of having an abnormally large nose.

macroscop′ic. Visible with the naked eye, without need of magnifying equipment.

mac′rospore. See megaspore.

macrosto′mia. Developmental malformation occurring when the embryonic maxillary and mandibular swellings fail to fuse, resulting in extension of the mouth toward the ear; the defect may be bilateral or unilateral.

macrostruc′ture. A structure visible with the unaided eye.

macro′tia. Abnormal largeness of the ears.

mac′ula, *pl.* **mac′ulae.** A small area differing in appearance from the surrounding tissue.

　corneal m., a moderately dense whitish opacity of the cornea.

　m. adherens, see desmosome.

　m. densa, that portion of the distal convoluted tubule of the kidney contacting the wall of the afferent arteriole just before the latter enters the glomerulus; part of the juxtaglomerular apparatus.

　m. lutea, see macula retinae.

　m. retinae, a small oval yellowish depression on the retina, lateral to and slightly below the optic disk; also called macula lutea and yellow spot.

　m. sacculi, the oval neuroepithelial sensory area in the medial wall of the saccule that houses the terminal arborizations of vestibular nerve fibers.

　m. utriculi, the neuroepithelial sensory area in the lateral wall of the utricle that houses the terminal arborizations of vestibular nerve fibers.

mac′ular, mac′ulate. Spotted; of the nature of macules.

macula′tion. The formation of macules or spots on the skin.

mac′ule. A nonelevated, discolored lesion on the skin; a spot on the skin.

maculocer′ebral. Relating to the brain and the macula lutea of the retina.

maculoerythe′matous. Both red and spotted; said of certain lesions.

maculopap′ular. Spotted and elevated.

maculopap′ule. A raised lesion (papule) on a discoloration or spot (macule) on the skin.

maculop′athy. Any disease of the macula retinae; also called macular retinopathy.

mad. 1. Suffering from a mental disorder. **2.** Rabid. **3.** Angry.

madaro′sis. Loss of the eyelashes or of the eyebrows.

Madurel′la. A genus of fungi (family Dematiaceae); some species cause maduromycosis.

maduromyco′sis. A chronic disease affecting chiefly the feet, marked by the formation of yellow, white, red, or black granules, draining sinuses, suppuration, and swelling; caused by fungi, especially *Madurella mycetomi*; formerly called Madura foot after a city in India where it was first observed; also called mycetoma.

Maffucci's syndrome. The combination of multiple cutaneous hemangiomas and dyschondroplasia; the vascular malformations are manifested by extensive birthmarks and dilatation of the veins (phlebectasias) in the form of soft, tender, purple tumors in subcutaneous tissue, lips, and palate; deformities of the hands and feet are usually evident.

mag′got. A legless, soft bodied grub that is the larva of various insects of the order Diptera, as the housefly; it develops usually in dead organic matter.

mag′ma. A soft inert mass composed of finely divided solids in an aqueous medium; a paste or salve.

magne′sia. Magnesium oxide.

　citrate of m., see magnesium citrate.

　m. magma, see milk of magnesia.

　milk of m., an aqueous suspension of magnesium hydroxide; used as a laxative and antacid; also called magnesia magma.

magne′sium. A light, moderately hard, metallic element with a silvery luster; symbol Mg, atomic number 12, atomic weight 24.32, valence 2; it is an essential nutritional substance.

　m. carbonate, a very light, white powdery compound, $MgCO_3$, used in gastric and intestinal acidity and as a laxative; it is insoluble in water.

　m. citrate, a colorless crystalline powder, $Mg_3(C_6H_5O_7)_2 \cdot 14\ H_2O$, used in solution as a laxative; also called citrate of magnesia.

　m. hydroxide, a white powdery compound, $Mg(OH)_2$, practically insoluble in water; used as an antacid and laxative.

　m. oxide, a white powdery compound, MgO, insoluble in water; used as an antacid and laxative; also called magnesia.

　m. sulfate, a colorless, crystalline compound, $MgSO_4$, soluble in water; effective cathartic, particularly useful in certain poisonings; the form $MgSO_4 \cdot 7H_2O$ is Epsom salt.

mag′netism. 1. The property of mutual attraction or repulsion produced by a magnet or by an electric current. **2.** The study of magnets and their properties. **3.** The force exhibited by a magnetic field.

mag′neton. A unit of measure of the magnetic movement of an atomic or subatomic particle.

magnifica′tion. An enlargement of an object by an optical element or instrument.

maieusiopho′bia. Abnormal fear of childbirth.

maim. To disable, mutilate, or cripple by an injury.

main. French for hand.

　m. d′accoucheur, accoucheur's hand; see under hand.

　m. en crochet, permanent flexure of the fourth

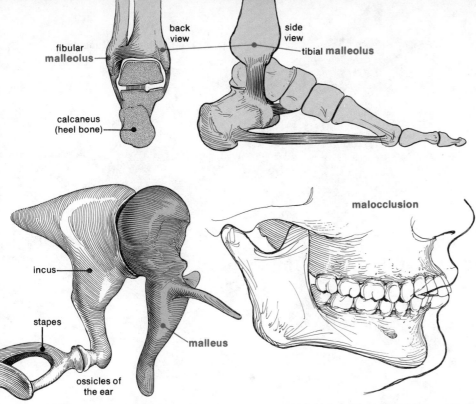
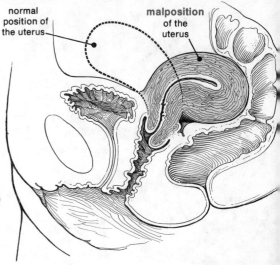
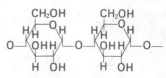

back view · side view

fibular **malleolus** · tibial **malleolus**

calcaneus (heel bone)

incus

stapes

malleus

ossicles of the ear

malocclusion

normal position of the uterus · **malposition** of the uterus

maltose

and fifth fingers, resembling the position of a person's hand while crocheting.

m. en griffe, griffin-claw hand; see under hand.

m. en lorgnette, opera glass hand; see under hand.

main′lining. Term used by drug addicts denoting intravenous injection of heroin or other drugs.

main′streaming. Placing of a handicapped child into a regular classroom by providing special, but not separate, services and barrier-free education.

Majocchi's disease. Annular telangiectatic purpura; see under purpura.

mal. French for disease.

grand m., generalized epilepsy; see under epilepsy.

m. de mer, seasickness.

petit m., petit mal epilepsy; see under epilepsy.

mala. Latin for cheekbone; the cheek.

malabsorp′tion. Inadequate or imperfect absorption.

m. syndrome, condition marked by weight loss, weakness, pallor, protuberant abdomen, bleeding tendency, and other symptoms and signs, caused by any disease which impairs the absorption of nutrients.

mala′cia. 1. Softening of tissues. **2.** Craving for highly seasoned food.

malacopla′kia. See malakoplakia.

maladie′. French for malady.

m. de Roger, see Roger's disease.

mal′ady. Illness; disease.

malaise′. A vague general discomfort or feeling of illness.

malakopla′kia. The formation of soft, fungus-like growths on the mucous membrane of a hollow organ, especially the urinary bladder; also written malacoplakia.

malalign′ment. The displacement of a tooth, or teeth, from normal position.

ma′lar. Of or relating to the cheek or cheek bone.

mala′ria. An infectious disease caused by any of four species of a protozoan parasite of the genus *Plasmodium;* transmitted by mosquitoes of the genus *Anopheles;* usual symptoms include anemia, fever, and enlargement of the spleen; the typical fever paroxysm has three stages—(1) chills and uncontrollable shaking, (2) high fever, (3) profuse sweating—and may occur on alternate days, every third day, or daily, depending on the time required for a new generation of parasites to complete its life cycle in the body. See also *Plasmodium.*

benign tertian m., see vivax malaria.

estivoautumnal m., see falciparum malaria.

falciparum m., a form caused by the most invasive of all malarial parasites, *Plasmodium falcipa-*

rum, causing infected blood cells to clump and block capillaries; the paroxysms of fever usually occur every other day but frequently at indefinite intervals; in severe cases cerebral, renal, gastrointestinal, or pulmonary complications may develop; also called malignant tertian or estivoautumnal malaria.

malariae m., a form caused by *Plasmodium malariae;* the paroxysms of fever usually occur every third day; also called quartan malaria.

malignant tertian m., see falciparum malaria.

quartan m., see malariae malaria.

quotidian m., a form in which the paroxysms occur daily; usually caused by two groups of *Plasmodium vivax* parasites reproducing alternately every 48 hr; may also be caused by a combination of *Plasmodium falciparum* and *Plasmodium vivax* or by two generations of *Plasmodium falciparum.*

relapsing m., a type in which exoerthrocytic forms of the parasite persist after the initial incubation period; if not destroyed, these forms act as a reservoir for repeated clinical episodes due to invasion of the red blood cells.

tertian m., see vivax malaria.

vivax m., a form caused by *Plasmodium vivax* or *Plasmodium ovale;* the paroxysms occur every other day; also called tertian or benign tertian malaria.

mala′rial. Relating to or caused by malaria.

Malassezia furfur. The fungus that causes tinea versicolor; the proper name for *Microsporon furfur.*

mal′ate. A salt of malic acid.

malathi′on. Substance used as an insecticide and, in veterinary medicine, against external parasites.

male. 1. Designating the sex of an individual containing organs that normally produce spermatozoa; symbol ♂ (the shield and spear zodiac sign for Mars). **2.** Masculine.

genetic m., an individual with a male karyotype that normally has one X and one Y chromosome.

malforma′tion. A defect or deformity.

congenital m., one evident at birth, either genetic or of environmental origin; commonly called birth defect.

malfunc′tion. Abnormal or inadequate function.

malic acid. An intermediate in carbohydrate metabolism; present in unripe apples, cherries, tomatoes, etc.

malig′nancy. The condition of being malignant or resistant to treatment.

malig′nant. Denoting any disease resistant to treatment and of a fatal nature; in the case of a tumor, having the property of uncontrollable growth and dissemination.

maling′er. To pretend to be ill to avoid work or an unpleasant situation, or for some other type of gain.

malin′gerer. One who pretends to be sick.

mal′leable. Capable of being made into thin sheets; said of certain metals.

mallea′tion. A spasmodic movement as of hammering of the hands.

malle′olar. Relating to one or both prominences on either side of the ankle.

malle′ollus. One of two projections (one on the tibia and one on the fibula) on either side of the ankle joint.

Malleomyces mallei. See *Pseudomonas mallei.*

Malleomyces pseudomallei. *Pseudomonas pseudomallei.*

mal′leus. The club-shaped and most lateral of the three auditory ossicles in the middle ear chamber which is firmly attached to the tympanic membrane and articulates with the incus; sometimes called hammer.

Mallory-Weiss syndrome. Lacerations of the lower esophagus with vomiting of blood, usually following protracted, severe, incoordinate vomiting and retching; commonly occurs following excessive alcohol ingestion.

malnutri′tion. Faulty nutrition due to inadequate diet or to a metabolic abnormality; wrong intake of nutrients, i.e., inadequate amounts or the wrong proportions of nutrients.

malocclu′sion. Abnormal contact of opposing teeth (mandibular and maxillary), so as to interfere with the efficient movement of the jaws during mastication.

close bite m., condition in which the edges of the anterior mandibular teeth extend lingually toward the gums of the opposing teeth when the jaws are closed.

open bite m., a condition marked by the failure of opposing teeth to establish contact when the jaws are closed.

mal′onyl. The bivalent radical of malonic acid.

malpighian body. Renal corpuscle; see under corpuscle.

malposi′tion. An abnormal or anomalous position of a part or of the body.

malprac′tice. Improper, unskillful, or negligent treatment of an individual by a health practitioner that results in injury.

malrota′tion. Failure of all or a portion of the intestines to rotate during embryonic development.

malt. Grain, especially barley, artificially made to sprout and then dried; it contains dextrin, maltose, glucose, and some enzymes.

mal′tase. A digestive enzyme that promotes the conversion of maltose into glucose.

mal′tose. $C_{12}H_{22}O_{11}$; a sugar formed by the action of a digestive enzyme on starch; it consists of two

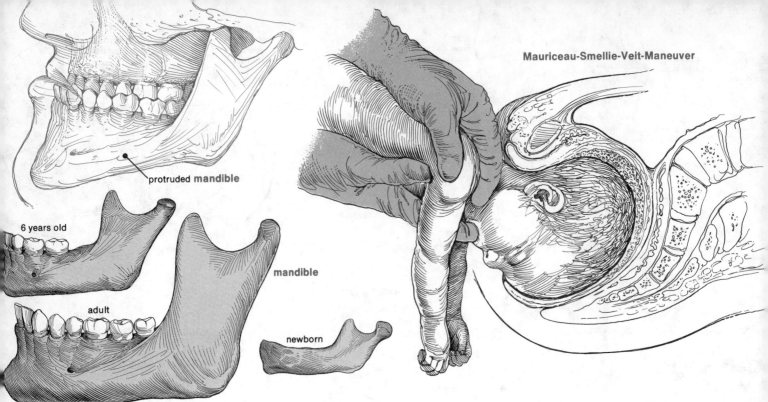

protruded **mandible**

6 years old

adult

mandible

newborn

glucose moieties; also called malt sugar.

ma'lum. Latin for disease.

malun'ion. Union of a fractured bone in a faulty alignment or position.

M + Am. Abbreviation for compound myopic astigmatism.

mam'elon, mam'melon. One of the three rounded prominences on the cutting edge of an erupting incisor tooth.

mam'ma, *pl.* **mam'mae.** The mammary gland or breast; rudimentary in the male but containing the milk-producing glands in the female.

mam'mal. A member of the class Mammalia.

Mamma'lia. A class of vertebrates that includes all animals that nourish their young with milk.

mam'maplasty. See mammoplasty.

mam'mary. Relating to the breast.

mammec'tomy. See mastectomy.

mam'melon. See mamelon.

mammil'la. 1. Nipple. **2.** Any nipple-like protuberance.

mam'millary. Relating to or resembling a nipple.

mam'millate, mam'millated. Having nipple-like projections.

mammi'tis. See mastitis.

mam'mogram. A roentgenogram of the mammary gland, usually done for the purpose of detecting cancers.

mammog'raphy. A soft tissue x-ray technique for visualization of the female breast; with this method, nonpalpable lesions within the breast can be identified.

zero m., a dry, totally photoelectric process of producing x-ray images of the female breast; also called xeromammography.

mam'moplasty, mam'maplasty. Plastic surgery of the breasts to improve their appearance; also called mastoplasty.

mammotroph'ic. Promoting the development, growth, and function of the mammary gland.

man'delate. A salt of mandelic acid.

mandelic acid. A crystalline substance, soluble in water; used as a urinary antibacterial agent; also called phenylglycolic acid.

man'dible. The horseshoe-shaped bone of the lower jaw which articulates with the skull at the temporomandibular joint; it lodges the lower teeth; also called jawbone.

mandib'ular. Relating to the lower jaw or mandible.

mandibulec'tomy. Surgical removal of the lower jaw.

mandibulopharyn'geal. Relating to the mandible and pharynx.

mandrag'ora. An herb long known and used in medieval medicine as a sedative, hypnotic, anesthetic, and poison; also called mandrake.

man'drake. See mandragora.

man'drel. A shaft on which a working tool is mounted, and by means of which it is rotated.

disk m., a mandrel designed to hold a polishing disk.

snap-on m., one with a split end that supports a rubber polishing cup.

maneu'ver. A procedure or movement requiring skill and dexterity.

Bracht's m., in obstetrics, maneuver used in breech extraction whereby the breech is allowed to deliver spontaneously up to the umbilicus, then the baby's body is held against the mother's symphysis and moderate suprapubic pressure is applied by an assistant.

Credé's m.'s, Credé's methods; see under method.

Heimlich m., a maneuver used to dislodge a piece of food stuck in a person's throat and obstructing the airway; standing in back of the victim, the rescuer places both arms around him; he makes a fist with one hand, grasps it with the other hand, and (with the thumb toward the victim) presses his fist sharply upward against the victim's abdomen, between the navel and the rib cage; this causes the diaphragm to elevate and the lungs to compress; the resulting increased air pressure forced through the trachea (windpipe) forces out the food particle.

Leopold's m.'s, in obstetrics, four methods of abdominal palpation to determine position of fetus in the uterus; in the first or fundal maneuver, the examiner gently palpates the uterine fundus with his fingers; this determines which fetal end occupies the fundus; in the second maneuver, placing the palms of his hands on each side of the abdomen, the examiner exerts gentle but deep pressure; this evaluates position of the fetal back and extremities; in the third maneuver or Pawlik grip, the examiner grasps the abdomen between the thumb and fingers of one hand, just above the pubic symphysis; this reveals degree of engagement of presenting part; in the fourth maneuver, with the first three fingers of each hand, the examiner palpates deeply into the pelvic brim; this reveals the direction of the head.

Mauriceau-Smellie-Veit m., in obstetrics, method of extracting the fetal head in breech presentation when the chin is directed posteriorly; the baby's body straddles the forearm of the operator, the middle finger is introduced into the baby's mouth and applied over the maxilla, and two fingers of the other hand are placed forklike over the fetal shoulder to exert traction.

Pinard's m., method of fetal extraction in a frank breech presentation; two fingers are passed along the fetal thigh to the knee to push it away from the midline and flex the leg; the foot is then readily grasped and brought down and out.

Ritgen's m., modified, delivery of a baby's head by applying forward pressure on the chin through the perineum with one hand while applying pressure on the head with the other hand; the maneuver is performed between contractions and allows for slow delivery of the head.

Scanzoni's m., rotation of fetal head with forceps followed by removal and reapplication of instrument for delivery to avoid injury to the maternal soft parts.

Valsalva m., (1) forced expiration against the closed glottis to increase pressure within the lungs; also called Weber's maneuver; (2) forced expiration with mouth closed and pinched nose to clear the auditory tube.

Weber's m., see Valsava maneuver (1).

man'ganese. A grayish or silvery metallic element; symbol Mn, atomic number 25, atomic weight 54.94; some of its salts are used in medicine.

man'ganous. Denoting a compound containing bivalent manganese.

man'ganum. Manganese.

mange. A contagious skin disorder of many animals due to the presence of burrowing itch mites, usually *Sarcoptes* or *Chorioptes*; in man the disease is called scabies.

-mania. Suffix denoting a pathological preoccupation with some thought or activity.

ma'nia. An emotional disorder characterized by a state of excitement, hyperactivity, and profuse and rapidly changing ideas.

ma'niac. A vague and misleading common term for an emotionally disturbed individual, usually implying violent behavior.

man'ic. Of or relating to mania.

manifesta'tion. The display of characteristic signs or symptoms of a disease.

neurotic m., the use of various defense mechanisms, such as depression, conversion, dissociation, etc., in an attempt to resolve emotional conflicts, handicapping the effectiveness of a person in daily living.

psychophysiologic m., symptoms which are primarily physical with a partial emotional origin.

psychotic m., the loss of contact with reality, impairing the ability of the person to function in society, indicating personality disintegration.

man'ikin, man'nikin. An anatomic model of the human body used for practicing certain manipulations, as those of obstetrics or dentistry; also called simulation model.

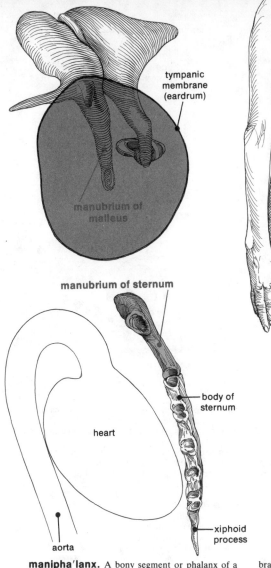

tympanic membrane (eardrum)

manubrium of malleus

manubrium of sternum

heart

body of sternum

aorta

xiphoid process

enlarged pistillate flower cluster

the source of **marijuana** (Cannabis sativa)

Marfan's syndrome long, thin extremities and digits

port-wine mark

manipha′lanx. A bony segment or phalanx of a finger.

manipula′tion. Treatment by the skillful use of the hands, as in reducing a dislocation or changing the position of the fetus.

man′na. The dried sugary exudate of the ash tree, *Fraxinus ornus*; formerly used as a mild laxative.

man′nerism. A distinctive characteristic or behavioral trait.

man′nikin. See manikin.

man′nitol. An alcohol, $C_6H_{14}O_6$, derived from fructose; used in the preparation of dietetic sweets and as an osmotic diuretic.

manom′eter. An instrument for measuring the pressure of gases and liquids.

manomet′ric. Relating to a manometer.

Manso′nia. A genus of mosquitoes in tropical Asia and Africa that transmit microfilaria to man.

manu′brium. A structure that resembles a handle; when used alone the term refers to the manubrium of the sternum.

m. of malleus, the process of the malleus attached to the inner surface of the tympanic membrane.

m. of sternum, the upper portion of the sternum articulating with the clavicles and the first and upper parts of the second costal cartilages on each side.

manus. Latin for hand.

m. extensa, backward deviation of the hand.

m. flexa, forward deviation of the hand.

m. valga, deviation of the hand toward the ulnar side.

m. vara, deviation of the hand toward the radial side.

MAO. Abbreviation for monoamine oxidase.

maple syrup urine disease. An autosomal recessive inherited disorder marked by deficient oxidative decarboxylation of α-keto acids; the urine has a characteristic maple syrup odor; hypotonia, hypoglycemia, and neurologic manifestations appear within the first week of life; also called branched-chain ketoaciduria.

maras′mus. Gradual, progressive wasting of the body, occurring mainly in young children; caused by protein and calorie depletion; also called athrepsia.

marble bone disease. See osteopetrosis.

Marchiafava-Micheli syndrome, Marchiafava-Micheli anemia. Paroxysmal nocturnal hemoglobinuria; see under hemoglobinuria.

Marcus Gunn's phenomenon. Gunn's phenomenon; see under phenomenon.

Marfan's syndrome. Disorder inherited as an autosomal dominant trait and marked by defective formation of elastic fibers which affects the skeleton, large arteries, suspensory ligaments of the crystalline lens, tendons, and joint capsules; the affected individuals have abnormally long slender extremities, spidery fingers, high palate, displacement of the lens, lax joints, and aneurysm of the aorta.

mar′gin. A border or edge.

ciliary m. of iris, the border of the iris attached to the ciliary body.

costal m., the curved lower portion of the thoracic wall, formed by the cartilages of the seventh through tenth ribs.

falciform m., the lower lateral border of the saphenous opening in the deep fascia (fascia lata) in front of the thigh; it lies anterior to the femoral vessels.

free gingival m., the edge of the gum tissue that is not directly attached to the tooth; also called free gum margin.

free gum m., see free gingival margin.

gingival m., the part of the gum, not attached to the tooth, facing either the lips, cheeks, or tongue.

infraorbital m., the lower border of the orbit.

orbital m., margin of the ocular orbit bounded by the frontal bone superiorly, the zygomatic bone laterally, the maxilla inferiorly, and the process of the maxilla and frontal bone medially.

pupillary m. of iris, the border of the iris forming the edge of the pupil.

right m. of heart, the border between the diaphragmatic and sternocostal aspects of the heart.

supraorbital m., the superior edge of the orbit.

margina′tion. Adhesion of leukocytes to the interior of capillary walls during early stages of inflammation.

margin′oplasty. Plastic surgery of the eyelid border.

Marie's disease. See acromegaly.

marijua′na, marihua′na. 1. A tall hemp plant. **2.** The dried, chopped leaves, flowers, and stems of the common hemp plant *Cannabis sativa* (family Moraceae); smoked or mixed into food to induce euphoria; the origin of the word is obscure, but may be a composite of the Spanish names Maria and Juana (Mary and Jane).

Marie-Strümpell disease. Ankylosing spondylitis; see under spondylitis.

mark. A visible impression on a surface; a blemish; a spot.

port-wine m., port-wine hemangioma; a congenital discoloration of the skin, usually on the face, varying from pink to purple.

mar′mot. A rodent that sometimes carries the plague bacillus and ticks that transmit Rocky Mountain spotted fever; also called groundhog and woodchuck.

marr′ow. Medulla of bone; the soft material filling the cavities of the bones.

red m., the marrow located in the cancellous (spongy) tissue of the ribs, the sternum, and the ends of the long bones; it is concerned with the formation of blood cells.

yellow m., the fatty material located in the center of long bones.

marsupializa′tion. Surgical procedure for eradication of a cyst, such as a pilonidal cyst, in which the sac is incised and emptied, then its edges are stitched to the edges of the external incision.

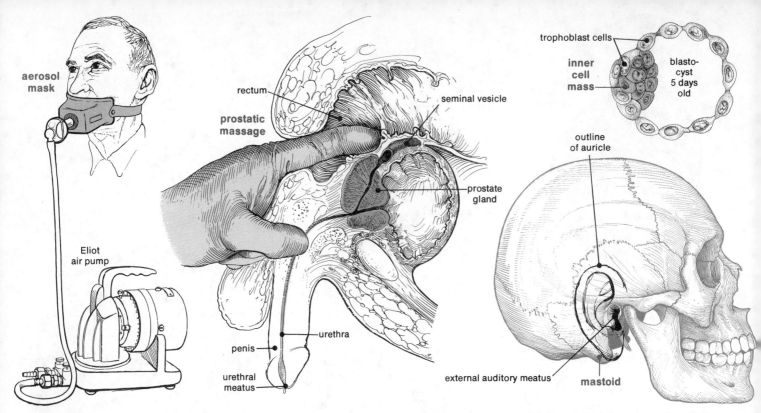

aerosol mask

Eliot air pump

rectum

prostatic massage

seminal vesicle

prostate gland

penis

urethra

urethral meatus

external auditory meatus

mastoid

trophoblast cells

inner cell mass

blastocyst 5 days old

outline of auricle

mas'culine. Relating to or marked by the characteristics of the male sex; mannish.

ma'ser. A device that converts incident electromagnetic radiation of various frequencies into a beam of highly amplified monochromatic radiation at a frequency within the microwave region; the term is an acronym for microwave amplification by stimulated emission of radiation.

optical m., see laser.

MASH. Abbreviation for mobile Army surgical hospital.

mask. 1. A covering for the face, or a portion of it, for the administration of anesthetics or oxygen, or as an antiseptic measure. **2.** An expressionless appearance or a pigmentation of the face characteristic of certain conditions. **3.** A facial bandage.

aerosol m., a face mask used in inhalation therapy.

m. of pregnancy, see chloasma.

surgical m., a covering for the mouth and nose, made of gauze or plastic material; used by hospital personnel in operating rooms or when caring for patients with communicable diseases.

masked. Concealed.

mask'ing. 1. The introduction of a noise in one ear for the purpose of excluding that ear from a hearing test given to the other ear. **2.** The opaque material placed over the metal or any other part of a dental prosthesis.

mas'ochism. 1. A form of sexual perversion in which satisfaction depends largely on being subjected to mistreatment or physical pain. **2.** The infliction of physical or psychological pain upon oneself to relieve guilt.

mas'ochist. 1. The passive partner in the practice of masochism. **2.** One who for psychological purposes exposes himself unnecessarily to suffering.

mass. 1. A body of coherent material. **2.** In pharmacology, a soft pasty mixture of drugs suitable for rolling into pills.

inner cell m., embryoblast; an aggregation of cells which stick together and collect at the embryonic pole of the blastocyst and which give rise to the tissues of the embryo.

lateral m. of atlas, the solid parts of the atlas (first vertebra) on either side, articulating above with the occipital condyles of the skull and below with the axis (second vertebra).

massage'. The rubbing, kneading, tapping, etc. of parts of the body for therapeutic purposes.

cardiac m., the application of manual rhythmic pressure to the ventricles of the heart to restore circulation; also called open chest massage.

closed chest m., the rhythmic compression of the heart between the sternum and the spine approxi-

mately 60 times a minute, in order to restore circulation; also called external cardiac compression.

gingival m., stimulation of the gums by rubbing or pressure.

prostatic m., a technique of pressing the prostate gland substance firmly with the pad of the index finger in order to express secretions into the prostatic urethra.

mas'seter. One of the muscles of mastication; its action is to close the jaw; see table of muscles.

massother'apy. The therapeutic use of massage.

mast-. Combining form denoting breast.

mastadeni'tis. See mastitis.

mastal'gia. Mastodynia.

mastatro'phia, mastat'rophy. Wasting or atrophy of the breasts.

mastec'tomy. Surgical removal of a breast; also called mammectomy.

masthelco'sis. Ulcers on the breast.

mas'ticate. To chew.

mastica'tion. The process of chewing food for swallowing.

mas'ticatory. Of or relating to mastication.

masti'tis. Inflammation of the breast; also called mammitis and mastadenitis.

chronic cystic m., see fibrocystic disease of breast.

interstitial m., inflammation of the connective tissue of the breast.

phlegmonous m., diffuse inflammation, sometimes accompanied by abscess formation.

plasma cell m., benign condition characterized chiefly by dilatation and occlusion of mammary ducts with indurated masses of secretion and plasma cells.

mastochrondro'ma. A benign breast tumor composed chiefly of cartilaginous tissue.

mas'tocyte. Mast cell; see under cell.

mastocytogen'esis. The formation of mast cells.

mastocyto'ma. A nodule resembling a tumor, composed chiefly of mast cells.

mastocyto'sis. See urticaria pigmentosa.

mastodyn'ia. Pain in the breast.

mas'toid. The downward projection of the temporal bone, located behind the ear.

mastoidec'tomy. Removal of the mastoid cells; formerly indicated in the presence of persistent or recurrent mastoiditis and otitis; rarely indicated since the advent of antibiotics.

mastoideocente'sis. Surgical creation of an opening into the mastoid cells or antrum of the temporal bone.

mastoidi'tis. Inflammation of the mastoid process.

mastoidot'omy. Surgical opening of the mastoid process of the temporal bone.

mastop'athy. Any disease of the breast; also called mazopathy.

mas'toplasty. See mammoplasty.

mastopto'sis. Sagging or pendulous breasts.

mastot'omy. Surgical incision of a breast.

masturba'tion. Self-manipulation of the genital organs to produce sexual excitement.

mate'ria. Latin for matter or substance.

m. alba, whitish, loosely adhered deposits on the teeth or dental appliances, composed of mucus, epithelial cells, food debris, and bacteria.

m. medica, (1) the science concerned with drugs used in medicine, their origin, preparation, and usage; (2) any substance used medically.

mater'nal. Relating to or derived from the mother.

mater'nity. 1. The state of being pregnant or a mother. **2.** A hospital for the care of women immediately before, during, and shortly after childbirth and for the care of newborn babies. **3.** Pertaining to pregnancy.

ma'ting. The pairing of male and female for reproduction.

assortative m., mating which is not random but involves individuals of specific characteristics, which may be similar (positive) or opposite (negative).

random m., mating without regard to the genetic constitution of the mate; also called panmixis.

matrilin'eal. Relating to inheritance of traits through the maternal line rather than the paternal.

ma'trix, pl. **ma'trices. 1.** The basic material from which anything (tooth, nail, etc.) develops. **2.** The homogeneous intercellular substance of any tissue. **3.** A mold in which a cast is made.

matrocli'nous. Inherited through the maternal line; derived from the mother. Cf. patroclinous.

mat'ter. 1. Substance. **2.** Waste from a living organism.

gray m., see substance, gray.

white m., see substance, white.

mat'urate. To mature.

matura'tion. 1. The process of becoming mature. **2.** A stage of cell division in which the number of chromosomes in the sex cells is reduced to one-half the number characteristic of the species. **3.** Pus formation.

mature. 1. Complete in natural development; ripe; e.g., the reproductive cell which has undergone the process of meiosis. **2.** Relating to or marked by full development, either mental or physical. **3.** To achieve full development.

matur'ity. The state of being mature.

Maurer's dots. Red-staining granules sometimes seen in the cytoplasm of red blood cells infected

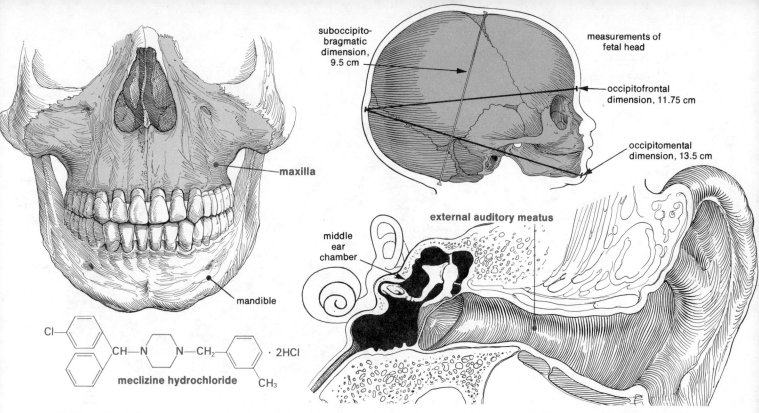

meclizine hydrochloride

measurements of fetal head

suboccipito-bragmatic dimension, 9.5 cm

occipitofrontal dimension, 11.75 cm

occipitomental dimension, 13.5 cm

maxilla

mandible

external auditory meatus

middle ear chamber

with *Plasmodium falciparum*.

maxil'la. One of a pair of irregularly shaped bones forming the upper jaw; it lodges the upper teeth.

max'illary. Relating to the upper jaw (maxilla).

maxilloden'tal. Relating to the upper jaw and the teeth.

maxillofac'ial. Pertaining to the upper jaw and the face.

max'imum. 1. The greatest quantity, value, or degree. 2. Fastigium; the height of a fever or any acute state.

  glucose transport m. (glucose Tm), the maximum rate at which the kidneys can reabsorb glucose (approximately 300 mg per minute).

  m. permissible concentration (MPC), the quantity of radiation considered to be relatively safe.

  tubular m. (Tm), the maximum ability of the renal tubules either to reabsorb or to secrete a given substance.

maze. An intricate labyrinth of walled pathways frequently used to study the learning process in experimental animals.

mazop'athy. See mastopathy.

M.b. Abbreviation in prescription writing for Latin *misce bene*, mix well.

Mb, MbCO, MbO₂. Abbreviations for myoglobin and its combinations with carbon monoxide and oxygen.

MBC. Abbreviation for maximum breathing capacity.

MBD. Abbreviation for minimal brain dysfunction.

M.C. Abbreviation for Medical Corps.

mc. Old abbreviation for millicurie; now mCi.

McArdle's syndrome. Type 5 glycogenosis; see under glycogenosis.

mcg, μg. Abbreviations for microgram.

mCi. Abbreviation for millicurie.

McNaughton rule. See rule, M'Naghten.

Md. Chemical symbol of the element mendelevium.

MD. Abbreviation for (a) muscular dystrophy, preferably called progressive muscular dystrophy; (b) the Latin *Medicinae Doctor*, Doctor of Medicine.

MDA. Abbreviation for 3,4-methylene dioxyamphetamine.

Me. Abbreviation for the methyl radical CH₃⁻.

meal. Food.

  Boyden m., one used to test the evacuation time of the gallbladder; it consists of flour, egg yolks, and milk mixed with sugar or port wine.

  test m., bland food, e.g., toast or crackers and tea, given before analysis of stomach secretions.

mean. The numerical average.

me'asle. The larva of the tapeworm.

mea'sles. An acute contagious viral disease marked by fever, inflammation of the mucous mem-

brane of the respiratory tract, and an eruption of red spots on the skin; the incubation period is usually 10 to 12 days; also called rubeola.

  German m., see rubella.

me'asly. Containing tapeworm larvae.

meas'ure. The dimensions, quantity, or capacity of something determined by measuring.

measures of central tendency. In biostatistics, the tendency of statistical data to group about an average value.

me'atal. Relating to a meatus or body opening.

meatom'eter. An instrument for measuring the size of a meatus, as that of the urethra.

meat'oscope. Instrument for visualization of the urethral meatus.

meatos'copy. Examination of the urethral meatus with a meatoscope.

meat'otome. Knife used in meatotomy.

meatot'omy. Incision for the enlargement of the urethral opening.

mea'tus, *pl.* **mea'tus, mea'tuses.** A body channel or its opening.

  external auditory m., external acoustic m., the auditory canal from the concha of the auricle to the tympanic membrane; it is approximately 25 mm in length on its superoposterior wall and 6 mm longer on its anteroinferior wall.

  inferior nasal m., the passageway with which the nasolacrimal duct communicates with the nasal cavity below the inferior nasal concha.

  internal acoustic m., internal auditory m., a canal through the petrous bone, about one cm in length, from the internal acoustic foramen to the medial wall of the vestibule and cochlea; it transmits the internal auditory artery, the vestibulocochlear nerve, and the motor and sensory roots of the facial nerve.

  middle nasal m., the passage from which the anterior ethmoidal cells and the frontal and maxillary sinuses communicate with the nasal cavity below the middle nasal concha.

  nasopharyngeal m., the passage in the posterior part of the nasal cavity from the back part of the turbinates to the choanae.

  superior nasal m., the passageway with which the posterior ethmoidal cells communicate with the nasal cavity below the superior nasal concha.

  urethral m., the external opening of the urethra.

mecap'ion. Device used to measure the output of an x-ray tube in roentgens.

mechan'ical. 1. Produced with the aid of a machine or apparatus. 2. Automatic.

mechanicorecep'tor. See mechanoreceptor.

mechan'ics. The branch of physics dealing with energy and forces acting on bodies (solid, liquid, or

gaseous) either in motion or at rest; divided into statics, dynamics, and fluid mechanics.

  body m., the study of the action of muscles on the body in motion and at rest.

mechanism. 1. An aggregation of parts that interact in order to perform a specific or common function. **2.** The means by which an effect is obtained.

  association m., mental process through which the memory of past experiences may be related to or compared with present ones.

  cough m., a mechanism for the removal of foreign material from the respiratory tract, consisting of a short inspiration, closure of the glottis, forcible expiratory effort, and then release of the glottis with a rush of air at flow rates of usually 3000–4000 ml/sec.

  countercurrent m., a mechanism essential to the production of an osmotically concentrated urine; it involves two basic processes, countercurrent multiplication in the nephronic (Henle's) loop and countercurrent exchange in the medullary blood vessels, the vasa recta.

  defense m., a psychic structure, usually unconscious, which serves as a protection against awareness of conflicts or anxiety.

  investing m., the structures that surround a tooth and provide retention, including the periodontal membrane, cementum of the tooth, alveolar bone, and gingiva.

  pressoreceptive m., mechanism whereby the pressoreceptive areas (especially the carotid sinuses and aortic arch) react to a stimulus such as a rise in arterial blood pressure.

  proprioceptive m., process by which the body regulates its muscular movements and maintains its equilibrium.

mechanocardio'graphy. The use of tracings that represent the mechanical effects of the heart beat.

mechanorecep'tor. A receptor that responds to the stimulation of mechanical pressure; also called mechanicoreceptor.

mechanother'apy. Treatment of disease or injury by mechanical means.

mechlorethamine hydrochloride. HN₂; an alkylating agent used in the treatment of Hodgkin's disease; Mustargen Hydrochloride®.

meclizine hydrochloride. Preparation used in the prevention and treatment of motion sickness; Bonine®.

mecom'eter. Instrument used to measure the newborn infant.

meconiorrhe'a. The passage of an abnormally large amount of meconium by the newborn infant.

meco'nium. The dark green intestinal contents

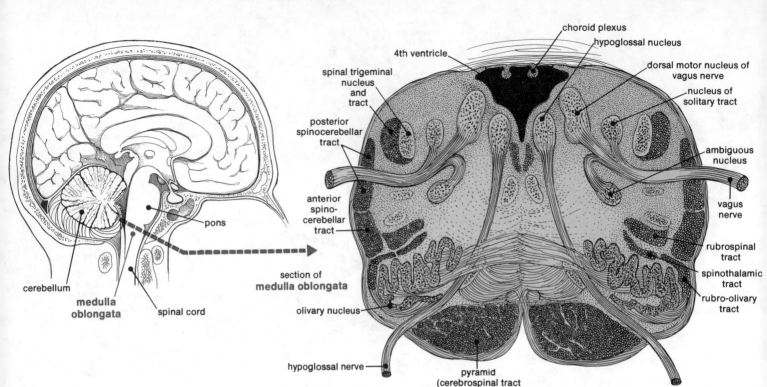

4th ventricle

choroid plexus
hypoglossal nucleus

spinal trigeminal
nucleus
and
tract

dorsal motor nucleus of
vagus nerve

nucleus of
solitary tract

posterior
spinocerebellar
tract

ambiguous
nucleus

anterior
spino-
cerebellar
tract

vagus
nerve

rubrospinal
tract

spinothalamic
tract

section of
medulla oblongata

rubro-olivary
tract

olivary nucleus

cerebellum

**medulla
oblongata**

pons

spinal cord

hypoglossal nerve

pyramid
(cerebrospinal tract

---

formed before birth and present in a newborn child.

meconium ileus. See ileus, meconium.

media. Plural of medium.

me′diad. Directed toward the midline.

me′dial. Relating to the middle; near the median plane of the body or an organ.

me′dian. 1. Central; situated in the middle, as certain nerves and blood vessels. **2.** In statistics, denoting the middle value in a distribution, i.e., the point in a series at which half of the plotted values are on one side and half on the other.

medias′tinal. Of or relating to the mediastinum.

mediastini′tis. Inflammation of the mediastinum.

mediastinog′raphy. Roentgenography or x ray of the mediastinum.

mediastinopericardi′tis. Inflammation of the sac enveloping the heart (pericardium) and the tissues and organs between the sternum and vertebral column (mediastinum).

mediastin′oscope. An instrument for visual inspection of the mediastinum through an incision above the suprasternal notch.

mediastinos′copy. Exploration of the mediastinum, under anesthesia, through a transverse suprasternal incision (usually 2 cm above the suprasternal notch); it allows access to the lymph nodes overlying the trachea for surgical biopsy.

mediastinot′omy. Incision into the mediastinum.

mediasti′num, *pl.* **mediasti′na. 1.** The central space in the chest bounded anteriorly by the sternum, posteriorly by the vertebral column, and laterally by the pleural sacs. **2.** A septum between two parts of an organ.

  anterior m., the division of the lower mediastinum located in front of the pericardium and behind the body of the sternum; it contains, among other structures, part of the thymus gland, a few lymph nodes, and loose areolar tissue.

  lower m., the part of the mediastinum below the plane which extends from the manubriosternal joint in front to the lower border of the fourth vertebra behind; it is subdivided into anterior, middle, and posterior mediastina.

  middle m., the broadest division of the lower mediastinum; it contains, among other structures, the pericardium and heart and the adjacent parts of the great vessels.

  posterior m., the division of the lower mediastinum located in back of the pericardium and in front of the vertebral column; it contains, among other structures, the esophagus, many lymph nodes, thoracic aorta, thoracic duct, and vagus nerves.

  superior m., the division of the mediastinum above the plane which extends from the manubriosternal joint in front to the lower border of the

fourth vertebra behind; it contains, among other structures, the aortic arch with its branches, the brachiocephalic veins and the upper half of the superior vena cava, the vagus, phrenic, cardiac, and left recurrent laryngeal nerves, the trachea, esophagus, thoracic duct, thymus gland, and some lymph nodes.

  upper m., the superior mediastinum.

med′icable. Potentially curable by drug therapy.

med′ical. 1. Relating to medicine. **2.** Medicinal.

medic′ament. A remedy; a healing agent.

medicamento′sus. Relating to or caused by a drug.

med′icate. 1. To treat disease with a medicinal substance. **2.** To impregnate with a medicinal substance.

med′icated. 1. Permeated with a medicinal substance. **2.** Treated medically.

medica′tion. 1. A medicine or drug. **2.** The act or process of administering remedies.

medic′inal. Having curative properties.

med′icine. 1. A drug. **2.** The science of diagnosing and treating general diseases or those involving the internal parts of the body, distinguished from surgery.

  clinical m., the study and practice of medicine at the bedside as opposed to theoretical and laboratory investigation.

  community m., the medical specialty dealing with the study and solution of in-depth community health problems.

  family m., the medical specialty dealing with first patient contact, long-term care, and a broad responsibility to all members of a family regardless of age.

  folk m., treatment of disease in the home with remedies and techniques passed on from generation to generation.

  forensic m., see jurisprudence, medical.

  internal m., the branch of medicine concerned with the nonsurgical aspects of diseases.

  legal m., see jurisprudence, medical.

  nuclear m., the application of nuclear energy in the diagnosis and treatment of disease; e.g., the use of radioisotopes as tracers.

  physical m., see physiatrics.

  preventive m., the study and practice of measures aimed at preventing disease.

  primary m., the care a patient receives during his initial contact with a health practitioner or health-service system; it implies an ongoing responsibility for the patient regardless of the presence or absence of disease and includes that aspect of preventive medicine that can be practiced at the family level.

  proprietary m., a medicinal preparation which is the property of the maker and, by patent or trade

mark, is protected against imitation.

  socialized m., state m., the control of medical practice by a branch of the government.

  space m., the branch of medicine concerned with disorders occurring in men and animals exposed to the hazards of space travel.

  state m., see socialized medicine.

  veterinary m., the diagnosis and treatment of the diseases of animals.

medicochirur′gical. Relating both to medicine and surgery.

medionecro′sis. Necrosis of the middle layer of an arterial wall.

  m. of the aorta, cystic medial necrosis; see under necrosis.

meditation, transcendental. An exercise of contemplation that induces a temporary hypometabolic state, a sense of well being, and a feeling of complete relaxation; this hypometabolic state is associated with changes in physiologic function including a reduction in oxygen consumption, a decrease in cardiac output, and altered brain wave activity.

me′dium, *pl.* **me′dia. 1.** A means. **2.** Any substance through which something is transmitted. **3.** Any substance used for the cultivation of bacteria; also called culture medium.

  clearing m., a substance used in histology to make specimens transparent.

  contrast m., any substance, e.g., barium, opaque to x rays, used to facilitate visual examination of internal organs; also called radiopaque medium.

  culture m., medium (3).

  radiopaque m., see contrast medium.

  rich m., culture medium containing various kinds of nutrients.

  selective m., culture medium containing components which limit growth to organisms of a specific type.

  separating m., a substance used in dentistry to coat impressions to facilitate removal of the cast.

MEDLARS. Medical Literature Analysis and Retrieval System, a computerized index of the U.S. National Library of Medicine for the search and retrieval of articles published in medical and related journals.

medroxyprogesterone acetate. Preparation used in combination with ethynyl estradiol as an oral contraceptive.

medul′la. Any centrally located soft tissue.

  adrenal m., the inner, reddish-brown portion of the adrenal gland which produces epinephrine and norepinephrine.

  m. oblongata, the oblong, caudal portion of the brain stem extending from the lower margin of the pons to, and continuous with, the spinal cord; also

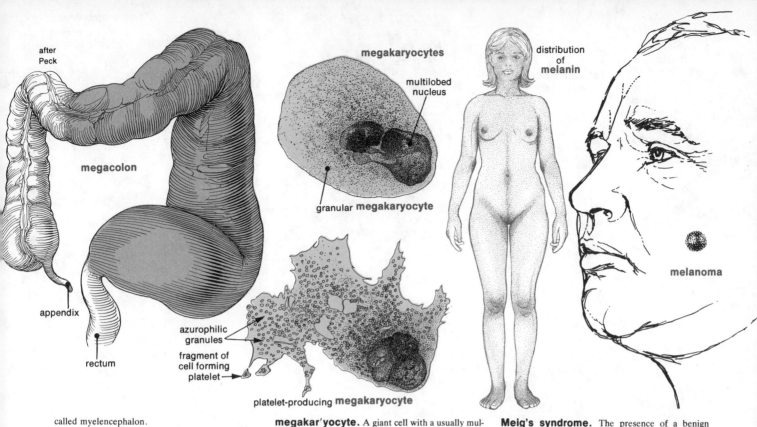

after Peck

megacolon

appendix

rectum

megakaryocytes

multilobed nucleus

granular **megakaryocyte**

azurophilic granules

fragment of cell forming platelet

platelet-producing **megakaryocyte**

distribution of **melanin**

melanoma

called myelencephalon.

m. of bone, the soft material filling the cavities of bones, composed of hemopoietic tissue; it produces most of the cells that circulate in the blood; also called marrow.

m. of kidney, the inner, darker portion of the kidney containing the vasa recta, loops of Henle, and collecting ducts.

m. of ovary, the inner part of the ovary composed of loose connective tissue containing lymphatics, nerves, and a mass of large contorted blood vessels.

m. spinalis, spinal cord; see under cord.

med´ullary. Relating to or resembling the medulla or marrow.

med´ullated. Containing or covered with a soft marrow-like substance.

medulla´tion. The formation of marrow or a medullary sheath.

medulliza´tion. The replacement of bone tissue by marrow, as in rarefying osteosis.

medul´loblast. An undifferentiated cell of the embryonic neural tube.

medulloblasto´ma. A rapidly growing tumor, usually of the vermis of the cerebellum, composed of undifferentiated preneurogliar cells.

mega-. Combining form meaning (a) one million; (b) large.

megablad´der. See megalocystis.

megaco´lon. Abnormally large colon.

congenital m., megacolon observed in young infants, resulting from absence of ganglion cells of the myenteric plexuses of the rectum and lower colon; the aganglionic area of the intestine is unable to relax during normal peristaltic activity, producing constriction and constipation; also called Hirschsprung's disease.

idiopathic m., a form having its onset in childhood, characterized chiefly by constipation and distention of colon (sometimes the entire colon) with feces, without constriction or absence of ganglion cells.

toxic m., marked dilatation of the colon in acute fulminating ulcerative colitis.

meg´adyne. Unit of force, equal to one million dynes.

mega electron volt (mev). One million electron volts.

megaesoph´agus. Abnormal enlargement of the lower esophagus.

megakar´yoblast. A primitive cell of the megakaryocyte series about 25 to 30 microns in diameter with a large oval or kidney-shaped nucleus and scanty cytoplasm; it develops into a promegakaryocyte before finally differentiating into a megakaryocyte.

megakar´yocyte. A giant cell with a usually multilobed nucleus, the precursor of platelets; the largest cell in the bone marrow (up to 100 microns in diameter).

megakaryophthi´sis. Deficiency of megakaryocytes in the bone marrow.

megalo-, megal-, -megaly. Combining forms meaning large.

meg´aloblast. An embryonic red blood cell of large size, found in the bone marrow in pernicious anemia and folic acid deficiency states.

megalocar´dia. See cardiomegaly.

megalochi´ria. Abnormally large size of the hands; also called macrochiria.

megalocor´nea. Developmental eye anomaly in which an otherwise normal cornea is abnormally large at birth and continues to grow in diameter; the pressure within the eye remains normal, which distinguishes this condition from buphthalmos; also called macrocornea.

megalocys´tis. An abnormally enlarged or distended bladder; also called megabladder.

meg´alocyte. See macrocyte.

megalodac´tylism. See macrodactylia.

megalogas´tria. Abnormally large size of the stomach.

megaloglos´sia. See macroglossia.

megaloma´nia. A psychopathologic condition in which the individual has unfounded conviction of his own great importance and power.

megalome´lia. See macromelia.

megalope´nis. Abnormally large penis.

megaloure´ter. Excessive dilatation of a ureter in the absence of obstruction.

megarec´tum. Abnormally dilated rectum.

megasig´moid. An extremely dilated sigmoid colon.

meg´aspore. The larger of the spores of certain protozoans or heterosporous plants; also called macrospore.

megavi´tamin. A vitamin far in excess of minimal daily requirement.

meg´avolt. (MV) A unit of electromotive force, equal to one million volts.

megavol´tage. Electromotive force in the range of two to 10 million electron volts (mev); used in radiotherapy.

meg´lumine. N-methylglucamine, a substance used in the preparation of radiopaque compounds.

meg´ohm. Unit of electric resistance, equal to one million ohms.

meibo´mian cyst. See chalazion.

meibomiani´tis, meibomi´tis. Inflammation of the meibomian (tarsal) glands on the inside of the eyelid.

Meig's syndrome. The presence of a benign ovarian fibroma associated with the formation of ascites and pleural effusion.

meio´sis. The special process of cell division during maturation of the sex cells in which two nuclear cell divisions occur in rapid succession, thus forming four gametes, each containing half the number of chromosomes found in the general body cells; when the ovum unites with the sperm in fertilization, the resulting cell then has the normal diploid number of chromosomes (46).

meiot´ic. Relating to meiosis.

mel-. Combining form related to (a) limb; (b) cheek; (c) honey or sugar.

mel. 1. Honey. **2.** A pharmaceutical preparation containing honey as an excipient.

melal´gia. Pain in the lower extremity.

melancho´lia. Severe depression.

mélangeur. A glass tube with an enlarged end used to collect and dilute blood specimens.

melan´ic. Having a dark color.

melanif´erous. Containing any dark pigment.

mel´anin. Black or dark brown pigment found in the skin, hair, and retina.

mel´anism. See melanosis.

melano-, melan-. Combining forms meaning an extremely dark or black hue; e.g., melanoma.

mel´anoamel´oblasto´ma. Benign tumor of the anterior maxilla, usually occurring in infants; it causes displacement of tooth buds.

mel´anoblast. A cell that when developed to maturity (melanocyte) is capable of producing melanin.

mel´anocyte. Mature pigment cell of the skin that produces melanin.

melanoder´ma. Any abnormal dark pigmentation of the skin predominantly resulting from accumulation of the pigment melanin; usually associated with other conditions.

melanodermati´tis. Excessive deposit of melanin in an area of dermatitis.

mel´anogen. Substance that may be transformed into melanin.

melanogene´mia. The presence in the blood of substances that produce melanin.

melanogene´sis. The formation or production of melanin by living cells.

melano´ma. A tumor or growth made up of melanin-pigmented cells.

malignant m., a malignant neoplasm derived from melanin-producing cells, occurring in the skin of any part of the body; formerly called melanosarcoma; also known as melanocarcinoma or simply as melanoma.

melanomato´sis. The presence of numerous

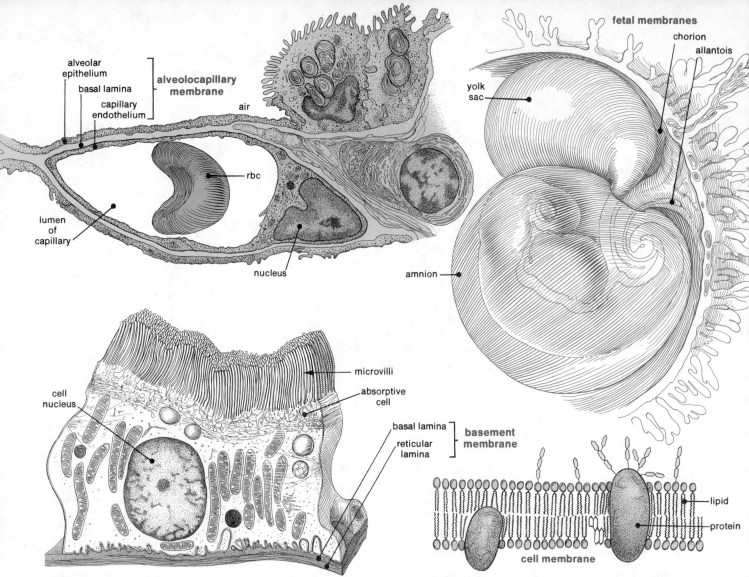

Labels in figure (top to bottom, left to right):
alveolar epithelium, alveolocapillary membrane, basal lamina, capillary endothelium, air, rbc, lumen of capillary, nucleus, fetal membranes, chorion, allantois, yolk sac, amnion, microvilli, absorptive cell, cell nucleus, basal lamina, reticular lamina, basement membrane, lipid, protein, cell membrane

melanomas.

melanony'chia. Black discoloration of the nails.

melanop'athy. Any disease characterized by black pigmentation of the skin.

melan'ophage. A phagocytic cell that engulfs particles of melanin; formerly called chromatophore.

mel'anophore. 1. In human histology and pathology, a pigment cell carrying melanin. **2.** In general biology, a cell that produces melanin.

melanopla'kia. Pigmented patches on the tongue and oral mucosa.

melanopro'tein. A protein complex with melanin.

melanorrhag'ia, melanorrhe'a. See melena.

melanosarco'ma. Malignant melanoma; see under melanoma.

melano'sis. Abnormal deposits of dark pigment in various organs or tissues; also called melanism.

mel'anosome. A single melanin-containing organelle that has finished synthesizing melanin.

melanot'ic. Pertaining to melanosis or to a darkened or blackened condition.

melanu'ria. Presence of melanin or other dark pigment in the urine; usually caused by malignant melanoma.

melas'ma. Cholasma.

melato'nin. A hormone believed to be secreted by the pineal gland.

mele'na. The passage of dark, tarry stools due to blood, usually originating in the upper intestinal tract; also called melanorrhagia and melenorrhea.

   m. spuria, melena in nursing babies in which the blood originates from fissures in the nipples of the mother.

melenem'esis. Vomiting of dark colored material.

melioido'sis. Infectious, glanders-like disease of wild rodents of Southeast Asia; caused by the bacillus *Pseudomonas pseudomallei* (*Actinobacillus*

pseudomallei); in man it may appear acutely or insidiously and is often associated with fever, cough, purulent sputum, and abscess formation.

meliten'sis. See brucellosis.

meli'tis. Inflammation of the cheek.

mel'itose. See raffinose.

melli'tum, *pl.* **melli'ta.** Any pharmaceutical preparation having honey as the excipient.

melli'tus. Latin for honeyed.

mel'oplasty, melonoplas'ty. Plastic surgery of the cheek.

mel'phalen. A compound, derivative of nitrogen mustard, sometimes used in the management of multiple myeloma.

membra'na, *pl.* **membra'nae.** Latin for membrane.

mem'brane. A thin sheet of tissue that covers a surface, envelopes a part, lines a cavity, divides a space, or connects two structures.

   abdominal m., peritoneum.

   alveolocapillary m., the blood-air barrier in the lung consisting of the alveolar epithelium, basal lamina, and the capillary endothelium.

   anterior limiting m., see Bowman's membrane.

   atlantooccipital m., any of two membranes (anterior and posterior) extending from the border of the foramen magnum to the atlas (first vertebra).

   basement m., a thin transparent noncellular layer under the epithelium of mucous membranes and secreting glands.

   basilar m. of the cochlear duct, one extending from the osseous spiral lamina to the basilar crest of the cochlea; it forms the floor of the cochlear duct and supports the spiral organ of Corti.

   Bowman's m., one of the five layers forming the cornea (between the epithelium and the substantia propria), consisting of fine, closely interwoven fibrils; also called anterior elastic lamina of cornea and anterior limiting membrane.

   Bruch's m., basal lamina of choroid; see under

lamina.

   cell m., a delicate structure about 90 Å in thickness that encloses the cell, separating the contents of the cell from the surrounding environment; it is comprised of lipids and proteins and regulates the passage of substances into and out of the cell; also called plasmalemma and unit or plasma membrane.

   cricothyroid m., a broad, thin membrane originating from the upper border of the cricoid cartilage, and extending to the vocal process of the arytenoid cartilage and to the thyroid cartilage.

   Descemet's m., one of the five layers of the cornea covering the posterior surface of the substantia propria; it is elastic, transparent, homogeneous, and extremely thin; also called posterior elastic lamina of cornea and posterior limiting membrane.

   diphtheritic m., the yellowish-gray, leathery exudate on the mucous membrane of the upper respiratory tract in diphtheria; also called false membrane.

   external limiting m., the third of ten layers of the retina; it has the form of chicken wire, allowing the ample passage of the rod and cone cells.

   false m., a tough fibrous exudate on a mucous membrane; also called pseudomembrane.

   fetal m.'s, extraembryonic membranes concerned with the respiration, excretion, nutrition, and protection of the embryo; they include the amnion, chorion, allantois, yolk sac, decidua, and placenta.

   glassy m., a prominent basal lamina in the ovary separating the epithelial layer of the follicle from the surrounding connective tissue of the stroma.

   glomerular filtration m., the capillary wall of the renal corpuscle; it allows ultrafiltration of the blood by delivering the plasma as primary urine to the urinary space within the nephronic (Bowman's) capsule; it does not allow the formed elements of the blood to pass through.

   hyaline m., basement membrane.

   hyaline-like m., the eosinophilic, homogeneous, transparent membrane lining the alveoli and air

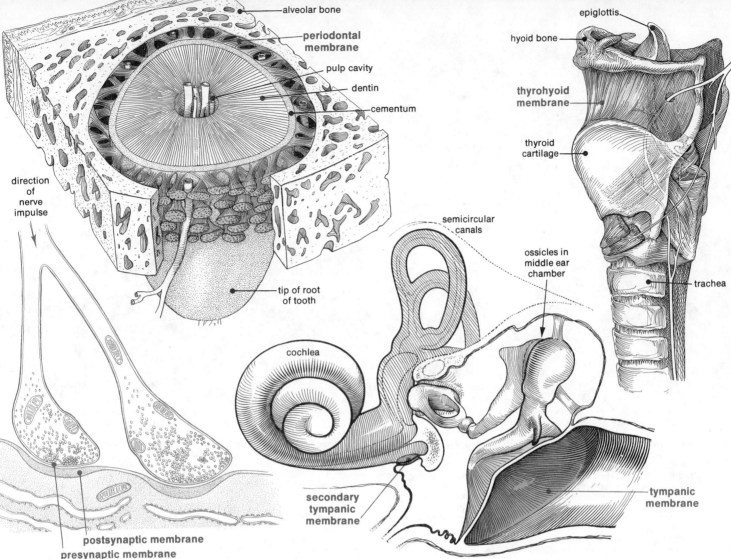

alveolar bone

periodontal membrane

pulp cavity

dentin

cementum

direction of nerve impulse

tip of root of tooth

postsynaptic membrane
presynaptic membrane

secondary tympanic membrane

cochlea

semicircular canals

ossicles in middle ear chamber

tympanic membrane

epiglottis

hyoid bone

thyrohyoid membrane

thyroid cartilage

trachea

passages of newborn (particularly premature) infants afflicted with hyaline membrane disease.

hyothyroid m., a thin, fibrous, membranous sheet extending from the hyoid bone to the thyroid cartilage.

internal limiting m., the last of ten layers of the retina forming both the inner limit of the retina and the outer boundary of the vitreous.

mucous m., one lining tubular structures and consisting of epithelium, basement membrane, lamina propria, and lamina muscularis; also called tunica mucosa.

Nasmyth's m., an extremely thin membrane covering the enamel of recently erupted teeth; it is soon abraded.

nuclear m., an ordered membrane interface regulating the exchange of material between the nucleus and cytoplasm of the cell.

obturator m., one that almost completely closes the obturator foramen of the hipbone; it leaves a small canal for the passage of structures from the pelvis to the thigh.

perineal m., the inferior layer of fascia of the urogenital diaphragm filling in the gap of the pubic arch of the pelvis.

periodontal m., dense white collagenous connective tissue fibers which surround the root of a tooth and attach it to the bone; also called periodontal ligament.

plasma m., see cell membrane.

posterior limiting m., see Descemet's membrane.

postsynaptic m., the portion of the cell membrane at the site of the synapse, sensitive to neurotransmitter substances; also called postjunctional membrane.

presynaptic m., the cell membrane of an axon at the site of the synapse, through which neurotransmitter substances pass into the synaptic cleft; also called prejunctional membrane.

Reissner's m., vestibular membrane of cochlear

duct.

secondary tympanic m., the membrane which closes the round window between the blind end of the scala tympani of the internal ear and the middle ear chamber.

semipermeable m., a membrane which permits the passage of water and small molecules but prevents the passage of large molecules or colloidal matter.

serous m., the outermost coat lining the external walls of the body cavities and reflected over the exposed surfaces of protruding organs.

suprapleural m., a dense, tent-shaped fascial layer attached from the inner part of the first rib and costal cartilage to the transverse process of the seventh cervical vertebra; it helps to close the thoracic inlet.

synaptic m., the cell membrane of a neuronal ending (presynaptic membrane) in relation to the postsynaptic membrane of the adjacent neuron, usually separated by a 200 Å synaptic cleft.

synovial m., the connective tissue membrane that lines the cavity of a synovial joint and produces the lubricating fluid.

tectorial m. of cochlear duct, a delicate gelatinous membrane positioned on the spiral organ of Corti of the internal ear.

thyrohyoid m., a broad fibroelastic sheet that fills in the interval between the hyoid bone and thyroid cartilage.

tympanic m., the membrane separating the external acoustic meatus from the middle ear chamber; it is kept tense for better reception of vibrations by the tensor muscle of the tympanum (tensor tympani); during ordinary conversation the tympanic membrane is displaced only the diameter of a molecule of hydrogen.

undulating m., an organelle of locomotion of certain flagellate parasites consisting of a finlike extension of the limiting membrane with a wavelike flag-

ellar sheath.

unit m., see cell membrane.

vestibular m. of cochlear duct, the delicate membrane in the internal ear separating the cochlear duct from the scala vestibuli; also called Reissner's membrane.

virginal m., hymen.

Zinn's m., the outermost layer of the iris.

membranelle. A minute membrane composed of fused cilia, seen in certain ciliate organisms.

membranocartilag'inous. Partly membranous and partly cartilaginous.

mem'branous. Relating to or of the nature of a membrane.

mem'ory. The process of neural mechanism involved in the storage and representation of an experience; the "read-in phase" of learning; the mental faculty of retaining in the subconscious an impression or idea of which the mind has once been conscious.

menac'me. The period of menstrual activity in a woman's life.

menadi'one. A synthetic preparation having vitamin K properties; used in the treatment of hemorrhagic disorders caused by low prothrombin content of blood.

menar'che. The first occurrence of the menses.

mendele'vium. Radioactive element; symbol Md, atomic number 101.

Menétrièr's disease, Menétrièr's syndrome. A disease of unknown etiology, characterized by huge gastric rugae and pseudopolyps, which may be associated with ulcer-like symptoms, bleeding, or idiopathic hypoproteinemia; also called giant hypertrophic gastritis.

Ménière's syndrome, Ménière's disease. Paroxysmal labyrinthine vertigo, characterized by recurrent episodes of severe vertigo associated with deafness and tinnitus, due to an unexplained increase in pressures of the endolymph; also called

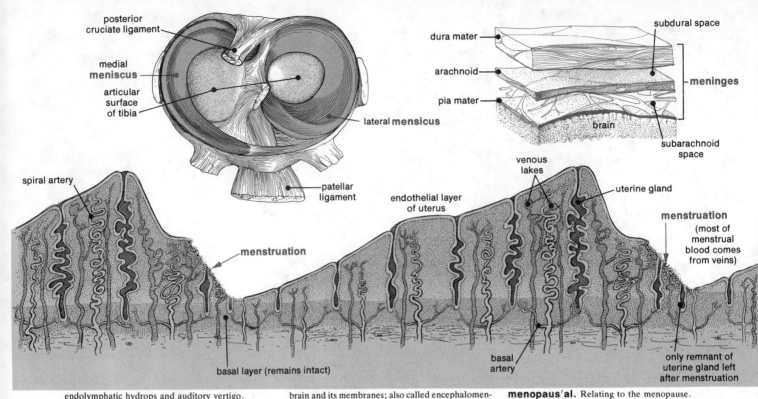

posterior cruciate ligament

medial meniscus

articular surface of tibia

lateral **mensicus**

patellar ligament

dura mater

arachnoid

pia mater

subdural space

meninges

brain

subarachnoid space

spiral artery

venous lakes

uterine gland

endothelial layer of uterus

menstruation

menstruation (most of menstrual blood comes from veins)

basal layer (remains intact)

basal artery

only remnant of uterine gland left after menstruation

---

endolymphatic hydrops and auditory vertigo.

menin′geal. Relating to the membranes that cover the brain and spinal cord.

meningeor′rhaphy. Surgical repair of a membrane, especially of those covering the brain and spinal cord (meninges).

menin′ges. Membranes; specifically the membranes that cover the brain and spinal cord (pia mater, arachnoid, and dura mater).

meningio′ma. An intracranial tumor arising from the arachnoid, usually occurring in adults over 30 years of age.

menin′gism, menin′gismus. Irritation of the brain or spinal cord producing symptoms similar to those of meningitis, but without inflammation of the meninges.

meningi′tis. Inflammation of the meninges (membranes covering the brain and spinal cord); the infection may occur via retrograde thrombophlebitis, via spinal fluid pathways, directly from a local infection, or by the blood stream.

  bacterial m., one caused by bacteria and generally marked by elevated protein, decrease in cerebrospinal fluid (CSF) sugar, and the presence of polymorphonuclear white blood cells in cloudy CSF.

  cerebrospinal m., meningococcal meningitis.

  meningococcal m., inflammation of the coverings of the brain and spinal cord caused by the bacterium *Neisseria meningitidis*; also called cerebrospinal meningitis and spotted fever.

  viral m., one caused by a virus and generally marked by lymphocytosis in cerebrospinal fluid (CSF).

meningo-, mening-. Combining forms relating to the membranes covering the brain and spinal cord.

menin′gocele. A congenital saclike, skin-covered protrusion of the meninges (membranes of the brain and spinal cord) through a defect in the skull or vertebral column; the most frequent sites are the midoccipital area of the head and the lumbosacral area of the spine.

meningococce′mia. Presence of meningococci in the blood; may be associated with petechial lesions, cardiovascular collapse, and/or meningitis; the causative agent is the gram-negative coccus *Neisseria meningitidis*.

meningococ′cus. *Neisseria meningitidis*; a microorganism that causes an infectious form of meningitis.

meningocor′tical. Relating to the membranes and the cortex of the brain.

menin′gocyte. A mesenchymal epithelial cell of the subarachnoid space.

menin′goencephali′tis. Inflammation of the brain and its membranes; also called encephalomeningitis.

menin′goenceph′alocele. Congenital defect consisting of an outpouching of the brain and its coverings (meninges) through a large gap in the skull, usually in the midoccipital area.

menin′goenceph′alomyeli′tis. Inflammation of the brain and spinal cord and their membranes.

menin′goencephalop′athy. Any disease of the brain and its membranes.

menin′gohy′droenceph′alocele. Congenital defect consisting of a saclike protrusion of the brain and its membranes (meninges) containing part of a ventricle filled with cerebrospinal fluid; the outpouching occurs through a large gap in the skull, usually in the midoccipital area.

menin′gomala′cia. Softening of the meninges.

menin′gomyeli′tis. Inflammation of the spinal cord and its membranes, most commonly the arachnoid and pia mater.

menin′gomy′elocele. An outpouching of the meninges (membranes covering the brain and spinal cord), containing spinal cord and/or nerve roots, through an abnormal gap in the vertebral column (spina bifida); the protrusion is devoid of a skin cover; also called myelomeningocele.

menin′goradiculi′tis. Inflammation of the meninges and nerve roots.

meningovas′cular. Concerning the meninges and adjacent blood vessels.

me′ninx, *pl.* **menin′ges.** A membrane, especially one of the membranes covering the brain and spinal cord.

meniscec′tomy. Surgical removal of an interarticular cartilage, especially from the knee joint.

menisci′tis. Inflammation of any interarticular cartilage.

menis′cocyte. Sickle cell; see under cell.

menis′cus, *pl.* **menis′ci.** A crescent-shaped structure, as the fibrocartilage that serves as a cushion between two bones meeting in a joint.

  lateral m. of knee joint, a nearly circular, crescent-shaped fibrocartilage attached to the lateral articular surface of the superior end of the tibia.

  medial m. of knee joint, a crescent-shaped fibrocartilage attached to the medial articular surface of the superior end of the tibia.

  m. tactus, tactile disk; see under disk.

  temporomandibular m., articular disk; see under disk.

meno-. Combining form relating to menstruation.

menolip′sis. The temporary cessation of menstruation.

menometrorrha′gia. Abnormal bleeding during or between menstrual periods.

menopaus′al. Relating to the menopause.

men′opause. The normal termination of the menses, occurring usually between the ages of 45 and 50; frequent symptoms include hot flushes, headache, vulvar discomfort, painful sexual intercourse, and mental depression; the symptoms correlate with the diminution of ovarian function and hormone production; commonly known as the "change of life."

  artificial m., cessation of menstruation by irradiation or surgical removal of ovaries.

  premature m., an abnormally early termination of menstruation.

menorrhag′ia. Excessive or prolonged menstruation; also called hypermenorrhea.

menorrhe′a. 1. Normal menstruation. **2.** Menorrhagia.

menos′chesis. Suppression of the menses.

menos′tasis, menosta′sia. Amenorrhea.

menother′mal. Relating to the hot flashes of menopause.

men′ses. Menstruation; periodic bloody discharge from the uterus.

men′strual. Relating to the menses.

  m. cycle, see cycle, menstrual.

men′struate. To discharge a bloody fluid from the uterus at regular intervals.

menstrua′tion. The periodic discharge from the uterus of a normally nonclotting bloody fluid, usually occurring at approximately a four-week interval and lasting from three to five days; approximately 35 ml of blood and 35 ml of serous fluid are lost; also called menses.

men′sual. Monthly.

mensura′tion. Measurement.

men′tal. 1. Relating to the mind. **2.** Relating to the chin.

  m. deficiency, see retardation, mental.

menta′tion. Mental activity.

men′thol. Peppermint camphor, an organic compound derived from peppermint oil or prepared synthetically; on the skin or in the respiratory tract (e.g., in cigarette smoke) it provides a sensation of coolness by selective stimulation of nerve endings sensitive to cold.

mento-. Combining form meaning chin.

men′ton. The lowermost point of the median plane of the lower jaw.

men′toplasty. Plastic surgery of the chin.

men′tum. Latin for chin.

meper′idine hydrochlo′ride. A widely used narcotic and analgesic which may produce addiction; Demerol®.

mepro′bamate. A minor tranquilizer used to allay anxiety; Equanil®; Miltown®.

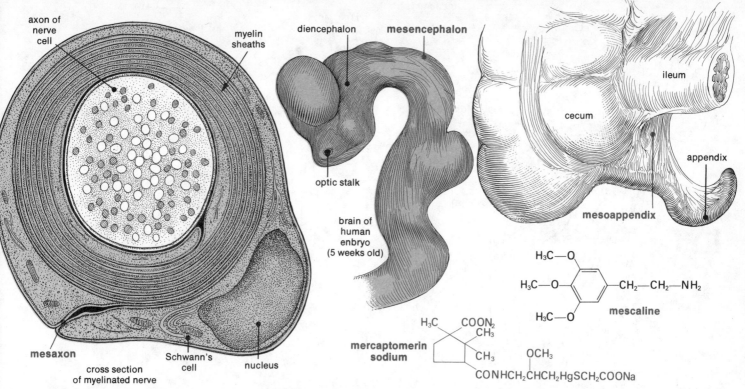

axon of nerve cell · **myelin sheaths** · **mesaxon** · Schwann's cell · cross section of myelinated nerve · nucleus

diencephalon · **mesencephalon** · optic stalk · brain of human enbryo (5 weeks old)

cecum · ileum · **mesoappendix** · appendix

$$H_3C-O \qquad CH_2-CH_2-NH_2$$
$$H_3C-O$$
$$H_3C-O \qquad \textbf{mescaline}$$

mercaptomerin sodium
$$H_3C \qquad COON_2$$
$$CH_3$$
$$CH_3 \qquad OCH_3$$
$$CONHCH_2CHCH_2HgSCH_2COONa$$

mepyr′apone. See metyrapone.

mEq. Abbreviation for milliequivalent; also written meq.

-mer. In chemistry, combining form denoting the smallest unit of a repeating structure.

meral′gia. Pain in the thigh.

m. paresthetica, burning, tingling, pricking, or numbness of the lateral side of the thigh due to compression of the lateral femoral cutaneous nerve.

meral′luride. An organic mercurial diuretic.

merbro′min. A green crystalline compound, used in aqueous solution as a germicide and antiseptic; Mercurochrome®.

mercap′tan. Any substance containing the radical —SH bound to carbon; analogous to alcohols and phenols but containing sulfur instead of oxygen; the basic ingredient of the polysulfide polymer in rubber-based materials; used in dentistry as an elastic impression compound; also called thioalcohol and thiol.

mercapto-. Combining form indicating the presence of a thiol group.

2-mercap′to-4-hydroxyprim′idine. See thiouracil.

mercaptomerin sodium. A mercurial diuretic used parenterally in the treatment of congestive heart failure, nephrotic syndrome, or ascites associated with disorders of the liver; Thiomerin®.

mercaptopu′rine. A yellow crystalline compound which is an analogue of purine; Purinethol®.

mercu′rial. 1. Relating to mercury. **2.** Denoting any pharmaceutical preparation of mercury.

mercurialen′tis. An early sign of mercurial poisoning, marked by a brown discoloration of the anterior capsule of the lens of the eye.

mercu′rialism. Poisoning by mercury or its compounds.

mercu′ric. Denoting a compound containing bivalent mercury.

mer′curous. Relating to or containing monovalent mercury.

m. chloride, HgCl; compound formerly used as a laxative and intestinal antiseptic; also called calomel, mercury monochloride, and mild mercury chloride.

mer′cury. A heavy, silvery, poisonous metallic element, liquid at room temperature; symbol Hg, atomic number 80, atomic weight 200.59, specific gravity 13.546; used in thermometers, barometers, manometers, vapor lamps, and batteries, and in the preparation of some pharmaceuticals; also called quicksilver and hydrargyrum.

mer′cury-197. (^{197}Hg). A radioactive mercury isotope used in brain tumor localization and in the study of renal function.

merid′ian. A line surrounding a spherical body, passing through both poles, or half of such a circle, containing both poles.

m. of cornea, any line bisecting the cornea through the apex.

m. of eye, any line surrounding the surface of the eyeball and passing through both poles.

mero-. Combining form meaning part or segment.

mer′ocrine. Denoting secreting cells that remain intact during discharge of the secretory products, as those in the salivary glands.

merot′omy. Cutting into parts.

merozo′ite. The product of asexual division (schizogeny) of a protozoan in the body of the host; in malaria, one of several small round cells which, on rupture of the red blood cells, reinfect other erythrocytes or liver cells, or form gametocytes (the sexual forms in man, infective for the mosquito).

mer′salyl. $C_{13}H_{16}HgNNaO_6$; a mercurial compound used as a diuretic.

mes-. See meso-.

mes′ad. Toward the middle.

mes′al. Median.

mesan′gial. Relating to the mesangium.

mesan′gium. The supporting stalk of the glomerulus; a specialized form of connective tissue present in the renal glomerulus (in the center of each lobule); it stabilizes the capillary loops both physically and chemically and consists of a few cells and a small amount of matrix produced by the cells.

mesaorti′tis. Inflammation of the muscular coat of the aorta.

mesarteri′tis. Inflammation of the muscular coat of an artery.

mesa′xon. A supporting cell membrane that completely encloses the axon, resulting from the fusion of two encircling arms; it generally elongates and encircles the axon like a jelly roll, forming the myelin lamellae.

mes′caline. A hallucinatory, addictive alkaloid derived from the peyote cactus; also prepared synthetically.

mes′calism. Addiction to mescaline.

mesenceph′alon. The embryonic midbrain; the second cephalic dilatation of the neural tube which develops into the corpora quadrigemina, the cerebral peduncles, and the cerebral aqueduct (aqueduct of Sylvius).

mes′enchyme. Embryonic connective tissue consisting of an aggregation of cells in contact with one another by means of long processes, thus forming a loose network; the space between the cells is filled with a ground substance; the mesenchymal cell is multipotential, i.e., it can develop into many kinds of connective tissue.

mesenter′ic. Of or relating to the mesentery.

mesenteri′tis. Inflammation of the mesentery.

mes′entery. A double layer of peritoneum attaching various organs to the body wall and conveying to them their blood vessels and nerves; commonly used in reference to the peritoneal fold attaching the small intestine to the posterior body wall.

mesh′work. Network.

me′sial. Situated in, near, or toward the middle, as toward the middle line or apex of the dental arch.

mesiobuc′cal. Pertaining to the mesial and buccal surfaces of a tooth; usually denoting the line angle formed by the junction of the two surfaces.

mesiobuc′co-occlu′sal. Relating to the mesial, buccal, and occlusal surfaces of a posterior tooth; usually denoting the point angle formed by the junction of the three surfaces.

mesiocer′vical. Relating to the mesial surface of the neck of a tooth; also called mesiogingival.

mesioclu′sion. Malocclusion in which the lower dental arch is anterior to the upper.

me′siodens. An accessory tooth located between the two upper incisors.

mesiodis′tal. Denoting the plane of a tooth from its mesial surface across to its distal surface.

mesiolabioinci′sal. Relating to the mesial, labial, and incisal surfaces of an anterior tooth; usually denoting the point angle formed by the junction of the three surfaces.

mesiolin′gual. Relating to the mesial and lingual surfaces of a tooth; usually denoting the line angle formed by the junction of the two surfaces.

mesiolinguoinci′sal. Relating to the mesial, lingual, and incisal surfaces of an anterior tooth; usually denoting the point angle formed by the junction of the three surfaces.

mesiolin′guo-occlu′sal. Relating to the mesial, lingual, and occlusal surfaces of a posterior tooth; usually denoting the point angle formed by the junction of the three surfaces.

mesio-occlu′sal. Relating to the mesial and occlusal surfaces of a posterior tooth; usually denoting the line angle formed by the junction of the two surfaces.

mesiover′sion. 1. Position of a tooth closer to the midline than normal. **2.** Position of a jaw (upper or lower) anterior to its normal position.

mes′merism. Treatment based on the method of Mesmer; thought to be primarily a form of hypnosis.

meso-, mes-. Prefixes denoting middle or intermediate; e.g., mesoblast.

mesoappen′dix. The mesentery of the appendix; the small, double-layered fold of peritoneum connecting the appendix to the mesentery of the ileum.

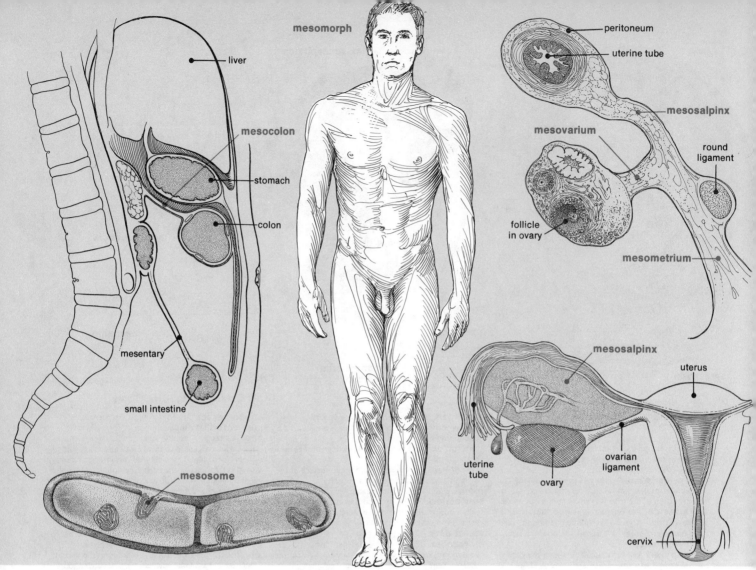

mesomorph

liver

mesocolon

stomach

colon

mesentary

small intestine

mesosome

peritoneum

uterine tube

mesosalpinx

mesovarium

round ligament

follicle in ovary

mesometrium

mesosalpinx

uterus

uterine tube

ovary

ovarian ligament

cervix

mes'oblast. The mesoderm in its early stage of development; the middle of the three germinal layers of the embryo.

mesoblas'tic. Relating to the mesoblast.

mesobronchi'tis. Inflammation of the middle or muscular layer of the bronchi.

mesocar'dium, *pl.* **mesocar'dia.** The double layer of mesoderm attaching the embryonic heart to the wall of the pericardial cavity.

mesoce'cum. The mesentery of the cecum; it is frequently absent.

mesocephal'ic. Denoting a skull having a cephalic index between 75 and 80; also called normocephalic.

mesocol'ic. Relating to the mesocolon.

mesoco'lon. The double layer of peritoneum attaching the colon to the posterior abdominal wall.

mes'oderm. The middle layer of embryonic cells, between the ectoderm and the endoderm; it gives rise to the dermis, connective tissues, the vascular and urogenital systems, and most skeletal and smooth muscles.

mesoepithe'lium. See mesothelium.

mesogas'trium. The broad primitive mesentery which encloses the enteric canal (future stomach) in the embryo, and from which the greater omentum is developed; also called mesogaster.

mesognath'ic. Having a slightly projecting upper jaw with a gnathic index between 98 and 103.

mesognath'ion. The part of the maxilla bearing the lateral incisor tooth.

mesome'trium. The broad ligament of the uterus below the attachment of the ovary; it extends to the lateral wall of the pelvis.

mes'omorph. A person having a body build with prominent musculature and heavy bony structure.

mes'on. 1. The median anteroposterior plane of the human body. **2.** Subatomic particle with a mass between that of the electron and the proton; formerly called mesotron.

mesonephro'ma. Rare ovarian tumor believed to be formed from displaced mesonephric tissue.

mesoneph'ros. An intermediate excretory organ of the embryo; it is replaced by the more permanent kidney (metanephros) while its duct system is retained in the male as the epididymis and ductus deferens; also called wolffian body.

mesor'chium. 1. The fold of peritoneum in the fetus which attaches the developing testis to the mesonephros and holds it in place. **2.** A fold of peritoneum in the adult between the testis and epididymis.

mesorec'tum. The short peritoneal fold investing the upper part of the rectum and connecting it to the sacrum.

mesorop'ter. The normal position of the eyes at rest.

mes'orrhine. Having a nose of moderate width with a nasal index from 47 to 51 on the skull.

mesosal'pinx. The upper free portion of the broad ligament, above the attachment of the ovary and investing the uterine tube.

mesosig'moid. Denoting the portion of peritoneum attaching the sigmoid colon to the posterior abdominal wall.

mes'osome. A structure present in some bacterial cells, 2500 to 5000 Å in diameter, derived from the invagination of the plasma membrane; thought to play a role in the formation of a membrane septum and a crosswall.

mesoster'num. The body or main portion of the sternum.

mesoten'don, mesotendin'eum. The connective tissue fold of synovial membrane extending from a tendon to the wall of its synovial tendon sheath.

mesothelio'ma. A neoplasm composed of cells similar to those forming the lining of the pleura, peritoneum, or pericardium; pleural mesothelioma has been associated with exposure to asbestos.

m. of genital tract, adenomatoid tumor.

m. of meninges, meningioma.

mesothe'lium. A single layer of large flattened cells, derived from the mesoderm, which forms the epithelium lining the internal surface of closed body cavities, such as the pericardium, pleura, and peritoneum; also called mesoepithelium.

mesova'rium. The short fold of peritoneum attaching the ovary to the posterior wall of the broad ligament.

Mes'ozoa. A group of parasitic organisms, intermediate between multicellular and unicellular animals, or possibly degenerate descendants of more organized forms.

messenger RNA. See under ribonucleic acid.

mes'tranol. Estrogen used in the preparation of certain oral contraceptives.

meta-, met-. Prefix indicating: **1.** Situated behind; e.g., metanephros. **2.** Occurring later in a series; e.g., metazoan. **3.** Transformation; e.g., metamorphosis. **4.** The 1,3 position in the benzene ring (two positions separated by a carbon atom). **5.** A less hydrous acid (one formed by loss of water); e.g., metaphosphoric acid. **6.** A derivative of a complex compound; e.g., metaprotein.

metabio'sis. The dependence of an organism upon the pre-existence (and influence on the environment) of another for its development and flourishing.

metab'olism. A general term applied to the chemical processes taking place in living tissues, necessary for the maintenance of the living organism. See also catabolism and anabolism.

basal m., the minimum amount of energy required to maintain vital functions in an individual at complete physical and mental rest; also called basal metabolic rate (BMR).

metab'olite. Any product of metabolism.

essential m., the substrate of an essential metabolic reaction.

mesoblast | **metabolite**

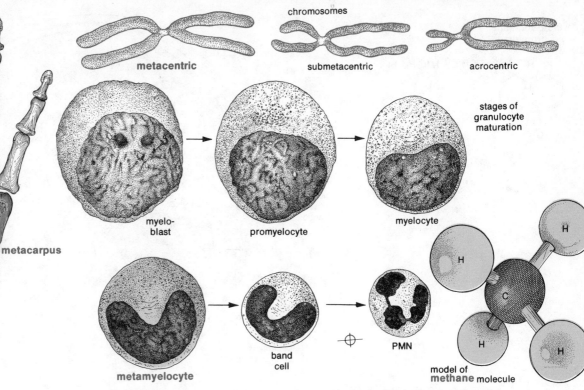

phalanges

metacarpus

carpus →

chromosomes

metacentric | submetacentric | acrocentric

stages of granulocyte maturation

myelo-blast | promyelocyte | myelocyte

metamyelocyte | band cell | PMN

model of **methane** molecule

metacarpophalan′geal. Relating to the articulations between the metacarpal bones and the phalanges.

metacar′pus. The five bones of the hand between the carpus and the phalanges.

metacen′tric. Pertaining to a chromosome with the centromere in the middle.

metachroma′sia. 1. The property by which certain cells stain in a color different from the dye with which they are stained. **2.** The property through which a single dye stains different tissue elements in different colors.

metachromat′ic. Term applied to cells and dyes exhibiting metachromasia.

metachro′sis. The ability to change color, possessed by certain animals.

metacre′sol (m-Cresol). $CH_3C_6H_4$; a local antiseptic.

met′acryptozo′ite. A member of a second or subsequent generation of the exoerythrocytic, tissue-dwelling malarial parasite; it develops from the sporozoite, without intervening blood-parasitic generations.

metacye′sis. Extrauterine pregnancy.

metafe′male. A female with three X chromosomes and two sets of autosomes, characterized by short stature and a certain degree of obesity; many are mildly retarded; also called superfemale and trisomy X.

Metagon′imus. A genus of small flukes which may infect man upon his eating fish containing the larvae.

metakine′sis. The separation of the two chromatids of a chromosome during the anaphase of mitosis.

met′al. Any of a group of substances that have a characteristic luster, are usually malleable, ductile, and conductors of electricity and heat, and, in chemical reactions, tend to lose electrons.

alkali-earth m., alkaline earth; see under earth.

noble m., one that cannot be oxidized by heat alone, nor readily dissolved by acid.

rare-earth m., any metallic element of atomic number 57 through 71.

metalloen′zyme. An enzyme having a metal ion as an integral part of its active structure.

metallophil′ia. Having an affinity for metal salts; said of certain cells.

metallopor′phyrin. Compound containing a porphyrin and a metal; e.g., hematin (iron), chlorophyll (magnesium), etc.

metallopro′tein. A protein containing a more or less tightly bound metal ion or ions; e.g., hemoglobin.

metallother′apy. Treatment of disease by the use of metals or metal compounds.

met′amale. A male with one X chromosome and two Y chromosomes, usually tall and somewhat lean in stature, and often having a tendency toward aggressive behavior; also called supermale and XYY syndrome.

met′amere. One of a series of homologous body segments.

metam′erism. The state of having a series of structures arranged in a repetitive pattern.

metamor′phosis. A change in form and/or function, as the phase in the development of certain insects from larva to adult.

retrograde m., the gradual degeneration of certain structures through lack of use, as the eyes of certain deep sea-dwelling fish.

metamy′elocyte. An immature granulocyte; an early stage of a granulocyte derived from a myelocyte; its cytoplasm contains fine specific granules, as well as azurophilic granules, and its nucleus is indented or kidney-shaped.

metaneph′rine. One of the products of catabolism of epinephrine excreted in the urine.

metaneph′ros. The permanent kidney in the human fetus, possessing a high degree of excretory function; it is formed caudal to the mesonephros, close to the termination of the cloaca, and develops following the regression of the mesonephros; it is composed of the metanephric duct (primitive ureter) and the metanephrogenic tissue.

metaneu′trophil, metaneu′trophile. Not staining normally with neutral dyes.

met′aphase. The second stage of cell division by mitosis, during which the chromatids are aligned along the equatorial plate of the cell and attached by spindle fibers to the centromere.

metaph′ysis. The line of junction of the epiphysis with the shaft (diaphysis) of a long bone.

metapla′sia. The development of adult tissue from cells that normally produce a different type of tissue.

metapsychol′ogy. A systematic, but usually speculative, attempt to state the underlying general laws of psychology.

metaraminol bitartrate. A sympathomimetic compound used to elevate the blood pressure in acute hypotensive conditions.

metaru′bricyte. Orthochromatic normoblast; see under normoblast.

metasta′ble. Denoting an intermediate, unstable, or transient state, as of a supersaturated solution or the excited state of an atomic nucleus.

metas′tasis. Transfer of a disease from its primary site to a distant location; metastasis can be accomplished by the transfer of microorganisms or by the transfer of cells as in malignant tumors.

metas′tasize. To pass or spread from one organ or tissue to another.

metatar′sal. Of or relating to the metatarsus.

metatarsophalan′geal. Relating to the metatarsus and the bones of the toes.

metatar′sus. The anterior portion of the foot between the toes and the instep, composed of five bones.

m. adductus, common deformity in which only the front part of the foot (at the tarsometatarsal joints) is drawn toward the midline; a common cause of the toe-in gait; also called metatarsus varus.

m. varus, see metatarsus adductus.

metathal′amus. The part of the thalamencephalon comprising the medial and lateral geniculate bodies.

Metazo′a. The subkingdom of animals comprised of multicellular individuals in which cells are differentiated into tissues; includes all animals except the protozoa.

metenceph′alon. The portion of the embryonic brain from which develop the pons, cerebellum, and pontine part of the fourth ventricle; together with the myelencephalon it makes up the hindbrain or rhombencephalon.

me′teorism. Tympanites; distention of the intestines with gas.

meter (M). **1.** Measure of length, equal to 39.37 inches. **2.** A measuring instrument.

rate m., device that indicates the magnitude of events averaged over differing time intervals.

total solids m., a calibrated refractometer used for determining the total solids in a drop of fluid, such as urine or serum.

mete′strus, mete′strum. The period of regression immediately following the period of sexual desire (estrus) in the mating season, prior to diestrus.

methacrylic acid. Compound present in oil of Roman camomile; usually obtained by reaction of acetone cyanohydrin and sulfuric acid; used to manufacture methacrylate resins and plastics.

meth′adone. A synthetic narcotic compound, used as an analgesic and in the treatment of heroin addiction.

methamphetamine hydrochloride. A potent sympathomimetic agent that stimulates the central nervous system and depresses the motility of the digestive tract, thus allaying hunger; taken orally or intravenously by drug abusers; produces strong psychic dependence; also known by the slang terms meth and speed.

meth′ane. An odorless, colorless gas, CH_4; produced by the decomposition of organic matter; it is

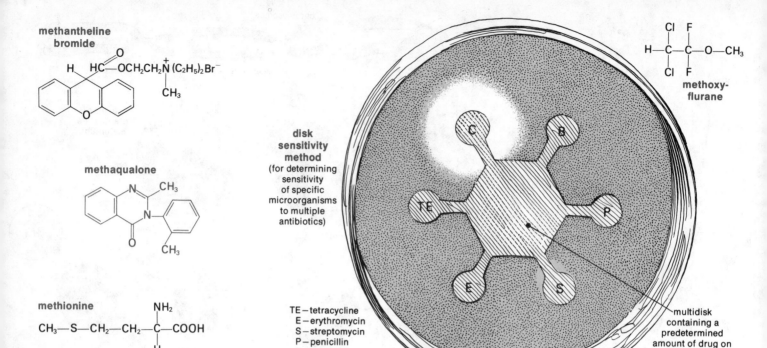

methantheline bromide

methaqualone

methionine

$$CH_3-S-CH_2-CH_2-\underset{\underset{H}{|}}{\overset{\overset{NH_2}{|}}{C}}-COOH$$

methoxy-flurane

disk sensitivity method
(for determining sensitivity of specific microorganisms to multiple antibiotics)

TE—tetracycline
E—erythromycin
S—streptomycin
P—penicillin
B—bacitracin
C—chloramphenicol

multidisk containing a predetermined amount of drug on each segment

---

the smallest and lightest hydrocarbon, and with its next-larger relative, ethane, makes up as much as 90 per cent of natural gas; also called marsh gas.

methanol. Methyl alcohol; see under alcohol.

methan′theline bromide. Drug used in the treatment of peptic ulcer; Banthine®.

methaq′ualone. A short-acting sedative; Quaalude®.

MetHb. Abbreviation for methemoglobin.

methemalbu′min. Compound formed by the combination of heme with plasma albumin; found in the blood of individuals with malarial hemoglobinuria or paroxysmal nocturnal hemoglobinuria.

methemoglo′bin (MetHb). A dark brown compound sometimes formed in the red blood corpuscles by the action of certain drugs on hemoglobin; equivalent to but chemically different from oxygenated hemoglobin; its oxygen is in firm union with iron and is not available to the tissues.

methemoglobine′mia. An excessive amount of methemoglobin in the blood.

methen′amine. $C_6H_{12}N_4$; a urinary antiseptic that acts by releasing formaldehyde in an acid medium; effective against *Escherichia coli,* a common cause of urinary tract infections.

　m. hippurate, a compound of methenamine and hippuric acid.

　m. mandelate, a compound of methenamine and mandelic acid.

methi′onine. An organic compound, $C_5H_{11}NO_2S$; one of the protein-derived amino acids, present in proteins such as egg albumin, which on hydrolysis yields about five per cent its weight of methionine; it is essential in the diet.

meth′od. A set form or mode of procedure, especially a systematic way of performing an examination, test, operation, etc.

　activated sludge m., a method of treating sewage waste by adding 15 per cent bacterially active liquid sludge; it causes the colloidal material of the sewage to coagulate and undergo sedimentation.

　aristotelian m., a method of study that emphasizes the relation between a general category and a specific object.

　copper-sulfate m., a method for the determination of specific gravity of blood or plasma; solutions of copper sulfate graded in specific gravity by increments of 0.004 are placed in a series of small containers; a drop of blood or plasma is placed into each container; the specific gravity of the copper sulfate solution, in which the drop of blood or plasma remains suspended indefinitely, indicates the specific gravity of the sample.

　Credé's m.'s, (1) a method of expressing the placenta in which the body of the uterus is vigor-
ously squeezed in order to produce placental separation; it usually traumatizes the placental site and is not generally recommended; (2) the application of one drop of a two per cent solution of silver nitrate onto each eye of the newborn infant to prevent gonococcal conjunctivitis; (3) use of manual pressure on the bladder, particularly a paralyzed bladder, to express urine.

　direct m., in dentistry, a technique of fabricating a wax pattern of lost tooth structure directly in the prepared cavity in the tooth; an inlay technique.

　disk sensitivity m., a procedure for determining the relative effectiveness of various antibiotics; small disks of paper are impregnated with known antibiotics and then placed in a Petri dish, on the surface of the medium that was inoculated with the organism being tested; after a period of incubation the lack of growth in areas around the various disks indicates the relative effectiveness of the antibiotics.

　flash m., a method of pasteurizing milk by quickly heating it to a temperature of 178°F, holding it there for a short time, and then reducing it rapidly to 40°F.

　immunofluorescence m.'s, any method in which a fluorescent labeled antibody is used to detect the presence or determine the location of the corresponding antigen.

　indirect m., in dentistry, the fabrication of a wax pattern of lost tooth structure formed on a cast or model that was made from an impression of prepared cavity.

　Kjeldahl m., a method of determining the amount of nitrogen in an organic compound by heating it with strong sulfuric acid in the presence of appropriate catalysts; the nitrogen is thereby converted to ammonia which is distilled off, titrated, and measured, and from this the amount of nitrogen is estimated.

　Lee-White m., a method of determining the coagulation time of venous blood by placing it in tubes of standard bore at body temperature.

　micro-Kjeldahl m., a modified Kjeldahl procedure designed for the analysis of nitrogenous compounds in relatively small quantities such as one or two milligrams.

　Nielsen m., a method of artificial respiration with the individual in a prone position; the elbows are raised for inspiration and then released; to induce expiration, pressure is applied over the scapulas.

　Ouchterlony m., double diffusion, a method of double immunodiffusion using a Petri dish of agar in which antigen and antibody are placed in separate wells cut into the gel; during incubation, both antigen and antibody diffuse from the wells and interact to form precipitins in the agar; as diffusion
progresses, concentration gradients are established; distinct bands or lines of precipitate form where diffused specific antigen and antibody meet in optimal proportions; the precipitin reaction is a useful analytic technique for the identification of unknown antibodies or antigens.

　rhythm m., birth control by avoiding sexual intercourse for several days before and after the approximate day of ovulation.

　Schafer-Nielsen-Drinker m., a method of artificial respiration in which the individual is placed face downward with hands under the forehead followed by someone's raising and lowering the elbows while another person exerts intermittent pressure upon the lower part of the ribs about 15 times a minute.

　Schick's m., a method of producing immunity to diphtheria by the injection of a mixture of toxin and antitoxin of that disease.

　silver cone m., the method in which a prefitted silver cone is placed into the apex of the root canal of a tooth and then sealed.

　Sippy's m., a method of treating peptic ulcer by neutralizing the free acid of the gastric juice with foods (milk and cream especially) administered frequently in small amounts.

　split cast m., a method of indexing dental casts on an articulator to facilitate their removal and replacement on the instrument.

　Westergren m., a method for estimating the sedimentation rate of red blood cells in blood; after mixing 4.5 ml of venous blood with 0.5 ml of 3.8 per cent aqueous solution of sodium citrate, a standard pipet (2-mm bore, 300 mm in length, and graduated at 1-mm intervals from zero to 200) is filled to the zero mark and kept in an upright position; in one hour the fall of the red blood cells is recorded; the average rate for males is zero to 15 millimeters and for females, zero to 20 millimeters.

　Wintrobe m., a method of determining the sedimentation rate of red cells in blood mixed with an anticoagulant, by the use of the narrow-bore Wintrobe tube; the amount of sedimentation is noted after one hour, then the sample is centrifuged and the measured volume of packed red cells is used to modify the first reading using a standard table; corrected normal value for males is zero to 10 millimeters and for females zero to 20 millimeters in one hour.

methotrex′ate. A folic acid antagonist used in the treatment of choriocarcinoma.

methoxyflu′rane. 2,2-Dichloro-1,1-difluoroethyl methyl ether; a clear, colorless liquid with a fruity odor; nonflammable and nonexplosive in air or oxygen; used as a slow anesthetic; Penthrane®.

methscopolamine bromide. A gastrointestinal antispasmodic agent of prolonged action (about

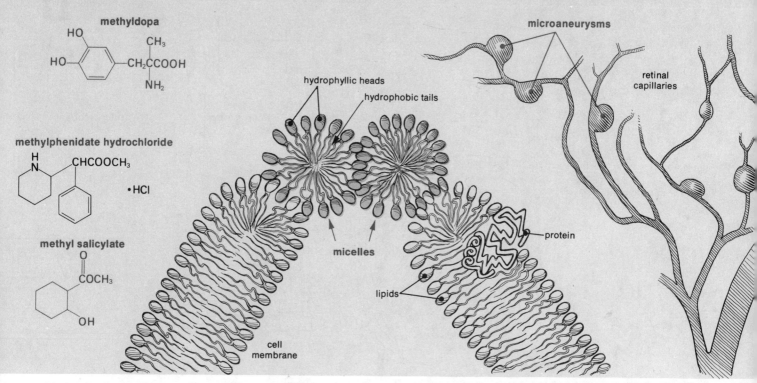

methyldopa

methylphenidate hydrochloride

methyl salicylate

hydrophyllic heads
hydrophobic tails
micelles
cell membrane
lipids
protein

microaneurysms
retinal capillaries

eight hours); used chiefly in the treatment of gastrointestinal diseases; Pamine Bromide®.

meth′yl. The radical —CH₃.

m. benzene, see toluene.

m. chloride, CH₃Cl; the hydrochloric acid ester of methyl alcohol; a refrigerant, used in spray form as a local anesthetic; also called chloromethane.

m. iodide, CH₃I; a somewhat colorless liquid used as a local anesthetic.

m. methacrylate, an acrylic resin; a plastic material.

m. salicylate, a colorless liquid, insoluble in water; used as an antipyretic and antiseptic; also called artificial wintergreen oil.

m. sulfoxide, see dimethyl sulfoxide.

meth′ylate. 1. To combine with methyl alcohol or the methyl radical. **2.** A compound of methyl alcohol and a metal.

meth′ylated. Combined with or containing methyl alcohol.

meth′ylcel′lulose. A bulk-forming cellulose derivative with laxative properties; available in powder, granules, or capsule forms and used for constipation and occasionally as an appetite depressant in the management of obesity; the synthetic form is used to prolong the duration of contact in ophthalmic drops.

meth′ylcholan′threne. A cancer-producing hydrocarbon.

methyldo′pa. A hypotensive drug used in the treatment of hypertension.

meth′ylene. The organic radical CH₂.

m. blue, see under blue.

3,4-methylene dioxyamphetamine (MDA). A hallucinogen commonly referred to as the love drug.

methylglu′camine diatrizo′ate. An organic compound used as a contrast medium in the making of x-ray transparencies.

methylmalon′ic acidu′ria. Excretion of excessive amounts of methylmalonic acid in urine.

methylpar′aben. An antifungal preservative; Niapagin®.

methylphen′idate hydrochlo′ride. A mild central nervous system stimulant similar to amphetamine; used in the management of children with hyperkinetic syndrome and in the treatment of narcolepsy; Ritalin®.

methylpred′nisolone. An anti-inflammatory agent, usually administered orally; commonly used immune suppressant.

methyltestos′terone. A methyl derivative of testosterone.

methyltrans′ferase. An enzyme that transfers a methyl group from one compound to another; also called transmethylase.

methyp′rylon. Compound having sedative and hypnotic properties.

methyser′gide malea′te. Compound used in the prophylactic treatment of migraine; prolonged use may be associated with retroperitoneal fibrosis; Sansert®.

MetMb. Abbreviation for metmyoglobin.

metmy′oglobin (MetMb). A reddish brown pigment resulting from the oxidation of myoglobin.

metopy′rone. See metyrapone.

Metor′chis. A genus of flukes; some of its species are found in cats, dogs, and occasionally in man.

metox′enous. Heteroecious.

metr-. Combining form meaning the uterus.

me′tra. Greek for uterus.

metrato′nia. Lack of tone of the uterine wall after childbirth.

metrec′tomy. Hysterectomy.

me′tria. Any inflammatory condition following childbirth.

met′ric. Relating to or based on the meter as a standard of measurement.

metri′tis. Inflammation of the uterus.

metrodynamom′eter. Instrument used to measure the strength of uterine contractions.

metromala′cia. Abnormal softening of the uterus.

metron′oscope. Device that exposes printed material at short intervals; used to test and develop reading speed.

metropath′ia hemorrhag′ica. Excessive, prolonged bleeding from the uterus, associated with cyst formation of the endometrium.

metropath′ic. Related to or caused by disease of the uterus.

metrop′athy. Any disease of the uterus.

metrophlebi′tis. Inflammation of the uterine veins, usually occurring only while bearing a child or immediately thereafter.

metropto′sia, metropto′sis. Prolapse of the uterus.

metrorrha′gia. Irregular bleeding from the uterus, especially during the intermenstrual period.

metrorrhe′a. Discharge of pus or mucus from the uterus.

metrorrhex′is. Rupture of the uterus.

metrosalpingi′tis. Inflammation of the uterus and the uterine (fallopian) tubes.

me′troscope. Instrument for viewing the uterine cavity.

metrostax′is. A slight continuous bleeding from the uterus.

metrosteno′sis. Constriction of the uterine cavity.

metrot′omy. Hysterotomy.

M. et sig. Abbreviation for Latin *misce et signa*.

metyr′apone. C₁₄H₁₄N₂O; 2-methyl-1,2-di-3-pyridyl-1-propanone; an inhibitor of adrenocortical steroid C-11 β hydroxylation; administered orally or intravenously as a diagnostic test to determine the capability of the pituitary gland to increase its production of corticotropin; also called mepyrapone and metopyrone.

mev. Symbol for a mega electron volt.

MG. Abbreviation for myasthenia gravis.

Mg. Chemical symbol of the element magnesium.

mg. Abbreviation for milligram.

mi′asm, mias′ma. Noxious vapors, as from a swamp; formerly thought to cause certain diseases such as malaria.

micelle. 1. A formation of approximately 50 to 100 amphipathic molecules arranged spherically, usually with the hydrophobic moiety on the inside and the hydrophilic groups on the outside. **2.** A hypothetical submicroscopic particle thought to be the unit of living matter, capable of growth and division.

Micheli's anemia, Micheli's syndrome. Paroxysmal nocturnal hemoglobinuria; see under hemoglobinuria.

micro-. Combining form meaning (a) small; (b) one-millionth; e.g., a microcurie is one-millionth of a curie.

microab′scess. A minute collection of leukocytes in solid tissues; a very small abscess.

microaer′ophil, microaer′ophile. A microorganism that requires very little free oxygen.

microaer′osol. A suspension in air of particles between one and 10 microns in diameter.

microanal′ysis. Special analytic technique involving quantities weighing one milligram or less.

microanat′omy. See histology.

microan′eurysm. A minute aneurysm of a small vessel as seen in diabetic retinopathy.

microangiog′raphy. The making of x-ray transparencies of the smallest blood vessels.

microangiop′athy. Any disorder of the small blood vessels.

thrombotic m., a combination of arteriolar thrombosis and capillary wall thickening resulting in a narrow lumen.

systemic diabetic m., the thickening of capillary basement membranes in many organs.

microbal′ance. A scale designed to weigh minute amounts of materials.

mi′crobe. A microorganism; a one-celled animal or plant, especially one that causes disease.

micro′bial, micro′bic. Relating to a microorganism.

micro′bicide. Anything that destroys microorganisms; a germicide; an antiseptic.

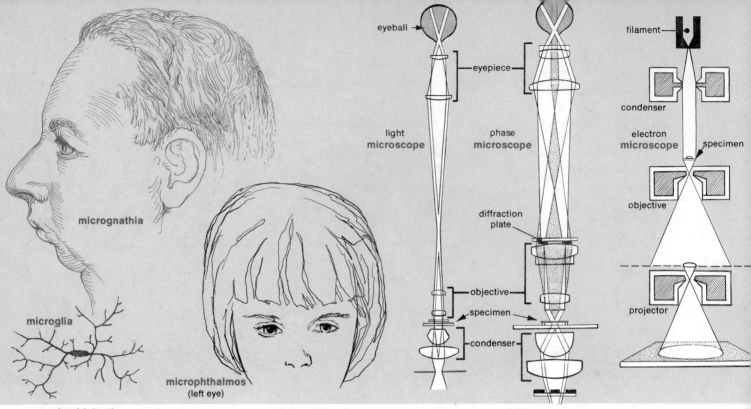

microscope

eyeball

eyepiece

light microscope

phase microscope

filament

condenser

electron microscope

specimen

diffraction plate

objective

objective

objective

specimen

condenser

projector

microbiolog'ic. Relating to microbiology.

microbiol'ogist. A specialist in microbiology.

microbiol'ogy. The branch of science concerned with the study of microorganisms and their effect on other living organisms.

microbio'ta. A general term denoting both plant and animal organisms that live in streams, as algae and protozoa.

mi'croblast. A small nucleated red blood cell.

mi'crobody. See peroxisome.

microbra'chia. Abnormal smallness of the arms.

microcar'dia. Abnormal smallness of the heart.

microceph'aly. Abnormal smallness of the head.

microchem'istry. The use of minute amounts (in the range of one milligram) of substances in chemical reactions.

microcircula'tion. Blood circulation in the capillaries, arterioles, and venules.

Micrococca'ceae. A family of gram-positive spherical or elliptical bacteria which divide in two or three planes, forming pairs, tetrads, or masses of cells; includes some pathogenic species; the type genus is *Micrococcus*.

micrococ'cus. One of several species of bacteria (genus *Micrococcus*) characterized by a spherical shape and occurring singly, in pairs, and (most frequently) in irregular clusters.

microcor'ia. Congenital smallness of the pupil.

microcor'nea. Abnormal smallness of the cornea.

microcou'lomb. A microunit of electric quantity; one-millionth of a coulomb.

mi'crocurie (μCi). A measure of radioactivity, one-millionth of a curie.

mi'crocyst. A tiny cyst, usually undetected by the unaided eye.

mi'crocyte. A small red blood cell at least two microns smaller than normal; can be seen in the blood of individuals with iron deficiency anemia.

microcyto'sis, microcythe'mia. Condition in which the red blood cells are abnormally small.

microdac'tyly. Abnormal smallness of the fingers or toes.

microden'tism. See microdontia.

microdissec'tion. Dissection with the aid of a microscope or enlarging lens.

microdon'tia, microden'tism. Abnormal smallness of the teeth.

microelec'trode. A fine caliber electrode used in physiologic experiments.

microfar'ad. A microunit of electrical capacity; one-millionth of a farad.

microfilare'mia. The presence of microfilariae in the blood.

microfila'ria. The prelarval or embryonic forms of filarial worms.

microgam'ete. The smaller male element in conjugation of cells of unequal size.

microgam'etocyte. The mother cell that produces microgametes.

microg'amy. Conjugation between two young cells in certain protozoans.

microgas'tria. Congenital smallness of the stomach.

microgen'ia. Abnormal smallness of the chin.

microgen'italism. Abnormal smallness of the external genital organs.

microg'lia. The smallest neuroglial cells; the macrophages of the brain and spinal cord; they help remove the cellular debris of the central nervous system.

microglos'sia. Abnormal smallness of the tongue.

microgna'thia. Abnormal smallness of the jaw, especially the lower jaw, usually resulting in a recessive, birdlike profile.

   primary m., see Pierre Robin syndrome.

microgo'nioscope. Instrument used to measure minute angles, as the filtration angle of the anterior chamber of the eye.

mi'crogram (mcg, μg). A unit of weight equivalent to one-millionth of a gram.

microgy'ria. Abnormal narrowness of the convolutions of the brain.

mi'crohm. A microunit of electrical resistance equivalent to one-millionth of an ohm.

microincinera'tion. The process of heating a tissue section to about 525°C and then observing the mineral ashes under a dark field microscope; also called spodography.

microincis'ion. See micropuncture (2).

microinva'sion. The earliest stage in the spread of a carcinoma to the adjacent tissues.

microkymatother'apy. Treatment of disease with high frequency radiation; also called microwave therapy.

mi'croliter (μl). One-millionth of a liter.

mi'crolith. A minute calculus.

microlithi'asis. The presence of minute concretions (gravel).

micromanipula'tion. Dissection, teasing, etc. of microscopic structures under the microscope.

micromanip'ulator. An instrument used in the dissection and injection of microscopic specimens and in isolation of single cells.

microme'lia. The state of having abnormally small limbs.

microm'eter. An instrument used to measure microscopic objects.

micrometh'od. Chemical analysis or techniques involving minimal amounts of material or the use of a microscope.

microm'etry. Measurement with a micrometer.

micromicro-. See pico-.

micromi'crogram. ($\mu\mu$g). Picogram; one-millionth of one-millionth (10^{-12}) of a gram.

micromi'cron ($\mu\mu$). One millionth of a micron.

micromo'lar. Having a concentration of one millionth of a mole.

mi'cromole (μmole). One-millionth of a mole.

micromye'lia. Congenital smallness or shortness of the spinal cord.

mi'cron (μ). A unit of length in the metric system equal to one-thousandth of a millimeter.

micron'ic. Having the size of one micron (μ).

micronu'cleus. 1. The smallest of the nuclei in a multinuclear cell. **2.** The smaller (reproductive) of the two nuclei in ciliates dividing mitotically, the larger being the vegetative nucleus.

micronu'trients. Essential compounds required by the body only in minute amounts; e.g., vitamins.

microorgan'ic. Relating to a microorganism.

microor'ganism. A microscopic animal or plant.

micropathol'ogy. 1. The microscopic study of disease-caused changes in the tissues. **2.** The study of disease caused by microorganisms.

mi'crophage. A small neutrophil that leaves the blood stream to phagocytose bacteria and small particles; contrasted with the larger macrophage that characteristically engulfs larger particles.

micropho'bia. Abnormal fear of microorganisms.

microphthal'mos, microphthal'mia. Abnormal smallness of the eyeballs.

micropipette, micropipet. Any variously shaped, calibrated glass tubes designed to transfer minute volumes of liquid.

micropla'sia. Arrested growth.

microplethysmog'raphy. The recording of changes in the size of a bodily part resulting from the flow of blood into and out of it.

micropunc'ture. 1. A technique for studying the function of the kidney by placement of a micropipette within a tubule and/or blood vessel of the kidney in order to sample the composition of fluid, measure the pressure, or determine the electric potential at different sites. **2.** Destruction of the organelles of a cell by a ruby laser beam; also called microincision.

mi'croscope. An instrument with a combination of lenses used to observe small objects or substances under magnification.

   binocular m., a microscope with two eyepiece tubes, permitting observation with both eyes simultaneously.

   bright field m., a microscope that makes an object visible by passing light through it (transillumina-

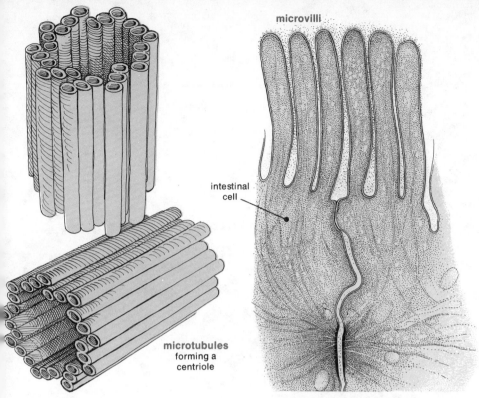

microvilli

intestinal cell

microtubules forming a centriole

	Human	Cow's
protein	2 g	3.5 g
carbohydrate	7 g	5 g
fat	4 g	3.5 g
calcium	25 mg	120 mg
phosphorus	16 mg	95 mg
iron	0.1 mg	0.1 mg
thiamine	17 µg	40 µg
riboflavin	30 µg	150 µg
nicotinic acid	170 µg	80 µg
ascorbic acid	3.5 µg	2.0 µg
vitamin A	170 IU	150 IU
vitamin D	1.0 IU	1.5 IU
calories	70	66

tion).

compound m., a microscope having an objective and an eyepiece at opposite ends of an adjustable cylinder.

dark field m., a microscope that uses a method of illumination by means of which the object structure is made to appear luminous against a dark field.

electron m., a microscope that uses electrons rather than visible light to irradiate clear, magnified images; capable of magnifying objects having dimensions smaller than the wavelengths of visible light.

interference m., one in which the emerging light is split into two beams which pass through the object and are recombined in the image plane, where transparent and refractile specimen details become visible as intensity differences; useful in the examination of living or unstained cells.

laser m., one in which a laser beam is focused on a microscopic field, causing it to vaporize; the emitted radiation is analyzed by means of a microspectrophotometer.

operating m., one used in the operating room for magnifying the surgical field.

phase m., phase contrast m., a microscope that makes use of the relationship between two paths of light: (1) light which enters the microscope objective directly through the specimen and (2) light which enters the objective after being diffracted by the specimen; all points of divergence between these two paths of light reveal a specimen or object whose lack of contrast would make it invisible under other types of illumination.

scanning electron m., a microscope in which the specimen is examined point by point by an electron beam and an image may be viewed on a television screen or photographed.

stereoscopic wide field m., a binocular form of microscope with double objectives, designed to give a three-dimensional view of the specimen; magnifying power is usually limited to about 150 diameters.

x ray m., a microscope that produces magnified images by recording the differences in the structure's absorption or emission of x rays.

microscop′ic. 1. Visible only with the aid of a microscope. **2.** Relating to the microscope.

micros′copy. The study of minute objects or organisms by means of a microscope.

mi′crosecond. One-millionth of a second; 10^{-6} second.

mi′crosome. See ribosome.

microspher′ocyte. A smaller than normal red blood cell having a spherical shape; present in hemolytic diseases.

microspherocyto′sis. Presence in the blood of a large number of small spherical red blood cells (spherocytes); associated with hemolysis.

Micros′porum. A genus of fungi causing skin infections.

M. audouini, fungus causing ringworm in humans, especially ringworm of the scalp.

microsto′mia. Congenital smallness of the mouth.

microsur′gery. Surgery aided by stereoscopic magnification which permits precise observation, differentiation, and delicate manipulation of tissues.

microsyr′inge. A hypodermic syringe specifically designed to measure accurately minute amounts of fluid to be injected.

mi′crotome. An instrument for slicing thin sections of tissue for microscopic examination.

microt′omy. The slicing of tissue into thin sections with a microtome.

microtonom′eter. Instrument designed to determine the tensions of oxygen and carbon dioxide in arterial blood.

microtu′bules. Long, slender, delicate cylindrical organelles, about 250 Å in diameter, made up of a protein, the amino acid of which resembles the muscle protein actin; they are scattered throughout the cytoplasm of almost every cell type; during cell division they increase greatly in number to form the mitotic spindle; they also form the framework of the basal body and the centriole, and the cores of cilia, flagella, and sperm tails; they play an important role in intracellular movements and in maintaining cell shape.

microvil′li. Submicroscopic finger-like projections on the surface of the cell membrane which greatly increase the surface area.

mi′crovolt. One-millionth of a volt; 10^{-6} volt.

mi′crowave. Any electromagnetic radiation having a very short wavelength between one millimeter and 30 centimeters; wavelengths shorter than one millimeter are in the infrared region, while those above 30 centimeters are radiowaves; also called microelectric wave.

mi′crurgy. Manipulative procedures performed on microscopic specimens with the aid of a microscope and often a micromanipulator.

mic′turate. To urinate.

micturi′tion. Urination; the act of urinating.

MID. Abbreviation for minimal infecting dose.

mid′brain. The part of the brain that develops from the embryonic mesencephalon; divided into three parts: the tectum (quadrigeminal plate), the tegmentum (cephalic continuation of the pontine tegmentum) and the crus cerebri (containing massive bundles of cortifugal fibers passing through to the lower brain stem and spinal cord).

middle lobe syndrome. A form of chronic ate-

lectasis marked by collapse of the middle lobe of the lung resulting from compression of the bronchus by surrounding lymph nodes, often due to tumor involvement; symptoms include chronic cough, wheezing, recurrent respiratory infections, and chest pains; also called Brock's syndrome.

mid′foot. The middle portion of the foot consisting of the navicular, cuboid, and cuneiform bones.

mid′gut. 1. The middle portion of the embryonic digestive tract between the foregut and the hindgut from which the ileum and the jejunum develop. **2.** The small intestine.

midmens′trual. Occurring midway between two menstrual periods.

midpel′vis. The area of the pelvis extending from the posterior inferior aspects of the symphysis in a line through the ischial spines to the sacrum intersecting it at about the second and third vertebrae.

mid′riff. The diaphragm.

midsec′tion. A section or division through the center of an organ or a part.

mid′wife. A woman who attends women at delivery.

midwif′ery. Practical obstetrics.

mi′graine. A recurrent, intense headache, usually confined to one side of the head and associated with nausea, vomiting, and visual disturbances.

migra′tion. Passing from one part of the body to another.

Mikulicz's disease. Benign bilateral swelling of the lacrimal and salivary glands associated with dryness of the mouth and reduced or absent lacrimation; believed by some clinical investigators to be identical to Sjögren's syndrome.

Mikulicz's syndrome. Painless enlargement of the salivary and lacrimal glands, usually bilateral, accompanied by dryness of mouth and decreased lacrimation; thought to be a complication of tuberculosis, leukemia, lymphoma, or sarcoidosis.

milia′ria. A skin eruption due to retention of sweat in the sweat follicles.

m. rubra, prickly heat; see under heat.

mil′iary. Having nodules of millet seed size (above 2 mm).

m. tuberculosis, see tuberculosis, acute miliary.

mil′ieu. French for environment or surroundings.

m. intérieur, the internal environment; the fluids bathing the tissue cells of multicellular animals.

mil′ium. A minute whitish or yellowish papule on the skin caused by the retention of fatty material (sebum).

milk. 1. A white or yellowish liquid secreted by the mammary glands of female mammals for the nourishment of the young, containing proteins, sugar, and lipids. **2.** An emulsion or suspension; formerly

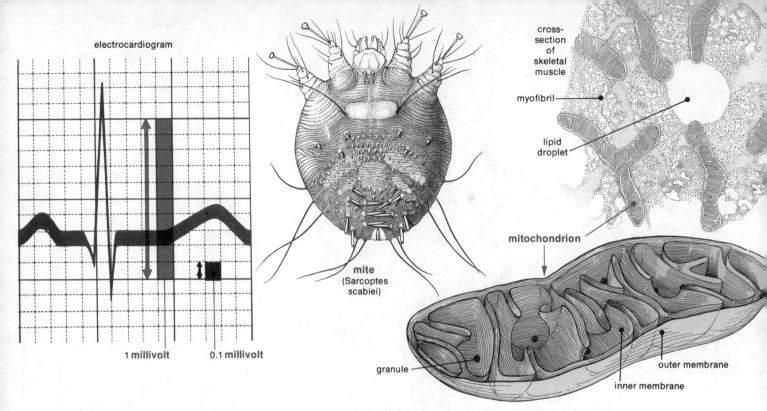

electrocardiogram

1 millivolt   0.1 **millivolt**

mite
(Sarcoptes
scabiei)

cross-
section
of
skeletal
muscle

myofibril

lipid
droplet

mitochondrion

granule

inner membrane

outer membrane

---

called magma. **3.** A milklike liquid.

  m. leg, colloquial term for a painful swelling of the leg resulting from clotting and inflammation of the great saphenous or femoral veins; occurring sometimes in women after childbirth.

  m. of magnesia, see under magnesia.

  m. sugar, see lactose.

  m. teeth, deciduous teeth; see under tooth.

  uterine m., secretion produced by uterine glands.

  witch's m., the milklike fluid sometimes secreted by the breasts of newborn babies of either sex.

milk-alkali syndrome. Hypercalcemia without hypercalcuria or hypophosphaturia, induced by the prolonged ingestion of large amounts of milk and soluble alkali, usually as therapy for peptic ulcer; it is reversible in its early stages, but if undetected leads to renal failure; also called Burnett's syndrome.

milk'ing. The removal of the contents of a tubular structure by gently running a finger along its length; also called stripping.

Milkman's syndrome. Osteoporosis causing multiple fractures; seen most frequently in postmenopausal women.

Millard-Gubler syndrome. Paralysis of facial muscles on one side and of the extremities on the opposite side, produced by a unilateral lesion of the brain stem.

milli-. A prefix used in the metric system indicating one-thousandth; e.g., one milliroentgen is one-thousandth of a roentgen.

milliam'pere (ma). One-thousandth of an ampere.

mil'licurie (mCi). A measure of radioactivity, one-thousandth of a curie.

milliequiv'alent (mEq). An expression of concentration of substance per liter of solution, calculated by dividing the concentration in milligrams per 100 milliliters by the molecular weight.

mil'ieu. The immediate surroundings of an individual.

mil'ligram (mg). One-thousandth of a gram.

mil'liliter (ml). One-thousandth of a liter; one cubic centimeter.

mil'limeter (mm). One-thousandth of a meter.

millimicro-. Prefix meaning one-billionth; equivalent of nano-.

millimi'crogram. One-billionth of a gram; preferred term is nanogram (ng).

millimi'cron (mμ). One-thousandth of a micron; preferred term is nanometer (nm).

mil'limole (mм). One-thousandth of a mole (gram-molecule).

mil'ling-in. The placing of abrasives between the occlusal surfaces of dentures while rubbing them together in the mouth or on the articulator; used to perfect the occlusion.

millios'mole (mOsm). One-thousandth of an osmole; the osmotic pressure exerted by the concentration of a substance in solution; expressed as milligrams per kilogram divided by atomic weight for an ionized substance, or divided by molecular weight for nonionized solutes; normal plasma osmolality is 280 to 300 mOsm/kg.

mil'lirad (mrad). One-thousandth of a rad.

mil'lirem (mrem). One-thousandth of a rem.

mil'liroentgen (mr). One-thousandth of a roentgen.

mil'lisecond (msec). One-thousandth of a second.

mil'livolt (mv). One-thousandth of a volt.

Milroy's disease. Familial and congenital swelling of subcutaneous tissues (usually confined to the extremities) with large accumulation of lymph.

mime'sis. Imitation; state in which one disease presents the symptoms of another.

mind. The psyche; the totality of conscious and unconscious processes serving to adjust the individual to the demands of the environment.

min'eral. Any naturally occurring homogeneous inorganic substance, having a characteristic crystalline structure and chemical composition.

mineralocor'ticoid. One of the steroids in the adrenal cortex that controls salt metabolism.

min'im. A unit of fluid measure; in the United States, $^1/_{60}$ of a fluid dram; about a drop.

minimal brain dysfunction syndrome. A complex of symptoms that involves impairment of some or all of the following functions: learning, language, perception, memory, concentration, and motor; neurologic examination usually yields minor abnormalities if any; diagnosis rests on psychological assessment of cognitive function. See also disability, learning.

mio'sis. 1. Reduction in size of the pupil of the eye. **2.** Phase of a disease in which the severity of the symptoms begins to diminish.

miot'ic. Denoting any agent that causes contraction of the pupil.

miracid'ium, *pl.* **miracid'ia.** A free-swimming ciliated larva of a trematode that penetrates a small intermediate host where it develops into a sporocyst.

mire. One of the luminous objects in the ophthalmometer (used to measure the anterior curvature of the cornea).

mir'ror. A polished surface that forms optical images by reflection.

  head m., a circular concave mirror attached to a headband, used to illuminate a bodily cavity.

misan'thropy. Aversion to people.

miscar'riage. Spontaneous abortion.

miscar'ry. To give birth to a nonviable fetus.

mis'ce (M). Latin for mix; used in prescription writing.

misce et signa. Latin for mix and label; used in prescription writing.

misc'ible. Capable of being mixed.

misdiagno'sis. A wrong diagnosis.

misog'yny. Hatred of women.

misopho'bia. An abnormal fear of contamination.

MIT. Abbreviation for monoiodotyrosine.

mite. Any of various minute arachnids that are often parasitic on man and animals; they may infest food and carry disease.

  harvest m., see chigger.

  hay itch m., see *Pyemotes ventricosus.*

  itch m., see *Sarcoptes scabiei.*

  northern fowl m., *Ornithonyssus sylviarum.*

mith'ridatism. Immunity to a poison achieved by taking gradually increased doses of it.

mi'ticide. An agent that kills mites.

mi'tis. Latin for mild; opposite of immitis.

mit'ochondria, *sing.* **mit'ochondrion.** Compartmentalized, double membrane, self-reproducing organelles present in the cytoplasm of almost all living cells, responsible for generating usable energy by the formation of ATP (adenosine triphosphate); in the average cell there are several hundred mitochondria, each about 15,000 Å in length.

mi'togen. A substance that stimulates cell mitosis.

mitogen'esis. The induction of mitosis in a cell.

mitogen'ic. Causing or inducing cell mitosis.

mito'sis. Multiplication or division of a cell which results in the formation of two daughter cells normally receiving the same chromosome and deoxyribonucleic acid (DNA) content as that of the original cell; also called karyokinesis.

mitot'ic. Relating to mitosis or cell division.

mi'tral. Relating to the left atrioventricular valve of the heart.

mitraliza'tion. In roentgenography, straightening of the left border of the heart shadow with protrusion of the atrial appendage and/or the pulmonary salient.

mit'telschmerz. Intermenstrual pain, specifically at the time of ovulation.

mix'ture. 1. An aggregation of two or more substances which are not chemically combined. **2.** A pharmaceutical preparation consisting of an insoluble substance suspended in a liquid by a viscid material such as sugar, glycerol, etc.

  binary m., one containing two substances.

  explosive m., one capable of instantaneous com-

---

milk | mixture

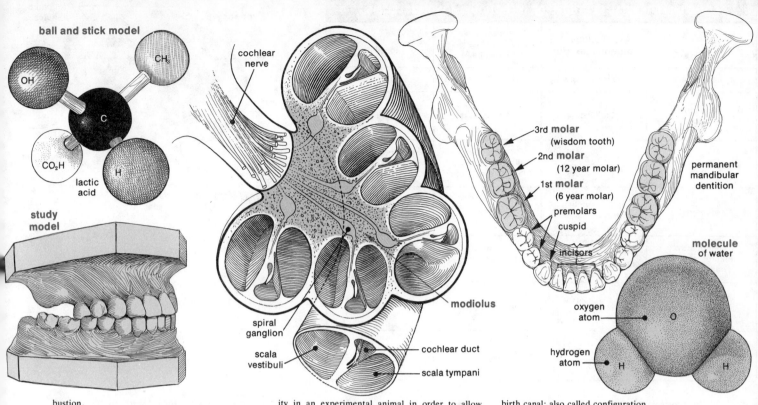

ball and stick model

OH, CH₃, C, CO₂H, H
lactic acid

study model

cochlear nerve

3rd **molar** (wisdom tooth)
2nd **molar** (12 year molar)
1st **molar** (6 year molar)
premolars
cuspid
incisors

permanent mandibular dentition

molecule of water

oxygen atom — O
hydrogen atom — H H

modiolus

spiral ganglion
scala vestibuli
cochlear duct
scala tympani

---

bustion.

ml. Abbreviation for milliliter.

MLD, mld. Abbreviation for minimal lethal dose.

MLD₅₀. Abbreviation for the minimal dose that is lethal for 50 per cent of the experimental animals tested for assay of a toxic substance.

mM. Abbreviation for millimole.

mm. 1. Abbreviation for millimeter. **2.** Sometimes used as an abbreviation for muscles.

Mn. Chemical symbol of the element manganese.

mnemon′ic. Relating to or assisting the memory.

mnemon′ics. A system for improving the memory.

MNSs blood group. A system of erythrocyte antigens determined by the allelic genes M, N, and S,s; first demonstrated by injecting human blood into rabbits, which developed antibodies against it; originally defined to include antigens to antibodies anti-M and anti-N and later extended to include those reacting to antibodies anti-S and anti-s; the group is primarily used to solve identification problems such as disputed paternity and for genetic linkage population studies.

M.O. Abbreviation for Medical Officer.

Mo. Chemical symbol of the element molybdenum.

mobiliza′tion. 1. Making a part movable. **3.** Starting a sequence of physiologic activity.

  stapes m., surgical procedure through which the footplate of the stapes is liberated from adhesions or overlapping bony tissue caused by otosclerosis or middle ear infection.

mo′bilize. To cause stored substances in the body to participate in physiologic activity; to liberate material from storage sites.

Möbius′ sign. Convergence weakness of the eyes occurring in exophthalmic goiter.

Möbius′ syndrome. A congenital disorder characterized by bilateral paralysis of both external rectus muscles and face muscles and sometimes associated with other musculoskeletal anomalies or neurologic disorders; also called congenital facial diplegia and congenital oculofacial paralysis.

MOD. Abbreviation for mesio-occlusodistal.

modal′ity. 1. Any of several forms of therapy; e.g., diathermy. **2.** An apparatus used to apply such therapy. **3.** Any of the main forms of sensation; e.g., hearing.

mode. In statistics, the value occurring most often.

mod′el. 1. A replica; a three-dimensional shape representing a likeness of some existing structure. **2.** In dentistry, a cast; a positive reproduction of the dentition and adjoining structures.

  ball and stick m., a three-dimensional schematic representation of a molecular structure.

  disease m., the artificial creation of an abnormal-

ity in an experimental animal in order to allow further study of the entity.

  study m., a replica of the teeth and adjoining oral structures used as a diagnostic aid; also called diagnostic cast.

mod′ifier. Agent that alters form or character without transforming; e.g., in genetics, a gene which alters the phenotypic effect of another gene.

modi′olus. The central pillar or column of bone around which the spiral canals of the cochlea turn.

modula′tion. The changes that take place in response to changes in the environment, such as the temporary change of osteoblasts into osteocytes and back to osteoblasts in response to altered conditions in the environment.

mogigraph′ia. Writer's cramp; see under cramp.

moi′ety. 1. One of two more or less equal parts. **2.** A part or portion of indefinite size.

mol. See gram-molecule.

mo′lal. Containing one mole of solute per 1000 grams of solvent. Cf molar (2).

molal′ity. The concentration of a solution expressed as the number of moles of solute per 1000 grams of solvent.

mo′lar. 1. A posterior tooth for grinding and pulverizing food. **2.** Containing one gram-molecular weight (1 mole) of solute per 1000 milliliters of solution. Cf molal. **3.** Relating to a body of matter; not molecular.

  deciduous m., one of eight posterior teeth in the deciduous (primary) dentition.

  first permanent m., largest permanent tooth in the mouth; first permanent tooth to erupt usually at the age of six years; also called six-year molar.

  impacted m., a molar unable to erupt properly.

  permanent m., one of 12 posterior teeth in the permanent (secondary) dentition.

  second permanent m., a permanent molar immediately distal to the first molar which usually erupts at the age of 12 years; also called 12 year molar.

  third permanent m., last permanent posterior tooth in the mouth which erupts usually between the ages of 17 and 21 years; also called wisdom tooth.

molar′ity. The concentration of a solution expressed as the number of moles of solute per liter of solution.

mold. 1. Any of a group of fungi usually growing on decaying organic matter. **2.** A receptable for shaping any cast material (wax, plastic, etc.). **3.** To shape.

  m. guide, a guide for specifying the shape of artificial teeth.

mold′ing. 1. The process of shaping. **2.** The change in shape of the fetal head as it passes through the

birth canal; also called configuration.

mole. 1. Pigmented cellular nevus; a circumscribed pigmented growth on the skin. **2.** Gram-molecule.

  hydatidiform m., a developmental anomaly of the placenta consisting of a nonmalignant mass of clear vesicles (which resembles a bunch of grapes), formed from cystic swelling of the chorionic villi; the mole may grow to fill the uterus and cause it to enlarge to the size of a six-month pregnancy; usually there is no embryo present; also called hydatid mole and hydatid degeneration.

molec′ular. Relating to or consisting of molecules.

molecular weight. The sum of the atomic weights of all the atoms making up a molecule; e.g., hydrogen (H) has an atomic weight of one and chlorine (Cl) has an atomic weight of 35.5; thus, a molecule of hydrochloric acid (HCl) has a molecular weight of 36.5.

mol′ecule. The smallest unit of a substance (composed of two or more atoms) which can exist in a free state and still retain the chemical properties of the substance.

  cyclic m., one which appears in organic compounds, and whose atoms are arranged in a ring or polygon.

moli′men, *pl.* **molim′ina.** The effort required by a normal physiologic function, especially the menstrual flow.

mollus′cum. A skin disease marked by the presence of soft rounded tumors.

  m. contagiosum, an infectious disease of the skin, marked by small wartlike lesions containing a substance resembling curds; caused by a virus.

molt. To cast off.

mol. wt. Abbreviation for molecular weight; also commonly abbreviated MW.

molyb′date. A salt of molybdic acid.

molyb′denum. Metallic element; symbol Mo, atomic number 42, atomic weight 95.95; it has several isotopes.

molyb′dic. Denoting a salt of trivalent or hexavalent molybdeum.

molybdic acid. Any of two acids, H₂MoO₄ (colorless needles), or H₂MoO₄·4H₂O, a yellow crystalline substance, soluble in ammonia and used as a reagent.

MOM. Abbreviation for milk of magnesia.

mom′ism. The state of being excessively dependent on or subordinate to one's mother or her substitute.

mon′ad. 1. A univalent element, radical, or atom. **2.** A unicellular organism. **3.** The single chromosome formed after the second division in meiosis.

monarthri′tis. Arthritis of one joint.

monartic′ular. Denoting a single joint.

SOME DIFFERENTIAL FEATURES OF INFECTIOUS MONONUCLEOSIS			
	infectious mononucleosis	infectious hepatitis (hepatitis A)	tonsillitis
usual age	15 to 25 years	15 to 25 years	5 to 20 years
incubation period	30 to 50 days	15 to 45 days	usually 3 to 5 days
fever	irregular; usually about 2 weeks	moderate; disappears when jaundice develops	moderate to high; usually under 5 days
sore throat	marked; whitish-gray exudate	none	constant; yellow or white exudate
adenopathy (enlargement of lymph nodes)	most commonly: anterior and posterior cervical chains; often generalized	minimal; usually cervical	submandibular; anterior cervical
splenomegaly (enlargement of spleen)	approximately 50%	less than 10%	none
hepatomegaly (enlargement of liver)	approximately 10%	over 80%	none

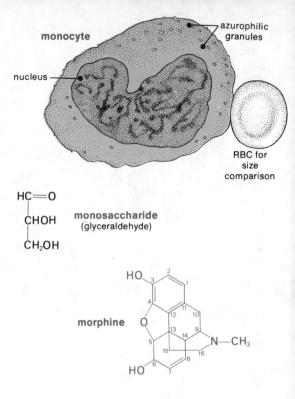

monosaccharide
(glyceraldehyde)

morphine

monau'ral. Relating to one ear.

Monday disease. The return of symptoms after a weekend away from work, as in the case of an allergic reaction to a substance encountered while at work.

Mondor's disease. Inflammation of the subcutaneous veins of the chest and breast, usually extending from the epigastric region to the axilla and occurring in both males and females.

mon'golism. Down's syndrome; congenital defect caused by an abnormal chromosome 21.

mon'goloid, mongo'lian. Having characteristics resembling mongolism (Down's syndrome).

monil'ethrix. Beaded hair, an anomalous condition in which the hair shafts exhibit nodosities or points of thickening alternating with normal or constricted girth, giving the appearance of a string of fusiform beads.

Monil'ia. A genus of molds or fungi, commonly known as "fruit molds;" formerly included in this genus was a similar group of organisms now called *Candida*.

monili'asis. Infection with any fungi of the genus *Monilia*.

monil'iform. Beaded; having the shape of a necklace.

mon'itor, car'diac. An electronic device used for observation of each heart beat of a person.

mon'itoring. Constant observation.

    constant cardiac m., prolonged observation of the electrocardiogram with the aid of an oscilloscope to detect irregularities in the heart rhythm.

mono-. Combining form meaning single.

mono. Colloquial abbreviation for mononucleosis.

mon'oam'ine. Compound containing only one amine group.

    m. oxidase, an enzyme that catalyzes the oxidation of a wide variety of physiologic amines to the corresponding aldehydes and NH_3.

    m. oxidase inhibitors (MAOI), derivatives of hydrazine and hydrazide that inhibit the action of certain enzymes.

mon'oblast. An immature cell of the monocytic series, from 18 to 22 μ in diameter, which has several nucleoli; formed primarily in the spleen and lymphoid tissues.

monochromat'ic. 1. Having one color. **2.** Indicating a spectral color of a single wavelength.

monocrot'ic. Forming a smooth single crest on the downward line of a curve; said of a pulse.

monoc'ular. Relating to, having, or used by one eye.

mon'ocyte. A large mononuclear white blood cell, generally 15 to 25 microns in diameter, with a round, kidney-shaped, or lobulated nucleus and a cytoplasm that stains a gray-blue color with Wright's stain; it is the largest cell found in normal blood; when it leaves the blood stream it becomes a macrophage (phagocyte).

monocytope'nia. Reduction of monocytes in the blood; also called monocytic leukopenia and monopenia.

monocyto'sis. Abnormal increase in the number of monocytes in the blood; at least 15 or more monocytes per 100 white blood cells.

monodac'tylism. The presence of only one finger on the hand or one toe on the foot.

monogamet'ic. See homogametic.

monog'enous. Produced asexually.

mon'ograph. A detailed written account of one particular subject, one class of subjects, or a small area of a special field of learning.

monohy'brid. A cross between parents that differ in one character.

mon'oiodoty'rosine (MIT). An amino acid formed by the iodination of tyrosine; an initial step in the formation of thyronin.

monolay'er. A film which consists of a single layer of molecules, formed on a water surface by certain substances, as proteins and fatty acids, in which some atoms are soluble in water while others are insoluble in water.

monoma'nia. Pathologic preoccupation with one idea.

mon'omer. A simple molecule of low molecular weight which when repeated in a chain forms a polymer; e.g., ethylene is the monomer of polyethylene.

monomor'phic. Having but one shape; unchangeable in size and form.

mononeuri'tis. Inflammation or degeneration of a single nerve trunk or some of its branches.

mononu'clear. Uninuclear.

mononucleo'sis. Abnormal increase of mononuclear white blood cells (monocytes) in the blood.

    infectious m., an infectious febrile disease caused by the Epstein-Barr virus (EBv); marked by fever, sore throat, enlargement of the spleen and lymph nodes, and the presence in the blood of an abnormally large number of atypical lymphocytes that resemble monocytes; the virus can be carried in the mouth and throat of afflicted individuals for several months after the disappearance of clinical illness; popularly known as kissing disease and sometimes called glandular fever.

monopha'sia. Disorder in which the individual's vocabulary is limited to a single word or sentence.

monople'gia. Paralysis of only one limb or part.

monor'chid. An individual with only one visible testicle.

mon'orchism, monor'chidism. The condition of having or appearing to have only one testicle, the other being absent or undescended.

monosacch'aride. A carbodydrate which is not further broken down by hydrolysis; a simple sugar.

mon'osome. A chromosome without its homologous chromosome.

monos'omy. Condition in which one chromosome of a pair of homologous chromosomes is missing.

monosub'stituted. Having only one atom in each molecule replaced.

monot'richous. Denoting a unicellular organism having a single flagellum.

monova'lent. See univalent.

monox'ide. An oxide containing only one oxygen atom.

monozygot'ic. Denoting identical twins, or twins formed by the division into two of the embryo derived from a single fertilized egg.

mons, *pl.* **mon'tes.** In anatomy, a slight prominence or elevation.

    m. pubis, the fleshy prominence formed by a pad of fatty tissue over the pubic symphysis in the female.

    m. ureteris, a slight prominence on the wall of the bladder at the entrance of the ureter.

mood. A prevailing emotional state of mind.

Moraxel'la. A genus of bacteria containing gram-negative, short, rod-shaped cells; aerobic and parasitic; sometimes found on the mucous membranes of man.

mor'bid. Of, pertaining to, or affected by disease; diseased; pathologic.

morbid'ity. 1. The condition of being diseased. **2.** The ratio of disease to the population of a given area.

morbil'li. Measles.

morbil'liform. Resembling measles.

morbil'lous. Relating to measles.

mor'bus. Latin for disease.

mor'dant. A substance used in bacteriology to fix a dye or stain.

morgue. A place where the dead are kept pending autopsy and burial.

mor'ibund. Dying.

mor'ioplasty. Surgical restoration of parts lost through injury or disease.

mo'ron. A mentally retarded individual with an IQ from 50 to 69.

morphe'a. A skin disease marked by indurated white or yellow lesions surrounded by a violet ring; occurring chiefly on the chest, face, or neck.

morphine'. An alkaloid compound extracted from opium, used in medicine as an analgesic; prolonged use causes addiction.

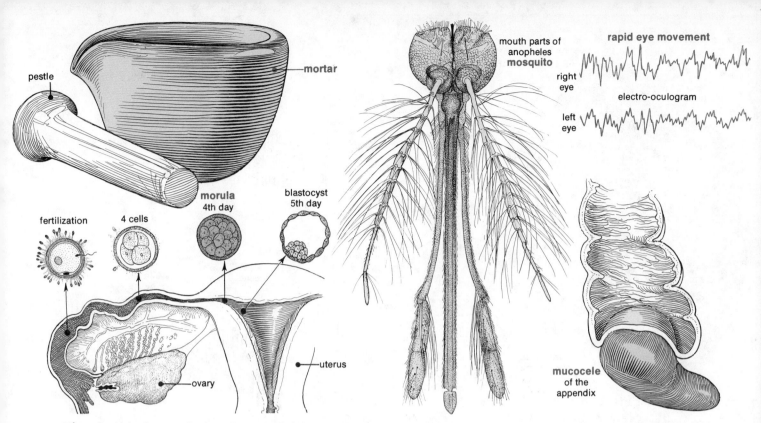

pestle

mortar

morula
4th day

blastocyst
5th day

fertilization

4 cells

ovary

uterus

mouth parts of
anopheles
mosquito

rapid eye movement

right
eye

electro-oculogram

left
eye

mucocele
of the
appendix

morpho-. Combining form meaning form, figure, or structure.

morphogen′esis. The embryonic differentiation of cells leading to the establishment of the characteristic structure and form of the organism or its parts.

morpholog′ic. Relating to the structure or form of organisms.

morphol′ogy. 1. The study of the configuration or structure of living organisms. **2.** The form or structure of an organism, exclusively.

Morquio's syndrome. Dwarfism with osteoporosis, knock-knees, abnormalities of the femoral heads, and flaccid ligaments; transmitted through an autorecesssive inheritance; also called mucopolysaccharidosis IV.

mors. Latin for death.

mor′tal. 1. Subject to death. **2.** Deadly.

mortal′ity. 1. The quality of being mortal. **2.** The death rate; the whole sum of deaths in a given population or a given time.

mor′tar. A small receptacle in which substances are crushed or pulverized with a pestle.

mortifica′tion. Gangrene.

mortinatal′ity. Natimortality.

mor′tuary. A funeral home where bodies of the deceased are prepared for burial.

mor′ula. A cluster of cleaving blastomeres resulting from the early division of the zygote; a stage in the development of the embryo prior to the blastula.

morula′tion. The formation of a morula.

mosa′ic. 1. Resembling inlaid work or a pattern consisting of numerous small pieces. **2.** An individual or tissue affected with mosaicism.

mosa′icism. Genetic condition in which an individual has two or more cell populations differing in genetic composition; the differing cells originate from a single cell type through an error (either genetic mutation or chromosomal aberration) occurring during early cell division of the fertilized egg.

Moschowitz's disease. Thrombotic thrombocytopenic purpura; see under purpura.

mOsm, mosm. Abbreviation for milliosmole.

mosqui′to. Any of various blood-sucking, winged insects (family Culicidae), some species of which are responsible for the transmission of various diseases such as malaria and yellow fever.

moth′er-sur′rogate. One who replaces an individual's mother in his emotional feelings.

mot′ile. Having the capacity to move spontaneously.

mo′tion. 1. Movement. **2.** A bowel movement.

motion sickness. A condition marked by nausea, dizziness, and often vomiting and headache, induced by some movement, as in travel by airplane, ship, car, etc. See under sickness.

motiva′tion. An incentive to act or the reason for an attitude.

mo′tor. Producing movement; denoting nerves that convey impulses from the nerve centers to the muscles.

m. oculi, the oculomotor nerve; the third cranial nerve; see table of nerves.

plastic m., an artificial point of attachment on an amputation stump through which motion is provided to an artificial limb.

mot′tling. 1. A condition marked by spotty coloration. **2.** Macular lesions of varying shades or hues.

moulage′. The making of a mold of a bodily structure, especially for identification, prosthetics, and teaching models.

mount. To prepare slides of tissues for microscopic examination.

mount′ing. Dental laboratory procedure in which a maxillary and/or mandibular cast is attached to an articulator.

mouse, *pl.* **mice.** Any of numerous small rodents of the genus *Mus*.

cancer-free white m. (CFW), a mouse used in cancer research.

New Zealand black m. (NZB), an inbred strain exhibiting (in the adult form) immune hemolytic anemia and renal disease.

mouse′pox. Ectromelia (2); a viral disease of mice.

mouth. The body opening through which an individual takes in food; the upper portion of the digestive tract, including the lips, tongue, teeth, and related parts; the oral cavity.

dry m., see sialoschesis.

trench m., necrotizing ulcerative gingivitis; see under gingivitis.

mouth′wash. A somewhat antiseptic solution for rinsing the mouth and teeth; it generally contains sodium borate, thymol, potassium bicarbonate, eucalyptol, methyl salicylate, alcohol, glycerin, and water; also called collutorium.

move′ment. 1. Change of place or position. **2.** The act of defecation.

Brownian m., erratic motion of microscopic particles suspended in a liquid or gas, resulting from collision with molecules in the suspending medium.

ciliary m., rhythmic motion of the cilia of epithelial cells or protozoa.

circus m., the movement of an excitation wave continuing uninterrupted around a ring of muscle or through the wall of the heart; also called circus rhythm.

conjugate m. of the eyes, movement of the two eyes in one direction.

passive m., movement of the body or any of its parts effected by an external force.

rapid eye m.'s (REM), the short, quick movements of the eyes during sleep which last from five to 60 minutes and are associated with dreaming. See under sleep.

saccadic m., a rapid, abrupt movement of the eyes, as occurs in changing fixation from one point to another.

streaming m., the characteristic movement of the protoplasm of certain white cells or unicellular organisms.

mox′a. 1. A small mass of combustible material placed on the skin and ignited to produce a counterirritation; used in Japanese popular medicine. **2.** A heated button-shaped metal device applied as a cautery.

moxibus′tion. Counterirritation by means of a moxa.

m.p. Abbreviation for melting point.

MPD. Abbreviation for maximal permissible dose.

mppcf. Abbreviation for millions of particles per cubic foot.

mr. Abbreviation for milliroentgen.

mrad. Abbreviation for millirad.

mrem. Abbreviation for millirem.

mRNA. Abbreviation for messenger RNA.

MS. Abbreviation for multiple sclerosis.

msec. Abbreviation for millisecond.

MSH. Abbreviation for melanocyte-stimulating hormone.

M.T. Abbreviation for major tranquilizer.

mu. 1. The twelfth letter of the Greek alphabet, μ. **2.** A micron.

mu′cid. Slimy.

mucif′erous. Secreting or producing mucus.

mu′ciform. Resembling mucus.

mu′cilage. In pharmacology, a thick viscous liquid; a water solution of the mucilaginous principles of certain vegetable substances.

mu′cin. A substance secreted by mucous membranes, containing an organic compound (mucopolysaccharide); the main constituent of mucus.

mu′cinase. Any enzyme, such as lysozyme, that acts on mucin.

mu′cinoid. Resembling mucin.

mucino′sis. A condition in which mucin is present in abnormal amounts.

mu′cinous. Relating to or containing mucin.

mu′cocele. 1. An intrasinus cyst which arises from the mucosal lining. **2.** An enlarged cavity that contains mucus. **3.** Mucous polyp.

mucocuta′neous. Relating to both mucous

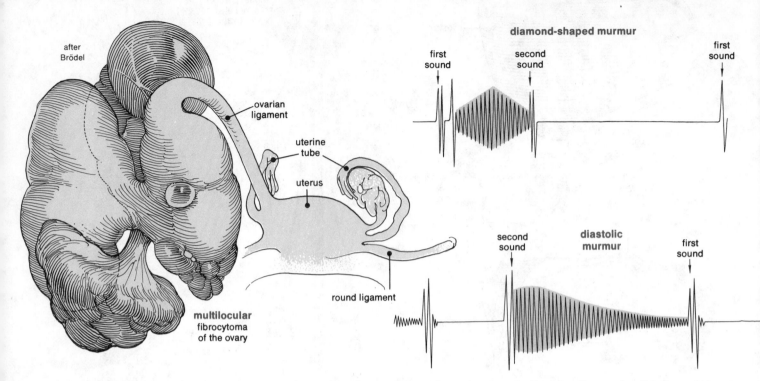

after Brödel

ovarian ligament

uterine tube

uterus

round ligament

multilocular fibrocytoma of the ovary

diamond-shaped murmur

first sound / second sound / first sound

diastolic murmur

second sound / first sound

---

membrane and skin, especially the line of meeting of those tissues as in the nasal, oral, vaginal, and anal orifices.

mucoenteri′tis. Inflammation of the intestinal mucous membrane; also called acute catarrhal enteritis.

mu′coid. 1. Resembling mucus. **2.** A mucus-like conjugated protein or polysaccharide of animal origin.

mucolyt′ic. Capable of dissolving mucus.

mucomem′branous. Relating to a mucous membrane.

mucoperios′teum. Periosteum with a closely adhered mucous membrane.

mucopolysacch′aride. Polysaccharide components, such as hyaluronic acid and chondroitin sulfate, attached to a polypeptide component through weak chemical bonding; a ubiquitous macromolecular complex that forms the amorphous component of intercellular material in the body.

mucopolysaccharido′sis. Any disease characterized by defective metabolism of mucopolysaccharides.
 m. 1, see Hurler's syndrome.
 m. 2, see Hunter's syndrome.

mucopro′tein. A group of organic compounds containing proteins and mucopolysaccharides.

mucopu′rulent. Containing mucus and pus.

mu′coupus′. Discharge composed of mucus and pus.

Mucora′ceae. A family of molds (order Mucorales) having a branching, nonsegmented mycelium; some species destroy food products (bread, fruits, and vegetables).

mucormyco′sis. An acute systemic disease characterized primarily by inflammation, necrosis, and suppuration, initially involving the paranasal sinuses, orbit, bronchi, or intestines and spreading to the brain, heart, kidney, or lungs; attributed to fungi of the order Mucorales.

muco′sa. The inner lining of a cavity, as the lining of the oral cavity.

mucosanguin′eous. Containing mucus and blood; said of a discharge.

mucose′rous. Relating to or containing serum or plasma and mucus.

mu′cosin. A mucin peculiar to the more tenacious, adhesive variety of mucus, as that of the nasal cavity.

mu′cous. Relating to, resembling, consisting of, or producing mucus.

mucoviscido′sis. See cystic fibrosis of pancreas.

mu′cus. The slippery, viscous suspension of mucin, desquamated cells, leukocytes, inorganic salt, and water secreted by glands in the mucous membranes;

the secretion moistens and protects the membrane.

mulieb′rity. The state of being a woman; any quality characteristic of women; the change of character in the female at puberty.

multan′gular. Having many angles; said of certain bones.

multi-. Combining form meaning many.

multiartic′ular. Relating to or affecting many joints.

multicel′lular. Composed of numerous cells.

multifacto′rial. Determined by several genetic and nongenetic factors. Cf polygenic.

mul′tifid. Composed of many segments or lobes formed by several clefts.

mul′tiform. Having many forms or shapes.

multigrav′ida. A woman who has been pregnant more than once.

multilob′ular. Having many lobules.

multiloc′ular. Having several cells or compartments.

multimam′mae. Polymastia; the presence of more than two breasts in the human.

multinu′clear. Having more than one nucleus; also called polynuclear.

multip′ara. A woman who has completed two or more pregnancies to the stage of viability, regardless of whether the fetuses were live or stillborn.

multipar′ity. The condition of having had two or more children; also called pluriparity.

multip′arous. 1. Having borne two or more offspring in separate pregnancies; relating to multipara. **2.** Giving birth to two or more children at one birth.

mul′tiple. 1. Having more than one part or component. **2.** Occurring in several sites at the same time.

multipo′lar. Having more than two poles, as certain nerve cells.

multiva′lence. The property of having the capacity to combine with two or more hydrogen atoms; also called polyvalence.

multiva′lent. Having the capacity to combine with more than one hydrogen atom, usually more than two; also called polyvalent.

mummifac′tion. 1. Cold gangrene; see under gangrene. **2.** Drying and compression of a dead retained fetus, so that it resembles parchment.

mumps. An acute contagious disease caused by an RNA myxovirus, affecting primarily the parotid glands and less often the sublingual and submaxillary glands; characterized by glandular swelling and fever; incubation period is about three weeks; secondary complications may involve the pancreas, testes, or central nervous system; also called epidemic parotitis.

Münchausen's syndrome. The fabrication by

an itinerant malingerer of a clinically convincing simulation of disease; it may include self-induced fits, faints, anesthesias, hallucinations, or delusions; the individual's history usually shows a long record of hospitalization.

mu′ral. Relating to the wall of any cavity.

muram′ic acid. A component of the murein molecule of bacterial cell walls.

muram′idase. Mucopeptide glucohydrolase, an enzyme that promotes the hydrolysis of muramic acid-containing mucopeptides in bacterial cell walls; e.g., lysozyme.

murein. The bag-shaped macromolecule that encases a bacterial cell.

muriat′ic. Hydrochloric.

muriatic acid. Hydrochloric acid.

mu′rine. Relating to animals of the family Muridae, especially rats and mice.

mur′mur. A relatively prolonged series of auditory vibrations resulting from turbulent blood flow.
 aortic m., one occurring at the aortic orifice.
 Austin-Flint m., a mid-diastolic or presystolic rumble, similar to the murmur of mitral stenosis, which appears to originate at the anterior leaflet of the mitral valve when the normal and abnormal streams of blood enter the left ventricle in cases of aortic incompetence; also called Flint's murmur.
 cardiac m., one arising in the heart.
 cardiopulmonary m., one believed to be caused by movement of air through a portion of the lung compressed by the contracting heart.
 continuous m., one that begins in systole and continues without interruption into all or part of the diastole.
 crescendo m., one that increases in intensity and stops suddenly; the opposite of a decrescendo murmur.
 crescendo-decrescendo m., one that increases to a peak and then decreases; also called diamond-shaped murmur.
 Cruveilhier-Baumgarten m., one heard on the abdominal wall over collateral veins connecting portal and caval venous systems.
 decrescendo m., one that progressively decreases in intensity; the opposite of a crescendo murmur.
 diamond-shaped m., named after the shape of its frequency intensity curve. See crescendo-decrescendo murmur.
 diastolic m., one beginning with or after the second heart sound and ending before the first heart sound, i.e., during diastole.
 Duroziez's m., a double murmur heard over the femoral artery in cases of aortic insufficiency.
 early diastolic m., one beginning with the second

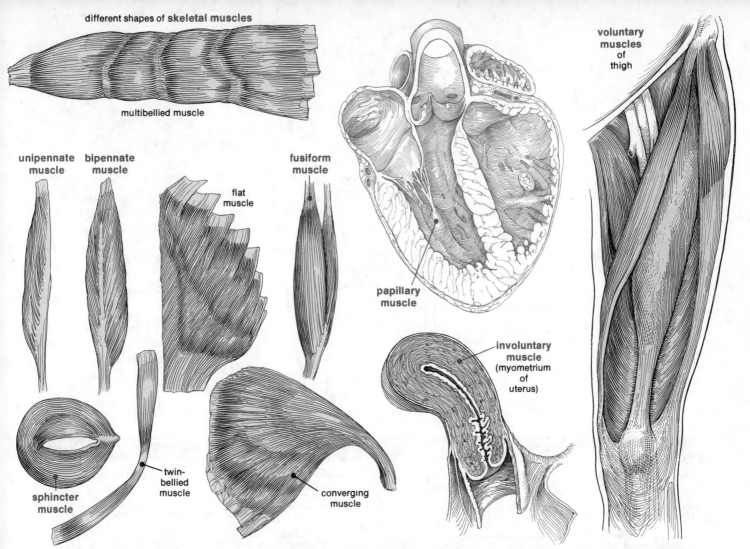

different shapes of **skeletal muscles**

multibellied muscle

unipennate muscle

bipennate muscle

flat muscle

fusiform muscle

papillary muscle

voluntary muscles of thigh

sphincter muscle

twin-bellied muscle

converging muscle

involuntary muscle (myometrium of uterus)

heart sound (at the time of aortic valve closure); the typical murmur of aortic incompetence.

ejection m., a crescendo-decrescendo murmur occurring when blood is ejected across the aortic or pulmonary valves; the murmur starts with the beginning of ejection; as ejection increases, so does the murmur (crescendo); as ejection decreases, the murmur decreases (descrecendo); it ends before the second heart sound.

extracardiac m., one heard over the heart area but originating from other structures.

Flint's m., Austin-Flint murmur.

functional m., one due to causes other than cardiac disorders; also called inorganic murmur.

Graham-Steell's m., an early diastolic, high-pitched, usually decrescendo murmur; caused by pulmonary incompetence due to pulmonary hypertension.

hemic m., a cardiac or vascular murmur occurring in anemic individuals without heart disease.

holosystolic m., see pansystolic murmur.

innocent m., one which is not caused by cardiovascular disease.

inorganic m., see functional murmur.

late diastolic m., see presystolic murmur.

machinery m., the continuous murmur typical of patent ductus arteriosus.

mid-diastolic m., one beginning soon, but at a clear interval, after the second heart sound; originating at the atrioventricular valves, usually due either to constriction of the orifices or to abnormal patterns of atrioventricular blood flow.

mitral valve m., a murmur produced at the mitral valve; caused by either constriction of the valve orifice or backward flow of blood through the valve.

musical m., one having a musical quality.

organic m., one caused by organic disease, i.e., a valvular deformity or a septal defect, in contrast to a functional murmur.

pansystolic m., holosystolic m., one beginning with the first heart sound, occupying all of systole, and ending with the second heart sound.

plateau m., one having a relatively constant intensity throughout its duration.

presystolic m., late diastolic m., a short, usually crescendo murmur heard during atrial systole, due most often to obstruction of one of the atrioventricular orifices.

pulmonary m., pulmonic m., one heard at the pulmonary orifice of the heart.

regurgitant m., one originating at the valvular orifices of the heart, due to leakage or backward flow of blood.

Roger's m., a loud pansystolic murmur with maximal intensity at the left sternal border caused by a small ventricular septal defect; also called bruit de Roger.

sea gull m., a musical murmur similar to the cry of a gull.

seesaw m., see to-and-fro murmur.

systolic m., one beginning with or after the first heart sound and ending at or before the second sound, i.e., during systole.

to-and-fro m., murmurs heard in both systole and diastole; also called seesaw murmur.

tricuspid m., one originating at the tricuspid orifice.

Mus'ca. A genus of flies.

M. domestica, see housefly.

muscae volitantes. Small spots observed on viewing a bright area which move away when an attempt is made to focus on them; believed to be remnants of embryonic structures in the vitreous body; also called "flitting flies."

mus'carine. A poisonous alkaloid present in certain mushrooms, causing inhibition of the heart action and gastrointestinal stimulation.

muscarin'ic. 1. Producing postganglionic parasympathetic stimulation, an effect resembling that of muscarine. **2.** An agent that produces such an effect.

mus'cle. Tissue that serves to produce motion, composed primarily of contractile cells. For individual muscles see table of muscles.

antagonistic m.'s, muscles with opposing actions.

antigravity m.'s, those maintaining the posture characteristic of a given species.

bipennate m., muscle with a central tendon; e.g., rectus muscle of thigh.

cardiac m., muscle of the heart (myocardium), composed of striated fibers.

fusiform m., one with a fleshy belly tapering at either extremity; also called spindle-shaped muscle.

hamstring m.'s, three muscles at the back of the thigh; the biceps muscle of the thigh (biceps femoris), the semitendinous muscle, and the semimembranous muscle; they flex the leg and rotate it medially and laterally at the knee joint, and extend the thigh at the hip joint; also called posterior femoral muscles.

involuntary m., one that is not under voluntary control; smooth muscle which responds to the autonomic nervous system.

papillary m.'s, the fleshy columns in the ventricles of the heart to which the chordae tendinae are attached.

skeletal m., a striated voluntary muscle that is attached to bones.

smooth m., unstriated, involuntary muscle.

sphincter m., a circular band of muscle; e.g., sphincter muscle of anus.

spindle-shaped m., see fusiform muscle.

strap m., any flat muscle, especially those of the neck associated with the hyoid bone and thyroid cartilage.

striated m., skeletal and cardiac muscle in which cross striations occur in the fibers; with the exception of the cardiac muscle, striated muscles are voluntary, as opposed to the smooth muscles under autonomic control.

synergistic m.'s, muscles having a mutually helpful action.

unipennate m., muscle with a tendon attached along one side; e.g., extensor muscle of little finger.

voluntary m., one whose action is under voluntary control.

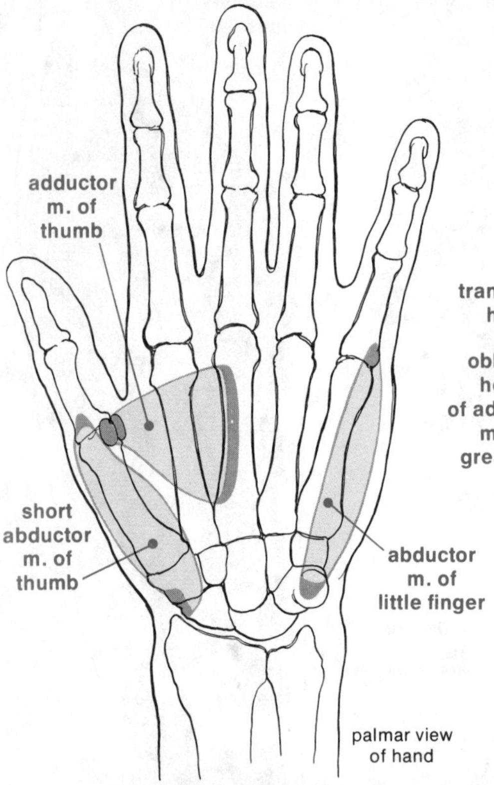

adductor m. of thumb

short abductor m. of thumb

abductor m. of little finger

palmar view of hand

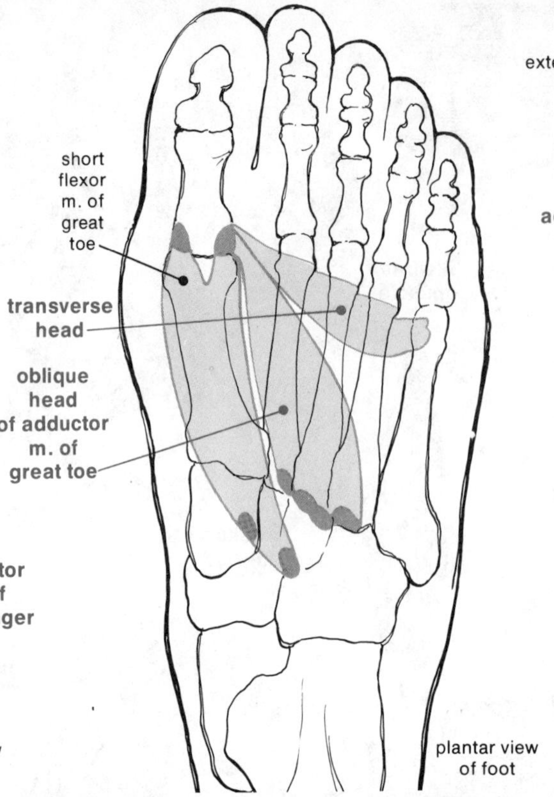

short flexor m. of great toe

transverse head

oblique head of adductor m. of great toe

plantar view of foot

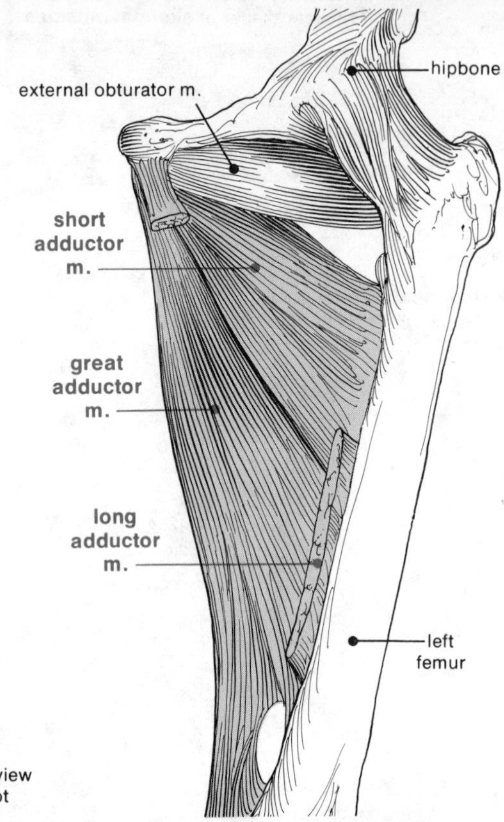

external obturator m.

hipbone

short adductor m.

great adductor m.

long adductor m.

left femur

MUSCLE	ORIGIN	INSERTION	ACTION
abductor m. of great toe *m. abductor hallucis*	calcaneus, plantar aponeurosis	proximal phalanx of great toe (joined by flexor muscle of great toe)	abducts and aids in flexion of great toe
abductor m. of little finger *m. abductor digiti minimi manus*	pisiform bone, tendon of ulnar flexor muscle of wrist	proximal phalanx of fifth digit	abducts little finger
abductor m. of little toe *m. abductor digiti minimi pedis*	lateral tubercle of calcaneus	proximal phalanx of little toe	abducts little toe
abductor m. of thumb, long *m. abductor pollicis longus*	posterior surface of ulna, middle third of radius	first metacarpal bone	abducts thumb and hand
abductor m. of thumb, short *m. abductor pollicis brevis*	flexor retinaculum of hand, scaphoid and trapezium	proximal phalanx of thumb	abducts and aids in flexion of thumb
adductor m., great *m. adductor magnus*	adductor part: inferior ramus of pubis, ramus of ischium; extersor part: ischial tuberosity	adductor part: linea aspera of femur; extensor part: adductor tubercle of femur	adducts, flexes, and laterally rotates thigh
adductor m., long *m. adductor longus*	pubis, below pubic crest	linea aspera of femur	adducts, flexes, and rotates thigh laterally
adductor m., smallest *m. adductor minimus*	the proximal portion of the great adductor muscle when it forms a distinct muscle		
adductor m., short *m. adductor brevis*	pubis, below origin of the long adductor muscle	upper part of linea aspera of femur	adducts, flexes, and rotates thigh laterally
adductor m. of great toe *m. adductor hallucis*	oblique head: long plantar ligament; transverse head: capsules of metacarpophalangeal joints	proximal phalanx of great toe (joined by flexor muscle of great toe)	oblique head: adducts and flexes great toe; transverse head: supports transverse arch, adducts great toe
adductor m. of thumb *m. adductor pollicis*	capitate, second, and third metacarpal bones	proximal phalanx of thumb	adducts and aids in apposition of thumb
anconeus m. *m. anconeus*	back of lateral epicondyle of humerus	olecranon process, posterior surface of ulna	extends forearm, abducts ulna in pronation of wrist
antitragus m. *m. antitragicus*	outer surface of antitragus of ear	caudate process of helix and anthelix	thought to be vestigial
arrector m.'s of hair *mm. arrectores pilorum*	dermis	hair follicles	elevate hairs of skin
articular m. of elbow *m. articularis cubiti*	posterior distal surface of humerus	posterior aspect of elbow joint	elevates capsule in extension of elbow joint
articular m. of knee *m. articularis genus*	lower part of anterior surface of femur	synovial membrane of knee joint	elevates capsule of knee joint

muscle | **muscle**

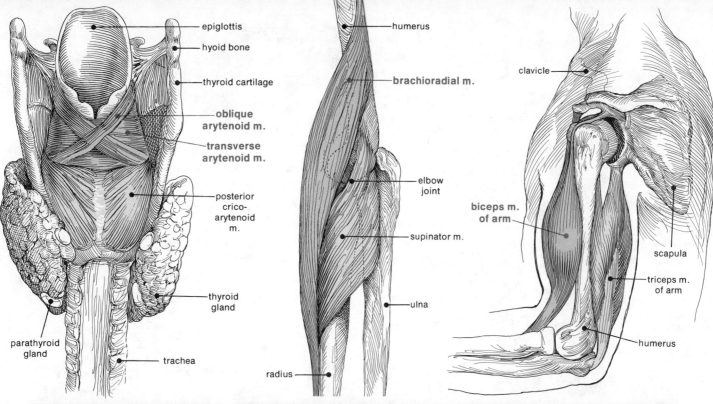

MUSCLE	ORIGIN	INSERTION	ACTION
aryepiglottic m. *m. aryepiglotticus*	apex of arytenoid cartilage	lateral margin of epiglottis	closes inlet of larynx
arytenoid m., oblique *m. arytenoideus obliquus*	muscular process of arytenoid cartilage	apex of opposite arytenoid cartilage, prolonged as aryepiglottic muscle	approximates vocal cords
arytenoid m., transverse (only unpaired muscle of the larynx) *m. arytenoideus transversus*	medial surface of arytenoid cartilage	medial surface of opposite arytenoid cartilage	approximates arytenoid cartilages; constricts the entrance to the larynx during swallowing
auricular m., anterior *m. auricularis anterior*	epicranial aponeurosis	cartilage of ear	feeble movement of auricle forward
auricular m., posterior *m. auricularis posterior*	mastoid process	cartilage of ear	feeble movement of auricle backward
auricular m., superior *m. auricularis superior*	epicranial aponeurosis	cartilage of ear	feeble elevation of auricle
auricular m., transverse *m. auricularis transversus*	upper surface of auricle	circumference of auricle	retracts helix
biceps m. of arm *m. biceps brachii*	long head: supraglenoid tubercle of scapula; short head: apex of coracoid process	tuberosity of radius	flexes forearm and arm, supinates hand
biceps m. of thigh *m. biceps femoris*	long head: ischial tuberosity (in common with semitendinous muscle); short head: supracondylar ridge of femur	head of fibula, lateral condyle of tibia	flexes knee, rotates leg laterally; long head extends thigh
brachial m. *m. brachialis*	distal two-thirds of humerus	coronoid process of ulna	flexes forearm
brachioradial m. *m. brachioradialis*	lateral supracondylar ridge and intermuscular septum of humerus	styloid process of radius	flexes forearm
bronchoesophageal m. *m. bronchoesophageus*	muscle fibers arising from the wall of the left bronchus	musculature of esophagus	reinforces esophagus
buccinator m. *m. buccinator*	pterygomandibular raphe, alveolar processes of jaws	orbicular muscle (*orbiculuaris oris*) at angle of mouth	retracts angle of mouth by compressing cheek; accessory muscle of mastication
bulbocavernous m. *m. bulbospongiosus*	female: central tendon of perineum; male: median raphe over bulb of penis, central tendon of perineum	female: dorsum of clitoris, urogenital diaphragm; male: corpus cavernosus, root of penis	female: compresses vaginal orifice; male: compresses urethra

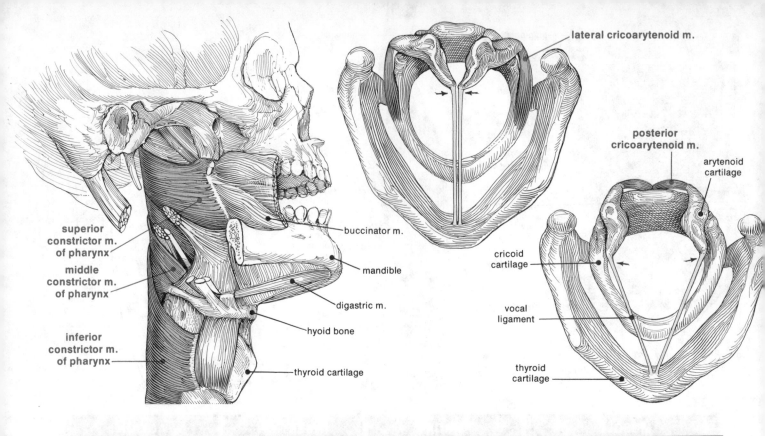

MUSCLE	ORIGIN	INSERTION	ACTION
caninus m. **canine m.**	*see levator muscle of angle of mouth*		
ceratocricoid m. *m. ceratocricoideus*	muscle fibers arising from posterior cricoarytenoid muscle	the inferior horn (cornu) of thyroid cartilage	helps posterior cricoarytenoid muscle separate vocal cords
chin m. *m. mentalis*	incisive fossa of mandible	skin of chin	wrinkles skin of chin
chondroglossus m. *m. chondroglossus*	lesser horn (cornu) of hyoid bone	side of tongue	depresses tongue
ciliary m. *m. ciliaris*	meridional part: scleral spur; circular part: sphincter of ciliary body	ciliary process	makes lens more convex in visual accommodation
coccygeus m. **ischiococcygeus m.** *m. coccygeus*	ischial spine and sacrospinous ligament	coccyx, lower part of lateral border of sacrum	aids in raising and supporting pelvic floor
constrictor m. of pharynx, inferior *m. constrictor pharyngis inferior*	cricoid and oblique line of thyroid cartilages	median raphe of posterior wall of pharynx	narrows lower part of pharynx in swallowing
constrictor m. of pharynx, middle *m. constrictor pharyngis medius*	stylohyoid ligament and horns of hyoid bone	median raphe of posterior wall of pharynx	narrows pharynx in swallowing
constrictor m. of pharynx, superior *m. constrictor pharyngis superior*	medial pterygoid plate, hamulus, pterygomandibular ligament, base of skull	median raphe of posterior wall of pharynx	narrows pharynx in swallowing
coracobrachial m. *m. coracobrachialis*	coracoid process of scapula (shoulder blade)	inner side of humerus	flexes, adducts arm
corrugator m. *m. corrugator*	brow ridge of frontal bone	skin of eyebrow	draws eyebrows together, wrinkles forehead
cremaster m. *m. cremaster*	inferior border of internal oblique abdominal muscle	pubic tubercle	elevates testis
cricoarytenoid m., lateral *m. cricoarytenoideus lateral*	upper margin of arch of cricoid cartilage	muscular process of arytenoid cartilage	approximates vocal cords so they meet in the midline for phonation
cricoarytenoid m., posterior *m. cricoarytenoideus posterior*	posterior surface of lamina of cricoid cartilage	muscular process of arytenoid cartilage	separates vocal cords, opening the glottis
cricothyroid m. *m. cricothyroideus*	anterior surface of arch of cricoid cartilage	lamina and inferior horn of thyroid cartilage	lengthens, stretches, and tenses vocal cords
deltoid m. *m. deltoideus*	lateral third of clavicle, acromion process, and	deltoid tuberosity of humerus	abductor of arm; aids in flexion and extension

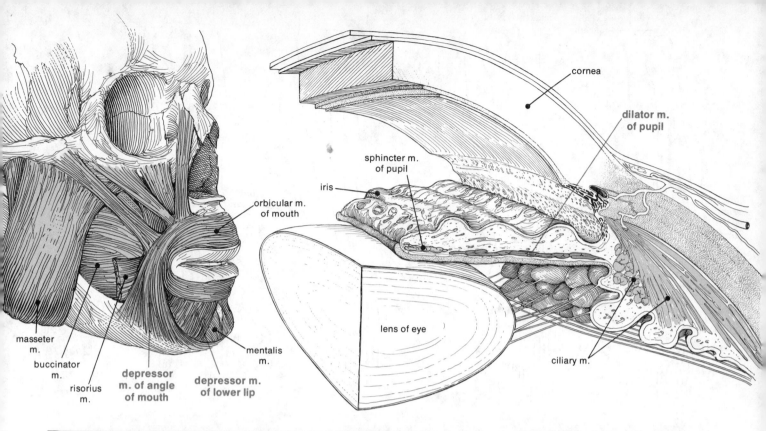

cornea

dilator m.
of pupil

sphincter m.
of pupil

iris

orbicular m.
of mouth

lens of eye

masseter
m.

buccinator
m.

risorius
m.

depressor
m. of angle
of mouth

depressor m.
of lower lip

mentalis
m.

ciliary m.

MUSCLE	ORIGIN	INSERTION	ACTION
depressor m., superciliary *m. depressor supercilii*	spine of scapula orbicular fibers of the eye (*orbicularis oculi*)	eyebrow	facial expression
depressor m. of angle of mouth triangular m. *m. depressor anguli oris*	oblique line of mandible	angle of mouth	pulls corner of mouth downward
depressor m. of lower lip quadrate m. of lower lip *m. depressor labii inferior*	mandible adjacent to mental foramen	lower lip	draws lower lip downward
depressor m. of nasal septum *m. depressor septi nasi*	incisor fossa of maxilla	ala and septum of nose	constricts nostrils and draws septum inferiorly
detrusor m. of urinary bladder detrusor urinae m. *m. detrusor vesicae*	in wall of urinary bladder		empties urinary bladder
detrusor urinae m.	see detrusor muscle of urinary bladder		
diaphragm diaphragmatic m. *diaphragma*	xiphoid process, six lower costal cartilages, four lower ribs, lumbar vertebrae, lateral arcuate ligaments	central tendon of diaphragm	increases capacity of thorax in inspiration (main muscle of inhalation)
diaphragm m., pelvic	composed of the coccygeus and levator ani muscles		forms floor to support pelvic viscera
digastric m. *m. digastricus*	digastric notch at mastoid process	mandible near symphysis	raises hyoid bone and base of tongue, lowers mandible
dilator m. of nose *m. dilator naris*	margin of piriform aperture of maxilla	margin of nostril	widens nostril
dilator m. of pupil *m. dilator pupillae*	circumference of iris	margin of pupil	dilates pupil
epicranial m. *m. epicranius*	the muscular and tendinous layer of the scalp composed of the occipitofrontal and temporoparietal muscles connected by an extensive intermediate aponeurosis (*galea aponeurotica*)		elevates eyebrows, draws scalp forward and backward
erector m. of penis	see ischiocavernous muscle		
erector m. of spine *m. erector spinae*	see sacrospinal muscle		
extensor m. of fingers, common *m. extensor digitorum communis*	lateral epicondyle of humerus	forms extensor expansion over fingers	extends fingers, hand, and forearm
extensor m. of great toe, long *m. extensor hallucis longus*	middle of fibula, interosseous membrane	distal phalanx of great toe	extends great toe, dorsiflexes foot

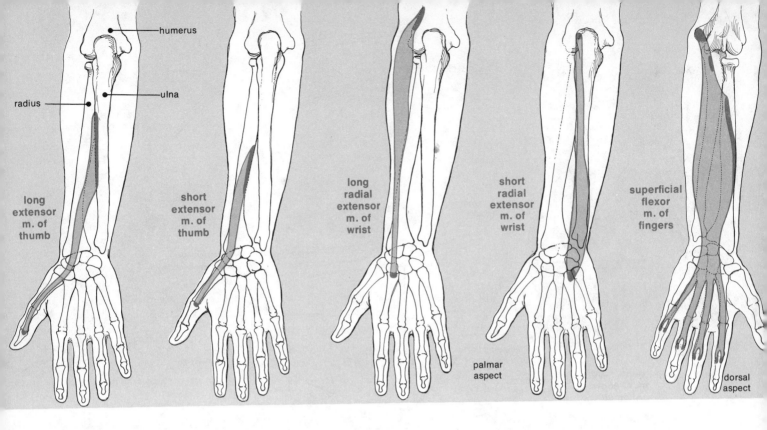

| long extensor m. of thumb | short extensor m. of thumb | long radial extensor m. of wrist | short radial extensor m. of wrist | superficial flexor m. of fingers |

palmar aspect

dorsal aspect

MUSCLE	ORIGIN	INSERTION	ACTION
extensor m. of great toe, short *m. extensor hallucis brevis*	dorsal surface of calcaneus	base of proximal phalanx of great toe	dorsiflexes great toe
extensor m. of index finger *m. extensor indicis*	posterior surface of ulna	extensor expansion of index finger	extends index finger and hand
extensor m. of little finger *m. extensor digiti minimi manus*	lateral epicondyle of humerus	extensor expansion of little finger	extends little finger
extensor m. of thumb, long *m. extensor pollicis longus*	middle third of ulna, adjacent interosseous membrane	distal phalanx of thumb	extends distal phalanx of thumb, abducts hand
extensor m. of thumb, short *m. extensor pollicis brevis*	middle third of radius	proximal phalanx of thumb	extends and abducts hand
extensor m. of toes, long *m. extensor digitorum longus pedis*	lateral condyle of tibia, upper three-fourths of fibula, interosseous membrane	extensor expansion of four lateral toes (by four slips)	extends toes
extensor m. of toes, short *m. extensor digitorum brevis pedis*	dorsal surface of calcaneus	extensor tendons of first, second, third, and fourth toes	extends toes
extensor m. of wrist, radial, long *m. extensor carpi radialis longus*	lateral supracondylar ridge of humerus	second metacarpal bone	extends and abducts wrist
extensor m. of wrist, radial, short *m. extensor carpi radialis brevis*	lateral epicondyle of humerus, radial collateral ligament	third metacarpal	extends and abducts wrist
extensor m. of wrist, ulnar *m. extensor carpi ulnaris*	humeral head: lateral epicondyle of humerus; ulnar head: posterior border of ulna	fifth metacarpal bone	extends and abducts wrist
fibular m.	see peroneal muscle		
flexor m. of fingers, deep *m. flexor digitorum profundus manus*	proximal three-fourths of ulna and adjacent interosseous membrane	distal phalanges of fingers	flexes terminal phalanges and hand
flexor m. of fingers, superficial *m. flexor digitorum superficialis manus*	humeroulnar head: medial epicondyle of humerus, coronoid process of ulna; radial head: anterior border of radius	middle phalanges of fingers	flexes phalanges, hand, and forearm
flexor m. of great toe, long *m. flexor hallucis longus*	lower two-thirds of posterior surface of fibula, intermuscular septum	distal phalanx of great toe	flexes great toe

muscle | muscle

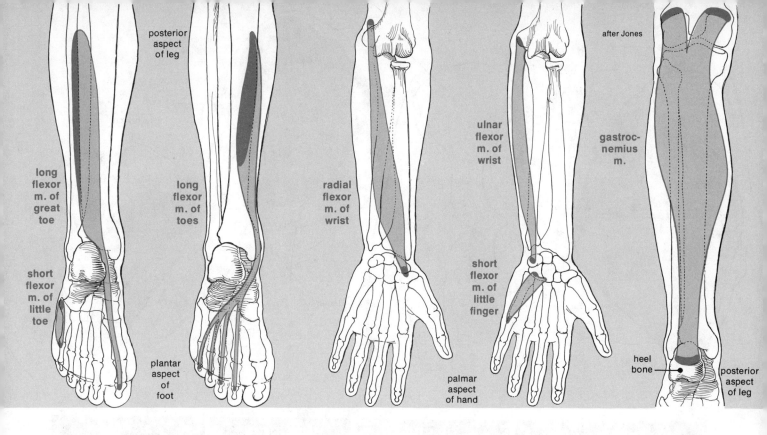

MUSCLE	ORIGIN	INSERTION	ACTION
flexor m. of great toe, short *m. flexor hallucis brevis*	cuboid and third cuneiform bones	both sides of proximal phalanx of great toe	flexes great toe
flexor m. of little finger, short *m. flexor digiti minimi brevis manus*	hook of hamate, flexor retinaculum	proximal phalanx of little finger	flexes proximal phalanx of little finger
flexor m. of little toe, short *m. flexor digiti minimi brevis pedis*	base of fifth metatarsal and plantar fascia	lateral surface of proximal phalanx of little toe	flexes little toe
flexor m. of thumb, long *m. flexor pollicis longus*	radius, adjacent interosseous membrane, coronoid process of ulna	distal phalanx of thumb	flexes thumb
flexor m. of thumb, short *m. flexor pollicis brevis*	tubercle of trapezium, flexor retinaculum	proximal phalanx of thumb	flexes and adducts thumb
flexor m. of toes, long *m. flexor digitorum longus pedis*	middle half of tibia	distal phalanges of lateral four toes (by four tendons)	flexes second to fifth toes
flexor m. of toes, short *m. flexor digitorum brevis pedis*	calcaneus and plantar fascia	middle phalanges of four lateral toes	flexes four lateral toes
flexor m. of wrist, radial *m. flexor carpi radialis*	medial epicondyle of humerus	bases of second and third metacarpal bones	flexes hand and forearm, aids in pronation and abduction of hand
flexor m. of wrist, ulna *m. flexor carpi ulnaris*	humeral head: medial epicondyle of humerus; ulnar head: olecranon and posterior border of ulnar	pisiform, hamate, and fifth metacarpal bones	flexes and adducts hand
frontal m.		see occipitofrontal muscle	
gastrocnemius m. *m. gastrocnemius*	medial head: popliteal surface of femur, upper part of medial condyle of femur; lateral head: lateral condyle of femur	calcaneus via calcaneal tendon (tendo calcaneus) (in common with soleus muscle)	flexes foot and leg
gemellus m., inferior *m. gemellus inferior*	lower margin of lesser sciatic notch	internal obturator tendon	rotates thigh laterally
gemellus m., superior *m. gemellus superior*	upper margin of lesser sciatic notch	internal obturator tendon	rotates thigh laterally
genioglossus m. *m. genioglossus*	mental spine of the mandible	ventral surface of tongue, body of hyoid bone and epiglottis	protrudes, retracts, and depresses the tongue, elevates the hyoid bone
geniohyoid m. *m. geniohyoideus*	mental spine (genial tubercle) of the mandible	body of the hyoid bone	elevates hyoid bone

muscle | muscle

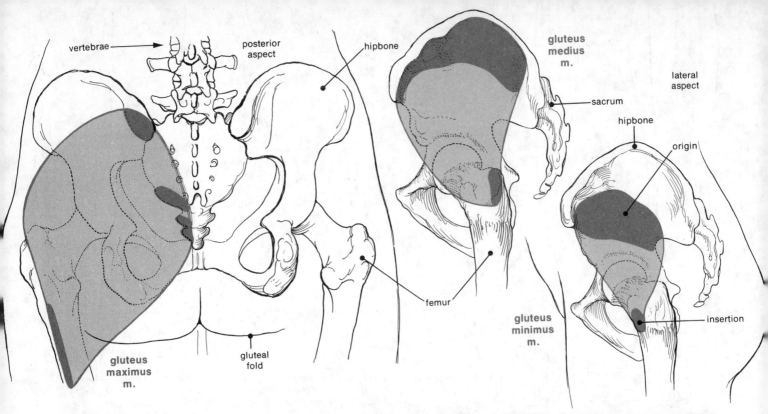

vertebrae — posterior aspect — hipbone — gluteus medius m. — lateral aspect — sacrum — hipbone — origin — femur — gluteus minimus m. — insertion — gluteus maximus m. — gluteal fold

MUSCLE	ORIGIN	INSERTION	ACTION
glossopalatine m.	see palatoglossus muscle		
gluteus maximus m. greatest gluteal m. *m. gluteus maximus*	upper portion of ilium, sacrum and coccyx, sacrotuberous ligament	gluteal tuberosity of femur, iliotibial tract (band of fascia lata)	chief extensor, powerful lateral rotator of thigh
gluteus medius m. middle gluteal m. *m. gluteus medius*	midportion of ilium	greater trochanter and oblique ridge of femur	abducts, rotates thigh medially
gluteus minimus m. least gluteal m. *m. gluteus minimus*	lower portion of ilium	greater trochanter of femur, capsule of hip joint	abducts, rotates thigh medially
gracilus m. *m. gracilus*	lower half of pubis	upper part of tibia	adducts thigh, flexes and rotates leg medially
helix m., smaller *m. helicis minor*	anterior rim of helix	crux of helix	thought to be vestigial
hyoglossus m. hyoglossal m. *m. hyoglossus*	body and greater horn (cornu) of hyoid bone	side of tongue	retracts, depresses tongue
iliac m. *m. iliacus*	iliac fossa, lateral aspect of sacrum	greater psoas tendon, lesser trochanter of femur	flexes and rotates thigh medially
iliococcygeus m. *m. iliococcygeus*	pubic symphysis and arching tendon over the internal obturator muscle	coccyx and perineal body	supports pelvic viscera
iliocostal m. *m. iliocostalis*	the lateral division of the sacrospinal muscle	inferior borders of the angles of the last six or seven ribs	extends vertebral column and assists in lateral movements of trunk
iliocostal m. of loins *m. iliocostalis lumborum*	iliac crest and sacrospinal aponeurosis	lumbodorsal fascia, transverse processes of lumbar vertebrae, angles of lower six ribs	extends lumbar spine
iliocostal m. of neck *m. iliocostalis cervicis*	upper six ribs	transverse processes of fourth, fifth, and sixth cervical vertebrae	extends cervical vertebral column
iliocostal m. of thorax *m. iliocostalis thoracis*	lower seven ribs, medial to the angles of the ribs	angles of upper seven ribs, transverse process of seventh cervical vertebra	keeps thoracic spine erect
iliopsoas m. *m. iliopsoas*	a compound muscle consisting of the iliac and greater psoas muscles, which join to form the iliopsoas tendon		
incisive m.'s of lower lip *mm. incisivi labii inferior*	portion of orbicular muscle of mouth (*orbicularis oris*)	angle of mouth	make vestibule of mouth shallow

muscle | muscle

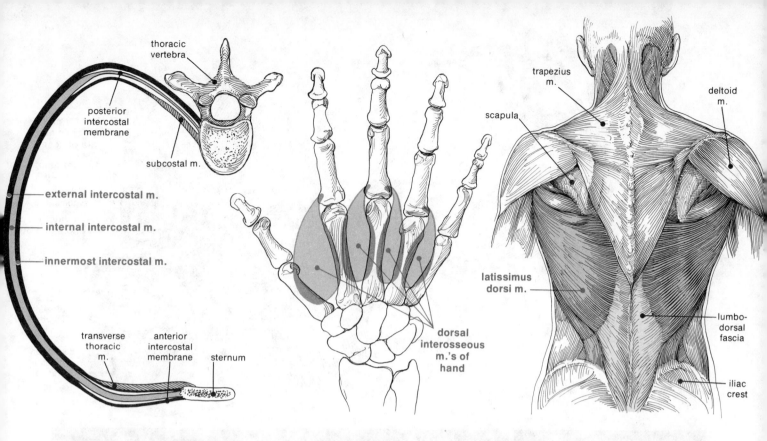

MUSCLE	ORIGIN	INSERTION	ACTION
incisive m.'s of upper lip *mm. incisivi labii superior*	portion of orbicular muscle of mouth (*orbicularis oris*)	angle of mouth	make vestibule of mouth shallow
infrahyoid m.'s *mm. infrahyoidei*	the ribbon-like muscles below the hyoid bone including the omohyoid, sternohyoid, sternothyroid, and thyrohyoid muscles		
infraspinous m. *m. infraspinatus*	infraspinous fossa of scapula	midportion of greater tubercle of humerus	rotates arm laterally
intercostal m.'s, external *mm. intercostales externi*	inferior border of rib	superior border of rib below origin	draw ribs together
intercostal m.'s, innermost *mm. intercostales intimi*	superior border of rib	inferior border of rib above origin	draw ribs together
intercostal m.'s, internal *mm. intercostales interni*	superior border of rib	inferior border of rib above origin	draw ribs together
interosseous m.'s, palmar (three in number) *mm. interossei palmares*	medial side of second, lateral side of fourth and fifth metacarpals	base of proximal phalanx in line with its origin	adduct index, ring, and little fingers; aid in extension of fingers
interosseous m.'s, plantar (three in number) *mm. interossei plantares*	medial side of third, fourth, and fifth metatarsal bones	medial side of proximal phalanges of third, fourth, and fifth toes	adduct three lateral toes toward second toe
interosseous m.'s of foot, dorsal (four in number) *mm. interossei dorsales pedis*	adjacent sides of metatarsal bones	proximal phalanges of both sides of second toe, lateral side of third and fourth toes	abduct lateral toes, move second toe from side to side
interosseous m.'s of hand, dorsal (four in number) *mm. interossei dorsales manus*	adjacent sides of metacarpal bones	extensor tendons of second, third, and fourth fingers	abduct, flex proximal phalanges
interspinal m.'s *mm. interspinales*	superior surface of spinous process of each vertebra	inferior surface of spinous process of vertebra above vertebra of origin	extend vertebral column
intertransverse m.'s *mm. intertransversarii*	extend between transverse processes of adjacent vertebrae		bend vertebral column laterally
ischiocavernous m. *m. ischiocavernosus*	ramus of ischium adjacent to crus of penis or clitoris	crus near pubic symphysis	maintains erection of penis or clitoris
ischiococcygeus m.	see coccygeus muscle		
latissimus dorsi m. *m. latissimus dorsi*	spinous processes of lower six thoracic vertebrae, lumbodorsal fascia, crest of ilium	floor of intertubercular groove of humerus	adducts, extends, medially rotates arm

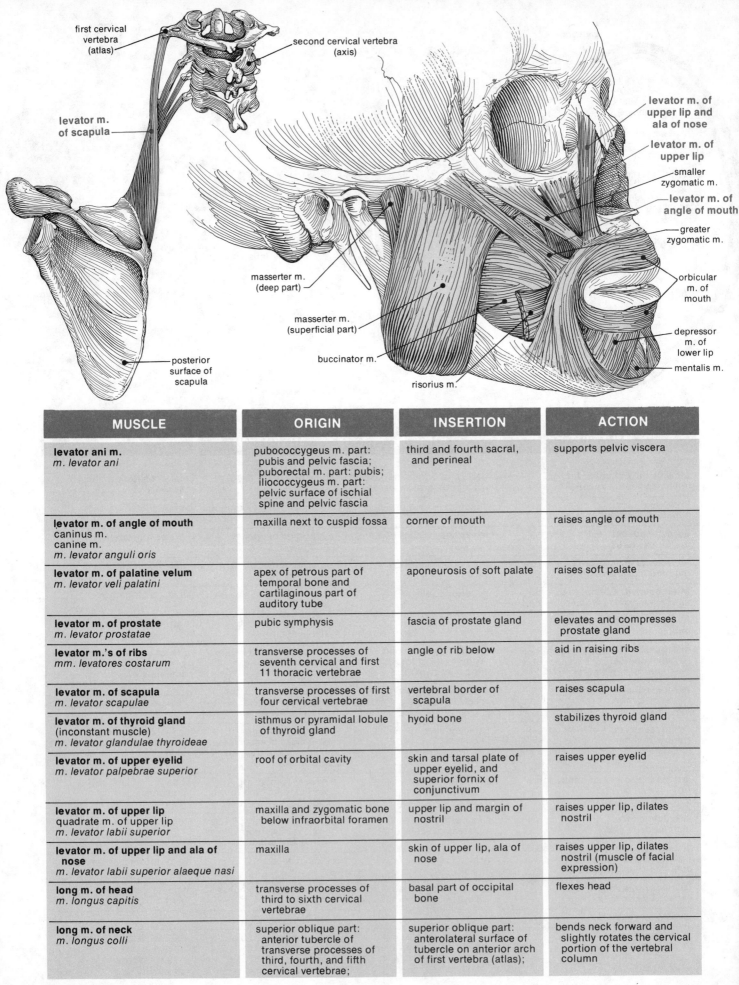

first cervical vertebra (atlas)

second cervical vertebra (axis)

levator m. of scapula

posterior surface of scapula

masserter m. (deep part)

masserter m. (superficial part)

buccinator m.

risorius m.

levator m. of upper lip and ala of nose

levator m. of upper lip

smaller zygomatic m.

levator m. of angle of mouth

greater zygomatic m.

orbicular m. of mouth

depressor m. of lower lip

mentalis m.

MUSCLE	ORIGIN	INSERTION	ACTION
levator ani m. *m. levator ani*	pubococcygeus m. part: pubis and pelvic fascia; puborectal m. part: pubis; iliococcygeus m. part: pelvic surface of ischial spine and pelvic fascia	third and fourth sacral, and perineal	supports pelvic viscera
levator m. of angle of mouth caninus m. canine m. *m. levator anguli oris*	maxilla next to cuspid fossa	corner of mouth	raises angle of mouth
levator m. of palatine velum *m. levator veli palatini*	apex of petrous part of temporal bone and cartilaginous part of auditory tube	aponeurosis of soft palate	raises soft palate
levator m. of prostate *m. levator prostatae*	pubic symphysis	fascia of prostate gland	elevates and compresses prostate gland
levator m.'s of ribs *mm. levatores costarum*	transverse processes of seventh cervical and first 11 thoracic vertebrae	angle of rib below	aid in raising ribs
levator m. of scapula *m. levator scapulae*	transverse processes of first four cervical vertebrae	vertebral border of scapula	raises scapula
levator m. of thyroid gland (inconstant muscle) *m. levator glandulae thyroideae*	isthmus or pyramidal lobule of thyroid gland	hyoid bone	stabilizes thyroid gland
levator m. of upper eyelid *m. levator palpebrae superior*	roof of orbital cavity	skin and tarsal plate of upper eyelid, and superior fornix of conjunctivum	raises upper eyelid
levator m. of upper lip quadrate m. of upper lip *m. levator labii superior*	maxilla and zygomatic bone below infraorbital foramen	upper lip and margin of nostril	raises upper lip, dilates nostril
levator m. of upper lip and ala of nose *m. levator labii superior alaeque nasi*	maxilla	skin of upper lip, ala of nose	raises upper lip, dilates nostril (muscle of facial expression)
long m. of head *m. longus capitis*	transverse processes of third to sixth cervical vertebrae	basal part of occipital bone	flexes head
long m. of neck *m. longus colli*	superior oblique part: anterior tubercle of transverse processes of third, fourth, and fifth cervical vertebrae;	superior oblique part: anterolateral surface of tubercle on anterior arch of first vertebra (atlas);	bends neck forward and slightly rotates the cervical portion of the vertebral column

muscle | **muscle**

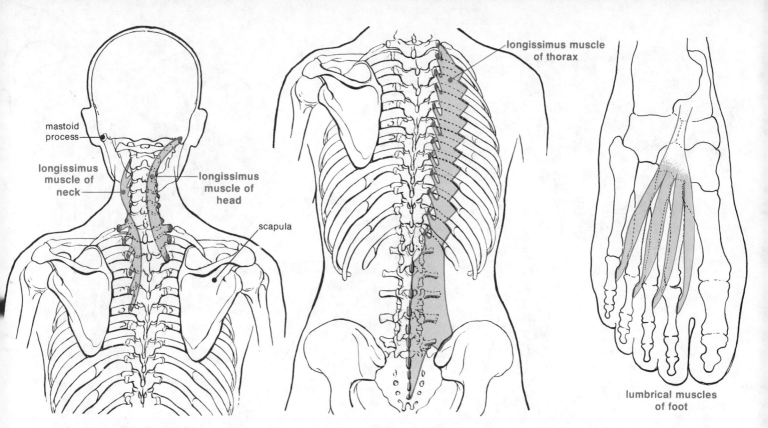

longissimus muscle of thorax

mastoid process

longissimus muscle of neck

longissimus muscle of head

scapula

lumbrical muscles of foot

MUSCLE	ORIGIN	INSERTION	ACTION
	inferior oblique part: front of bodies of first two or three thoracic vertebrae; vertical part: front of bodies of first three thoracic and last three cervical vertebrae	inferior oblique part: anterior tubercle of transverse processes of fifth and sixth cervical vertebrae vertical part: front of bodies of second, third, and fourth cervical vertebrae	
longissimus m. of head trachelomastoid m. *m. longissimus capitis*	transverse processes of cervical vertebrae	mastoid process of temporal bone	draws head backward, rotates head
longissimus m. of neck *m. longissimus cervicis*	transverse processes of upper six thoracic vertebrae	transverse processes of second through sixth vertebrae	extends cervical vertebrae
longissimus m. of thorax *m. longissimus thoracis* *m. longissimus dorsi*	sacrospinal aponeurosis, transverse processes of lower six thoracic and first two lumbar vertebrae	transverse processes of lumbar and thoracic vertebrae, inferior borders of ribs	extends thoracic vertebrae
longitudinal m. of tongue, inferior *m. longitudinalis inferior linguae*	undersurface of tongue at base	tip of tongue	acts to alter shape of tongue
longitudinal m. of tongue, superior *m. longitudinalis superior linguae*	submucosa and septum of tongue	margins of tongue	acts to alter shape of tongue
lumbrical m.'s of foot *m. lumbricales pedis*	tendons of long flexor muscle of toes	medial side of proximal phalanges of four lateral toes	aid in flexion of toes
lumbrical m.'s of hand (four in number) *mm. lumbricales manus*	tendons of deep flexor muscle of fingers	extensor tendons of four lateral fingers	flex proximal, extend middle and distal phalanges
masseter m. *m. masseter*	superficial part: zygomatic process and arch; deep part: zygomatic arch	superficial part: ramus and angle of lower jaw; deep part: upper half of ramus, coronoid process of lower jaw	closes mouth, clenches teeth (muscle of mastication)
mentalis m. *m. levator menti*	incisor fossa of mandible	skin of chin	raises and protrudes lower lip
multifidus m. *m. multifidus*	sacrum and transverse processes of lumbar, thoracic, and lower cervical vertebrae	spinous processes of lumbar, thoracic, and lower cervical vertebrae	extends, rotates vertebral column

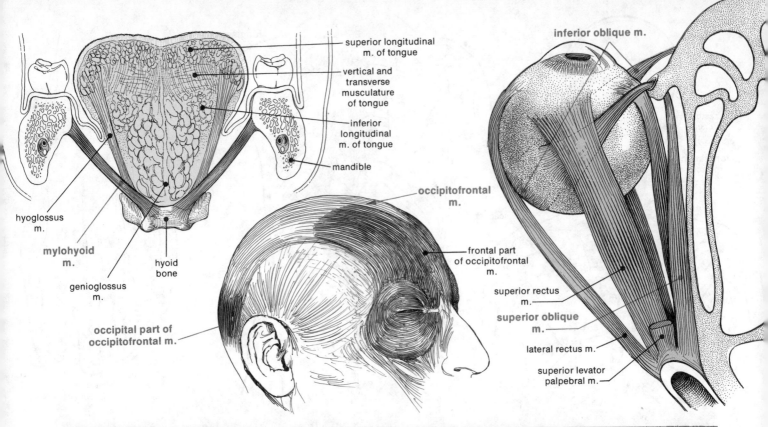

MUSCLE	ORIGIN	INSERTION	ACTION
m. of Treitz	see suspensory muscle of duodenum		
mylohyoid m. *m. mylohyoideus*	mylohyoid line of mandible	median raphe and hyoid bone	elevates floor of mouth and tongue, depresses mandible
nasal m. *m. nasalis*	maxilla adjacent to cuspid and incisor teeth	side of nose above nostril	draws margin of nostril toward septum
oblique m. of abdomen, external *m. obliquus externus abdominis*	external surface of lower eight ribs at costal cartilages	anterior half of crest of ilium, linea alba through rectus sheath	flexes and rotates vetebral column, tenses abdominal wall
oblique m. of abdomen, internal *m. oblique internus abdominis*	iliac crest, lumbodorsal fascia, inguinal ligament	lower three or four costal cartilages, linea alba by conjoint tendon to pubis	flexes and rotates vertebral column, tenses abdominal wall
oblique m. of auricle *m. obliquus auriculae*	eminence of concha	convexity of the helix	thought to be vestigial
oblique m. of eyeball, inferior *m. obliquus inferior bulbi*	floor of orbital cavity at anterior margin	between insertion of superior and lateral recti	rotates eyeball upward and outward
oblique m. of eyeball, superior *m. obliquus superior bulbi*	lesser wing of sphenoid above the optic foramen	after passing through a fibrous pulley, it reverses direction to insert on the sclera deep to the superior rectus muscle	rotates eyeball downward and outward
oblique m. of head, inferior *m. obliquus capitis inferior*	spine of axis vertebra	transverse process of atlas vertebra	rotates head
oblique m. of head, superior *m. oblique capitis superior*	transverse process of atlas vertebra	outer third of inferior curved line of occipital bone	rotates head
obturator m., external *m. obturatorius externus*	margin of obturator foramen of pelvis, obturator membrane	intertrochanteric fossa of femur	flexes and rotates thigh laterally
obturator m., internal *m. obturatorius internus*	pelvic surface of hipbone and obturator membrane, margin of obturator foramen	greater trochanter of femur	abducts and laterally rotates thigh
occipital m.	see occipitofrontal muscle		
occipitofrontal m. *m. occipitofrontalis*	frontal part: epicranial aponeurosis; occipital part: highest nuchal line of occipital bone	frontal part: skin of eyebrow, root of nose occipital part: epicranial aponeurosis	frontal part: elevates eyebrows; occipital part: draws scalp backward

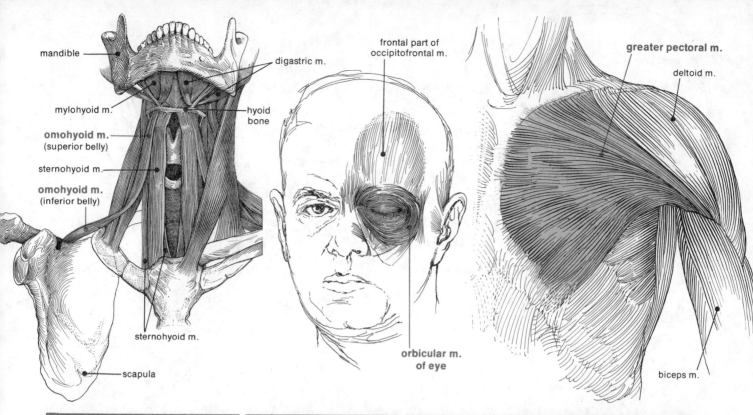

Labels on illustration:

- mandible
- mylohyoid m.
- omohyoid m. (superior belly)
- sternohyoid m.
- omohyoid m. (inferior belly)
- sternohyoid m.
- scapula
- digastric m.
- hyoid bone
- frontal part of occipitofrontal m.
- orbicular m. of eye
- greater pectoral m.
- deltoid m.
- biceps m.

MUSCLE	ORIGIN	INSERTION	ACTION
omohyoid m. *m. omohyoideus*	medial tip of suprascapular notch	lower border, body of hyoid bone	depresses and retracts hyoid bone
opposing m. of little fingers *m. opponens digiti minimi manus*	hook of hamate bone, flexor retinaculum	fifth metacarpal	draws fifth metacarpal bone toward palm
opposing m. of thumb *m. opponens pollicis*	tubercle of trapezium, flexor retinaculum	lateral border of first metacarpal bone	draws first metacarpal bone toward palm, opposes thumb
orbicular m. of eye *m. orbicularis oculi*	orbital part: frontal process of maxilla, adjacent portion of frontal bone; palpebral part: medial palpebral ligament; lacrimal part: posterior lacrimal ridge of lacrimal bone	near origin after encircling orbit — orbital tubercle of zygomatic bone	closes eyelids, tightens skin of forehead, compresses lacrimal sac
orbicular m. of mouth *m. orbicularis oris*	muscles adjacent to mouth	muscles interlace to encircle mouth	closes and purses lips
orbital m. *m. orbitalis*	bridges inferior orbital groove and sphenomaxillary fissure		thought to be rudimentary; may feebly protrude the eyeball
palatoglossus m. glossopalatine m. *m. palatoglossus* *m. glossopalatinus*	undersurface of soft palate	dorsum and side of tongue	elevates tongue and narrows fauces
palatopharyngeus m. *m. palatopharygeus* *m. pharyngeopalatus*	soft palate	posterior wall of thyroid cartilage and wall of pharynx	elevates pharynx, helps shut nasopharynx, narrows fauces, aids in swallowing
palmar m., long *m. palmaris longus*	medial epicondyle of humerus	flexor retinaculum, palmar aponeurosis	flexes hand
palmar m., short *m. palmaris brevis*	flexor retinaculum	skin of palm	aids in deepening hollow of palm, wrinkles skin of palm
pectinate m.'s *mm. pectinati*	a number of muscular columns projecting from the inner walls of the auricles of the heart		contract in systole of heart
pectineal m. *m. pectineus*	pectineal line of pubis	pectineal line of femur between lesser trochanter and linea aspera	adducts and aids in flexion of thigh
pectoral m., greater *m. pectoralis major*	medial half of clavicle, sternum, and costal cartilages; aponeurosis of external oblique muscle of abdomen	lateral lip of intertubercular groove of humerus	flexes, adducts, and rotates arm medially

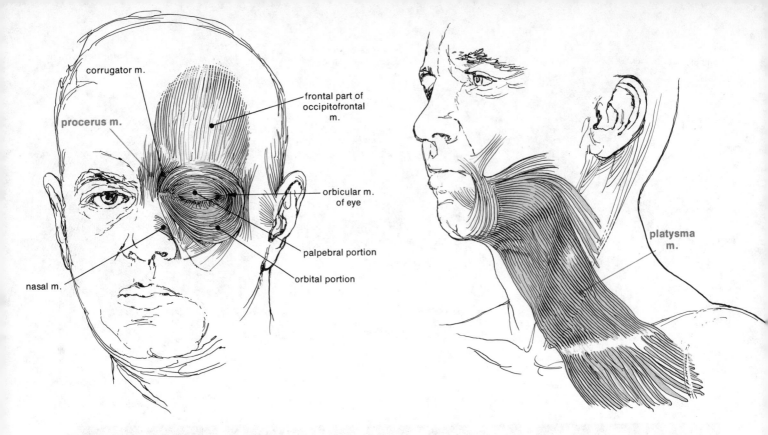

MUSCLE	ORIGIN	INSERTION	ACTION
pectoral, m., smaller *m. pectoralis minor*	anterior aspect of second through fifth ribs	coracoid process of scapula	draws scapula downward, elevates ribs
pectoralis major m.		see pectoral muscle, greater	
pectoralis minor m.		see pectoral muscle, smaller	
peroneal m., long fibular m., long *m. peroneus longus*	upper aspects of tibia and fibula	first metatarsal bone, first cuneiform bone	aids in flexion and everts foot
peroneal m., short fibular m., short *m. peroneus brevis*	lower two-thirds of fibula	tuberosity of fifth metatarsal bone	aids in flexion of and everts foot
peroneal m., third *m. peroneus tertius*	distal fourth of fibula, interosseous membrane	fascia of fifth metatarsal bone on dorsum of foot	extends and everts foot
piriform m. *m. piriformis*	internal aspect of sacrum, sacrotuberous ligament	upper portion of greater trochanter of femur	rotates thigh laterally
plantar m. *m. plantaris*	popliteal groove of lateral condyle of femur	medial side of calcaneal tendon	extends foot (plantar flexion)
platysma m. *m. platysma myoides*	superficial fascia of upper chest	skin over mandible, cheek, and mouth	depresses lower jaw and lower lip, wrinkles skin of neck and upper part of chest
pleuroesophageal m. *m. pleuroesophageus*		muscle fibers from left mediastinal pleura to esophagus	reinforces musculature of esophagus
popliteal m. *m. popliteus*	popliteal groove of lateral condyle of femur	medial two-thirds of popliteal line on posterior surface of tibia	flexes leg and rotates it medially
procerus m. *m. procerus* *m. pyramidalis nasi*	fascia covering bridge of nose	skin between eyebrows	wrinkles skin over bridge of nose (assists frontal muscle)
pronator m., quadrate *m. pronator quadratus*	distal fourth of shaft of ulna	distal fourth of shaft of radius	pronates forearm
pronator m., round *m. pronator teres*	humeral part: medial epicondyle of humerus; ulnar part: coronoid of ulna	lateral aspect of radius bone	pronates and flexes forearm
psoas m., greater *m. psoas major*	transverse processes of bodies of lumbar vertebrae	lesser trochanter of femur	flexes and medially rotates thigh
psoas m., smaller *m. psoas minor*	bodies of last thoracic and first lumbar vertebrae	pectineal line of hipbone	flexes vertebral column

muscle | **muscle**

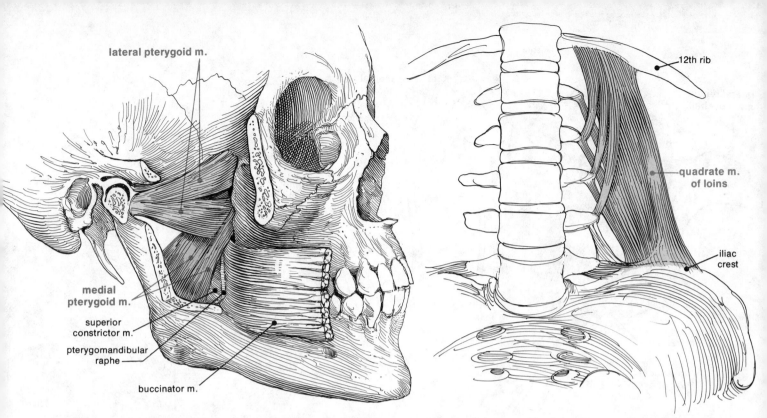

lateral pterygoid m.

12th rib

quadrate m. of loins

iliac crest

medial pterygoid m.

superior constrictor m.

pterygomandibular raphe

buccinator m.

MUSCLE	ORIGIN	INSERTION	ACTION
pterygoid m., lateral external pterygoid m. *m. pterygoideus lateralis*	pterygoid plate and greater wing of sphenoid	condyle of mandible, capsule of temporomandibular joint	opens and protrudes mandible and moves it side to side
pterygoid m., medial internal pterygoid m. *m. pterygoideus medialis*	maxillary tuberosity and lateral pterygoid plate	medial surface of ramus and angle of mandible	closes and protrudes mandible
pubococcygeus m. *m. pubococcygeus*	pubic symphysis	coccyx and perineal body	supports pelvic floor
puborectal m. *m. puborectalis*	pubic symphysis	interdigitates to form a sling which passes behind the rectum	holds anal canal at right angle to rectum
pubovaginal m. *m. pubovaginalis*	part of levator ani muscle in the female		
pubovesical m. *m. pubovesicalis*	posterior surface of body of pubis	female: around fundus of bladder to front of vagina; male: around fundus of bladder to prostate gland	strengthens musculature of urinary bladder
pyramidal m. *m. pyramidalis*	pubic symphysis	linea alba	tenses abdominal wall
quadrate m. of loins *m. quadratus lumborum*	iliac crest, lumbodorsal fascia, lumber vertebrae	12th rib, transverse processes of upper lumbar vertebrae	draws rib cage inferiorly, bends vertebral column laterally
quadrate m. of lower lip *m. quadratus labii inferior*	see depressor muscle of lower lip		
quadrate m. of sole *m. quadratus plantae*	calcaneus and plantar fascia	tendons of long flexor muscle of toes (*m. flexor digitorum longus*)	straightens pull of tendon of the long flexor muscle of toes
quadrate m. of thigh *m. quadratus femoris*	proximal part of the external border of the tuberosity of the ischium	proximal part of the linea quadrata (line extending vertically and distally from the intertrochanteric crest of femur)	rotates thigh laterally
quadrate m. of upper lip *m. quadratus labii superior*	see levator muscle of upper lip		
quadratus lumborum m.	see quadrate muscle of loins		
quadriceps m. of thigh *m. quadriceps femoris*	the large fleshy mass which covers the front and side of the femur, consisting of the rectus muscle of thigh (*m. rectus femoris*), lateral vastus muscle (*m. vastus lateralis*), medial vastus muscle (*m. vastus medialis*), and intermediate vastus muscle (*m. vastus intermedius*)		great extensor muscle of leg

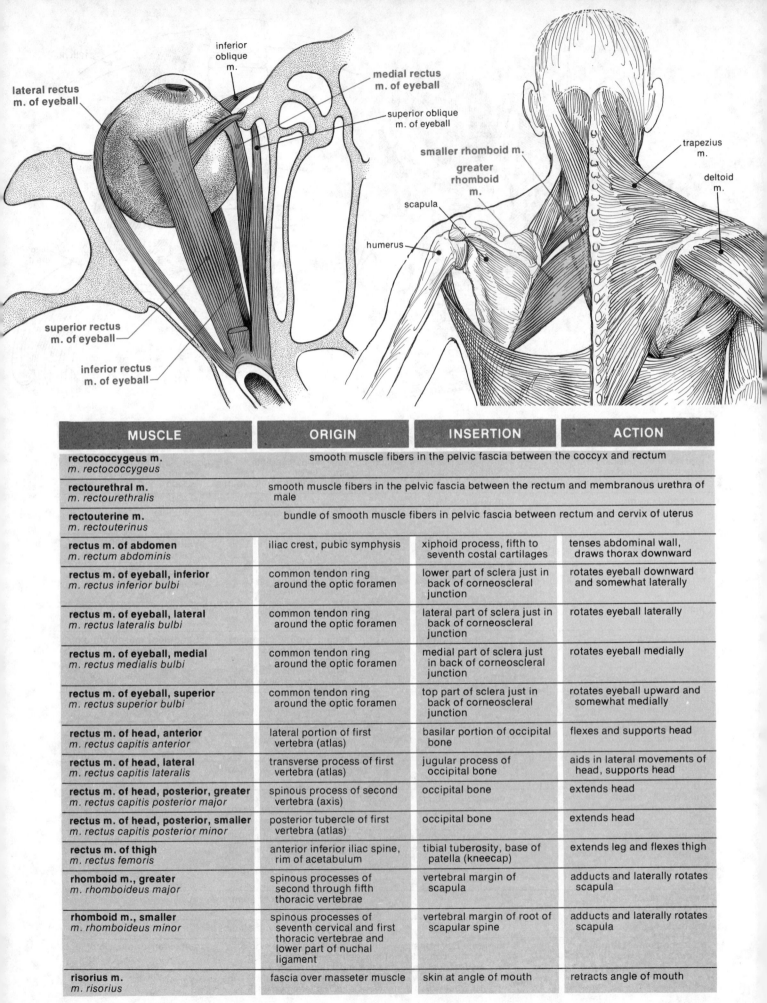

inferior oblique m.

lateral rectus m. of eyeball

medial rectus m. of eyeball

superior oblique m. of eyeball

smaller rhomboid m.

greater rhomboid m.

scapula

humerus

trapezius m.

deltoid m.

superior rectus m. of eyeball

inferior rectus m. of eyeball

MUSCLE	ORIGIN	INSERTION	ACTION
rectococcygeus m. *m. rectococcygeus*	smooth muscle fibers in the pelvic fascia between the coccyx and rectum		
rectourethral m. *m. rectourethralis*	smooth muscle fibers in the pelvic fascia between the rectum and membranous urethra of male		
rectouterine m. *m. rectouterinus*	bundle of smooth muscle fibers in pelvic fascia between rectum and cervix of uterus		
rectus m. of abdomen *m. rectum abdominis*	iliac crest, pubic symphysis	xiphoid process, fifth to seventh costal cartilages	tenses abdominal wall, draws thorax downward
rectus m. of eyeball, inferior *m. rectus inferior bulbi*	common tendon ring around the optic foramen	lower part of sclera just in back of corneoscleral junction	rotates eyeball downward and somewhat laterally
rectus m. of eyeball, lateral *m. rectus lateralis bulbi*	common tendon ring around the optic foramen	lateral part of sclera just in back of corneoscleral junction	rotates eyeball laterally
rectus m. of eyeball, medial *m. rectus medialis bulbi*	common tendon ring around the optic foramen	medial part of sclera just in back of corneoscleral junction	rotates eyeball medially
rectus m. of eyeball, superior *m. rectus superior bulbi*	common tendon ring around the optic foramen	top part of sclera just in back of corneoscleral junction	rotates eyeball upward and somewhat medially
rectus m. of head, anterior *m. rectus capitis anterior*	lateral portion of first vertebra (atlas)	basilar portion of occipital bone	flexes and supports head
rectus m. of head, lateral *m. rectus capitis lateralis*	transverse process of first vertebra (atlas)	jugular process of occipital bone	aids in lateral movements of head, supports head
rectus m. of head, posterior, greater *m. rectus capitis posterior major*	spinous process of second vertebra (axis)	occipital bone	extends head
rectus m. of head, posterior, smaller *m. rectus capitis posterior minor*	posterior tubercle of first vertebra (atlas)	occipital bone	extends head
rectus m. of thigh *m. rectus femoris*	anterior inferior iliac spine, rim of acetabulum	tibial tuberosity, base of patella (kneecap)	extends leg and flexes thigh
rhomboid m., greater *m. rhomboideus major*	spinous processes of second through fifth thoracic vertebrae	vertebral margin of scapula	adducts and laterally rotates scapula
rhomboid m., smaller *m. rhomboideus minor*	spinous processes of seventh cervical and first thoracic vertebrae and lower part of nuchal ligament	vertebral margin of root of scapular spine	adducts and laterally rotates scapula
risorius m. *m. risorius*	fascia over masseter muscle	skin at angle of mouth	retracts angle of mouth

muscle | muscle

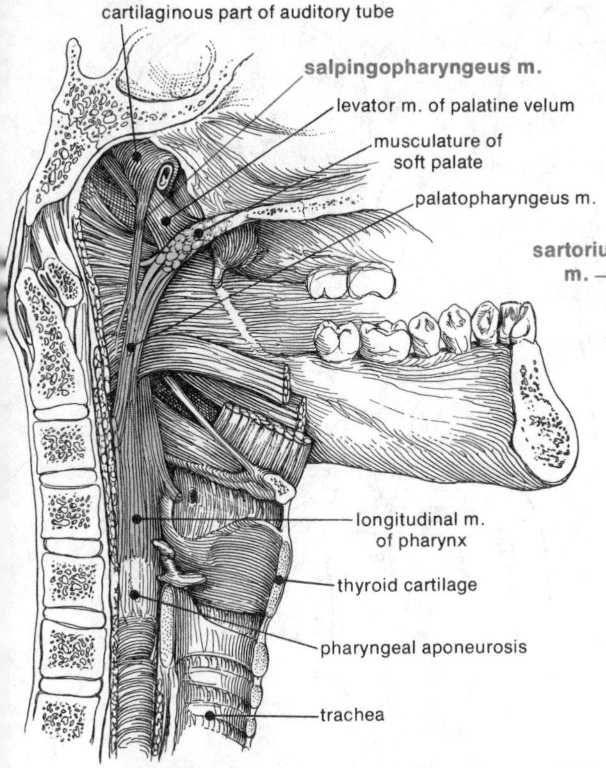

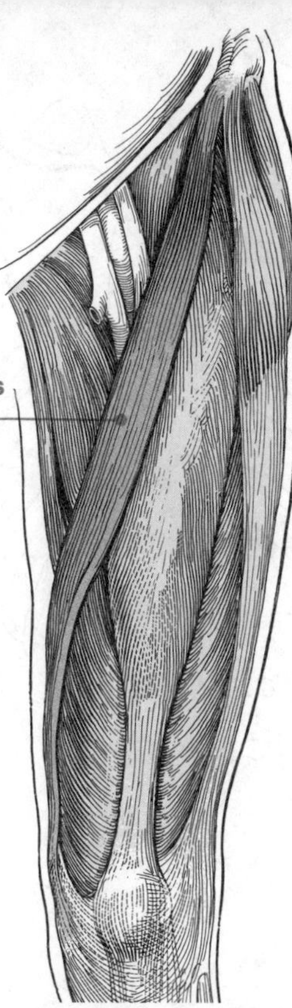

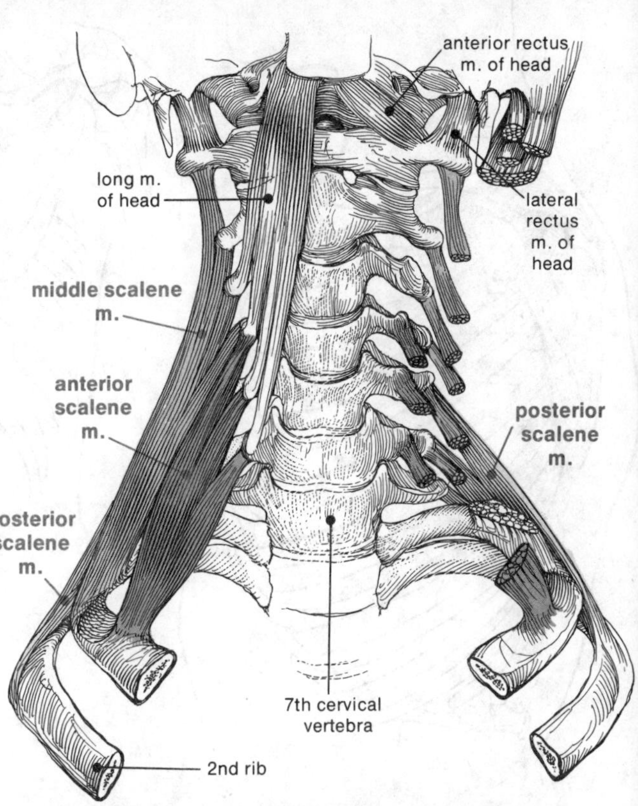

MUSCLE	ORIGIN	INSERTION	ACTION
rotator m.'s *mm. rotatores*	transverse processes of all vertebrae below second cervical	lamina above vertebra of origin	extend and rotate the vertebral column toward opposite side
sacrococcygeus m., dorsal *m. sacrococcygeus dorsalis*	a muscular or tendinous slip from the dorsal aspect of the sacrum to the coccyx		
sacrococcygeus m., ventral *m. sacrococcygeus ventralis*	a muscular or tendinous slip from the lower sacral vertebrae to the coccyx		
sacrospinal m. erector m. of spine *m. erector spinae*	deep muscle arising from the broad and thick tendon attached to the middle crest of sacrum, spinous processes of lumbar and 11th and 12th thoracic vertebrae, and back part of the iliac crest; it splits in the upper lumbar region into three columns of muscles: iliocostal (lateral division), longissimus (intermediate division), and spinal (medial division)		extends vertebral column and bends trunk to one side
salpingopharyngeus m. *m. salpingopharyngeus*	cartilage of auditory (pharyngotympanic) tube	wall of pharynx	opens auditory tube
sartorius m. *m. sartorius*	anterior superior iliac spine	upper medial surface of tibia	flexes thigh and leg
scalene m., anterior *m. scalenus anterior*	transverse processes of third to sixth cervical vertebrae	scalene tubercle of first rib	raises first rib, stabilizes or inclines neck to the side
scalene m., middle *m. scalenus medius*	transverse processes of first six cervical vertebrae	upper surface of first and second ribs	raises first rib, stabilizes or inclines neck to the side
scalene m., posterior *m. scalenus posterior*	transverse processes of fifth to seventh cervical vertebrae	outer surface of upper border of second rib	raises second rib, stabilizes or inclines neck to the side
scalene m., smallest *m. scalenus minimus*	occasional extra muscle fibers or slip of posterior scalene muscle		
semimembranous m. *m. semimembranosus*	tuberosity of ischium	upper portion of tibia, lateral condyle of femur	extends thigh, flexes and rotates leg medially
semispinal m. of head *m. semispinalis capitis*	transverse processes of six upper thoracic and four lower cervical vertebrae	occipital bone between superior and inferior nuchal lines	rotates head and draws it backward
semispinal m. of neck *m. semispinalis cervicis*	transverse processes of upper six thoracic vertebrae	spinous processes of second through sixth cervical vertebrae	extends and rotates vertebral column
semispinal m. of thorax *m. semispinalis thoracis*	transverse processes of lower six thoracic vertebrae	spinous processes of upper six thoracic and lower two cervical vertebrae	extends and rotates vertebral column

muscle | **muscle**

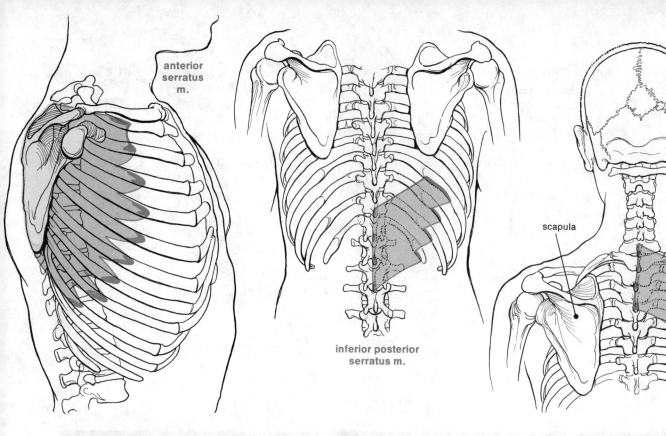

anterior
serratus
m.

inferior posterior
serratus m.

scapula

superior
posterior
serratus
m.

MUSCLE	ORIGIN	INSERTION	ACTION
semitendinous m. *m. semitendinosus*	tuberosity of ischium (in common with biceps muscle of thigh)	upper part of tibia	flexes and rotates leg medially, extends thigh
serratus m., anterior *m. serratus anterior*	lateral surface of eight or nine uppermost ribs	vertebral border of scapula	draws scapula forward and laterally, rotates scapula in raising arm
serratus m., posterior, inferior *m. serratus posterior inferior*	spinous processes of last two thoracic and first two or three lumbar vertebrae, supraspinal ligament	inferior borders of the last four ribs, slightly beyond their angles	draws the ribs outward and downward (counteracting the inward pull of the diaphragm)
serratus m. posterior, superior *m. serratus posterior superior*	caudal part of nuchal ligament, spinous processes of the seventh cervical and first two or three thoracic vertebrae, supraspinal ligament	upper borders of the second, third, fourth, and fifth ribs, slightly beyond their angles	raises the ribs
soleus m. *m. soleus*	upper third of fibula, soleal line of tibia, tendinous arch	calcaneous by calcaneal tendo (*tendon calcaneus*)	flexes foot
sphincter m. of anus, external *m. sphincter ani externus*	tip of coccyx, anococcygeal ligament	central tendon of perineum	closes anus
sphincter m. of anus, internal *m. sphincter ani internus*	muscular ring surrounding approximately 2.5 cm of the anal canal, about 6 mm from the orifice of the anus		aids in occlusion of anal aperture and expulsion of feces
sphincter m. of bile duct *m. sphincter choledochus*	a circular muscle around lower part of the bile duct within the wall of the duodenum (part of the sphincter muscle of hepatopancreatic ampulla)		constricts lower part of bile duct
sphincter m. of hepatopancreatic papilla sphincter of Oddi *m. sphincter papillae hepatopancreaticae*	circular muscle around terminal part of main pancreatic duct and common bile duct including duodenal papilla (papilla of Vater)		constricts both lower part of common bile duct and main pancreatic duct
sphincter m. of pupil *m. sphincter pupillae*	circular fibers of iris arranged in a narrow band about 1 mm in width		constricts pupil
sphincter m. of pylorus *m. sphincter pylori*	thick muscular ring at the end of the stomach		acts as valve to close lumen
sphincter m. of urethra external urethral sphincter m. *m. sphincter urethrae*	ramus of pubis	fibers interdigitate around urethra	closes urethra
sphincter m. of urinary bladder *m. sphincter vesicae urinariae*	thick muscular ring toward the lower part of bladder around internal urethral orifice		acts as valve to close internal urethral orifice

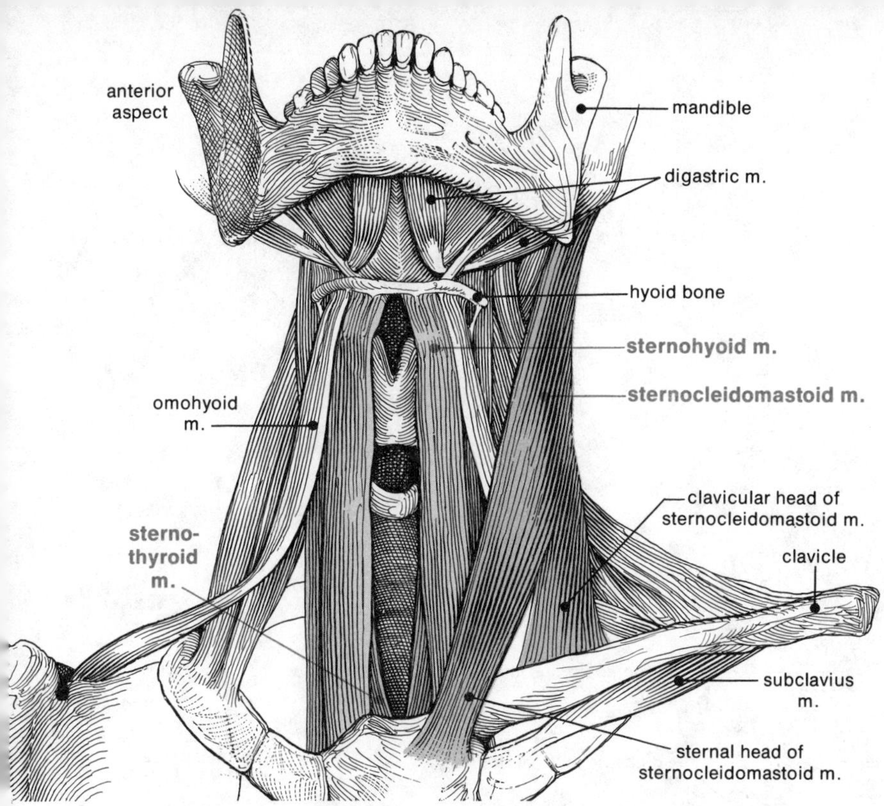

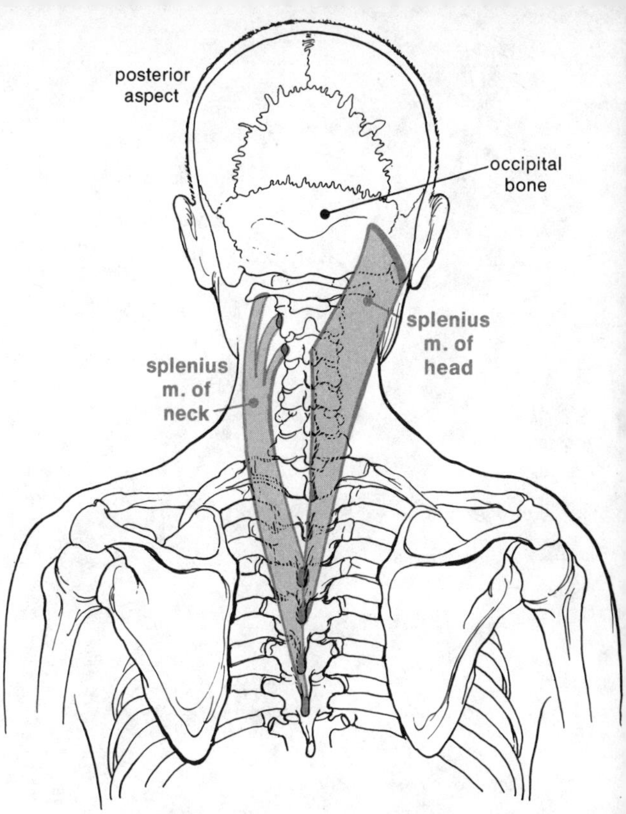

anterior aspect

mandible

digastric m.

hyoid bone

sternohyoid m.

sternocleidomastoid m.

omohyoid m.

clavicular head of sternocleidomastoid m.

clavicle

sterno-thyroid m.

subclavius m.

sternal head of sternocleidomastoid m.

posterior aspect

occipital bone

splenius m. of head

splenius m. of neck

MUSCLE	ORIGIN	INSERTION	ACTION
sphincter m. of vagina *m. sphincter vaginae*	pubic symphysis	interdigitates around and interlaces into vaginal barrel	constricts vaginal orifice
sphincter of Oddi	see sphincter muscle of hepatopancreatic papilla		
spinal m. of head *m. spinalis capitis* *m. biventer cervicis*	usually inseparably connected with semispinal muscle of head		
spinal m. of neck *m. spinalis cervicis*	transverse processes of upper six thoracic and seventh cervical vertebrae	spinous processes of second, third, and fourth cervical vertebrae	extends vertebral column
spinal m. of thorax *m. spinalis thoracis*	spinous processes of upper two lumbar and lower two thoracic vertebrae	spinous processes of second through ninth thoracic vertebrae	extends vertebral column
splenius m. of neck *m. splenius cervicis* *m. splenius colli*	nuchal ligament, spinous processes of third to sixth thoracic vertebrae	posterior tubercles of the transverse processes of upper two or three cervical vertebrae	extends head and neck, turns head toward the same side
splenius m. of head *m. spenius capitis*	spinous processes of upper thoracic vertebrae	mastoid process and superior nuchal line	inclines and rotates head
stapedius m. *m. stapedius*	wall of the conical cavity inside the pyramid of the middle ear chamber	posterior surface of neck of stapes	pulls head of stapes posteriorly, tilting the baseplate
sternal m. *m. sternalis*	small superficial muscular band at sternal end of greater pectoral muscle (*m. pectoralis major*), parallel with the margin of sternum		
sternocleidomastoid m. *m. sternocleidomastoideus*	sternal head: anterior surface of manubrium; clavicular head: medial third of clavicle	mastoid process, superior nuchal line of occipital bone	rotates and extends head, flexes vertebral column
sternocostal m.	see transverse muscle of thorax		
sternohyoid m. *m. sternohyoideus*	medial end of clavicle, posterior surface of manubrium, first costal cartilage	lower border of body of hyoid bone	depresses hyoid bone and larynx
sternothyroid m. *m. sternothyroideus*	dorsal surface of upper part of sternum and medial edge of first costal cartilage	oblique line on lamina of thyroid cartilage	draws thyroid cartilage downward
styloglossus m. *m. styloglossus*	lower end of styloid process, stylomandibular ligament	longitudinal part: side of tongue near dorsal surface; oblique part: over hyoglossus muscle	raises and retracts tongue

muscle | muscle

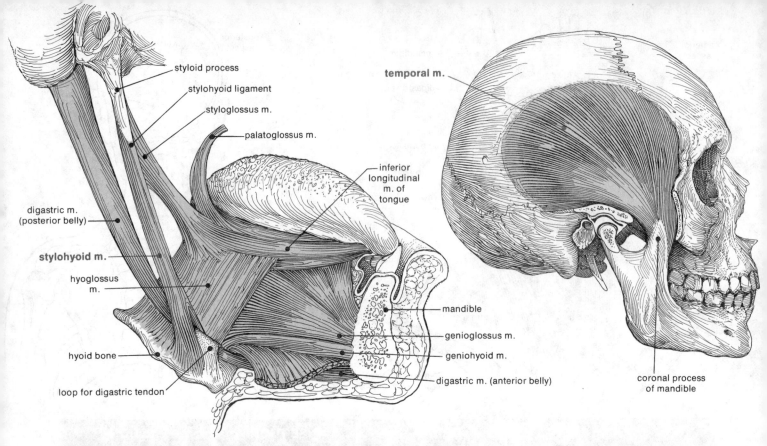

styloid process
stylohyoid ligament
styloglossus m.
palatoglossus m.
inferior longitudinal m. of tongue
digastric m. (posterior belly)
stylohyoid m.
hyoglossus m.
hyoid bone
loop for digastric tendon
temporal m.
mandible
genioglossus m.
geniohyoid m.
digastric m. (anterior belly)
coronal process of mandible

MUSCLE	ORIGIN	INSERTION	ACTION
stylohyoid m. *m. stylohyoideus*	posterior and lateral surfaces of the styloid process near the base	body of hyoid bone at its junction with the greater horn (cornu)	draws hyoid bone upward and backward
stylopharyngeus m. *m. stylopharyngeus*	root of styloid process	borders of thyroid cartilage, wall of pharynx	elevates and opens pharynx
subclavius m. *m. subclavius*	junction of first rib and costal costilages	lower surface of clavicle	depresses lateral end of clavicle
subcostal m.'s *mm. subcostales*	inner surface of ribs near angle	lower inner surface of second or third rib below rib of origin	draw adjacent ribs together
subscapular m. *m. subscapularis*	subscapular fossa	lesser tubercle of humerus	rotates arm medially
supinator m. *m. supinator*	lateral epicondyle of humerus, supinator crest of ulna	upper third of radius	supinates the forearm
suprahyoid m.'s *mm. suprahyoidei*	the group of muscles attached to the upper part of the hyoid bone including the digastric, stylohyoid, mylohyoid, and geniohyoid muscles		
supraspinous m. *m. supraspinatus*	supraspinous fossa	superior aspect of greater tubercle of humerus	abducts arm
suspensory m. of duodenum ligament of Treitz m. of Treitz *m. suspensorius duodeni*	connective tissue around celiac artery and right crus of diaphragm	superior border of duodenojejunal curve, part of ascending duodenum	acts as suspensory ligament
tarsal m., inferior *m. tarsalis inferior*	inferior rectus muscle of eyeball	tarsal plate of lower eyelid	widens palpebral fissure
tarsal m., superior *m. tarsalis superior*	aponeurosis of levator muscle of upper eyelid	tarsus plate of upper eyelid	raises upper eyelid
temporal m. *m. temporalis*	temporal fossa	coronoid process of mandible	closes mouth, clenches teeth, retracts lower jaw
temporoparietal m. *m. temporoparietalis*	temporal fascia above ear	epicranial aponeurosis	tightens scalp
tensor m. of fascia lata *m. tensor fasciae latae*	iliac crest	iliotibial tract of fascia lata	tenses fascia lata
tensor m. of palatine velum *m. tensor veli palatini*	spine of sphenoid, scaphoid fossa of internal pterygoid process, cartilage of the auditory tube	midline of aponeurosis of soft palate, wall of auditory tube	elevates palate

muscle | muscle

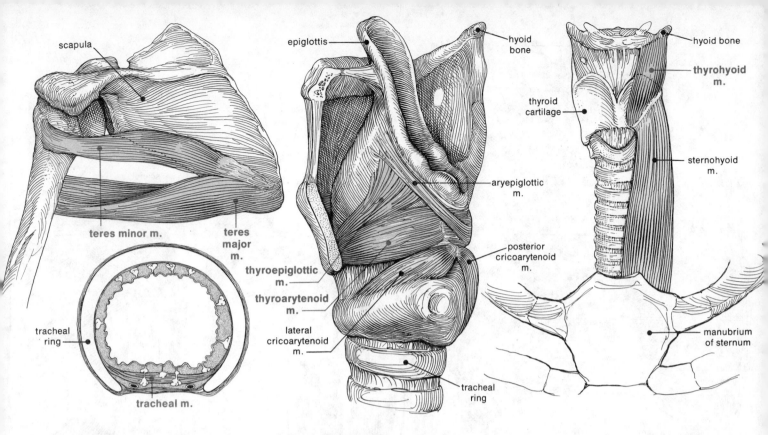

Labels on illustrations:

scapula

teres minor m.

teres major m.

tracheal ring

tracheal m.

epiglottis

thyroepiglottic m.

thyroarytenoid m.

lateral cricoarytenoid m.

hyoid bone

aryepiglottic m.

posterior cricoarytenoid m.

tracheal ring

hyoid bone

thyrohyoid m.

thyroid cartilage

sternohyoid m.

manubrium of sternum

MUSCLE	ORIGIN	INSERTION	ACTION
tensor m. of tympanum tensor m. of tympanic membrane (ear drum) *m. tensor tympani*	cartilaginous portion of auditory (eustachian) tube and adjoining part of great wing of sphenoid bone	manubrium of malleus near its root	draws tympanic membrane medially, thus increasing its tension
teres major m. *m. teres major*	inferior axillary border of scapula	crest of lesser tubercle of humerus	adducts and rotates arm medially
teres minor m. *m. teres minor*	axillary border of scapula	inferior aspect of greater tubercle of humerus	rotates arm laterally
thyroarytenoid m. *m. thyroarytenoideus*	inside of thyroid cartilage	base of arytenoid cartilage	aids in closure of laryngeal inlet
thyroepiglottic m. *m. thyroepiglotticus*	inside of thyroid cartilage	margin of epiglottis	depresses the epiglottis
thyrohyoid m. *m. thyrohyoideus*	oblique line of thyroid cartilage	greater horn (*cornu*) of hyoid bone	elevates larynx, depresses hyoid bone
tibial m., anterior *m. tibialis anterior*	upper two-thirds of tibia, interosseous membrane	first metatarsal bone, first cuneiform bone	extends and inverts foot
tibial m., posterior *m. tibialis posterior*	interosseous membrane adjoining tibia and fibula	navicular, with slips to three cuneiform bones; cuboid, second, third, and fourth metatarsals	principal inverter of foot, aids in flexion of foot
tracheal m. *m. trachealis*	anastomosing transverse muscular bands connecting the ends of the tracheal rings		
trachelomastoid m.	see longissimus muscle of head		
tragus m. *m. tragicus*	a band of vertical muscular fibers on the outer surface of the tragus of the ear		
transverse m. of abdomen *m. transversus abdominis*	7th–12th costal cartilages, lumbar fascia, iliac crest, inguinal ligament	xiphoid process, linea alba, conjoint tendon to pubis	supports abdominal viscera
transverse m. of auricle *m. transversus auriculae*	see auricular muscle, transverse		
transverse m. of chin *m. transversus menti*	superficial muscular fibers of depressor muscle of angle of mouth (triangular muscle) which turn back and cross to the opposite side below the chin		
transverse m. of nape *m. transversus nuchae*	an occasional muscle passing between the tendons of the trapezius and sternocleidomastoid muscles		
transverse m. of perineum, deep *m. transversus perinei profundus*	inferior ramus of ischium	central tendon of perineum, external anal sphincter	fixes central tendon of perineum

muscle | muscle

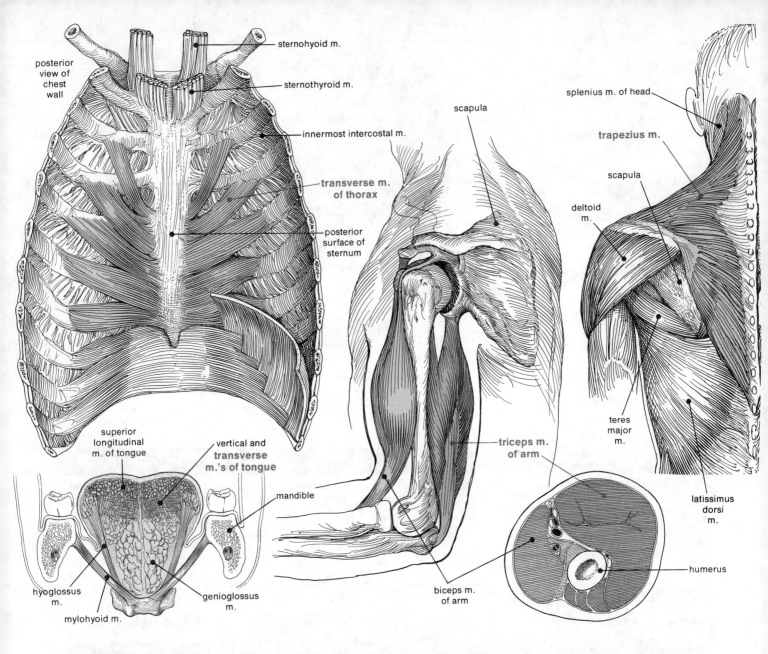

posterior view of chest wall

sternohyoid m.

sternothyroid m.

innermost intercostal m.

transverse m. of thorax

posterior surface of sternum

scapula

splenius m. of head

trapezius m.

scapula

deltoid m.

teres major m.

latissimus dorsi m.

triceps m. of arm

superior longitudinal m. of tongue

vertical and **transverse m.'s of tongue**

mandible

hyoglossus m.

genioglossus m.

mylohyoid m.

biceps m. of arm

humerus

MUSCLE	ORIGIN	INSERTION	ACTION
transverse m. of perineum, superficial *m. transversus perinei superficialis*	ramus of ischium near tuberosity	central tendon of perineum	supports central tendon of perineum
transverse m. of thorax sternocostal m. *m. transversus thoracis*	xiphoid process, posterior surface of lower part of sternum	second to sixth costal cartilages	narrows chest, draws costal cartilages downward
transverse m. of tongue *m. transversus linguae*	median fibrous septum of tongue	submucous fibrous tissue at sides of tongue	narrows and elongates tongue
trapezius m. *m. trapezius*	superior nuchal line of occipital bone, nuchal ligament, spinous processes of seventh cervical and all thoracic vertebrae	superior part: posterior border of lateral third of clavicle; middle part: median margin of acromion, superior lip of posterior border of scapular spine; inferior part: tubercle at apex of median end of scapular spine	elevates shoulder, rotates scapula to raise shoulder in full abduction and flexion of arm, draws scapula backward
triangular m.	see depressor muscle of angle of mouth		
triceps m. of arm *m. triceps brachii*	long head: infraglenoid tubercle of scapula; lateral head: proximal portion of humerus; medial head: distal half of humerus	olecranon process of ulna	extends arm and forearm

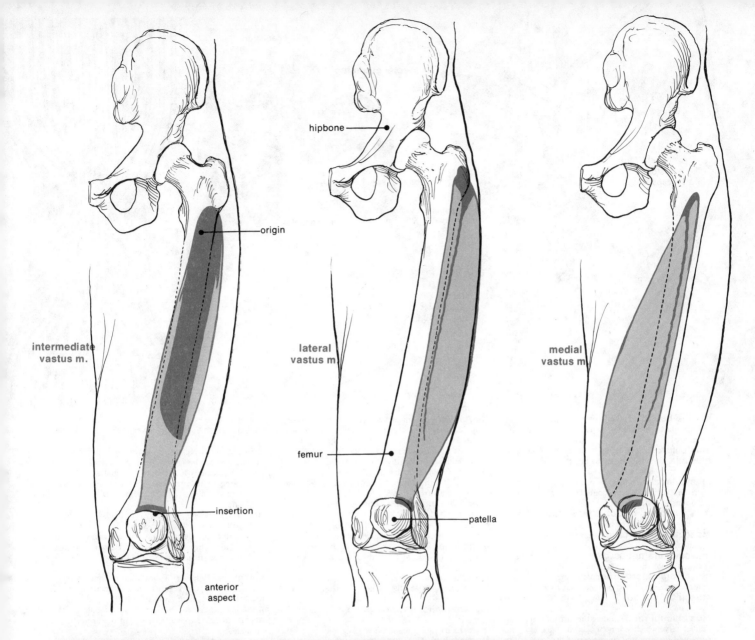

intermediate vastus m.

origin

insertion

anterior aspect

hipbone

lateral vastus m

femur

patella

medial vastus m

MUSCLE	ORIGIN	INSERTION	ACTION
triceps of calf *m. triceps surae*	combined gastrocnemius and soleus muscles; its tendon of insertion is the calcaneal tendon		
uvula m. *m. uvulae*	palatine aponeurosis and posterior nasal spine of palatine bone	mucous membrane of uvula	elevates uvula
vastus m., intermediate *m. vastus intermedius*	anterior and lateral surface of femur	common tendon of quadriceps muscle of thigh, patella	extends leg
vastus m., lateral *m. vastus lateralis*	lateral aspect of femur	common tendon of quadriceps muscle of thigh, patella	extends leg
vastus m., medial *m. vastus medialis*	medial aspect of femur	common tendon of quadriceps muscle of thigh, patella	extends leg
vertical m. of tongue *m. verticalis linguae*	dorsal fascia of tongue	sides and ventral surface of tongue	aids in mastication, swallowing, and speech by altering shape of tongue
vocal m. *m. vocalis*	lamina of thyroid cartilage	vocal process of arytenoid cartilage	adjusts tension of vocal cords
zygomatic m., greater *m. zygomaticus major*	zygomatic arch	angle of mouth	draws upper lip upward
zygomatic m., smaller *m. zygomaticus minor*	malar surface of zygomatic bone	upper lip	aids in forming nasolabial furrow, muscle of facial expression

muscle | **muscle**

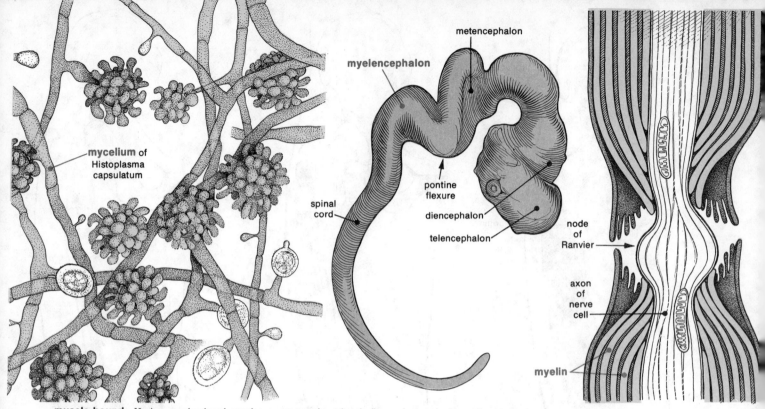

mycelium of Histoplasma capsulatum

myelencephalon
metencephalon
spinal cord
pontine flexure
diencephalon
telencephalon

node of Ranvier
axon of nerve cell
myelin

muscle-bound. Having overdeveloped muscles which limit movements, usually due to excessive exercise.

mus′cular. Of or relating to a muscle or muscles.

muscula′ris. The muscular layer of the wall of a tubular or hollow structure.

mus′cularize. To change into muscle, as the conversion of scar tissue into muscle tissue in a wound of a muscle.

mus′culature, muscula′tion. The system of muscles in the body or a body part.

musculoaponeurot′ic. Relating to muscle and aponeurosis.

musculocuta′neous. Relating to muscle and skin, as certain nerves that supply both structures.

musculomem′branous. Relating to or composed of muscular and membranous tissues.

musculoskel′etal. Relating to the muscles and skeleton.

mus′culospi′ral. Denoting the distribution of the radial nerve which innervates certain muscles of the arm and forearm and spirals across the back of the humerus.

musculotrop′ic. Acting upon muscular tissue.

Musset's sign. Rhythmic nodding of the head, occurring in incompetence of the aortic valve.

mu′tagen. Any agent that causes a permanent change in the genetic material (mutation), as radioactive substances, ultraviolet light, etc.

mutagen′esis. The formation of mutation.

mutagen′ic. Causing mutation.

mu′tant. An organism that differs from the parental strain as a result of having a gene that has undergone structural change.

mu′tase. One of various enzymes that promote the apparent migration of a phosphate group from one hydroxyl group to another of the same molecule.

muta′tion. 1. The process in which a gene undergoes a permanent, heritable, structural change. **2.** The modified gene.

mute. A person who is unable to speak.

mutila′tion. 1. Damaging or removing an essential part of the body. **2.** The state of being mutilated.

mu′tism. Inability to speak.

mu′tualism. A state in which two dissimilar organisms live together with mutual benefit; a form of symbiosis.

MV. Abbreviation for megavolt.

mv. Abbreviation for millivolt.

MW. Abbreviation for molecular weight.

My. Abbreviation for myopia.

myadeno′ma. A benign tumor derived from glandular epithelial tissue.

myal′gia. Muscle pain.

myasthe′nia. Weakness of muscle.

m. gravis, a chronic disease characterized by variable degrees of muscular weakness, which may progress to paralysis; it frequently begins in the muscles of the eyes and is often associated with abnormalities of the thymus gland; the disease attacks the point at which nerve meets muscle, stopping the electrical impulse before it can excite the muscle to contract.

myato′nia, myat′ony. Absence of muscle tone.

myat′rophy. See myoatrophy.

myce′lial. Relating to mycelium; having the filamentous appearance of a mold colony.

myce′lium. The network of threadlike filaments (hyphae) constituting the body or vegetative portion of a fungus.

my′cete. A fungus.

my′cetism, mycetis′mus. Mushroom poisoning.

mycetogen′ic, mycetogenet′ic. Caused by fungi.

myceto′ma. See maduromycosis.

Mycetozo′a. The slime animals; microscopic animal forms, similar to fungi and often regarded as such.

my′cid. A secondary lesion occurring in certain mycotic infections.

myco-, myc-. Combining forms denoting a relationship to fungus.

mycobacte′ria. Microorganisms of the genus *Mycobacterium*.

Mycobacte′rium. A genus (family Mycobacteriaceae) of aerobic gram-positive, acid-fast, nonmotile, rod-shaped bacteria; some of its species are called bacilli.

M. leprae, the causative agent of leprosy; also called Hansen's bacillus.

M. tuberculosis, the causative agent of tuberculosis in man and animals; formerly called *Bacillus tuberculosis.*

mycodermomyco′sis, mycodermati′tis. A fungal infection of the skin.

mycogastri′tis. Inflammation of the stomach caused by a fungus.

mycol′ogist. A specialist in fungi and fungal diseases.

mycol′ogy. The branch of science concerned with the study of fungi.

Mycoplas′ma. A genus of bacteria lacking a rigid cell wall, having instead a triple-layered membrane (thus occurring in many shapes); the smallest free-living organisms presently known, being intermediate in size between viruses and bacteria; some species are pathogenic.

M. pneumoniae, one of the main causes of primary atypical pneumonia in man; also called Eaton

agent.

mycoplas′ma. Any organism of the genus *Mycoplasma.*

T-m.'s, microorganisms known to inhabit the urinary tracts of a large percentage of individuals; they have the capacity to attach to mammalian cells and to aggregate mucoproteins; so called because they form tiny colonies in agar (about 20 microns in diameter).

myco′sis. Disease caused by a fungus.

deep m., see systemic mycosis.

systemic m., deep m., a serious disease, often fatal, caused by various fungi that can invade the subcutaneous tissues and spread throughout the organism.

mycot′ic. Relating to mycosis or any disease caused by fungi or vegetable microorganisms.

mydri′asis. Dilatation of the pupil.

mydriat′ic. Any agent that dilates the pupil.

myec′tomy. Surgical removal of a portion of a muscle.

myelenceph′alon. The portion of the embryonic brain from which develop the medulla oblongata and the bulbar part of the fourth ventricle; together with the metencephalon it makes up the hindbrain or rhombencephalon.

myel′ic. 1. Relating to the spinal cord. **2.** Relating to bone marrow.

my′elin. A fatty substance that forms a major component of the sheath that surrounds and insulates the axon of some nerve cells.

my′elinated. Possessing a myelin sheath.

myelina′tion. The formation of a medullary sheath around a nerve fiber; also called myelinization.

myelin′ic. Relating to myelin.

myeliniza′tion. See myelination.

myeli′tis. 1. Inflammation of the spinal cord. **2.** Inflammation of the bone marrow.

apoplectiform m., inflammation of the gray matter of the spinal cord, with sudden onset of paralysis.

compression m., a progressive form of myelitis due to pressure on the spinal cord, as from a hemorrhage or tumor.

concussion m., inflammation following concussion of the spinal cord.

disseminated m., inflammation of several distinct areas of the spinal cord; also called multiple focal myelitis.

radiation m., myelitis caused by excessive exposure to x rays.

transverse m., inflammation extending across the whole thickness of the spinal cord.

myelo-. Combining form indicating a relationship

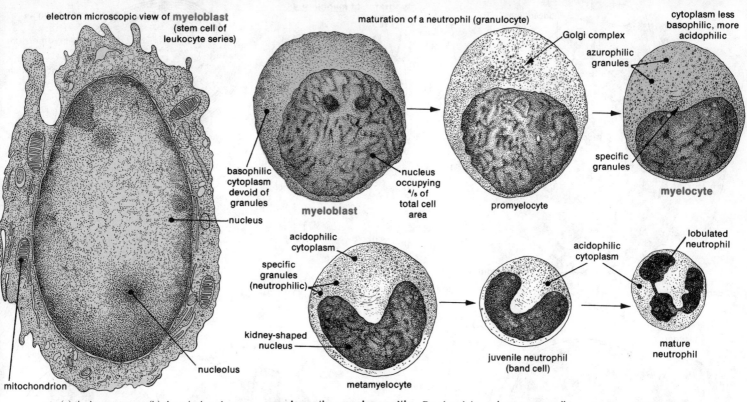

electron microscopic view of **myeloblast** (stem cell of leukocyte series)

mitochondrion

nucleolus

nucleus

basophilic cytoplasm devoid of granules

myeloblast

nucleus occupying ⁴/₅ of total cell area

maturation of a neutrophil (granulocyte)

Golgi complex

promyelocyte

cytoplasm less basophilic, more acidophilic

azurophilic granules

specific granules

myelocyte

acidophilic cytoplasm

specific granules (neutrophilic)

kidney-shaped nucleus

metamyelocyte

acidophilic cytoplasm

juvenile neutrophil (band cell)

lobulated neutrophil

mature neutrophil

to (a) the bone marrow, (b) the spinal cord.

myeloarch'itecton'ics. The study of the arrangement of nerve fibers in the cerebral cortex.

my'eloblast. A cell in the early stage of development, occurring normally in bone marrow; the first recognizable cell of the granulocytic (myeloid) series; it has a large, oval nucleus that occupies about four-fifths of the cell, usually containing two to five nucleoli; it can differentiate into a neutrophilic, eosinophilic, or basophilic granulocyte; also called granuloblast.

myeloblaste'mia. The presence of myeloblasts in the blood.

myeloblasto'ma. Malignant tumor composed chiefly of myeloblasts, occurring in certain diseases such as myeloblastic leukemia.

myeloblasto'sis. The presence of a large number of myeloblasts in the blood or tissues, as in acute leukemia.

my'elocele. Developmental defect in which the vertebral arches are absent, leaving an open groove lined with imperfect spinal cord tissue and through which cerebrospinal fluid drains; also called rachischisis and spondyloschisis.

my'elocyst. A cyst originating from a rudimentary medullary canal in the central nervous system.

myelocyst'ic. Relating to or of the nature of a myelocyst.

myelocys'tocele. The hernial protrusion of spinal cord substance through a defect in the vertebral column.

my'elocyte. 1. A young cell of the granulocytic (myeloid) series, developed from the promyelocyte and occurring normally in red bone marrow; its main characteristics are: a cytoplasm containing specific neutrophilic granules, an oval nucleus with the nuclear chromatin appearing as thick strands, and no discernible nucleoli. 2. A nerve cell in the gray matter of the brain or spinal cord.

myelocyto'sis. The increase of myelocytes in the circulating blood above the normal range.

myeloencephal'ic. Relating to the spinal cord and brain.

myeloencephali'tis. Encephalomyelitis; acute inflammation of the brain and spinal cord.

myelofibro'sis. A myeloproliferative disorder marked by fibrosis of the bone marrow, associated with abnormal proliferation of blood-forming elements, myeloid metaplasia of the spleen and liver, and anemia; also called myelosclerosis with myeloid metaplasia, agnogenic myeloid metaplasia, osteomyelofibrotic syndrome, and megakaryocytic splenomegaly.

myelogen'esis. Development of the bone marrow.

myelogen'ic, myelogenet'ic. Developed in the bone marrow.

myelog'raphy. Roentgenography of the spinal cord after introduction of a radiopaque substance into the spinal arachnoid space.

my'eloid. 1. Relating to, derived from, or of the nature of bone marrow. 2. Of or relating to the spinal cord.

myelo'ma. A tumor composed of cell types normally found in bone marrow.

multiple m., disease characterized by the appearance of scattered malignant tumors in various bones of the body; associated with the production of abnormal globulins and the presence of Bence Jones protein in the urine; the condition occurs mostly in persons in the sixth to eighth decade of life and affects males more often than females; also called myelomatosis and plasma cell myeloma.

plasma cell m., a general term applied to a number of disorders having in common the proliferation of plasma cells or the formation of abnormal proteins, such as multiple myeloma, soft tissue plasmacytomas, and plasma cell leukemia.

myelomala'cia. Softening of the spinal cord.

myelomato'sis. See myeloma, multiple.

myelomeningi'tis. Inflammation of the spinal cord and its membranes.

myelomenin'gocele. See meningomyelocele.

my'elon. The spinal cord.

myeloneuri'tis. Inflammation of the spinal cord and one or more peripheral nerves.

myelon'ic. Of or relating to the spinal cord.

myelop'athy. Any disease of the spinal cord.

myeloph'thisis. 1. Atrophy or wasting of the spinal cord. 2. Insufficiency of the cell-forming activity of the bone marrow.

my'eloplast. A leukocyte of the bone marrow.

myelopoie'sis. The formation of bone marrow or the blood cells derived from it.

myeloprolif'erative. Relating to proliferation of blood-forming elements.

myeloproliferative syndrome. A group of disorders characterized by abnormal proliferation of one or more types of bone marrow cells; includes myelofibrosis, polycythemia vera, and idiopathic thrombocytosis.

myeloradiculi'tis. Inflammation of the spinal cord and the roots of the spinal nerves.

myeloradic'ulodyspla'sia. Congenital abnormal development of the spinal cord and spinal nerve roots.

myeloradic'ulop'athy. Disease involving the spinal cord and spinal nerve roots.

myelorrha'gia. Bleeding into the spinal cord.

myelosarco'ma. Malignant tumor derived from bone marrow cells.

myelos'chisis. Cleft spinal cord resulting from failure of the normal closing of the neural tube.

myelosclero'sis. Induration of the spinal cord with overdevelopment of the interstitial connective tissue resulting from chronic inflammation; also called sclerosing myelitis and spinal sclerosis.

myelo'sis. Condition marked by abnormal proliferation of blood-forming cells in bone marrow and other organs.

chronic nonleukemic m., condition characterized primarily by undue proliferation of elements giving rise to white blood cells, the total count remaining normal; a variant of myelofibrosis.

erythremic m., disorder marked chiefly by abnormal proliferation of erythroid and myeloid precursors in bone marrow, bizarre red blood cell morphology, anemia, hemorrhagic disorders, and enlargement of the spleen and liver; also called Di-Guglielmo's syndrome.

myelot'omy. The cutting of nerve fibers in the spinal cord.

myelotox'ic. 1. Destructive to bone marrow. 2. Relating to diseased bone marrow.

myelyt'ic. Relating to or marked by inflammation of the spinal cord or of the bone marrow.

myenter'ic. Relating to the muscular layer (myenteron) of the intestine.

myen'teron. The muscular layer of the intestine.

myesthe'sia. Muscular sensibility; sensation felt within a muscle.

my'iasis. Any infection resulting from infestation of human tissue by fly maggots or flies, usually by deposition of ova by flies in open wounds.

mylohy'oid. Relating to the posterior portion of the lower jaw and to the hyoid bone.

myo-, my-. Combining forms meaning muscle.

myoarchitecton'ic. Relating to the structure of muscles.

myoat'rophy. Wasting away of muscles due to lack of use; also called myatrophy.

my'oblast. The embryonic cell which becomes a muscle cell.

myoblasto'ma. Granular cell tumor; see under tumor.

myocar'dial. Pertaining to the heart muscle (myocardium).

myocar'diograph. An instrument for graphically recording the action of the heart muscle.

myocardiop'athy. Cardiomyopathy.

primary m., myocardiopathy of unknown cause.

myocardior'raphy. Surgical suture of the muscular wall of the heart.

myocardi'tis. Inflammation of the heart muscle.

acute isolated m., an acute form of unknown

303

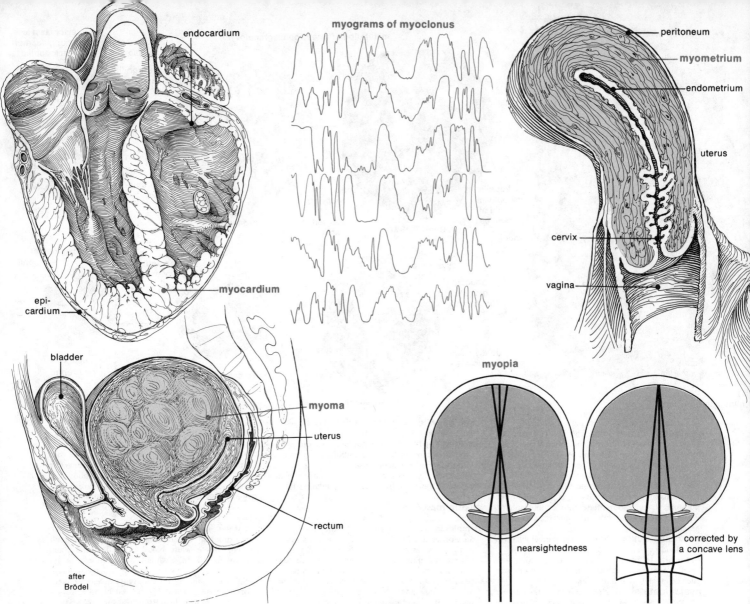

endocardium

myocardium

epi-cardium

myograms of myoclonus

peritoneum

myometrium

endometrium

uterus

cervix

vagina

bladder

myoma

uterus

rectum

after Brödel

myopia

nearsightedness

corrected by a concave lens

---

cause; also called Fiedler's myocarditis.

Fiedler's m., see acute isolated myocarditis.

myocar′dium. The middle and thickest layer of the heart wall composed of specialized striated muscle cells and intervening connective tissue; each cell possesses a central nucleus, a plasma membrane (sarcolemma), and numerous contractile myofibrils that are separated by varying amounts of sarcoplasm.

infarcted m., dead heart muscle resulting, usually, from an occluded artery.

my′ocele. Herniation of a muscle.

myocelluli′tis. Inflammation of muscle (myositis) and cellular tissue (cellulitis).

myoclo′nia. Any disorder characterized by twitching or spasmodic contraction of muscles.

myoclon′ic. Marked by myoclonus.

myoc′lonus. A sudden rapid twitch resulting from the sudden contraction of one or more muscle groups.

my′ocyte. A muscle cell.

myodynamom′eter. An instrument used to measure muscular strength.

myodys′tony. A succession of minute contractions during slow relaxation of a muscle following electrical stimulation.

myoede′ma. The localized contraction of a degenerating muscle when struck; also called mounding.

myoelec′tric. Relating to the electric attributes of muscles.

myoendocardi′tis. Inflammation of the wall and lining of the cardiac cavities.

myoepithe′lium. Tissue composed of contractile epithelial cells that resemble smooth muscle cells.

myofascial syndrome. A painful condition of skeletal muscles characterized by the presence of one or more discrete hyperesthetic areas termed

trigger points, located within muscles or tendons; when stimulated by pressure, these trigger points produce pain in the area of the patient's symptoms.

myofi′bril. One of the fine longitudinal fibrils present in muscle fiber; each myofibril is divided into a series of repeating units, the sarcomeres, which are the fundamental structural and functional units of contraction.

myofibro′ma. A benign tumor containing fibrous and muscular tissues.

myofibro′sis. Chronic inflammation of a muscle with excessive formation of connective tissue, resulting in atrophy of the muscular tissue.

myofil′aments. The microscopic structures that make up the fibrils of striated muscle.

my′ogen. A mixture of proteins, extractable from skeletal muscle with cold water, consisting largely of glycolytic enzymes.

myogen′ic. Of muscular origin.

myog′lia. A fine network of fibrils formed by muscle cells; also called muscle cement.

myoglo′bin. An oxygen-transporting protein found in muscle fibers, similar to hemoglobin.

myoglobinu′ria. The presence of myoglobin in the urine, usually after crush injuries or occasionally after very vigorous exercise.

paroxysmal idiopathic m., see rhabdomyolysis.

myoglob′ulin. A globulin present in muscle tissue.

myoglobulinu′ria. Myoglobinuria.

my′ogram. A tracing produced by myography.

my′ograph. An instrument for graphically recording muscular contractions.

myog′raphy. A technique used to record muscular activity.

my′oid. Resembling muscle.

myoky′mia. A twitching or tremor of individual fasciculi (bundles of fibers) of a muscle.

myolipo′ma. A benign tumor composed chiefly of adipose and muscle tissues.

myol′ogy. The branch of science concerned with the study of muscles.

myol′ysis. Disintegration of muscle tissue.

myo′ma. A benign tumor consisting of muscle tissue.

myomala′cia. Abnormal softening and degeneration of muscular tissue.

myomatec′tomy. Removal of a myoma.

myo′matous. Resembling a myoma.

myomec′tomy. Surgical removal of a myoma, specifically of a myoma of the uterus.

myom′eter. An apparatus for determining the strength of a muscular contraction.

myometri′tis. Inflammation of the muscular layer of the uterine wall.

myome′trium. The thick, smooth muscle forming the middle layer of the wall of the uterus.

my′on. A functional unit consisting of a muscle fiber with its basal membrane, together with the associated blood capillaries and nerves.

myonecro′sis. Death of muscle tissue.

myoneu′ral. Relating to muscle and nerve, as the nerve endings which terminate in muscular tissue.

myop′athy. Any disease of muscular tissue.

myopericardi′tis. Inflammation of the muscle tissue of the heart and the enveloping membrane (pericardium).

myo′pia. A condition of the eye in which light rays entering the eyeball from a distance focus in front of the retina, causing only near objects to be seen in focus; also called nearsightedness and shortsightedness.

myop′ic. Relating to or afflicted with myopia.

my′oplasm. The contractile part of a muscle cell.

my′oplasty. Surgical repair of a muscle.

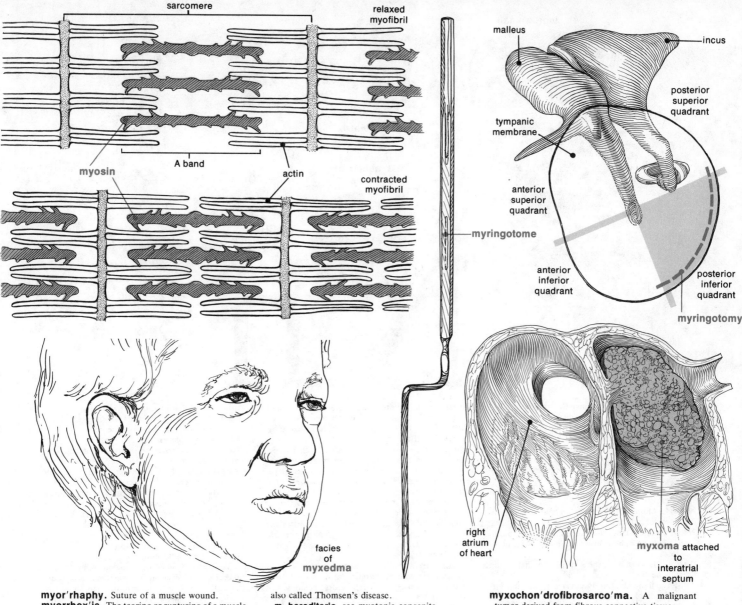

sarcomere

relaxed
myofibril

myosin

A band

actin

contracted
myofibril

malleus — incus

tympanic
membrane

posterior
superior
quadrant

anterior
superior
quadrant

myringotome

anterior
inferior
quadrant

posterior
inferior
quadrant

myringotomy

facies
of
myxedma

right
atrium
of heart

myxoma attached
to
interatrial
septum

myor′rhaphy. Suture of a muscle wound.

myorrhex′is. The tearing or rupturing of a muscle.

myosarco′ma. A general term for a malignant neoplasm or sarcoma derived from muscular tissue.

myosclero′sis. Chronic inflammation of a muscle with overgrowth of the interstitial connective tissue, resulting in hardening of the muscle.

my′osin. The thick filaments of polymerized protein molecules in the myofibril which, along with the protein actin, are responsible for muscular contraction; they comprise the dark A bands seen microscopically; called "A" bands because they are anisotropic to polarized light. See also actin.

myo′sis. Miosis.

myosi′tis. Inflammation of a muscle, usually a voluntary muscle.

m. ossificans, condition in which muscular tissue is replaced by bone; it may be localized following an injury or, rarely, it may be generalized, progressive (beginning in childhood), and due to unknown causes.

my′ospasm. Spasmodic contraction of a muscle or group of muscles.

my′otome. 1. Knife used in surgery to divide muscle. **2.** In embryology, the portion of the mesodermic somite from which skeletal muscle develops.

myot′omy. 1. Dissection of muscles. **2.** Surgical division of a muscle.

myoto′nia. Temporary rigidity of a muscle or group of muscles.

m. atrophica, disease marked by stiffness and eventual atrophy of the muscles, associated with cataract and slurred speech; also called myotonic dystrophy and Steinert's disease.

m. congenita, m. hereditaria, hereditary disease marked by temporary tonic spasm of certain muscles whenever a voluntary movement is attempted;

also called Thomsen's disease.

m. hereditaria, see myotonia congenita.

myoton′ic. Characterized by myotonia.

myringec′tomy. Surgical removal of the tympanic membrane (eardrum).

myringi′tis. Inflammation of the tympanic membrane.

myringo-, myring-. Combining forms denoting the tympanic membrane (eardrum).

myrin′goplasty. A surgical procedure performed to close a perforation of the eardrum acquired through injury or infection; also called type I tympanoplasty.

myringorup′ture. The tearing or rupturing of the tympanic membrane (eardrum).

myring′otome. A knife used for puncturing the tympanic membrane.

myringot′omy. Surgical incision of the tympanic membrane (eardrum) to allow drainage of the middle ear chamber; also called tympanic paracentesis.

mysopho′bia. Morbid fear of contamination, manifested by constant hand washing.

mythoma′nia. An abnormal compulsion to tell lies.

myx-, myxo-. Combining forms denoting mucus.

myxadeno′ma. Benign tumor derived from glandular epithelial tissue.

myxede′ma. A severe form of hypothyroidism occurring in juveniles and adults; caused by insufficient circulating thyroid hormone; marked by dry skin, brittle hair, swelling of the face, puffy eyelids, dull expression, and muscle weakness.

pretibial m., a bulging over the lateral aspect of the lower leg above the lateral malleolus, found in some cases of thyrotoxicosis, usually associated with exophthalmic goiter (Graves' disease).

myxedem′atous. Relating to myxedema.

myxochon′drofibrosarco′ma. A malignant tumor derived from fibrous connective tissue.

myx′ochondro′ma. A benign tumor composed chiefly of cartilaginous tissue.

myx′ocyte. One of the stellate or polyhedral cells found in mucous tissue.

myx′ofibro′ma. A benign tumor of connective tissue containing portions that resemble primitive mesenchymal tissue.

myx′oid. Resembling or containing mucus.

myx′olipo′ma. A benign tumor of adipose tissue containing portions that resemble primitive mesenchymal tissue.

myxo′ma. A benign tumor composed of connective tissue embedded in a soft, mucoid matrix; also called mucoid tumor.

atrial m., a benign primary tumor arising from the lining of the atria and resembling a polyp; it may cause murmurs which change with shifts in body position or simulate mitral or tricuspid stenosis.

myx′omato′sis. Fatal disease of rabbits marked by the presence of multiple myxomatous growths of the skin and mucous membranes.

myx′omyce′te. Fungus or slime mold found in rotting vegetation.

myx′oneuro′ma. Tumor resulting from proliferation of Schwann cells in which degenerative changes produce areas that resemble primitive mesenchymal tissue.

myx′opoie′sis. The formation of mucus.

myx′osarco′ma. A malignant tumor derived from connective tissue.

myx′ospore. A spore embedded in a gelatinous mass.

myx′ovi′rus. One of a group of RNA viruses that have an affinity for certain mucins and cause influenza or infections resembling influenza.

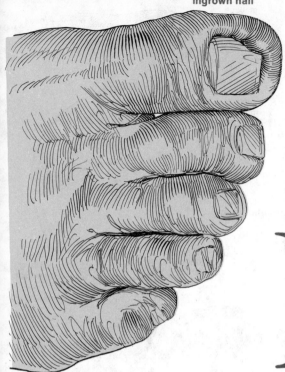

ingrown nail

nail root

eponychium

nail

nail matrix

nail bed

nalidixic acid

nalorphine

naloxone

Nn

N. 1. Abbreviation for normal. **2.** Symbol for nitrogen.

n. 1. Abbreviation for nasal. **2.** Symbol for (a) refractive index; (b) neutron.

Na. Chemical symbol of the element sodium.

NA. Abbreviation for *Nomina Anatomica.*

na′creous. Having a mother-of-pearl luster; iridescent.

NAD. Abbreviation for nicotinamide adenine dinucleotide.

NADH. Abbreviation for nicotinamide adenine dinucleotide, reduced.

NADP. Abbreviation for nicotinamide adenine dinucleotide phosphate; also abbreviated NAD phosphate.

nafcil′lin. A semisynthetic penicillin that is not readily destroyed by gastric acids.

nail. The flattened, translucent structure on the dorsal surface of the distal end of a finger or toe, composed of several layers of flat, clear cells; also called unguis.

  hippocratic n., a deformed overhanging fingernail associated with the clubbing of terminal phalanges in certain pulmonary and cardiac conditions.

  ingrown n., a toenail with its edges growing abnormally into the soft tissues; also called onychocryptosis.

  n. bed, the portion of tissue to which the nail is firmly adhered.

  n. matrix, the thick portion of nail bed beneath the nail root from which the nail develops.

  n. root, the portion of nail which is implanted into a groove of the skin.

nail′ing. The fastening of a fractured bone with a nail.

nail-patella syndrome. Hereditary condition characterized by bilateral underdevelopment of the kneecap, deformity and dislocation of the head of the radius, and dystrophy of fingernails.

nal′buphine. A non-narcotic potent pain reliever with a duration of action as long as or longer than that of morphine.

nalidix′ic acid. An antibacterial preparation effective against infections of the urogenital tract; NegGram®.

nal′orphine. $C_{19}H_{21}NO_3$; narcotic antagonist used as an antidote to narcotic overdosage; capable of causing withdrawal symptoms in narcotic addicts; Nalline®.

nalox′one. Narcotic antagonist used in treating respiratory depression suspected of being produced by a narcotic; Narcan®.

name. A word that designates and distinguishes one entity from another.

  brand n., see trade name.

  chemical n., systematic n., a scientific name that indicates a precise chemical structure; e.g., 2-(diphenylmethoxy)-*N,N*-dimethylethylamine hydrochloride (Benadryl®).

  generic n., strictly defined, a name that designates a family relationship among drugs; e.g., antihistamine, barbiturate, etc.; often used as a synonym for nonproprietary name; e.g., diphenhydramine (Benadryl®).

  nonproprietary n., one assigned to a drug (by the United States Adopted Name Council) when it is found to have therapeutic value; it indicates the chemical composition of the drug and is not protected by trademark registration; e.g., diphenhydramine (Benadryl®).

  proprietary n., see trade name.

  semisystematic n., semitrivial n., a name used in the sciences, especially chemistry, composed of two parts, one of which relates to a scientific (systematic) name, the other to a common (trivial) name; e.g., cortisone, derived from cortex and the suffix -one (indicating an aldehyde group).

  systematic n., see chemical name.

  trade n., brand n., proprietary n., name selected by the pharmaceutical company that manufactures and sells the drug; it is registered and protected by a trademark and is usually followed by an encircled superscript R; e.g., Benadryl®.

  trivial n., a common name that tells nothing about the structure of the organism or chemical it designates; e.g., water, caffeine, etc.

nano-. Combining form meaning small size; used with metric units of measure to denote one-billionth (10^{-9}).

nanoceph′aly. Abnormal smallness of the head.

nanocor′mia. Abnormal smallness of the body in relation to the head and extremities.

nanocu′rie (nCi). A unit of radioactivity equal to one-billionth of a curie; 10^{-9} curie.

na′nogram (ng). A unit of weight equal to one-billionth of a gram; 10^{-9} gram.

nan′oid. Dwarfish.

nanome′lia. Abnormal smallness of the extremities.

nanom′elus. Individual characterized by nanomelia.

nanome′ter (nm). A unit of linear measure equal to one-thousandth of a micron; 10^{-9} meter; also called millimicron.

nanosec′ond (nsec). A unit of time equal to one-billionth of a second; 10^{-9} second.

nanoso′ma, nanoso′mia. Dwarfism.

na′nus. A dwarf.

nape. The back of the neck; also called nucha.

naph′thalene. Tar camphor, a crystalline hydro-carbon derived from coal tar, insoluble in water, and soluble in alcohol; used as an insecticide (mothballs) and antiseptic, and in the manufacture of indigo and lampblack.

naph′thol. A crystalline, antiseptic derivative of naphthalene.

α-naph′thol. Alpha-naphthol; colorless crystals, soluble in water; used in microscopy.

N.A.P.N.E.S. Abbreviation for National Association for Practical Nurse Education and Services.

nar′cissism. Self-love, as opposed to object-love or love of another person; the term is derived from Narcissus, a figure in Greek mythology who fell in love with his own reflected image.

narco-. Combining form denoting stupor.

nar′colepsy. Condition characterized by paroxysmal episodes of sleep lasting from minutes to hours; frequently accompanied by transient muscular weakness, sleep paralysis, and hallucinations during the period between sleep and wakefulness; also called paroxysmal sleep and sleep epilepsy.

narco′ma. See narcosis.

narcoma′nia. An uncontrollable craving for narcotics.

narco′sis. A deep stuporous state produced by some narcotic drugs; also called narcoma.

narcosyn′thesis. Psychotherapeutic treatment conducted with the aid of a partial anesthetic.

narcother′apy. Psychotherapy conducted after a state of complete relaxation is induced by injecting a barbiturate drug intravenously (either sodium amytal or sodium pentothal); under this therapy some individuals have a capacity to communicate thoughts previously repressed.

narcot′ic. A drug intended for the relief of pain that also produces insensibility, stupor, and sleep; with prolonged use it may become addictive.

nar′cotism. Addiction to a habit-forming drug.

nar′cotize. To subject to the influence of a narcotic.

na′ris, *pl.* **na′res.** See nostril.

  posterior n., the opening connecting the nasal cavity with the nasopharynx on either side; also called choana.

na′sal. Relating to the nose.

nas′cent. Beginning to exist; denoting an atom or element at the moment it is liberated from a compound.

na′sion. A craniometric point; the midline of the nasofrontal suture.

NAS-NRC. Abbreviation for National Academy of Science-National Research Council.

naso-. Combining form meaning nose.

nasoan′tral. Relating to the nose and the maxillary sinus (antrum).

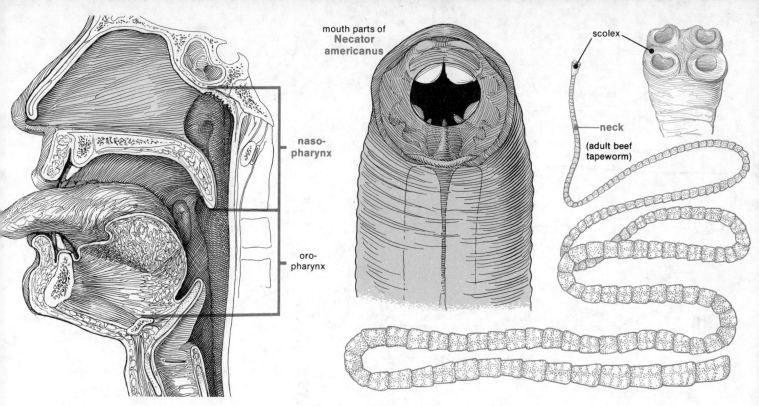

mouth parts of
**Necator
americanus**

naso-
pharynx

oro-
pharynx

scolex

neck

(adult beef
tapeworm)

nasofron'tal. Of or relating to the nose and the frontal bones.

nasola'bial. Relating to the nose and lip.

nasolac'rimal. 1. Relating to the nasal and the lacrimal bones. **2.** Relating to the nose and the structures producing and conveying tears.

na'so-o'ral. Concerning the nose and the mouth.

nasopal'atine. Concerning the nose and the palate.

nasopharyn'geal. Relating to the nasopharynx.

nasopharyngi'tis. Inflammation of the nasopharynx.

nasopharyn'goscope. An instrument for visual examination of the nasal passages and the nasopharynx.

nasophar'ynx. The uppermost part of the pharynx, located above the level of the soft palate immediately behind the nasal cavity; also called rhinopharynx and pars nasalis pharyngis.

na'soscope. See rhinoscope.

nasosepti'tis. Inflammation of the lining of the nasal septum.

nasosinusi'tis. Inflammation of the lining of the nasal cavity and adjacent sinuses.

na'sus. Latin for nose.

na'tal. Relating to birth.

natal'ity. The birth rate.

na'tes. The buttocks.

natimortal'ity. The proportion of stillbirths and newborn deaths to the birth rate.

National Formulary (NF). An official publication of the American Pharmaceutical Association which provides authoritative information on drugs.

na'trium. Latin for sodium (Na).

natriure'sis. Increased sodium excretion in the urine.

natriuret'ic. 1. Of or relating to the excretion of sodium in the urine. **2.** An agent promoting excretion of sodium.

na'turopath. One who practices naturopathy.

naturop'athy. The treatment of the sick by the exclusive use of physical forces such as sunlight, heat, etc., supplemented with massage and diet.

nau'sea. A feeling of the need to vomit.

  n. gravidarum, nausea occurring in pregnant women.

nau'seant. 1. Nauseating; inducing a feeling of the need to vomit. **2.** Any agent that induces nausea.

nau'seate. To cause a desire to vomit.

nau'seous. Relating to or causing nausea.

na'vel. Umbilicus; the depressed area of the abdominal wall, marking the site of attachment of the umbilical cord to the fetus.

navic'ular. Boat-shaped; see table of bones.

Nb. Chemical symbol of the element niobium.

NCI. Abbreviation for National Cancer Institute.

Nd. Chemical symbol of the element neodymium.

NE. Abbreviation for norepinephrine.

Ne. Chemical symbol of the element neon.

nearsight'edness. See myopia.

neb'ula. A slight opacity of the cornea.

nebuliza'tion. The process of converting a liquid into a fine spray.

neb'ulize. 1. To create a fine spray from a liquid. **2.** To medicate through a fine spray.

nebuliz'er. An apparatus for dispersing a liquid in the form of a fine spray.

Neca'tor. A genus of hookworms of the class Nematoda.

  N. americanus, a nematode parasite that produces the human hookworm disease (necatoriasis); also called "New World" hookworm, *Uncinaria americana,* and American hookworm.

necatori'asis. A human hookworm disease caused by the nematode parasite *Necator americanus.*

neck. 1. The part of the body between the head and the trunk. **2.** Any relatively constricted portion of a structure or organ. **3.** The germinative portion of an adult tapeworm; the region of cestode segmentation behind the scolex. **4.** The portion of a tooth between the crown and root.

  n. of womb, uterine cervix; see under cervix.

  stiff n., see torticollis.

  webbed n., one with lateral folds extending from the head to the clavicles, giving it a broad, short appearance.

necro-, necr-. Combining forms meaning dead.

necrobio'sis. The natural death of tissue with the concurrent replacement thereof.

  n. diabeticorum, a condition characterized by patchy degeneration of the skin in which fat tissue is extensively involved in the concurrent destructive and reparative process; usually, but not exclusively, associated with diabetes.

necrocyto'sis. The abnormal decomposition and death of cells.

necrogen'ic. Originating in dead matter.

necrol'ogy. 1. A record of people who have died, especially during a specific period of time. **2.** Obituary.

necrol'ysis. Loosening or separation of tissue due to death and decay of cells.

necroma'nia. Morbid interest in death or dead bodies.

necropar'asite. See saprophyte.

nec'rophile. One afflicted with necrophilia.

necrophil'ia. An abnormal fascination with the dead; especially erotic attraction on contact with

dead bodies, usually of males with female corpses.

necroph'ilous. Feeding on dead tissue; said of certain bacteria.

necropho'bia. A morbid fear of death or dead bodies.

nec'ropsy. See autopsy.

necros'copy. Autopsy.

nec'rose, nec'rotize. To cause or undergo irreversible damage, decomposition, and death; said of cells, tissues, and organs.

necro'sis. Death of tissue within a circumscribed area.

  acute tubular n. (ATN), a form of acute renal failure usually caused by a toxic agent or associated with a hypotensive period, especially from shock, sepsis, or trauma; characterized classically by absent or scanty urine followed by gradually increasing flow of dilute urine, often reaching very large amounts.

  aseptic n., necrosis occurring without infection. See also epiphyseal aseptic necrosis.

  caseous n., one in which the tissue becomes soft, dry, and cheeselike, as in the lesions of tuberculosis.

  central n., one involving the inner portion of a part, as necrosis in the cells surrounding the central veins of the liver.

  coagulation n., one induced by loss of arterial blood supply to a tissue, leading to denaturation and coagulation of cell protein.

  colliquative n., see liquefactive necrosis.

  cystic medial n., accumulation of mucopolysaccharide ground substance between connective tissue fibers of the middle layer of the aorta; also called medionecrosis of aorta and mucoid medial degeneration.

  epiphyseal aseptic n., a form of bone destruction most commonly occurring in the head of the femur (Legg-Perthes disease); also seen in the medial femoral condyle, the humeral head, and the tibial tubercle (Osgood-Schlatter disease); associated with systemic corticosteroid therapy, sickle cell disease, alcoholism, and other disorders; also called avascular necrosis.

  fat n., death of fatty tissue, characterized by the formation of small, white, chalky areas.

  liquefactive n., complete and rapid dissolution of cells (including cell membranes) by enzymes, forming circumscribed areas of softened tissue with a semifluid exudate; characteristic of abscesses and infarcts of the brain; also called colliquative necrosis.

  renal papillary n., ischemic necrosis of the renal papillae, usually occurring in patients with diabetes and pyelonephritis, in individuals who have habitually ingested large quantities of analgesic medicines,

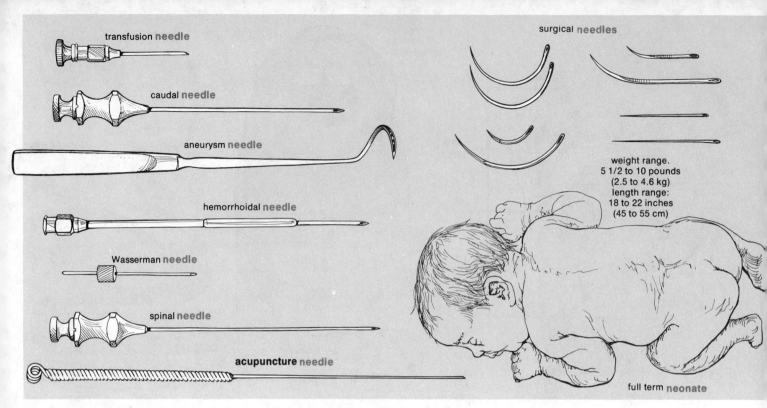

transfusion **needle**

caudal **needle**

aneurysm **needle**

hemorrhoidal **needle**

Wasserman **needle**

spinal **needle**

acupuncture needle

surgical **needles**

weight range.
5 1/2 to 10 pounds
(2.5 to 4.6 kg)
length range:
18 to 22 inches
(45 to 55 cm)

full term **neonate**

in sickle cell disease, and in the presence of obstructive uropathy and infection; also called necrolizing papillitis.

necrosper'mia. A condition in which the semen contains a high percentage of nonmotile sperm.

necrot'ic. Relating to dead tissue.

nec'rotize. See necrose.

necrot'omy. Surgical removal of a dead portion of a bone (sequestrum); also called necrectomy.

needle. 1. A slender, pointed implement for stitching or puncturing. 2. To separate tissues. 3. To puncture the lens capsule to allow absorption of the lens substance; a surgical procedure for the treatment of soft cataract.

  acupuncture n., a fine needle, usually three to five inches in length, used to perform acupuncture.

  atraumatic n., an eyeless surgical needle.

  exploring n., a grooved needle which is thrust into a tumor or cavity to determine the presence or absence of fluid.

  hypodermic n., a hollow needle for injecting fluids beneath the skin.

  lumbar puncture n., one designed for entering the spinal canal to remove cerebrospinal fluid or to introduce medication.

  Menghini n., one designed to obtain tissue, especially from the liver, for biopsy; the tissue core is obtained and held in with the aid of suction applied to the end of the needle.

  Vim-Silverman n., one provided with a stylet and tweezer-like cutters used to obtain tissue for biopsy.

need'ling. A surgical technique in which the lens capsule is punctured to permit absorption of a soft cataract.

NEFA. Abbreviation for nonesterified fatty acids.

neg'ative. 1. Absent; nonreactive; not indicative of the presence of a specific abnormal condition, such as a disorder, anomaly, or microorganism. 2. Denoting a quantity less than zero.

neg'ativism. Persistent opposition to suggestions or advice; a symptom of certain psychiatric disorders which also occurs normally in late infancy.

neg'atron. Electron.

Neisse'ria. A genus of bacteria (family Neisseriaceae) composed of small, gram-negative organisms occurring in pairs, each having a coffee-bean shape, flattened at the site of contact with its mate; parasitic (some pathogenic) in man.

  N. catarrhalis, nonpathogenic species found in the respiratory tract and saliva.

  N. gonorrhoeae, the cause of gonorrhea and ophthalmia neonatorum; formerly called *Diplococcus gonorrhoeae.*

  N. meningitidis, intracellular species, the cause of meningococcal meningitis.

nemathel'minth. A member of the phylum Nemathelminthes.

Nemathelmin'thes. A phylum of round worms, including the class Nematoda; characterized by cylindrical bodies with pointed ends.

nemato-. Combining form denoting (a) a threadlike structure; (b) a relationship to a nematode worm.

nemat'ocide. An agent that kills roundworms.

nem'atocyst. One of many minute stinging organelles in various marine coelenterates, such as sea nettle, Portuguese man-of-war, and hydra; when stimulated it ejects a potent venom.

Nemato'da. A class of round worms of the phylum Nemathelminthes, some species of which are parasitic in man.

ne'matode, ne'matoid. Any parasitic worm of the class Nematoda; also called roundworm.

nematodi'asis. Infestation with nematode or roundworm parasites.

ne'matoid. 1. Relating to a nematode worm. 2. Resembling a thread.

nematol'ogy. The science that deals with nematode worms.

neo-. Combining form meaning new.

neoarthro'sis. See pseudarthrosis.

neoblas'tic. Relating to or originating in new tissue.

neocerebel'lum. The lateral lobes of the cerebellum; so called because it is the last part of the cerebellum to develop.

neocinet'ic. Neokinetic.

neocor'tex. See isocortex.

neocystos'tomy. Surgical procedure whereby a ureter or a segment of the ileum is inserted into the bladder.

neocyto'sis. The presence of immature cells in the blood; also called skeocytosis.

neodym'ium. A silvery, rare-earth metallic element; symbol Nd, atomic number 60, atomic weight 144.27.

neogen'esis. Regeneration; new formation of tissue.

neokinet'ic. Denoting the area of the cerebral cortex that regulates motor activities.

neolal'ism. The use of neologisms.

neol'ogism. Any new word or phrase or old word used in a new way; the coining of bizarre neologisms is a common symptom among psychotic individuals.

neomem'brane. False membrane; see under membrane.

ne'omorph. 1. New formation; a part or organ that is not evolved from a similar structure in an ancestor. 2. A mutant gene producing an effect not produced by any nonmutant gene in the same locus.

ne'omycin. An antibacterial substance comprised of a group of organic complexes produced by the metabolism of the bacteria *Streptomyces fradiae*.

ne'on. A rare, inert, gaseous element in the atmosphere; symbol Ne, atomic number 10, atomic weight 20.183.

neona'tal. Pertaining to the first month of life.

ne'onate, neona'tus. A newborn.

neonatol'ogist. A specialist in neonatology.

neonatol'ogy. The study of the newborn; a subspecialty related to obstetrics, pediatrics, and fetal biology.

neopal'lium. See isocortex.

neopla'sia. The formation and growth of a tumor or new tissue.

ne'oplasm. The abnormal, excessive, and uncontrolled multiplication of cells with the formation of a mass or new growth of tissue; it may be localized (benign) or spreading and invasive (malignant); also called tumor. Cf hyperplasia and hypertrophy.

ne'oplasty. 1. Neoplasia. 2. Plastic surgery.

neos'tomy. Surgical creation of a new artificial opening.

nephelom'eter. An instrument for measuring the concentration of particles in suspension by means of reflected or transmitted light.

nephelom'etry. The estimation of the number of particles in a suspension with the aid of a nephelometer.

nephr-. See nephro-.

nephrecta'sia, nephrec'tasy. Dilatation of the pelvis of the kidney.

nephrec'tomy. Surgical removal of a kidney.

neph'ric. Renal; relating to the kidney.

nephrid'ium. One of the excretory tubules of invertebrates.

nephrit'ic. Afflicted with nephritis.

nephri'tis. Inflammation of the kidneys; a nonspecific term, often used to indicate glomerulonephritis or Bright's disease.

  acute n., acute glomerulonephritis; see under glomerulonephritis.

  acute interstitial n., acute inflammation of the interstitial tissues of the kidney, generally with involvement of the tubules and relative sparing of the glomeruli; commonly caused by reaction to a drug.

  Balkan n., a chronic progressive nephritis most commonly seen in Bulgaria, Rumania, and Yugoslavia.

  chronic n., chronic renal disease having a variety of etiologies; the term is most often used to refer to a form of chronic glomerulonephritis.

  chronic interstitial n., fibrotic interstitial tissue accompanied by chronic inflammatory cells; thought to be caused by many different agents,

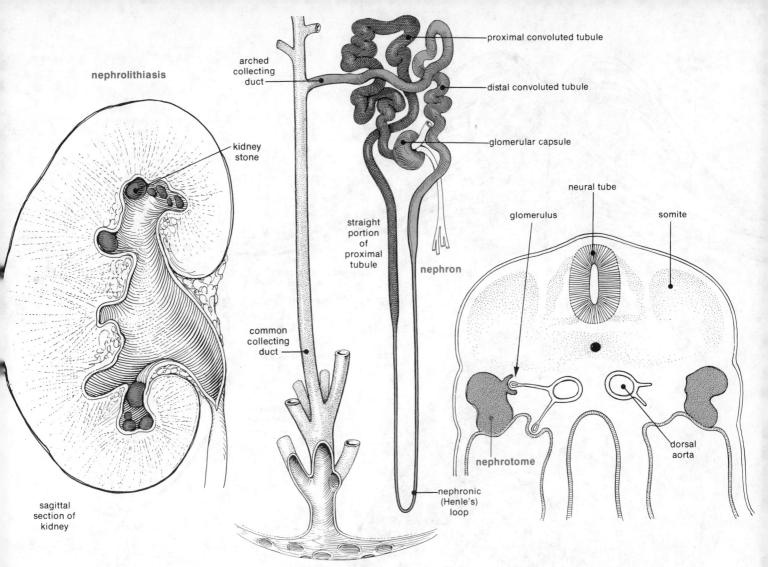

nephrolithiasis

kidney stone

sagittal section of kidney

arched collecting duct

proximal convoluted tubule

distal convoluted tubule

glomerular capsule

straight portion of proximal tubule

nephron

common collecting duct

nephronic (Henle's) loop

neural tube

glomerulus

somite

nephrotome

dorsal aorta

including chronic drug reaction, heavy metal toxicity, and gout.

Ellis type 1 n., acute glomerulonephritis; see under glomerulonephritis.

Ellis type 2 n., membranous glomerulonephritis; see under glomerulonephritis.

hereditary n., familial renal disease progressing to chronic renal failure; associated with nerve deafness; also called Alport's syndrome.

potassium-losing n., unusual potassium loss in the urine; may be seen, uncommonly, as a manifestation of renal tubular acidosis and chronic pyelonephritis.

salt-losing n., tendency of some individuals with chronic renal disease to excrete a high percentage of filtered sodium; most likely to occur with chronic pyelonephritis, polycystic kidneys, analgesic nephropathy, or medullary cystic disease.

nephritogen'ic. Producing nephritis.

nephro-, nephr-. Combining forms meaning kidney.

nephroblasto'ma. Wilm's tumor; see under tumor.

nephrocalcino'sis. Condition marked by calcifications scattered throughout the kidneys; also called renal calcinosis.

nephrogen'ic, nephrogenet'ic. Originating in the kidney.

neph'rogram. Roentgenogram of the kidney.

nephrog'raphy. Roentgenography of the kidney.

nephrohydro'sis. See hydronephrosis.

neph'roid. Resembling a kidney.

neph'rolith. Kidney stone.

nephrolithi'asis. Condition marked by the presence of stones in the kidney.

nephrolithot'omy. Cutting through the kidney for the removal of kidney stones.

nephrol'ogy. The study of the kidney and its diseases.

nephrol'ysin. An antibody that causes specific

destruction of kidney cells.

nephromala'cia. Softening of the kidneys.

neph'romere. In embryology, portion of the intermediate mesoderm from which the kidney develops.

neph'ron. The functional unit of the kidney, located mostly within the renal cortex; it consists of the glomerulus and its tubules up to the point where the tubule enters the common collecting duct; the parts include the glomerular (Bowman's) capsule, the proximal convoluted tubules, the straight portion of the proximal tubule (pars recta), the descending and ascending limbs of the nephronic (Henle's) loop, the distal convoluted tubule, and the arched collecting duct.

nephrop'athy. Any disease of the kidney.

neph'ropexy. Surgical fixation of a displaced kidney.

nephroph'thisis. 1. Suppurative inflammation with wasting of kidney substance. 2. Tuberculosis of the kidney.

nephropto'sia, nephropto'sis. Downward displacement of a kidney.

nephropyeli'tis. Inflammation of the renal pelvis.

nephropyeloplas'ty. Reparative surgery of the kidney pelvis.

nephropyo'sis. Suppuration of a kidney.

nephrorrhag'ia. Hemorrhage from or into the kidney.

nephrosclero'sis. Renal impairment secondary to arteriosclerosis or hypertension.

arteriolar n., renal changes associated with hypertension in which the arterioles thicken and the areas they supply undergo ischemic atrophy and interstitial fibrosis.

malignant n., rapid deterioration of renal function caused by inflammation of renal arterioles; it accompanies malignant hypertension.

nephrosclerot'ic. Relating to nephrosclerosis.

nephro'sis. General term denoting diseases of the

kidneys which were thought to involve primarily the tubules; noninflammatory disease of the kidneys.

lipoid n., a form of nephrotic syndrome in which minimal or no glomerular abnormalities are noted by light microscopy and the major abnormality on electron microscopy is fusion of epithelial foot processes; also called minimal change disease and idiopathic nephrotic syndrome.

lower nephron n., acute tubular necrosis.

sclerosing n., a condition marked by tubular necrosis, interstitial fibrosis, and sclerosis.

nephrospa'sia, nephros'pasis. Floating kidney; see under kidney.

neph'rostome, nephros'toma. In embryology, one of the ciliated funnels connecting the embryonic uriniferous tubules with the celomic cavity.

nephros'tomy. The creation of an opening in the kidney pelvis into which a tube is inserted to drain the kidney.

nephrot'ic. Of, relating to, or caused by nephrosis.

nephrotic syndrome. A clinical symptom complex caused by various kidney diseases; characterized by generalized edema, low plasma albumin concentration, and severe proteinuria; by far the most common cause is glomerulonephritis, a primary renal disease.

neph'rotome. The plate of embryonic mesenchyme of the somites of a vertebrate embryo from which the kidney tubules develop.

nephrotom'ogram. Sectional x rays (tomogram) of the kidney following injection of radiopaque material.

nephrotomog'raphy. X-ray examination of the kidney by means of tomography.

nephrot'omy. Incision of the kidney.

nephrotox'ic. Destructive to the cells of the kidney.

nephrotox'in. A particular substance (cytotoxin) that is destructive to kidney cells.

nephrotrop'ic. See renotrophic.

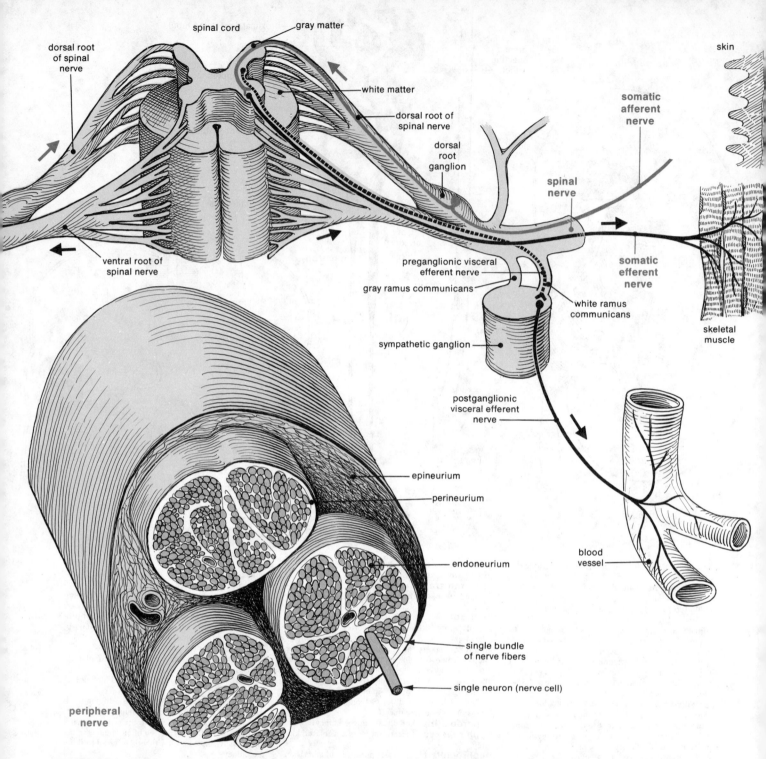

spinal cord

gray matter

dorsal root of spinal nerve

dorsal root of spinal nerve

dorsal root ganglion

white matter

skin

somatic afferent nerve

spinal nerve

ventral root of spinal nerve

preganglionic visceral efferent nerve

gray ramus communicans

sympathetic ganglion

somatic efferent nerve

white ramus communicans

skeletal muscle

postganglionic visceral efferent nerve

epineurium

perineurium

endoneurium

blood vessel

single bundle of nerve fibers

single neuron (nerve cell)

peripheral nerve

nephrotuberculo′sis. Tuberculosis of the kidney.

nephroureterec′tomy. Removal of a kidney with complete or partial removal of its ureter.

neptu′nium. A radioactive metallic element; symbol Np, atomic number 93, atomic weight 237; prepared artificially by the neutron bombardment of uranium atoms.

nerve. A cordlike structure of one or more fascicles of nerve tissue that carries impulses (messages) from the central nervous system (brain and spinal cord) to the various structures of the body and from the structures to the central nervous system. For specific nerves, see table of nerves.

accelerator n.'s, nerve fibers arising from the hypothalamus and brain stem which reach the heart via the cardiac nerves and increase the rate of its beat; they are part of the sympathetic division of the autonomic nervous system.

afferent n., a nerve that carries an impulse from the periphery to the central nervous system where it is interpreted into the consciousness of sensation; those arising from the skin, muscles, and joints are called somatic afferent; those from the viscera are known as visceral afferent.

augmentor n.'s, nerves that increase the force as well as the rate of the heart beat.

autonomic n., a bundle of nerve fibers relating to the activity of cardiac muscle, smooth muscle, and glands; they belong to the autonomic nervous system.

cranial n.'s, nerves directly connected with the brain. See table of nerves.

dead n., a misnomer for a functionless tooth pulp.

depressor n., a nerve which causes depression of a motor center, or one that reduces the function of an organ.

efferent n., a nerve that conveys impulses from the central nervous system to the periphery; those that terminate at skeletal muscles are called somatic efferent nerves; those that terminate at smooth muscles, cardiac muscles, and gland cells are called visceral efferent (autonomic) nerves.

inhibitory n., one that carries impulses which diminish functional activity of a structure.

mixed n., a nerve comprised both of afferent and efferent fibers.

motor n., efferent nerve.

peripheral n.'s, the cranial and spinal nerves with their branches; in general, they carry both afferent and efferent fibers.

pressor n., an afferent nerve which when stimulated excites vasoconstriction, thereby increasing blood pressure.

sensory n., afferent nerve.

somatic n., the afferent (sensory) and efferent (motor) nerves that innervate skeletal muscle and somatic tissue.

spinal n.'s, the thirty-one pairs of nerves directly connected with the spinal cord. See table of nerves.

vasomotor n., an efferent nerve that can cause blood vessels to dilate (vasodilator nerve) or to constrict (vasoconstrictor nerve).

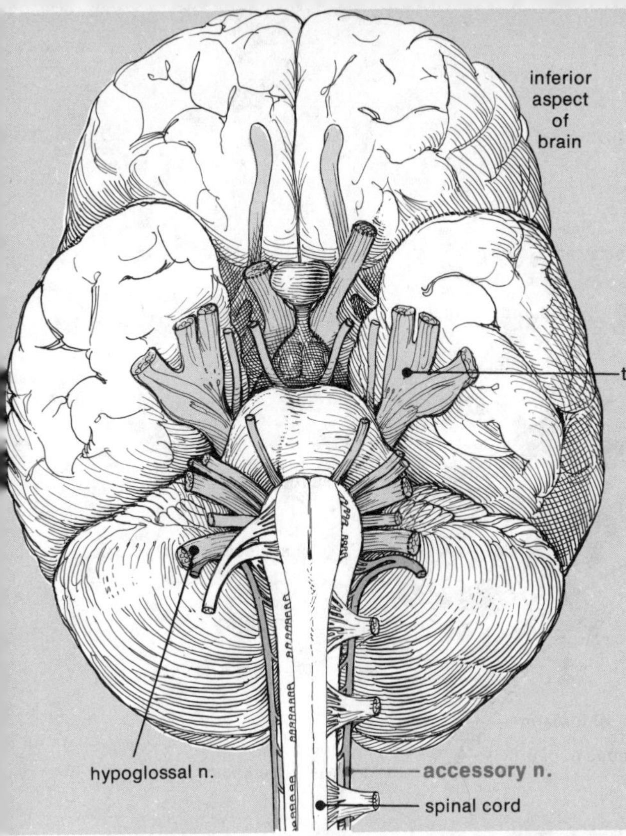

inferior aspect of brain

middle superior alveolar nn.

posterior superior alveolar nn.

infraorbital n.

trigeminal n.

maxillary n.

anterior superior alveolar nn.

mandibular n.

trigeminal n.

lingual n.

inferior alveolar n.

mylohyoid n.

hypoglossal n.

accessory n.

spinal cord

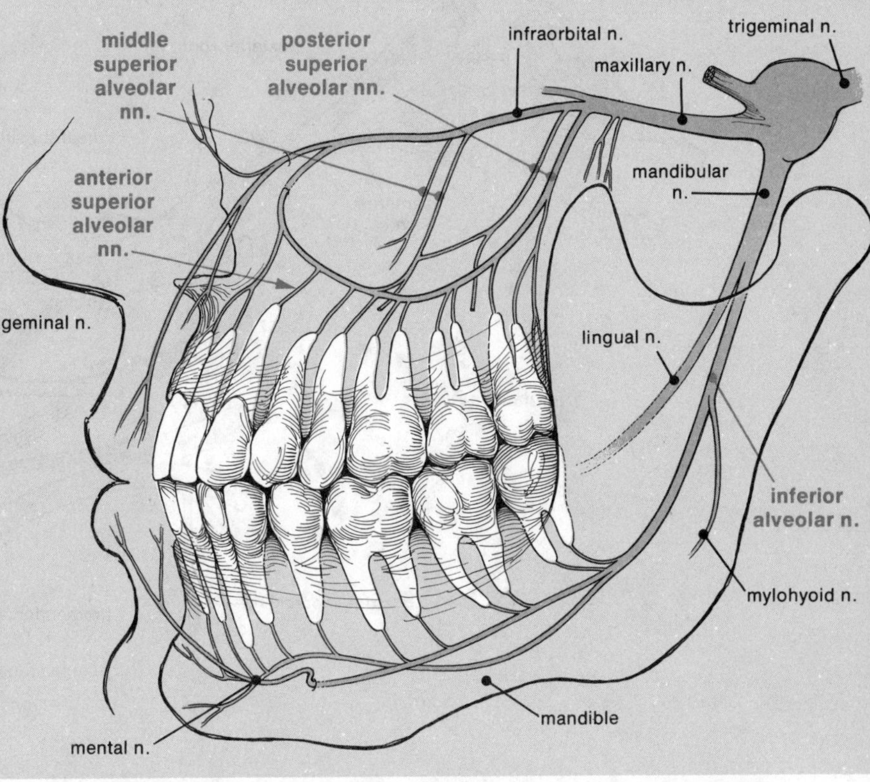

mental n.

mandible

NERVE	ORIGIN	BRANCHES	DISTRIBUTION
abducent n. sixth cranial n. *n. abducens*	brainstem at inferior border of pons	filaments	lateral rectus muscle of eyeball
accessory n. spinal accessory n. eleventh cranial n. *n. accessorius*	cranial part: side of medulla oblongata; spinal part: first five cervical segments of spinal cord	internal branch to vagus external branched to cervical plexus	striate muscles of larynx and pharynx sternocleidomastoid and trapezius muscles
acoustic n.	*see vestibulocochlear nerve*		
acoustic meatus n., external *n. meatus acustici externi*	auriculotemporal n.	filaments	external acoustic meatus
alveolar n.'s, anterior superior anterior superior dental n.'s *nn. alveolares anterior superior*	infraorbital n.	filaments	maxillary sinus, cuspid and incisors, superior dental plexus, floor of nose
alveolar n., inferior inferior dental n. *n. alveolaris inferior*	mandibular n.	mylohyoid, dental, incisive, mental	mylohyoid and anterior belly of digastric muscles, lower teeth, skin of chin, mucous membrane of lower lip
alveolar n.'s, middle superior middle superior dental n.'s *nn. alveolares superior medius*	infraorbital n.	filaments	maxillary sinus, superior dental plexus
alveolar n.'s, posterior superior posterior superior dental n.'s *nn. alveolares superior posterior*	maxillary	filaments	maxillary sinus, cheek, gums, molar and bicuspid teeth, superior dental plexus
ampullary n., anterior	*see ampullary nerve, superior*		
ampullary n., lateral *n. ampullaris lateralis*	vestibular n.	filaments	ampulla of lateral semicircular duct
ampullary n., posterior inferior ampullary n. *n. ampullaris posterior*	vestibular n.	filaments	ampulla of posterior semicircular duct
ampullary n., superior anterior ampullary n. *n. ampullaris superior*	vestibular n.	filaments	ampulla of superior semicircular duct
anococcygeal n.'s *nn. anococcygei*	coccygeal plexus	filaments	skin over the coccyx
ansa cervicalis ansa hypoglossi *ansa cervicalis*	branch from first cervical uniting with branches from second and third cervical segments of spinal cord	filaments	omohyoid, sternohyoid, and sternothyroid muscles

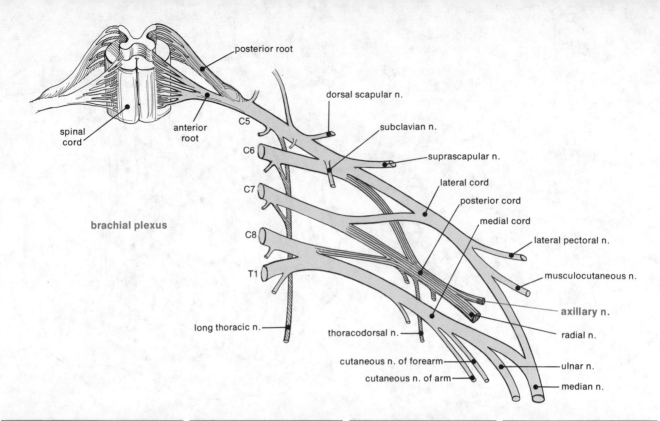

posterior root

dorsal scapular n.

subclavian n.

spinal cord

anterior root

C5

C6

suprascapular n.

C7

lateral cord

posterior cord

medial cord

brachial plexus

C8

lateral pectoral n.

T1

musculocutaneous n.

axillary n.

long thoracic n.

thoracodorsal n.

radial n.

cutaneous n. of forearm

ulnar n.

cutaneous n. of arm

median n.

NERVE	ORIGIN	BRANCHES	DISTRIBUTION
auditory n.	see vestibulocochlear nerve		
auricular n.'s, anterior (usually two in number) *nn. auriculares anterior*	auriculotemporal n.	filaments	skin of anterosuperior part of external ear, principally the helix and tragus
auricular n., great *n. auricularis magnus*	second and third cervical nerves	anterior, posterior	skin about ear, mastoid process and parotid gland
auricular n., posterior *n. auricularis posterior*	facial n.	auricular, occipital	posterior auricular and occipital muscles, skin of external ear
auriculotemporal n. *n. auriculotemporalis*	mandibular division of trigeminal n.	anterior auricular, external acoustic meatus, articular, parotid, superficial temporal, branches communicating with otic ganglion and facial n.	external meatus and skin of anterior superior part of auricle, temporomandibular joint, parotid gland, skin of temporal region
axillary n. circumflex n. *n. axillaris*	posterior cord of brachial plexus	posterior, anterior	deltoid and teres minor muscles, and neighboring skin
brachial plexus *plexus brachialis*	fifth to eighth cervical and first thoracic nerves	from cervical nerves: phrenic, muscular, accessory phrenic; from roots: dorsal scapular, long thoracic; from trunks: subclavius, suprascapular; from cords: pectoral, subscapular, thoracodorsal, axillary, medial cutaneous of forearm, medial cutaneous of arm; terminal nerves: musculocutaneous, median, ulnar, radial	upper limb
buccal n. buccinator n. long buccal n. *n. buccalis*	mandibular division of trigeminal n.	filaments, branches communicating with buccal branches of facial n.	skin of cheek, mucous membranes of mouth and gums
buccinator n.	see buccal nerve		
cardiac n., inferior cervical *n. cardiacus cervicalis inferior*	inferior cervical ganglion, first thoracic ganglion, stellate ganglion, or ansa subclavia	to cardiac plexus	heart

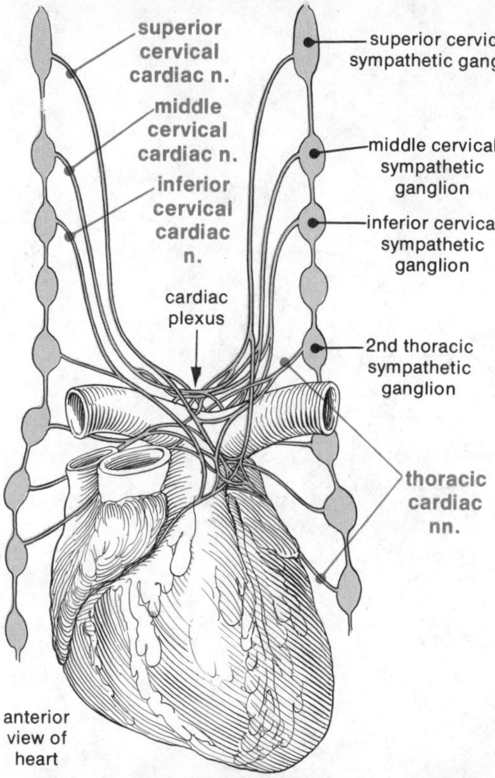

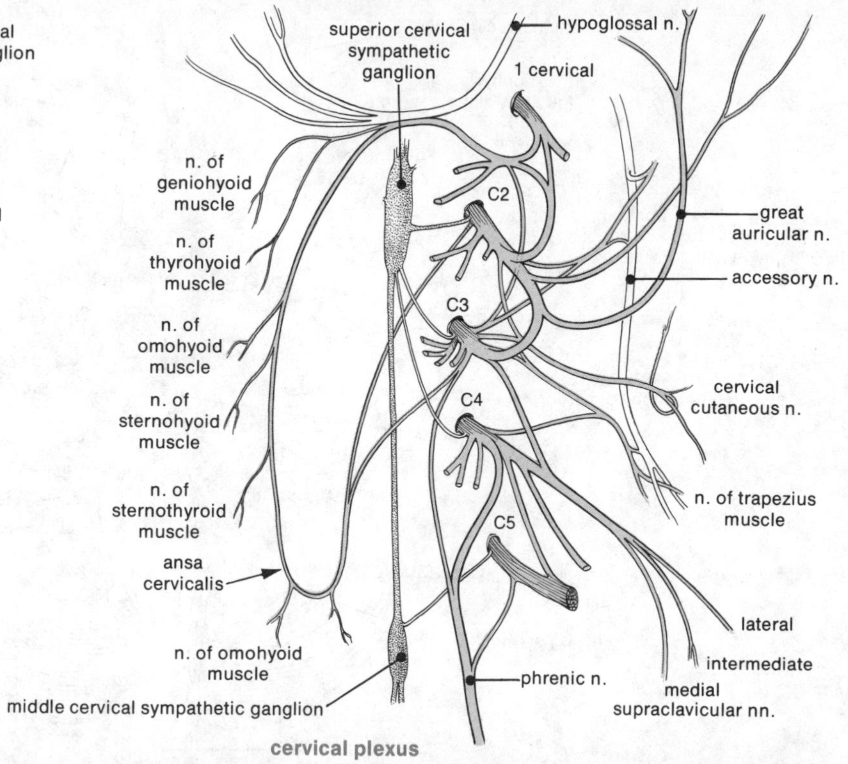

anterior view of heart

cervical plexus

NERVE	ORIGIN	BRANCHES	DISTRIBUTION
cardiac n., middle cervical great cardiac n. *n. cardiacus cervicalis medius*	middle cervical ganglion	to deep part of cardiac plexus	heart
cardiac n., superior cervical *n. cardiacus cervicalis superior*	lower part of superior cervical ganglion	to cardiac plexus	heart
cardiac n.'s, thoracic *nn. cardiaci thoracici*	second to fifth thoracic ganglion	to cardiac plexus	heart
caroticotympanic n.'s *nn. caroticotympanici*	superior cervical sympathetic ganglion	filaments	middle ear chamber, auditory tube
carotid n.'s, external *nn. carotici externi*	superior cervical ganglion	filaments	external carotid plexus, cranial blood vessels, smooth muscles and glands of head
carotid n., internal *n. caroticus internus*	cephalic end of superior cervical ganglion	medial, lateral	internal carotid plexus, cranial blood vessels, smooth muscle glands of head, cavernous plexus
carotid sinus n. carotid n. *n. caroticus*	glossopharyngeal n. just beyond its emergence from the jugular foramen	filaments	nodose ganglion, carotid sinus, carotid body
cavernous n. of clitoris, greater *n. cavernosus clitoridis major*	uterovaginal plexus	filaments	corpus cavernosum of clitoris
cavernous n.'s of clitoris, lesser *nn. cavernosi clitorides minor*	uterovaginal plexus	filaments	erectile tissue of clitoris
cavernous n. of penis, greater *n. cavernosus penis major*	prostatic plexus	filaments	corpus cavernosum of penis
cavernous n.'s of penis, lesser *nn. cavernosi penis minor*	prostatic plexus	filaments	corpus spongiosum of penis and penile urethra
cervical n.'s (eight pairs of spinal nerves) *nn. cervicales*	cervical segments of spinal cord	filaments	cervical plexus and brachial plexus
cervical plexus *plexus cervicalis*	first to fourth cervical nerves	cutaneous branches: lesser occipital, great auricular, anterior cutaneous, supraclavicular; muscular branches: anterior and lateral rectae of head, long muscles of head and neck, geniohyoid, thyrohyoid, and omohyoid (superior belly), sternohyoid, and	muscles and skin of neck and upper back; diaphragm

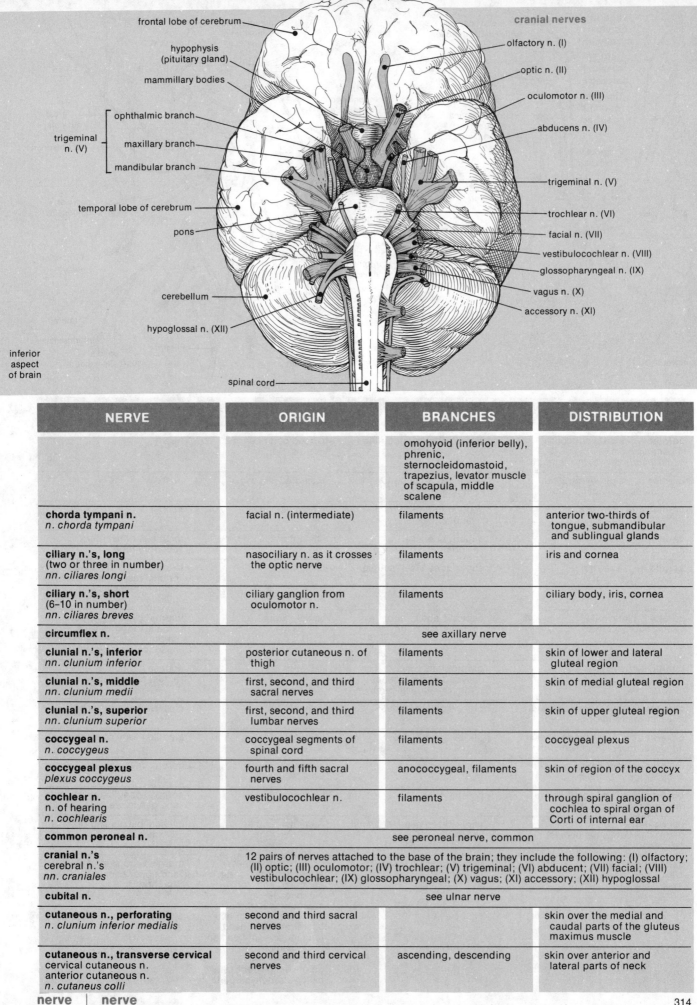

frontal lobe of cerebrum

cranial nerves

hypophysis
(pituitary gland)

mammillary bodies

olfactory n. (I)

optic n. (II)

oculomotor n. (III)

abducens n. (IV)

trigeminal
n. (V)
- ophthalmic branch
- maxillary branch
- mandibular branch

trigeminal n. (V)

temporal lobe of cerebrum

trochlear n. (VI)

pons

facial n. (VII)

vestibulocochlear n. (VIII)

glossopharyngeal n. (IX)

cerebellum

vagus n. (X)

accessory n. (XI)

hypoglossal n. (XII)

inferior
aspect
of brain

spinal cord

NERVE	ORIGIN	BRANCHES	DISTRIBUTION
		omohyoid (inferior belly), phrenic, sternocleidomastoid, trapezius, levator muscle of scapula, middle scalene	
chorda tympani n. *n. chorda tympani*	facial n. (intermediate)	filaments	anterior two-thirds of tongue, submandibular and sublingual glands
ciliary n.'s, long (two or three in number) *nn. ciliares longi*	nasociliary n. as it crosses the optic nerve	filaments	iris and cornea
ciliary n.'s, short (6–10 in number) *nn. ciliares breves*	ciliary ganglion from oculomotor n.	filaments	ciliary body, iris, cornea
circumflex n.	see axillary nerve		
clunial n.'s, inferior *nn. clunium inferior*	posterior cutaneous n. of thigh	filaments	skin of lower and lateral gluteal region
clunial n.'s, middle *nn. clunium medii*	first, second, and third sacral nerves	filaments	skin of medial gluteal region
clunial n.'s, superior *nn. clunium superior*	first, second, and third lumbar nerves	filaments	skin of upper gluteal region
coccygeal n. *n. coccygeus*	coccygeal segments of spinal cord	filaments	coccygeal plexus
coccygeal plexus *plexus coccygeus*	fourth and fifth sacral nerves	anococcygeal, filaments	skin of region of the coccyx
cochlear n. n. of hearing *n. cochlearis*	vestibulocochlear n.	filaments	through spiral ganglion of cochlea to spiral organ of Corti of internal ear
common peroneal n.	see peroneal nerve, common		
cranial n.'s cerebral n.'s *nn. craniales*	12 pairs of nerves attached to the base of the brain; they include the following: (I) olfactory; (II) optic; (III) oculomotor; (IV) trochlear; (V) trigeminal; (VI) abducent; (VII) facial; (VIII) vestibulocochlear; (IX) glossopharyngeal; (X) vagus; (XI) accessory; (XII) hypoglossal		
cubital n.	see ulnar nerve		
cutaneous n., perforating *n. clunium inferior medialis*	second and third sacral nerves		skin over the medial and caudal parts of the gluteus maximus muscle
cutaneous n., transverse cervical cervical cutaneous n. anterior cutaneous n. *n. cutaneus colli*	second and third cervical nerves	ascending, descending	skin over anterior and lateral parts of neck

nerve | nerve

314

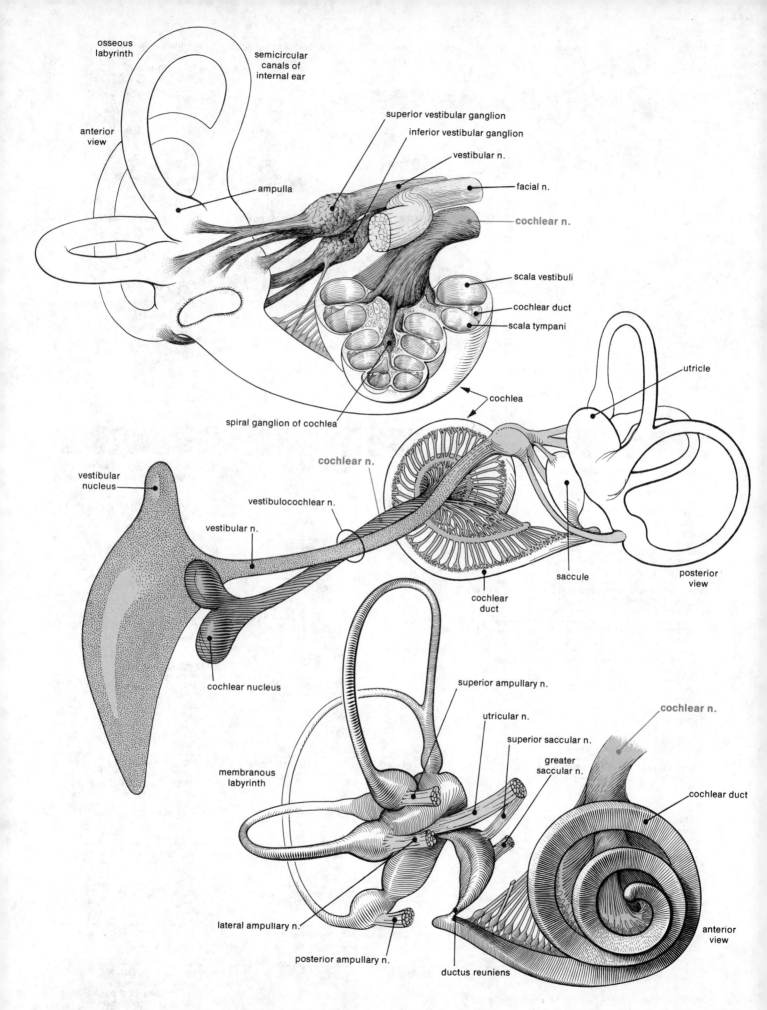

osseous labyrinth

semicircular canals of internal ear

anterior view

ampulla

superior vestibular ganglion

inferior vestibular ganglion

vestibular n.

facial n.

cochlear n.

scala vestibuli

cochlear duct

scala tympani

cochlea

spiral ganglion of cochlea

utricle

vestibular nucleus

cochlear n.

vestibulocochlear n.

vestibular n.

saccule

posterior view

cochlear nucleus

cochlear duct

superior ampullary n.

utricular n.

superior saccular n.

greater saccular n.

cochlear n.

cochlear duct

membranous labyrinth

lateral ampullary n.

posterior ampullary n.

ductus reuniens

anterior view

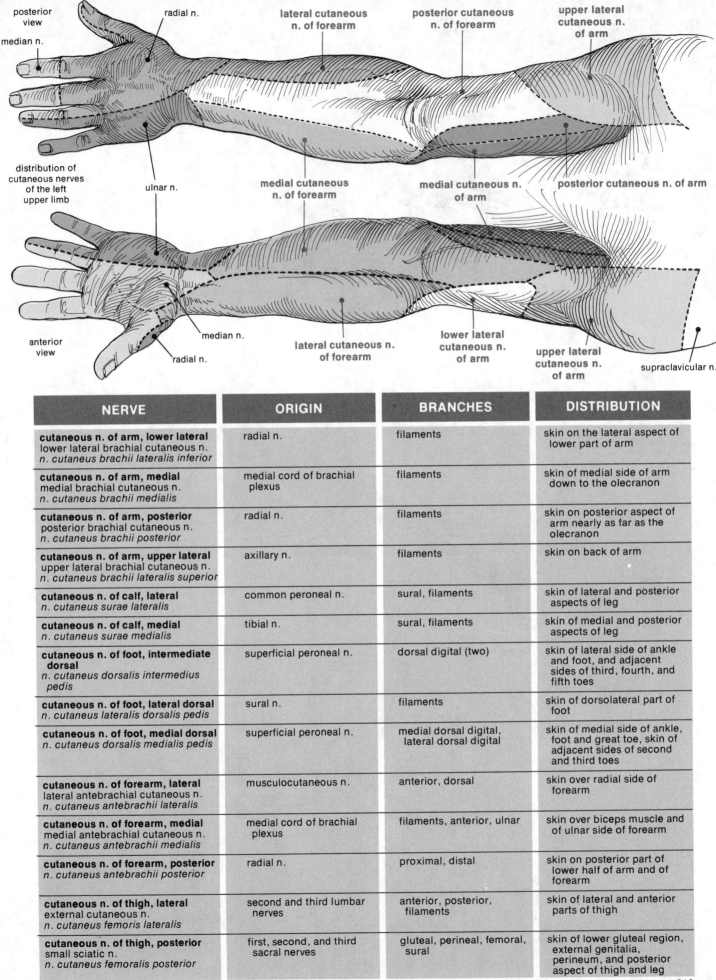

posterior view

median n.

radial n.

lateral cutaneous n. of forearm

posterior cutaneous n. of forearm

upper lateral cutaneous n. of arm

distribution of cutaneous nerves of the left upper limb

ulnar n.

medial cutaneous n. of forearm

medial cutaneous n. of arm

posterior cutaneous n. of arm

anterior view

median n.

radial n.

lateral cutaneous n. of forearm

lower lateral cutaneous n. of arm

upper lateral cutaneous n. of arm

supraclavicular n.

NERVE	ORIGIN	BRANCHES	DISTRIBUTION
cutaneous n. of arm, lower lateral lower lateral brachial cutaneous n. *n. cutaneus brachii lateralis inferior*	radial n.	filaments	skin on the lateral aspect of lower part of arm
cutaneous n. of arm, medial medial brachial cutaneous n. *n. cutaneus brachii medialis*	medial cord of brachial plexus	filaments	skin of medial side of arm down to the olecranon
cutaneous n. of arm, posterior posterior brachial cutaneous n. *n. cutaneus brachii posterior*	radial n.	filaments	skin on posterior aspect of arm nearly as far as the olecranon
cutaneous n. of arm, upper lateral upper lateral brachial cutaneous n. *n. cutaneus brachii lateralis superior*	axillary n.	filaments	skin on back of arm
cutaneous n. of calf, lateral *n. cutaneus surae lateralis*	common peroneal n.	sural, filaments	skin of lateral and posterior aspects of leg
cutaneous n. of calf, medial *n. cutaneus surae medialis*	tibial n.	sural, filaments	skin of medial and posterior aspects of leg
cutaneous n. of foot, intermediate dorsal *n. cutaneus dorsalis intermedius pedis*	superficial peroneal n.	dorsal digital (two)	skin of lateral side of ankle and foot, and adjacent sides of third, fourth, and fifth toes
cutaneous n. of foot, lateral dorsal *n. cutaneus lateralis dorsalis pedis*	sural n.	filaments	skin of dorsolateral part of foot
cutaneous n. of foot, medial dorsal *n. cutaneus dorsalis medialis pedis*	superficial peroneal n.	medial dorsal digital, lateral dorsal digital	skin of medial side of ankle, foot and great toe, skin of adjacent sides of second and third toes
cutaneous n. of forearm, lateral lateral antebrachial cutaneous n. *n. cutaneus antebrachii lateralis*	musculocutaneous n.	anterior, dorsal	skin over radial side of forearm
cutaneous n. of forearm, medial medial antebrachial cutaneous n. *n. cutaneus antebrachii medialis*	medial cord of brachial plexus	filaments, anterior, ulnar	skin over biceps muscle and of ulnar side of forearm
cutaneous n. of forearm, posterior *n. cutaneus antebrachii posterior*	radial n.	proximal, distal	skin on posterior part of lower half of arm and of forearm
cutaneous n. of thigh, lateral external cutaneous n. *n. cutaneus femoris lateralis*	second and third lumbar nerves	anterior, posterior, filaments	skin of lateral and anterior parts of thigh
cutaneous n. of thigh, posterior small sciatic n. *n. cutaneus femoralis posterior*	first, second, and third sacral nerves	gluteal, perineal, femoral, sural	skin of lower gluteal region, external genitalia, perineum, and posterior aspect of thigh and leg

nerve | nerve

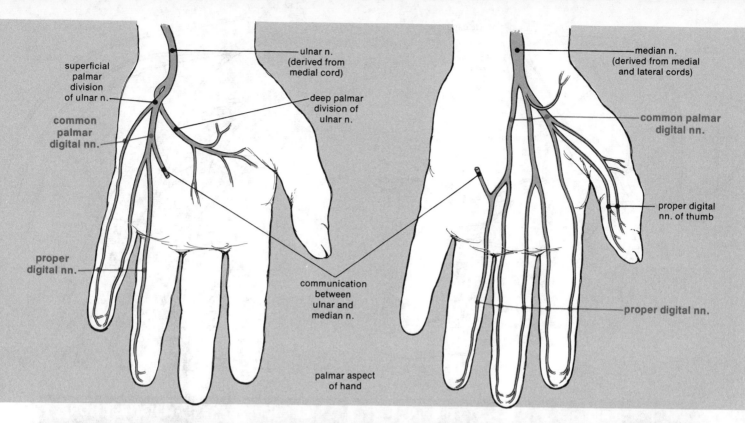

superficial
palmar
division
of ulnar n.

common
palmar
digital nn.

proper
digital nn.

ulnar n.
(derived from
medial cord)

deep palmar
division of
ulnar n.

communication
between
ulnar and
median n.

palmar aspect
of hand

median n.
(derived from medial
and lateral cords)

common palmar
digital nn.

proper digital
nn. of thumb

proper digital nn.

NERVE	ORIGIN	BRANCHES	DISTRIBUTION
dental n.'s		see alveolar nerves	
digital n.'s, common palmar *nn. digitales palmares communes*	median n. ulnar n.	proper digitals	palmar skin of palmar surface and sides of digits, lumbrical muscles
digital n.'s, proper digital collaterals *nn. digitales proprii*	common palmar digital nerves		skin of palmar surface and dorsal surface over terminal phalanx of the digits
digital n.'s of foot, dorsal *nn. digitales dorsales pedis*	intermediate dorsal cutaneous n. of foot	filaments	dorsal aspect of toes
digital n.'s of lateral plantar n., common plantar *nn. digitales plantares communes nervi plantaris lateralis*	superficial branch of lateral plantar n.	proper plantar	plantar aspect of lateral toes
digital n.'s lateral plantar n., proper plantar *nn. digitales plantares proprii nervi plantaris lateralis*	common plantar digital nerves of lateral plantar nerve	filaments	plantar aspect of lateral toes
digital n.'s of lateral side of great toe and medial side of second toe *nn. digitales dorsales hallucis lateralis et digiti secundi medialis*	deep peroneal n.	filaments	adjacent sides of great and second toes
digital n.'s of medial plantar n. common plantar *nn. digitales plantares communes nervi plantaris medialis*	medial plantar n.	proper plantar	plantar aspect of medial toes
digital n.'s of medial plantar n., proper plantar *nn. digitales plantares proprii nervi plantaris medialis*	common plantar	filaments	plantar aspect of medial toes
digital n.'s of radial n., dorsal *nn. digitales dorsales nervi radialis*	superficial branch of radial n.	filaments	skin of dorsum of lateral fingers
digital n.'s of ulnar n., common palmar *nn. digitales palmares communes nervi ulnaris*	superficial branch of palmar branch of ulnar n.	proper palmar	skin of palmar surface of little and ring fingers
digital n.'s of ulnar n., dorsal *nn. digitales dorsales nervi ulnaris*	dorsal branch of ulnar n.	filaments	skin of dorsum of medial fingers
digital n.'s of ulnar, proper palmar *nn. digitales palmares proprii nervi ulnaris*	common palmar digital nerves of ulnar	filaments	palmar surface of little and ring fingers

nerve | nerve

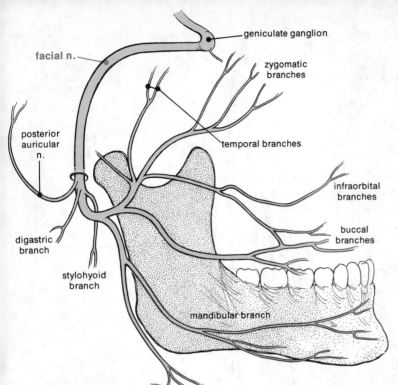

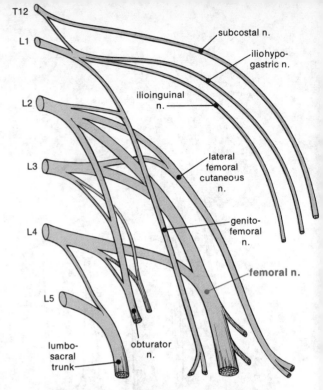

NERVE	ORIGIN	BRANCHES	DISTRIBUTION
dorsal n. of clitoris n. dorsalis clitoridis	pudendal n.	filaments	urethra and clitoris
dorsal n. of penis n. dorsalis penis	pudendal n.	filaments	urethra and penis
dorsal scapular n.	see scapular nerve, dorsal		
eighth cranial n.	see vestibulocochlear nerve		
eleventh cranial n.	see accessory nerve		
ethmoid n., anterior n. ethmoidalis anterior	nasociliary n.	internal, external, lateral, and medial nasal	mucous membrane of nasal cavity
ethmoid n., posterior n. ethmoidalis posterior	nasociliary n.	filaments	mucous membrane of posterior ethmoidal and sphenoidal sinuses
facial n. seventh cranial n. n. facialis	lower border of pons	petrosal, to tympanic plexus, stapedial, chorda tympani, muscular, auricular, temporal zygomatic, buccal, mandibular, cervical	motor part: muscles of facial expression, scalp, external ear, buccinator, platysma, stapedius, stylohyoid, and posterior belly of digastric; sensory part: anterior two-thirds of tongue, parts of external acoustic meatus, soft palate, and adjacent pharynx; parasympathetic part: secretomotor fibers of submandibular, sublingual, lacrimal, nasal, and palatine glands
femoral n. anterior crural n. n. femoralis	second, third, and fourth lumbar nerves	articular, muscular, saphenous, anterior cutaneous	skin of anterior and medial side of leg, hip and knee joint, quadriceps muscle of thigh, pectineal, sartorius, and iliac muscles
fifth cranial n.	see trigeminal nerve		
first cranial n.	see olfactory nerve		
fourth cranial n.	see trochlear nerve		
frontal n. n. frontalis	ophthalmic n.	supraorbital, supratrochlear, frontal sinus	conjunctiva, skin of upper eyelid and forehead, corrugator and frontal muscles, scalp, frontal sinus
n. of geniohyoid n. geniohyoideus	hypoglossal n.	filaments	geniohyoid muscle

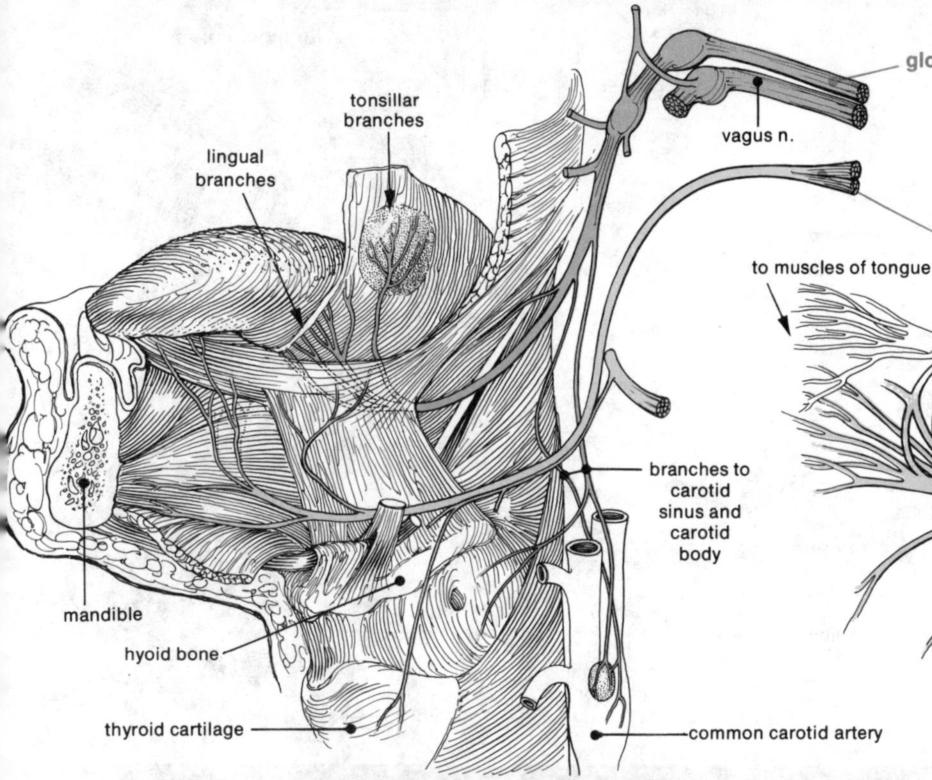

tonsillar branches
lingual branches
glossopharyngeal n.
vagus n.
hypoglossal canal through occipital bone
hypoglossal n.
to muscles of tongue
lingual n.
C1
C2
cervical ventral rami
C3
branches to carotid sinus and carotid body
mandible
hyoid bone
thyroid cartilage
common carotid artery
ansa cervicalis

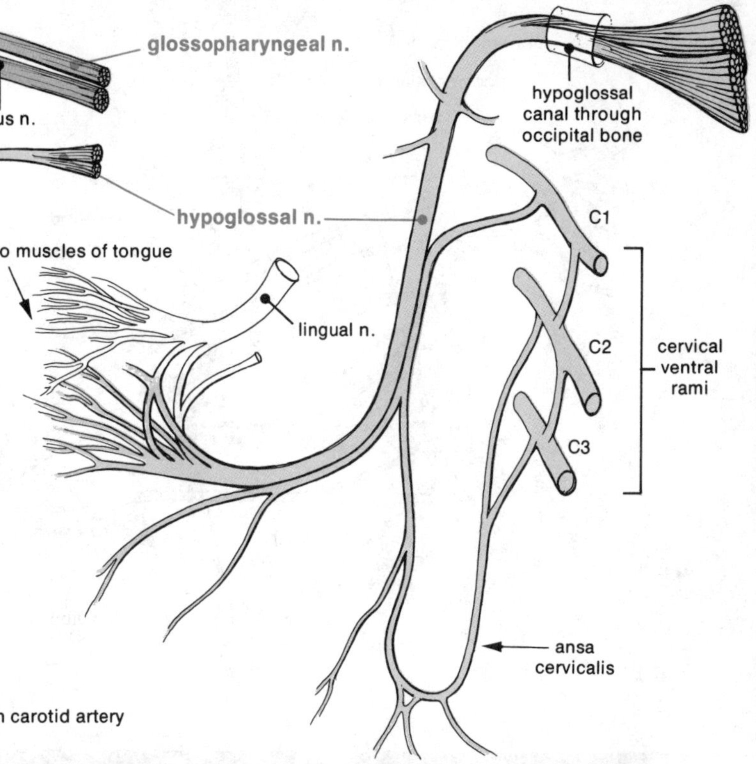

NERVE	ORIGIN	BRANCHES	DISTRIBUTION
genitofemoral n. genitocrural n. *n. genitofemoralis*	first and second lumbar nerves	genital, femoral	cremaster muscle, skin of scrotum or labium major and adjacent thigh, proximal part of anterior surface of thigh
glossopalatine n.	see intermediate nerve		
glossopharyngeal n. ninth cranial n. *n. glossopharyngeus*	upper part of medulla oblongata	tympanic, carotid sinus, pharyngeal, stylopharyngeal, tonsillar, lingual	tongue and pharynx, fauces, palatine tonsil, blood pressure receptor of the carotid sinus, stylopharyngeus muscle
gluteal n., inferior *n. gluteus inferior*	fifth lumbar nerve and first and second sacral nerves		gluteus maximus muscle
gluteal n., superior *n. gluteus superior*	fourth and fifth lumbar nerves and first sacral nerve	superior, inferior, filaments	gluteus minimus and medius muscle, tensor muscle of fascia lata
hemorrhoidal n.	see rectal nerve, inferior		
hemorrhoidal n., middle *n. hemorrhoidalis medius*	pudendal plexus	filaments	rectum
hemorrhoidal n., superior *n. hemorrhoidalis superior*	hypogastric plexus	filaments	rectum
hypogastric n. *n. hypogastricus*	a single large nerve (or several parallel bundles) which interconnects the superior hypogastric plexus with the inferior hypogastric plexus		
hypoglossal n. twelfth cranial n. *n. hypoglossus*	series of rootlets between the pyramid and olive of the medulla oblongata	meningeal, descending hypoglossal, thyrohyoid, geniohyoid, muscular	intrinsic and extrinsic muscles of the tongue; dura mater
hypoglossal n., small	see lingual nerve		
iliohypogastric n. *n. iliohypogastricus*	first lumbar n.	lateral, anterior cutaneous, muscular	abdominal muscles, skin of lower part of abdomen and gluteal region
ilioinguinal n. *n. ilioinguinalis*	first lumbar n.	anterior scrotal (male), anterior labial (female), muscular, filaments	muscles of abdominal wall, skin of proximal and medial part of thigh, root of penis (male), mons pubis and labium major (female)
infraoccipital n.	see suboccipital nerve		
infraorbital n. *n. infraorbitalis*	maxillary n.	inferior palpebral, external nasal, superior labial, middle and superior alveolar	upper teeth, skin of face, mucous membrane of mouth and floor of nasal cavity

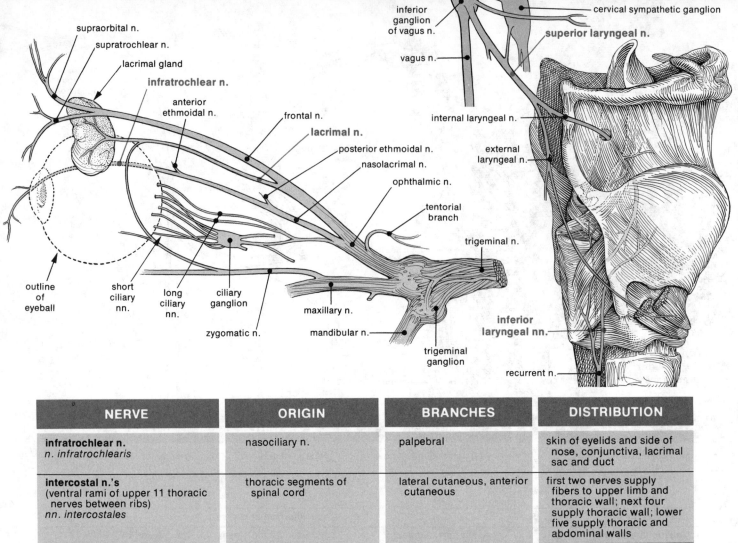

NERVE	ORIGIN	BRANCHES	DISTRIBUTION
infratrochlear n. *n. infratrochlearis*	nasociliary n.	palpebral	skin of eyelids and side of nose, conjunctiva, lacrimal sac and duct
intercostal n.'s (ventral rami of upper 11 thoracic nerves between ribs) *nn. intercostales*	thoracic segments of spinal cord	lateral cutaneous, anterior cutaneous	first two nerves supply fibers to upper limb and thoracic wall; next four supply thoracic wall; lower five supply thoracic and abdominal walls
intercostobrachial n. *n. intercostobrachialis*	second and frequently third intercostal n.	filaments	skin of medial and posterior part of arm; axilla
intermediate n. glossopalatine n n. of Wrisberg *n. intermedius*	brainstem at inferior border of pons	greater petrosal, chorda tympani	taste buds of anterior two-thirds of tongue, glands of soft palate and nose, submandibular and sublingual glands, skin of external acoustic meatus and mastoid process
interosseous n. of forearm, anterior *n. interosseus antebrachii anterior*	median n.		most of the deep anterior muscles of forearm
interosseous n. of forearm, posterior *n. interosseus antebrachii posterior*	deep branch of radial n.	muscular, articular	wrist and intercarpal joints, deep extensor muscles of forearm, long abductor and extensor muscles of thumb
interosseous n. of leg *n. interosseus cruris*	tibial n.	filaments	ankle joints
jugular n. *n. jugularis*	superior cervical ganglion	filaments	to glossopharyngeal and vagus nerves
labial n.'s, anterior *nn. labiales anterior*	ilioinguinal n.	filaments	skin of anterior labial area of female genitalia
labial n.'s, posterior *nn. labiales posterior*	perineal n.	filaments	skin of posterior portion of labia and vestibule of vagina
lacrimal n. *n. lacrimalis*	ophthalmic n.	superior palpebral, glandular, filaments	lacrimal gland and adjacent conjunctiva, skin of upper eyelid
laryngeal nn., inferior *nn. laryngeii inferior*	recurrent laryngeal n.	filaments	all intrinsic muscles of larynx except cricothyroid muscle
laryngeal n., superior *n. laryngeus superior*	vagus n. near the inferior ganglion	external, internal	mucous membrane of the larynx and epiglottis; inferior pharyngeal and cricothyroid muscles

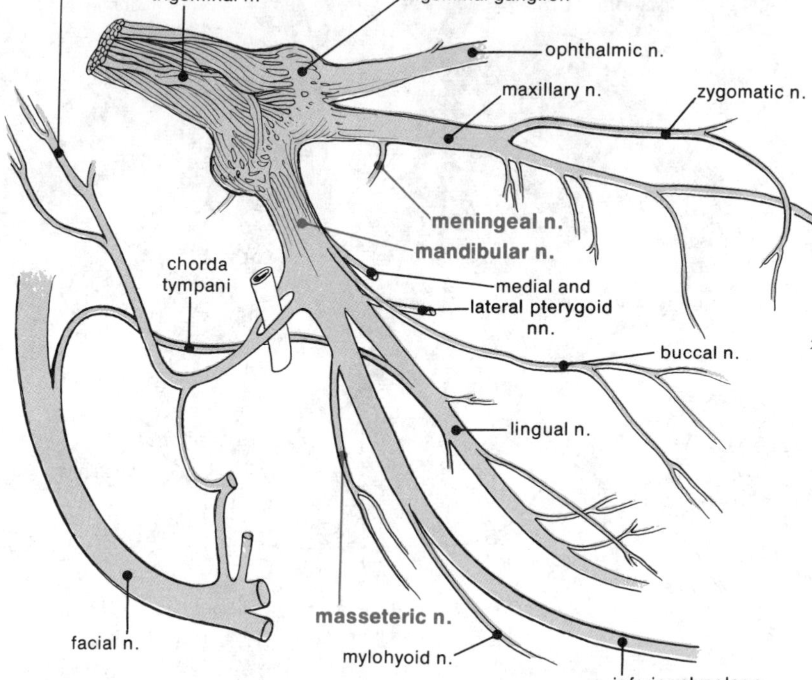

auriculotemporal n.
trigeminal n.
trigeminal ganglion
ophthalmic n.
maxillary n.
zygomatic n.
meningeal n.
mandibular n.
chorda tympani
medial and lateral pterygoid nn.
buccal n.
lingual n.
facial n.
masseteric n.
mylohyoid n.
inferior alveolar n.
median n. 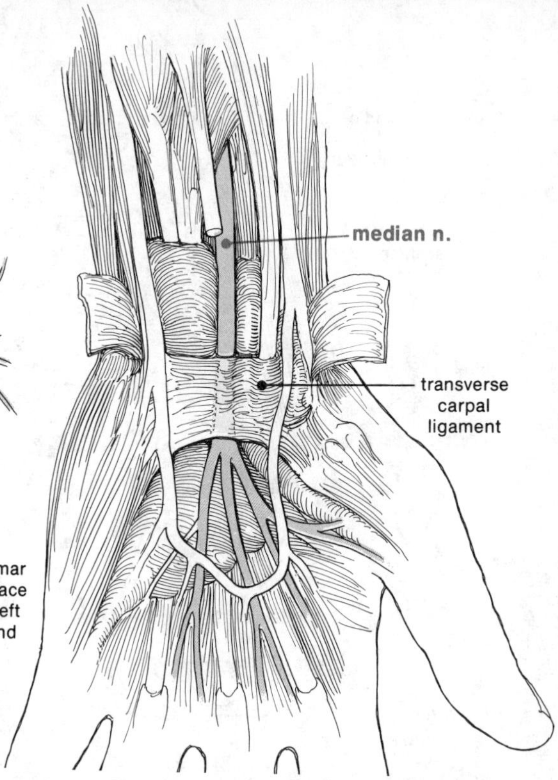
transverse carpal ligament
palmar surface of left hand

NERVE	ORIGIN	BRANCHES	DISTRIBUTION
laryngeal recurrent n.	see recurrent nerve		
lingual n. small hypoglossal n. *n. lingualis*	mandibular division of trigeminal n.	sublingual, branches communicating with hypoglossal n., chorda tympani, and submandibular ganglion	mucous membranes of anterior two-thirds of tongue, floor of mouth, gums, and sublingual glands
lumbar n.'s (five pairs of spinal nerves) *nn. lumbales*	lumbar segments of spinal cord	ventral, dorsal	lumbar plexus, deep muscles and skin of lower back
mandibular n. inferior maxillary n. *n. mandibularis*	trigeminal ganglion	masseteric, medial pterygoid, lateral pterygoid, deep temporal, buccal, auriculotemporal, lingual, inferior alveolar, meningeal	muscles of mastication, tensor tympani, palatal velum, anterior belly of digastric, and mylohyoid muscles, mandible, lower teeth and gums, anterior two-thirds of tongue, cheek, lower face, meninges, temporomandibular joint, skin of temporal region, external ear
masseteric n. *n. massetericus*	mandibular n.	filaments	masseter muscle, temporomandibular joint
maxillary n. superior maxillary n. *n. maxillaris*	trigeminal ganglion	middle meningeal, zygomatic, pterygopalatine, posterior superior alveolar, middle superior alveolar, anterior superior alveolar, inferior palpebral, external nasal, superior labial, infraorbital	skin of middle part of face, nose, lower eyelid, and upper lip; upper teeth and gums, tonsil and roof of mouth, soft palate, maxillary sinus, mucous membrane of nasopharynx
median n. *n. medianus*	by two roots from the medial and lateral cords of the brachial plexus	muscular, digital, articular, anterior interosseous, common palmar digitals, proper digital	most of flexor muscles of forearm, short muscles of thumb, lateral lumbricals, skin of hand, hand joints, elbow joint, pulp under nails
meningeal n. *n. meningeus*	vagus	filaments	meninges
meningeal n., middle *n. meningeus medius*	maxillary n.	filaments	meninges, especially the dura mater
mental n. *n. mentalis*	inferior alveolar n.	filaments	skin of chin, mucous membrane of lower lip

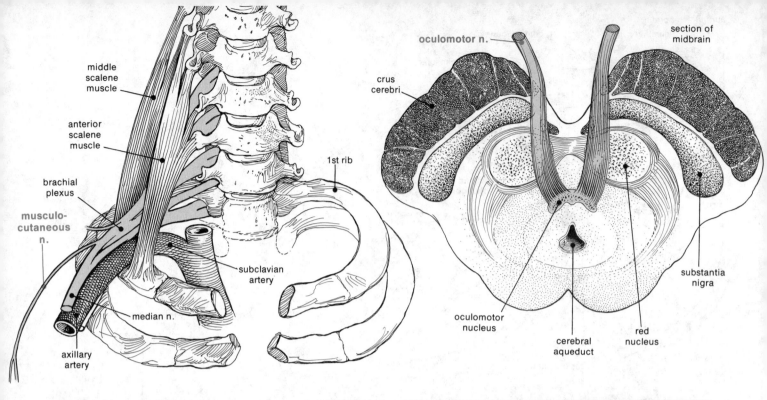

Labels for the first illustration: middle scalene muscle, anterior scalene muscle, brachial plexus, **musculo-cutaneous n.**, median n., axillary artery, 1st rib, subclavian artery.

Labels for the second illustration: oculomotor n., crus cerebri, section of midbrain, oculomotor nucleus, cerebral aqueduct, red nucleus, substantia nigra.

NERVE	ORIGIN	BRANCHES	DISTRIBUTION
musculocutaneous n. *n. musculocutaneus*	lateral cord of brachial plexus	muscular, articular filament, humeral filament, lateral cutaneous n. of forearm	coracobrachialis, brachialis and biceps muscles; skin of lateral side of forearm
musculospiral n.	see radial nerve		
mylohyoid n. *n. mylohyoideus*	inferior alveolar n. just before it enters mandibular foramen	filaments	mylohyoid and anterior belly of digastric muscles
nasal n.'s, external *nn. nasales externi*	infraorbital n.	filaments	skin on side of nose
nasociliary n. nasal n. *n. nasociliaris*	ophthalmic n.	long ciliary, anterior ethmoidal, posterior ethmoidal, infratrochlear, communication with ciliary ganglion	mucous membranes of nasal cavity, anterior ethmoidal and frontal sinuses; iris, cornea, conjunctiva, lacrimal sac, skin of eyelids and side of nose
nasopalatine n. Scarpa's n. *n. nasopalatinus*	pterygopalatine ganglion	filaments	mucous membrane of hard palate and nasal septum
ninth cranial n.	see glossopharyngeal nerve		
obturator n. *n. obturatorius*	second, third, and fourth lumbar nerves	anterior, posterior, filaments	hip and knee joints, skin of medial side of thigh, gracilis muscle, great, long, and short adductor muscles
obturator n., accessory *n. obturatorius accessorius*	third and fourth lumbar nerves	muscular, articular	pectineal muscle, hip joint
n. of obturator, internal and gemellus, superior *n. obturator internus et gemellus superior*	fifth lumbar and first and second sacral nerves	filaments	muscles of internal obturator and superior gemellus
occipital n., large *n. occipitalis major*	median branch of dorsal division of second cervical n.	muscular, filaments	scalp over top and back of head; semispinal muscle of head
occipital n., small *n. occipitalis minor*	second cervical n.	auricular, filaments	skin of side of head and behind ear
occipital n., third least occipital n. *n. occipitalis tertius*	cutaneous part of third cervical n.	filaments	skin of lower part of back of head
oculomotor n. third cranial n. *n. oculomotorius*	midbrain at medial side of cerebral peduncle	superior, inferior	levator muscle of upper eyelid, most intrinsic and extrinsic muscles of eye

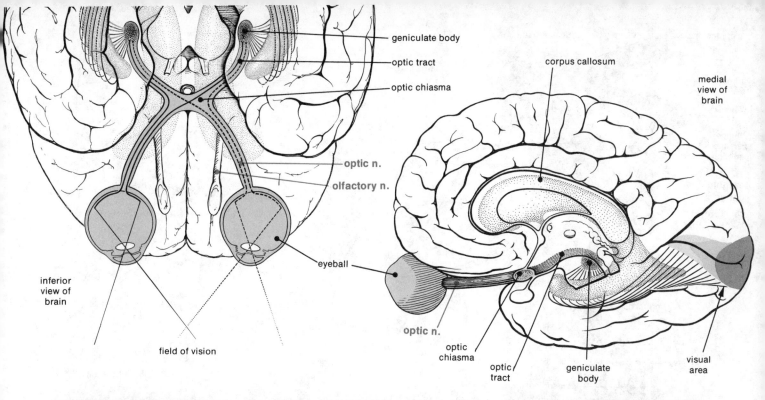

NERVE	ORIGIN	BRANCHES	DISTRIBUTION
olfactory n. first cranial n. *n. olfactorius*	olfactory bulb	filaments	nasal mucosa
ophthalmic n. *n. ophthalmicus*	trigeminal ganglion	tentorial, lacrimal, frontal, nasociliary	dura mater, eyeball, conjunctiva, lacrimal gland, mucous membrane of nose and paranasal sinuses, skin of the forehead, eyelids, and nose
optic n. second cranial n. n. of sight *n. opticus*	optic chiasm	filaments	rod and cone cells of retina
palatine n., large anterior palatine n. *n. palatinus anterior*	pterygopalatine ganglion	posterior inferior nasal, lesser palatine	gums, mucous membrane of hard and soft palates
palatine n.'s, small *nn. palatini medius et posterior*	pterygopalatine ganglion	filaments	soft palate, uvula, palatine tonsil
palpebral n., inferior *n. palpebralis inferior*	infraorbital n.	filaments	lower eyelid
palpebral n., superior *n. palpebralis superior*	lacrimal n.	filaments	upper eyelid
pectoral n., lateral *n. pectoralis lateralis*	lateral cord of brachial plexus	filaments	greater pectoral muscle
pectoral n., medial *n. pectoralis medialis*	medial cord of brachial plexus	filaments	smaller pectoral muscle and caudal part of greater pectoral muscle
perineal n. *n. perinei*	pudendal n.	superficial (two), deep	urogenital diaphragm, skin of external genitalia, perineal muscles, mucous membrane of urethra
peroneal n., common external popliteal n. peroneal n. *n. peroneus communis*	sciatic n.	articular (three), lateral cutaneous n. of calf, deep peroneal, superficial	knee joint, skin of posterior and lateral surfaces of leg, short head of biceps muscle of thigh, leg muscles
peroneal n., deep anterior tibial n. *n. peroneus profundus*	common peroneal n.	muscular, articular, lateral terminal, medial terminal	anterior tibial, long extensor of great toe, long extensor of toes, short extensor of toes, third peroneal, ankle joint, tarsal and tarsophalangeal joints of second, third and fourth toes

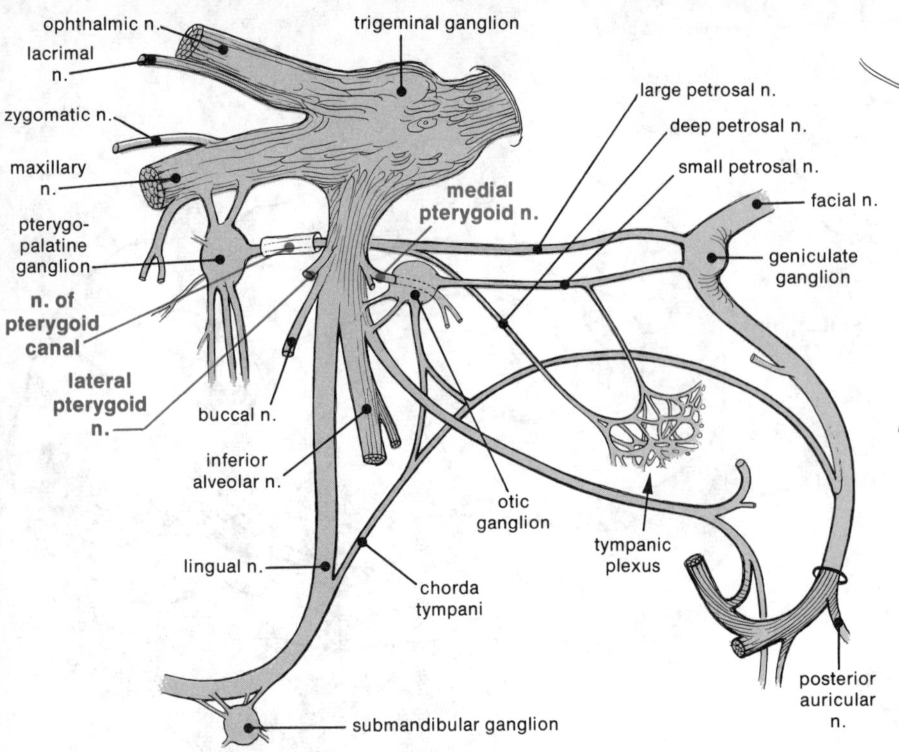

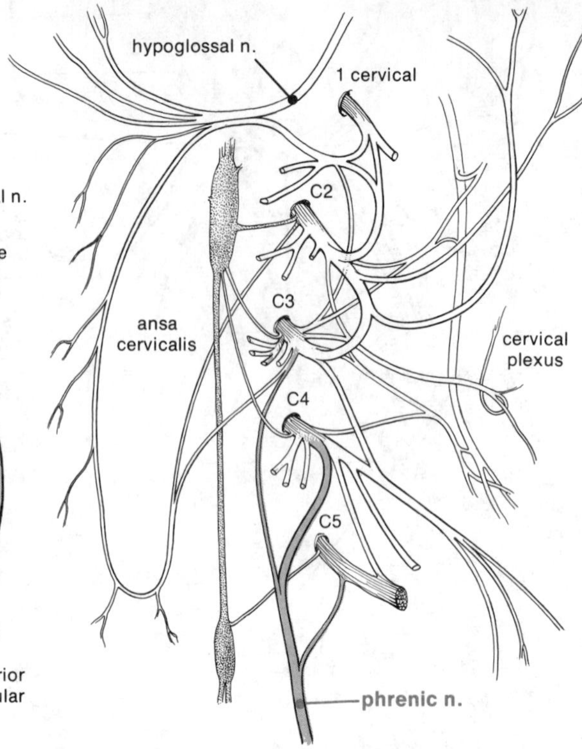

NERVE	ORIGIN	BRANCHES	DISTRIBUTION
peroneal n., superficial musculocutaneous n. *n. peroneus superficialis*	common peroneal n.	muscular, cutaneous filaments, medial dorsal cutaneous, intermediate dorsal cutaneous	long and short peroneal muscles, skin of lower part of leg, skin of medial side of foot, ankle, and side of great toe, skin of adjacent sides of second, third, fourth, and fifth toes
petrosal n., deep *n. petrosus profundus*	internal carotid plexus	joins greater petrosal nerve to form nerve of the pterygoid canal	glands and blood vessels of the pharynx, nasal cavity, and palate
petrosal n., large greater superficial petrosal n. *n. petrosus major*	geniculate ganglion of facial n.	filaments	mucous membrane and glands of palate, nose, and nasopharynx
petrosal n., small lesser superficial petrosal n. *n. petrosus minor*	tympanic n.	ganglionic, filaments	otic ganglion, parotid gland
phrenic n. internal respiratory n. of Bell *n. phrenicus*	third, fourth and fifth cervical nerves	pleural, pericardial, terminal	diaphragm, pericardium
phrenic n.'s, accessory *nn. phrenici accessorii*	inconstant branch from fifth cervical n. which arises with subclavian n.	joins phrenic	diaphragm
n. of piriform *n. piriformis*	second sacral n.	filaments	piriform muscle
plantar n., lateral external plantar n. *n. plantaris lateralis*	tibial n.	muscular, superficial, deep	skin of fifth and lateral half of fourth toes, deep muscles of foot
plantar n., medial internal plantar n. *n. plantaris medialis*	tibial n.	proper plantar digital, common digitals (three), plantar cutaneous, muscular, articular	skin of sole of foot, skin of adjacent sides of great, second, third and fourth toes, joints of tarsus and metatarsus, short flexor muscle of great toe, lumbrical muscles of foot
pterygoid canal, n. of; Vidian n. *n. canalis pterygoidei*	formed by union of large petrosal and deep petrosal nerves	filaments	glands of nose, palate, and pharynx; pterygopalatine ganglion
pterygoid n., lateral *n. pterygoideus lateralis*	mandibular n.		deep surface of lateral pterygoid muscle
pterygoid n., medial *n. pterygoideus medialis*	mandibular n.	tensor veli palatini, tensor tympani	tensor veli palatini, tensor tympani and medial pterygoid muscles

nerve | nerve

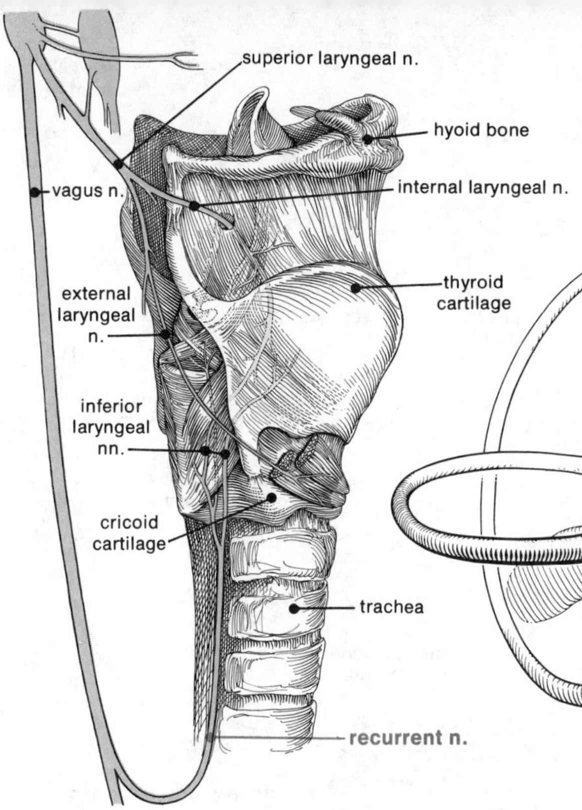

Labels in figure: superior laryngeal n., hyoid bone, internal laryngeal n., vagus n., external laryngeal n., thyroid cartilage, inferior laryngeal nn., cricoid cartilage, trachea, recurrent n., semicircular canals of internal ear, ampulla, utricular n., superior saccular n., utricle, saccule, greater saccular n., ampullary n., pudendal n., dura mater, 4 lumbar, L5, 1 sacral, S2, S3, S4, S5, sacral nn., sciatic n.

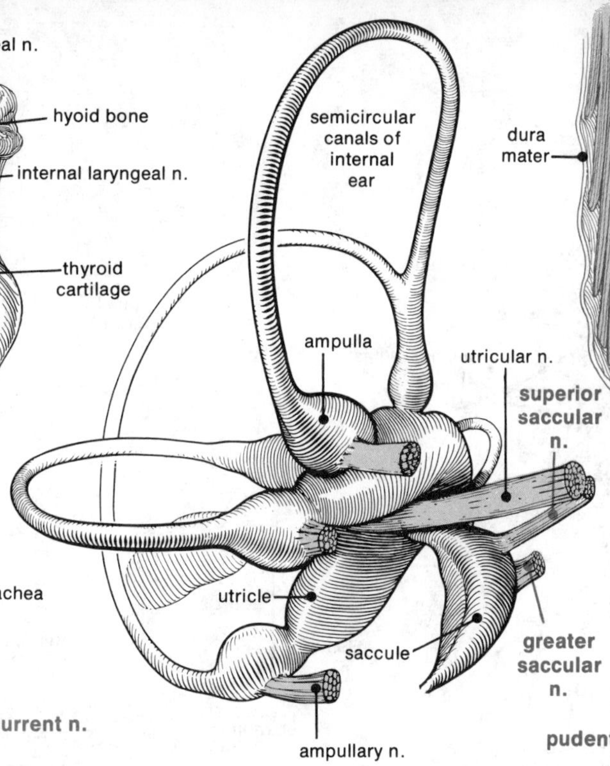

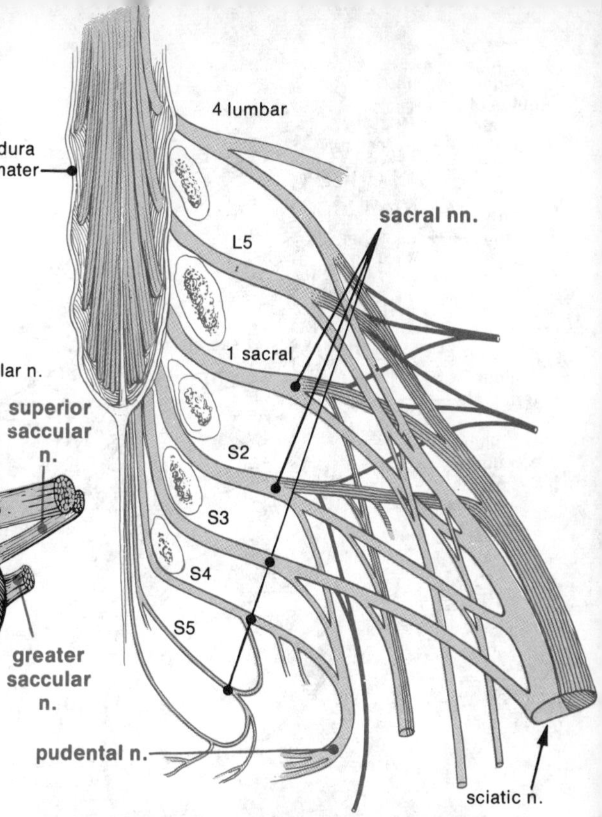

NERVE	ORIGIN	BRANCHES	DISTRIBUTION
pterygopalatine n.'s sphenopalatine n.'s *nn. pterygopalatine*	maxillary n.	orbital, greater palatine, posterior superior nasal, pharyngeal	mucous membranes of posterior ethmoidal and sphenoidal sinuses, nasal part of pharynx, and hard palate; periosteum of orbit, gums, nasal septum
pudendal n. internal pudic n. *n. pudendus*	second, third, and fourth sacral nerves	inferior rectal, perineal	urogenital diaphragm, skin around anus, skin of scrotum or labium major, external sphincter of anus
pudendal plexus *plexus pudendus*	second, third and fourth sacral nerves	visceral, muscular, pudendal, dorsal nerve of penis or clitoris	bladder, prostate, seminal vesicles, external genitalia, rectum, urogenital diaphragm, skin and muscles of anus, scrotum, and labium major
n. of quadrate muscle of thigh and gemellus, inferior *n. quadratus femoris et gemellus inferior*	fourth and fifth lumbar and first sacral nerves	filaments	quadrate muscle of thigh and inferior gemellus muscle
radial n. musculospiral n. *n. radialis*	posterior cord of brachial plexus	muscular, articular, superficial, deep, proximal, deep, cutaneous	extensor muscles of arm and forearm, and skin covering them
rectal n., inferior inferior hemorrhoidal n. *n. rectalis inferior*	pudendal n.	filaments	external sphincter of anus, skin around anus
recurrent n. recurrent laryngeal n. inferior laryngeal n. *n. recurrens*	vagus n.	pharyngeal, inferior laryngeal, tracheal, esophageal, cardiac	all muscles of larynx except cricothyroid; cardiac plexus, trachea, esophagus
saccular n., greater *n. saccularis major*	vestibular n.	filaments	the larger of two nerves that innervate the saccule of the internal ear
saccular n., superior *n. saccularis superior*	vestibular n.	filaments	the smaller of two nerves that innervate the saccule of the internal ear
sacral n.'s (five pairs of spinal nerves) *nn. sacrales*	sacral segments of spinal cord	dorsal, ventral	deep muscles and skin of lower back, pelvic viscera, sacral and pudendal plexuses
sacral plexus *plexus sacralis*	fourth and fifth lumbar and first, second and third sacral nerves	superior and inferior gemellae, internal obturator, superior and	muscles and skin of perineum and lower limb; hip joint

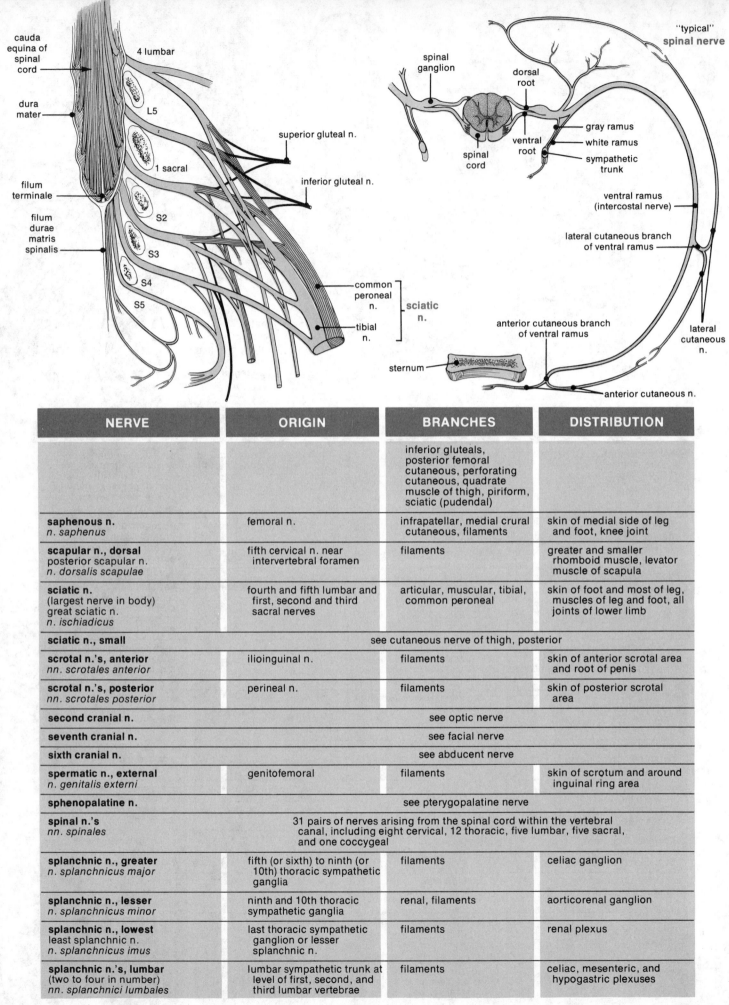

NERVE	ORIGIN	BRANCHES	DISTRIBUTION
		inferior gluteals, posterior femoral cutaneous, perforating cutaneous, quadrate muscle of thigh, piriform, sciatic (pudendal)	
saphenous n. *n. saphenus*	femoral n.	infrapatellar, medial crural cutaneous, filaments	skin of medial side of leg and foot, knee joint
scapular n., dorsal posterior scapular n. *n. dorsalis scapulae*	fifth cervical n. near intervertebral foramen	filaments	greater and smaller rhomboid muscle, levator muscle of scapula
sciatic n. (largest nerve in body) great sciatic n. *n. ischiadicus*	fourth and fifth lumbar and first, second and third sacral nerves	articular, muscular, tibial, common peroneal	skin of foot and most of leg, muscles of leg and foot, all joints of lower limb
sciatic n., small	see cutaneous nerve of thigh, posterior		
scrotal n.'s, anterior *nn. scrotales anterior*	ilioinguinal n.	filaments	skin of anterior scrotal area and root of penis
scrotal n.'s, posterior *nn. scrotales posterior*	perineal n.	filaments	skin of posterior scrotal area
second cranial n.	see optic nerve		
seventh cranial n.	see facial nerve		
sixth cranial n.	see abducent nerve		
spermatic n., external *n. genitalis externi*	genitofemoral	filaments	skin of scrotum and around inguinal ring area
sphenopalatine n.	see pterygopalatine nerve		
spinal n.'s *nn. spinales*	31 pairs of nerves arising from the spinal cord within the vertebral canal, including eight cervical, 12 thoracic, five lumbar, five sacral, and one coccygeal		
splanchnic n., greater *n. splanchnicus major*	fifth (or sixth) to ninth (or 10th) thoracic sympathetic ganglia	filaments	celiac ganglion
splanchnic n., lesser *n. splanchnicus minor*	ninth and 10th thoracic sympathetic ganglia	renal, filaments	aorticorenal ganglion
splanchnic n., lowest least splanchnic n. *n. splanchnicus imus*	last thoracic sympathetic ganglion or lesser splanchnic n.	filaments	renal plexus
splanchnic n.'s, lumbar (two to four in number) *nn. splanchnici lumbales*	lumbar sympathetic trunk at level of first, second, and third lumbar vertebrae	filaments	celiac, mesenteric, and hypogastric plexuses

nerve | nerve

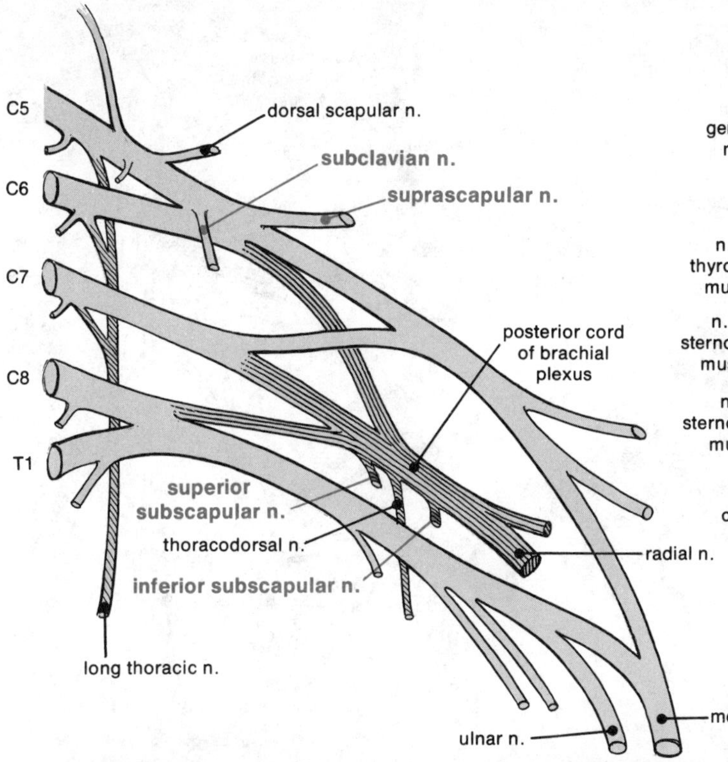

C5
dorsal scapular n.
subclavian n.
suprascapular n.
C6
C7
posterior cord of brachial plexus
C8
T1
superior subscapular n.
thoracodorsal n.
radial n.
inferior subscapular n.
long thoracic n.
median n.
ulnar n.

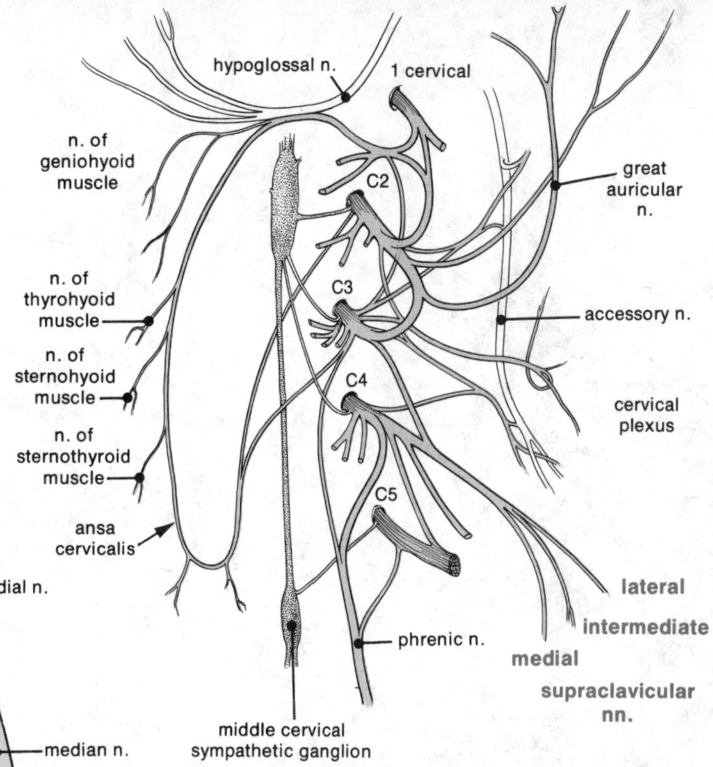

hypoglossal n.
1 cervical
n. of geniohyoid muscle
C2
great auricular n.
n. of thyrohyoid muscle
C3
accessory n.
n. of sternohyoid muscle
C4
cervical plexus
n. of sternothyroid muscle
C5
ansa cervicalis
lateral
intermediate
phrenic n.
medial
supraclavicular nn.
middle cervical sympathetic ganglion

NERVE	ORIGIN	BRANCHES	DISTRIBUTION
splanchnic n.'s, sacral *nn. splanchnici sacrales*	sacral sympathetic ganglion	filaments	inferior hypogastric plexus
splanchnic n.'s, pelvic *nn. splanchnici pelvini*	second to fourth sacral segments of spinal cord	filaments	inferior hypogastric plexus, sigmoid colon, pelvic viscera
n. of stapedius *n. stapedius*	facial n.	filaments	stapedius muscle
n. of sternohyoid *n. sternohyoideus*	convexity of ansa cervicalis	filaments	sternohyoid muscle
n. of sternothyroid *n. sternothyroideus*	convexity of ansa cervicalis	filaments	sternothyroid muscle
subclavian n. *n. subclavius*	superior trunk of brachial plexus	articular, filaments	subclavius muscle, sternoclavicular joint
subcostal n. *n. subcostalis*	12th thoracic n.	filaments	skin of lower abdominal wall and gluteal region; some abdominal muscles
sublingual n. *n. sublingualis*	lingual n.	filaments	sublingual gland and mucous membrane of floor of mouth
suboccipital n. infraoccipital n. *n. suboccipitalis*	first cervical	filaments	deep muscles of back of neck
subscapular n.'s (usually two in number) *nn. subscapulares*	posterior cord of brachial plexus	superior, inferior	subscapular and teres major muscles
supraclavicular n.'s intermediate middle supraclavicular n.'s *nn. supraclaviculares intermedii*	third and fourth cervical nerves	filaments	skin over pectoral and deltoid muscles
supraclavicular n.'s, lateral posterior supraclavicular n.'s supra-acromial n.'s *nn. supraclaviculares laterales*	third and fourth cervical nerves	filaments	skin of upper and dorsal parts of shoulder
supraclavicular n.'s, medial anterior supraclavicular n.'s *nn. supraclaviculares mediales*	third and fourth cervical nerves	filaments	skin of medial infraclavicular region as far as the midline, sternoclavicular joint
supraorbital n. *n. supraorbitalis*	frontal n.	medial, lateral	skin of upper eyelid and forehead, frontal muscle, scalp
suprascapular n. *n. suprascapularis*	superior trunk of brachial plexus	supraspinous, infraspinous, articular, filaments	supraspinous and infraspinous muscles, shoulder joint

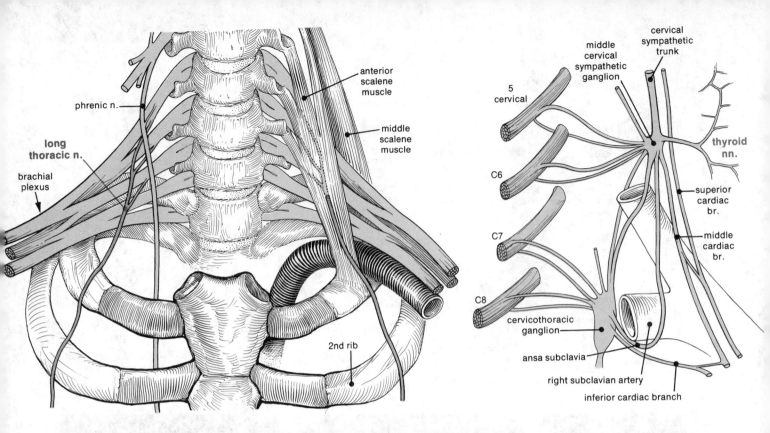

NERVE	ORIGIN	BRANCHES	DISTRIBUTION
supratrochlear n. *n. supratrochlearis*	frontal n.	filaments	conjunctiva, skin of upper eyelid and forehead, corrugator and frontal muscles
sural n. short saphenous n. *n. suralis*	medial and lateral cutaneous nerves of calf	lateral dorsal cutaneous, lateral calcaneal	skin of back of leg and lateral side of foot
temporal n.'s, deep (usually two in number) *nn. temporales profundi*	mandibular division of trigeminal n.	filaments	temporal muscle
n. to tensor tympani *n. tensoris tympani*	medial pterygoid n.	filaments	tensor muscle of tympanum
n. to tensor veli palatini *n. tensoris veli palatini*	medial pterygoid n.	filaments	tensor muscle of palatine velum
tenth cranial n.	see vagus nerve		
tentorial n. *n. tentorii*	ophthalmic n.	filaments	meninges
terminal n. *n. terminalis*	cerebral hemispheres near olfactory trigone	filaments	dura mater, mucous membrane of nasal septum
third cranial n.	see oculomotor nerve		
thoracic n.'s (12 pairs of spinal nerves) *nn. thoracici*	thoracic segments of spinal cord	dorsal, ventral	thoracic and abdominal walls (parietes) and skin of the buttock
thoracic n., long n. of serratus anterior *n. thoracicus longus*	fifth, sixth, and seventh cervical nerves	filaments	all digitations of serratus anterior muscle
thoracoabdominal intercostal n.'s *nn. thoracoabdominales intercostales*	ventral primary divisions of 7th–11th thoracic nerves beyond the intercostal spaces	filaments	anterior abdominal wall
thoracodorsal n. long subscapular n. n. of latissimus dorsi *n. thoracodorsalis*	posterior cord of brachial plexus	filaments	latissimus dorsi muscle
n. of thyrohyoid *n. thyrohyoideus*	hypoglossal n. and first cervical n.	filaments	thyrohyoid muscle
thyroid n.'s *nn. thyroideus*	middle cervical ganglion		thyroid gland

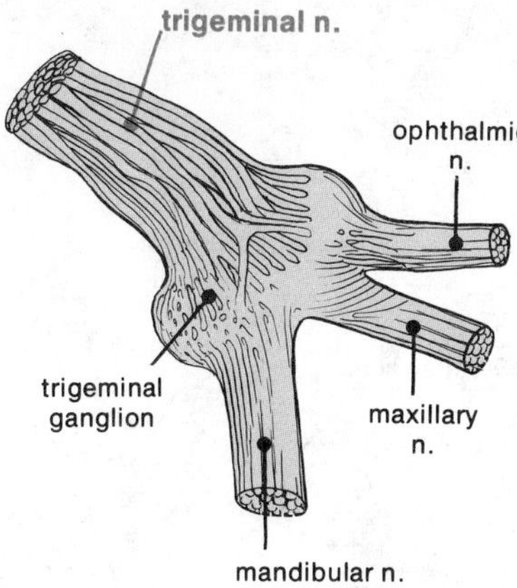

trigeminal n.

ophthalmic n.

trigeminal ganglion

maxillary n.

mandibular n.

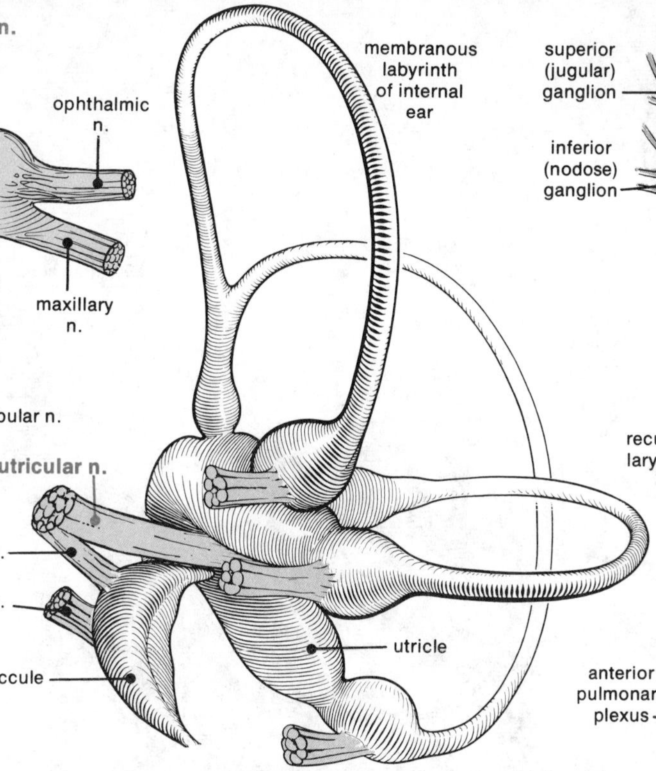

membranous labyrinth of internal ear

utricular n.

superior saccular n.

greater saccular n.

saccule

utricle

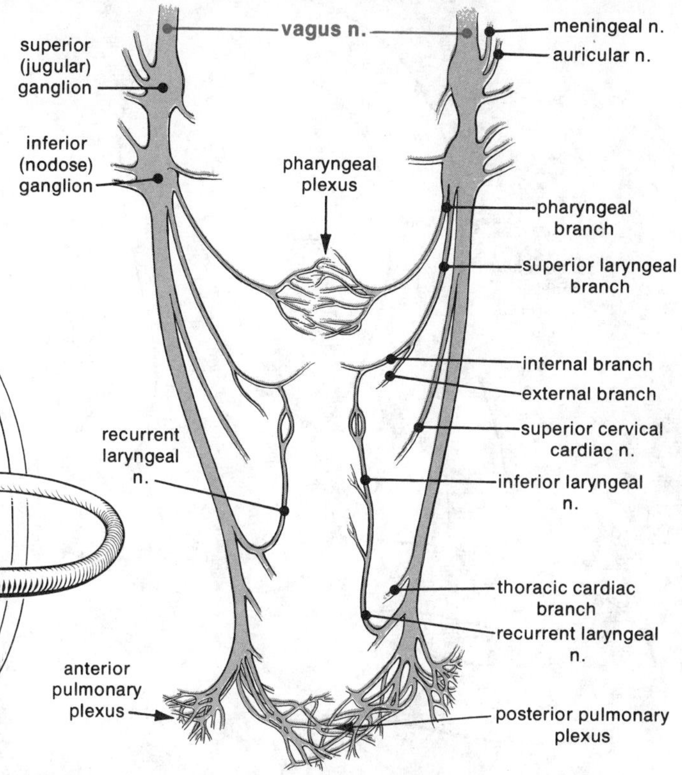

superior (jugular) ganglion

inferior (nodose) ganglion

vagus n.

meningeal n.

auricular n.

pharyngeal plexus

recurrent laryngeal n.

anterior pulmonary plexus

pharyngeal branch

superior laryngeal branch

internal branch

external branch

superior cervical cardiac n.

inferior laryngeal n.

thoracic cardiac branch

recurrent laryngeal n.

posterior pulmonary plexus

NERVE	ORIGIN	BRANCHES	DISTRIBUTION
tibial n. internal popliteal n. *n. tibialis*	sciatic n.	articular, medial and lateral plantar, medial calcaneal, medial sural cutaneous	knee and ankle joints, muscles of posterior leg
tibial n., anterior	see peroneal nerve, deep		
trigeminal n. (largest of the cranial nerves) fifth n. trifacial n. *n. trigeminus*	brainstem at inferior surface of pons	the three roots (motor, sensory, and intermediate) expand into the trigeminal ganglion near the apex of the petrous portion of the temporal bone, from which the ophthalmic, maxillary, and mandibular nerves arise	skin of face, mucous membranes and internal structures of the head, muscles of mastication
trochlear n. (smallest of the cranial nerves) fourth cranial n. *n. trochlearis*	midbrain immediately posterior to the inferior colliculus	filaments	superior oblique muscle of eyeball
twelfth cranial n.	see hypoglossal nerve		
tympanic n. n. of Jacobson *n. tympanicus*	glossopharyngeal n.	lesser petrosal, filaments	middle ear chamber, tympanic membrane, mastoid air cells, auditory tube, parotid gland
ulnar n. cubital n. *n. ulnaris*	medial cord of brachial plexus	articular, muscular, dorsal, palmar, palmar cutaneous	intrinsic muscles of hand, elbow, wrist and hand joints, skin of medial side of hand
utricular n. *n. utricularis*	vestibular n.	filaments	utricle of the internal ear
utriculoampullary n. *n. utriculoampullaris*	a division of the vestibular portion of the vestibulocochlear n.; it innervates the macula of the utricle and the ampullae of the anterior and lateral semicircular ducts		
vaginal n.'s *nn. vaginales*	pelvic plexus	filaments	vagina
vagus n. tenth cranial n. pneumogastric n. *n. vagus*	side of medulla oblongata	meningeal, auricular, pharyngeal, superior laryngeal, superior and inferior cardiac, anterior and posterior bronchial, recurrent, esophageal, gastric, hepatic, celiac	dura mater, skin of posterior surface of external ear, voluntary muscles of larynx and pharynx, heart, nonstriated muscles and glands of esophagus, stomach, trachea, bronchi,

nerve | nerve

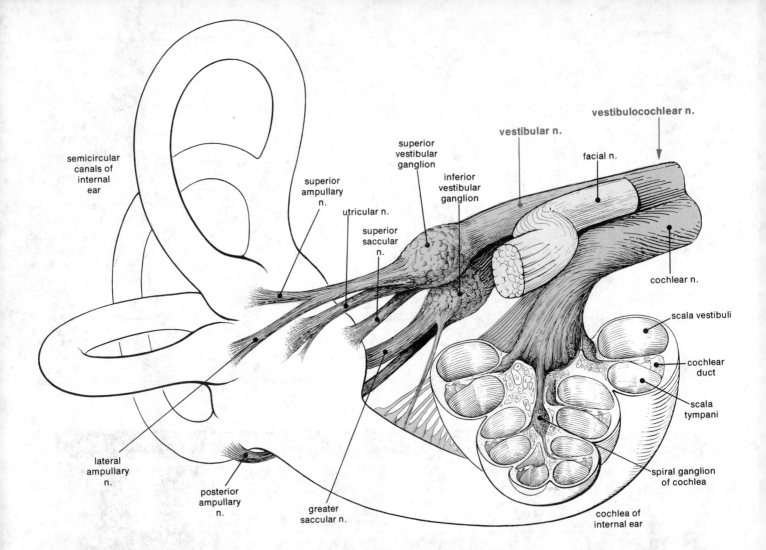

NERVE	ORIGIN	BRANCHES	DISTRIBUTION
			biliary tract, and intestines, mucous membranes of pharynx, larynx, bronchi, lungs, digestive tract, and kidney
vertebral n. *n. vertebralis*	cervicothoracic ganglion	meningeal, filaments	meninges, joins cervical n.'s
vestibular n. n. of equilibration *n. vestibularis*	vestibulocochlear n.	utricular, saccular, ampullary	through the vestibular ganglion (ganglion of Scarpa) to maculae of utricle and saccule, and to ampullae of semicircular ducts
vestibulocochlear n. eighth cranial n. auditory n. acoustic n. otic n. *n. vestibulocochlearis*	brainstem between pons and medulla oblongata formed by union of vestibular and cochlear nerves	vestibular (medial), cochlear (lateral)	receptor organs in the membranous labyrinth of internal ear
Vidian n.	see pterygoid canal, nerve of		
vomernasal n. *n. vomernasalis*	present in the nasal septum of the fetus but disappears before birth		
zygomatic n. orbital n. temporomalar n. *n. zygomaticus*	maxillary n.	zygomaticotemporal, zygomaticofacial	temporal muscle, skin of side of forehead, orbicular muscle of eye, skin on prominence of cheek
zygomaticofacial n. *n. zygomaticofacialis*	zygomatic n.	filaments	skin over prominence of cheek (zygoma), orbicular muscle of eye
zygomaticotemporal n. *n. zygomaticotemporalis*	zygomatic n.	filaments	temporal muscle and skin on side of forehead

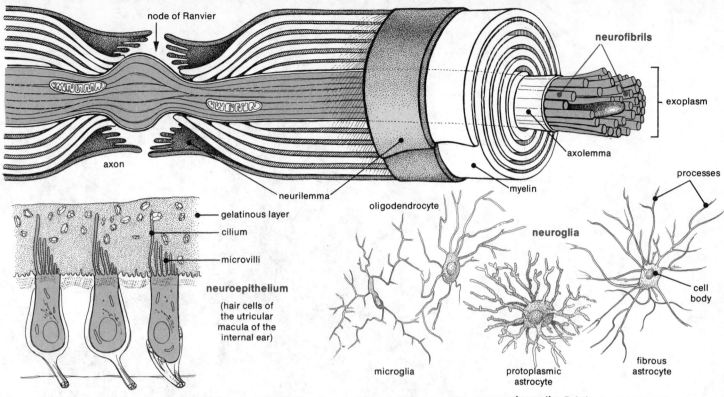

node of Ranvier

neurofibrils

exoplasm

axolemma

axon

neurilemma

myelin

neuroglia

processes

oligodendrocyte

cell body

gelatinous layer

cilium

microvilli

neuroepithelium

(hair cells of the utricular macula of the internal ear)

microglia

protoplasmic astrocyte

fibrous astrocyte

ner'vous. 1, Relating to nerves. **2.** Highstrung; excitable.

ner'vousness. Undue irritability and excitability.

ner'vus, *pl.* **ner'vi.** Latin for nerve.

nes'slerize. To treat with Nessler's reagent in order to determine the level of urea nitrogen in the blood and in the urine.

nest. A collection of similar cells.

cell n.'s, small collections of a different type of cell in a tissue.

epithelial n.'s, small aggregations of neoplastic tissue composed of compressed polygonal cells, frequently seen in squamous cell carcinoma; also called epithelial pearls and onion bodies.

net. Reticulum; network.

net'work. A structure composed of interlocking filaments; also called reticulum and rete.

chromatin n., basophilic network in the nuclei of many cells, appearing after fixation.

Purkinje's n., network of muscle fibers beneath the endocardium of the cardiac ventricles.

neur-. See neuro-.

neu'ral. 1. Relating to the nervous system. **2.** Referring to the dorsal region of an embryo.

neural'gia. Severe pain along the course of a nerve.

trigeminal n., tic douleureux; severe facial pain in the area of the trigeminal nerve.

neural'gic. Relating to neuralgia.

neuranagen'esis. Regeneration of a nerve.

neuraprax'ia. Injury to a nerve resulting in temporary paralysis.

neurasthe'nia. Condition marked by fatigue, irritability, and poor concentration; originally considered to be due to exhaustion of the nervous system.

neuratroph'ia, neurat'rophy. Atrophy of the nerves.

neurax'is. 1. The central nervous system. **2.** Axon.

neurax'on. See axon.

neurec'tomy. Surgical removal of a nerve segment.

neurecto'pia, neurec'topy. Abnormal location of a nerve.

neurer'gic. Of or relating to the action of nerves.

neurilem'ma. The thin cytoplasmic membrane of a Schwann cell enwrapping the axon of an unmyelinated nerve fiber and also the myelin layers of a myelinated nerve fiber; also called sheath of Schwann.

neurilemmi'tis. Inflammation of the neurilemma.

neurilemo'ma. A benign encapsulated tumor originating from a peripheral or sympathetic nerve or from the facial nerve; also called neurinoma and schwannoma.

Antoni type A n., a relatively solid tumor consisting of Schwann cells (arranged in twisting bundles) and reticulum fibers.

Antoni type B n., a relatively soft tumor consisting of Schwann cells (arranged in a haphazard way), reticulum fibers, and minute cysts.

neuri'tis. Inflammation or degeneration of a nerve.

intraocular optic n., see papillitis.

multiple n., polyneuritis; neuritis that involves several nerves.

optic n., neuritis of the optic nerve.

pseudo-optic n., (1) congenital abnormal elevation of the optic disk; (2) mild hyperemia of the optic disk.

toxic n., neuritis resulting from a chemical toxin as in arsenic or lead poisoning.

traumatic n., neuritis following an injury.

neuro-, neur-. Combining forms denoting nerve or nervous system.

neuroanastomo'sis. Surgical union of nerves.

neuroanat'omy. The branch of anatomy concerned with the study of the nervous system.

neurobiol'ogy. The integrated study of neuroanatomy and neurophysiology, i.e., of the structure and the normal vital processes of the nervous system.

neurobiotax'is. The tendency of nerve cells to move in the direction of the area where most of the impulses originate.

neu'roblast. An embryonic nerve cell.

neuroblasto'ma. A highly malignant tumor arising most frequently from the medulla of the adrenal gland; it is the most common malignant tumor of childhood and infancy; also called sympathoblastoma and sympathogonioma.

neurocar'diac. 1. Relating to the nerve supply of the heart. **2.** Relating to a cardiac neurosis.

neu'rocele. The ventricles of the brain and the central canal of the spinal cord.

neurochem'istry. The study of the chemical activity of nervous tissues.

neurochoroidi'tis. Inflammation of the optic nerve and the middle, vascular coat of the eye (choroid).

neuroc'ladism. Regeneration of a cut nerve by the outgrowth of axonal branches from the proximal stump which grow toward, and make contact with, the distal stump to bridge the gap.

neuroclon'ic. Relating to or marked by nervous spasm.

neurocra'nium. The portion of the skull containing the brain, distinguished from the facial bones.

neurocyto'ma. See ganglioneuroma.

neurodermati'tis. Localized inflammation of the skin, of nervous or psychological origin.

neurodynam'ic. Relating to nervous energy.

neurodyn'ia. Neuralgia.

neuroec'toderm. In embryology, the part of the ectoderm that gives rise to the neural tube.

neuroendocrinol'ogy. The study of the interactions of the nervous system with the endocrine glands.

neuroepithelio'ma. A type of glioma consisting primarily of cells that resemble the precursors of specialized sensory epithelium or of the brain and spinal cord.

neuroepithe'lium. 1. The specialized epithelium composed of cells that act as receptors of external stimuli, as the hair cells of the internal ear. **2.** The layer of the ectoderm from which the neural tube develops.

neurofi'bril. A nerve fibril; one of numerous aggregates of slender filaments running parallel with one another in the axon and dendrite but crossing and intermingling in the cell body.

neurofibro'ma. A nonmalignant tumor originating in the connective tissues of nerves; it occurs most frequently in the skin, where nodules are formed; the overlying epidermis may become pigmented. See also neurofibromatosis.

neurofibromato'sis. An inherited disorder transmitted as a dominant trait and characterized by the development of multiple, pedunculated, soft tumors (neurofibromas) in various sites, especially the skin, and the presence of light brown (café au lait) spots on the skin; present in from five to 20 per cent of patients with pheochromocytoma; also called von Recklinghausen's or Recklinghausen's disease.

neurogen'esis. The formation of the nervous system.

neurogen'ic, neurogenet'ic. Originating in the nervous system.

neurog'lia. The nonneuronal tissue of the brain and spinal cord that performs supportive and other ancillary functions; composed of various types of cells collectively called neuroglial cells or glial cells; also called glia.

neurog'liocyte. One of the cells composing the supporting, non-nervous portion of the nervous system.

neurogliomato'sis. The presence of tumors of neuroglial cells in the brain or spinal cord.

neuroglio'sis. 1. Abnormal proliferation of neuroglial cells. **2.** The presence of several gliomas in the brain or spinal cord.

neu'rogram. The hypothesized imprint left on the brain by each mental experience, stimulation of which produces memory; also called brain residual.

neurohistol'ogy. Microscopic study of the ner-

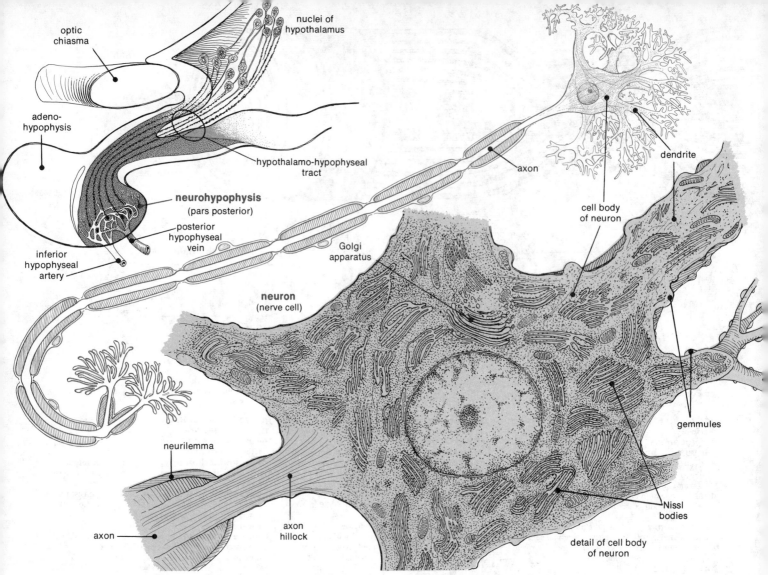

optic chiasma

nuclei of hypothalamus

adeno-hypophysis

hypothalamo-hypophyseal tract

neurohypophysis (pars posterior)

posterior hypophyseal vein

inferior hypophyseal artery

axon

cell body of neuron

dendrite

neuron (nerve cell)

Golgi apparatus

gemmules

neurilemma

axon

axon hillock

Nissl bodies

detail of cell body of neuron

---

vous system.

neurohor'mone. A hormone whose secretion is controlled by the nervous system.

neurohu'mor. An active chemical substance that effects the passage of nerve impulses from one cell to another at the synapse.

neurohypophy'seal. Relating to the posterior lobe of the pituitary gland; also written neurohypophysial.

neurohypoph'ysis. The posterior or nervous lobe of the hypophysis; developed from the floor of the diencephalon.

neu'roid. Resembling a nerve.

neuroker'atin. 1. A proteolipid network in the myelin sheath of axons. **2.** The pseudokeratin present in brain tissue.

neurolem'ma. Neurilemma.

neurolep'tic. Any major tranquilizer which acts on the nervous system and has therapeutic effects on psychoses and other types of psychiatric disorders; also called antipsychotic.

neurol'ogist. A specialist in the nervous system and its diseases.

neurol'ogy. The branch of medicine that deals with the nervous system and its diseases.

neu'rolymph. Cerebrospinal fluid.

neurol'ysin. An agent that causes destruction of nerve cells; also called neurotoxin.

neurol'ysis. 1. Destruction of nerve tissue. **2.** The removal of adhesions from a nerve.

neuro'ma. Old term denoting any neoplasm derived from nerve tissue; more specific terms are generally preferred.

  acoustic n., a tumor of the eighth cranial nerve (vestibulocochlear nerve).

  amputation n., one located at the proximal end of an injured nerve; also called traumatic neuroma.

  traumatic n., see amputation neuroma.

neuromala'cia. Abnormal softening of nervous tissue.

neuromech'anism. The part of the nervous system that controls the function of an organ.

neuromus'cular. Relating to nerve and muscle, such as the nerve endings in a muscle, or the interaction of nerve and muscle.

neuromyasthe'nia. Muscular weakness, especially of emotional origin.

  epidemic n., an epidemic febrile disorder generally affecting only adults, marked by stiffness of the neck and back, fever, headache, diarrhea, and localized muscular weakness; also called Iceland disease and benign myalgic encephalomyelitis.

neuromyeli'tis. Inflammation of the nerves and spinal cord.

  n. optica, inflammation of the optic nerves and spinal cord; considered a type of multiple sclerosis; also called Devic's disease.

neuromyop'athy. A disorder of muscle that indicates a disease of the nerve supplying the muscle.

neuromyosi'tis. Nerve inflammation complicated by inflammation of the muscles with which the affected nerve is in relation.

neu'ron. A nerve cell; the basic functional and anatomic unit of the nervous system, concerned with the conduction of impulses; structurally it is the most complex cell of the body; the human nervous system contains about 28 billion neurons.

  afferent n., one that conducts impulses toward the spinal cord and brain; also called sensory neuron.

  bipolar n., a neuron possessing two separate axons as in the retina, olfactory mucosa, internal ear, and taste buds.

  central n., one entirely within the spinal cord or brain.

  efferent n., one that conducts impulses away from the brain and spinal cord; also called motor neuron.

  internuncial n., one that connects afferent and efferent neurons; also called association neuron.

  multipolar n., a neuron with several short processes (dendrites) and a single long axon.

  pyramidal n., pyramidal cell; a multipolar neuron whose cell body lies in the cerebral cortex.

  unipolar n., a neuron having a single process (axon) attached to its cell body.

neu'ronal. Of or relating to a nerve cell.

neuron'ic. Relating to a nerve cell.

neuroni'tis. Inflammation of nerve cells, especially those of the roots of spinal nerves.

neuron'ophage. A phagocyte that devours injured or diseased nerve cells.

neuronopha'gia. Destruction of unwanted nerve cells by neuronophages.

neuronyx'is. See acupuncture.

neuro-ophthalmol'ogy. The branch of ophthalmology concerned with the part of the nervous system related to the eye; also written neurophthalmology.

neuropapilli'tis. See papillitis.

neuroparal'ysis. Paralysis due to disease of the nerve supplying the affected part.

neuropath'ic. Relating to a disease of the nervous system.

neuropathogen'esis. The origin of diseases of the nervous system.

neuropathol'ogy. Study of diseases of the nervous system.

neurop'athy. Any disease of the nervous system.

  diabetic n., a complication of diabetes mellitus in which the peripheral nerves and the innervation of the bladder and bowel may be affected.

  peripheral n., a disorder of the peripheral nerves characterized by motor and sensory changes in the extremities; most commonly associated with alcoholism and/or poor nutrition.

neuropharmacol'ogy. Study of drugs that affect the nervous system.

neurophthalmol'ogy. See neuro-ophthalmology.

neuroph'thisis. Wasting of nervous tissue.

neurophys'ine. A huge endocrine gland molecule

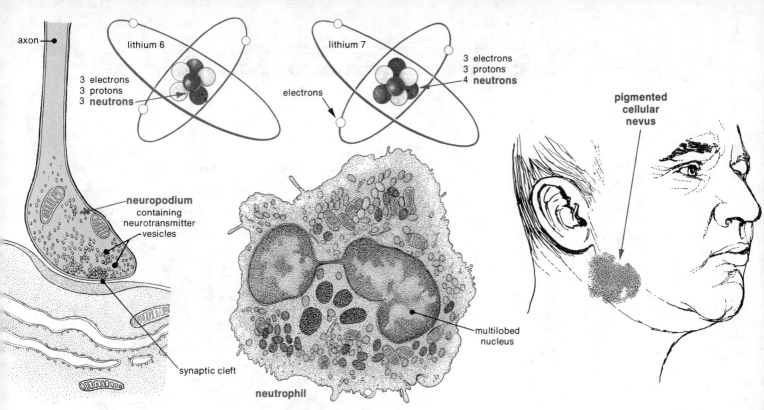

axon

lithium 6

3 electrons
3 protons
3 **neutrons**

lithium 7

3 electrons
3 protons
4 **neutrons**

electrons

neuropodium
containing
neurotransmitter
vesicles

**pigmented
cellular
nevus**

multilobed
nucleus

synaptic cleft

neutrophil

produced in nerve cell bodies at the base of the brain and stored in the pituitary gland; this macromolecule with a 92-step chemical sequence is thought to be a transporter of the hormones vasopressin and oxytocin.

neurophysiol′ogy. Study of the normal vital processes of the nervous system.

neu′ropile. A dense net of interwoven glia and nerve cells and their processes.

neu′roplasm. The protoplasm of a nerve cell.

neu′roplasty. Reparative surgery of the nerves.

neuroplex′us. A network (plexus) of nerves. See also plexus.

neuropo′dium, *pl.* **neuropo′dia.** The enlarged, rounded termination of an axon at the site of a synapse.

neu′ropore. The opening at the ends of the neural tube of the developing embryo prior to complete closure around the 20–25 somite stage.

neuropsychi′atry. The study of both organic and functional diseases of the nervous system.

neuropsychol′ogy. The study of the relationship between the mind and the nervous system.

neuropsychop′athy. Functional nervous disease accompanied by mental symptoms.

neuropsycho′sis. Obsolete term; see psychosis.

neuroradiol′ogy. Study of the nervous system with the aid of x rays.

neuroretini′tis. Inflammation of the head of the optic nerve and adjacent retina.

neuror′rhaphy. Surgical suturing of the ends of a divided nerve.

neurosarcoclei′sis. Operative removal of the bony canal surrounding a nerve for the relief of neuralgia.

neurosclero′sis. Hardening of nerves.

neurosecre′tion. Any of several secretory products of nerve cells (e.g., of the neurohypophysis and those of the base of the hypothalamus) which enter the blood stream and act as hormones.

neuro′sis, *pl.* **neuro′ses.** Emotional maladjustment which may impair thinking and judgement but causes minimal loss of contact with reality.

  anxiety n., neurosis marked by exaggerated uncontrollable anxiety and apprehension of either acute or gradual onset.

  battle n., war n., disorder induced by conditions of warfare; formerly called shell-shock.

  cardiac n., neurosis marked by exaggerated concern with the state of one's heart in the absence of heart disease; also called cardioneurosis.

  obsessive-compulsive n., disorder marked by the persistent intrusion of unwanted ideas and the compulsion to perform repetitive acts, e.g., repeated hand-washing or touching; anxiety develops when

the individual is prevented from performing his ritual.

  war n., see battle neurosis.

neuroskel′eton. The part of the skeleton surrounding the brain and spinal cord.

neu′rosome. 1. One of the minute granules in the protoplasm of a nerve cell. **2.** The body of a nerve cell.

neurosplanch′nic. Relating to the autonomic nervous system.

neurosur′geon. A specialist in surgery of the nervous system.

neurosur′gery. Surgery of the nervous system.

  stereotactic n., neurosurgery involving the use of a mechanically directed probe introduced into the brain through a small hole in the skull using precise topographical coordinates to arrive at the desired location.

neurosyph′ilis. Syphilis of the nervous system.

neurot′ic. Relating to or affected with a neurosis.

neurotiza′tion. Nerve regeneration.

neurot′omy. Surgical division of a nerve.

neuroton′ic. 1. Stimulating impaired nervous function. **2.** An agent having such an effect.

neurotox′in. See neurolysin.

neurotransmit′ter. Any substance that aids in transmitting impulses between two nerve cells or between a nerve and a muscle; e.g., acetylcholine.

neurotrophasthe′nia. Condition due to undernourishment and marked by fatigue, poor concentration, and feelings of inadequacy.

neurotrop′ic. Having an affinity for nervous tissue; said of certain histologic dyes and microorganisms.

neu′rula. The early vertebrate embryo during the stages when it possesses a neural plate.

neurula′tion. The formation and closure of the neural plate in the early vertebrate embryo.

neutraliza′tion. 1. The chemical reaction between an acid and a base that yields a salt and water. **2.** The process of rendering something ineffective.

neu′tralize. 1. To render ineffective, as in counteracting the effect of a drug or toxin. **2.** To make neutral.

neutri′no. An uncharged subatomic particle emitted from a radioactive nucleus when an electron is emitted from, or captured by, the nucleus; believed to have zero mass when at rest; it travels at the speed of light and interacts with matter only in the reverse process by which it is produced.

neu′trocyte. Neutrophil.

neutrocytope′nia. See neutropenia.

neu′tron. An uncharged subatomic particle existing along with the protons in the nucleus of an atom; slightly heavier than a proton.

neutrope′nia. Abnormally small number of neutrophils in the blood; also called neutrocytopenia and neutrophilic leukopenia.

neu′trophil. A mature white blood cell having a nucleus of three to five lobes joined by thin strands of chromatin; the most numerous of the white blood cell population (50 to 75 per cent in normal individuals); its primary function is the ingestion and digestion of particulate matter, especially highly virulent bacteria; after it migrates from the blood stream to a site of infection, it may be called a microphage; also called neutrophilic or polymorphonuclear leukocyte.

  toxic n., one having large dark granules (toxic granules) due to severe infection or to a drug reaction.

neutrophil′ia. Increased number of neutrophils in the blood; also called neutrocytosis and neutrophilic leukocytosis.

ne′void. Resembling a nevus.

nevoxan′thoendothelio′ma. Single or multiple reddish papules, usually seen in young children; also called juvenile xanthogranuloma.

ne′vus, *pl.* **ne′vi.** A benign lesion of the skin; may be pigmented or nonpigmented, flat or elevated, smooth or warty; may become malignant.

  blue n., a circumscribed, blue to black nodule beneath the skin, occurring anywhere in the body but most commonly on the dorsum of the hand and foot; chiefly composed of dopa-positive melanocytes (pigment-producing cells) containing a high concentration of melanin pigment; becomes malignant only rarely.

  hairy pigmented n., a pigmented cellular nevus (mole) containing hairs.

  intradermal n., one occurring in the dermis (layer of the skin deep to the epidermis).

  junctional n., one occurring in the area between the dermis and epidermis (layers of the skin).

  n. flammeus, port-wine hemangioma; see under hemangioma.

  n. vasculosus, strawberry hemangioma; see under hemangioma.

  pigmented cellular n., a circumscribed nevus composed of melanocytes (pigment-producing cells) and varying from smooth to rough (depending on the amount of keratin present) and from nonpalpable to nodular; commonly known as a mole.

  port-wine n., port-wine hemangioma; see under hemangioma.

  spider n., see spider, arterial.

  systematized n., a widely distributed congenital nevus exhibiting a pattern.

new′born. 1. A recently born infant. **2.** Just born.

Newcastle disease. An acute contagious dis-

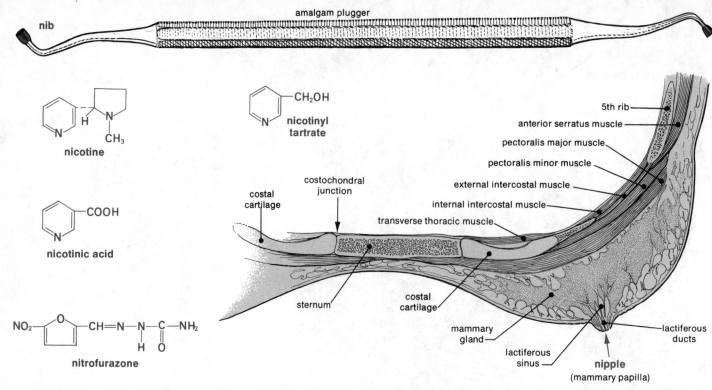

nib

amalgam plugger

nicotine

nicotinyl tartrate

nicotinic acid

nitrofurazone

5th rib
anterior serratus muscle
pectoralis major muscle
pectoralis minor muscle
external intercostal muscle
internal intercostal muscle
transverse thoracic muscle
costochondral junction
costal cartilage
sternum
costal cartilage
mammary gland
lactiferous sinus
nipple
(mammary papilla)
lactiferous ducts

ease of fowl caused by an RNA virus; transmissible to man, causing respiratory and nervous symptoms.

new'ton. A unit of force in the meter-kilogram-second system; the force required to accelerate a mass of one kilogram one meter per second per second.

ng. Abbreviation for nanogram.

NHLBI. Abbreviation for National Heart Lung and Blood Institute.

Ni. Chemical symbol of the element nickel.

ni'acin. The official designation for nicotinic acid in its role as a vitamin; see nicotinic acid.

ni'acinam'ide. See nicotinamide.

NIAMDD. Abbreviation for National Institute of Arthritis, Metabolism and Digestive Diseases.

nib. In dentistry, the working part of a condensing instrument corresponding to the blade of a cutting instrument.

NICHD. Abbreviation for National Institute of Child Health and Human Development.

niche. A small recess or eroded area, especially in the wall of a hollow organ, usually detected by contrast radiography.

nick'el. A metallic element, symbol Ni, atomic number 28, atomic weight 58.71.

nick'ing. constriction of a blood vessel of the retina.

  A-V n., depression of a retinal vein into the tissue of the retina at the point where it is crossed by an artery; usually caused by elevated arterial blood pressure; also called arteriovenous nicking.

nicotin'amide. White crystalline compound, soluble in water; a B-complex vitamin used to treat pellagra; also called nicotinic acid amide and niacinamide.

nicotinamide adenine dinucleotide (NAD). One of the coenzymes of the vitamin niacin (nicotinic acid); in association with any of a number of proteins, it acts as an oxidation-reduction catalyst; formerly called diphosphopyridine nucleotide (DPN); also called coenzyme I and codehydrogenase I.

nicotinamide adenine dinucleotide phosphate (NADP). A coenzyme that participates in biological oxidation reactions; structurally and functionally similar to NAD; formerly known as triphosphopyridine nucleotide; also called coenzyme II; Furacin®.

nic'otine. An alkaloid derived from tobacco (*Nicotiana tabacum*); small doses stimulate and large doses depress autonomic ganglia.

nicotin'ic. Resembling nicotine; denoting the action of certain agents on the nervous system.

nicotinic acid. Niacin; an odorless, white crystalline compound, part of the vitamin B complex; used in the prevention and treatment of pellagra.

nicotinic acid amide. See nicotinamide.

nicotinomimet'ic. Simulating the action of nicotine.

nicotinyl tartrate. Compound used as a peripheral vasodilator in certain peripheral vascular diseases; Roniacol Tartrate®.

nictita'tion. Winking.

nida'tion. The embedding or implantation of the fertilized ovum in the uterine mucosa during pregnancy.

ni'dus. 1. A nest. **2.** The point of focus of a morbid process. **3.** The point of origin or nucleus of a nerve.

  n. avis, a cerebellar depression between the biventral lobe and the uvula, which accommodates the cerebellar tonsil.

  n. lienis, the nest of the spleen, formed by part of the phrenicocolic ligament.

  n. hirundinis, nidus avis.

NIEHS. Abbreviation for National Institute of Environmental Health Science.

Niemann-Pick disease. A rare form of lipidosis marked by an accumulation of foam cells in the reticuloendothelial system, spleen, liver, kidneys, and pancreas; at a late stage, deposits of sphingomyelin, gangliosides, and cholesterol may be found in the brain and spinal cord; a familial disorder most commonly seen in Jewish infants.

night'mare. A dream accompanied by intense anxiety, fear, oppression, and helplessness.

NIH. Abbreviation for National Institutes of Health.

ni'hilism. In psychiatry, a delusion of nonexistence; it may be total (including the patient and the world as a whole) or selective (referring to a part of the patient or his environment).

  therapeutic n., a disbelief in the value of any type of therapy.

Nikolsky's sign. A peculiar vulnerability of the skin in pemphigus vulgaris; the superficial layer of the skin is easily rubbed off with slight friction.

ninhy'drin. Triketohydrindene hydrate, an important reagent widely used in the analytical determination of amino acids and related substances.

nio'bium. A rare metallic element, symbol Nb, atomic number 41, atomic weight 92.906; formerly called columbium (Cb).

nip'ple. The conical protuberance at the apex of the mammary gland on which the outlets of the milk ducts are located; also called mamilla and teat.

  inversion of n., congenital failure of nipple to protrude from the breast.

nit. 1. The egg of a louse. **2.** A unit of luminance.

ni'ter. See potassium nitrate.

ni'trate. A salt of nitric acid.

ni'tric. Relating to, derived from, or containing nitrogen.

  n. acid, a colorless or yellowish corrosive liquid, HNO_3.

nitrida'tion. Formation of nitrides through the combination with nitrogen.

ni'tride. A compound containing nitrogen and one other element, usually a more electropositive one.

nitrifica'tion. 1. The conversion of nitrogenous matter into nitrates by the action of bacteria. **2.** The treatment of a material with nitrogen or nitrogen compounds.

ni'trile, ni'tril. A compound containing trivalent nitrogen (N^{-3}) in a cyanogen group.

ni'trite. A salt or ester of nitrous acid.

ni'tritoid. Resembling the reaction caused by a nitrite, such as the reaction following the intravenous administration of arsphenamine.

nitro-. Combining form denoting a compound containing the univalent group NO_2.

nitrobacte'ria. Bacteria that cause the conversion of nitrogenous matter into nitrates.

nitrofu'ran. Furan derivative containing a nitro group; used as antibacterial agent.

nitrofurant'oin. Bitter crystals, slightly soluble in water, used as a urinary antibacterial agent; Furadantin®.

nitrofu'razone. 5-Nitro-2-furaldehyde semicarbazone; a topical antibacterial agent; Furacin®.

ni'trogen. A colorless, odorless, gaseous element forming about 47 per cent of the atmosphere by weight; symbol N, atomic number 7, atomic weight 14.008.

  blood urea n. (BUN), a constituent of normal whole blood. See nitrogen, urea.

  filtrate n., see nonprotein nitrogen.

  n. balance, the difference between the amounts of nitrogen taken into and released by the body.

  n. cycle, the continuous process in which nitrogen is deposited in the soil, assimilated by bacteria and plants, transferred to animals, and returned to the soil.

  n. equivalent, the nitrogen content of protein.

  n. lag, the time elapsed between the ingestion of protein and the excretion in the urine of an equal amount of nitrogen.

  n. monoxide, see nitrous oxide.

  n. mustards, toxic compounds similar in composition to mustard gas but with nitrogen replacing sulfur; some have been used to treat neoplastic diseases.

  nonprotein n., the nitrogen content of the blood exclusive of the protein bodies; normally urea contains about half of the nonprotein nitrogen in the blood; also called filtrate nitrogen.

  urea n., the portion of nitrogen derived from the urea content of a biologic sample such as blood or

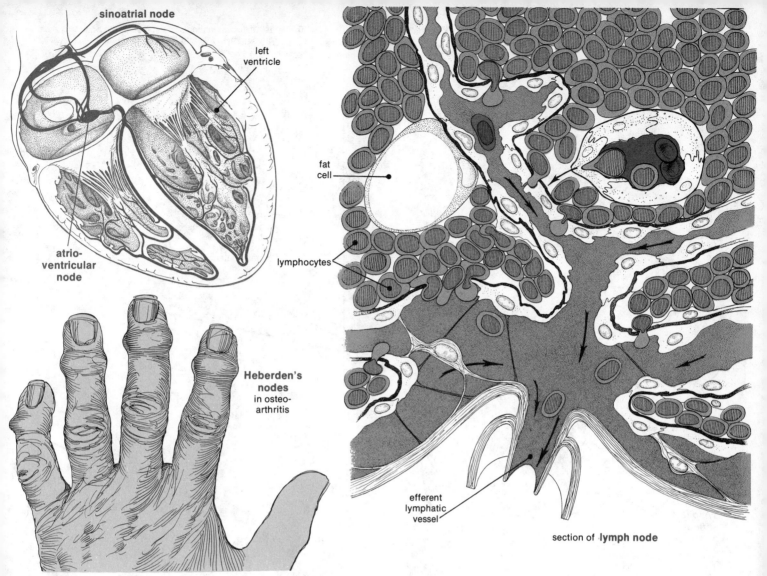

sinoatrial node

left ventricle

atrio-ventricular node

fat cell

lymphocytes

Heberden's nodes in osteo-arthritis

efferent lymphatic vessel

section of **lymph node**

urine.

nitrog′enous. Containing nitrogen.

nitroglyc′erin. A thick, yellow, explosive liquid, used in the production of dynamite; in medicine the solid form is used as a vasodilator in the treatment of angina; also called trinitroglycerin.

nitroprus′side. A salt containing the radical Fe(CN)₅NO; e.g., sodium nitroprusside.

nitroso-. Combining form indicating the presence of the radical – NO in a compound.

nitroso. The univalent radical or group – NO, especially when present in organic compounds.

ni′trosyl. The nitroso radical or group – NO, when attached to an electronegative element such as chlorine.

ni′trous. Denoting a compound of nitrogen containing the smallest possible number of oxygen atoms.

n. oxide, a colorless gas of sweet taste, N_2O, used as a mild anesthetic; also called nitrogen monoxide and laughing gas.

NLM. Abbreviation for National Library of Medicine.

nm. Abbreviation for nanometer.

n.m. Abbreviation for nuclear membrane.

NMET. Abbreviation for normetanephrine.

nn. Abbreviation for nerves.

No. Chemical symbol of the element nobelium.

no. Abbreviation for number.

nobe′lium. The tenth transuranium element to be discovered; symbol No, atomic number 102, atomic weight 253.

Nocar′dia. A genus (family Actinomycetes) that includes fungus-like bacteria; the organisms are delicate, branching, often beaded, intertwining filaments that break into rod-shaped or coccoid forms; they are soil-dwelling and some are pathogenic.

N. asteroides, a species isolated from diseases resembling pulmonary tuberculosis and brain abscesses.

N. madurae, a species that is the causative agent of maduromycosis.

nocardio′sis. Any of several conditions caused by any species of *Nocardia*.

noci-. Combining form indicating (a) an injury; (b) a harmful agent or influence.

nocicep′tor. A peripheral nerve organ that receives and transmits painful sensations.

nocipercep′tion. Perception of painful or injurious stimuli.

noctam′bulism. See somnambulism.

noctipho′bia. An abnormal fear of night and its accompanying darkness and silence.

noctu′ria. Voiding of urine during the night.

node. 1. A circumscribed mass of differentiated tissue. **2.** A swelling.

Aschoff and Tawara's n., atrioventricular node.

atrioventricular n., the A-V node; a small uncapsulated node made of thin strips of interwoven modified cardiac muscle and situated near the orifice of the coronary sinus; when normally activated by the sinoatrial node, it transmits the impulse, through the Purkinje fibers, to the ventricular muscles causing practically simultaneous contraction.

A-V n., see atrioventricular node.

Bouchard's n., a small, hard nodule located in the proximal interphalangeal joint of a finger in osteoarthritis.

Delphian n., a midline node encased in fascia and resting on the thyroid isthmus; also called prelaryngeal node.

Heberden's n., a small, hard nodule located in the distal interphalangeal joint of a finger in osteoarthritis; it is an enlargement of the tubercle at the articular extremity of the distal phalanx.

Hensen's n., primitive node.

lymph n., an oval structure located along the course of a lymphatic vessel; its functions are the filtration of foreign matter and the production of lymphocytes; when enlarged, it provides a sign of infection or malignancy.

Osler n., small, tender, and discolored node usually appearing on the pads of fingers and toes in subacute endocarditis.

primitive n., a local swelling or thickening of ectodermal cells at the cranial end of the primitive streak of the embryo from which a strand of cells grows toward the cranium, between the ectoderm and endoderm in the midline, until it is blocked at the prechordal plate.

Ranvier's n., an interruption or constriction occurring at regular intervals (of about one millimeter) in the myelin sheath of a nerve fiber; it is here that a collateral branch may leave the axon; the area between two nodes is occupied by a single Schwann cell.

S-A n., see sinoatrial node.

sentinel n., see signal node.

signal n., an enlarged, palpable, supraclavicular lymph node which is often the first sign of an abdominal neoplasm; also called sentinel node and Virchow's node.

singer's n., trachoma of the vocal bands; a small, whitish, beadlike enlargement of the vocal cords, caused by overuse or abuse of the voice, as in prolonged singing, especially of high notes; also called teacher's node.

sinoatrial n., the S-A node; the mass of interwoven strips of cardiac muscle fibers that normally acts as the pacemaker of the cardiac conduction system; situated in the wall of the right atrium at the upper end of the crista terminalis just at the point of entry of the superior vena cava; it receives fibers from both autonomic nervous systems and is the part of the heart that originates the heart beat.

Virchow's n., see signal node.

no′dose. Having nodes.

nodos′ity. 1. A knotlike swelling. **2.** The condition of having nodes.

nod′ular. Relating to or having nodes.

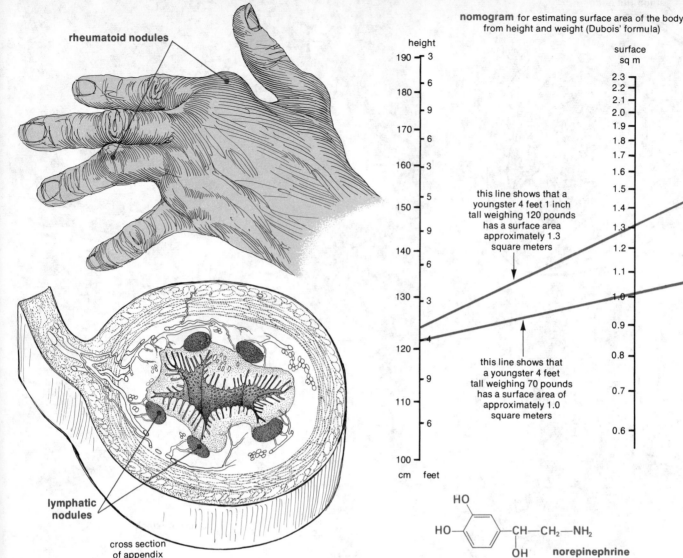

rheumatoid nodules

lymphatic nodules

cross section of appendix

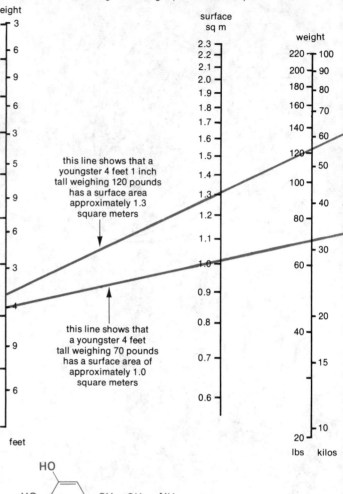

nomogram for estimating surface area of the body from height and weight (Dubois' formula)

height

surface sq m

weight

this line shows that a youngster 4 feet 1 inch tall weighing 120 pounds has a surface area approximately 1.3 square meters

this line shows that a youngster 4 feet tall weighing 70 pounds has a surface area of approximately 1.0 square meters

cm   feet

lbs   kilos

HO—

HO—⟨⟩—CH—CH₂—NH₂
         |
         OH   **norepinephrine**

---

nodula′tion. The presence or the formation of nodules.

nod′ule. A small node or closely packed collection of cells appearing distinct from the surrounding tissue.

  Aschoff n., see body, Aschoff.

  cold n., a thyroid nodule containing a lower concentration of an administered dose of radioactive iodine than the rest of the gland.

  hot n., a thyroid nodule containing a higher concentration of an administered dose of radioactive iodine than the rest of the gland; usually benign.

  lymphatic n., an aggregation of densely packed lymphocytes, seen in the submucosa of the intestines.

  rheumatoid n.'s, round or ovoid masses occurring most commonly subcutaneously over pressure points and near joints, in patients with rheumatoid arthritis.

  Schmorl's n., a localized protrusion of the central portion of an intervertebral disk through the cartilage plate and into the spongy bone of the vertebral body.

nod′ulus, *pl* **nod′uli.** Latin for nodule.

Nogu′chia. A genus of gram-negative, motile, encapsulated bacteria found in the conjunctiva of man and animals affected by a follicular type of disease.

no′ma. A rapidly destructive gangrenous disease of the mouth; seen in poorly nourished children and debilitated adults; also called gangrenous stomatitis.

Nomina Anatomica (NA). A system of anatomic terminology prepared by the International Congress of Anatomists.

nom′ogram, nom′ograph. A graph consisting of three coplanar graduated lines of different variables arranged in such a manner that a straight line connecting two known values on two of the graduated lines intersects the unknown value on the third graduated line; used generally to estimate the surface area of a body on the basis of an individual's height and weight.

nomotop′ic. Located in the normal or usual place.

no′nan. Recurring every ninth day; said of a fever.

nonapep′tide. A peptide possessing nine amino acids.

nonchro′mogens. Group III mycobacteria, mycobacteria that either are colorless or produce a light yellow pigment when grown in the presence of light.

non compos mentis. Latin for not having control of the mind; mentally not capable of managing one's affairs and hence legally not responsible.

nonconduc′tor. Anything that does not readily transmit electrical current, light, or heat.

nondis′ease. A disease suspected but not confirmed by further appropriate examinations.

nondisjunc′tion. Failure of paired chromosomes to separate at metaphase, so that both chromosomes are received by one daughter cell and none by the other.

nonelec′trolyte. A substance which, when in solution, does not conduct an electric current.

noninva′sive. Denoting diagnostic procedures that do not involve the use of instruments that penetrate the skin.

nonmet′al. Any electronegative element (e.g., iodine and fluorine) which forms oxides that produce acids and, in a solid state, is a poor conductor of heat and electricity.

non-nucleated. Without a nucleus.

nonocclu′sion. Condition in which a tooth of one arch fails to contact its opponent of the other arch.

non′ose. A sugar having nine carbon atoms.

nonpar′ous. Nulliparous; never having borne children.

nonpen′etrance. Failure of a genetic trait to be evident even though the genetic elements that usually produce the trait are present.

nonresec′table. Not capable of being cut off; said of a tumor not suitable for resection.

nonsecre′tor. A person whose body secretions do not contain antigens of the ABO blood group.

nonu′nion. Complication of a bone fracture in which healing stops short of firm union.

nonvi′able. Not capable of living.

Noonan's syndrome. Antimongoloid slant of the eyes and low set ears associated with valvular pulmonic stenosis.

nor-. 1. Combining form denoting nitrogen without a radical; e.g., norepinephrine is epinephrine minus the radical—CH₃ attached to the nitrogen atom. **2.** Indicating a change from a branched-chain compound into that of a straight-chain compound; e.g., leucine, norleucine.

noradren′aline. see norepinephrine.

norepineph′rine. A chemical substance (hormone) that produces constriction of practically all the blood vessels of the body; it is secreted by the postganglionic endings of the sympathetic nervous system; it is also produced and stored by the adrenal medulla and released upon stimulation of its sympathetic nerves; also called levarterenol and noradrenaline.

nor′ethan′drolone. C₂₀H₃₀O₂; an androgen used in protein anabolism; Nilevar®.

noreth′indrone. A progestational agent used in conjunction with estrogen as an oral contraceptive; Norlutin®.

norethyn′odrel. A steroid structurally similar to progesterone, used in combination with mestranol as an oral contraceptive.

norm. An ideal standard or pattern regarded as typical for a specific group.

nor′mal. 1. Conformed to an established norm, standard, or pattern. **2.** Perpendicular; a line or plane forming a right angle with another. **3.** In bacteriology, nonimmune; denoting an animal or serum that has not been experimentally exposed to or treated with any microorganism.

  n. solution, see under solution.

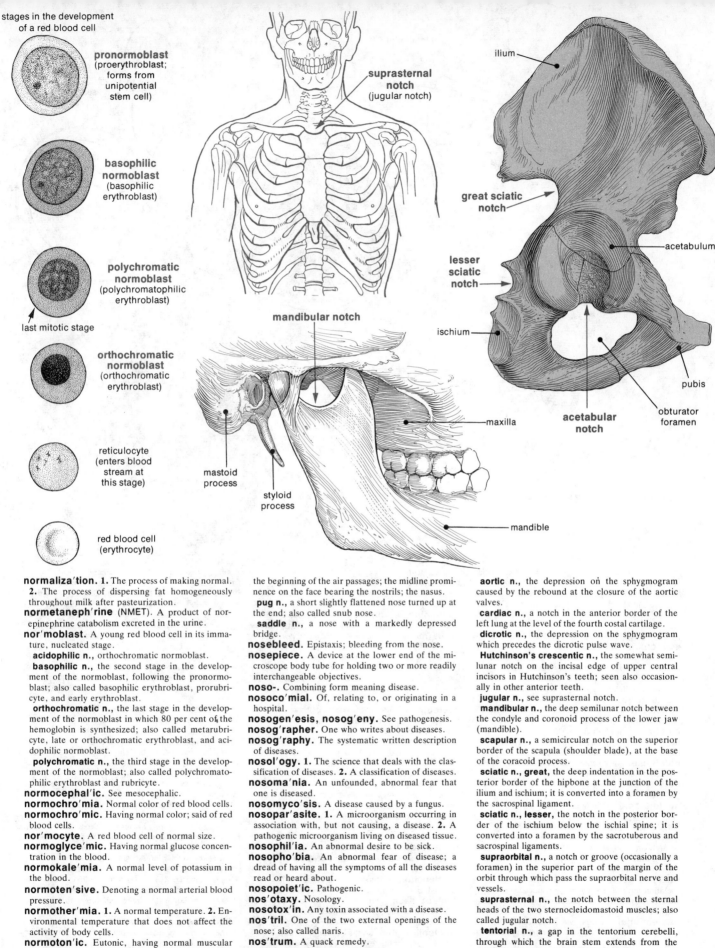

stages in the development of a red blood cell

pronormoblast (proerythroblast; forms from unipotential stem cell)

basophilic normoblast (basophilic erythroblast)

polychromatic normoblast (polychromatophilic erythroblast)

last mitotic stage

orthochromatic normoblast (orthochromatic erythroblast)

reticulocyte (enters blood stream at this stage)

red blood cell (erythrocyte)

suprasternal notch (jugular notch)

mandibular notch

mastoid process

styloid process

maxilla

mandible

ilium

great sciatic notch

lesser sciatic notch

acetabulum

ischium

acetabular notch

obturator foramen

pubis

---

normaliza′tion. 1. The process of making normal. **2.** The process of dispersing fat homogeneously throughout milk after pasteurization.

normetaneph′rine (NMET). A product of nor-epinephrine catabolism excreted in the urine.

nor′moblast. A young red blood cell in its imma-ture, nucleated stage.

acidophilic n., orthochromatic normoblast.

basophilic n., the second stage in the develop-ment of the normoblast, following the pronormo-blast; also called basophilic erythroblast, prorubri-cyte, and early erythroblast.

orthochromatic n., the last stage in the develop-ment of the normoblast in which 80 per cent of the hemoglobin is synthesized; also called metarubri-cyte, late or orthochromatic erythroblast, and aci-dophilic normoblast.

polychromatic n., the third stage in the develop-ment of the normoblast; also called polychromato-philic erythroblast and rubricyte.

normocephal′ic. See mesocephalic.

normochro′mia. Normal color of red blood cells.

normochro′mic. Having normal color; said of red blood cells.

nor′mocyte. A red blood cell of normal size.

normoglyce′mic. Having normal glucose concen-tration in the blood.

normokale′mia. A normal level of potassium in the blood.

normoten′sive. Denoting a normal arterial blood pressure.

normother′mia. 1. A normal temperature. **2.** En-vironmental temperature that does not affect the activity of body cells.

normoton′ic. Eutonic, having normal muscular tone.

normoto′pia. The state of being in the normal location.

normovole′mia. A normal blood volume.

nose. The external organ of the sense of smell and

the beginning of the air passages; the midline promi-nence on the face bearing the nostrils; the nasus.

pug n., a short slightly flattened nose turned up at the end; also called snub nose.

saddle n., a nose with a markedly depressed bridge.

nosebleed. Epistaxis; bleeding from the nose.

nosepiece. A device at the lower end of the mi-croscope body tube for holding two or more readily interchangeable objectives.

noso-. Combining form meaning disease.

nosoco′mial. Of, relating to, or originating in a hospital.

nosogen′esis, nosog′eny. See pathogenesis.

nosog′rapher. One who writes about diseases.

nosog′raphy. The systematic written description of diseases.

nosol′ogy. 1. The science that deals with the clas-sification of diseases. **2.** A classification of diseases.

nosoma′nia. An unfounded, abnormal fear that one is diseased.

nosomyco′sis. A disease caused by a fungus.

nosopar′asite. 1. A microorganism occurring in association with, but not causing, a disease. **2.** A pathogenic microorganism living on diseased tissue.

nosophil′ia. An abnormal desire to be sick.

nosopho′bia. An abnormal fear of disease; a dread of having all the symptoms of all the diseases read or heard about.

nosopoiet′ic. Pathogenic.

nos′otaxy. Nosology.

nosotox′in. Any toxin associated with a disease.

nos′tril. One of the two external openings of the nose; also called naris.

nos′trum. A quack remedy.

no′tal. Of or relating to the back.

notch. An indentation or depression.

acetabular n., a notch in the inferior margin of the acetabulum of the hipbone; it is bridged by the transverse acetabular ligament.

aortic n., the depression on the sphygmogram caused by the rebound at the closure of the aortic valves.

cardiac n., a notch in the anterior border of the left lung at the level of the fourth costal cartilage.

dicrotic n., the depression on the sphygmogram which precedes the dicrotic pulse wave.

Hutchinson's crescentic n., the somewhat semi-lunar notch on the incisal edge of upper central incisors in Hutchinson's teeth; seen also occasion-ally in other anterior teeth.

jugular n., see suprasternal notch.

mandibular n., the deep semilunar notch between the condyle and coronoid process of the lower jaw (mandible).

scapular n., a semicircular notch on the superior border of the scapula (shoulder blade), at the base of the coracoid process.

sciatic n., great, the deep indentation in the pos-terior border of the hipbone at the junction of the ilium and ischium; it is converted into a foramen by the sacrospinal ligament.

sciatic n., lesser, the notch in the posterior bor-der of the ischium below the ischial spine; it is converted into a foramen by the sacrotuberous and sacrospinal ligaments.

supraorbital n., a notch or groove (occasionally a foramen) in the superior part of the margin of the orbit through which pass the supraorbital nerve and vessels.

suprasternal n., the notch between the sternal heads of the two sternocleidomastoid muscles; also called jugular notch.

tentorial n., a gap in the tentorium cerebelli, through which the brain stem extends from the posterior into the middle cranial fossa.

trochlear n., a large concavity on the anterior surface of the olecranon process of the ulna which articulates with the trochlea of the humerus.

vertebral n., one of two notches above and below

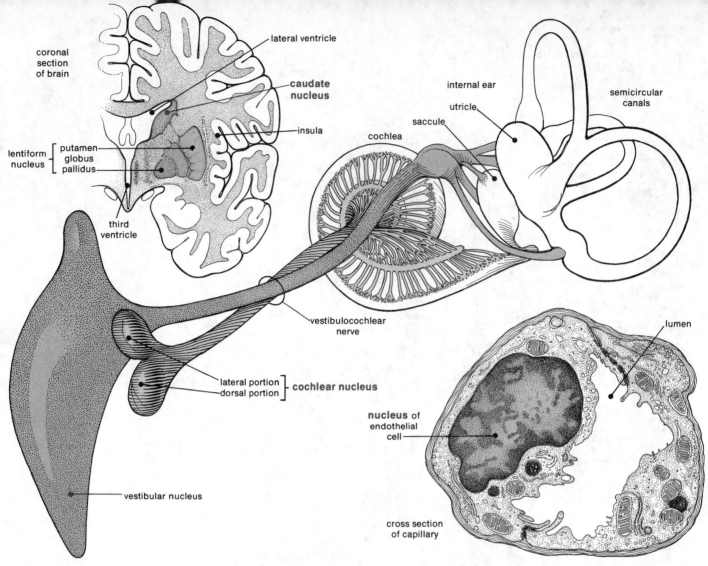

coronal section of brain

lateral ventricle

caudate nucleus

insula

lentiform nucleus { putamen globus pallidus }

third ventricle

internal ear

utricle

saccule

semicircular canals

cochlea

vestibulocochlear nerve

lateral portion
dorsal portion } cochlear nucleus

vestibular nucleus

lumen

nucleus of endothelial cell

cross section of capillary

---

the pedicle of a vertebra; the notches of two adjacent vertebrae form an intervertebral foramen.

no′tochord. A supporting rod of cells in the embryo of all chordates; in vertebrates it is replaced partially or wholly by the skull and vertebral column.

nox′a. Any harmful agent or influence.

nox′ious. Harmful to health.

Np. Chemical symbol of the element neptunium.

NPN. Abbreviation for nonprotein nitrogen.

nsec. Abbreviation for nanosecond.

nu. Thirteenth letter of the Greek alphabet, *ν*; symbol for kinematic viscosity.

nu′bile. Ready for marriage; said of a sexually mature young woman.

nu′cha. The back of the neck.

nu′chal. Relating to the back of the neck.

nu′clear. Of or relating to a nucleus.

nu′clease. An enzyme that promotes the breakdown of nucleic acid into nucleotides.

nu′cleated. Having a nucleus.

nu′clei. Plural of nucleus.

nucleic acids. Chemical compounds, of the utmost biologic importance, contained in all living organisms in the form of deoxyribonucleic acid (DNA) and ribonucleic acid (RNA); they consist mainly of a sugar moiety (pentose or deoxypentose), nitrogenous bases (purines and pyrimidines), and phosphoric acid.

nucleo-, nucle-. Combining forms indicating a relationship to (a) a nucleus; (b) nucleic acid.

nucleocap′sid. The protein coat (capsid) of a virus together with its enclosed nucleic acid.

nucleof′ugal. Moving away from a cell nucleus.

nu′cleogram. The data obtained through nucleography.

nucleog′raphy. A method of observing and recording the chemical composition, structure, size, etc., of a cell nucleus.

nucleohis′tone. A nucleoprotein derived from a histone; a salt between the basic protein and the nucleic acid.

nucleolone′ma. A dense, coarse strand that branches, forming a network within the nucleolus of a cell.

nucle′olus, *pl.* **nucle′oli.** A small, spherical organelle located in the nucleus of a cell; it contains RNA (ribonucleic acid) and protein and is an active center of protein and RNA synthesis, as well as an important center for the formation of ribosomes.

nu′cleon. One of the constituent particles of an atomic nucleus, i.e., a proton or a neutron.

nucleon′ics. The technology and application of nuclear energy.

nucleop′etal. Moving toward a cell nucleus.

nu′cleophil, nu′cleophile. The electron donor in a chemical reaction.

nu′cleoplasm. The protoplasm of the cell nucleus, composed mainly of proteins, metabolites, and ions; also called karyoplasm.

nucleopro′tein. A nondescript complex of compounds consisting of a simple protein and a nucleic acid; chromosomes and viruses are largely nucleoprotein in nature.

nucleoretic′ulum. Any structural network within the nucleus.

nucleorrhex′is. The breaking up of a cell nucleus.

nucleot′idase. An enzyme that catalyzes the splitting of a nucleotide into nucleosides and phosphoric acid.

nu′cleoside. A purine or pyrimidine base attached to a sugar (pentose, ribose, or deoxyribose).

nucleot′idase. An enzyme that catalyzes the splitting of a nucleotide into nucleosides and phosphoric acid.

nu′cleotide. One of the compounds into which nucleic acid splits on hydrolysis, consisting of a nitrogenous base (either a purine or a pyrimidine), a sugar (either ribose or deoxyribose), and a phosphate group; also called mononucleotide.

nucleoti′dyltrans′ferase. Enzymes that transfer nucleotide residues from nucleoside di- or tri-

phosphates into dimer or polymer forms.

nucleotox′in. A toxin affecting cell nuclei.

nu′cleus, *pl.* **nu′clei. 1.** The generally oval protoplasmic body in the center of the cell which contains the chromosomes and is surrounded by a nuclear membrane; an essential organelle that controls metabolism, growth, and reproduction. **2.** A localized mass of gray matter, composed of nerve cells, in the brain or spinal cord. **3.** The heavy, central, positively charged portion of the atom (composed of protons and neutrons) which contains the mass of the atom, about which the electrons revolve in orbit.

abducens n., a cranial nerve nucleus with fibers directed ventrally to supply the lateral rectus muscle of the eye.

amygdaloid n., an oval mass of gray matter in the anterior portion of the temporal lobe of the cerebrum, near the uncus; it is continuous with the cortex.

anterior horn n., a column of cells extending the entire length of the spinal cord and organized into medial and lateral groups, each with several subdivisions.

caudate n., a long horseshoe-shaped mass of gray matter consisting of an enlarged anterior portion which occupies most of the lateral wall of the anterior horn of the lateral ventricle, a narrower body extending along the floor of the lateral ventricle, and a tapered, curved tail which follows the curvature of the inferior horn of the lateral ventricle and enters the temporal lobe terminating in the amygdaloid complex.

cochlear n., a nucleus located on the surface of the inferior cerebellar peduncle at the junction of the medulla oblongata and the pons; it receives incoming fibers from the bipolar cells in the spiral ganglion of the cochlea.

dentate n. of the cerebellum, the largest of the central nuclei of the cerebellum embedded within the hemisphere of the cerebellum; its efferent fibers

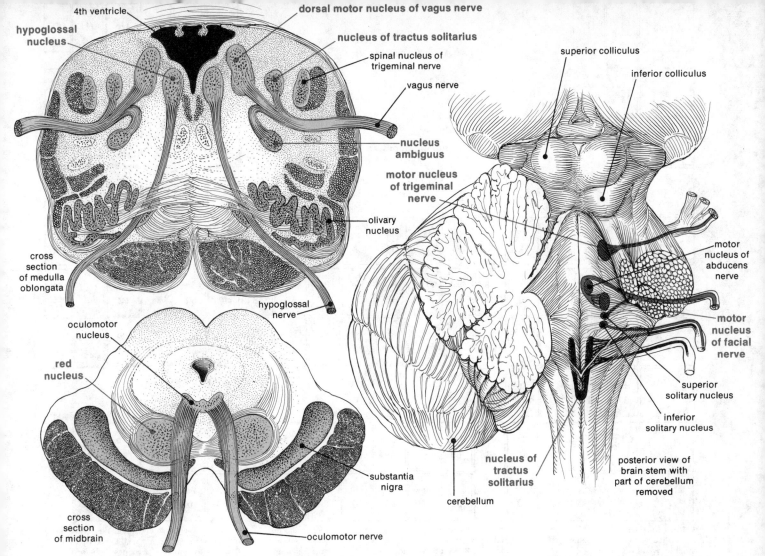

4th ventricle

hypoglossal nucleus

dorsal motor nucleus of vagus nerve

nucleus of tractus solitarius

spinal nucleus of trigeminal nerve

vagus nerve

nucleus ambiguus

motor nucleus of trigeminal nerve

olivary nucleus

cross section of medulla oblongata

hypoglossal nerve

oculomotor nucleus

red nucleus

cross section of midbrain

substantia nigra

oculomotor nerve

superior colliculus

inferior colliculus

motor nucleus of abducens nerve

motor nucleus of facial nerve

superior solitary nucleus

inferior solitary nucleus

nucleus of tractus solitarius

cerebellum

posterior view of brain stem with part of cerebellum removed

pass to the brain stem.

diploid n., a cell nucleus containing the diploid or normal double complement of chromosomes.

dorsal motor n. of vagus, a nucleus situated in the floor of the fourth ventricle which sends fibers through the medulla oblongata to the vagus and spinal accessory nerves which end in vagal sympathetic plexuses in the chest and abdomen.

Edinger-Westphal n., a circumscribed group of nerve cells whose fibers run to the oculomotor nerve and thence to the ciliary ganglion, innervating the intrinsic eye muscles.

hypoglossal n., a cranial nerve nucleus with fibers directed to the lower border of the pyramid to supply the tongue.

inferior colliculus n., an ovoid cellular mass surrounded by a thin cortex which serves as a relay in transmitting auditory impulses to thalamic levels and is involved in acoustic reflexes.

inferior salivatory n., a nucleus from which fibers pass via the small petrosal nerve to the optic ganglion to supply the parotid gland.

lenticular n., see lentiform nucleus.

lentiform n., a mass of gray matter the size and shape of a Brazil nut, deeply buried in the white matter of the cerebral hemisphere; a vertical plate of white matter divides the nucleus into a large lateral portion, the putamen, and a smaller medial portion, the globus pallidus; also called lenticular nucleus.

mesencephalic n. of trigeminal nerve, a cranial sensory nerve nucleus which receives fibers from extrinsic eye muscles and muscles of mastication; the mesencephalic root of the trigeminal nerve arises from it.

motor n. of facial nerve, a nucleus which gives rise to fibers that innervate the voluntary facial muscles.

motor n. of trigeminal nerve, a nucleus from which fibers run laterally with the mandibular nerve to innervate the muscles of mastication.

n. ambiguus, a motor nucleus composed of large multipolar cells which sends fibers through the glossopharyngeal, vagus, and spinal accessory nerves to supply the pharynx and larynx; also called ambiguous nucleus.

n. pulposus, the central gelatinous part of the intervertebral disk enclosed in several layers of fibrous tissue; it generally becomes fibrocartilaginous in old age.

n. of spinal accessory, a cranial nerve nucleus whose fibers form rootlets which join bulbar rootlets of the spinal accessory nerve to innervate the trapezius and sternocleidomastoid muscles.

n. of tractus solitaris, the nucleus of the solitary tract that receives visceral afferent fibers from the facial, glossopharyngeal, and vagus nerves; a slender nucleus extending the entire length of the medulla oblongata.

paraventricular n. of hypothalamus, a collection of nerve cells in the anterior part of the hypothalamus on either side of the third ventricle; it gives rise to the paraventriculohypophyseal tract which passes to the posterior lobe of the hypophysis (pituitary gland); related to the autonomic nervous system.

principal sensory n. of trigeminal nerve, a nucleus which receives fibers carrying impulses of touch, pain, and temperature from the head and face.

red n., a large oval nucleus situated in the midbrain, extending from the caudal margin of the superior colliculus to the subthalamic region; it receives fibers mainly from the deep cerebellar nuclei and the cerebral cortex; it is characterized by its pinkish-yellow color, its central position, and its capsule-like covering formed by the fibers of the superior cerebellar peduncle.

spinal n. of trigeminal nerve, a cranial sensory nerve nucleus which receives fibers that mediate pain and temperature for the head and face.

superior colliculus n., a laminated nucleus forming the top half of the tectum (roof of the midbrain) which serves as a primary relay in transmitting visual impulses.

superior salivatory n., scattered neurons in the dorsolateral reticular formation which send fibers through the chorda tympani to the submaxillary ganglion to supply the submaxillary and sublingual glands.

supraoptic n. of hypothalamus, one of two nuclei in the hypothalamus located on either side of the third ventricle near the optic tract; it gives rise to the supraopticohypophyseal tract which passes to the posterior lobe of the hypophysis (pituitary gland).

ventral posterolateral n. (VPL nucleus), a large mass of the thalamus which receives terminal fibers of the spinothalamic tract and medial lemniscus; it projects to the sensory cortex.

ventral posteromedial n. (VPM nucleus), a crescentic mass of the thalamus ventral to the centrum medianum that receives the secondary trigeminal tract; its axons project to the postcentral gyrus for the face.

vestibular n., a nucleus located in the floor of the fourth ventricle that receives fibers from the bipolar ganglion cells of the vestibular nerve.

nu′clide. An atom or a species of atom marked by its particular atomic number and atomic mass (A) or proton number (Z); nuclides with the same proton number are isotopes of a specific element; nuclides with the same atomic mass but different atomic numbers are isobars.

nulligrav′ida. A woman who has never been pregnant.

nullip′ara. A woman who has never given birth to children.

nullipar′ity. The condition of not having borne children.

nullip′arous. Never having borne children.

nulloso′mic. Lacking both members of a single pair of chromosomes.

Periodic Table

Group	I	II												III	IV	V	VI	VII	O
Period																			
1	H 1		METALS										NONMETALS						He 2
2	Li 3	Be 4		atomic numbers										B 5	C 6	N 7	O 8	F 9	Ne 10
3	Na 11	Mg 12												Al 13	Si 14	P 15	S 16	Cl 17	Ar 18
4	K 19	Ca 20	Sc 21	Ti 22	V 23	Cr 24	Mn 25	Fe 26	Co 27	Ni 28	Cu 29	Zn 30	Ga 31	Ge 32	As 33	Se 34	Br 35	Kr 36
5	Rb 37	Sr 38	Y 39	Zr 40	Nb 41	Mo 42	Tc 43	Ru 44	Rh 45	Pd 46	Ag 47	Cd 48	In 49	Sn 50	Sb 51	Te 52	I 53	Xe 54
6	Cs 55	Ba 56	* 57-71	Hf 72	Ta 73	W 74	Re 75	Os 76	Ir 77	Pt 78	Au 79	Hg 80	Ti 81	Pb 82	Bi 83	Po 84	At 85	Rn 86
7	Fr 87	Ra 88	** 89-103	Rf 104	Ha 105													

*	lanthanide elements (rare earth)	La 57	Ce 58	Pr 59	Nd 60	Pm 61	Sm 62	Eu 63	Gd 64	Tb 65	Dy 66	Ho 67	Er 68	Tm 69	Yb 70	Lu 71
**	actinide elements	Ac 89	Th 90	Pa 91	U 92	Np 93	Pu 94	Am 95	Cm 96	Bk 97	Cf 98	Es 99	Fm 100	Md 101	No 102	Lw 103

number (no). One of a series of symbols expressing a specified quantity or a definite value in a fixed order derived by counting.

atomic n., the number or position of an element in the periodic system; it represents the number of negative electrons outside the atomic nucleus.

Avogadro's n., the number of molecules or particles in one gram mole of any compound; it equals 6.022×10^{23}.

Brinell hardness n. (BHN), a number expressing the hardness of a dental material, derived by measuring the diameter of a dent made by pressing, with the aid of the Brinell tester, a standard carbide ball into the surface of the material under a specified load.

electronic n., the number of electrons in the outermost orbit (valence shell) of an element.

f-n., the number denoting the speed of a lens or its ability to gather light; rated by dividing the focal length of the lens or lens system by its effective aperture diameter; the smaller the f-number, the greater the exposure to light; also called f-stop.

Knoop hardness n. (KHN), a number representing the hardness of material (especially tooth structure and dental materials) determined by the penetration of a diamond indenting tool.

Mach n. (M), a number representing the ratio of the speed of an object to the speed of sound in the same surrounding medium.

mass n., the nearest integer to the number expressing the sum of the protons and neutrons in the atomic nucleus of an isotope; denoted as a prefix superscript, e.g., ^{16}O (oxygen-16).

num'bness. Insensibility of a part.

num'mular. 1. Shaped like a small coin; discoid; usually denoting the thick mucous sputum in certain respiratory disorders. **2.** Arranged like stacks of coins.

nummula'tion. Formation of disc-shaped masses.

nurse. 1. An individual trained to care for the sick, disabled, or enfeebled. **2.** To give nourishment to the breast; to suckle. **3.** To care for or tend one unable to provide for his own needs.

graduate n., one who is a graduate of an accredited school of nursing.

head n., one who is in charge of supervising the nursing staff of a hospital.

licensed practical n. (LPN), a practical nurse who is licensed to care for patients but has a range of allowable authority less than that of a registered nurse.

n.-anesthetist, a registered nurse who specializes in the administration of anesthetics.

practical n., an individual who is trained to provide certain nursing skills but has not graduated from a full nursing school program.

private duty n., one who is not a member of the hospital staff but is privately employed to provide nursing care to an individual patient.

public health n., a graduate nurse who has had special training in the techniques of preventing disease.

registered n. (RN), a graduate nurse who, having passed a state registration examination, is registered and licensed to practice.

scrub n., a nurse who dons a sterile gown and gloves to assist during a surgical procedure.

visiting n., one who provides nursing care to patients in their homes.

wet n., a woman who breast-feeds another woman's child.

nurs'ing. 1. Feeding at the breast. **2.** Activities that consitute the duties of a nurse.

n. home, a small private hospital for persons convalescing or people (especially aged persons) who require assistance in caring for and feeding themselves.

nu'trient. A nourishing component of food.

nutri'tion. The process in which a living organism utilizes food for growth and replacement of tissues through digestion, absorption, assimilation, and excretion.

nu'triture. The state of the body in regard to nourishment, especially in regard to a specific nutrient, such as protein.

nux'. Latin for nut.

n. vomica, a poisonous nut from *Strychnos nux-vomica*, a tree native to southeastern Asia; it is a source of two alkaloids, strychnine and brucine, and has been used as a bitter tonic, a tincture, and a central nervous system stimulant; also called strychnos seed, poison nut, and Quaker button.

nyctalo'pia. Impaired vision in subdued light, while daylight vision is normal; generally due to vitamin A deficiency; often used incorrectly instead of hemeralopia (day blindness); also called night blindness and day sight.

nycterohe'meral. See nyctohemeral.

nyctohem'eral. Indicating both night and day; also called nycterohemeral.

nyctopho'bia. Exaggerated and unreasonable fear of darkness.

nymph. The wingless stage in the development of certain insects immediately after hatching.

nymphola'bial. Relating to the labia minora and the labia majora.

nymphoma'nia. Excessive sexual desire in the female.

nymphoma'niac. A woman affected with nymphomania.

nymphon'cus. A swelling or enlargement of one or both labia minora.

nymphot'omy. Surgical incision of the clitoris or the labia minora.

nystag'mic. Relating to or affected with a jerky twitching of the eyeball.

nystag'mograph. Apparatus used to record graphically the movements of the eyeball in nystagmus.

nystagmog'raphy. The recording of nystagmic movements of the eyes.

electro-n., electronystagmography.

photoelectric n., procedure based on photosensor oculography.

nystag'moid. Resembling nystagmus.

nystag'mus. An involuntary movement of the eyes in either a rotatory, vertical, or horizontal direction; most commonly it is a rhythmic jerking with a fast and slow component, and is described by the direction of the quick component.

nys'tatin. An antibiotic agent obtained from cultures of *Streptomyces noursei;* used in the treatment of monilia infections.

nyx'is. A puncture.

NZB. Abbreviation for New Zealand black mouse.

objectives
housed in nosepiece
of microscope

vertex • sinciput • newborn skull • occiput

occipitomental
dimension

Oo

Ω. The Greek letter omega; symbol for ohm.

O. 1. Abbreviation for (a) octarius (pint); (b) oculus (eye). **2.** Symbol for (a) a blood type of the ABO group in which the serum does not contain agglutinogen; (b) oxygen.

o-. In chemistry, abbreviation for ortho-.

OAA. Abbreviation for oxaloacetic acid.

OB. Abbreviation for obstetrics.

obdormi′tion. Numbness of a bodily part due to pressure on the sensory nerve.

obe′lion. A craniometric point on the sagittal suture of the skull where it crosses the line, joining the two parietal foramina.

obese′. Very fat; corpulent.

obe′sity. Excessive accumulation of fat in the subcutaneous tissues.

  alimentary o., simple obesity.

  endogenous o., obesity attributed to endocrine and metabolic abnormalities.

  exogenous o., simple obesity.

  simple o., obesity that occurs when the caloric intake is greater than the energy expenditure.

o′bex. The small, triangular lamina at the caudal angle of the roof of the 4th ventricle.

obfusca′tion. 1. The process of rendering obscure or indistinct; a darkening. **2.** Confusion.

OB/GYN. Abbreviation for obstetrics and gynecology.

ob′ject. 1. Anything perceptible through any of the senses. **2.** A person or thing that arouses any type of emotion in an observer.

  sex o., a person or thing that arouses sexual feelings in another.

  test o., device used to determine the defining power of the objective lens of a microscope.

objec′tive. The lens or arrangement of lenses in a microscope or other optical system which receives light from the field of view and forms the first image; so named because it is nearest the object.

  immersion o., a high power objective designed to include oil or other liquid instead of air between its front lens and the cover glass.

ob′ligate. Capable of surviving in only one environment; said of certain parasites; opposite of facultative.

oblique′. Having a slanting or sloping direction; deviating from the perpendicular or the horizontal; inclined.

obliq′uity. Asynclitism.

obli′quus. Latin for oblique.

oblonga′ta. Having a long dimension; elongated; oblong.

obmutes′cence. Loss of speech; also called dumbness.

obnubila′tion. A confused state of mind.

OBS. Abbreviation for organic brain syndrome.

obser′verscope. A Y-shaped instrument which enables two observers to view simultaneously the interior of a canal or cavity.

obses′sion. A persistently recurring and unwanted idea that cannot be eliminated.

obses′sive-compul′sive. Having an obsessive-compulsive neurosis; see under neurosis.

obstet′ric, obstet′rical. Relating to obstetrics.

obstetric′ian. A physician who specializes in obstetrics.

obstet′rics. The branch of medicine concerned principally with the management of pregnancy, labor, and the phenomena following childbirth to complete involution of the uterus.

obstipa′tion. Constipation which does not respond to treatment; persistent failure to pass any stool.

obstruc′tion. An impedance; a blockage or clogging.

ob′struent. 1. Causing obstruction. **2.** An agent having such an effect.

obtund′. To diminish pain or touch sensations.

obtun′dent. An agent that dulls perception of pain or touch.

obtura′tion. A stoppage.

ob′turator. 1. Any structure that closes a bodily opening. **2.** A prosthetic device used to close a defect in the hard palate. **3.** An instrument used to occlude a hollow cannula during its insertion into the body.

obtu′sion. Dulling of normal sensibility.

occip′ital. Relating to the back of the head; see under bone.

occipitaliza′tion. Fusion or ankylosis between the atlas and occipital bone.

occipitoat′loid. Pertaining to the occipital bone and the first vertebra (atlas); applied to the articulation between the two bones.

occipitobregmat′ic. Pertaining to the occiput and the bregma (a measurement in craniometry).

occipitomen′tal. Relating to the back of the head and the chin.

occipitopari′etal. Relating to the occipital and parietal bones.

occipitotem′poral. Relating to the occipital and temporal bones.

oc′ciput. The lower back of the head.

occlud′e. 1. To close or obstruct. **2.** In dentistry, to bring together the upper and lower teeth.

occlu′der. 1. Device placed before an eye to block vision. **2.** Device placed on a blood vessel to prevent flow; used in certain physiologic experiments in animals.

occlu′sal. 1. Relating to a closure. **2.** In dentistry, relating to the contacting surfaces of teeth or occlusion rims.

occlu′sion. 1. The process of closing or the state of being closed. **2.** In dentistry, the contact of the mandibular teeth with the maxillary teeth in any functional relation. **3.** In chemistry, the absorption of a gas by a metal.

  abnormal o., malocclusion.

  afunctional o., malocclusion which prevents proper mastication.

  centric o., occlusion in which the upper and lower teeth are together in a normal, relaxed manner, and the mandible is in centric relation to the maxilla.

  coronary o., impedence of coronary circulation, usually by thrombosis.

  eccentric o., relating to teeth, any occlusion other than centric occlusion.

  enteromesenteric o., obstructed blood flow in the wall of the intestine and in the mesentery.

  hepatic vein o., a rare condition characterized by blocking of the hepatic veins, usually by tumor infiltration or by thrombosis of the vessels, causing enlargement of the liver, portal hypertension, and ascites; also called Budd-Chiari syndrome.

  pathogenic o., an occlusal relationship capable of incurring damage to supporting tissues.

  protrusive o., protrusion of the lower jaw from centric position.

occlu′sive. Covering; closing.

occlusom′eter. See gnathodynamometer.

occult′. Hidden, as a concealed hemorrhage.

ocel′lus, pl. **ocel′li.** A simple eye of many invertebrates.

OCG. Abbreviation for omnicardiogram.

ochrono′sis. A characteristic brown-black pigmentation of connective tissue occurring in certain metabolic disorders; a result of deposition of homogentisic acid.

octa-. Combining form meaning eight.

octamethyl pyrophosphoramide (OMPA). Chemical used as a plant insecticide; commonly called schradan.

oc′tan. Occurring every eighth day; said of certain fevers.

octapep′tide. A peptide compound of eight amino acid residues, such as the posterior pituitary hormones, oxytocin and vasopressin.

octav′alent. Having the combining power of eight hydrogen atoms.

oc′ular. 1. Relating to the eye. **2.** The eyepiece of a microscope.

oc′ulist. An obsolete term for ophthalmologist.

oculocerebrorenal syndrome. Hereditary syndrome consisting of congenital cataracts and glaucoma, mental retardation, and reabsorption

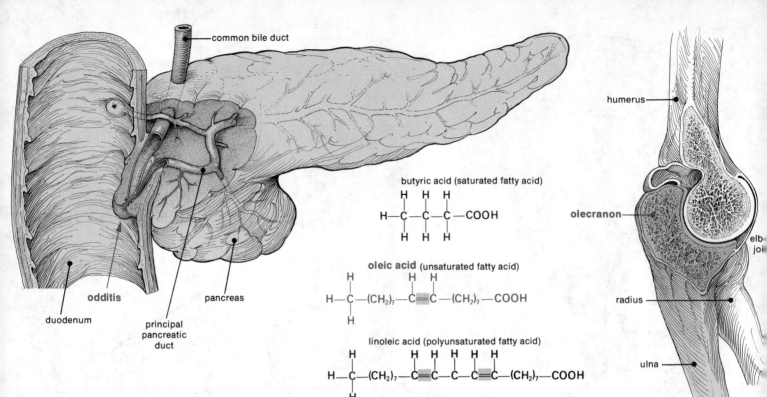

butyric acid (saturated fatty acid)

oleic acid (unsaturated fatty acid)

linoleic acid (polyunsaturated fatty acid)

common bile duct

odditis

pancreas

duodenum

principal pancreatic duct

humerus

olecranon

radius

ulna

elbow joint

---

dysfunction of the kidney tubules leading to proteinuria, glycosuria, aminoaciduria, and inability to concentrate and acidify the urine; also called cerebro-oculorenal dystrophy and Lowe's syndrome.

oculocuta'neous. Relating to the eyes and the skin.

oculogy'ria. Rotation of the eyeballs.

oculogy'ric. Relating to or causing rotation of the eyeballs.

oculomo'tor. 1. Relating to or causing movements of the eyeball. **2.** Relating to the oculomotor nerve (cranial nerve III).

oculomyco'sis. See ophthalmomycosis.

oculona'sal. Relating to the eye and the nose.

oculop'athy. Ophthalmopathy.

oc'ulus, *pl.* **oc'uli.** Latin for eye.

  o. dexter (O.D.), right eye.

  o. sinester (O.S.), left eye.

  o. uterque (O.U.), the two eyes.

O.D. Abbreviation for (a) optical density; (b) oculus dexter (right eye); (c) Doctor of Optometry.

oddi'tis. Inflammation of the sphincter of the hepatopancreatic duct (sphincter of Oddi), at the junction of the duodenum and common bile duct.

odontec'tomy. The removal of a tooth by the excision of bone around the root before it is extracted.

odontex'esis. The thorough scaling of teeth.

odon'tic. Of or relating to teeth; dental.

odonto-, odont-. Combining forms denoting a tooth or teeth; e.g., odontoblast.

odon'toblast. A specialized cell in the dental papilla of a developing tooth which produces the matrix that forms the dentin of the tooth; it lines the pulp cavity and may form secondary dentin throughout life.

odontoblasto'ma. 1. Tumor composed chiefly of epithelial and mesenchymal cells that may develop to produce calcified tooth substances. **2.** An odontoma in its early stage.

odon'tocele. Alveolodental cyst; see under cyst.

odon'toclast. A multinucleated cell believed to be involved in the absorption of the roots of primary teeth.

odontogen'ic. Derived from tissues involved in tooth formation; said of certain tumors.

odontog'eny. Development of teeth.

odon'toid. Shaped like a tooth, as the odontoid process of the second cervical vertebra.

odontol'ogy. Dentistry.

  forensic o., a branch of forensic medicine which applies knowledge of dentistry to civil and criminal problems.

odontol'ysis. Erosion of teeth.

odonto'ma. A tumor developed from tissues involved in tooth formation.

odontop'athy. Any disease of the teeth.

odontop'risis. Grinding of the teeth.

odontorrha'gia. Profuse bleeding from the socket after extraction of a tooth.

odon'toscope. A small circular mirror used for inspecting the teeth.

odontother'apy. Treatment of diseases of teeth.

odontot'omy. Cutting into a tooth.

o'dor. An emanation from any substance that stimulates the sense of smell; a smell or a scent.

odorif'erous. Odorous; giving off an odor.

odorim'eter. An instrument for determining the intensity of odors.

odorim'etry. Measurement of relative intensity of odors.

odor'iphore. See osmophore.

odyn-, -odynia. Combining forms indicating pain.

odynacu'sis. Hypersensitivity of the spiral organ of Corti (organ of hearing), so that noises cause actual discomfort; also called painful hearing.

odynom'eter. Instrument used to measure the degree of sensitivity to a painful stimulus; also called algesiometer.

odynopha'gia. Painful swallowing.

oer'sted (H). Unit of magnetic intensity, equal to the intensity of a magnetic field exerting a mechanical force of one dyne on a unit magnetic pole.

Oesophagos'tomum. A genus of nematode worms that form nodules in the intestinal wall of ruminants, swine, and man, especially in Africa.

oest'rid. A two-winged botfly, the larva of which is parasitic in man and animals.

Oes'trus. A genus of tissue-invading botflies.

of'fal. Waste parts of a butchered animal.

official. In pharmacology, authorized by or listed in the U.S. Pharmacopeia or the National Formulary.

offic'inal. Kept in stock; available without special preparation; said of pharmaceuticals.

OGTT. Abbreviation for oral glucose tolerance test.

ohm (Ω). A unit of electrical resistance equal to that of any conductor allowing one ampere of current to pass from a one volt potential across its terminals.

ohm'meter. An apparatus for direct measurement of the electric resistance (in ohms) of a conductor.

-oid. A combining form indicating a resemblance to the preceding element of the compound word; e.g., odontoid.

oid'iomyce'tes. Common name for a group of fungi that produce arthrospores (reproductive spores) through fragmentation of the mycelium.

oid'ium, *pl.* **oid'ia.** A free, thin-walled hyphal cell frequently called arthrospore.

oil. Any of several substances that are viscous, unctuous, flammable, and not miscible with water but soluble in several organic solvents; classified, according to their origin, as animal, mineral, or vegetable oils.

  arachis o., see peanut oil.

  castor o., oil obtained from castor-oil plant seeds (*Ricinus communis*); used as a laxative and externally as an emollient for skin disorders.

  cod liver o., oil obtained from fresh livers of cod fish; a rich source of vitamin A and D.

  mineral o., liquid petrolatum, a mixture of liquid hydrocarbons obtained from petroleum; also called white mineral oil and liquid paraffin.

  o. of gaultheria, oil of wintergreen.

  o. of wintergreen, a fragrant, volatile oil, rich in methyl salicylate, obtained from the macerated leaves of wintergreen; also called oil of gaultheria.

  peanut o., oil extracted from peanuts; used as a vehicle in pharmaceutical preparations; also called arachis oil.

  pine o., the volatile oil (crude turpentine) produced by the destructive distillation of pine wood; used as a deodorant and disinfectant.

  rectified tar o., oil obtained from pine tar; used in the treatment of certain skin disorders.

  red o., see oleic acid.

  safflower o., oil from seeds of the safflower, *Carthamus tinctorius*; rich in polyunsaturated fats; used as a dietary supplement and in the manufacture of cosmetics.

  wheat germ o., oil obtained from the embryo of the wheat kernel; a rich source of vitamin E.

oint'ment. Any of numerous soft, bland, highly viscous preparations used as a vehicle for external medication, as an emollient, or as a cosmetic; a salve.

  benzoic and salicylic acid o., one composed of benzoic acid and salicylic acid in a water-soluble base; used to treat athlete's foot and similar fungus infections; also called Whitfield's ointment.

  Whitfield's o., benzoic and salicylic acid oil.

-ol. Suffix indicating an alcohol or a phenol.

oleandomycin phosphate. Antibiotic substance elaborated by *Streptomyces antibioticus*; used in the treatment of streptococcal and staphylococcal infections.

o'leate. 1. A salt of oleic acid. **2.** A pharmaceutical preparation containing an alcohol or metallic base and oleic acid.

olec'ranon. Point of the elbow; the prominent curved process of the ulna forming the tip of the elbow.

o'lefin. An open-chain hydrocarbon having at least one double bond.

ole'ic. Of or relating to oil.

oleic acid. A colorless unsaturated fatty acid with

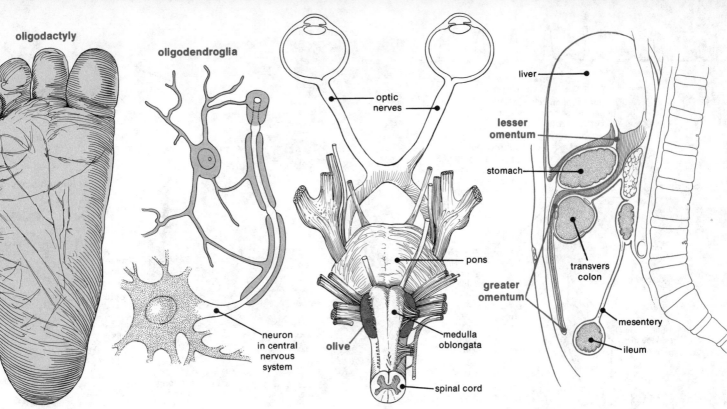

oligodactyly

oligodendroglia

optic nerves

liver

lesser omentum

stomach

transvers colon

greater omentum

mesentery

ileum

pons

olive

medulla oblongata

spinal cord

neuron in central nervous system

a lardlike aroma; a constituent of most of the common fats and oils; also called red oil.

o'lein. The glyceryl ester of oleic acid; a colorless oily substance occurring in many natural fats and oils; the main constituent of olive oil; also called triolein.

oleo-. Combining form meaning oil.

oleom'eter. Apparatus used to determine the specific gravity of oils.

oleores'in. 1. A natural compound of some plants (e.g., pines) containing resins and essential oils. **2.** An extract of a drug.

oleothor'ax. The therapeutic introduction of oil into the pleural cavity, as in the treatment of pulmonary tuberculosis and other disorders; also called eleothorax.

oleovi'tamin. A preparation containing an edible oil and a vitamin.

olfac'tie. See olfacty.

olfac'tion. 1. The sense of smell. **2.** The act of smelling.

olfactol'ogy. The science concerned with the study of the sense of smell.

olfactom'eter. A device for testing the sense of smell.

olfac'tory. Relating to the sense of smell; denoting the first cranial nerve or olfactory nerve.

olfac'ty, olfac'tie. An arbitrary unit of smell, used in olfactometry to determine the strength of a stimulus.

olig-, oligo-. Combining forms meaning few or little.

olige'mia. Deficient amount of blood in the body.

olighid'ria. A condition of scanty or diminished perspiration.

oligoam'nios. See oligohydramnios.

oligocho'lia. Abnormally low secretion of bile.

oligochy'lia. Hypochylia; deficiency of chyle.

oligochy'mia. A lack of chyme.

oligodac'tyly, oligodactyl'ia. Congenital absence of one or more digits of a hand or foot.

oligoden'drocyte. A cell of the oligodendroglia.

oligodendrog'lia. Non-nervous supportive tissue (neuroglia) surrounding nerve cells and fibers, with short, beaded processes and no fibrils.

oligodendroglio'ma. A relatively slow growing, solid tumor made up of oligodendroglia, usually found in the cerebrum of adults.

oligodip'sia. Abnormally reduced thirst.

oligodon'tia. Congenital absence of one or more teeth.

oligodynam'ic. Effective in very small quantities.

oligohydram'nios. Deficient amount of amniotic fluid in the pregnant uterus, sometimes represented by only a few milliliters of a thick viscid fluid; also

called oligoamnios.

oligomenorrhe'a. Reduction in the frequency of menstruation; occurring in intervals between the cycles from 38 days to three months.

oligonu'cleotide. A compound made up of a small number of nucleotides (2 to 10).

oligosac'charide. A compound made up of a small number of monosaccharide units (2 to 10).

oligosper'mia, oligosper'matism. Abnormally low concentration of spermatozoa in the semen.

oligotricho'sis. See hypotrichosis.

oligu'ria. Abnormally low excretion of urine; arbitrarily defined as less than 400 ml of urine per day for an adult of average size.

ol'ive. A smooth prominent oval mass on each side of the medulla oblongata; also called oliva.

Ollier's syndrome. A nonhereditary unilateral disorder marked by the presence of nonossified cartilage in the long bones, resulting in shortening of an extremity; also called dyschondroplasia, enchondromatosis, and hemichondrodysplasia.

-oma. Suffix denoting a morbid state, generally a tumor.

omal'gia. Pain in the shoulder area.

omega. Last letter of the Greek alphabet, Ω.

omen'tal. Of or relating to the omentum.

omentec'tomy. Surgical removal of the entire omentum, or of a portion of it.

omentofixa'tion. See omentopexy.

omen'topexy. Suturing of the omentum to the abdominal wall; also called omentofixation and epiplopexy.

omentor'rhaphy. Suturing of the omentum.

omen'tum. A peritoneal fold in the abdominal cavity which connects various viscera with each other or with the abdominal wall.

  greater o., a prominent double fold of peritoneum descending a variable distance from the greater curvature of the stomach to the front of the small intestine, where turning upon itself (thereby making four layers) it ascends to the top of the transverse colon; it resembles an apron and usually contains large deposits of fat.

  lesser o., the fold of peritoneum extending between the liver and the lesser curvature of the stomach and the beginning of the duodenum; the portion connecting the liver to the stomach is called the hepatogastric ligament, while the portion passing from the liver to the duodenum is named the hepatoduodenal ligament; the right border of the lesser omentum is free, forming the ventral margin of the epiploic foramen.

omn. hor. Abbreviation for Latin *omni hora*.

omni hora (omn. hor.). Latin for every hour; used

in prescription writing.

omniv'orous. Living on both plant and animal food.

omo-. Combining form meaning shoulder.

omoclavic'ular. Relating to the shoulder and the clavicle (collarbone).

omohy'oid. See table of muscles.

omomatol'ogy. The vocabulary of a science; also called nomenclature.

omothy'roid. See table of muscles.

omphal-, omphalo-. Combining forms denoting the umbilicus.

omphalec'tomy. Surgical removal of the navel.

omphal'ic. Umbilical.

omphali'tis. Inflammation of the navel.

om'phalocele. Congenital hernia at the umbilicus, either into the umbilical cord, or through a defect of the abdominal wall (omphalocele proper); also called exomphalos, umbilical eventration, and amniotic hernia.

omphalomesenter'ic. Relating to the umbilicus and the mesentery.

omphalophlebi'tis. Inflammation of the umbilical veins.

omphalorrha'gia. Bleeding from the navel.

omphalorrhe'a. A discharge from the navel.

om'phalos, om'phalus. The navel.

omphalot'omy. Cutting of the umbilical cord at birth.

om'phalotripsy. Crushing, instead of cutting, of the umbilical cord after childbirth.

o'nanism. Withdrawal of the penis just prior to ejaculation during sexual intercourse; the term is derived from the story of Onan, son of Judah (Genesis 38:9); commonly used as synonymous with male masturbation; also called coitus interruptus.

Onchocer'ca. A zoologic genus of elongated, parasitic filarial worms that inhabit the connective tissue of humans and animals; usually found coiled and entangled within firm nodules; two species, *Onchocerca caecutiens* and *Onchocerca volvulus*, can penetrate the skin.

onchocerci'asis, oncocerci'asis. Skin disease caused by infestation with a threadlike worm, *Onchocerca volvulus*; marked by irritation of the skin with corneal opacities and skin nodules; transmitted by the bite of infested flies; also called river blindness and volvulosis.

onco-, oncho-. Combining forms denoting a relationship to a tumor.

on'cocyte. An acidophilic, granular tumor cell.

oncogen'esis. The origin of a neoplasm.

oncogen'ic, oncog'enous. 1. Causing tumor formation. **2.** Originating from a tumor.

oncol'ogy. The scientific study of neoplasms.

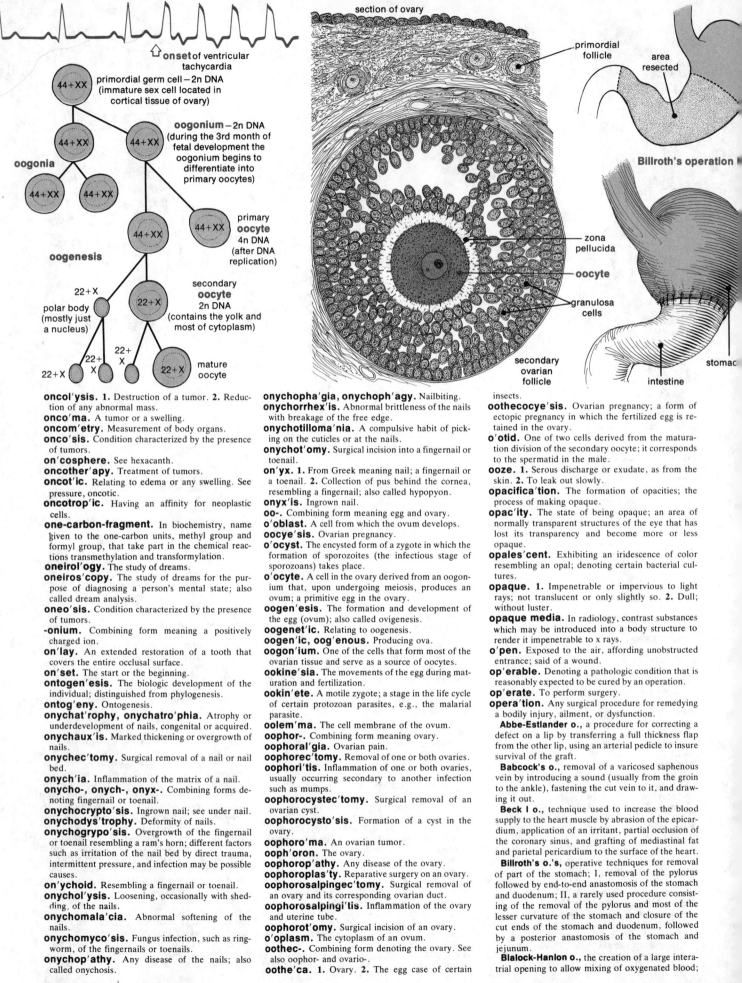

onset of ventricular tachycardia

primordial germ cell — 2n DNA (immature sex cell located in cortical tissue of ovary)

oogonia

44+XX

44+XX

44+XX

44+XX

oogonium — 2n DNA (during the 3rd month of fetal development the oogonium begins to differentiate into primary oocytes)

oogenesis

44+XX

44+XX

primary oocyte 4n DNA (after DNA replication)

polar body (mostly just a nucleus)

22+X

22+X

secondary oocyte 2n DNA (contains the yolk and most of cytoplasm)

22+X

22+X

22+X

22+X

22+X

mature oocyte

section of ovary

primordial follicle

zona pellucida

oocyte

granulosa cells

secondary ovarian follicle

area resected

Billroth's operation

stomach

intestine

---

oncol'ysis. 1. Destruction of a tumor. **2.** Reduction of any abnormal mass.

onco'ma. A tumor or a swelling.

oncom'etry. Measurement of body organs.

onco'sis. Condition characterized by the presence of tumors.

on'cosphere. See hexacanth.

oncother'apy. Treatment of tumors.

oncot'ic. Relating to edema or any swelling. See pressure, oncotic.

oncotrop'ic. Having an affinity for neoplastic cells.

one-carbon-fragment. In biochemistry, name given to the one-carbon units, methyl group and formyl group, that take part in the chemical reactions transmethylation and transformylation.

oneirol'ogy. The study of dreams.

oneiros'copy. The study of dreams for the purpose of diagnosing a person's mental state; also called dream analysis.

oneo'sis. Condition characterized by the presence of tumors.

-onium. Combining form meaning a positively charged ion.

on'lay. An extended restoration of a tooth that covers the entire occlusal surface.

on'set. The start or the beginning.

ontogen'esis. The biologic development of the individual; distinguished from phylogenesis.

ontog'eny. Ontogenesis.

onychat'rophy, onychatro'phia. Atrophy or underdevelopment of nails, congenital or acquired.

onychaux'is. Marked thickening or overgrowth of nails.

onychec'tomy. Surgical removal of a nail or nail bed.

onych'ia. Inflammation of the matrix of a nail.

onycho-, onych-, onyx-. Combining forms denoting fingernail or toenail.

onychocrypto'sis. Ingrown nail; see under nail.

onychodys'trophy. Deformity of nails.

onychogrypo'sis. Overgrowth of the fingernail or toenail resembling a ram's horn; different factors such as irritation of the nail bed by direct trauma, intermittent pressure, and infection may be possible causes.

on'ychoid. Resembling a fingernail or toenail.

onychol'ysis. Loosening, occasionally with shedding, of the nails.

onychomala'cia. Abnormal softening of the nails.

onychomyco'sis. Fungus infection, such as ringworm, of the fingernails or toenails.

onychop'athy. Any disease of the nails; also called onychosis.

onychopha'gia, onychoph'agy. Nailbiting.

onychorrhex'is. Abnormal brittleness of the nails with breakage of the free edge.

onychotilloma'nia. A compulsive habit of picking on the cuticles or at the nails.

onychot'omy. Surgical incision into a fingernail or toenail.

on'yx. 1. From Greek meaning nail; a fingernail or a toenail. **2.** Collection of pus behind the cornea, resembling a fingernail; also called hypopyon.

onyx'is. Ingrown nail.

oo-. Combining form meaning egg and ovary.

o'oblast. A cell from which the ovum develops.

oocye'sis. Ovarian pregnancy.

o'ocyst. The encysted form of a zygote in which the formation of sporozoites (the infectious stage of sporozoans) takes place.

o'ocyte. A cell in the ovary derived from an oogonium that, upon undergoing meiosis, produces an ovum; a primitive egg in the ovary.

oogen'esis. The formation and development of the egg (ovum); also called ovigenesis.

oogenet'ic. Relating to oogenesis.

oogen'ic, oog'enous. Producing ova.

oogon'ium. One of the cells that form most of the ovarian tissue and serve as a source of oocytes.

ookine'sia. The movements of the egg during maturation and fertilization.

ookin'ete. A motile zygote; a stage in the life cycle of certain protozoan parasites, e.g., the malarial parasite.

oolem'ma. The cell membrane of the ovum.

oophor-. Combining form meaning ovary.

oophoral'gia. Ovarian pain.

oophorec'tomy. Removal of one or both ovaries.

oophori'tis. Inflammation of one or both ovaries, usually occurring secondary to another infection such as mumps.

oophorocystec'tomy. Surgical removal of an ovarian cyst.

oophorocysto'sis. Formation of a cyst in the ovary.

oophoro'ma. An ovarian tumor.

ooph'oron. The ovary.

oophorop'athy. Any disease of the ovary.

oophoroplas'ty. Reparative surgery on an ovary.

oophorosalpingec'tomy. Surgical removal of an ovary and its corresponding ovarian duct.

oophorosalpingi'tis. Inflammation of the ovary and uterine tube.

oophorot'omy. Surgical incision of an ovary.

o'oplasm. The cytoplasm of an ovum.

oothec-. Combining form denoting the ovary. See also oophor- and ovario-.

oothe'ca. 1. Ovary. **2.** The egg case of certain insects.

oothecocye'sis. Ovarian pregnancy; a form of ectopic pregnancy in which the fertilized egg is retained in the ovary.

o'otid. One of two cells derived from the maturation division of the secondary oocyte; it corresponds to the spermatid in the male.

ooze. 1. Serous discharge or exudate, as from the skin. **2.** To leak out slowly.

opacifica'tion. The formation of opacities; the process of making opaque.

opac'ity. The state of being opaque; an area of normally transparent structures of the eye that has lost its transparency and become more or less opaque.

opales'cent. Exhibiting an iridescence of color resembling an opal; denoting certain bacterial cultures.

opaque. 1. Impenetrable or impervious to light rays; not translucent or only slightly so. **2.** Dull; without luster.

opaque media. In radiology, contrast substances which may be introduced into a body structure to render it impenetrable to x rays.

o'pen. Exposed to the air, affording unobstructed entrance; said of a wound.

op'erable. Denoting a pathologic condition that is reasonably expected to be cured by an operation.

op'erate. To perform surgery.

opera'tion. Any surgical procedure for remedying a bodily injury, ailment, or dysfunction.

  Abbe-Estlander o., a procedure for correcting a defect on a lip by transferring a full thickness flap from the other lip, using an arterial pedicle to insure survival of the graft.

  Babcock's o., removal of a varicosed saphenous vein by introducing a sound (usually from the groin to the ankle), fastening the cut vein to it, and drawing it out.

  Beck I o., technique used to increase the blood supply to the heart muscle by abrasion of the epicardium, application of an irritant, partial occlusion of the coronary sinus, and grafting of mediastinal fat and parietal pericardium to the surface of the heart.

  Billroth's o.'s, operative techniques for removal of part of the stomach; I, removal of the pylorus followed by end-to-end anastomosis of the stomach and duodenum; II, a rarely used procedure consisting of the removal of the pylorus and most of the lesser curvature of the stomach and closure of the cut ends of the stomach and duodenum, followed by a posterior anastomosis of the stomach and jejunum.

  Blalock-Hanlon o., the creation of a large interatrial opening to allow mixing of oxygenated blood;

---

oncolysis | operation

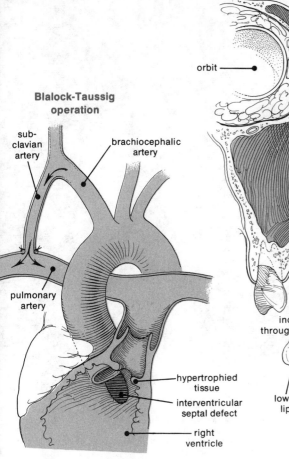

Blalock-Taussig operation

- subclavian artery
- brachiocephalic artery
- pulmonary artery
- hypertrophied tissue
- interventricular septal defect
- right ventricle

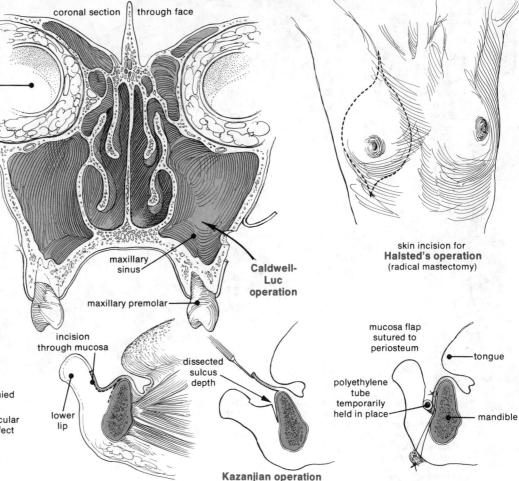

coronal section through face

- orbit
- maxillary sinus
- maxillary premolar
- **Caldwell-Luc operation**

incision through mucosa
- lower lip
- dissected sulcus depth

Kazanjian operation

skin incision for **Halsted's operation** (radical mastectomy)

- mucosa flap sutured to periosteum
- tongue
- polyethylene tube temporarily held in place
- mandible

---

a palliative measure for abnormality of the heart in which the aorta originates from the right ventricle and the pulmonary artery from the left ventricle.

Blalock-Taussig o., the anastomosing of the brachiocephalic trunk (innominate), a subclavian, or a carotid artery to the pulmonary artery to direct blood from the systemic circulation to the lungs, in cases of congenital pulmonary stenosis with septal defect.

blind o., one in which the surgeon operates by using his sense of touch and knowledge of surgical anatomy without full view of the operative field.

bloodless o., one performed with little or no blood loss.

Bricker's o., diversion of urine disposal from the bladder by connecting the ureter to a pouch of isolated ileum opening onto the abdominal wall.

Caldwell-Luc o., removal of the contents of a maxillary sinus through an opening on its facial wall above the root of the bicuspid tooth.

exploratory o., one used to establish a diagnosis by ascertaining the condition present.

fenestration o., an ear operation in which a sound pathway to the labyrinth is established to take the place of the oval window, occluded by otosclerotic stapes fixation; consists of creating a fistula into the osseous labyrinth of the horizontal semicircular canal or promontory and covering the opening with an elastic membrane or skin flap; the average opening or fenestra is generally the size of the oval window.

Gillies' o., reduction of fractures of the zygoma and zygomatic arch through an incision above the hairline.

Halsted's o.'s, (1) removal of a breast for carcinoma along with the greater and smaller pectoral muscles and adjacent lymphatic structures; (2) operation for the repair of a direct inguinal hernia.

Hofmeister o., reestablishment of intestinal continuity after partial removal of the stomach by closure of the lesser curvature side of the stomach and the duodenal stump, followed by anastomosis of the greater curvature side of the stomach and jejunum.

Huggins' o., removal of testes for cancer of the prostate gland.

Kazanjian's o., a surgical procedure for extend-

ing the vestibular sulcus of edentulous ridges to increase their height and to improve denture retention.

Manchester o., high amputation of the uterine cervix and suturing together of the broad ligament bases in front of the shortened cervix; devised to relieve first and second degree prolapse of the uterus.

Naffzinger's o., removal of the lateral and superior orbital walls for severe malignant exophthalmos.

open o., one in which the surgeon operates with full view of the operative field.

Pott's o., side-to-side connection between the aorta and the pulmonary artery; a palliative measure for tetralogy of Fallot.

plastic o., one intended to restore appearance, function, or lost parts.

radical o., a thorough one intended to effect a complete cure.

Roux-en-Y o., procedure in which the jejunum is cut about 15 cm below its origin, the distal end is sutured to the stomach, and the end of the proximal segment is sutured to the side of the jejunum farther down.

stapes mobilization o., freeing of stapes from overgrowth of bone to restore hearing in individuals with otosclerosis.

Whipple's o., removal of carcinoma of the head of the pancreas.

op′erative. 1. Relating to an operation. **2.** Active.

oper′culated. Having a caplike cover or operculum, as the eggs of certain parasitic worms.

oper′culum, pl. **oper′cula. 1.** In anatomy, any structure resembling a lid or cover. **2.** The mucus sealing the opening of the endocervical canal of the uterus during pregnancy. **3.** The caplike cover of the eggs of certain parasitic worms. **4.** The attached portion of a retinal detachment. **5.** The tissue covering (partly or completely) an unerupted tooth. **6.** One of the four gyri of the cerebrum that cover the insula (island of Reil).

o. oculi, the eyelid.

op′eron. A cluster of two or more structural genes and an operator gene on a chromosome governing the synthesis of the enzymes of a metabolic path-

way.

ophi′asis. Loss of hair occurring in bands partly or completely encircling the head.

ophidi′asis, ophidism. Poisoning by the venom of a snake.

ophid′ic. Relating to snakes.

ophidiopho′bia. A morbid fear of snakes.

ophryo′sis. Spasmodic twitching in the area of the eyebrow.

ophthalmal′gia. Pain in the eyeball.

ophthalmec′tomy. Surgical removal of the eyeball.

ophthal′mia. Inflammation of the eye.

gonorrheal o., acute purulent conjunctivitis caused by gonorrheal infection.

o. neonatorum, acute purulent conjunctivitis of the newborn infant acquired during passage through the birth canal when the mother has gonorrhea.

sympathetic o., bilateral inflammation of the uveal tracts following a perforating wound or retention of a foreign object in one eye, leading to bilateral blindness; also called metastatic, migratory, or transferred ophthalmia.

ophthal′mic. Pertaining to the eyeball.

ophthalmit′ic. Relating to inflammation of the eye.

ophthalmo-. Combining form meaning eye.

ophthal′moblenorrhe′a. Purulent conjunctivitis.

ophthal′mocente′sis. Surgical puncture of the eye.

ophthalmodi′aphan′oscope. Instrument used to inspect the interior of the eye by means of transmitted light.

ophthal′modone′sis. A trembling motion of the eyes.

ophthal′modynamom′eter. 1. Instrument for estimating the blood pressure of the retinal vessels. **2.** Instrument for measuring the power of convergence of the eyes, applied to a near point of vision.

ophthal′modynamom′etry. Measurement of the blood pressure in the retinal circulation within the eye by means of an ophthalmodynamometer; used to determine the presence of a stenotic lesion in the carotid artery system.

ophthal′modyn′ia. Ophthalmalgia.

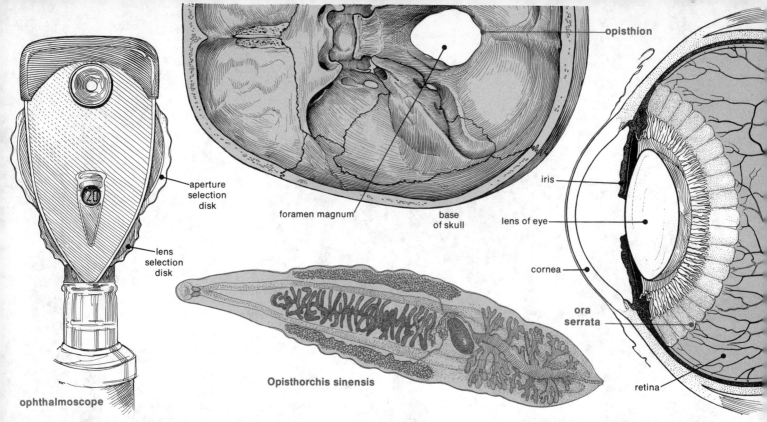

ophthalmoscope

aperture selection disk

lens selection disk

foramen magnum

base of skull

Opisthorchis sinensis

opisthion

iris

lens of eye

cornea

ora serrata

retina

---

ophthal'mo-eikonom'eter. Instrument for measuring the ocular disorder, aniseikonia.

ophthal'mograph. Instrument used to record eye movements during reading.

ophthal'moleu'koscope. Instrument used to test color perception; it controls color intensities by means of filters to produce a white mixture.

ophthalmol'ogist. A physician who specializes in treating diseases and refractive errors of the eye.

ophthalmol'ogy. The branch of medicine concerned with the eye, its diseases and refractive errors.

ophthal'momala'cia. Abnormally low intraocular pressure of the eyeball.

ophthalmom'eter. An instrument for measuring the curvature of the anterior surface of the cornea.

ophthalmom'etry. The measuring of the curvature of the anterior surface of the cornea with the ophthalmometer.

ophthal'momyco'sis. Any disease of the eye or its appendages caused by fungus; also called oculomycosis.

ophthal'momyi'asis. Infection of the eye with the larvae of flies; also called ocular myiasis.

ophthal'momyot'omy. Surgical division of any of the extrinsic (extraocular) eye muscles.

ophthal'moneuri'tis. Inflammation of the optic nerve.

opthalmop'athy. Any disease of the eye.

ophthal'mophacom'eter. Instrument used to measure the curvature of the cornea and lens of the eye.

ophthal'moplas'ty. Reparative surgery of the eye.

ophthal'mople'gia. Paralysis of one or more muscles of the eye.

  external hereditary o. see ophthalmoplegia progressiva.

  o. progressiva, external hereditary o., hereditary, progressive paralysis of the external muscles of the eye; also called Graefe's disease.

ophthal'mopleg'ic. 1. Relating to paralysis of the eye muscles. **2.** An agent causing such an effect.

ophthal'mopto'sia, **ophthal'mopto'sis.** Obsolete term for exophthalmos.

ophthal'morrha'gia. Bleeding from the eye.

ophthal'morrhe'a. Abnormal discharge from the eye.

ophthal'morrhex'is. Rupture of the eyeball.

ophthal'moscope. An instrument used in examination of the interior of the eye.

ophthalmos'copy. Examination of the interior of the eye by means of the ophthalmoscope.

ophthal'motonom'eter. An instrument for determining the tension of the eyeball; used for detection of glaucoma; tonometer.

ophthal'motonom'etry. Determination of the intraocular tension with the ophthalmotonometer.

ophthalmoto'nus. Intraocular tension; see under tension.

ophthal'motrope. A model of the two eyes designed to demonstrate the action of the extrinsic eye muscles.

ophthal'moxero'sis. See xerophthalmia.

-opia. Combining form denoting vision.

o'piate. Any preparation derived from opium.

o'pioid. Natural or synthetic compounds that have morphine-like pharmacologic activity; also called narcotic analgesic.

opis'thion. The middle point on the posterior margin of the foramen magnum of the occipital bone of the skull.

opisthochei'lia. Receding lips.

opisthocra'nium. The area in the midline of the cranium that protrudes farthest backward.

opisthorchi'asis. Infection with Asiatic flukes (*Opisthorchis viverrini* and *felineus*); transmitted through the ingestion of raw or undercooked infested fish.

Opisthor'chis. A genus of flukes characterized by having testes located near the posterior end of the lancet-shaped body.

  O. sinensis, a pathogenic variety of flukes transmitted to man through the ingestion of inadequately cooked infested fish.

opisthot'onos. A muscle spasm causing rigidity of the neck and back and arching of the back with convexity forward, as in acute cases of tetanus or meningitis.

o'pium. A bitter, brownish drug prepared from the dried gummy juice of unripe pods of a poppy, *Papaver somniferum*; used as an anesthetic; habitual use causes addiction and excessive use is fatal.

Oppenheim's sign. Dorsal extension of the big toe elicited by stroking the medial side of the tibia; seen in pyramidal tract disease.

oppo'nens. Opposing; a qualifying addition to the names of several muscles of the hand and foot whose function is to pull the lateral digits across the palm or sole.

op'sin. The protein constituent of the rhodopsin molecule (a retinal pigment).

op'sonin. A serum substance naturally present in blood (usually an antibody), which coats particulates, such as bacteria, and renders them susceptible to destruction by phagocytes (phagocytosis).

opsoniza'tion. The process by which antibody affects antigen so that it is more readily phagocytized.

op'sonize. To sensitize microorganisms with specific opsonin, thereby rendering them more susceptible to phagocytosis; also called opsonify.

op'sonocytopha'gic. Relating to the increased phagocytic activity of leukocytes in blood containing specific opsonin.

optesthe'sia. The ability to perceive a light stimulus.

op'tic. Pertaining to the eye.

op'tical. Relating to vision.

op'tical bench. An apparatus for ascertaining the physical properties and aberrations of a lens or lens system.

op'tical cen'ter. The point of a lens through which passing light rays suffer no angular deviation.

opti'cian. One who makes or sells lenses, eyeglasses, or other optical instruments; a person who adjusts eyeglasses after a prescription furnished by an ophthalmologist or optometrist.

opticocil'iary. Relating to the optic and ciliary nerves.

opticocine'rea. The gray substance of the optic nerve.

op'tics. The science concerned with the study of light and refracting media, especially of the eye.

op'timum. Denoting the most suitable or favorable conditions.

optom'eter. Any of several devices used to measure the refractive state of the eye; also called opsiometer and optimeter.

optom'etrist. An individual who specializes in examining, measuring, and treating visual defects by means of corrective lenses.

optom'etry. The measuring of visual acuity and correction of visual defects by glasses.

optomyom'eter. Instrument used to determine the relative strength of the extrinsic muscles of the eye.

OR. Abbreviation for operating room.

o'ra, pl. **o'rae.** A border.

  o. serrata, the serrated margin of the retina, situated in the anterior portion of the eyeball.

o'rad. Toward the mouth.

o'ral. Relating to the mouth.

oral'ity. In psychoanalysis, relating to the oral or earliest stage of sexual development.

or'ange. 1. An edible fruit, *Aurantii fructus*; its rind contains numerous oil glands and is used in producing pharmaceutical preparations. **2.** The hue in the spectrum between yellow and red; the color evoked by radiant energy of wavelengths from 575 to 625 nm.

  methyl o., sodium salt of helianthin; yellow-orange powder used as an indicator with a pH range from 3.2 to 4.4 (yellow at 3.2, pink at 4.4).

orbic'ular. Circular.

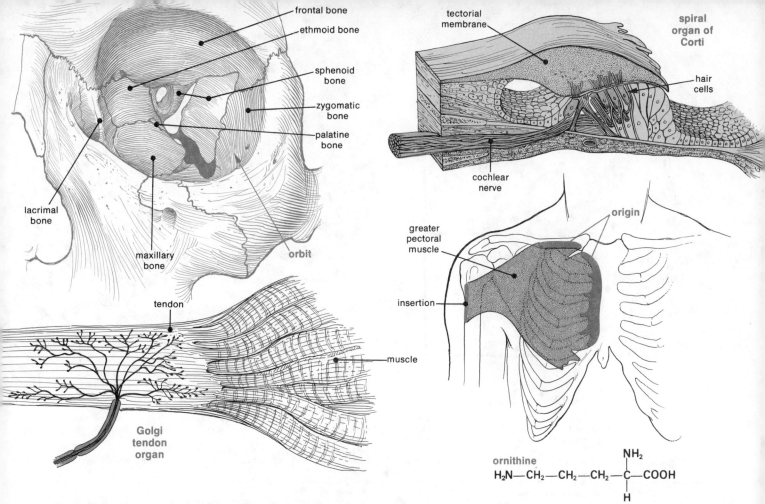

Labels in figure (top to bottom, left to right):

frontal bone
ethmoid bone
sphenoid bone
zygomatic bone
palatine bone
lacrimal bone
maxillary bone
orbit
tendon
Golgi tendon organ
muscle

tectorial membrane
spiral organ of Corti
hair cells
cochlear nerve
origin
greater pectoral muscle
insertion
muscle

ornithine
$$H_2N—CH_2—CH_2—CH_2—\overset{\overset{\displaystyle NH_2}{|}}{\underset{\underset{\displaystyle H}{|}}{C}}—COOH$$

orbit. One of two cavities in the skull that contains the eyeball and its associated structures; it is formed by portions of seven bones: frontal, maxillary, zygomatic, lacrimal, sphenoid, palatine, and ethmoid; commonly called eye socket.

or′bital. Relating to the orbit.

orbitog′raphy. The making of x-ray films of the orbit following injection of a radiopaque substance over the orbit floor; a diagnostic technique used when a blow-out fracture is suspected.

orbitonom′eter. Instrument used to measure the degree of resistance offered by the eyeball when pressed into the socket.

orbitot′omy. Surgical incision into the orbit.

or′cein. A purple dye used in cytology.

orchi-, orchid-, orchio-. Combining forms meaning testis.

orchial′gia. Pain in a testis; also called orchiodynia, orchidalgia, and testalgia.

orchichore′a. Involuntary twitching of the testis.

orchidor′rhaphy. See orchiopexy.

orchiec′tomy, orchidec′tomy. Surgical removal of one or both testes; also called castration.

orchiepididymi′tis. Inflammation of a testis and epididymis.

or′chiocele. A tumor of the testis.

or′chiodyn′ia. See orchialgia.

orchion′cus. A neoplasm or tumor of the testis.

orchiop′athy. Any disease of the testes.

orchiopex′y. Suturing of a testis to the scrotum as in the correction of an undescended testis; also called orchidorrhaphy and orchiorrhaphy.

or′chioplasty. Reparative surgery of the testes.

orchior′rhaphy. See orchiopexy.

orchioscir′rhus. Abnormal hardening of the testis.

orchiot′omy. Surgical incision into a testis.

or′chis. Greek for testis.

orchi′tis. Testitis; inflammation of the testis.

   o. parotidea, acute orchitis, usually unilateral, occurring as a complication of mumps; sometimes causes atrophy of the testis.

or′der. A biologic taxonomic category ranking just below class and above family.

or′derly. An attendant in a hospital ward whose responsibilities do not require professional training.

orexigen′ic. Stimulating the appetite.

orf. A viral disease of sheep occasionally transmitted to the skin of man, especially to sheepherders and veterinarians; the chancre-type lesions appear most frequently on the hands and face; also called ecthyma contagiosum.

or′gan. A differentiated structure of the body that performs some specific function.

   end o., the expanded termination of a nerve fibril as found in muscle tissue, skin, mucous membrane, or glands.

   Golgi tendon o., special bare nerve ending ramifying about bundles of collagen fibers of tendons, usually at the ends of muscles; the afferent fibers are among the largest fibers in peripheral nerve tissue.

   o. of Corti, see spiral organ of Corti.

   o.'s of Zuckerkandl, small masses of chromaffin tissue located along the abdominal aorta; they are more prominent in the fetus.

   sense o., any organ of special sense, as the eye, and the accessory structures associated with it.

   spiral o. of Corti, the sensory receptors for hearing, contained in the cochlear duct of the internal ear; also called organ of Corti.

   target o., the organ that is stimulated by a hormone.

or′ganelle. A specialized cytoplasmic structure of a cell performing a specific function, such as a mitochondrion.

organ′ic. 1. Relating to the organs of the body. **2.** Relating to living organisms. **3.** Organized; structural.

organic brain syndrome (OBS). **organic mental syndrome** (OMS). A syndrome resulting from diffuse or local impairment of brain tissue function, manifested by alteration of orientation, memory, comprehension, and judgment.

   acute o. b. s., acute confusional state, characterized by a sudden onset and a high degree of reversibility.

   chronic o. b. s., disorder marked by an insidious onset, a progressive course, and a high degree of irreversibility; always due to focal or diffuse brain lesions.

   psychotic o. b. s., acute or chronic organic brain syndrome associated with psychiatric symptoms.

or′ganism. Any living entity, plant or animal.

organiza′tion. 1. An arrangement of distinct but dependent parts with varied functions that contribute to the whole; the organic structure of an organism. **2.** The process of forming into organs.

or′ganizer. 1. A group of cells on the dorsal lip of the blastopore that stimulates the differentiation of cells in the embryo. **2.** Any group of cells having such an ability.

or′ganoid. 1. Resembling an organ. **2.** Composed of the cellular elements of an organ.

organolep′tic. 1. Stimulating an organ of sense. **2.** Capable of receiving a sensory stimulus.

organ′omercu′rial. An organic compound of mercury; some compounds of this type have diuretic properties.

organot′ropism. The predilection of microorganisms and chemicals for certain organs or tissues; e.g., viruses infecting primarily the central nervous tissue.

or′gasm. The climax of the sexual act.

orienta′tion. 1. Awareness of oneself in reference to time, place, and other individuals; the act of finding one's bearings. **2.** The relative position of atoms in a compound.

or′ifice. An opening.

or′igin. 1. The site of attachment of a muscle to a bone which is less movable than the one to which it is inserted. **2.** The starting point or beginning of a nerve.

or′nithine. $NH_2(CH_2)_3CHCH_2COOH$; an amino acid formed when urea is removed from arginine; an important intermediate in urea biosynthesis, it possesses one less carbon than its homologue lysine.

Ornithodo′ros. A genus of ticks (family Argasidae) some of which transmit the agents of relapsing fevers.

Ornithonyssus sylviarum. A species of mites parasitic on many domestic and wild fowl; they also infest man, producing a pruritic dermatitis; also called northern fowl mite.

ornitho′sis. An infectious disease of birds occasionally transmitted to man; when transmitted by parrots or other psittacine birds, the disease is known as psittacosis; in man, the disease may cause an influenza-like condition or pneumonia; the exact

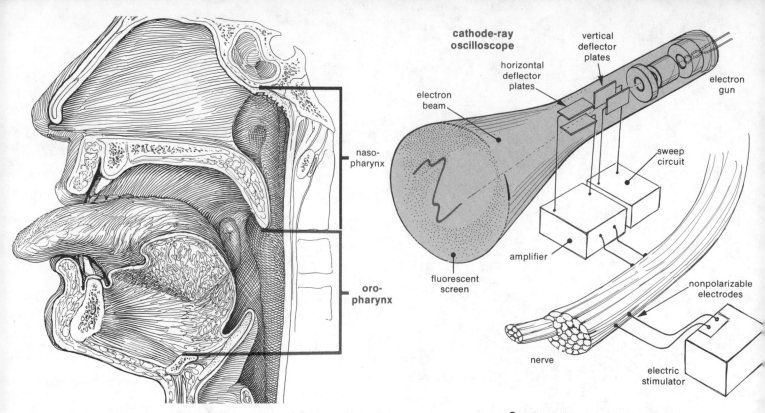

cathode-ray oscilloscope

electron gun

vertical deflector plates

horizontal deflector plates

electron beam

nasopharynx

oropharynx

sweep circuit

amplifier

fluorescent screen

nonpolarizable electrodes

nerve

electric stimulator

classification of the agent causing the disease is not settled, since it has features resembling a large virus on the one hand and *Rickettsia* or bacteria on the other.

oroling′ual. Relating to the mouth and tongue.

orona′sal. Relating to the mouth and the nose.

or′opharynx. The central portion of the pharynx directly behind the oral cavity, extending from the inferior border of the soft palate to the lingual surface of the epiglottis; it contains the palatine tonsils and the posterior faucial pillars.

orrhorrhe′a. Any condition in which a thin, watery fluid oozes from structures such as nasal membranes, urethra, etc.

orthet′ics. See orthotics.

ortho-. Combining form denoting (a) straight, normal; (b) correction of maladjustments or deformities; (c) an acid in its highest form of hydration; (d) the adjacent carbon positions in a benzene ring.

orthobio′sis. Living in a manner that promotes physical and mental health.

orthochromat′ic. Staining the color of the dye used; said of certain cells.

orthocra′sia. Condition in which the body reacts normally to drugs.

orthodig′ita. Correction of malformed fingers or toes.

orthodon′tics. A specialty of dentistry dealing with correction and prevention of irregularities of the teeth.

orthodon′tist. A dentist who specializes in orthodontics.

orthodrom′ic. Conducting impulses along a normal path.

orthogen′ics. The study and treatment of defects (physical and mental).

orthognath′ic. Having straight jaws and a straight profile; having a face with no projection of the lower jaw, one with a gnathic index below 98.

or′thograde. The erect posture of man; opposed to pronograde.

orthokinet′ics. A method of treatment for hypertrophic osteoarthritis in which a muscular action is transferred from one set of muscles to another in order to protect the affected joint.

orthom′eter. Instrument used to measure the degree of protrusion of the eyeballs.

orthopae′dics. See orthopedics.

orthopan′tograph. In radiology, a panoramic device that x-rays all the teeth on a single extraoral film.

orthope′dic. Relating to orthopedics.

orthope′dics, orthopae′dics. The surgically oriented branch of medicine concerned with the preservation and restoration of functions of the skeletal system and associated structures.

orthope′dist. One who practices orthopedics.

orthopercus′sion. Percussion in which the left middle finger is flexed at a right angle and the tip of the finger is placed on the chest wall; the flexed finger is then struck upon the knuckle.

orthopho′ria. Condition in which the visual axes of the two eyes are free from a tendency to deviate.

orthophos′phate. A salt of phosphoric acid (H_3PO_4).

orthopne′a. Difficulty in breathing except in an upright position.

orthopne′ic. Relating to or afflicted with orthopnea.

or′thopod. Slang for orthopedist.

orthopsychi′atry. The study and treatment of human behavior for the purpose of promoting healthy emotional growth and development.

Orthop′tera. An order of insects that includes grasshoppers, cockroaches, locusts, etc.

orthop′tics. The training process or techniques used for the improvement of visual perception and coordination of the two eyes for efficient binocular vision, or for the elimination of strabismus.

orthop′tist. One who is trained to treat ocular muscle imbalance, as strabismus, by reeducation of visual habits and exercise.

or′thoscope. An instrument that eliminates the refracting power of the cornea by means of a layer of water in a glass container held in contact with the eye.

orthoscop′ic. 1. Relating to the orthoscope. 2. Having normal vision. 3. Giving a correct and proportioned image.

orthos′copy. 1. Examination of the eye with an orthoscope. 2. The state of an optical system that produces images free of distortion.

orthostat′ic. Relating to or caused by the upright position.

orthothana′sia. 1. The science of natural death. 2. The deliberate discontinuance of artificial means of maintaining life.

orthot′ics. The making and fitting of orthopedic appliances; also called orthetics.

or′thotist. One who makes and fits orthopedic appliances.

orthot′onos, orthot′onus. Tetanic spasm in which the head, body, and limbs are fixed rigidly in a straight line.

orthotop′ic. Occurring in the normal position.

orthotrop′ic. Growing or extending along a vertical axis.

orthovol′tage. Medium electromotive force, from 200 to 300 kilovolts; used in radiotherapy.

O.S. Abbreviation for oculus sinister.

Os. Chemical symbol of the element osmium.

os, *pl.* **ora.** Latin for mouth; orifice, as the os of the cervix.

os, *pl.* **os′sa.** Latin for bone.

osche-. Combining form denoting a relationship to the scrotum.

os′cheocele. Indirect inguinal hernia; see hernia, inguinal.

os′cheoplasty. Reparative surgery of the scrotum; also called scrotoplasty.

oscilla′tion. 1. A backward and forward movement. 2. A stage of inflammation in which leukocytes accumulate in small vessels, blocking the flow of blood and causing a to-and-fro movement with each cardiac contraction.

oscil′logram. A graphic record traced by an oscillograph.

os′cillograph. An apparatus for graphically recording the oscillations of an electric current.

oscillom′eter. Instrument used to measure variations in blood pressure.

oscillop′sia. State in which observed objects seem to oscillate.

os′cilloscope. An electronic instrument that temporarily displays the variations of a fluctuating electrical quantity on the fluorescent screen of a cathode-ray tube.

os′citate. To gape; to yawn.

os′culum, *pl.* **os′cula.** A tiny opening.

-ose. Suffix denoting (a) a carbohydrate; e.g., sucrose, glucose; (b) a substance resulting from the digestion of a protein; e.g., albuminose.

Osgood-Schlatter disease. Epiphysial aseptic necrosis; see under necrosis.

Osiander's sign. Pulsation of the vagina in early pregnancy.

-osis. Suffix denoting (a) an abnormal or diseased condition; e.g., tuberculosis; (b) any increase; e.g., leukocytosis; (c) a process; e.g., osmosis.

Osler's disease. Hereditary hemorrhagic telangiectasia; see under telangiectasia.

Osler's sign. Small painful swellings in the skin and subcutaneous tissues of the hands and feet occurring in endocarditis.

Osler-Weber-Rendu syndrome. Hereditary hemorrhagic telangiectasia; see under telangiectasia.

osmat′ic. Relating to the sense of smell.

osmidro′sis. Condition marked by a fetid odor of sweat; also called bromidrosis.

osmiophil′ic. Easily fixed with osmium textroxide.

os′mium. Metallic element; symbol Os, atomic number 76, atomic weight 190.2.

 o. tetroxide, OsO_4; a crystalline compound com-

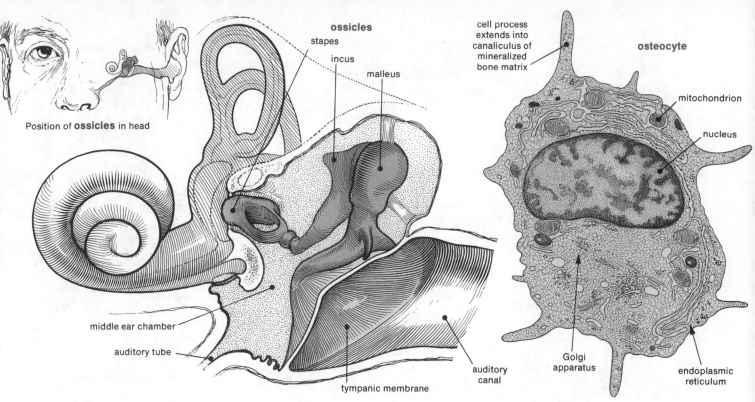

Position of ossicles in head

ossicles — stapes, incus, malleus

middle ear chamber
auditory tube
tympanic membrane
auditory canal

osteocyte — cell process extends into canaliculus of mineralized bone matrix, mitochondrion, nucleus, Golgi apparatus, endoplasmic reticulum

---

monly used as a tissue fixative for electron microscopy; it has an irritating odor.

osmo-. Combining form relating to (a) osmosis; (b) odors.

osmocep′tor. Osmoreceptor.

osmolal′ity. The osmotic concentration of a solution expressed as osmoles of the dissolved substance per kilogram of solvent (water).

osmo′lar. See osmotic.

osmolar′ity. The osmotic concentration of a solution expressed as osmoles of the dissolved substance per liter of solution.

os′mole. One gram-molecular weight of any non-dissociating compound; i.e., glucose, 6.023×10^{23} particles (molecules and ions) in solution.

osmom′eter. An instrument for determining osmolality of a liquid, such as urine, by measuring the freezing point depression.

osmom′etry. The measure of concentration of solute per kilogram of water; serum osmolality is normally from 280 to 300 mOs/kg.

os′mophil, osmophil′ic. Thriving in a solution of high osmotic pressure.

os′mophore. In chemistry, a radical or atomic group whose presence in a compound causes the particular odor of the compound; also called odoriphore and aromatophore.

osmorecep′tor, osmocep′tor. 1. A specialized sensory nerve ending in the hypothalamus which responds to changes in the osmotic pressure of the blood by regulating the secretion of the neurohypophyseal antidiuretic hormone (ADH). **2.** A receptor that responds to the sensation of odors (olfactory stimuli).

osmoreg′ulatory. 1. Regulating the osmolarity of the blood by acting to alter antidiuretic hormone release. **2.** Influencing osmosis.

osmo′sis. The passage of liquid from a concentrated solution to a diluted one through a semipermeable membrane that separates them.

osmot′ic. Relating to osmosis; also called osmolar. See also pressure, osmotic.

osphresiol′ogy. The study of odors and of the sense of smell.

os′seous. Bony.

os′sicle. A small bone.

auditory o.'s, the three bones of the ear; malleus, incus, and stapes; together they form a bony chain across the middle ear chamber for the conduction of sound waves from the tympanic membrane (eardrum) to the oval window; they are secured to the walls of the chamber by ligaments.

ossic′ular. Of or relating to an ossicle.

ossiculec′tomy. Surgical removal of one or more ossicles of the middle ear.

ossiculot′omy. Surgical incision of one of the ossicles of the middle ear or of adhesions that prevent their movements.

ossifica′tion. The replacement of cartilage by bone.

os′sify. To change into bone.

osteal′gia, ostal′gia. Pain in a bone.

ostei′tis. Inflammation of bone.

o. deformans, Paget's disease; a bone disease of unknown cause, characterized by localized, excessive destruction and repair with associated deformities.

o. fibrosa cystica, disease characterized chiefly by softening and resorption of bone and replacement with fibrous tissue; caused by excessive secretion of hormone from the parathyroid glands.

osteo-, oste-, ost-. Combining forms denoting bone or bones; e.g., osteology.

osteoarthri′tis. See degenerative joint disease.

osteoarthrop′athy. Disorder affecting the long bones of the extremities and joints, often accompanied by clubbing of the fingers; almost always associated with disease elsewhere in the body, usually the lungs, pleura, and mediastinum.

hypertrophic o., painful swelling and periosteal deposition of new bone in the long bones of the extremities, clubbing of the fingers, and swelling and tenderness of joints; occurs most commonly in association with pulmonary disease, especially pulmonary neoplasm; also seen with cyanotic heart disease, ulcerative colitis, regional enteritis, and liver disorders.

idiopathic hypertrophic o., osteoarthropathy that does not occur secondary to any disease; also called primary osteoarthropathy.

os′teoblast. A bone-forming cell; it arises from a fibroblast and is responsible for the formation of bone matrix; found on the advancing surface of developing bone.

osteoblasto′ma. A benign tumor derived from primitive bone tissue; occurs most frequently on the spine of young individuals; also called giant osteoid osteoma.

osteochondri′tis. Inflammation of both bone and its cartilage.

osteochondrodys′trophy. General term for a group of disorders involving bone and cartilage, including the Morquio syndrome.

osteochondro′ma. A single benign bony outgrowth capped by growing cartilage; most frequently occurring near the end of long bones of individuals between 10 and 25 years of age; also called solitary osteocartilagenous exostosis.

osteochondromato′sis. Multiple hereditary exostosis; see under exostosis.

osteochondrosarco′ma. A malignant tumor of cartilaginous tissue usually arising from a benign bone tumor.

osteochondro′sis. Any disorder of the ossification centers in children; characterized by death of tissues in the absence of infection.

osteoc′lasis, osteocla′sia. Surgical or manual fracture or refracture of a deformed bone for the purpose of resetting it in a more normal position.

os′teoclast. A large multinucleated cell which is formed in bone narrow and absorbs bone tissue.

osteoclasto′ma. Giant cell tumor of bone; see under tumor.

osteocra′nium. The fetal cranium after ossification has occurred.

os′teocyte. One of numerous flattened, nucleated bone cells arising from osteoblasts by modulation; it plays a role in maintaining the constituents of the intercellular matrix at normal levels; each is contained in a space (lacuna) and its processes extend through openings of the lacuna into minute canals within the bone tissue.

osteocyto′ma. Solitary bone cyst; see under cyst.

osteoden′tin. A hard substance, structurally intermediate between dentin and bone, which partially fills the pulp cavity of teeth of the aged.

osteoder′mia. The presence of bony deposits on the skin.

osteodesmo′sis. The conversion of tendons into bone.

osteodyn′ia. Ostealgia.

osteodys′trophy. Defective bone formation.

renal o., generalized bone changes resembling osteomalacia and rickets, occurring in children or adults with chronic renal failure.

osteofibro′ma. A benign tumor-like lesion composed chiefly of osseous and fibrous connective tissue.

os′teogen. The inner layer of periosteum from which new bone is formed.

osteogen′esis. The formation of bone.

o. imperfecta, a rare disease characterized by bone fragility, blue sclera, and otosclerotic deafness; thought to be transmitted as an autosomal dominant trait.

osteogen′ic, osteogenet′ic. Relating to bone formation; derived from bone.

os′teoid. Resembling bone; usually refers to the soft organic part of intercellular bone matrix produced by osteogenic and osteoblast cells.

osteol′ogy. The study of the structure of bones.

osteol′ysis. Destruction of bone.

osteo′ma. A benign tumor composed of bone tissue; it may develop on a bone (homoplastic osteoma) or on other structures (heteroplastic os-

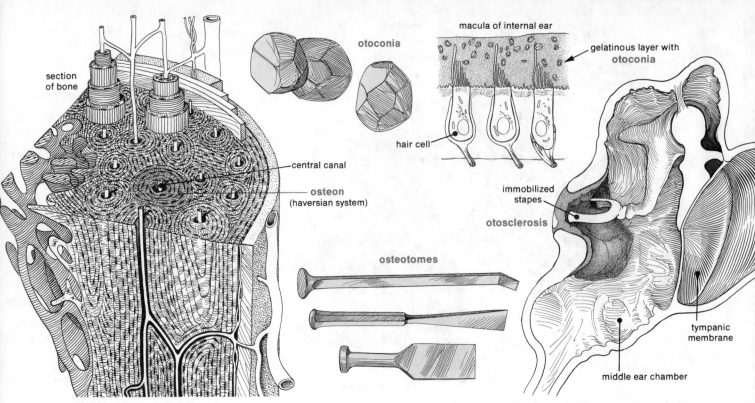

section of bone

otoconia

macula of internal ear

gelatinous layer with **otoconia**

hair cell

central canal

osteon (haversian system)

immobilized stapes

otosclerosis

osteotomes

tympanic membrane

middle ear chamber

teoma); also called osseous tumor.

   dental o., a bony growth projecting from the root of a tooth.

osteomala′cia. A disease marked by softening of the bones, due to faulty calcification; it usually affects adult females and is similar to rickets in children.

os′teomere. One of a series of bony structures, such as the vertebrae.

osteom′etry. The branch of anthropology concerned with the relative size of human bones.

osteomyeli′tis. Infection of bone, most commonly caused by a staphylococcus, affecting the metaphyseal regions of the long bones of children.

osteomyelodyspla′sia. Disease characterized by enlargement of the bone marrow cavities, thinning of the osseous tissue, and associated leukopenia and fever.

osteomyelofibrot′ic syndrome. See myelofibrosis.

osteomyelog′raphy. The examination of bone marrow with x rays.

os′teon. The basic unit of compact bone structure consisting of a central canal and the concentric bony lamellae around it; also called haversian system.

osteon′cus. Term sometimes used to denote a bony growth.

osteonecro′sis. Death of bone tissue, occurring most commonly in the head of the femur, less frequently in the medial femoral condyle, and occasionally in the head of the humerus.

os′teopath. A practitioner of osteopathy.

osteopatho′logy. The study of bone diseases.

osteop′athy. 1. Disease of bones. **2.** A system of medical practice based on the belief that the normal body is capable of making its own remedies against infection; therapeutics is mainly manipulative, although surgical, medicinal, and hygienic methods are used when indicated.

osteoperiosti′tis. Inflammation of a bone and its periosteum.

osteopetro′sis. An uncommon hereditary disorder transmitted as an autosomal recessive trait; characterized principally by overgrowth and denseness of bones and narrowing of the marrow, with resulting anemia, visual disturbances, deafness, and delayed tooth eruption; seen most frequently in children; also called Albers-Schönberg or marble bone disease.

osteophlebi′tis. Inflammation of the veins of a bone.

osteoph′ony. The conduction of sound by bone.

os′teophyte. A bony outgrowth.

os′teoplasty. Plastic surgery of bones; bone grafting.

osteoporo′sis. Disease of the bones due to deficiency of bone matrix, occurring most frequently in postmenopausal women.

osteoradionecro′sis. Death and degeneration of bone tissue caused by radiation.

osteorrha′gia. Bleeding from bone.

osteor′rhaphy. Wiring of a broken bone; also called osteosuture.

osteosarco′ma. Bone cancer, usually occurring in the shaft at either end of a long bone; also called osteoma sarcomatosum.

osteosarco′matous. Relating to or causing bone cancer.

osteosclero′sis. Abnormally increased density or hardness of bone.

osteosu′ture. See osteorrhaphy.

osteosyn′thesis. Fastening the ends of a fractured bone.

osteota′bes. Degeneration of bone marrow.

os′teotome. A chisel used for cutting bone.

osteotomoc′lasis, osteotomocla′sia. Operative procedure for straightening an abnormally curved bone.

osteot′omy. Cutting of a bone, usually with a saw or chisel.

os′tial. Relating to an orifice or ostium.

os′tium. A small opening into a hollow structure.

   o. primum, interatrial foramen primum; see under foramen.

   o. secundum, interatrial foramen secundum; see under foramen.

O.T. Abbreviation for occupational therapy.

ot-. See oto-.

otal′gia. See earache.

otal′gic. 1. Relating to earache. **2.** Any remedy for an earache.

OTC. Abbreviation for over the counter.

othelco′sis. 1. Ulceration of the external ear. **2.** Suppuration of the middle ear.

othemorrhe′a, othemorrha′gia. Bleeding from the ear.

o′tic. Of or relating to the ear.

otit′ic. Relating to inflammation of the ear.

oti′tis. Inflammation of the ear.

   chronic suppurative o. media, inflammation of the middle ear attended by a thick mucopurulent discharge from the mucous membrane; the infection may progress to involve the bone.

   o. externa, inflammation of the external auditory canal due to the presence of a furuncle or to a variety of skin infections.

   o. media, infection of the middle ear, usually secondary to upper respiratory infections, generally transmitted to the middle ear through the auditory tube.

oto-, ot-. Combining forms denoting a relationship to the ear.

otoantri′tis. Inflammation of the mastoid antrum.

otoblennorrhe′a. Chronic inflammation of the middle ear with perforation of the tympanic membrane (eardrum) and a mucopurulent discharge from the ear.

otoceph′aly. Defect characterized by extreme smallness of the chin and approximation of the ears toward the front of the neck.

otoclei′sis. 1. Closure of the auditory (eustachian) tube. **2.** Obstruction of the external auditory canal.

otoco′nia, sing. **otoco′nium.** Granular particles composed of calcium carbonate and protein normally embedded in the gelatinous layer that covers the maculae of the utricle and saccule of the internal ear; also called otoliths and statoconia.

otodecano′ic acid. See stearic acid.

otodyn′ia. Earache.

otoencephali′tis. Inflammation of the brain, secondary to inflammation of the middle ear and mastoid cells; also called otocerebritis.

otogan′glion. Otic ganglion; see under ganglion.

otolaryngol′ogist. A specialist in otolaryngology.

otolaryngol′ogy. The branch of medicine concerned with the study of the ear and the upper respiratory tract and the treatment of their diseases.

o′toliths. See otoconia.

otolog′ic. Relating to otology.

otol′ogist. A specialist in ear diseases.

otol′ogy. The branch of medicine concerned with diseases of the ear.

-otomy. Combining form meaning surgical incision.

otomyco′sis. Fungal infection of the external auditory canal.

otoneural′gia. Neuralgic earache.

otop′athy. Any disease of the ear.

o′toplasty. Plastic surgery of the auricle of the ear.

otopyorrhe′a. Purulent discharge from the middle ear through a perforated tympanic membrane.

otorhinolaryngol′ogy. The branch of medicine that deals with the ear, nose, and larynx, and their diseases.

otorhinol′ogy. Study of the ear and the nose.

otorrha′gia. Bleeding from the ear.

otorrhe′a. Discharge from the ear.

otosclero′sis. The formation and overgrowth of new spongy bone in the capsule of the middle ear, which immobilizes the stapes and interferes with the conduction of sound waves, resulting in slow, progressive hearing loss; surgical removal of the stapes and the sclerotic bone covering the oval window and replacement with prosthetic devices frequently restores hearing.

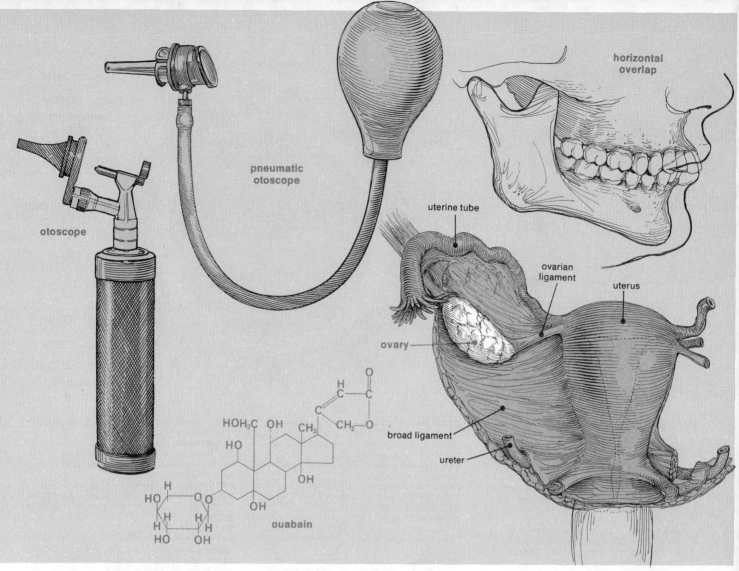

otoscope

pneumatic otoscope

ouabain

uterine tube

ovarian ligament

uterus

ovary

broad ligament

ureter

horizontal overlap

o′toscope. An instrument for examining the ear.
   pneumatic o., one that uses alternate positive and negative pressure to observe the degree of flaccidity of the tympanic membrane.

otos′copy. Examination of the tympanic membrane with an otoscope.

otot′omy. 1. Dissection of the ear. **2.** Myringotomy.

ototox′ic. Having a deleterious effect upon the ear.

ototoxic′ity. The capability of having a deleterious or harmful effect upon the ear, especially its neural parts.

O.U. Abbreviation for oculus uterque.

ouaba′in. A rapidly acting cardiac glycoside from the seeds of *Strophanthus gratus*; a constituent of African arrow poison.

ounce. 1. An avoirdupois unit of weight equal to 437.5 grains or 16 drams; $1/16$th of a pound. **2.** An apothecary unit of weight (used in the United States Pharmacopeia) equal to 480 grains or 1.097 avoirdupois ounces.
   fluid o., either of two units of liquid capacity: (1) in the U.S. Customary System, the equivalent of 1.804 cubic inches or $1/16$th of a pint; (2) in the British Imperial System (used in liquid or dry measure), the equivalent of 1.734 cubic inches or $1/20$th of a pint.

-ous. Suffix used in chemical nomenclature, meaning occurring in its lowest valency.

out′lay. A graft on the surface of a bone.

out′let. 1. A passage or exit. **2.** A means of releasing feelings and energies.
   pelvic o., the lower aperture of the pelvis, bounded by the pubic arch, the ischial tuberosities, the sacrotuberous ligaments, and the tip of the coccyx.

out′patient. A patient treated in a hospital or clinic without being hospitalized.

out′put. 1. The quantity of a substance produced by or eliminated from the body during a given span of time. **2.** The measure of performance by an organ or a system.
   cardiac o., the quantity of blood pumped by the heart per unit of time, usually per minute; the product of stroke volume and cardiac rate.
   minute o., the quantity of blood pumped by the heart during one minute, normally four to five liters at rest in an average sized individual.
   stroke o., the quantity of blood ejected with a single heart beat.
   urinary o., the quantity of urine excreted by the kidneys.

out′toed. Foot position in which the toes are turned outward to a marked degree.

ova. Plural of ovum.

ovalbu′min. Albumin from egg whites.

ovalocyto′sis. Elliptocytosis; an inherited disorder in which 25 to 90 per cent of red blood cells have an oval shape.

ovaral′gia, ovarial′gia. Pain in an ovary.

ova′rian. Of or relating to the ovary.

ovariec′tomy. Surgical removal of an ovary.

ovario-. Combining form denoting ovary.

ova′riocente′sis. Puncture of an ovarian cyst.

ovariocye′sis. Ovarian pregnancy.

ovariohysterec′tomy. Surgical removal of the ovaries and uterus.

ovariop′athy. Disease of the ovary.

ovariorrhex′is. Rupture of an ovary.

ovariosalpingec′tomy. Surgical removal of an ovary and the corresponding uterine tube.

ovariot′omy. An incision into an ovary.

ova′rium. Latin for ovary.

ov′ary. One of the paired sexual glands in which the ova are formed; it produces the hormones progesterone and estrogen.

o′verbite. Vertical overlap; see under overlap.

overclosure, reduced interarch distance. A condition in which the mandible rises too far before the teeth make contact, due to modification of tooth shape (through grinding), drifting of teeth, or loss of teeth, resulting in a shortened face length.

overcompensa′tion. A type of behavior in which an overwhelming feeling of inadequacy inspires exaggerated correction, e.g., overaggressiveness and the striving for power at all costs.

overdetermina′tion. In psychiatry, the multiple causation of a single event, behavior, or emotional symptom.

overdose′. 1. An excessive dose; too great a dose. **2.** To give, prescribe, or take an excessive dose.
   barbiturate o., an overdose of barbiturates causing severe poisoning; a common mode of suicide.
   narcotic o., an excessive dose of a narcotic drug producing the clinical triad of stupor (or coma), respiratory depression, and pinpoint pupils (miosis); treatment generally consists of ventilatory and circulatory care and administration of narcotic antagonists.

overhang′. An excess of dental filling material beyond the normal tooth contour; also called gingival margin excess.

overhydra′tion. Excess of fluids in the body; may result from the intravenous administration of unduly large amounts of glucose solution; also called water intoxication and hyperhydration.

o′verjet, o′verjut. Horizontal overlap; see under overlap.

overlap′. To extend over; e.g., the suturing of a layer of tissue over another to insure added strength.
   horizontal o., excessive projection of the upper anterior and/or posterior teeth beyond their antagonists of the lower jaw in a horizontal direction; also called overjet, overjut, and buck teeth.
   vertical o., the overlapping of the lower incisors by the upper incisors when the posterior teeth are in normal contact; also called overbite.

o′verlay. Any condition which is superimposed on an already existing one.

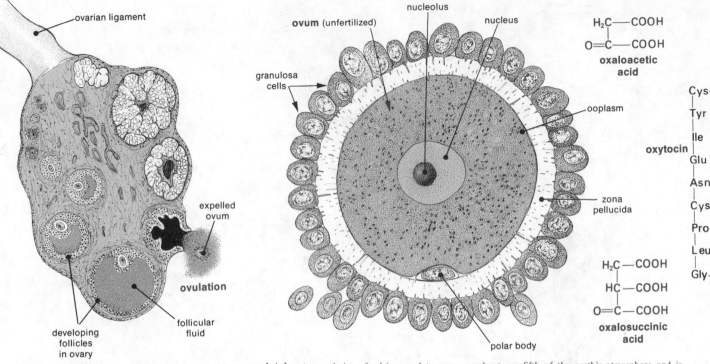

ovarian ligament

ovum (unfertilized)

nucleolus

nucleus

granulosa cells

ooplasm

expelled ovum

ovulation

follicular fluid

developing follicles in ovary

zona pellucida

polar body

$$H_2C—COOH$$
$$O{=}C—COOH$$

oxaloacetic acid

Cys
Tyr
Ile
Glu
Asn
Cys
Pro
Leu
Gly—N

oxytocin

$$H_2C—COOH$$
$$HC—COOH$$
$$O{=}C—COOH$$

oxalosuccinic acid

---

emotional o., an emotional disturbance resulting from, or added to, an organic disease.

overnutri'tion. Overeating; excessive caloric intake.

overri'ding. The slipping of one fragment of a broken bone alongside the other.

over the counter (OTC). Denoting a medication not requiring a prescription for purchase.

overventila'tion. See hyperventilation.

ovi-. Combining form meaning egg.

ovici'dal. Causing destruction of the ovum.

o'viduct. Uterine tube; see under tube.

ovif'erous. Containing or conveying eggs.

ovigen'esis. See oogenesis.

o'vine. Relating to sheep.

ovip'arous. Egg-laying; producing eggs that hatch outside the body of the maternal organism. Cf ovoviviparous and viviparous.

ovipos'it. To lay eggs, especially with the aid of an ovipositor; characteristic of insects.

oviposi'tion. The act of laying or depositing eggs; said especially of insects.

ovipos'itor. A specialized tubular structure at the end of the abdomen of many female insects for boring holes to house their eggs.

ovo-. Combining form meaning egg.

o'void. Egg-shaped.

ovomu'coid. Mucoprotein of egg white.

ovotes'tis. A gonad in which both testicular and ovarian tissues are present; a form of hermaphroditism.

ovovivip'arous. Bearing young that develop from eggs retained within the maternal body, as certain fish, reptiles, and insects.

ovula'tion. The discharge of an ovum from the mature (graafian) follicle of the ovary.

o'vule. 1. The ovum in the ovarian follicle. **2.** Any small egglike structure.

ovulocy'clic. Denoting any periodic occurrence that is associated with and takes place within the ovulatory cycle; e.g., ovulocyclic porphyria.

o'vum, *pl.* **o'va.** An egg; the female sexual cell which, when fertilized by union with the male element, develops into a new individual.

oxa-. Combining form denoting an oxygen bridge; e.g., −CH·O·CH−.

oxacillin sodium. Preparation used in the treatment of penicillin-resistant staphylococcal infections; Prostaphlin®.

ox'alate. A salt of oxalic acid.

oxalic acid. A compound produced by oxidation of glyoxylate; it is present in excessive amounts in persons afflicted with primary hyperoxaluria.

oxaloacetic acid. An intermediate in the tricarboxylic acid cycle; also called ketosuccinic acid.

oxalo'sis. Accumulation of calcium oxalate crystals in the kidneys, bones, arteries, and myocardium; a feature of primary hyperoxaluria, usually leading to death by renal failure.

oxalosuccinic acid. An intermediate in the tricarboxylic acid cycle.

oxalu'ria. The presence of abnormally large quantities of calcium oxalate in the urine.

oxa'zepam. A tranquilizer; Serax®.

ox'idase. One of a group of oxidizing enzymes which promote either the addition of oxygen to a metabolite or the removal of hydrogen or of electrons.

ox'idation. 1. A chemical reaction in which electrons from one reactant (the reducing agent) are transferred to the other reactant (the oxidizing agent); the atoms in the element losing electrons increase their valence correspondingly. Cf reduction. **2.** The combination of a substance with oxygen.

oxida'tion-reduc'tion. Any chemical reaction in which electrons are transferred from one atom or molecule to another; also called redox.

ox'ide. A binary compound of oxygen with another element or radical; e.g., mercuric oxide.

  acid o., an oxygen compound of nonmetals; e.g., SO_2.

  basic o., an oxygen compound of metals; e.g., Al_2O_3.

ox'idize. To combine or to cause combination with oxygen.

ox'idoreduc'tase. An enzyme that promotes an oxidation-reduction reaction.

ox'ime. A condensation product of the action of hydroxylamine on a ketone or an aldehyde.

oxim'eter. Instrument used to measure photoelectrically the degree of oxygen saturation in the circulating blood.

oxo-. Combining form meaning containing oxygen.

oxy-. Combining form meaning (a) pointed; (b) acute; (c) shrill; (d) the presence of oxygen in a molecule.

oxyacid. An acid containing oxygen; also called oxacid.

oxyblep'sia. Acute vision; also called oxyopia.

ox'ycel'lulose. Cellulose in which all or most of the glucose residues have been converted to glucoronic acid residues.

oxyceph'aly. Peaked, conical skull.

oxychromat'ic. Staining brightly with eosin and other acid dyes.

oxychro'matin. Oxyphil chromatin; chromatin that stains with acid dyes.

ox'ygen. An odorless and colorless gas, symbol 0, atomic number 8, atomic weight 16; it constitutes about one-fifth of the earth's atmosphere and is essential to animal and plant life.

ox'ygenase. One of several enzymes catalyzing the activation of molecular oxygen and the subsequent incorporation of both atoms of the oxygen molecule into the substrate.

ox'ygenate. To saturate or infuse with oxygen.

oxygena'tion. The combination of hemoglobin with oxygen; provision of oxygen to a tissue or individual.

ox'ygenize. Oxidize.

oxyhemoglo'bin (HbO_2). The bright red hemoglobin combined with oxygen, present in arterial blood; also called oxygenated hemoglobin.

oxyla'lia. Abnormally rapid speech.

oxyo'pia. See oxyblepsia.

ox'yphil, ox'yphile. Eosinophilic leukocyte; see under leukocyte.

oxypho'nia. Abnormal shrillness of voice.

oxypu'rine. An oxygen-containing purine.

17-oxyster'oid. 17-Ketosteroid.

ox'ytetracyc'line. Antibiotic produced by *Streptomyces rimosus*; Terramycin®.

oxyto'cia. Rapid childbirth.

oxyto'cic. 1. Relating to rapid childbirth. **2.** An agent that hastens the process of childbirth, especially by stimulating contraction of the uterine muscle.

oxyto'cin. A hormone formed in the base of the brain (hypothalamus) and stored in the posterior lobe of the hypophysis (pituitary gland); it stimulates smooth muscle, causing primarily strong contractions of the uterus and ejection of milk from the breast (distinguished from prolactin, which stimulates milk production).

oxyuri'asis. Infestation with pinworms.

oxyu'ricide. 1. An agent which kills pinworms. **2.** Destructive to pinworms.

oxyu'rid. Pinworm.

Oxyu'ris. A genus of nematode worms commonly known as pinworms.

oz. Abbreviation for ounce.

oze'na. A fetid discharge from the nose in patients with certain forms of chronic rhinitis.

o'zone (O_3). A blue, poisonous, gaseous triatomic form of oxygen formed naturally from an electric discharge through oxygen or by exposure of oxygen to ultraviolet radiation; made commercially by passing oxygen over 10,000 volt charged aluminum plates; used chiefly as an antiseptic, disinfectant, and bleaching agent.

ozonom'eter. An apparatus that estimates the amount of ozone in the atmosphere by the use of a series of test papers.

ozosto'mia. Bad breath.

---

overlay | ozostomia

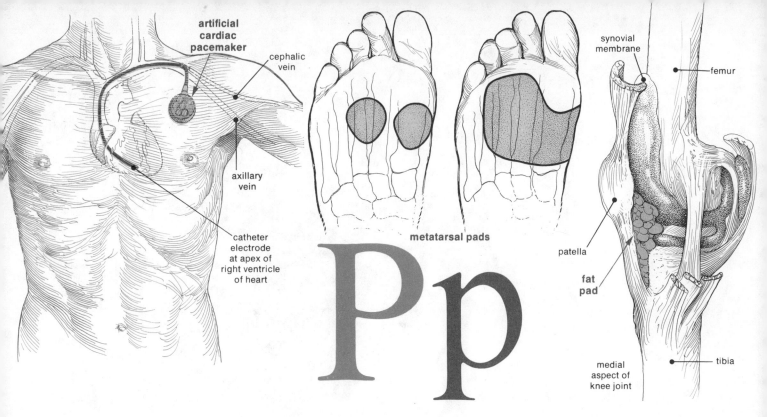

artificial cardiac pacemaker

cephalic vein

axillary vein

catheter electrode at apex of right ventricle of heart

metatarsal pads

Pp

synovial membrane

femur

patella

fat pad

tibia

medial aspect of knee joint

P. 1. Abbreviation for Pharmacopeia. **2.** Symbol for the element phosphorus.

p. 1. Abbreviation for (a) optic; (b) papilla; (c) pulse; (d) pupil. **2.** Symbol for proton.

p-. Abbreviation for para- (2). For terms beginning with *p-*, see under specific term.

P₁. Symbol for the first parental generation; P_1 individuals are the parents of the F_1 generation. See filial generation, under generation.

Pa. Symbol for the element protactinium.

PA. Abbreviation for (a) pulmonary artery; (b) posterior-anterior.

PABA. Abbreviation for *p*-aminobenzoic acid.

pab′lum. A precooked food, usually for infants, made from wheat, oat, and corn meals, wheat embryo, alfalfa leaves, brewers' yeast, iron, and salt.

pab′ulum. Any nourishing substance.

pacchionian granulations. See granulation, arachnoid.

pace′maker. 1. Any bodily structure that serves to establish and maintain a rhythmic pace, as the sinoatrial node of the heart which regulates the heartbeat. **2.** A substance whose rate of reaction regulates a series of chain or related reactions.

artificial cardiac p., any of several usually miniaturized and surgically implanted electronic devices that substitute for the normal cardiac pacemaker and regulate the heartbeat; used in treating individuals with chronic heart block who have (1) episodes of syncope or convulsions owing to ventricular bradycardia, (2) cardiac failure secondary to the bradycardia, and (3) unstable ventricular rhythms associated with the heart block.

brain p., a pacemaker implanted on the surface of the cerebellum which is primarily used to bring intractable epilepsy under control; also called cerebellar electrical stimulator.

demand p., one in which the stimulus is only fired when the ventricular contraction does not occur within a specified period of time; a signal from the heart's previous ventricular depolarization inhibits the pulse generator from firing for an additional second.

ectopic p., any cardiac pacemaker other than the sinus node.

external p., artificial pacemaker with electrodes placed externally on the chest wall.

fixed-rate p., an artificial pacemaker that discharges electrical stimuli at a uniform and uninterrupted rate.

shifting p., see wandering pacemaker.

wandering p., phenomenon in which the point of origin of the heart beat shifts back and forth from one center to another, usually between the sinus and AV nodes; also called shifting pacemaker.

pachy-. Combining form meaning thick.

pachybleph′aron. Thickening of the border of an eyelid.

pachyceph′aly, pachycepha′lia. Abnormal thickening of the skull.

pachycho′lia. Abnormal viscousness of the bile.

pachychromat′ic. Having a thick chromatin network.

pachydac′tyly. Abnormal enlargement of the fingers or toes.

pachyder′ma. Abnormally thick skin.

p. laryngis, a form of chronic laryngitis, marked by the formation of warty thickening of the epithelium, usually on the vocal cords; it is caused by chronic irritation.

pachydermat′ocele. 1. Congenital looseness of the skin, which hangs in folds; also called cutis laxa. **2.** A large neurofibroma.

pachydermato′sis. Pachyderma of long duration.

pachyder′matous. Characterized by pachyderma.

pachyder′moperiosto′sis. Inherited condition marked by osteoarthropathy, coarseness of facial features with thickening and oiliness of the skin, excessive sebaceous gland secretion, and enlargement of hands with clubbing of fingers.

pachygy′ria. Abnormally thick convolutions of the cerebral cortex.

pachyleptomeningi′tis. Inflammation of the membranes of the brain and spinal cord.

pachylo′sis. A dry, thickened, scaly state of the skin, especially on the lower extremities.

pachymeningi′tis. Inflammation and thickening of the dura mater.

pachymeningop′athy. Any disease of the dura mater.

pachym′eter. Instrument used to measure the thickness of membranes or thin plates.

pachyonych′ia. Excessive thickness of the fingernails or toenails.

p. congenita, a congenital deformity characterized by abnormalities of the skin (bullae and papular hyperkeratoses) and mucous membranes (leukokeratoses) and excessively thick nails.

pachyperiosti′tis. Proliferative thickening of the membrane enveloping bones due to inflammation.

pachyperitoni′tis. Inflammation and thickening of the peritoneum.

pachypleuri′tis. Inflammation of the pleura accompanied by thickening of the membrane; also called productive pleurisy.

pachysalpingi′tis. Chronic interstitial inflammation of the muscular layer of the uterine tube, producing thickening; also called chronic parenchyma-

tous salpingitis.

pachyso′mia. Abnormal thickening of the soft parts of the body, as in acromegaly.

pach′ytene. The stage of prophase in meiosis in which each paired chromosome separates into its two component sister chromatids, so that each homologous chromosome pair becomes a set of four intertwined chromatids called a bivalent.

pack. 1. To fill or stuff. **2.** To wrap a patient in hot, cold, wet, or dry blankets or sheets. **3.** The blankets or sheets so used. **4.** In dentistry, the application of a dressing to a surgical site. **5.** The dressing so used.

pack′er. Instrument for inserting an absorbent dressing or tampon into a bodily cavity, such as the vagina.

pack′ing. The material used to fill a cavity or a wound, such as gauze, sponge, etc.

PA_{CO₂}. Symbol denoting partial pressure of carbon dioxide (CO_2) in arterial blood; normal value is approximately 40 mmHg.

pad. A cushion of soft material.

abdominal p., a large pad used for absorbing discharges from surgical abdominal wounds.

buccal fat-p., an encapsulated mass of fat on the outer side of the cheek situated superficial to the buccinator muscle and pierced by the parotid duct; in infants it is prominent and is called sucking or suctorial pad because it is thought to help prevent the cheeks from being sucked inward while nursing.

fat p., a circumscribed cushion-like mass of fat.

infrapatellar fat-p., a large pad of fat which separates the patellar ligament and part of the patella (kneecap) from the synovial membrane of the knee joint.

ischiorectal fat-p., a pad of fat in the anal region extending upward on both sides of the anus; it contains many fibrous septa that support the anal canal.

metatarsal p., one of various shaped pads worn inside the shoe under the metatarsal bones to shield painful weight-bearing areas from pressure.

Passavant's pad., Passavant's ridge; see under ridge.

retropubic fat-p., a large quantity of fat in the U-shaped retropubic space located between the pubic symphysis and the bladder and extending backward on each side of the bladder; it is limited above by the peritoneum.

P.ae. Abbreviation of the Latin *partes aequales*.

Paget's disease. A bone disease of unknown cause; characterized by localized areas of bone destruction followed by replacement with overdeveloped, light, soft, porous bone and associated with deformities, such as thickening of portions of the skull and bending of weight-bearing bones; Bee-

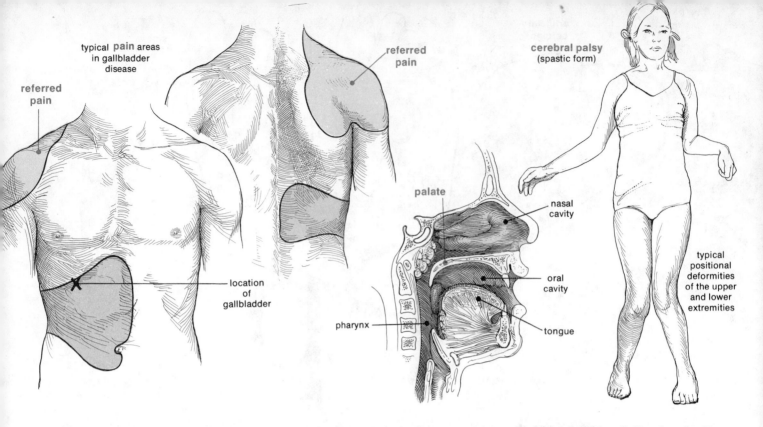

typical pain areas
in gallbladder
disease

referred
pain

referred
pain

location
of
gallbladder

palate

nasal
cavity

oral
cavity

pharynx

tongue

cerebral palsy
(spastic form)

typical
positional
deformities
of the upper
and lower
extremities

thoven is believed to have been afflicted with this disease; also called osteitis deformans.

pagopha′gia. The ingestion of abnormally large quantities of ice.

-pagus. Combining form denoting a conjoined twin; the first part of the word indicates the attached parts.

PAH. Abbreviation for *p*-aminohippuric acid.

pain. A physical or mental sensation of distress or suffering.

   bearing-down p., one accompanying the contractions of the uterus during the second stage of labor.
   false p's., those resembling true labor pains.
   girdle p., a painful sensation encircling the waist like a tight belt, occurring in some diseases of the spinal cord.
   growing p's., pains in the limbs of children, usually felt at night and resembling rheumatism; attributed to growth, faulty posture, or fatigue.
   labor p's., rhythmic pains of increasing severity, frequency, and duration, caused by contraction of the uterus during childbirth.
   phantom limb p., the sensation of pain felt in a limb, although that limb has been amputated.
   referred p., paint felt in an area other than the site of origin, such as the pain near the shoulder associated with biliary disease.

paint. A pharmaceutical preparation in a liquid vehicle which is applied to the skin with a brush or large applicator; upon evaporation, it leaves a coating on the skin.

pair′ing. Attachment of two homologous chromosomes in a sideward direction, prior to crossing over.

pal′atal. Relating to the palate.

pal′ate. The roof of the mouth; it consists of a bony anterior part (hard palate) and a solft muscular posterior portion (soft palate).

   cleft p., a congenitally malformed palate, with a fissure along the midline, usually associated with a harelip.

palat′iform. Resembling the palate or roof of the mouth.

pal′atine. Relating to the palate or roof of the mouth.

palato-. Combining form denoting palate.

palatoglos′sal. Relating to the palate and the tongue.

pal′atograph. Instrument for recording the movements of the soft palate during speech and respiration; also called palate myograph and palatomyograph.

palatopharyn′geal. Relating to the palate and the pharynx.

palatopharyn′goplasty. Operative procedure

to correct a shortened soft palate (sometimes necessary in plastic repair of a cleft palate).

pal′atoplasty. Reparative surgery of the palate, especially a cleft palate.

palatople′gia. Paralysis of the muscles of the soft palate.

palatos′chisis. Cleft palate.

paleenceph′alon. The phylogenetically older part of the brain which includes all of it except the cerebral cortex and closely related parts.

paleo-, pale-. Combining forms meaning ancient or prehistoric.

paleobiol′ogy. The study of evolution of life from a non-oxygen dominated environment.

paleocerebel′lum. The earlier developed parts of the cerebellum, i.e., vermis and flocculus.

paleocor′tex. The earlier developed parts of the cerebral cortex, i.e., the olfactory cortex.

paleokinet′ic. Denoting the primitive nervous motor mechanism concerned with automatic movements.

paleopathol′ogy. The study of disease of ancient man as revealed in mummies, bones, and art forms such as paintings, statues, etc.

paleostria′tum. See globus pallidus.

palila′lia. See paliphrasia.

palindro′mia. Recurrence of a pathologic condition.

palindrom′ic. Recurring.

palingen′esis. The reappearance of ancestral structural features.

paliphra′sia. The involuntary repetition of phrases in speaking; may be caused by encephalitis; also called palilalia.

palla′dium. Metallic element resembling platinum; symbol Pd, atomic number 46, atomic weight 106.4.

pallesthe′sia. The perception of vibration, especially through bones; also called vibratory sensibility.

pal′liate. To mitigate.

pal′liative. 1. Alleviating. **2.** A medicine or treatment that affords temporary relief but does not effect a cure.

pallidec′tomy. Surgical removal or destruction of the globus pallidus.

pallidot′omy. Cutting of nerve fibers from the globus pallidus in the brain for the relief of pathologic involuntary movements.

pal′lium. The cerebral cortex and subadjacent white substance.

pal′lor. Paleness; lack of color.

palm. The anterior or inner surface of the hand.

pal′mar. Relating to the palm of the hand.

palmitic acid. A saturated fatty acid found in

various fats and oils; also called hexadecanoic acid.

pal′pable. Perceptible by palpation; tangible.

pal′pate. To examine by touching or pressing with the fingers or the palms of the hands.

palpa′tion. Examination by touch or pressure of the hand, over an organ or area of the body, as a diagnostic aid.

palpe′bra, *pl.* **palpe′brae.** Latin for eyelid.

pal′pebral. Of or relating to the eyelids.

palpita′tion. Rapid or forceful heartbeat, of which the patient is conscious.

pal′sy. Paralysis.

   ataxic cerebral p., cerebral palsy characterized by inability to coordinate voluntary muscular movements.
   Bell's p., see facial palsy.
   cerebral p., condition marked by disturbances of voluntary motor function caused by damage to the brain's motor control centers; it is characterized primarily by spastic paralysis or impairment of control or coordination over voluntary muscles; it is often accompanied by mental retardation, seizures, and disorders of vision and communication; it may be either congenital or acquired.
   dyskinetic cerebral p., cerebral palsy characterized by uncontrolled and purposeless movements which disappear during sleep.
   facial p., Bell's p., paralysis of the facial muscles on one side, caused by a usually self-limited lesion of the facial (VII) nerve.
   shaking p., see paralysis agitans.
   spastic cerebral p., cerebral palsy characterized by increased muscle tension and exaggerated reflex activity in an arm and a leg of the same side (hemiplegia) or arms and legs on both sides (tetraplegia or quadriplegia).
   trembling p., paralysis agitans.

pal′udism. Malaria.

pan-. Prefix meaning all.

panace′a. A remedy which is supposed to cure all diseases; a cure-all.

panagglu′tinin. An agglutinin that reacts with all human erythrocytes.

panangii′tis. Inflammation of all layers of a blood vessel.

panarthri′tis. 1. Inflammation of an entire joint. **2.** Inflammation of all the body joints.

panat′rophy. A generalized wasting away of the body.

pancardi′tis. Inflammation of all layers of the heart; i.e., myocarditis, endocarditis, and pericarditis.

Pancoast's syndrome. Carcinoma of the apex of the lung or upper mediastinum (Pancoast's tumor) invading the brachial plexus and the cervical

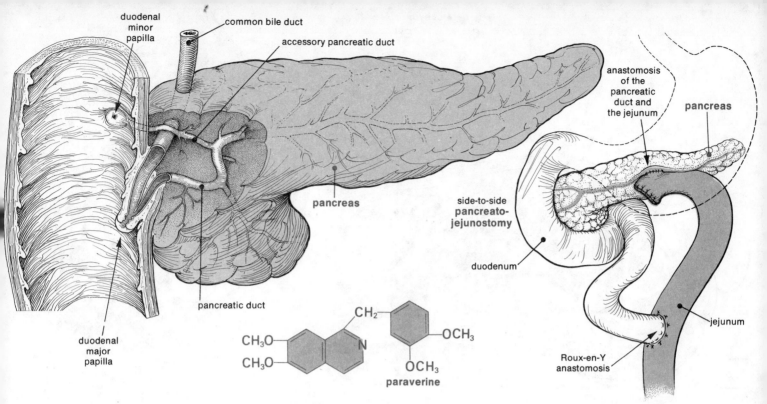

duodenal minor papilla

common bile duct

accessory pancreatic duct

anastomosis of the pancreatic duct and the jejunum

pancreas

pancreas

side-to-side pancreato-jejunostomy

duodenum

pancreatic duct

duodenal major papilla

Roux-en-Y anastomosis

jejunum

CH_3O

CH_3O

CH_2

N

OCH_3

OCH_3

paraverine

sympathetic chain and resulting in pain, weakness, and atrophy of the arm and hand muscles; also called pulmonary sulcus, Ciuffini-Pancoast, or Horner's syndrome.

pancolec'tomy. The removal of the entire colon.

pan'creas. A soft gland, 4 to 6 inches long, lying behind the stomach and extending transversely from the concavity of the duodenum to the spleen; it secretes enzymes (amylase, lipase), which aid in digestion of food, into the small intestine and hormones (glucagon, insulin) which, when taken up by the bloodstream, help regulate carbohydrate metabolism by controlling blood sugar levels.

pancreat-, pancreatico-, pancreato-, pancreo-. Combining forms denoting a relationship to the pancreas.

pancreatec'tomy. Surgical removal of the pancreas.

pancreathelco'sis. The presence of abscesses of the pancreas.

pancreaticoduodenos'tomy. Surgical joining of the pancreatic duct into the duodenum.

pancreaticogastros'tomy. The surgical anastomosis of the pancreatic duct to the stomach.

pancreaticojejunos'tomy. Surgical inplantation of the pancreatic duct into the jejunum.

pan'creatin. A mixture of pancreatic enzymes extracted from hogs or cattle; used as a digestive aid.

pancreati'tis. Inflammation of the pancreas.

pancreatoduodenec'tomy. Surgical removal of the pancreas and the adjacent portion of the duodenum.

pancreatog'enous. Originating in the pancreas.

pancreatog'raphy. The making of x-ray films of the pancreas.

pancreat'olith. A pancreatic stone; also called pancreolith.

pancreatolithec'tomy. Surgical removal of pancreatic stones.

pancreatolithi'asis. Stones in the pancreas.

pancreatolithot'omy. Incision of the pancreas for the removal of a stone; also called pancreolithotomy.

pancreat'omy. See pancreatotomy.

pancreatot'omy. Incision of the pancreas; also called pancreatomy.

pancreatrop'ic. Exerting an effect on the pancreas.

pan'creolith. See pancreatolith.

pancreolithot'omy. See pancreatolithotomy.

pancreozy'min. A hormone secreted by the mucosa of the small intestine that stimulates the secretion of pancreatic enzymes.

pancytope'nia. Reduction of all the cell components of the blood (red blood cells, white blood cells, and blood platelets).

pandem'ic. Denoting an epidemic that affects the population of a wide geographic area.

panen'doscope. A cystoscope which offers a wide view of the interior of the urinary bladder.

panesthe'sia. The sum of all sensations experienced at one time.

panhypopitu'itarism. Condition characterized by absence of all the recognized anterior pituitary hormones; also called Simmond's disease.

panhysterec'tomy. Surgical removal of the entire uterus, including the cervix.

panhys'terosalpingec'tomy. The removal of the entire uterus and uterine tubes (the ovaries are left intact).

panhys'terosalpingo-oophorec'tomy. Removal of the entire uterus, uterine tubes, and ovaries.

pan'ic. A sudden, overpowering anxiety and fear.

panmix'is. Random mating.

panniculi'tis. Inflammation of the subcutaneous layer of connective tissue and fat (superficial fascia) of the abdominal wall.

  relapsing febrile nodular nonsuppurative p., see Weber-Christian disease.

pannic'ulus. A layer of membranous tissue.

  p. adiposus, the subcutaneous layer of connective tissue and fat (superficial fascia).

pan'nus. A superficial vascularization of the cornea with a membrane-like infiltration of granulation tissue; it may occur in several degrees of denseness and may cover part or all of the cornea; a common complication of trachoma.

panophthal'mia, panophthalmi'tis. Generalized infection and inflammation of the eyeball.

Panorex'. In dentistry, a radiographic machine that rotates the film holder and x-ray tube around the patient's head and shifts the patient to change the axis of rotation of the tube-film assembly relative to his head.

panostei'tis, panosti'tis. Inflammation of a bone in its entirety.

panoti'tis. General inflammation of the ear.

pansystol'ic. Occurring throughout systole, from first to second heart sound.

pantothenic acid. $HOCH_2-C(CH_3)_2-CHOH-CO-NH-CH_2-CH_2-COOH$; a colorless liquid component of the vitamin B complex, widely distributed in plant and animal tissues especially the liver; part of coenzyme A.

PA_{O_2}. Symbol denoting partial pressure of oxygen in arterial blood.

pap. Any soft or semiliquid food, as bread soaked in milk.

papa'in. A proteolytic enzyme obtained from the unripe fruit of the papaya; used as a meat tenderizer and also in medicine as a protein digestant.

papav'erine. A non-narcotic alkaloid of opium which has vasodilator properties.

pa'per. A thin sheet substance made of the cellulose pulp of wood or other fibrous material; used for writing, filtering, medicating, and testing.

  biuret p., a strip of filter paper dipped in biuret reagent and allowed to dry.

  filter p., porous unsized paper suitable for filtering solutions.

  litmus p., white blotting paper impregnated with litmus; used as an acid-base indicator; it turns red in a slightly acidic solution and blue in an alkaline one.

  p. point, in dentistry, a cone of absorbent paper than can be inserted into the entire length of a root canal of a tooth; used to medicate the canal or to absorb fluid.

papil'la. A small, nipple-like protrusion.

pap'illary. Relating to or resembling a papilla or nipple.

papillec'tomy. Surgical removal of any papilla.

papillede'ma. Swelling of the optic nerve head caused by increased intracranial pressure.

papillif'erous. Containing papillae.

papil'liform. Resembling a papilla.

papilli'tis. Inflammation of the optic nerve head; also called neuropapillitis and intraocular optic neuritis.

  necrotizing p., renal papillary necrosis; see under necrosis.

papilloadenocysto'ma. A lobulated benign tumor derived from epithelium, characterized by glands or glandlike structures, formation of cysts, and finger-like projections of neoplastic cells enveloping a core of fibrous connective tissue.

papillocarcino'ma. 1. A malignant tumor originating from a papilloma. **2.** A malignant tumor with papillary projections.

papillo'ma. An overgrowth of the papillae of the skin or mucous membrane; also called papillary tumor and villoma.

  hard p., one derived from squamous epithelium, such as corns or warts.

  villous p., one composed of numerous slender outgrowths, usually found in the bladder, within the mammary gland, or arising from the choroid plexus in the lateral ventricle of the brain.

papillomato'sis. The development of several papillomas.

papillo'matous. Resembling a papilloma.

papilloretini'tis. Inflammation of the optic disk and neighboring parts of the retina; also called retinopapillitis.

pap'ovavi'ruses. A group of DNA viruses repli-

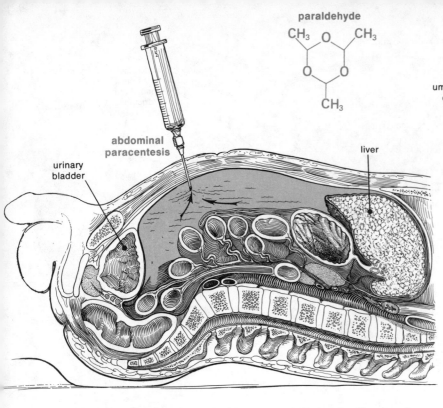

abdominal
paracentesis

urinary
bladder

liver

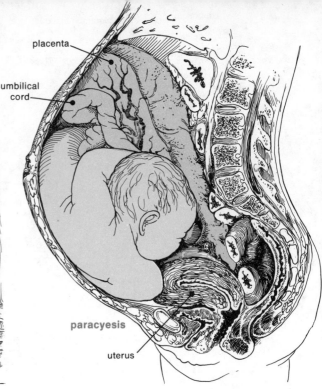

paraldehyde

CH_3 O CH_3

O   O

CH_3

placenta

umbilical
cord

paracyesis

uterus

cating in the nuclei of vertebrate cells; some members of this group cause warts in man, others have produced malignant tumors in laboratory animals.

pap′ula. Papule.

pap′ular. Relating to papules.

papula′tion. The formation of papules.

pap′ule. A superficial solid elevation on the skin, ranging in size up to one centimeter.

papulopus′tular. Denoting an eruption composed of papules (small elevations on the skin) and pustules (elevations on the skin containing pus).

papulo′sis. The occurrence of numerous papules, usually widespread.

papulosquam′ous. Denoting a skin eruption composed of small elevations (papules) and loose scaly lesions.

papulovesic′ular. Having both papules and vesicles.

para-. Prefix denoting (1) alongside, against, accessory to, deviation from normal; (2) a compound derived from two symmetrically arranged substitutions in the benzene ring; abbreviated *p-* in chemical terms.

para. Denoting past pregnancies that have reached the period of viability, regardless of whether the child is dead or alive at the time of delivery; the term refers to pregnancies, not fetuses; thus, a woman who gives birth to twins at the end of her first pregnancy is still para I.

parabio′sis. 1. Union of two organisms, either natural (e.g., conjoined twins) or artificially produced. **2.** Temporary loss of conductivity of a nerve.

parablep′sia, parablep′sis. False vision, as in visual illusion or hallucination.

paraca′sein. Compound produced when the enzyme rennin acts upon casein (the protein of milk); it reacts with calcium, resulting in the curdling of milk.

paracente′sis. The surgical puncture of a cavity for the purpose of removing fluid.

  abdominal p., paracentesis of the abdomen.

  tympanic p., myringotomy; incision of the tympanic membrane (eardrum) in order to drain the middle ear chamber.

paracen′tral. Located near a central structure.

parachor′dal. In embryology, located near and anterior to the notochord.

parachromatop′sia. See dichromatism.

paracoccid′ioidomyco′sis. A chronic systemic fungal disease caused by a yeastlike fungus (*Paracoccidioides brasiliensis*), characteristically causing gastrointestinal symptoms, painful ulcers of the mouth and nose, and inflammation and suppuration of the lymph nodes of the neck; the infection disseminates to the skin and other organs; also called

South American blastomycosis.

paracol′pium. Tissues near the vagina.

paracu′sis. 1. Impaired hearing. **2.** Auditory hallucination.

paracye′sis. Extrauterine pregnancy.

paracys′tic. Near the bladder.

paraden′tal. Periodontal.

paradid′ymis. A small body made up of a few convoluted tubules attached to the lower part of the spermatic cord above the head of the epididymis; considered to be a remnant of the mesonephros (wolffian body); also called parepididymis and organ of Giraldès.

paradip′sia. Abnormal craving for fluids.

par′affin. 1. A waxy, somewhat transparent purified mixture of solid hydrocarbons derived from petroleum; also called paraffin wax. **2.** One of the methane or alkane series of saturated aliphatic hydrocarbons having the general formula C_nH_{2n+2}.

paraformal′dehyde. A water-soluble, white, crystalline polymer of formaldehyde; used in treating various skin disorders.

paragang′lia, *sing.* paragang′lion. Collection of chromaffin cells forming globular or ovoid bodies present about the ganglia of the sympathetic chain; also called chromaffin bodies.

paraganglio′ma. A tumor composed of chromaffin tissue in a paraganglion or the medulla of the adrenal gland; also called chromaffinoma.

par′agene. Any extrachromosomal replicating unit or hereditary determinant; also called plasmid.

parageu′sia. Any abnormality in the sense of taste.

paragglutina′tion. Group agglutination; see under agglutination.

paraglob′ulin. A globulin present in blood plasma and lymph.

paragonimi′asis. Infection with a worm of the genus *Paragonimus*, especially the lung fluke species *Paragonimus westermani*.

Paragon′imus. A genus of trematode worms which includes the lung worms of man and animals.

parahepat′ic. Located near the liver.

parakerato′sis. The retention of nuclei in the cells of the stratum corneum of the epithelium, as seen in psoriasis.

parakine′sia, parakine′sis. Any abnormality of motor function.

parala′lia. Speech defect in which one letter is substituted for another.

paralbu′min. Albuminous substance usually present in ovarian cysts and ascites.

paral′dehyde. A polymer of acetaldehyde, $(CH_3CHO)_3$; colorless liquid of pungent odor, used as a hypnotic and sedative.

paralge′sia. Any abnormal painful sensation.

par′allax. The apparent displacement of an object caused by a change in the observation position.

parallelepiped, corneal. The section of cornea illuminated by the light beam of the slit lamp.

paral′ysis. 1. Loss of voluntary muscular function. **2.** Loss of sensation. **3.** Loss of any organic function.

  acute ascending p., paralysis, often fatal, beginning in the lower extremities and ascending rapidly to involve the trunk, arms, and neck; sometimes called Landry's paralysis.

  ascending p., paralysis progressing from the periphery to the nerve centers, or from the lower limbs upward.

  Brown-Séquard's p., (1) paralysis of the lower extremities occurring in certain disorders of the urinary tract; (2) see Brown-Séquard's syndrome.

  congenital oculofacial p., see Möbius' syndrome.

  Duchenne's p., childhood muscular dystrophy; see under dystrophy.

  Duchenne-Erb p., a form affecting the deltoid, biceps, anterior brachial, and long supinator muscles.

  familial periodic p., periodic paralysis.

  global p., paralysis affecting both sides of the body completely.

  hyperkalemic p., periodic paralysis associated with abnormally high serum potassium concentrations; attacks start in infancy, are frequent, and relatively mild, and last a few minutes to a few hours; autosomal dominant inheritance.

  hypokalemic p., periodic paralysis in which serum potassium level drops sharply during attacks, which start in late childhood or adolescence, are relatively severe, and last for a day or more; autosomal dominant inheritance.

  infantile p., see poliomyelitis.

  jake p., a form induced by drinking Jamaica ginger (jake); also called ginger paralysis.

  Landry's p., see acute ascending paralysis.

  p. agitans, Parkinson's disease, a disorder characterized, in its fully developed form, by stiffness and slowness of voluntary movement, stooped posture, propulsive gait, rigidity of facial expression, and rhythmic tremor of the limbs; usually has an insidious onset in individuals between 50 and 65 years old; cause is unknown; changes in the melanin-containing nerve cells in the brain stem are regularly observed; also called shaking palsy.

  periodic p., recurrent abrupt episodes of paralysis or extreme muscular weakness lasting from a few minutes to a few days, occurring in otherwise healthy individuals.

papula | **paralysis**

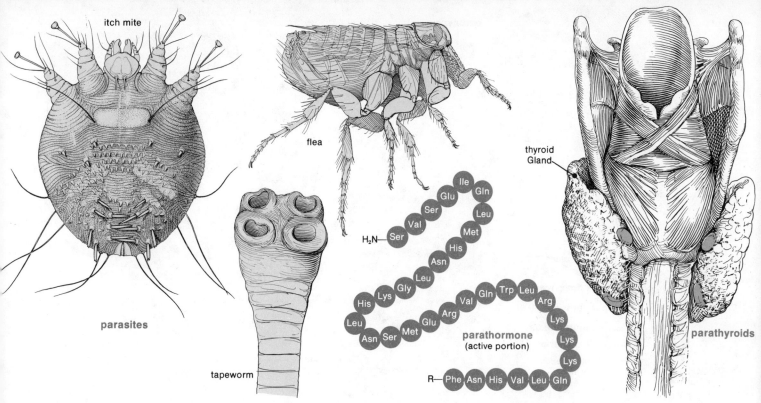

itch mite

flea

tapeworm

parasites

thyroid Gland

parathyroids

H_2N — Ser — Val — Ser — Glu — Ile — Gln — Leu — Met — His — Asn — Leu — Gly — Lys — His — Leu — Asn — Ser — Met — Glu — Arg — Val — Gln — Trp — Leu — Arg — Lys — Lys — Lys

parathormone (active portion)

R — Phe — Asn — His — Val — Leu — Gln

postictal p., see Todd's paralysis.

progressive bulbar p., progressive paralysis and atrophy of the muscles of the tongue, lips, palate, larynx, and pharynx, due to degeneration of the neurons that innervate them.

pseudobulbar p., paralysis of the tongue and lips, resulting in difficulty in speech and swallowing, often accompanied by spasmodic laughter; caused by brain lesions in the upper motor neurons; also called laughing sickness.

tick p., a rapidly progressive, usually symmetrical paralysis following a tick bite; symptoms include numbness of the extremities, throat, and face, progressing quickly to inability to stand, paralysis of the extremities and trunk, slurred speech, and impaired vision.

Todd's p., temporary paralysis sometimes occurring after a grand mal epileptic convulsion and usually lasting from several minutes to hours after the seizure; also called postictal paralysis.

vasomotor p., see vasoparalysis.

paralyt'ic. 1. Relating to paralysis. **2.** A person afflicted with paralysis.

parame'cium. Any of many ciliate protozoans of the genus *Paramecium,* usually slipper-shaped with an oral groove for feeding.

parame'dian. Near the midline.

paramed'ical. Adjunctive to or relating indirectly to the practice of medicine.

parame'nia. Any disorder or irregularity of menstruation.

param'eter. In statistics, a characteristic of the population.

paramet'ric. Relating to the structures adjacent to the uterus (parametrium).

parametri'tis. Inflammation of the connective tissue adjacent to the uterus and the veins and lymphatics contained in it; also called pelvic cellulitis.

parame'trium. The connective tissue near the uterine cervix, extending upward along the sides of the uterus, between the two layers of the broad ligaments.

param'yloido'sis. Accumulation of the protein amyloid in lymph nodes; seen in some chronic nonspecific inflammations.

paramyoto'nia. An atypical form of myotonia; abnormal muscular tonicity and spasms.

paramyx'ovi'ruses. Spherical or filamentous RNA viruses; all members cause respiratory tract infections, some cause mumps; the measles virus has tentatively been placed in this group.

parana'sal. Located near the nose.

paranoi'a. A rare, slowly progressive mental disorder characterized by convincing and logical delusions of persecution and grandeur without any other

signs of personality deterioration; some features of true paranoia, such as feelings of persecution, may be found in other psychiatric illnesses.

paranoi'ac. Relating to or suffering from paranoia.

par'anoid. Resembling paranoia; overly suspicious.

paranu'clear. Located near the nucleus.

paranu'cleus. An accessory nucleus or a small chromatin body resembling a nucleus, sometimes seen in the cell protoplasm lying just outside of the nucleus.

parapar'esis. Slight or partial paralysis of both lower limbs.

paraperitone'al. Near or alongside the peritoneum.

parapha'sia. A disturbance of speech marked by substitution of words and disorganized sentence formation; a mild form of aphasia.

literal p., substitution of words that are similar in sound to the correct one.

verbal p., substitution of words that are similar in meaning to the correct one.

paraphimo'sis. Tightness of the prepuce or foreskin, which when retracted behind the glans penis cannot be returned to its normal position.

p. palpebrae, a turning outward of the margin of an eyelid (usually the upper one) due to spastic contraction of the orbicularis oculi muscle; usually it is of short duration.

paraple'gia. Paralysis of both legs and lower part of the body.

paraprocti'tis. Inflammation of the tissues surrounding the rectum and anus.

parapro'tein. An abnormal serum protein, such as macroglobulin, cryoglobulin, and myeloma protein, characterized by a well defined peak on electrophoresis.

paraproteine'mia. A disorder marked by the presence of abnormal proteins in the blood as seen in multiple myeloma.

parapsychol'ogy. The study of extrasensory phenomena.

parasalpingi'tis. Inflammation of the tissues surrounding a uterine tube.

par'asite. Any organism which in its natural habitat feeds and lives on or in a different organism.

parasit'ic. Of, relating to, or characteristic of a parasite.

parasit'icide. Any agent that destroys parasites.

par'asitism. 1. The mode of existence between a parasite and its host. **2.** An abnormal condition resulting from infestation with parasites.

par'asitize. To live as a parasite.

parasitol'ogy. The scientific study of parasites

and parasitism; a branch of microbiology.

parasitos'is. Infestation with parasites.

paraspa'dia, paraspa'dias. The presence of a lateral opening into the male urethra.

parasympathet'ic. Relating to the part of the autonomic nervous system concerned with conserving and restoring energy, as by slowing the heart rate.

parasympatholyt'ic. Denoting an agent that neutralizes the actions of acetylcholine on structures and smooth muscles innervated by the parasympathetic nerves; also called anticholinergic, anti-muscarinic, spasmolytic, atropinic, and parasympathoparalytic.

parasympathomimet'ic. Producing effects similar to those caused by stimulation of the parasympathetic system.

parasympathoparalyt'ic. See parasympatholytic.

parasys'tole. A second automatic cardiac rhythm existing simultaneously with normal sinus rhythm and firing at a regular and uninterrupted rate.

intermittent p., a parasystolic rhythm that is interrupted and subsequently resumes.

parathi'on. A highly poisonous organic phosphate insecticide; an inhibitor of cholinesterase.

parathor'mone. Parathyroid hormone; a polypeptide produced and secreted into the bloodstream by the four parathyroid glands; its main function is to maintain a constant concentration of calcium in the blood.

parathy'roid. 1. Located beside the thyroid gland. **2.** A parathyroid gland.

parathyroidec'tomy. Surgical removal of the parathyroid glands.

parathyrotrop'ic, parathyrotroph'ic. Having an effect on the parathyroid glands.

par'atope. The region of the surface of an antibody that combines with an antigen. Cf. epitope.

paratricho'sis. Any disorder affecting hair growth.

paraty'phoid. Resembling typhoid (fever or bacillus).

paraumbil'ical. Situated near the navel (umbilicus).

paraung'ual. Alongside or near a fingernail or toenail.

paravag'inal. Near or next to the vagina.

paraver'tebral. Alongside the vertebral column.

parecta'sia, parec'tasis. Excessive distention of a part or organ.

paregor'ic. An antiperistaltic compound consisting of powdered opium, anise oil, benzoic acid, camphor, and glycerin in diluted alcohol; principally used in relieving abdominal cramps and diarrhea;

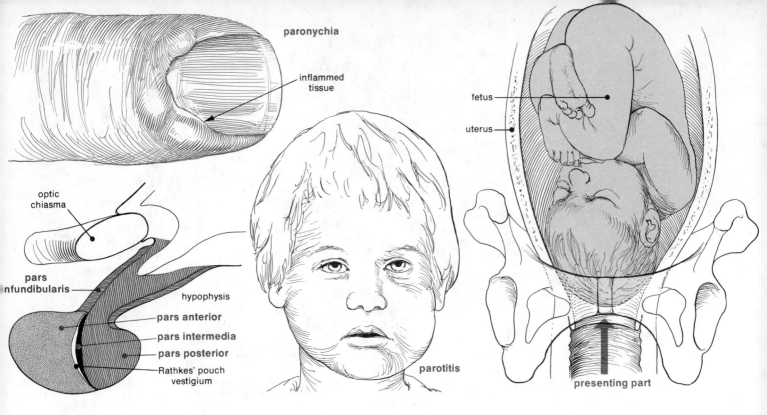

paronychia

inflammed tissue

optic chiasma

pars infundibularis

hypophysis

pars anterior

pars intermedia

pars posterior

Rathkes' pouch vestigium

parotitis

fetus

uterus

presenting part

also called camphorated opium tincture.

parenceph′alon. Cerebellum.

paren′chyma. The characteristic tissue of an organ or gland, as distinguished from connective tissue.

paren′chymal, paren′chymatous. Relating to the parenchyma.

paren′teral. 1. Situated outside the alimentary tract. **2.** Taken into the body in a way other than through the alimentary canal, as by intravenous or intramuscular injection.

pare′sis. Partial paralysis; weakness.

paresthe′sia. An abnormal sensation, as burning, tingling, or numbness.

paresthet′ic. Characterized by paresthesia.

paret′ic. Relating to or suffering from paresis.

par′ies, pl. **pari′etes.** A wall of a body cavity, as of the chest.

pari′etal. Pertaining to the wall of a cavity.

parieto-. Combining form denoting a relationship to any wall of a body cavity.

parieto-occipital. Relating to the parietal and occipital bones of the skull or lobes of the cerebrum.

par′ity. The state of a woman in respect to having given birth to children.

parkinso′nian. 1. Relating to paralysis agitans (Parkinson's disease). **2.** One who suffers from paralysis agitans.

par′kinsonism. A group of nervous disorders (including paralysis agitans) marked by muscular rigidity, tremors, lack of facial expression, akinesia, and postural abnormalities.

Parkinson's disease. See paralysis agitans.

paroni′ria. Morbid dreaming; terrifying dreams causing sleep disturbance.

p. ambulans, morbid dreaming while sleepwalking.

paronych′ia. Inflammation of the tissues around a nail; also called whitlow.

parooph′oron. A group of coiled, vestigial tubules situated in the broad ligament between the epoophoron and the uterus; best seen in the child, the tubules are remnants of the excretory part of the mesonephros or wolffian body.

paros′mia. Any disorder of the sense of smell, especially a perverted sense of smell as may occur in some cases of schizophrenia, uncinate gyrus lesions, and hysterias.

parot′id. Situated near the ear, as the parotid salivary gland.

parotidec′tomy. Surgical removal of the parotid gland.

paroti′tis, parotidi′tis. Inflammation of the parotid gland.

epidemic p., mumps; an acute contagious disease

caused by a virus present in discharges of the nose and in saliva; complications usually involve the ovaries and the testes, sometimes causing sterility in men.

par′ous. Having borne one or more children.

parova′rium. The lateral part of the vestigial remains of the mesonephric tubules located in the mesosalpinx between the ovary and the uterine tube.

par′oxysm. 1. A sudden onset or recurrence of symptoms of a disease. **2.** A convulsion.

paroxys′mal. Occurring in or of the nature of paroxysms.

pars, pl. **par′tes.** A particular portion of a structure; a part.

p. abdominalis esophagi, the portion of the esophagus between the diaphragm and the stomach.

p. anterior hypophyseos, the anterior lobe of the hypophysis (pituitary gland).

p. cartilaginea septi nasi, the cartilaginous portion of the nasal septum.

p. flaccida membranae tympani, the small, flaccid, somewhat triangular upper part of the tympanic membrane (eardrum); also called Shrapnell's membrane.

p. infundibularis hypophyseos, the infundibular part of the anterior lobe of the hypophysis that extends upward and wraps around the infundibular stalk.

p. intermedia hypophyseos, the intermediate part of the hypophysis, between the posterior and anterior lobes.

p. membranacea septi nasi, the membranous anterior portion of the nasal septum.

p. membranacea urethrae masculinae, the membranous part of the male urethra extending about half an inch or one and a quarter centimeters from the prostate gland.

p. muscularis septi interventricularis, the muscular portion of the interventricular septum of the heart.

p. nasalis pharyngis, see nasopharynx.

p. posterior hypophyseos, the posterior lobe of the hypophysis (pituitary gland).

p. prostatica urethrae, the portion of the male urethra that transverses the prostate gland; it is about two and a half centimeters in length.

p. radiata lobuli corticalis renis, medullary ray; see under ray.

part. A portion.

presenting p., in obstetrics, the portion of the fetus closest to the birth canal and which is felt through the cervix on vaginal examination; the presenting part determines the presentation.

partes aequales (P.ae.). Latin for equal parts;

used in prescription writing.

parthenogen′esis. Reproduction of organisms in which the female reproduces without fecundation by the male.

par′ticle. 1. An extremely small part, portion, or division of matter. **2.** One of the minute subdivisions of matter; e.g., an electron.

alpha p., a positively charged particle ejected from the nucleus of a radioactive atom and consisting of two neutrons and two protons (helium nucleus).

beta p., an electron, either positively (positron) or negatively (negatron) charged, which is emitted from an atomic nucleus during beta decay of a radionuclide.

Dane p., a double-shelled particle about 42 nm (millimicrons) in diameter, thought to represent the hepatitis B virus (HBV); the core, containing nucleic acids, is 28 nm in diameter and the lipoprotein outer coat is 7 nm thick.

elementary p., (1) the fundamental or simplest unit of matter that so far has defied subdivision; (2) platelet; (3) one of many knoblike repeating units attached to the matrix side of the inner membrane of the mitochondrion; it has a 90 Å spherical head, spaced at approximately 100 Å intervals, and is connected by a 50 Å-long stalklike structure to a baseplate in the membrane itself; formerly called F_1 particle; also called elementary transport particle and elementary body.

partic′ulate. Relating to or composed of fine particles.

partu′rient. 1. Relating to childbirth. **2.** About to give birth; in labor.

parturifa′cient. 1. Inducing or accelerating childbirth. **2.** An agent that induces or accelerates childbirth.

parturi′tion. The act of giving birth; also called childbirth.

par′tus. Childbirth; parturition.

parvicel′lular. Pertaining to or composed of exceptionally small cells.

PAS, PASA. Abbreviations for p-aminosalicylic acid.

pas′sage. 1. The act of passing. **2.** A channel, duct, pore, opening, or path along which something may pass. **3.** A bowel movement.

Passavant's cushion. See ridge, Passavant's.

pas′sion. 1. An intense emotion or appetite, such as love or greed. **2.** Fervent sexual desire; also called lust. **3.** Suffering.

pas′sive. Nonresponsive; submissive; inert; not initiating or participating.

passiv′ity. 1. The inertness exhibited by certain metals under conditions in which chemical activity

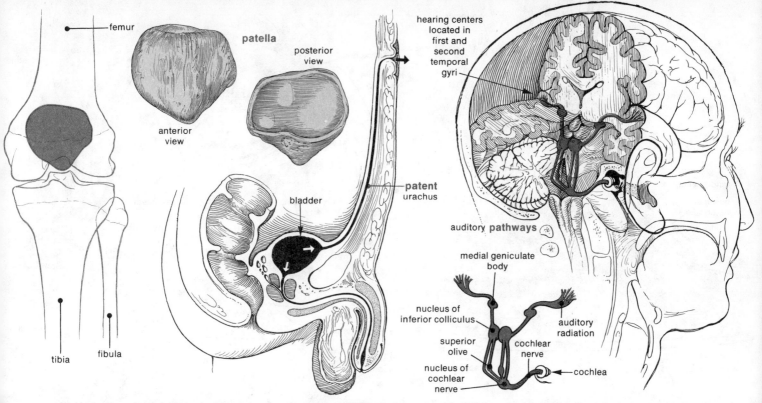

femur

patella

anterior view

posterior view

hearing centers located in first and second temporal gyri

patent urachus

bladder

auditory **pathways**

medial geniculate body

nucleus of inferior colliculus

superior olive

nucleus of cochlear nerve

auditory radiation

cochlear nerve

cochlea

tibia

fibula

should take place, due to the formation of a coating of peroxide, oxygen, or salt. **2.** In dentistry, the state of inactivity of the oral structures when a removable partial denture is in place but not used in mastication. **3.** Passivism, a passive or submissive attitude or behavior.

paste. A soft semisolid substance.

  dermatologic p., pharmaceutical preparation composed of starch, sulfur, dextrin, zinc oxide, or calcium carbonate mixed with glycerin, petrolatum, or soft soap and containing antiseptics for external use.

  p. filler, a mixture of slow-hardening materials used in dentistry to fill root canals.

  resorcinol p., mild, a bactericidal and fungicidal composed of 10 per cent resorcinol, 25 per cent zinc oxide, 25 per cent starch, and 40 per cent light liquid petrolatum; also called Lassar's mild resorcin paste.

  zinc oxide p. with salicylic acid, mixture of two per cent salicylic acid in paste of zinc oxide; used as an antiseptic and soothing agent; also called Lassar's zinc paste with salicylic acid.

Pasteurel´la. A genus (family Brucellaceae) of round, ellipsoidal, or rod-shaped gram-negative bacteria which usually occur singly.

  P. multocida, a gram-negative coccobacillus species prevalent in the oral cavities of dogs and cats; it often causes infection following dog and cat bites; although complications are rare, septicemia and tendinitis can occur if therapy is not instituted.

  P. pestis, the species causing plague in rodents and man, transmitted by the infected rat flea.

  P. tularensis, the species causing tularemia in man and rodents.

pasteurello´sis. Infection with bacteria of the genus *Pasteurella*; it includes hemorrhagic septicemia, tularemia, plague, and pseudotuberculosis.

pasteuriza´tion. The process of destroying or retarding the growth of bacteria in milk and other liquids, without destroying the flavor of the product, by heating the liquid to a moderate degree (60–70°C) for a sustained period of time (30 minutes) rather than by boiling it quickly.

pas´teurize. To subject milk or other liquids to pasteurization.

patch. A small area or section of a surface differing from or contrasting with the whole.

  cotton wool p.'s, coagulated exudates from the retinal capillaries, appearing as white fluffy areas on the retina.

  herald p., a solitary large lesion appearing before (sometimes days or weeks) the general eruption of pityriasis rosea.

  mucous p., a moist, yellowish lesion on the mu-

cous membrane of the mouth or external genitalia, usually seen in secondary syphilis.

  Peyer's p.'s, small whitish masses of lymphoid tissue situated in the mucous and submucous layers of the small intestine.

  smoker's p., see leukoplakia.

patel´la. A somewhat flattened triangular bone, embedded in the combined tendons of the extensor muscles of the leg, located at the front of the knee joint; the largest sesamoid bone of the body; also called kneecap.

patel´lapexy. The surgical fixation of the patella to the distal end of the femur.

patel´lar. Of or relating to the patella.

patellec´tomy. Surgical removal of the patella.

pa´tency. The state of being open.

pa´tent. 1. Open or exposed. **2.** Apparent.

path. The course taken by a nervous impulse.

path´finder. A filiform bougie for passage through a narrow stricture, such as the urethra; it serves as a guide for the introduction of a larger sound or catheter.

patho-, -pathy. Combining forms meaning disease.

path´ogen. Any microorganism or substance capable of causing disease.

pathogen´esis, pathogen´esy. The origin and development of disease; also called nosogenesis and nosogeny.

pathogen´ic, pathogenet´ic. Causing disease.

pathogenic´ity. Disease-producing capability.

pathogen´ism. The relationship between a pathogen and its host.

pathognomon´ic. A special characteristic of a disease; denoting one or more typical symptoms of a disease.

patholog´ic. Pertaining to or caused by disease.

pathol´ogist. A specialist in pathology.

pathol´ogy. The branch of medicine concerned with the study of disease in all its aspects (its nature, causes, development, and consequences).

pathomime´sis. Imitation of disease, whether intentional or unconscious.

pathoneuro´sis. Abnormal preoccupation with disease.

pathopho´bia. An abnormal fear of disease.

pathophysiol´ogy. The study of pathologic alteration in bodily function, as distinguished from structural defects.

pathopsychol´ogy. The study of abnormal psychic processes from the point of view of general psychology.

path´way. A path or course; specifically, the linked neurons through which an impulse is conducted to the cerebral cortex (afferent pathway), or

from the brain to the skeletal musculature (efferent pathway).

pa´tient. A person who is under medical treatment.

patrocli´nous. Inherited through the paternal line; derived from the father. Cf matroclinous.

pat´ten. A support worn under one shoe to equalize the length of both legs.

pat´tern. 1. An arrangement or design. **2.** In dentistry, a form used to develop a mold from which a restoration is produced, such as an inlay or denture.

  juvenile p., precordial T-wave inversion in the electrocardiogram; a persistent juvenile pattern sometimes seen in healthy adults, especially young Negroes.

  wax p., an exact wax model of lost tooth structure which, when invested and burned out, will produce a mold in which a casting may be made.

pat´ulous. Freely open; spread widely apart; expanded; patent.

pause. 1. Temporary stop. **2.** To suspend activity for a time.

  compensatory p., the pause following a premature beat, usually a ventricular extrasystole; the short cycle ending with the premature beat plus the compensatory pause together equal two of the regular cardiac cycles.

  sinus p., a spontaneous interruption in the regular sinus rhythm of the heart marked by a long-lasting absence of sinus P waves; thought to result from a high degree of S-A block or sinus arrest.

Pb. Symbol for lead; from Latin *plumbum*.

PBI. Abbreviation for protein-bound iodine.

p.c. Abbreviation of Latin *post cibum*, after meals.

PCG. Abbreviation for phonocardiogram.

Pco₂, pCO₂. Symbol for partial pressure of carbon dioxide.

PCP. Abbreviation for (a) phencyclidine (hallucinogen); (b) pulmonary capillary pressure.

PCV. Abbreviation for packed cell volume.

Pd. Chemical symbol for the element palladium.

PDM. Abbreviation for periodontal membrane.

PDR. Abbreviation for *Physicians' Desk Reference*.

pearl. 1. A small hard mass of mucus found in the sputum in asthma. **2.** A small sphere of thin glass containing a fluid meant to be inhaled after crushing of the sphere in a handkerchief.

  enamel p., a spherical nodule of enamel attached to a tooth, usually on the root; also called enameloma.

  Epstein's p., minute white masses of epithelium seen on the palate of the newborn.

  gouty p., sodium urate concretion, seen on the ear cartilage of individuals with gout.

peau. French for skin.

  p. d'orange, a dimpled appearance of the skin,

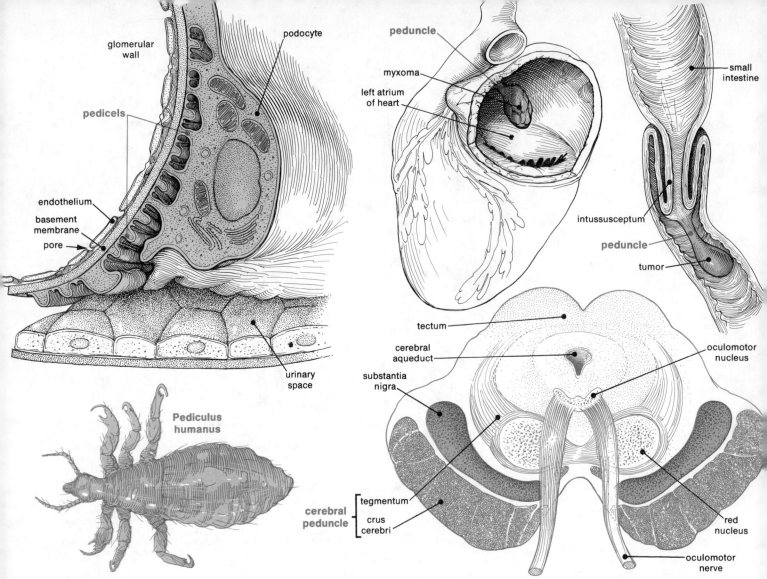

glomerular wall

podocyte

pedicels

endothelium

basement membrane

pore

urinary space

Pediculus humanus

peduncle

myxoma

left atrium of heart

small intestine

intussusceptum

peduncle

tumor

tectum

cerebral aqueduct

substantia nigra

oculomotor nucleus

cerebral peduncle

tegmentum

crus cerebri

red nucleus

oculomotor nerve

---

like that of an orange; seen in some cases of cancer of the breast.

pec'ten. 1. Any anatomic structure resembling a comb. **2.** A narrow area in the middle of the anal canal.

pec'tinate. Comb-shaped.

pectine'al. Relating to any comb-shaped structure.

pec'toral. Pertaining to the chest.

pectoral'gia. Pain in the chest.

pectora'lis. Relating to the chest.

pectoril'oquy. Transmission of the articulate voice through the chest wall, audible by use of the stethoscope; indicative of a cavity when present alone; indicative of consolidation when accompanied by bronchophony; also called pectorophony.

pectoroph'ony. See pectoriloquy.

pec'tus, *pl.* **pec'tora.** The chest; especially the anterior wall.

Ped. Abbreviation for pediatrics.

ped'al. Relating to the feet.

pederas'ty. Anal intercourse, especially between a man and boy.

pediat'ric. Relating to the study and treatment of children's diseases.

pediatric'ian. A physician who specializes in pediatrics.

pediat'rics. The branch of medicine concerned with the care and development of children and the treatment of their diseases.

ped'icel. Foot process or plate; the secondary process of a podocyte which helps form the visceral capsule of a renal corpuscle.

ped'icle. 1. A stem or stalk, as of a tumor. **2.** A tubed or narrow stalk by means of which a skin graft remains attached temporarily to the donor site.

pedic'ular. Relating to lice.

pedic'ulicide. Any agent or chemical capable of destroying lice.

pediculo'sis. The state of being infested with lice.

p. capitis, infestation of the hair of the head with lice.

p. corporis, the presence of lice on the body or clothes; they usually infest the clothes until feeding time.

p. pubis, the presence of lice on the pubic hair or neighboring parts of the body; the infesting louse is usually a species of *Phthirus,* not *Pediculus;* therefore, the condition is more correctly termed phthiriasis pubis.

Pedic'ulus. A genus of lice of the family Pediculidae.

P. humanus capitis, the head louse; a species that infests the scalp of man and attaches its eggs to hair.

P. humanus corporis, the body louse; one that infests the body of man (as distinguished from his head and extremities).

P. humanus, the sucking species infesting man and feeding on his blood; a vector of relapsing fever, typhus, and trench fever.

P. pubis, *Phthirus pubis.*

pedic'ulus, *pl.* **pedic'uli. 1.** Louse; parasite of the genus *Pediculus.* **2.** Pedicle; stalk.

ped'icure. 1. Care and treatment of the feet. **2.** Cosmetic care of the feet, especially of the toenails.

ped'igree. Family tree; a diagram setting forth a line of an individual's ancestors.

pedodon'tics. The branch of dentistry dealing with the preventive care and treatment of children's teeth.

pedodon'tist. A specialist in pedodontics.

pedol'ogy. A branch of biology and of sociology that studies the behavior and development of children.

pedophil'ia. Love of children; in psychiatry, it denotes the love of children by an adult for sexual purposes.

ped'uncle. 1. A large stalklike mass of nerve fibers connecting a suprasegmental structure to other

portions of the nervous system. **2.** The narrow part of a structure serving as support or attachment.

cerebellar p., inferior, a bundle of largely afferent nerve fibers on either side of the medulla oblongata, connecting the medulla and spinal cord with the cerebellum; also called restiform body.

cerebellar p., middle, one of a pair of large bundles of nerve fibers originating in the pontine nuclei and distributed to all parts of the cerebellar cortex; also called brachium pontis.

cerebellar p., superior, a large bundle of largely efferent nerve fibers extending from each cerebellar hemisphere upward over the pons and reaching the tegmentum of the midbrain, where it decussates; the fibers originate in the dentate and emboliform nuclei and terminate chiefly in the opposite red nucleus and thalamus.

cerebral p., the part of the midbrain in front of the cerebral aqueduct, composed of the tegmentum (dorsal part) and crus cerebri (ventral part).

p. of the pineal body, the dorsal stalk of the pineal body; also called habenula.

thalamic p., the fibers passing between the thalamus and cerebral cortex (subdivided into anterior, posterior, superior, and inferior peduncles).

pedun'culate, pedun'culated. Having a stalk or peduncle.

pedunculot'omy. Surgical incision of the cerebral puduncle.

pelio'sis. Purpura.

pellag'ra. A condition caused by vitamin (nicotinic acid) deficiency, marked by skin lesions, gastrointestinal disturbances, and nervous disorders.

pella'grin. An individual afflicted with pellagra.

pellag'roid. Resembling pellagra.

pellag'rous. Relating to pellagra.

pel'licle. 1. Thin membrane or cuticle. **2.** A film on the surface of a liquid. **3.** A firm mass formed by some fungi on the surface of a liquid medium.

pel'vic. Of or relating to a pelvis.

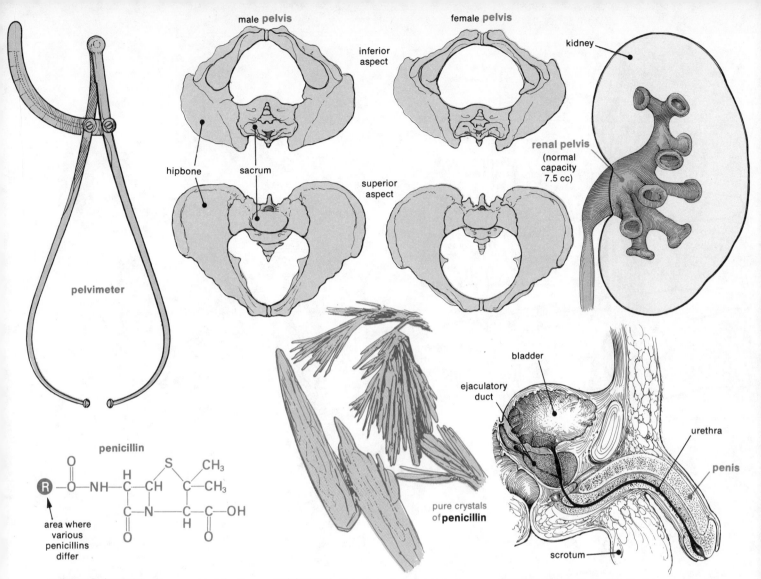

male pelvis

female pelvis

inferior aspect

superior aspect

kidney

hipbone

sacrum

renal pelvis (normal capacity 7.5 cc)

pelvimeter

bladder

ejaculatory duct

urethra

penis

penicillin

$$R-O-NH-C-CH \begin{matrix} & S & CH_3 \\ & & CH_3 \end{matrix}$$
$$C-N-C-COOH$$

area where various penicillins differ

pure crystals of **penicillin**

scrotum

pelvicephalom´etry. Measurement of the diameters of the fetal head in relation to those of the mother's pelvis.

pelvic inflammatory disease (PID). Inflammation in the pelvic cavity, especially of the female genital organs.

pelvilithot´omy. Pyelolithotomy.

pelvim´eter. A caliper-shaped instrument for measuring the diameters and capacity of the pelvis.

pelvim´etry. The measurement of the dimensions and capacity of the inlet and the outlet of the pelvis (birth canal).

  x-ray p., pelvimetry performed by application of a grid to roentgenograms of the pelvic bones.

pelviot´omy. 1. Division of the pubic joint. **2.** Incision into the pelvis of the kidney.

pel´vis, *pl.* **pel´ves. 1.** A basin-like skeletal structure that supports the spinal column and rests on the lower limbs. **2.** A funnel-shaped structure, as the pelvis of the kidney.

  android p., a female pelvis with characteristics of a male pelvis.

  brim of the p., the circumference of the plane dividing the major and minor pelves.

  cavity of the minor p., see cavity, pelvic.

  contracted p., one in which any of the important diameters is shorter than normal.

  false p., see major pelvis.

  funnel-shaped p., one with a normal inlet and a greatly narrowed outlet.

  inlet of p., the upper opening of the true pelvis; the space within the pelvic brim.

  major p., false p., the expanded portion of the pelvis situated above and in front of the pelvic brim.

  minor p., true p., the portion of the pelvis situated below and behind the pelvic brim.

  renal p., the funnel-shaped structure, formed by the junction of two tubes (greater calices), into which the urine is discharged from the kidney.

  true p., see minor pelvis.

pelvisa´cral. Relating to the pelvis and the sacrum.

pel´viscope. An illuminated instrument for examining the interior of the pelvis.

pelvospondyli´tis. Inflammation of the sacral vertebrae (pelvic portion of spinal column), usually resulting in hardening of the sacroiliac and apophyseal joints.

  p. ossificans, ankylosing spondylitis; see under spondylitis.

pem´phigoid. An eruption of soft blebs resembling those of pemphigus vulgaris.

pem´phigus. Any skin disease characterized by severe blistering.

  familial benign chronic p., a blistering dermatosis; recurrent eruption of vesicles and bullae that become scaling and crusted lesions with vesicular borders, predominantly of the neck, groin, and axillary regions; autosomal dominant inheritance; also called Hailey-Hailey disease.

  p. erythematosus, see Senear-Usher disease.

  p. foliaceus, a form of pemphigus characterized by widespread leaf-like scaliness and slightly exudative lesions, resembling exfoliative dermatitis; histologically the blisters are high in the epidermis.

  p. vegetans, a form of pemphigus characterized by exuberant overgrowth or vegetations in or about the eroded surfaces left by ruptured blisters; also called Neumann's disease.

  p. vulgaris, a serious systemic illness of unknown etiology, characterized by an eruption of flaccid vesicles over the entire body, with erosion on the mucous membranes; if left untreated, it is inevitably fatal.

Pendred's syndrome. Congenital deafness and goiter with or without hypothyroidism; inherited as a simple recessive trait.

pen´etrance. The frequency with which a heritable trait is manifested in individuals known to carry the gene that causes it.

penetrom´eter. Device for measuring the penetrating power of a given x-ray beam.

-penia. Combining form denoting a deficiency or scarcity; e.g., leukopenia.

penicil´lamine. A degradation product of penicillin; a chelating agent used in the treatment of hepatolenticular degeneration (Wilson's disease) and lead poisoning.

penicil´lin. Any of a family of antibiotic compounds obtained from cultures of the mold *Penicillium notatum* and related species, or produced biosynthetically; it inhibits bacterial cell wall synthesis, resulting in eventual death to the cell when the penicillin-poisoned bacteria outgrows its cell wall.

penicil´linase. 1. Enzyme produced by certain bacteria (e.g., some strains of staphylococcus) that render penicillin inactive. **2.** Enzyme obtained from cultures of *Bacillus cereus*; used to treat delayed penicillin reactions.

Penicil´lium. A genus of fungi; a saprophytic mold that yields several antibiotic substances.

  P. notatum, an ascomycete fungus from which penicillin and notatin are derived.

pen´ile. Relating to the penis.

pe´nis. The male organ of copulation and of urinary excretion; composed of three columns of erectile tissue, two dorsolateral (corpora cavernosa) and one medial (corpus spongiosum) which contains the urethra and expands at the end forming the glans penis.

pen´nate. Resembling a feather; feathered or winged; also called penniform and pinnate.

pen´niform. See pennate.

pentaba´sic. Denoting an acid that has five hydrogen atoms replaceable by a metal or radical.

pental´ogy. Any condition having five components.

pentatom´ic. 1. Denoting a molecule comprised of five atoms. **2.** Denoting a compound possessing five atoms in a ring. **3.** Denoting a chemical with

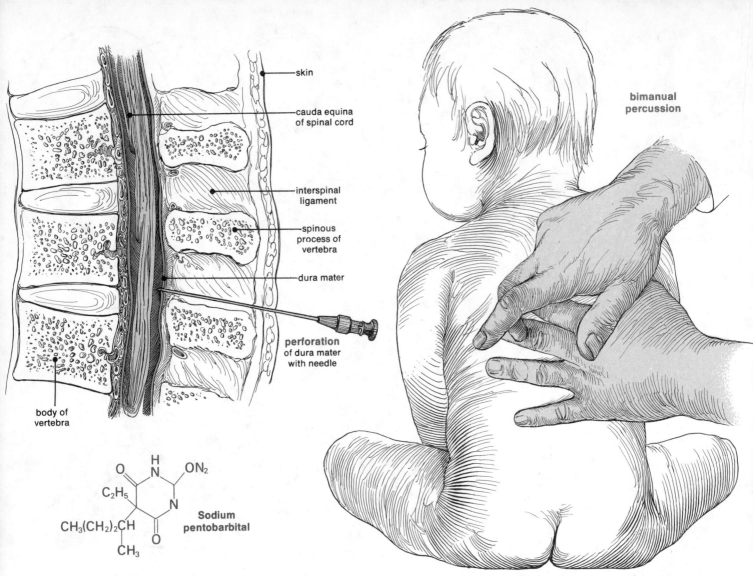

skin

cauda equina
of spinal cord

interspinal
ligament

spinous
process of
vertebra

dura mater

perforation
of dura mater
with needle

body of
vertebra

**bimanual
percussion**

Sodium
pentobarbital

five replaceable hydrogen atoms. **4.** Denoting an alcohol containing five hydroxyl groups.

pentav′alent. An atom or group of atoms having a valence of five; capable of combining with five atoms of hydrogen.

pentobarb′ital. A short-acting barbiturate, $C_{11}H_{12}N_2O_3$, generally used for sleep induction; Nembutal®.

  sodium p., the sodium salt of pentobarbital, a short-acting hypnotic that reduces apprehension and produces drowsiness; used for sedation during labor, and prior to surgery and various diagnostic procedures.

pen′tose. Any one of a class of monosaccharides containing five carbon atoms in the molecule ($C_5H_{10}O_5$); e.g., arabinose, lyxose, ribose, and xylose.

pentosu′ria. The presence of any of the pentoses in the urine.

pep′sin. An enzyme present in gastric juice; it converts proteins into peptones and proteoses.

pepsin′ogen. The precursor of pepsin, present in the lining of the stomach; an inert substance that is converted into pepsin during digestion by the action of hydrochloric acid.

pepsinog′enous. Producing pepsin.

pepsinu′ria. The presence of pepsin in the urine.

pep′tic. 1. Of or relating to digestion. **2.** Relating to pepsin.

pep′tidase. An enzyme that catalyzes the hydrolysis of peptide bonds of a protein or peptide.

pep′tide. One of various compounds which yield two or more amino acids on hydrolysis; one of the compounds into which the protein molecule is split during digestion.

pep′tize. To transform a gel into a sol.

peptol′ysis. The hydrolysis or splitting up of peptones.

pep′tone. Any of various protein derivatives obtained by the action of an enzyme or an acid on a natural protein.

peptone′mia. The presence of peptone in the blood.

pep′tonize. To convert protein into peptone.

peptonu′ria. The presence of peptones in the urine.

Pep′tostreptococ′cus. A genus of spherical gram-positive, nonmotile bacteria found normally in the intestinal, respiratory, and female genital tracts, oral cavity, and certain pyogenic infections.

per-. 1. Prefix meaning throughout. **2.** In chemistry, containing the largest possible amount of a specified chemical element or radical.

per anum. Latin for through the anus.

per′cept. A mental impression of something perceived by the senses that forms an image in the mind.

percep′tion. The process of becoming aware of something through any of the senses.

  depth p., the ability to detect by sight the three dimensional quality of objects and their position in space; perception of the third dimension; also called stereoscopic vision.

  extrasensory p. (ESP), perception through other than the five senses.

  light p. (LP), the ability to distinguish light from dark.

perceptiv′ity. The ability or faculty of perception.

perchlor′ide. A chloride having the largest possible amount of chlorine.

percola′tion. Extraction of the soluble parts of a solid mixture by passing a liquid solvent slowly through it.

percuss′. 1. To tap the surface of specific areas of the body to determine the degree of density of the structures beneath by the sound produced. **2.** To tap a bodily part as a therapeutic measure.

percuss′ion. The act of tapping the body, especially the chest, back, and abdomen, to determine the condition of underlying structures by the sounds produced.

  auscultatory p., auscultation for the purpose of listening to sounds produced by percussion.

  bimanual p., one in which the finger of one hand taps a finger of the other hand which is placed on the patient.

  palpatory p., percussion combined with palpation in order to perceive tactile as well as auditory impressions.

percus′sor. 1. A device that sends vibrations through the chest wall to aid in freeing mucus deposits and improve bronchial drainage. **2.** A hammer for use in percussion.

percuta′neous. 1. Having the ability to pass through unbroken skin, as in absorption by inunction. **2.** Denoting procedures such as biopsies or intravenous or intra-arterial catheterizations performed with needle puncture without incision.

perfec′tionism. A propensity for setting extremely high standards of performance for oneself.

perfla′tion. The forcing of air into a cavity or canal to expel any contained material.

per′forans. Denoting certain anatomic structures which pass through other structures.

perfora′tion. 1. A small hole or series of holes through an organ or organelle. **2.** The act of piercing a body part.

perfu′sate. A fluid that has been poured (1) over a special surface, e.g., a charged plate, or (2) through a tissue or semipermeable membrane.

perfu′sion. The passage of a fluid through the vessels of an organ.

peri-. Prefix meaning around.

periadeni′tis. Inflammation of the tissues around a gland.

peria′nal. Adjacent to or around the anus; also called circumanal.

periangi′tis. Inflammation of the tissues surrounding a blood vessel or a lymphatic vessel.

periantri′tis. Antral gastritis; see under gastritis.

Labels: lung, pericardium, sternum, heart

Labels: Schwann's cell, nucleus of neuron, perikaryon, axon, dendrites

periaor'tic. Surrounding or located near the aorta.

periaorti'tis. An inflammatory condition affecting the adventitia of the aorta and the tissues around it.

periap'ical. Relating to the tissues surrounding the tip of a dental root, including the alveolar bone.

periappendici'tis. Inflammation of the tissues near or surrounding the vermiform appendix.

periarte'rial. Surrounding an artery.

periarteri'tis. Inflammation of the outer coat of an artery.

   p. nodosa, see polyarteritis nodosa.

periarthri'tis. Inflammation of the tissues near a joint.

periax'ial. Surrounding an axis.

peribron'chial. Surrounding a bronchus or bronchi.

peribuc'cal. Situated around the mouth.

peribul'bar. Surrounding any anatomic bulb, especially of the eye and the urethra.

peribur'sal. Situated around a bursa.

pericardec'tomy. See pericardiectomy.

pericar'dial, pericar'diac. 1. Situated around the heart. **2.** Of or relating to the pericardium.

pericardicente'sis,   **pericardiocente'sis.** Surgical puncture of the membrane covering the heart (pericardium) for the purpose of aspirating a pericardial effusion.

pericardiec'tomy. Surgical removal of a portion of the pericardium; also called pericardectomy.

pericardios'tomy. The making of an opening into the pericardium.

pericardiot'omy. See pericardotomy.

pericardi'tis. Inflammation of the pericardium.

   adhesive p., the presence of dense fibrous tissue which fixes the pericardium to the heart or to other structures in the chest.

pericar'dium. The thin, double-layered, membranous sac that encloses the heart; the layers are separated by a small amount of tissue fluid which lubricates the constantly rubbing surfaces; they fuse

as they attach to the great vessels and diaphragm.

pericardot'omy. Surgical incision of the pericardium; also called pericardiotomy .

perice'cal. Surrounding the cecum.

pericel'lular. Surrounding or situated around a cell.

pericementi'tis. Periodontitis.

pericholangi'tis. Inflammation of the tissues around the bile ducts or interlobular bile capillaries.

pericholecysti'tis. Inflammation of the tissues surrounding the gallbladder.

perichon'drial. Relating to or composed of perichondrium.

perichondri'tis. Inflammation of the perichondrium.

perichon'drium. A fibrous membrane which covers cartilage except at joint endings, composed of an outer dense irregular connective tissue and an inner layer which is responsible for production of new cartilage.

per'ichord. The sheath covering the notochord.

perichor'dal. Relating to the sheath of the notochord.

pericolpi'tis. Inflammation of the tissues surrounding the vagina.

pericor'onal. Surrounding the crown of a tooth.

pericoroni'tis. Inflammation of the gums around a partially erupted tooth.

pericra'nial. Relating to the fibrous membrane covering the skull.

pericrani'tis. Inflammation of the membrane covering the skull.

pericra'nium. The fibrous membrane covering the skull; also called periosteum of the skull.

pericys'tic. 1. Surrounding the urinary bladder. **2.** Around the gallbladder. **3.** Surrounding a cyst.

per'icyte. One of the elongated connective tissue cells located around the capillaries.

peridendrit'ic. Surrounding the dendrites of a nerve cell or neuron.

periden'tal. Periodontal; surrounding a tooth.

peridenti'tis. Periodontitis.

periden'tium. See periodontium.

perides'mic. Surrounding a ligament; relating to the membrane surrounding a ligament (peridesmium).

peridesmi'tis. Inflammation of the connective tissue surrounding a ligament.

perides'mium. The connective tissue membrane covering a ligament.

periendothelio'ma. See perithelioma.

periesopha'geal. Surrounding the esophagus.

periesophagi'tis. Inflammation of the tissues around the esophagus.

periganglion'ic. Surrounding a nerve ganglion.

perigas'tric. Surrounding the stomach.

perihepat'ic. Occurring around the liver.

perihepati'tis. Inflammation of the peritoneum and tissues around the liver; a complication in women with gonococcal inflammation of the pelvic organs, resulting from the spread of gonococci to the upper abdomen; also called Fitz-Hugh-Curtis syndrome and hepatitis externa.

perikar'yon. The main cytoplasmic matrix surrounding the nucleus of the cell body of the neuron; it is crowded with granular organelles including neurofibrils, chromidial substance (Nissl bodies), Golgi apparatus, mitochondria, and a centrosome; also called neuroplasm.

per'ilymph. The fluid contained in the bony labyrinth, surrounding the membranous labyrinth of the internal ear.

perilymphat'ic. 1. Relating to the perilymph. **2.** Surrounding a lymphatic vessel.

perim'eter. 1. An edge or border. **2.** A device to determine the extent and characteristics of the visual field.

perimet'ric. 1. Surrounding the uterus. **2.** Relating to the measuring of the visual field.

perimetri'tis. Inflammation of the outer coat of

INCUBATION PERIODS OF VARIOUS DISEASES		
Disease	Incubation Period	Rash
gastroenteritis	6–24 hours	—
diphtheria	2–5 days	—
scarlet fever	1–5 ''	1st day
measles	10–15 ''	4th ''
rubella	14–21 ''	1st ''
chicken-pox	14–21 ''	1st ''
mumps	7–26 ''	—
smallpox	7–16 ''	3rd ''
whooping cough	2–21 ''	—
poliomyelitis	7–21 ''	—
virus influenza	1–4 ''	—
gonorrhea	1–8 ''	—
typhus	8–16 ''	5th ''
yellow fever	3–6 ''	—
infectious hepatitis	15–35 ''	—
brucellosis	7–14 ''	—
typhoid fever	3–38 ''	—
syphilis	1–6 weeks	—

GESTATION PERIODS OF SOME ANIMALS	
Species	Range
mouse	18–20 days
rabbit	30–32 ''
cat	56–65 ''
dog	58–63 ''
swine	111–116 ''
cow	273–291 ''
horse	329–346 ''

the uterus (perimetrium).

perime'trium. The serous membrane covering the uterus.

perim'etry. The determination of the extent of the visual field with the aid of a perimeter, usually for the purpose of diagnosing disturbances in the visual pathways.

perimys'ial. Relating to the perimysium.

perimys'ium. Connective tissue that surrounds the fasciculi (bundles of muscle fibers) and also forms the fibrous septa throughout the muscle.

perina'tal. Occurring or relating to, immediately before, during, or shortly after birth; applied to the time that usually starts with completion of 20 weeks of gestation and generally ends 28 days after birth.

perine'al. Relating to the perineum.

perine'oplasty. Reparative surgery of the perineum, as for the correction of a relaxed condition; sometimes called perineorrhaphy.

perineor'rhaphy. Suture of the perineum, usually performed for the repair of a laceration occurring during childbirth. See also perineoplasty.

perineot'omy. See episiotomy.

perineph'ric. Perirenal; surrounding or located about the kidney.

perinephri'tis. Inflammation of the tissues around the kidney.

perineph'rium. The connective tissue and fat around the kidney.

perine'um. 1. The area bounded by the pubis, the coccyx, and the thighs. **2.** The area between the external genitalia and the anus.

perineu'ral. Surrounding a nerve.

perineuri'tis. Inflammation of the perineurium.

perineu'rium. A layer of connective tissue surrounding and supporting each separate bundle of nerve fibers in a peripheral nerve; it consists of a variable number of layers of squamous epithelial cells.

perinu'clear. Surrounding or situated near a nucleus.

pe'riod. 1. An interval of time. **2.** An occurrence of menstruation.

　absolute refractory p., (1) the period in the cardiac cycle when the heart muscle does not respond to even a high-intensity stimulus; it corresponds to the contraction phase; (2) the time immediately following the passage of an impulse through a nerve.

　gestation p., time between conception and parturition; period of pregnancy.

　incubation p., time between infection with a pathogenic microorganism and appearance of first symptoms.

　latent p., (1) time elapsed between application of

a stimulus and the resulting response; (2) the incubation period of an infectious disease.

　missed p., the failure of menstruation to occur in a month.

　neonatal p., the first 30 days of infant life.

　puerperal p., time between termination of labor and return of the uterus to its original state (approximately six weeks).

　relative refractory p., (1) time during relaxation of heart muscle in which a stronger than ordinary stimulus is required to elicit a response; (2) time, following the absolute refractory period of a nerve, in which a stronger than ordinary stimulus is necessary to transmit an impulse.

　Wenckebach p., the progressively lengthened P-R interval in successive cardiac cycles preceding a dropped beat, due to an atrioventricular (A-V) block.

period'ic. 1. Happening or recurring at regular intervals of time; appearing in cycles, as a disease with regularly recurring symptoms. **2.** Intermittent; appearing now and then.

period'ic acid. A colorless, water-soluble, inorganic acid, $HIO_4 \cdot 2H_2O$, resulting from the action of concentrated hydrochloric acid on iodine.

period'ical. A journal published at regular intervals.

periodic'ity. 1. Recurrence of a phenomenon at regular intervals of time. **2.** Recurrence of similar properties in a group of elements, as seen in the periodic system.

periodon'tal. Surrounding a tooth; also called peridental.

periodontal disease. Any disease of the tissues surrounding and supporting the teeth; there are two principal groups: disease confined to the gingiva (gingivitis) and disease affecting the underlying supporting periodontal tissue (periodontitis).

periodon'tics. The branch of dentistry concerned with the study of the tissues surrounding the teeth and with the treatment of their diseases.

periodon'tist. A specialist in periodontics.

periodonti'tis. A disease of the periodontium manifested by inflammation of the gums, loss of bone tissue around the teeth, degeneration of the periodontal membrane or ligament, and the formation of pockets between the teeth and the surrounding bone; also called pyorrhea.

periodon'tium. The tissues surrounding and supporting the teeth, including the cementum, periodontal membrane or ligament, alveolar bone, and gingiva (gums); also called peridentium.

periodontocla'sia. A general term denoting destruction or degenerative changes of the supporting tissues of teeth.

periodonto'sis. A rare condition of unknown cause marked by noninflammatory degeneration of the periodontal tissues, resulting in premature tooth loss.

perio'ral. Situated about the mouth.

perior'bita. Periosteum lining the interior of the orbit.

perior'bital. Related to or situated about the orbit or periorbita.

periorchi'tis. Inflammation of the tunica vaginalis testis.

perios'teal. Relating to or of the nature of the periosteum.

periosteo'ma. A tumor surrounding a bone; also called periostoma.

periosteomyeli'tis. Inflammation of the entire bone and the surrounding periosteum.

periosteot'omy, periostot'omy. The surgical cutting of the periosteum.

perios'teum. A thick fibrous membrane covering the surface of bones except at points of articulation; it consists, in adults, of two layers: the external layer of dense connective tissue conveying blood vessels and nerves to the bone, and the internal layer of loose connective tissue.

periosti'tis. Inflammation of the periosteum.

periosto'ma. See periosteoma.

periostot'omy. See periosteotomy.

peripap'illary. Surrounding the optic disk.

periph'eral. Pertaining to the outer surface of the body or situated away from the center.

periph'ery. The area of the body away from the center; the outer surface of the body.

peripor'tal. Surrounding or situated around the portal vein, especially in the liver substance.

periprocti'tis. Inflammation of the tissues situated around the rectum and anus.

perirec'tal. Adjacent to or around the rectum.

perire'nal. Surrounding the kidney in whole or part; also called perinephric.

perisal'pinx. The peritoneal covering of the uterine tube.

perispleni'tis. Inflammation of the peritoneum covering the spleen and of the structures surrounding that organ.

peristal'sis. The alternate contraction and relaxation of the walls of a tubular structure by means of which its contents are moved onward, characteristic of the intestinal tract, ureter, etc.

peris'tole. The ability of the walls of the stomach to contract about its contents following the ingestion of food.

perisyno'vial. Situated around a synovial membrane.

peritec'tomy. See peritomy.

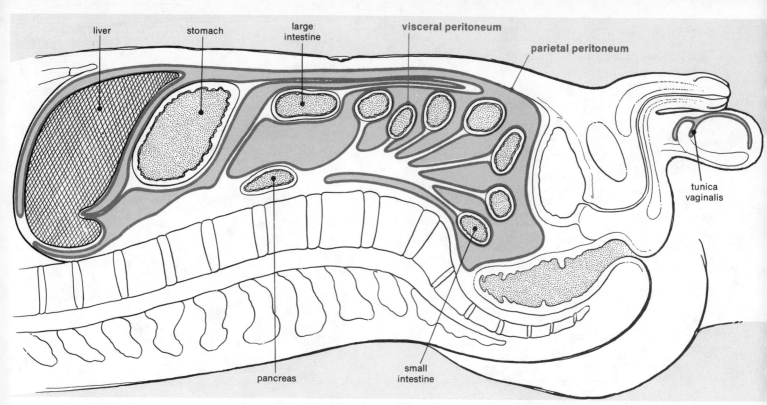

Labels on diagram: liver, stomach, large intestine, visceral peritoneum, parietal peritoneum, tunica vaginalis, pancreas, small intestine

peritendini′tis. Inflammation of the sheath around a tendon.

perithelio′ma. A tumor which appears to be derived from the tissues surrounding blood vessels (perithelium); also called periendothelioma.

perithe′lium. Thin layer of connective tissue surrounding the small vessels.

perit′omy, peritec′tomy. 1. The cutting of the conjunctiva at the edge of the cornea; a preliminary step in various surgical procedures. **2.** Circumcision.

peritone′al. Of or relating to the peritoneum.

perito′neocente′sis. Paracentesis or tapping of the peritoneal cavity for the purpose of removing fluid.

peritoneoc′lysis. Irrigation of the peritoneal cavity.

perito′neoscope. An illuminated tubular instrument for visual examination of the peritoneum through an abdominal wall incision.

peritoneos′copy. Direct inspection of the peritoneal cavity by means of a lighted tubular instrument inserted through the abdominal wall.

peritoneot′omy. Incision of the peritoneum.

peritone′um. The serous membrane lining the walls of the abdominal and pelvic cavities and enclosing the viscera.

   parietal p., the layer of peritoneum lining the walls of the abdominal and pelvic cavities.

   visceral p., the layer of peritoneum investing the abdominal and pelvic organs.

peritoni′tis. Inflammation of the peritoneum, usually attended by abdominal pain, constipation, vomiting, and fever; it may be caused by perforation of the digestive tract, by infection of an organ, such as the appendix, or by a blood-borne infection.

   benign paroxysmal p., periodic abdominalgia; see under abdominalgia.

per′itonize. To cover with peritoneum.

periton′sillar. Around a tonsil.

peritonsilli′tis. Inflammation affecting the peritonsillar tissues.

peritra′cheal. Situated about the trachea.

perit′richous. 1. Relating to cilia or any projections from the surface of a cell. **2.** Having flagella uniformly distributed throughout the body; applied to bacteria. **3.** Having modified cilia arranged in a spiral fashion around the mouth opening; said of certain protozoa.

periumbil′ical. Situated around or near the umbilicus; also called periomphalic.

periung′ual. Around a nail.

periuret′eral, periureter′ic. Located around one or both ureters.

periureteri′tis. Inflammation of tissues adjacent to the ureter.

periurethri′tis. Inflammation of the tissue around the urethra.

perivas′cular. Around a vessel.

per′iwinkle. Any of several attractive evergreen shrubs or small trees with glossy blue-green leaves and fragrant flowers of the genus *Vinca*, especially *Vinca minor* and *Vinca rosea*; they contain active dimeric alkaloids including vinblastine, vincristine, vinleurosine, and vinrosidine; also called myrtle.

PERLA. Acronym for pupils equal and reactive to light and accommodation.

perlèche. A form of oral candidiasis marked by inflammation at the angles of the mouth, with an accumulation of whitish macerated epithelium; it occurs mainly among undernourished children, especially those who have a habit of licking the angles of the mouth.

perman′ganate. Any of the salts of permanganic acid.

permangan′ic acid. An unstable inorganic acid, $HMnO_4$, derived from manganese.

permeabil′ity. The condition of being permeable.

per′meable. Being of a substance that allows the passage of another substance; also called pervious.

per′mease. A specific protein in the cell membrane of microorganisms that facilitates passage of nutrients, such as sugar, across the membrane in the direction of the concentration gradient; part of the active transport system.

perni′cious. Highly destructive; tending to cause death.

per′nio. See chilblain.

perome′lia. Severe congenital malformation of the extremities, including absence of a hand or a foot.

perone′al. Relating to the fibula or the lateral portion of the leg.

perone′us. See table of muscles.

pero′ral. Administered through the mouth.

per os (p.o.). Latin for by mouth.

perox′idase. Enzyme found in plant and animal tissues; it causes the decomposition of peroxides which liberate oxygen, thus facilitating oxidation.

perox′ide. The oxide of a series containing the greatest number of oxygen atoms.

   hydrogen p., hydrogen dioxide, H_2O_2; an unstable compound, used in solution as an antiseptic, bleaching agent, and oxidizing agent.

perox′isome. A membrane-bounded organelle in cells about 0.5 μ in diameter that contains oxidase and peroxidase; formerly called microbody.

peroxy-. Combining form indicating the presence of an additional oxygen atom; e.g., hydrogen peroxide, peroxyformic acid.

peroxyace′tyl ni′trate. The main pollutant of smog, responsible for the irritation of the eyes and the nose.

per primam, per primam intentionem. Latin terms meaning by first intention, a way in which a wound heals; see under intention.

per rec′tum. By way of the rectum.

persalt′. In chemistry, any salt containing the maximum amount of the acid radical.

per secundum, per secundum intentionem. Latin terms meaning by second intention, a way in which a wound heals; see under intention.

persevera′tion. 1. The pathologic, involuntary repetition of a single response to various questions, as seen in organic brain disease. **2.** The duration of a mental image.

personal′ity. The sum total of an individual's patterns of reaction to his environment.

   cyclothymic p., a personality disorder characterized by frequent alternation between moods of elation and depression; also called affective personality.

   inadequate p., a personality characterized by inept responses to emotional, social, and intellectual demands.

   multiple p., condition in which the individual adopts two or more different identities with total intervening amnesia.

   obsessive-compulsive p., behavior pattern characterized by excessive self-imposed orderliness, rigid adherence to perfectionism, and undue concern with trifles; distinguished from obsessive-compulsive neurosis.

   passive-aggressive p., character disorder characterized by aggressiveness expressed passively in such ways as procrastination, stubbornness, obstructionism, or intentional inefficiency; this behavior usually indicates hostility which the person does not dare express openly.

   psychopathic p., an outdated term for sociopathic behavior.

   schizoid p., personality type characterized by avoidance of close or competitive relationships and by a detached reaction to life experiences.

   split p., an outdated term for schizophrenia.

perspira′tion. 1. Sweat; the fluid secreted by the sweat glands, consisting of water, sodium chloride and phosphate, urea, ammonia, creatinine, fats, and other waste products. **2.** The process of sweating.

   insensible p., perspiration that evaporates before it can be perceived on the skin; the term sometimes denotes evaporation from the lungs.

   sensible p., perspiration that is perceived as moisture on the skin.

persua′sion. In psychiatry, a therapeutic ap-

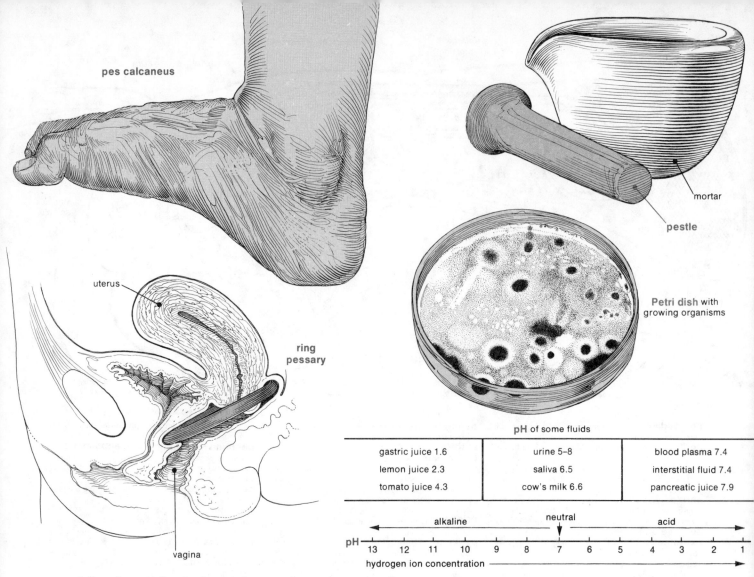

pes calcaneus

mortar

pestle

uterus

ring pessary

vagina

Petri dish with growing organisms

pH of some fluids

gastric juice 1.6	urine 5–8	blood plasma 7.4
lemon juice 2.3	saliva 6.5	interstitial fluid 7.4
tomato juice 4.3	cow's milk 6.6	pancreatic juice 7.9

alkaline ← neutral → acid

pH 13 12 11 10 9 8 7 6 5 4 3 2 1

hydrogen ion concentration

proach directed toward influencing the mind of another by authority, argument, reason, or entreaty.

pertus'sis. An acute respiratory illness of infants and young children usually caused by *Bordetella pertussis*, a gram-negative coccobacillus; in a typical case, the patient manifests paroxysmal coughing with a terminal whoop; a pertussis vaccine is available and is generally administered to infants together with diphtheria and tetanus toxoids; also called whooping cough.

pervapora'tion. The concentration of a colloidal solution by placing the solution in a bag of semipermeable material and suspending it over a hot plate; only the colloid remains in the bag while the rest of the substances pass through.

perver'sion. A deviation from what is considered normal.

per'vert. A person who practices perversions, usually sexual.

per'vious. Permeable; being of a substance that is capable of being penetrated.

pes. **1.** Latin for foot. **2.** Any footlike or basal bodily structure.
  p. anserinus, (1) the goosefoot-like plexiform branching of the facial nerve in, and in front of, the parotid gland; (2) the combined insertions of the tendons of the sartorius, gracilis, and semitendinosus muscles at the medial border of the tibial tuberosity.
  p. calcaneus, foot deformity characterized by dorsiflexion of the foot and prominence of the heel; the weight of the body rests on the heel.
  p. cavus, see clawfoot.
  p. corvinus, crow's foot, the wrinkles radiating from the outer corner (lateral canthus) of the eye, seen in many adults.
  p. equinus, foot deformity characterized by plantar flexion; the weight of the body rests on the ball of the foot.
  p. planus, see flatfoot.

pes'sary. **1.** A device used to support a displaced uterus when surgery is contraindicated, or as a contraceptive. **2.** A medicated vaginal suppository.
  diaphragm p., see diaphragm, contraceptive.
  Menge p., a ring pessary with a cross bar and a detachable knob, used when the uterus is markedly prolapsed.
  ring p., a ring of plastic, rubber, or metal, used to support the uterus in cases of slight prolapse.
  Smith-Hodge p., one used to hold the retroposed uterus in anteposition after it has been brought forward manually.

pes'ticide. Any agent that is used to destroy pests, especially insects, rodents, and fungi.

pes'tilence. An epidemic of a usually deadly disease, especially of the bubonic plaque.

pes'tis. Latin for plague.

pes'tle. A club-shaped tool, used for breaking and grinding substances in a mortar.

pete'chia. A small hemorrhage, appearing as a nonraised, purplish-red spot of the skin, nail beds, or mucous membranes.

pet'iole. A slender stalk-like structure; a stem or pedicle; also called petiolus.
  epiglottic p., the pointed lower end of the epiglottic cartilage which is connected by the thyroepiglottic ligament to the back of the thyroid cartilage.

peti'olus. See petiole.

petit' mal. See epilepsy, petit mal.

Pe'tri dish. A shallow circular container made of glass or plastic with a loose-fitting cover, used for the cultivation of microorganisms; also called Petri plate.

petrifac'tion. The conversion of an organic substance into stone; also called fossilization.

pétrissag'e. A kneading of the muscles in massage.

petrola'tum. A pale yellow to amber semisolid mixture of hydrocarbons from petroleum; used as a soothing and lubricant agent and in the preparation

of ointments; also called petroleum jelly, soft paraffin, and Vaseline®.
  hydrophilic p., a mixture of cholesterol, stearyl alcohol, and white wax.
  liquid p., mineral oil; a liquid mixture of hydrocarbons from petroleum; used as an internal lubricant.
  white p., white, purified, and deodorized petrolatum.

petro'sal. Relating to the petrous part of the temporal bone.

petrosi'tis. Inflammation of the petrous portion of the temporal bone.

pe'trous. **1.** Denoting hardness. **2.** Relating to the petrous portion of the temporal bone.

Peutz-Jeghers syndrome, Peutz syndrome. A familial disorder characterized chiefly by the presence of numerous polyps in the intestinal tract, especially the jejunum, and dark brown spots of the lips, oral mucosa, and fingers.

-pexy. Combining form indicating surgical fixation.

peyo'te, peyo'tl. A small gray-brown cactus, *Lophophora williamsii*, with a carrot-shaped root and a small mushroom-like spineless head ("button"); it has hallucinatory properties.

Peyronie's disease. The formation of dense fibrous tissue in the corpus cavernosum of the penis causing painful erection; associated with sclerosis of other parts of the body; also called fibrous cavernitis.

PG. Abbreviation for prostaglandins.

PGA₁, PGB, etc. Abbreviations for prostaglandins A, B, etc.

pg. Abbreviation for picogram.

PGH. Abbreviation for (a) pituitary growth hormone; (b) prostaglandin H.

pH. The symbol expressing the degree of alkalinity or acidity of a solution; it denotes the negative logarithm to the base 10 of the hydrogen-ion concentration [$pH = -\log(H^+)$]; a solution with pH 7 is neutral; values below 7 indicate a degree of acidity;

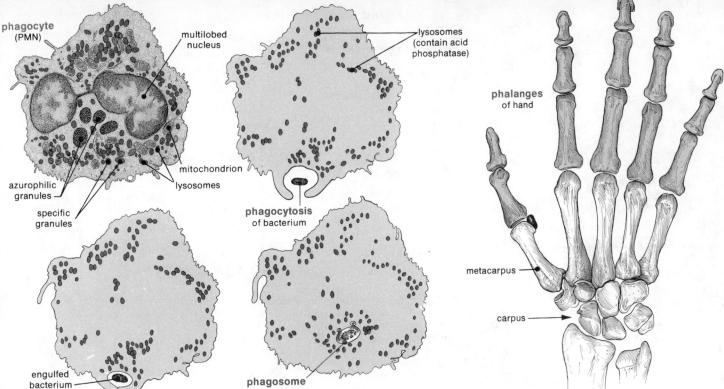

phagocyte (PMN) — multilobed nucleus — azurophilic granules — specific granules — mitochondrion — lysosomes

lysosomes (contain acid phosphatase) — phagocytosis of bacterium

engulfed bacterium — phagosome

phalanges of hand — metacarpus — carpus

values above 7 indicate a degree of alkalinity; the normal pH of blood serum is approximately 7.4.

PHA. Abbreviation for phytohemagglutinin.

phaci'tis. Inflammation of the crystalline lens.

phaco-. Combining form meaning lens.

phacoanaphylax'is. Intraocular inflammation due to hypersensitivity to the protein of the crystalline lens, usually following cataract surgery of one eye.

phac'ocele. Hernia of the crystalline lens, as through a ruptured sclera.

phac'ocyst. Capsule enclosing the crystalline lens.

phacocystec'tomy. Partial removal of the capsule of the crystalline lens.

phacocysti'tis. Inflammation of the capsule of the crystalline lens.

phacoemulsifica'tion. Removal of a cataractous lens by means of a low frequency ultrasonic needle.

phacoery'sis. Removal of the crystalline lens by suction.

phac'oid. Shaped like a lentil.

phacol'ysis. 1. Dissolution of the crystalline lens. **2.** Operative procedure to allow dissolution and absorption of the lens.

phacomala'cia. Softening of the crystalline lens, as may occur in a soft cataract.

phacometachore'sis. Dislocation of the crystalline lens, either complete or partial.

phacometece'sis. Displacement of the crystalline lens into the anterior chamber of the eye.

phacoplane'sis. A free-floating crystalline lens.

phac'osclero'sis. Hardening of the lens of the eye, especially a cataractous lens.

phac'oscope. An instrument for observing the lens of the eye, especially its changes during accommodation.

-phage. Combining form meaning ingesting, devouring, or destroying; e.g., macrophage.

phage. See bacteriophage.

phageden'ic. Rapidly spreading; said of certain ulcers.

phago-. Combining form meaning ingesting, devouring, or destroying; e.g., phagocyte.

phag'ocyte. Any cell that ingests bacteria, foreign particles, or other cells.

phagocyt'ic. Pertaining to phagocytes or phagocytosis.

phagocy'tin. A basic bactericidal protein found in neutrophils which plays a role in the intracellular destruction of phagocytized gram-negative bacteria.

phag'ocytize. Phagocytose.

phagocy'toblast. A primitive cell which develops into a phagocyte.

phagocytol'ysis. Destruction of phagocytes.

phag'ocytose. To engulf and digest bacteria and other foreign bodies; denoting the action of phagocytic cells.

phagocyto'sis. A process in which a substance is engulfed and then held or digested by a cell, as the leukocyte engulfs and destroys pathogens; phagocytosis plays a nutritive and defensive role in cell function.

phagoma'nia. A morbid compulsion to eat.

phag'osome. A compound entity of a phagocytic vesicle combined with a lysosome; formed when a cell ingests a particle by invaginating its cytoplasmic membrane (plasmalemma) and is joined by a lysosome during the process of phagocytosis.

phagother'apy. 1. Treatment of infectious disease by a bacteriophage. **2.** Treatment by feeding, especially overfeeding.

phag'otype. In microbiology, a strain of bacteria which differs from other strains of the same species by its vulnerability to the action of a specific virus (bacteriophage).

phalan'geal. Relating to a phalanx.

phalangec'tomy. 1. Amputation of a finger. **2.** Removal of one or more phalanges of a finger or toe.

phal'anx, *pl.* **phalan'ges.** Any bone of a finger or toe.

phallec'tomy. Amputation of the penis.

phal'lic. 1. Of, relating to, or resembling a phallus or penis. **2.** In psychoanalysis, relating to the penis during the phase of infantile sexuality.

phal'licism, phal'lism. Worship of the male genital.

phallocamp'sis. Any curvature of the penis during erection.

phallodyn'ia. Pain in the penis.

phal'loplasty. Reparative surgery of the penis.

phal'lus. Penis.

phanero'sis. The process of becoming visible.

phan'tom. 1. A teaching model of a bodily part, especially the female pelvis. **2.** Something seemingly sensed, but having no physical reality; also called phantasm and specter.

  p. pain, see under pain.

phantos'mia. The intermittent or persistent odor, pleasant or unpleasant, perceived when no apparent odorant is inhaled.

pharmaceu'tic, pharmaceu'tical. Relating to pharmacy.

pharmaceu'tics. The branch of science concerned with the preparation and dosage of medicinal products.

phar'macist. A druggist; one who is trained in the preparation and dispensing of drugs.

pharmacodiagno'sis. Use of drugs in diagnosis of disease.

pharmacodynam'ic. Relating to the effects of drugs.

pharmacodynam'ics. The study of the effects of drugs on healthy experimental animals; also called pharmacokinetics.

pharmacogenet'ics. The branch of biochemical genetics concerned with the genetically determined variations in responses to drugs in man and laboratory animals.

pharmacog'nosist. A practitioner of pharmacognosy.

pharmacog'nosy, pharmacognos'tics. The branch of pharmacology concerned with the study of medicinal substances in their natural, unprepared, or crude state.

pharmacog'raphy. A description of drugs in their crude state.

pharmacokinet'ics. See pharmacodynamics.

pharmacol'ogist. One who specializes in pharmacology.

pharmacol'ogy. The branch of science concerned with the unified study of all aspects of the interactions of drugs and their effect on living organisms.

pharmacoma'nia. A morbid impulse to take drugs.

pharmacope'dia. The total knowledge of crude drugs and medicinal preparations.

pharmacoped'ics. Obsolete term; see pharmacy (1).

pharmacope'ia, pharmacopoe'ia. A book containing a list of medicinal drugs, description of their preparation and use, and chemical tests for identifying them and for determining their purity; the first edition of the *U.S. Pharmacopeia* (USP) was published in 1820.

pharmacopho'bia. Abnormal fear of taking medicines.

phar'macotherapeu'tics. The administration of drugs in the prevention or treatment of disease and their use in planned alteration of normal function.

phar'macy. 1. The preparing and dispensing of medicines. **2.** Drugstore.

pharyngal'gia. Pharyngodynia; pain in the pharynx.

pharyn'geal. Relating to the pharynx.

pharyngec'tomy. Surgical removal of a portion of the pharynx.

pharyngis'mus. Involuntary convulsive contractions of the pharyngeal muscles; also called pharyngospasm.

pharyngi'tis. Inflammation of the pharynx.

  atrophic p., chronic pharyngitis with wasting of the mucous glands; also called pharyngitis sicca.

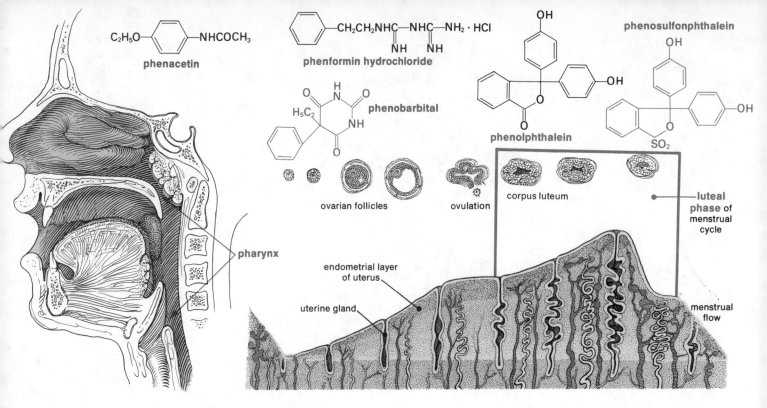

phenacetin

phenformin hydrochloride

phenobarbital

phenolphthalein

phenosulfonphthalein

pharynx

ovarian follicles

ovulation

corpus luteum

luteal phase of menstrual cycle

endometrial layer of uterus

uterine gland

menstrual flow

fusospirochetal p., sore throat, foul breath, and pharyngeal ulcers covered with a gray film, occasionally accompanied by fever; also called Vincent's angina and gangrenous pharyngitis.

gangrenous p., see fusospirochetal pharyngitis.

granular p., pharyngitis with enlargement of the lymphoid follicles of the mucous membrane, which appears granular; also called clergyman's sore throat.

membranous p., pharyngitis with a fibrous exudate forming a false membrane.

streptococcal p., group A streptococcal respiratory infection, characterized by some or all of the following signs and symptoms: sore red throat, sometimes associated with abdominal pain, swelling and tenderness of the lymph nodes of the neck, and high fever; also called hemolytic streptococcal sore throat and strep throat.

pharyngo-, pharyng-. Combining forms indicating a relationship to the pharynx.

pharyn'gocele. Hernial protrusion of the pharyngeal wall into the pharynx.

pharyngodyn'ia. Pain in the pharynx; also called pharyngalgia.

pharyn'goesopha'geal. Relating or belonging to the pharynx and the esophagus.

pharyn'goglos'sal. Relating to the pharynx and the tongue.

pharyn'golaryn'geal. Relating to both the pharynx and the larynx.

pharyn'golaryngi'tis. Inflammation of both the pharynx and the larynx.

pharyn'gomyco'sis. A fungal invasion of the mucous membrane of the pharynx.

pharyn'gopal'atine. Referring to both the pharynx and the palate.

pharyn'goplasty. Plastic surgery of the pharynx.

pharyngople'gia. Paralysis of the muscles of the pharynx.

pharyngorrhinos'copy. Visual examination of the nasal portion of the pharynx by means of an instrument (rhinoscope).

pharyngosclero'ma. A circumscribed area of hard tissue in the mucous membrane of the pharynx.

pharyn'goscope. An instrument used for inspecting the pharynx.

pharyngos'copy. Visual examination of the pharynx.

pharyn'gospasm. Pharyngismus; the sudden involuntary contraction (spasm) of the pharyngeal muscles.

pharyngosteno'sis. Constriction of the pharynx.

pharyngot'omy. Surgical incision of the pharynx.

pharyngotonsilli'tis. Inflammation of the pharynx and tonsils.

pharyngoxero'sis. Dryness of the mucous membrane of the pharynx.

phar'ynx. A musculomembranous cavity located behind the nasal cavities, mouth, and larynx; it is approximately five inches long and connects the nose with the larynx and the mouth with the esophagus; the part of the pharynx above the soft palate is the nasopharynx, the portion that lies directly posterior to the mouth is the oropharynx, and the portion behind the larynx and continuous with the esophagus is the laryngopharynx.

phase. 1. A stage in a development or cycle. **2.** A homogeneous substance (solid, liquid, or gaseous), physically distinct and mechanically separable, present in a heterogeneous chemical system; e.g., the components of an emulsion.

anal p., see stage, anal.

aqueous p., the water portion of a mixture of water and an immiscible liquid.

continuous p., the surrounding or dispersion medium in a heterogeneous mixture; also called external or dispersion phase.

dispersed p., the insoluble particles in a colloidal solution; also called internal or enclosed phase.

dispersion p., see continuous phase.

enclosed p., see dispersed phase.

genital p., see stage, genital.

internal p., see dispersed phase.

lag p., the period in the growth of a bacterial culture following inoculation into a medium; there is no increase in cell numbers and very little increase in cell size.

logarithmic p., period in the development of a bacterial culture in which there is most rapid multiplication.

luteal p., interval (about 14 days long) of menstrual cycle from formation of corpus luteum to beginning of menstrual flow.

meiotic p., stage during formation of sexual cells in which the number of chromosomes per cell is halved; also called reduction phase.

Oedipal p., see stage, Oedipal.

oral p., see stage, oral.

reduction p., see meiotic phase.

supernormal recovery p., interval during recovery of heart muscle following excitation, corresponding to the U wave of the electrocardiogram.

phas'mid. 1. One of a pair of minute lateral postanal chemoreceptors present in roundworms of the class Phasmidia. **2.** A roundworm possessing such organs.

Ph.D. Abbreviation for Doctor of Philosophy.

Phe. Symbol for phenylalanine or its radical.

phenacetin. A bitter compound used as an analgesic and to reduce temperature in fever; when combined in a preparation with aspirin and caffeine, it is commonly known as APC (aspirin, phenacetin, and caffeine); also called acetophenetidin.

phenan'threne. Compound derived from coal; used in the manufacture of dyes and drugs.

phency'clidine (PCP). A hallucinogen that has a pressor effect upon the cardiovascular system; commonly called angel's dust and peaCe pill.

phenethicillin potassium. White powder, soluble in water, insoluble in acidic solutions; used orally as an antibiotic.

phenformin hydrochloride. Hypoglycemic agent used alone or in conjunction with sulfonylurea or with insulin in the management of diabetes.

pheniramine maleate. An antihistaminic agent.

phenobar'bital. Phenylethylbarbituric acid, $CO(NHCO)_2C(C_2H_5)(C_6H_5)$; used as a sedative and hypnotic; also called phenobarbitone.

phenobar'bitone. See phenobarbital.

phe'necop'y. Condition that resembles a genetic disorder but is not inherited; it results from environmental influences.

phe'nol. Carbolic acid; a caustic crystalline compound, C_6H_5OH, derived from coal tar; used as an anesthetic and disinfectant.

phenolphthal'ein. A colorless, crystalline compound, slightly soluble in water; derived from heating phenol with phthalic anhydride in the presence of concentrated sulphuric acid; used as a hydrogen ion indicator (pH 8.2–10.0) and as a cathartic (laxative).

phenolsulfonphthal'ein (PSP). A dye used by parenteral injection as a test for measuring renal tubular function; also used as an indicator, being yellow at pH 6.8 and red at pH 8.4; also called phenol red.

phenomenol'ogy. The study, description, and classification of all possible phenomena in human experience, without attempting to explain or interpret them.

phenom'enon, *pl.* **phenom'ena.** An event, manifestation, or fact that is perceptible by the senses.

Arthus p., an inflammatory and, eventually, necrotic lesion produced on the skin of a sensitized animal by the injection of antigen into the skin.

Bell's p., the normal upward turning of the eyes on bilateral closure.

Bordet-Gengou p., the removal of complement from fresh serum, when the serum is incubated with red blood cells or bacteria that have been sensitized with specific lysin.

declamping p., shock occurring after the removal

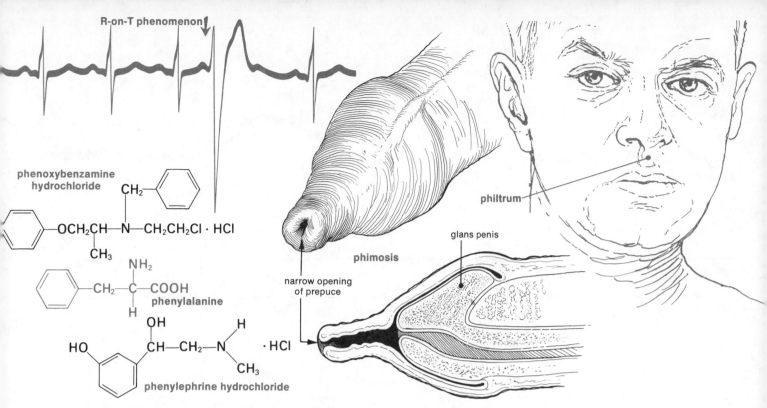

R-on-T phenomenon

phenoxybenzamine hydrochloride

phenylalanine

phenylephrine hydrochloride

philtrum

phimosis

narrow opening of prepuce

glans penis

of clamps from a large blood vessel (e.g., aorta); also called declamping shock.

déjà vu p., the feeling that an experience, occurring for the first time, has been experienced before.

Donath-Landsteiner p., destruction of red blood cells, occurring in a sample of blood from a person affected with paroxysmal cold hemoglobinuria, when cooled to about 5°C and then returned to about 37°C.

escape p., (1) the increase in excretion of sodium and water which occurs after two or three days of excessive mineralocorticoid activity (endogenous, as in primary aldosteronism, or due to administration of exogenous mineralocorticoid); after the initial phase of sodium and fluid retention there is an "escape" from the sodium-retaining effects and a new equilibrium is established; (2) after initial constriction, failure of the pupil of an eye to constrict upon repeated and alternate stimulation of both eyes; seen in retrobulbar neuritis.

Goldblatt p., arterial hypertension caused by partial occlusion of a renal artery; also called Goldblatt's hypertension.

Gunn's p., exaggerated opening of the eyes when the mouth is opened and closing of the eyes when the mouth is closed; also called jaw-winking syndrome.

immune adherence p., the adherence of a cell (platelet, red blood cell, leukocyte, or microorganism), coated with antibody and complement, to normal cells (platelets, etc.), resulting in agglutination; also called immune adherence.

Pfeiffer's p., destruction of bacteria when introduced into the peritoneal cavity of an immunized guinea pig, or into that of a normal guinea pig when immune serum is introduced at the same time.

Raynaud's p., numbness and pallor of the fingers occurring secondary to another disease.

R-on-T p., in electrocardiography, a premature ventricular complex (QRS) interrupting the T wave of the previous beat; predisposes to ventricular tachycardia and/or fibrillation.

Shwartzman p., a reaction elicited when (1) two small subcutaneous doses of endotoxin are given 24 hours apart to an experimental animal; the second injection will cause a localized hemorrhagic necrosis and inflammation of blood vessels; called localized Shwartzman phenomenon or reaction; (2) if the injections are given intravenously, widespread hemorrhages and bilateral necrosis of kidney cortex will occur; the animal dies within 24 hours; called generalized Shwartzman phenomenon or reaction.

Wenckebach p., progressive lengthening of the A-V conduction time (P-R interval) in successive cycles until a beat is dropped.

phe'notype. In genetics, the visible appearance of an organism, produced by the interaction of its genetic constitution with the environment.

phenotyp'ic. Relating to a phenotype.

phenoxybenzamine hydrochloride. An α-adrenergic blocking agent that blocks the response of smooth muscle and endocrine glands to the action of epinephrine; used to treat peripheral vascular diseases; Dibenzyline®.

phentol'amine. An α-adrenergic blocking agent used in the diagnosis of pheochromocytoma; Regitine®.

phen'yl. The univalent radical of phenol, C_6H_5.

phenylal'anine. An essential amino acid occurring as a constituent of many proteins.

phenylalanine hydroxylase. An enzyme that, with NAD (nicotine adenine dinucleotide) as coenzyme, promotes the oxidation of phenylalanine to tyrosine; absence of this enzyme produces phenylketonuria.

phen'ylbu'tazone. A derivative of pyrazoline, used primarily to relieve pain in musculoskeletal disorders; an anti-inflammatory agent.

phenylephrine hydrochloride. A sympathomimetic amine closely related chemically to epinephrine; a powerful vasoconstrictor of sustained action, used as a nasal decongestant, as a mydriatic, and in preventing hypotension during spinal anesthesia; Neo-Synephrine®.

phenylethylbarbituric acid. See phenobarbital.

phenylglycolic acid. See mandelic acid.

phenylhy'drazine. Colorless liquid used in the detection of sugars, aldehydes, and ketones.

phenylketonu'ria (PKU). Condition in which metabolism of the amino acid phenylalanine (phe) is deficient, producing increased phenylalanine in the body with resulting nerve and brain cell damage and severe mental retardation; originally known as phenylpyruvic oligophrenia.

phenylpropanolamine hydrochloride. Preparation used as a nasal decongestant and bronchodilator.

phenylthiocar'bamide. See phenylthiourea.

phenylthioure'a. A substance that is tasteless to those individuals (taste-blind) who are homozygous for an autosomal recessive gene, but tastes bitter to those individuals (tasters) who carry the dominant allele; also called phenylthiocarbamide.

phe'ochrome. Staining a brownish yellow with chromic salts.

pheochro'moblast. A young chromaffin (one of the cells forming the medulla of the adrenal gland).

pheochro'mocyte. A chromaffin cell forming the medulla of an adrenal gland, a sympathetic

paraganglion, or a pheochromocytoma.

pheochromocyto'ma. A catecholamine-producing tumor of the chromaffin cells of the sympathoadrenal system, usually the adrenal medulla; the symptoms are due to increased secretion of epinephrine and norepinephrine and consist of headache, palpitation, tachycardia, and constant or paroxysmal hypertension of moderate to severe grade.

pher'omones. Substances secreted externally by an organism that influences the behavior of other organisms of the same species.

Ph.G. Abbreviation for Graduate in Pharmacy.

phi'al. Vial.

phiala prius agitate (ppa). Latin for shake bottle first.

phil'trum. The middle vertical groove of the upper lip, below the nose.

phimo'sis. Tightness of the foreskin, so that it cannot be retracted over the glans penis.

phlebal'gia. Pain originating in a venule or vein.

phlebarte'riecta'sia. General dilatation of the veins and arteries.

phlebecta'sia. Dilatation or varicosity of a vein.

phlebec'tomy. Surgical removal of a segment of a vein.

phlebemphrax'is. Venous thrombosis; arrest of circulation in a vein by a thrombus.

phlebi'tis. Inflammation of a vein.

phlebo-, phleb-. Combining forms indicating a vein; e.g., phlebitis.

phleboc'lysis. Injection of medicinal liquids into a vein.

phleb'ogram. A tracing of the venous (usually jugular) pulse made by the phlebograph.

phleb'ograph. A device for recording venous pulsations.

phlebog'raphy. 1. The making of phlebograms. **2.** Venography; x-ray photography of a vein after intravenous injection with a radiopaque substance.

phleb'olith. A concretion in a vein resulting from the calcification of an old thrombus; also called vein stone.

phleboplas'ty. Repair of a vein.

phleborrha'gia. Bleeding from a vein.

phlebor'rhaphy. Suture of a vein; also called venisuture.

phleborrhex'is. Rupture of a vein.

phlebosclero'sis. Fibrous hardening of the veins, especially the inner coats.

phlebosta'sis. Compression of veins of the extremities for the temporary removal of blood from the circulation; also called bloodless phlebotomy and venostasis.

phlebothrombo'sis. Clotting of blood within a vein without inflammation of its walls. Cf thrombo-

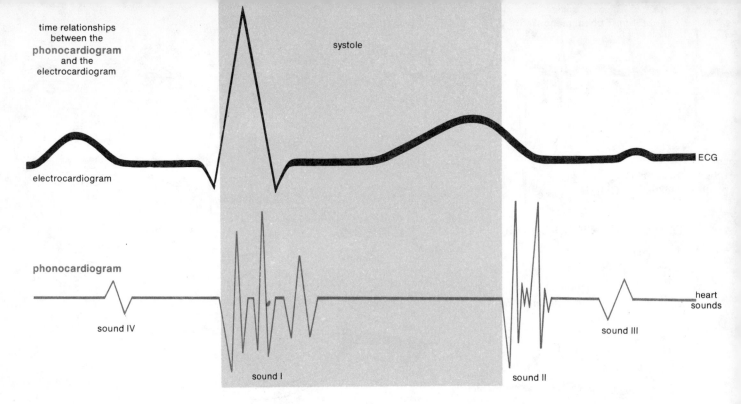

time relationships
between the
phonocardiogram
and the
electrocardiogram

systole

electrocardiogram

ECG

phonocardiogram

heart sounds

sound IV

sound I

sound II

sound III

phlebitis.

phlebot'omize. To perform a phlebotomy.

Phlebot'omus. A genus of bloodsucking sandflies of the family Psychodidae.

P. papatasii, the species that is the vector of sandfly fever (phlebotomus or pappataci fever).

phlebot'omy. Withdrawal of blood from a vein; also called venesection.

phlegm. 1. Mucus secreted by the mucosa of the respiratory tract. **2.** According to ancient Greek physiology, one of the four humors of the body.

phlegma'sia. Inflammation.

p. alba dolens, puerperal thrombophlebitis; see under thrombophlebitis.

p. cerulea dolens, severe pain, swelling, and cyanosis of a limb, followed by circulatory collapse and shock, due to thrombosis of the limb.

phlegmat'ic. Apathetic; calm.

phleg'mon. Acute inflammation of the subcutaneous connective tissue.

phleg'monous. Relating to inflammation of subcutaneous tissues.

phlogis'tis. Inflammatory.

phlogis'ton. A hypothetical substance of negative mass which, before the discovery of oxygen, was believed to be given off by substances undergoing combustion.

phlor'izin. Substance extracted from the roots of apple, pear, plum, and cherry trees; injected into experimental animals to produce glycosuria by inhibiting the renal tubular reabsorption of glucose.

phlycte'na, *pl.* **phlycte'nae.** One of several small blisters caused by a burn of the first degree.

phlycten'ule. A minute red nodular pustule occurring in the conjunctiva or cornea.

-phobia. Combining form denoting irrational, abnormal fear of a specific object or situation; e.g., hypnophobia, claustrophobia, etc.

pho'bia. Any abnormal, irrational fear.

pho'bic. Relating to abnormal fear.

pho'bism. The state of being affected by a phobia.

phocome'lia. Gross underdevelopment of extremities, particularly the upper limbs; the hands and feet are attached close to the body, resembling the flippers of a seal.

phocom'elus. An individual with phocomelia.

phon-. See phono.

pho'nal. Related to the voice.

phonasthe'nia. Difficult or abnormal production of the voice.

phona'tion. The utterance of vocal sounds which are culturally appropriate for human communication.

pho'natory. Relating to the utterance of vocal sounds.

phonau'tograph. Instrument designed to produce a visible record of a sound.

pho'neme. The smallest distinctive group of speech sounds in a language.

phone'mic. Relating to the discrimination of distinctive speech sounds.

phonet'ic. Relating to speech sounds.

phonet'ics. The branch of linguistics concerned with the study of the sounds of speech in all their aspects (their production, combination, and representation by written symbols); also called phonology.

phoniat'rics. The study and treatment of speech defects.

phon'ic. Relating to sound or to the voice; also called phonetic.

pho'nism. A subjective sensation of sound created by, and in addition to, unrelated stimuli, such as light, taste, touch, etc.

phono-, phon-. Combining forms denoting sound or voice; e.g., phonocardiogram.

phonoangiog'raphy. The recording and subsequent analysis of sound produced by the blood passing through an artery; useful in determining the extent of narrowing of the lumen by atherosclerosis.

phonocar'diogram. (PCG). A graphic representation of the heart sounds made with the phonocardiograph.

phonocar'diograph. An instrument that makes graphic records of the heart sounds.

phonocardiog'raphy. The recording of the sounds produced by the action of the heart.

phonocath'eter. A catheter-microphone combination for recording cardiac sounds from within the heart and great vessels.

phono-electrocar'dioscope. A dual-beam oscilloscope that displays both heart sounds and electrocardiographic tracings.

pho'nogram. A symbol representing a sound; e.g., a letter or a syllable in a phonetic alphabet.

phonol'ogy. The science of speech sounds and their organization into patterns.

phonomassag'e. The application of loud noises to the external auditory canal in order to cause movement of the ear ossicles.

phonom'eter. Apparatus used to measure the intensity and pitch of sounds.

phonop'athy. Any disease of the organs involved in speech.

pho'nophore. A funnel- or bell-shaped stethoscope.

phonophotog'raphy. The photographic recording of sound-vibration curves.

phonopneumomassag'e. The application of loud noises and a jet of air into the external auditory

canal to produce movement of the ear ossicles.

phonop'sia. Subjective visual sensations, as of color, induced by the hearing of certain sounds.

phonorecep'tor. A receptor for sound stimuli.

-phoresis. Combining form meaning transmission.

pho'resy. The nonparasitic association of one animal with another for the purpose of obtaining transportation.

pho'ria. The line of direction assumed by one eye in relation to the other eye.

-phoria. Combining form denoting a constant tendency of an eye to turn from the normal position during binocular vision; e.g., hyperphoria, exophoria, etc.

phorom'eter. An instrument for detecting the presence and degree of imbalance of the eye muscles (heterophoria).

phorop'ter. Instrument used to determine the refractive state of the eyes, phorias, amplitude of accommodation, etc.

phos-. Combining form meaning light.

phose. A subjective visual sensation, as of a bright light or color.

phos'gene. Carbonyl chloride, $COCl_2$; a poisonous gas that condenses to a liquid at temperatures below 8°C.

phosgen'ic. Light-producing.

pho'sis. Any condition that produces subjective visual sensations.

phosphagen'ic. Phosphate-producing.

phos'phatase. Any of a group of enzymes that promote the hydrolysis of phosphoric esters.

acid p., one active in an acid medium; present in all cells except erythrocytes.

alkaline p., one active in an alkaline medium; found in bone, blood, kidneys, and other tissues.

phos'phate. A salt or ester of phosphoric acid.

phospha'ted. Containing phosphates.

phosphat'ic. Relating to phosphates.

phosphatidic acid. An acid which results from the partial hydrolysis of a phospholipid and which on hydrolysis yields two fatty acid molecules and one molecule each of glycerol and phosphoric acid.

phosphat'idylcho'line. A phospholipid compound resulting from condensation of phosphatidic acid and choline; also called lecithin.

phosphat'idyleth'anolam'ine. A phospholipid, the product of condensation of phosphatidic acid and ethanolamine; also called cephalin.

phosphatu'ria. The presence of a high percentage of phosphates in the urine.

phos'phene. A sensation of light experienced upon pressure on, or electrical stimulation of, the eyeball.

phos'phide. A compound containing trivalent

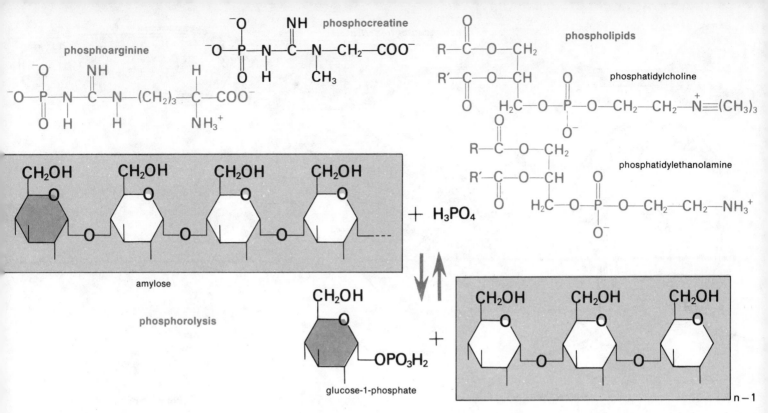

phosphoarginine

phosphocreatine

phospholipids

phosphatidylcholine

phosphatidylethanolamine

amylose

phosphorolysis

glucose-1-phosphate

$n-1$

phosphorus; e.g., sodium phosphide, Na_3P.

phos'phine. PH_3; a colorless, poisonous gas of characteristic odor; also called hydrogen phosphide and phosphorated hydrogen.

phos'phite. A salt of phosphorous acid.

phosphoar'ginine. Compound serving as a store of energy for muscle contraction in invertebrates; it corresponds to phosphocreatine in muscles of vertebrates.

phosphocre'atine. Creatine phosphate; see under creatine.

phosphodi'ester. A diesterified orthophosphoric acid; $RO - PO_2H - OR -$, as in the nucleic acids.

phosphodies'terase. One of a group of enzymes that split phosphodiester bonds, as those between nucleotides.

phosphoenolpyruvic acid. A high-energy compound, intermediate in the conversion of glucose to pyruvic acid.

phosphofructoki'nase. An enzyme of the glycolytic pathway that catalyzes the phosphorylation of fructose-6-phosphate to fructose-1,6-diphosphate in the presence of ATP and Mg^{++}; it controls the rate of glucose-6-phosphate utilization.

phosphoglu'comu'tase. Enzyme that promotes the reaction glucose-6-phosphate ⇌ glucose-1-phosphate.

phosphoki'nase. See phosphotransferase.

phospholip'ase. Any enzyme that catalyzes the hydrolysis of a phospholipid; also called lecithinase.

phospholip'id. A class of waxy or greasy compounds containing phosphoric acid; most of them occur in plant and animal tissues, especially in membranes, such as the myelin sheath of nerve cells and red blood cell membranes; phosphatidylcholine, phosphatidylethanolamine, and sphingomyelin are examples.

phosphopro'tein. One of a group of conjugated proteins containing a simple protein combined with a phosphorous compound; e.g., casein.

phos'phor. A substance that glows when stimulated by external radiation; used in the detection of radioactivity.

phos'phorated, phos'phoretted. Combined with phosphorus; also called phosphureted.

phosphores'cence. 1. The afterglow or continuous emission of light from a substance, without temperature rise, after exposure to light, heat, or electric current; distinguished from fluorescence, in which light is emitted essentially only when the exciting source is present. **2.** The faint greenish glow of white phosphorus in the presence of air, due to slow oxidation. **3.** The luminescence of certain living organisms such as fire flies.

phosphores'cent. Having the capacity to glow, especially in the dark.

phos'phoretted. See phosphorated.

phosphorib'osyltrans'ferase. One of a group of enzymes (important in nucleotide biosynthesis) that transfer ribose 5-phosphate from 5-phospho-α-D-ribosyl 1-pyrophosphate to a purine, pyrimidine, or pyridine acceptor.

phosphoric acid. H_3PO_4; colorless crystals that are soluble in water and important as a source of phosphate groups in metabolism; the principal component of silicate and zinc phosphate dental cement liquids.

phos'phorism. Chronic poisoning with phosphorus.

phos'phorized. Phosphorated.

phosphorol'ysis. A reaction analogous to hydrolysis in which the elements of phosphoric acid, rather than of water, are added in the course of splitting a bond; the conversion of glycogen to glucose 1-phosphate is an example.

phos'phorous. 1. Relating to or containing phosphorus. **2.** Phosphorescent.

phos'phorus. A poisonous nonmetallic element, symbol P, atomic number 15, atomic weight 30.975; it occurs in nature always in combined form, as inorganic phosphates in minerals and water and as organic phosphates in all living cells.

phos'phorus-32 (^{32}P). A β-emitting radioactive phosphorus isotope with atomic weight 32 and with a half-life of 14.3 days; used in brain, eye, skin, and stomach tumor localization, as a tracer to study metabolism, and in the treatment of certain osseous and hematopoietic disorders.

phosphor'ylase. An enzyme that triggers the splitting of the glycogen molecule to form glucose.

phosphoryla'tion. The addition of phosphate to an organic compound through the action of a phosphorylase.

phosphotrans'ferase. An enzyme that catalyzes the transfer of phosphorous-containing groups; also called phosphokinase.

phosphotungstic acid. Green crystals, soluble in water, used as a reagent for alkaloids and for albumin.

phos'phureted. See phosphorated.

phot. A unit of illumination equal to one lumen per square centimeter of surface.

phot-. See photo-.

photal'gia. Pain in the eyes caused by light; also called photodynia.

photesthe'sia. Perception of light.

phot'ic. Relating to light.

pho'tism. Production of a visual sensation by stimulation of another sense organ.

photo-, phot-. Combining forms meaning light.

photoactin'ic. Producing luminous and chemical effects, said of radiation.

photoal'lergy. See photosensitization.

photobiol'ogy. The study of the effect of light on organisms (plants or animals).

photobiot'ic. Capable of living only in the light.

photocat'alyst. A substance that brings about a light-stimulated reaction; e.g., chlorophyll.

photocep'tor. See photoreceptor.

photochem'istry. The branch of chemistry concerned with chemical changes caused by light.

photochro'mogens. Group I mycobacteria, mycobacteria that produce a bright yellow pigment when grown in the presence of light.

photocoagula'tion. Coagulation of protein material in the tissues with the heat generated by an intense, precisely focused beam of light from a carbon arc or laser; used in the treatment of retinal detachment and other intraocular conditions.

photocoag'ulator. Apparatus used in photocoagulation.

photodermati'tis. 1. Development of skin lesions in areas exposed to sunlight; seen in individuals who have developed a sensitivity to certain drugs; e.g., tetracycline. **2.** Any inflammatory skin condition in which light is an important causative factor.

photodisintegra'tion. Nuclear deterioration due to absorption of high-energy radiation.

photodynam'ic. Relating to the energy-producing effects of light.

photody'nia. See photalgia.

photoelectric'ity. Electricity resulting from the action of light.

photoelectrom'eter. Device used to measure concentration of substances in solution by means of a photoelectric cell.

photoelec'tron. An electron which has been set free (ejected from its orbit) by collision with a high energy photon.

pho'togen. A bacterium producing luminescence.

photogen'esis. The production of light.

photogen'ic, photog'enous. Producing light.

photokines'is. In biology, movement in response to light.

photolumines'cent. Having the ability to emit light at room temperature after exposure to radiant energy of a different wavelength.

photol'ysis. Decomposition of a chemical compound by the action of radiant energy, especially light.

pho'tolyte. A product of chemical decomposition caused by light.

photomacrog'raphy. The photographic recording of images of gross specimens at low magnification using photomacro lenses mounted on a camera.

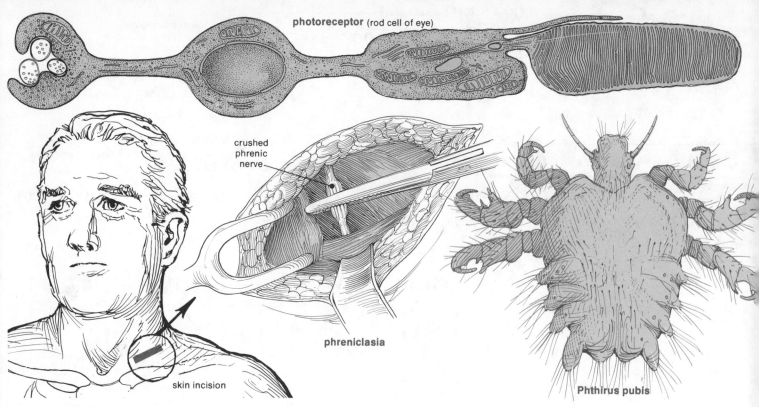

photoreceptor (rod cell of eye)

crushed phrenic nerve

phreniclasia

skin incision

Phthirus pubis

photom′eter. Instrument used to measure the intensity of a light source; also called illuminometer.

photom′etry. The measurement of the intensity of a light source.

photomi′crograph. Photograph of an object as viewed through the microscope.

photomicrog′raphy. The photographic recording of images seen through a microscope.

pho′ton. A unit or quantum of energy of a light wave or other electromagnetic wave, regarded as a minute particle of no electric charge and zero mass.

photopercep′tive. See photoreceptive.

photoper′iod. The varying length of exposure of a living organism to light.

photoper′iodism. The physiologic response of living organisms to varying periods of exposure to light (photoperiod).

photopho′bia. Abnormal intolerance or fear of light.

photopho′bic. Relating to abnormal intolerance or fear of light.

photophthal′mia. Inflammation of the eyes caused by exposure to intense light, as in snow blindness.

photop′sia, photop′sy. A subjective sensation of flashing light and sparks experienced with certain diseases of the retina, optic nerve, or brain.

photop′sin. The protein constituent (opsin) of the pigment (iodopsin) in the retinal cones.

photoreactiva′tion. The reversal of a photochemical reaction by exposure to light; e.g., reversal of the effect of ultraviolet rays on cells by exposure to visible light rays.

photorecep′tive. Capable of perceiving light rays; also called photoperceptive.

photorecep′tor. A nerve end-organ capable of being stimulated by light, as the rods and cones of the retina; also called photoceptor.

photoretini′tis. Inflammation of the retina caused by exposure to intense light.

pho′toscan. A photograph of the distribution and concentration of an internally administered radiopaque substance.

photosensitiza′tion. Hypersensitization of skin to sunlight or ultraviolet rays; caused by ingestion of certain plants or drugs; also called photoallergy.

photosta′ble. Unchanged upon exposure to light.

photosyn′thesis. The process by which green plants, using chlorophyll and the energy of sunlight, turn carbon dioxide and water into food substance (carbohydrate); molecular oxygen is liberated in the process.

phototax′is, phototax′y. Movement of an organism (as a whole) toward or away from a light source. Cf phototropism.

photother′apy. Treatment of disease with light.

photother′mal. 1. Relating to both light and heat. **2.** Relating to heat produced by light.

phototox′ic. Relating to an injurious effect produced or promoted by overexposure to light, ultraviolet rays, or x rays.

photot′ropism, photot′ropy. Movement of parts of an organism toward or away from a light source. Cf phototaxis.

phren. 1. Greek for diaphragm. **2.** The mind.

phrenec′tomy. See phrenicectomy.

phrenemphrax′is. See phreniclasia.

-phrenia. Combining form denoting a relationship to (a) the diaphragm, (b) the mind.

phren′ic. Relating to the diaphragm.

phrenicec′tomy. Surgical removal of a portion of the phrenic nerve; also called phrenectomy.

phrenicla′sia. Crushing of a portion of the phrenic nerve; also called phrenemphraxis.

phrenicot′omy. Division of a phrenic nerve in order to paralyze one-half of the diaphragm.

phrenocol′ic. Relating to the diaphragm and the colon.

phrenogas′tric. Relating to the diaphragm and the stomach.

phrenohepat′ic. Relating to the diaphragm and the liver.

phrenol′ogy. An obsolete doctrine concerned with the study of mental capacity and traits of character based upon the external configuration of the skull.

phrenople′gia. Paralysis of the diaphragm.

phren′osin. A cerebroside present in the white matter of the brain; also called cerebron.

phrenotrop′ic. Exerting its foremost effect upon the mind or brain.

phrynoder′ma. A dry eruption of the skin thought to be due to vitamin A deficiency.

PHS. Abbreviation for Public Health Service.

phthal′ein. Any of various dyes, such as phenolphthalein, derived from the condensation of phthalic anhydride with the phenols; some are used as indicators and occasionally as purgatives.

phthiri′asis. Infestation with the species of lice *Phthirus pubis,* more commonly known as crabs.

Phthi′rus. A genus of sucking lice of the order Anoplura.

  P. pubis, a parasite of man infesting areas of coarse hair, particularly in the pubic region, but also the hair of the chest, axillae, eyebrows, and eyelashes; also called pubic or crab louse.

phthis′ic. Relating to or afflicted with phthisis.

phthisiol′ogy. The study and treatment of pulmonary tuberculosis.

phthi′sis. 1. Tuberculosis. **2.** A wasting away of

tissue.

  black p., miners′ p., anthracosis.

  marble cutters′ p., see calcicosis.

  potters′ p., see silicosis.

  stonecutters′ p., pneumoconiosis.

phycomyco′sis. General term for acute and chronic systemic diseases caused by fungi of the class Phycomycetes (Zygomycetes), usually occurring in debilitated individuals.

phylax′is. Protection against infection.

phylogen′esis. The evolutionary development or racial history of the species; distinguished from ontogenesis; also called phylogeny.

phylog′eny. See phylogenesis.

phy′lum. One of the first divisions of the animal or vegetable kingdom; below subkingdom and above subphylum.

phy′ma. A small skin tumor.

phymato′sis. Disorder marked by the presence of small nodules (phymas) in the skin.

physiat′rics. The branch of medicine concerned with diagnosis and treatment of disease of the neuromusculoskeletal systems with physical elements (heat, cold, water, electricity, etc.) to bring about maximal restoration of physical, physiological, social, and vocational function; also called physical medicine or rehabilitation.

physi′atrist. A physician who specializes in physiatrics (physical medicine or rehabilitation).

phys′ic. Any medicine, especially a cathartic.

phys′ical. Relating to the body.

physicochem′ical. Relating to both physics and chemistry.

phys′ics. The science concerned with the study of matter and energy and the interactions between the two.

physio-, phys-. Combining forms indicating a relationship to nature or to the physical.

physiog′nomy. 1. The art of judging human character and mental qualities from facial features and general bodily carriage. **2.** The countenance, especially regarded as an indication of the character.

physiolog′ic, physiolog′ical. 1. Relating to physiology. **2.** Denoting the various normal processes of a living organism.

physiol′ogist. A specialist in physiology.

physiol′ogy. The science concerned with the normal functions and activities of the living organism.

physiother′apy. Physical therapy; see under therapy.

physique′. The structure of the body with reference to its proportions, muscular development, and appearance; also called biotype.

physo-. Combining form indicating (a) a tendency to swell; (b) a relationship to air or gas.

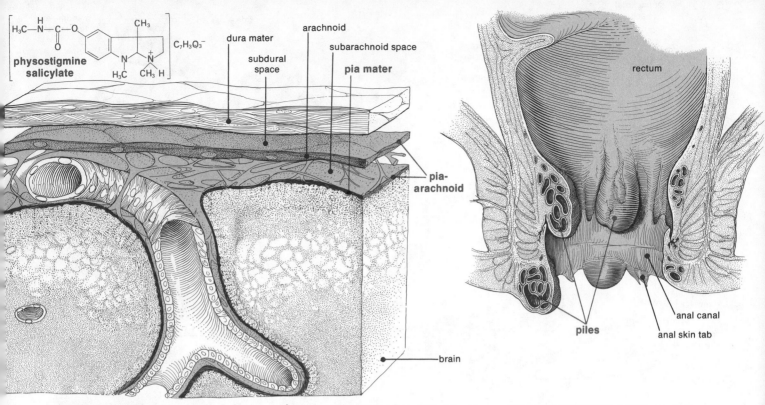

physohematome'tra. Distention of the uterine cavity with gas and blood.

physostig'mine, physostig'min. A poisonous crystalline compound, $C_{15}H_{21}N_3O_2$, extracted from the Calabar bean; it is a reversible inhibitor of the cholinesterases, and prevents destruction of acetylcholine; also called eserine.

p. salicylate, used to reduce intraocular tension in glaucoma, in the treatment of postoperative intestinal atony and urinary retention, and in the management of myasthenia gravis; also called eserine salicylate.

phy'tin. The mixed magnesium-calcium salt of phytic acid; used as a dietary supplement.

phyto-, phyt-. Combining forms indicating a relationship to plants; e.g., phytobezoar.

phytoaggglu'tinin. See lectin.

phytobe'zoar. An undigested concretion remaining in the stomach over a long period, composed mostly of vegetable fibers, seeds and skins of fruits, and sometimes starch granules and fat globules.

phytohemagglu'tinin (PHA). An extract derived from the stringbean; originally used as a red blood cell agglutinating reagent; it stimulates human lymphoid cells to divide, replicate their DNA, and transcribe RNA.

phy'toid. Resembling a plant.

phy'tol. An unsaturated alcoholic fragment obtained on hydrolysis of chlorophyll; an open-chain terpene; used for the synthesis of vitamins E and K_1.

phytopathol'ogy. The study of plant diseases.

phytotox'ic. Having a poisonous effect on plant life; inhibiting plant growth.

phytotox'in. A toxin produced by certain higher plants.

pI. Symbol for isoelectric point; see under point.

pi'a-arach'noid. The pia mater and arachnoid as one functional unit.

pi'al. Relating to the pia mater.

pi'a ma'ter. A delicate membrane, innermost of the three membranes enveloping the brain and spinal cord.

pian'. See yaws.

piarach'noid. Pia-arachnoid.

pi'ca. Perverted appetite marked by a craving for unnatural food or substances.

pick'ling. In dentistry, the method of removing impurities and oxides from the surface of metals by immersion in acid.

pickwickian syndrome. A condition characterized by extreme obesity, breathlessness on exertion, and somnolence similar to primary alveolar hypoventilation; arterial Pco_2 is elevated; cyanosis, tachycardia, and evidence of heart failure are common; named for the fat boy in Dickens' *Pickwick Papers.*

pico-. A combining form used in the metric system to indicate one-trillionth (10^{-12}); e.g., picogram, one-trillionth of a gram; also called micromicro-.

pi'cogram (pg). a unit of weight equal to one trillionth of a gram $(10^{-12}$ g); also called micromicrogram $(\mu\mu g)$.

picornavi'ruses. A large group of RNA viruses infecting vertebrate cells and multiplying in the cytoplasm; the group represents the smallest of known viruses and includes those causing poliomyelitis, meningitis, myocarditis, and the common cold.

pic'rate. A salt of picric acid.

pic'ric acid. Crystalline compound used as a reagent and in dyes and antiseptics; also called trinitrophenol and carbazotic acid.

picrocar'mine. Solution containing ammonia and picric acid, used to stain tissues in histology.

picrofor'mol. Substance containing formalin and picric acid; used as a fixative.

picrotox'in. The bitter powder obtained from the fruit of *Anamirta cocculus;* a central nervous system stimulant formerly used as an antidote for barbiturate poisoning.

PID. Abbreviation for pelvic inflammatory disease.

piebald'ness. Localized areas of depigmented scalp and hair; also called albinismus conscriptus.

pie'dra. Spanish for stone; a fungal disease of the hair characterized by formation of numerous small, hard, waxy concretions on extruded hairshafts; also called trichosporosis.

Pierre Robin syndrome. A syndrome characterized by respiratory obstruction in infants with a receding jaw and glossoptosis; frequently accompanied by cleft palate; also called primary micrognathia and Robin syndrome.

piesesthe'sia. Sensitivity to different degrees of pressure; also called pressure sense.

piezochem'istry. The study of the effects of extremely high pressures on chemical reactions.

piezoelectricity. Electricity generated by pressure applied to certain crystals.

PIF. Abbreviation for prolactin-inhibiting factor.

pigeon-toe, in-toeing. The turning in of the feet on walking; may be a physical sign of other disorders such as metatarsus adductus, medial torsion of the tibia, bowlegs, and congenital contraction of the internal rotators of the hip.

pig'ment. 1. Any colored material present in skin, whether deposited in the tissue proper or present in the blood passing through the skin. **2.** Any substance that produces a characteristic color in tissue, such as hemoglobin.

hepatogenous p., bile pigment derived from the destruction of hemoglobin in the liver.

malarial p., denatured hemoglobin products, in rods or granules within the malarial parasite.

melanotic p., melanin.

visual p., the photosensitive pigment in the rod and cone cells of the retina that initiates vision by the absorption of light.

pigmenta'tion. Coloration by deposition of pigment.

pigmentum nigrum. The dark pigment lining the choroid layer of the eye.

pii'tis. Inflammation of the pia mater.

pi'lar, pilar'is, pil'ary. Pertaining to or covered with hair.

pilas'ter. An abnormally prominent linea aspera on the femur, resulting in a backward concavity.

pile. 1. A single hemorrhoid. **2.** A vertical series of alternate plates of two different metals separated by layers of cloth or paper moistened with a dilute acid solution for producing a current of electricity; also called voltaic or Volta's pile. **3.** A battery consisting of cells similarly constructed.

atomic p., apparatus containing alternate layers of uranium and graphite in which a chain reaction is initiated and controlled, for the production of heat for power or for the production of plutonium; also called nuclear reactor and atomic furnace.

piles. Hemorrhoids.

pi'leus. A nipple shield.

p. ventriculi, the first portion of the duodenum as seen in an x-ray picture; also called duodenal cap.

pi'li. Plural of pilus.

pill. 1. A small tablet of medicine. **2.** An oral contraceptive, commonly referred to as *the pill.*

enteric coated p., a pill coated with a substance, such as salol, which prevents its disintegration until it has reached the intestine.

pep p., colloquialism for an amphetamine or a related pharmaceutical with a pronounced stimulant effect on the central nervous system.

pil'lar. Any vertical anatomic structure somewhat resembling a supporting column.

Corti's p.'s, the pillars forming the center and inner walls of the tunnel in the spiral organ of Corti.

p.'s of the fauces, anterior, a pair of mucous membrane folds which pass downward from the soft palate to the side of the tongue; also called glossopalatine arch.

p.'s of the fauces, posterior, a pair of mucous membrane folds which pass downward from the posterior margin of the soft palate to the lateral wall of the pharynx; also called pharyngopalatine arch.

pil'lion. A temporary artificial leg.

pill-rolling. The circular motion of the tips of the thumb and index finger, characteristic of paralysis agitans.

pilo-, pili-. Combining forms denoting a relation-

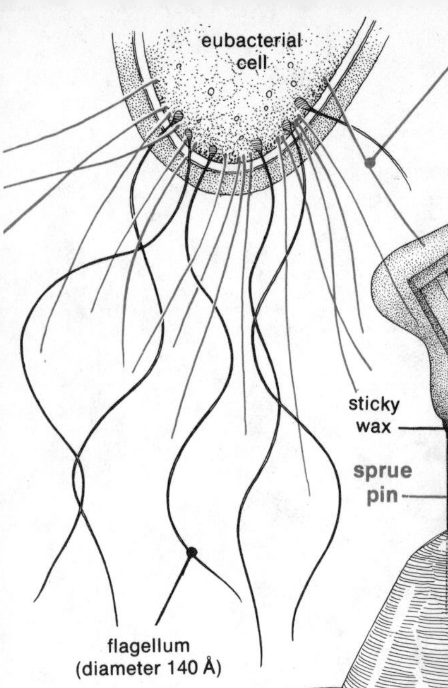
eubacterial cell
pilum
(diameter 70 Å)
flagellum
(diameter 140 Å)

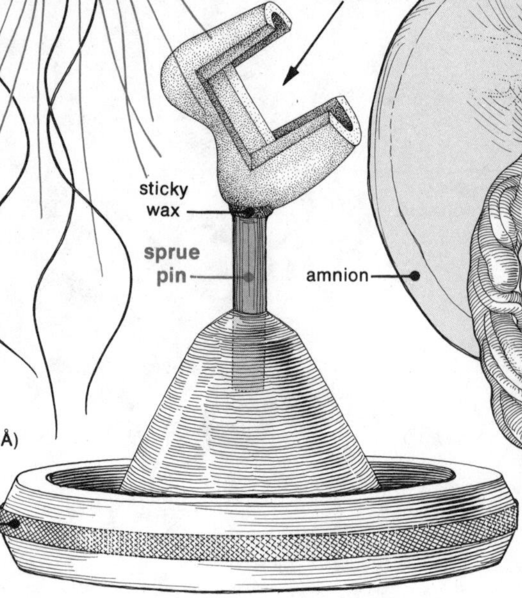
inlay wax impression of tooth restoration
sticky wax
sprue pin
crucible former

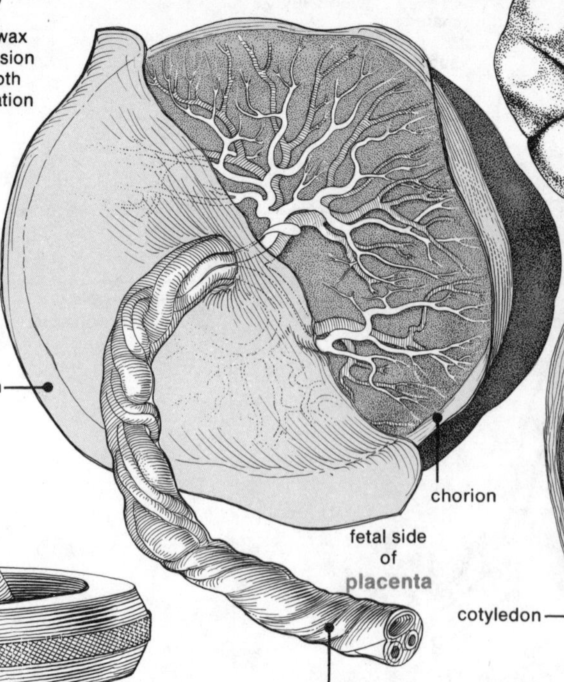
amnion
chorion
fetal side of placenta
umbilical cord

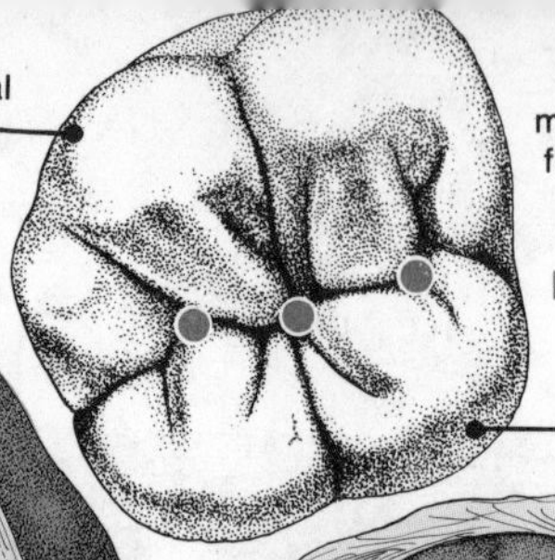
buccal side
left mandibular first molar
pits
lingual side

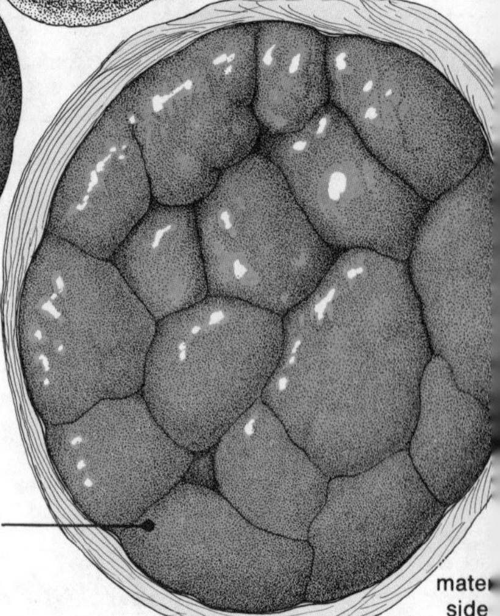
cotyledon
mate
side
place

ship to hair.

pilocar′pine. An alkaloid obtained from the leaves of the jaborandi tree; a parasympathomimetic agent used to induce sweating or to increase salivary secretion; also acts topically to contract the pupils and reduce intraocular pressure.

pilocar′pus. A small genus of shrubs (family Rutaceae) native to the West Indies and tropical America; source of the alkaloid, pilocarpine.

pilocys′tic. Denoting a cyst, usually dermoid, containing hair.

piloerec′tion. Erection of hairs.

pilomatrixo′ma. A benign tumor of the growing portion of the hair apparatus; also called Malherbe's calcifying epithelioma.

pilomo′tor. Relating to muscles or nerves in the skin that control the movement of hairs, as in the formation of goose pimples.

piloni′dal. Denoting the presence of hairs in a dermoid cyst or ingrown hairs in the deep layers of skin.

pi′lose. Covered with hair.

piloseba′ceous. Relating to the sebaceous glands that open into the hair follicles.

pilo′sis. Hirsutism.

pi′lus, *pl.* **pi′li. 1.** One of the fine hairs covering almost the entire surface of the human body. **2.** A fine, hollow, strawlike filamentous appendage, somewhat analogous to the flagellum, that occurs on some bacteria; it serves to anchor the bacterial cell to the substrate on which it is growing; pili are shorter, straighter, and more numerous than flagella; also called fimbria.

pimelo′sis. 1. Obesity. **2.** Fatty degeneration.

pi-meson. See pion.

pim′ple. A papule or pustule; a small inflamed swelling of the skin.

pin. A short, straight, cyclindrical piece of metal.

retention p.'s, small griplike pegs extending from a metal casting into the tooth's dentin.

sprue p., a short metal pin used to attach a dental wax pattern to the crucible former; it provides the entrance through the investment, permitting the molten metal to flow into the mold.

Steinman's p., a firm metal pin used for the internal fixation of fractured bones.

pincement. In massage, a manipulation in which the skin is gently nipped or pinched.

pin′eal. 1. Shaped like a pine cone. **2.** Relating to the pineal body.

pinealec′tomy. Surgical removal of the pineal body.

pin′ealocyte. One of the cells forming the substance of the pineal body.

pinealo′ma. A relatively rare tumor derived from the pineal gland.

pinguec′ula. A small, slightly raised, yellowish, nonfatty thickening of the conjunctiva of the eye near the sclerocorneal junction, usually on the nasal side.

pin′iform. Pineal (1).

pink disease. See acrodynia.

pink′eye. Acute contagious inflammation of the conjunctiva.

pin-lay. In dentistry, a veneer containing parallel pins for retention.

pin′ledge. In dentistry, vertical parallel pins placed in a tooth or teeth to aid in retention of a restoration.

pin′na. The projecting portion of the external ear; also called auricle.

pin′ocyte. A cell that engulfs liquids in a way that resembles the engulfment of solid particles by a phagocyte.

pinocyto′sis. The engulfment of liquid droplets by a cell through minute invaginations formed on the surface, which close to form fluid-filled vacuoles (vesicles); by this process, protein is reabsorbed from the filtrate by tubular cells of the kidney; the phenomenon is similar to phagocytosis (the engulfing of solid particles).

pi′nosome. A membrane-bounded vesicle containing pinocytosed fluid.

Pins' sign. See Ewart's sign.

pint. 1. A unit of liquid measure equal to 16 fluid ounces or 28.875 cubic inches. **2.** A unit of dry measure equal to 33.6 cubic inches.

imperial p., a British unit of liquid or dry measure equal to 34.659 cubic inches; 20 fluid ounces.

pin′ta. A nonvenereal infection caused by the spirochete *Treponema carateum;* endemic in Mexico, Colombia, Cuba, and the Philippines.

pin′worm. A nematode worm, *Enterobius vermicularis,* that infests the intestines, especially in children; also called seat worm (because it may cause pruritus ani) and threadworm.

pi′on. A small particle found in the nuclei of atoms; it constitutes the force that holds neutrons and protons together; also called pi-meson.

piperaz′ine. Compound used effectively against the intestinal worms *Ascaris* and *Oxyuris.*

pipette′, pipet′. A calibrated glass tube, open at both ends, used for transferring and/or measuring small quantities of liquids in laboratory work.

automatic p., an instrument for transferring small amounts of liquid repetitively and automatically.

pir′iform. Pear-shaped.

pi′siform. Pea-shaped or pea-sized; e.g., one of the carpal bones.

pit. 1. Any natural depression on the surface of the body. **2.** A pockmark. **3.** A pointed depression in dental enamel at the junction of two or more developmental grooves, as in the occlusal and buccal surfaces of molars.

pitch. One of three important properties of sound (others are intensity and quality) denoting the function of the number of vibrations of sound waves per second; the greater the number of vibrations per unit time, the higher the pitch; commonly called tone.

pitch′blende. A brownish-black mineral containing a large proportion of uranium oxide; it is the principal source of radium.

pith. 1. The center of a hair. **2.** To pierce the medulla of a laboratory animal, usually by the insertion of a needle or a knife at the base of the skull, to render the animal nonfeeling.

pito′cin. See oxytocin.

pitu′icyte. The dominant type of cell (fusiform) of the posterior lobe of the pituitary gland.

pitu′itary. 1. Relating to the pituitary gland (hypophysis). **2.** A preparation obtained from either the anterior or posterior lobe of the pituitary gland of domesticated animals; used therapeutically by man.

pityri′asis. A skin disease marked by fine scaly desquamation.

p. rosea, an eruption of papules of unknown cause usually involving the trunk and the extremities; it begins as an oval patch (herald patch) six to eight cm in diameter, followed in a few days by a generalized eruption which disappears spontaneously in one to two months.

pit′yroid. Scaly.

Pityros′porum. A genus of nonpathogenic, yeastlike fungi which produce extremely fine spores and no mycelium; generally found in dandruff and seborrheic dermatitis.

piv′ot. A part about which a related structure rotates or swings.

PK. Abbreviation for psychokinetics.

PKU. Abbreviation for phenylketonuria.

place′bo. An inert substance containing no medication but prescribed as medicine, given especially to satisfy a patient; also used in controlled studies to determine the efficacy of drugs.

placen′ta. The organ within the pregnant uterus through which the fetus derives its nourishment; at term it averages one-sixth the weight of the fetus; it is disk-shaped, about one inch thick, and seven inches in diameter.

accessory p., a mass of placental tissue distinct from the main placenta.

p. previa, condition in which the placenta is implanted in the lower segment of the uterus and

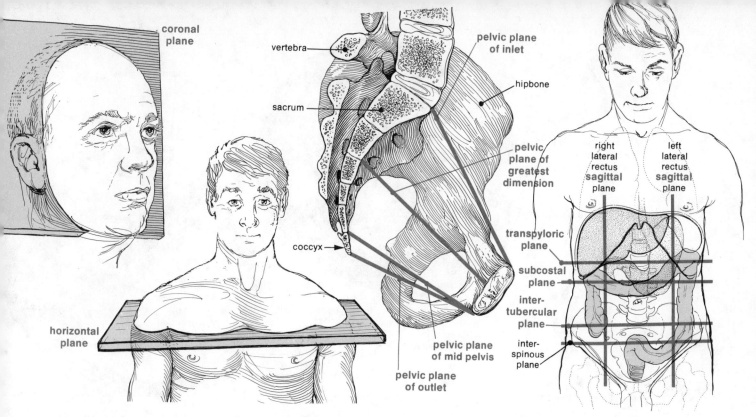

coronal plane

vertebra

pelvic plane of inlet

hipbone

sacrum

right lateral rectus sagittal plane

left lateral rectus sagittal plane

pelvic plane of greatest dimension

transpyloric plane

subcostal plane

inter- tubercular plane

coccyx

horizontal plane

pelvic plane of mid pelvis

pelvic plane of outlet

inter- spinous plane

covers the cervical opening, partly or completely.

retained p., one which is not expelled after childbirth.

placen′tal. Relating to the placenta.

placen′tascan. Determination of the location of the placenta by the use of ultrasound or by means of a scintillation detector after injection of a radioactive substance; also called placental scan.

placenta′tion. The development and organization of the placenta after attachment of the blastocyst to the uterine wall or other structures.

placenti′tis. Inflammation of the placenta; usually limited to the fetal surface, involving especially the zone between the amnion and chorion.

placentog′raphy. The making of roentgenograms of the placenta following injection of a radiopaque substance.

plac′ode. An ectodermal thickening in the early embryo from which a sense organ or structure develops; e.g., lens placode.

pladaro′sis, pladaro′ma. A soft, wartlike tumor on the eyelid.

plagioceph′aly. Malformation of the skull in which one side is more developed anteriorly and the other side posteriorly.

plagioproso′pia. In obstetrics, an oblique facial presentation of the fetus.

plague. 1. Acute infectious disease caused by *Pasteurella pestis* and marked by high fever, prostration, glandular swelling, or pneumonia; transmitted to humans by fleas that have bitten infected rodents. **2.** Any widespread disease or one causing excessive mortality.

bubonic p., a form marked by buboes (inflammatory enlargement of lymphatic glands).

hemorrhagic p., bubonic plague in which bleeding may occur into an organ or from the nose and alimentary, respiratory, or urinary tracts.

pneumonic p., a fatal form accompanied by pneumonia with abundant bloodstained sputum.

septicemic p., a variant of bubonic plague leading to death so quickly that localized lesions do not become clinically apparent.

sylvatic p., bubonic plague in wild animals, especially rodents.

plan′chet. A flat metal disk container on which a radioactive sample is placed while its activity is measured.

plane. 1. A flat or level surface. **2.** An imaginary surface formed by extension through any axis or two definite points. **3.** A particular level, as a stage in surgical anesthesia.

bite p., a dental appliance that covers the palate and has an inclined or flat plane at the front border that offers resistance to the upper incisors when

they make contact.

coronal p., a vertical plane that passes from side to side at right angles to the sagittal plane, dividing the head into anterior and posterior portions; often used interchangeably with frontal plane.

frontal p., a vertical plane passing at right angles to the sagittal plane, dividing the body into anterior and posterior portions. Cf coronal plane.

guide p., a plane formed in the occlusal surfaces of occlusion rims to position the lower jaw in centric relation.

horizontal p., the plane extending across the long axis of the body separating an upper portion from the lower part; also called traverse plane.

intercristal p., a horizontal plane passing through the highest points of the iliac crests; it lies on the level of the fourth lumbar vertebra.

intertubercular p., a horzontal plane passing through the tubercles of the iliac crests; it lies on the level of the fifth lumbar vertebra.

median sagittal p., a sagittal plane that passes through the midline.

parasagittal p., any vertical plane parallel to the sagittal plane.

pelvic p. of greatest dimension, the roomiest portion of the pelvic cavity extending from the middle of the posterior surface of the pubic symphysis to the junction of the second and third sacral vertebrae, passing laterally through the ischial bone over the middle of the acetabulum; its anteroposterior diameter is approximately 12.75 cm and its transverse diameter is around 12.5 cm.

pelvic p. of inlet (superior strait), the heart-shaped upper opening of the true pelvis, bounded anteriorly by the upper border of the pubis, laterally by the iliopectineal line, and posteriorly by the sacral promontory.

pelvic p. of midpelvis, plane of least pelvic dimension extending from the lower margin of the pubic symphysis through the ischial spines to the sacrum; the anteroposterior diameter measures approximately 11.5 cm and its transverse diameter is around 10.0 cm.

pelvic p. of outlet (inferior strait), the lower opening of the true pelvis bounded anteriorly by the pubic arch, laterally by the ischial tuberosities, and posteriorly by the tip of the coccyx.

p.'s of reference, planes that serve as a guide for the location of other planes.

sagittal p., a vertical plane extending in an anteroposterior direction.

subcostal p., a horizontal plane passing through the lowest point of the costal margin on each side, generally the inferior border of the 10th costal cartilage.

transpyloric p., a horizontal plane passing through the tips of the ninth costal cartilages; the plane passes through the pylorus, the neck of the pancreas, and the hili of the kidneys.

transverse p., see horizontal plane.

planig′raphy. Tomography.

planim′eter. A device that measures the area of any surface by tracing its boundaries with a mechanically coupled pointer.

plano-, plani-. Combining form denoting flatness.

pla′no. Having a flat surface; said of an afocal lens, i.e., one without refractive power.

planocon′cave. Flat on one side and curved inward on the other; denoting a lens of that shape.

planocon′vex. Flat on one side and curved outward on the other; denoting a lens of that shape.

plan′ta, *pl.* **plan′tae.** Latin for the sole of the foot.

planta′go. Any plant of the genus *Plantago*.

p. seed, see seed, plantago.

Planta′go. A large genus of herbs (family Plantaginaceae) comprised chiefly of roadside weeds.

P. psyllium, species producing seeds which are used as a mild laxative; also called Spanish psyllium and Old World plantain. See also seed, plantago.

plan′tain. 1. Any plant of the genus *Plantago*. **2.** A type of banana plant (*Musa paradisiaca*). **3.** The starchy fruit of such a plant, resembling a large banana; a staple food in tropical regions.

p. seed, see seed, plantago.

plantal′gia. Pain in the sole of the foot.

plan′tar. Relating to the sole of the foot.

plaque. A small flat growth.

atherosclerotic p., arteriosclerotic p., a deposit of cholesterol on the intimal surface of the blood vessels.

dental p., a deposit of bacteria and other materials on the surface of a tooth which contributes to tooth decay and to the development of periodontal disease.

-plasia. Combining form denoting formation.

plas′ma. 1. The clear fluid of blood and lymph in which cells are suspended; it also contains dissolved proteins. **2.** Protoplasm.

antihemophilic p. (human), human plasma in which the antihemophilic components have been preserved; used for the temporary arrest of bleeding in hemophilia.

dried p., preparation consisting of vacuum-dried frozen plasma which contains no added dextrose; it may be preserved at room temperature almost indefinitely, but usually is provided with a five-year expiration date.

frozen p., preparation made by prompt freezing of liquid plasma and stored at a constant tempera-

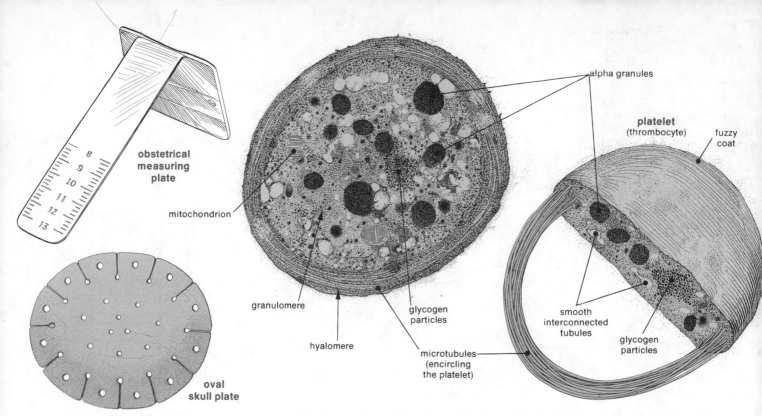

obstetrical
measuring
plate

mitochondrion

granulomere

hyalomere

glycogen
particles

microtubules
(encircling
the platelet)

alpha granules

platelet
(thrombocyte)

fuzzy
coat

smooth
interconnected
tubules

glycogen
particles

oval
skull plate

ture of −18°C or below; usually provided with a five-year expiration date.

liquid p., preparation made by adding five per cent dextrose to normal plasma and preserved at temperatures between 15° and 30°C; usually provided with a two-year expiration date.

p. expander, plasma substitute.

p. substitute, a solution of a substance such as dextran, administered intravenously as a substitute for plasma; used in hemorrhage and shock.

p. thromboplasmin antecedent, see factor XI.
p. thromboplasmin component, see factor IX.
plas'mablast. The precursor of the plasma cell.
plas'macyte. Plasma cell; see under cell.
plasmacyto'ma. A solitary tumor made up primarily of plasma cells, usually occurring in the skeleton; almost invariably a precursor of disseminated plasma cell myeloma.
plasmacyto'sis. 1. The presence of plasma cells in the blood. **2.** Abnormally large percentage of plasma cells in the tissues.
plasmalem'ma. Cell membrane; see under membrane.
plasmal'ogen. One of a group of phospholipids present in the brain and muscle.
plasmaphere'sis. A method of obtaining plasma without waste of blood components; blood is drawn, plasma is separated, and the blood cells are returned to the donor suspended in a suitable medium (e.g., Ringer's solution); also called plasmopheresis.
plas'mid. See paragene.
plas'min. A proteolytic enzyme derived from plasminogen; essential in blood clot dissolution (fibrinolysis).
plasmin'ogen. A globulin present in tissues, body fluids, circulating blood, and within clots; the inactive precursor of plasmin.
plasmo'dium, *pl.* **plasmo'dia.** A mass of protoplasm with multiple nuclei.
plas'mocyte. Plasma cell; see under cell.
Plasmo'dium. A genus of the class Sporozoa; some species cause malaria. See also malaria.

P. falciform, the parasitic species causing falciparum (malignant tertian) malaria, with fever recurring irregularly every 36 to 48 hours; it invades mature red blood cells which retain normal size and frequently contain basophilic granules and cytoplasmic precipitates (Maurer's dots); reproduction takes place in the visceral capillaries; except in severe fatal cases, only very young forms are seen in peripheral blood; multiple infection of red blood cells is extremely frequent.

P. malariae, the species causing quartan malaria, with fever recurring every 72 hours; invades mature

red blood cells and never fills the cell completely; infected cells occasionally show fine granules (Ziemann's dots).

P. ovale, a rare parasitic species in man; the cause of ovale (benign tertian) malaria, with fever recurring every 48 hours; infected cells are irregular and fimbriated with abundant acidophilic granules (Schüffner's dots).

P. vivax, the species causing vivax (benign tertian) malaria, with fever recurring every 48 hours; invades young red blood cells; young forms are ameboid and one-third the size of the cell; mature forms almost fill the distended cell; infected cell appears enlarged, deficient in hemoglobin, and contains acidophilic granules (Schüffner's dots).
plasmo'dium, *pl.* **plasmo'dia.** A mass of protoplasm with multiple nuclei.
plas'mogen. Protoplasm.
plasmol'ysis. Process in which the cytoplasm of a bacterial cell shrinks away from the cell wall when the cell is immersed in a hypertonic solution.
plasmophere'sis. See plasmapheresis.
plasmorrhex'is. See erythrocytorrhexis.
plas'ter. 1. A white powder, essentially gypsum, which forms a paste when mixed with water and sets to a smooth solid; used for immobilization and impressions of bodily parts. **2.** A pastelike material for application to the surface of the body.

adhesive p., a pressure-sensitive, sticky mixture of rubber, resins, and waxes with an absorbent powder filler, spread upon a cotton fabric.

mustard p., a pastelike mixture of powdered mustard seed, flour, and water, spread on cloth and applied to the skin as a poultice; it exerts an emollient, relaxing effect upon the skin and underlying tissues.

p. of Paris, β-hemihydrate; gypsum or calcium sulfate from which water of crystallization has been calcined or expelled by heat in the open air.
plas'tic. 1. Capable of being shaped or molded; pliable. **2.** In dentistry, a restorative substance that is soft enough to be molded, after which it will harden or set. **3.** Any of a large group of synthetic or semisynthetic organic compounds of high molecular weight produced by polymerization. **4.** Well-formed.
plasticity. The capability of being molded.
plas'tid. A self-replicating organelle in the cytoplasm of plant cells and in some plantlike organisms which serves as a center of special physiologic activities.
-plasty. Combining form denoting shaping or plastic repair of.
plate. 1. In anatomy, any flattened, relatively thin structure. **2.** In dentistry, an artificial denture, espe-

cially the portion to which artificial teeth are anchored. **3.** In microbiology, a glass culture container such as the Petri dish. **4.** A smooth, flat device of uniform thickness.

axial p., the primitive streak of an embryo.

bone p., a metal bar with perforations for immobilization of fractured bones.

chorionic p., the portion of the chorion that is attached to the uterus at an early stage in the formation of the placenta; the primordium of the chorion frondosum.

epiphysial p., the plate or disk of cartilage between the shaft and the epiphysis of a long bone during its growth.

Ishihara p.'s, a series of plates designed as tests for color blindness; they consist of numbers made of primary colored dots printed on a background of many dots of various sizes and in confusing colors; individuals who are color blind are unable to read the numbers.

medullary p., the middle ectodermal thickening in the embryo from which the neural tube develops; the anlage of the central nervous system; also called neural plate.

motor p., a motor end-plate.

neural p., see medullary plate.

obstetrical measuring p., one for calculating the digital measurements of internal conjugata without a pelvimeter.

occlusal plane p., in dentistry, a metal plate used to establish the occlusal plane of the teeth.

pterygoid p.'s, a short, broad lateral plate and a long, narrow medial plate that project inferiorly from the sphenoid bone; the pterygoid fossa lies between them.
plate'let. A disc-shaped, colorless protoplasmic body, from two to four microns in diameter (smaller than a red blood cell), derived from a megakaryocyte; a constituent of the blood of mammals; it plays an important role in the process of coagulation: shortly after bleeding begins (before the platelets aggregate to form a plug), a lipoprotein on its surface, platelet factor 3, is activated and reacts with plasma factors to promote prothrombin activation, leading ultimately to the arrest of bleeding (hemostasis); normal level ranges from 150,000 to 300,000 platelets per cubic millimeter of blood.
plateletphere'sis. The removal of platelets from the drawn blood of a healthy donor, thereby permitting the transfusion of this blood fraction to individuals who have platelet deficiency disorders; the remainder of the blood (white and red blood cells and plasma) is immediately returned to the donor.
pla'ting. 1. The planting or streaking of bacteria in a Petri dish or similar container. **2.** The application

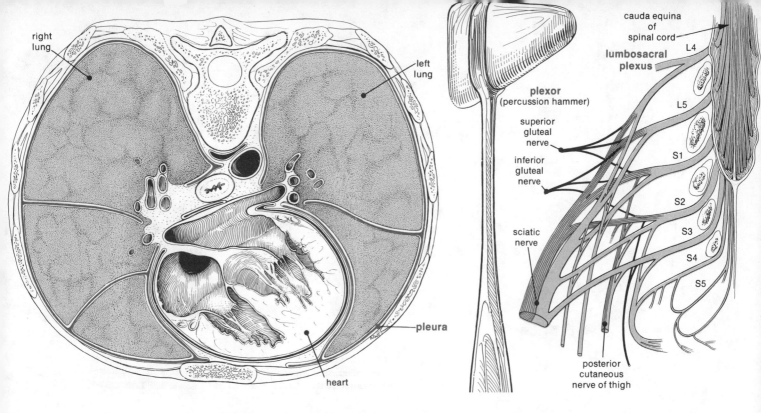

right lung

left lung

pleura

heart

plexor (percussion hammer)

superior gluteal nerve

inferior gluteal nerve

sciatic nerve

posterior cutaneous nerve of thigh

cauda equina of spinal cord

lumbosacral plexus

L4

L5

S1

S2

S3

S4

S5

of a metal strip to the fractured ends of a bone to keep them in place. **3.** The electrolytic deposition of a metal.

plat'inum. A silver-white metallic element, symbol Pt, atomic number 78, and atomic weight 195.09.

platy-. Combining form denoting flatness.

platyba'sia. A developmental deformity in which the floor of the occipital bone of the skull bulges upward, as if pushed by the cervical spine.

platyceph'alous, platycephal'ic. Having a wide flat head with a vertical cranial index below 70.

platyhel'minth. Common name for a worm of the phylum Platyhelminthes; any tapeworm or fluke.

Platyhelmin'thes. A phylum of flatworms characterized by bilaterally symmetrical, flat bodies without a true body cavity; some are parasitic, such as tapeworms and flukes.

platyhier'ic. Having a broad sacral bone with an index greater than 100.

platypel'ic, platypel'loid. Having a broad, flat pelvis with a pelvic inlet index of less than 90.

plat'yrrhine. 1. Having a broad nose, generally with nostrils directed to the sides. **2.** Denoting a skull with a nasal index greater than 53.

platys'ma. See table of muscles.

platyspondyl'ia, platyspondyl'isis. Having broad, flat vertebral bodies.

pledg'et. A small, flattened tuft, usually of cotton or gauze.

pleio-. Combining form meaning many.

pleiotrop'ic. In genetics, producing many effects; having several phenotypic expressions; also called polyphenic.

pleiot'ropism, pleiot'ropy. Phenomenon in which a single gene is responsible for several distinct and apparently unrelated observable effects, such as a hereditary syndrome.

pleo-. Combining form meaning more.

pleochro'matism. The property of crystals by which they show different colors when illuminated from different angles.

pleocyto'sis. An increase in the number of leukocytes, especially lymphocytes, in the body; usually the term is applied to an increase in the number of lymphocytes in the spinal fluid.

pleomas'tia. The presence of more than two breasts or nipples.

pleomor'phic. Occurring in more than one structural form.

pleomor'phism. 1. The assumption of two or more forms by a single organism during its life cycle. **2.** The occurrence of various shapes in the same species.

pleop'tics. Any type of orthoptic method of treat-

ing amblyopia (dimness of vision).

plerocer'coid. The larval stage of a tapeworm, occurring in an intermediate host.

plesiother'apy. See brachytherapy.

ples'sor. See plexor.

plethys'mograph. Device for measuring variation in size of a part or organ.

plethysmog'raphy. The recording of the variation in the size of a part produced by changes in the circulation of the blood within it.

plethysmom'etry. Measurement of the fullness of a hollow structure such as a blood vessel.

pleur- See pleuro-.

pleur'a. The serous membrane enveloping the lungs and lining the walls of the chest cavity.

   parietal p., the layer lining the walls of the chest cavity.

   visceral p., the layer covering the lungs.

pleuracot'omy. Incision into the pleural cavity, as for the introduction of a drainage tube.

pleural'gia. Pain in the pleura.

pleur'isy. Inflammation of the pleura.

pleuri'tis. Pleurisy.

pleuro-, pleur-. Combining forms denoting (a) the side; (b) the pleura; (c) a rib.

pleurocente'sis. Puncture and drainage of the pleural cavity.

pleurodyn'ia. Pain in the intercostal muscles, usually affecting one side only.

   epidemic p., acute infectious disease caused by the Coxsackie B virus; characterized chiefly by seizures of chest pain augmented by movement; also called devil's grip, benign dry pleurisy, and Bornholm disease.

pleurogen'ic, pleurog'enous. 1. Originating in the pleura. **2.** Originating in a rib.

pleurog'raphy. Roentgenography of the pleura and lungs.

pleu'rolith. A calculus in the pleural cavity.

pleuropericardi'tis. Inflammation of the membranes enveloping the lungs and the heart.

pleuropul'monary. Relating to the pleura and the lungs.

pleurot'omy. Incision into the pleural cavity.

plex'al. Relating to a plexus.

plexec'tomy. Surgical removal of a plexus.

plex'iform. Resembling or forming a network of nerves, veins, or lymphatics.

plex'or. A small rubber-headed hammer used in percussion; also called plessor.

plex'us, *pl.* **plex'uses** or **plex'us.** A network of nerves, veins, or lymphatics.

   Auerbach's p., see myenteric plexus.

   brachial p., a plexus of the ventral primary divisions of the fifth to eighth cervical and the first

thoracic nerves; it lies in the lateral part of the neck and extends into the axilla, supplying nerves to the upper limb.

   celiac p., a large plexus of sympathetic nerves and ganglia located in the peritoneal cavity at the level of the first lumbar vertebra; it contains two large ganglionic masses and a dense network of fibers surrounding the roots of the celiac and superior mesenteric arteries; it supplies nerves to the abdominal viscera; also called solar plexus.

   cervical p., a plexus of the ventral primary divisions of the first four cervical nerves which sends out numerous cutaneous, muscular, and communicating branches.

   choroid p., a vascular proliferation in a cerebral ventricle which regulates the intraventricular pressure by secretion or absorption of cerebrospinal fluid.

   lumbar p., a plexus of the ventral primary divisions of the first three and the larger portion of the fourth lumbar nerves; located ventral to the transverse processes of the lumbar vertebrae.

   lumbosacral p., the combined lumbar, sacral, and pudendal plexuses.

   Meissner's p., see submucosal plexus.

   myenteric p., a network of nerves and ganglia situated between the circular and longitudinal muscular fibers of the esophagus, stomach, and intestines; also called Auerbach's plexus.

   pampiniform p., a venous plexus in the spermatic cord which drains the testis and empties into the testicular vein.

   pudendal p., one formed from the ventral branches of the second and third sacral nerves and all of the fourth sacral nerve; considered by some to be part of the sacral plexus.

   sacral p., a plexus of the ventral primary divisions of the fourth lumbar to the third sacral nerves; it lies on the posterior wall of the pelvis and supplies the buttocks, perineum, lower extremities, and pelvic viscera.

   solar p., see celiac plexus.

   submucosal p., a plexus of autonomic nerve fibers which ramifies in the submucosal coat of the intestine; it also has ganglia from which nerve fibers pass to the muscles and mucous membrane of the intestine; also called Meissner's plexus.

   tympanic p., a plexus of nerves on the promontory of the middle ear chamber which supplies the mucous membrane of the middle ear, mastoid air cells, and the auditory tube; it also gives off a small branch to the otic ganglion.

pli'ca, *pl.* **pli'cae. 1.** A fold, as of skin or membrane. **2.** A matted state of the hair, resulting from filth and parasites.

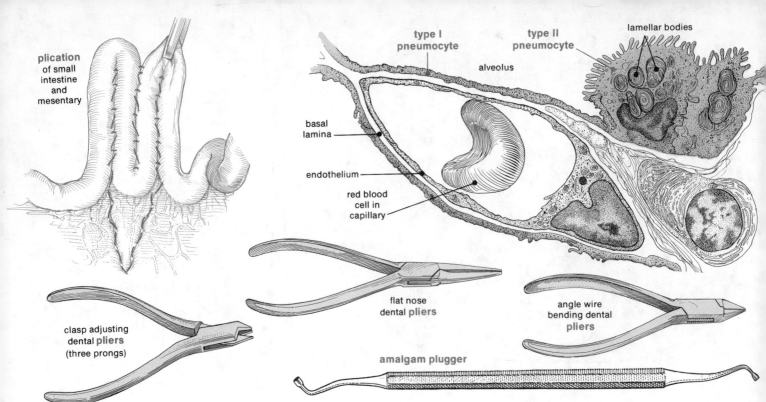

plication of small intestine and mesentary

type I pneumocyte
type II pneumocyte
lamellar bodies
alveolus
basal lamina
endothelium
red blood cell in capillary

clasp adjusting dental **pliers** (three prongs)

flat nose dental **pliers**

angle wire bending dental **pliers**

amalgam plugger

p. circularis, one of the transverse folds of mucous membrane of the small intestine; also called circular fold and valve of Kerckring.

p. semilunaris conjunctiva, the crescent-shaped fold formed by the conjunctiva at the inner angle of the eye.

p. triangularis, a fold of mucous membrane covering the anteroinferior part of the palatine tonsil and projecting from the glossopalatine arch.

pli′cate. Arranged in folds; folded.

plica′tion. The surgical folding of a muscle or of the wall of a hollow organ.

plicot′omy. Surgical section of the posterior fold of the tympanic membrane (eardrum).

pli′ers. Any of several tools of varying shapes used in dentistry and orthopedic surgery for bending, cutting, contouring, etc.

-ploid. Suffix meaning multiple in form; e.g., in genetics it designates a specific multiple of the chromosome set of an organism's nucleus, as 16-ploid, 32-ploid, etc.

plombage′. The surgical filling of a bodily space with inert material, as the filling of part of the thoracic cavity with plastic balls to compress the lung in the treatment of pulmonary tuberculosis.

plo′sive. Designating a speech sound whose articulation requires retaining the air stream for a moment and then suddenly releasing it.

plug. 1. Any mass that occludes a bodily passage or opening. **2.** A lumpy mass.

cervical p., see mucous plug.

epithelial p., a mass of epithelial cells that temporarily closes the external nares of the fetus.

mucous p., a plug formed by secretions of mucous glands, especially the mass of cervical mucus secreted by the endocervix which provides a mechanical and antibacterial barrier to the uterine cavity during pregnancy; also called cervical plug.

plug′ger. An instrument used to compress or condense filling material, such as amalgam, in a tooth cavity.

root canal p., a fine-tapered instrument with a blunt tip, used for packing dental material, such as gutta percha, into a root canal.

plum′bic. Relating to lead.

plum′bism. Lead poisoning; see under poisoning.

plum′bum. Latin for lead.

Plummer's disease. Hyperthyroidism resulting from toxic adenoma of the thyroid gland.

Plummer-Vinson syndrome. Postcricoid esophageal web usually seen in middle-aged women with severe iron deficiency and associated with atrophy of the oral and pharyngeal mucosa, inflammation of the lips, spoon-shaped nails, and splenomegaly; symptoms usually include dysphagia, sore tongue, and dry mouth; also called sideropenic dysphagia and Paterson-Kelly webs.

plu′mose. Feathery.

pluri-. Combining form meaning several. For words beginning thus, but not found here, see multi- and poly-.

pluricaus′al. Having two or more causes; applied to a disease that develops in the presence of two or more causative factors.

plurigland′ular. Denoting several glands; also called polyglandular.

plurip′ara. Multipara.

pluripar′ity. Multiparity.

plurip′otent. 1. Capable of affecting more than one organ. **2.** Denoting embryonic tissue that may develop in any of several ways.

pluto′nium. A transuranian radioactive element having 15 isotopes with half-lives from 20 minutes to 76 million years; symbol Pu, atomic number 94, atomic weight (chemical scale) 239.11.

Pm. Chemical symbol of the element promethium.

PMI. Abbreviation for point of maximal impulse; see impulse, cardiac.

P-mitrale. A pattern in the electrocardiogram consisting of wide, notched P waves in leads I and II, with flat, inverted P waves in III; occurring in mitral valve disease.

PMN. Abbreviation for polymorphonuclear leukocyte.

pneo-. Combining form indicating a relationship to breath or respiration; e.g., pneometer.

pneum-, pneuma-, pneumat-, pneumato-. Combining forms denoting (a) the presence of air or gas (e.g., pneumatocele); (b) a relation to breath or breathing (e.g., pneumatoscope).

pneuma. In ancient Greek philosophy and medicine, (a) a life-giving principle (now identified as oxygen); (b) the soul or spirit of God.

pneumarthro′sis. Air in a joint.

pneumat′ic. 1. Relating to air. **2.** Relating to breathing.

pneumatiza′tion. The development of air cells or cavities, especially those of the temporal and ethmoid bones.

pneumat′ocele. 1. An air-filled cyst in the lung, characteristic of staphylococcal pneumonia. **2.** A swelling of the scrotum with gas; also called gas tumor. **3.** Herniation of lung tissue; also called pneumonocele.

pneumat′ograph. Pneumograph.

pneumator′rhachis. The presence of gas or air in the vertebral column.

pneumatu′ria. The passage of gas through the urethra during urination, usually due to the entering of air into the bladder from the bowel through a vesicocolic fistula.

pneumo-, pneumon-, pneumono-. Combining forms denoting relationship to the lungs.

pneumoarthrog′raphy. The making of an x-ray film of a joint after injection of air.

pneumobacil′lus. See *Klebsiella pneumoniae.*

pneu′mocele. Pneumatocele.

pneumoceph′alus. The presence of air within the skull.

pneumocho′lecysti′tis. Inflammation of the gallbladder with gas-producing organisms.

pneumococce′mia. The presence of pneumococci in the blood.

pneumococ′ci. Collective name for the many serologic types of the bacterium *Streptococcus pneumoniae,* formerly known as *Diplococcus pneumoniae.*

pneumoconio′sis, *pl.* **pneumoconio′ses.** Fibrosis of the lungs caused by prolonged inhalation of foreign material, particularly silica, coal, and asbestos, as occurs in coal mining, stone cutting, etc; the main symptoms are chronic dry cough and shortness of breath; specific forms are named according to the offending agent; e.g., silicosis, asbestosis, and anthracosis.

Pneumocystis carinii. A parasitic, basophilic microorganism measuring one micron or less in diameter, occurring singly or in aggregates within a cystlike structure; the causative agent of pneumocystosis.

pneumocysto′sis. Interstitial pneumonia caused by *Pneumocystis carinii,* which invade the walls of the alveoli; occurs in premature and debilitated infants during the first three months of life or in individuals receiving immunosuppressive drugs.

pneu′mocyte, pneumon′ocyte. Any of the alveolar epithelial cells of the lungs.

granular p., type II pneumocyte.

membranous p., type I pneumocyte.

type I p., a thin squamous epithelial cell lining the inside of the pulmonary alveolar wall; it has a large attenuated cytoplasm that may extend up to 100 microns; also called membranous pneumocyte and respiratory or type I cell.

type II p., a secretory cuboidal epithelial cell in the niches of the pulmonary alveolar wall; it possesses large, oval lamellar bodies thought to store surfactant, a surface-active phospholipid, which when secreted reduces the surface tension of the alveoli; also called granular pneumocyte, and great alveolar, septal, or type II cell.

pneumodynam′ics. The mechanism of respiration.

pneumoencephalog′raphy. The making of x-ray films of the brain after replacing the cerebrospi-

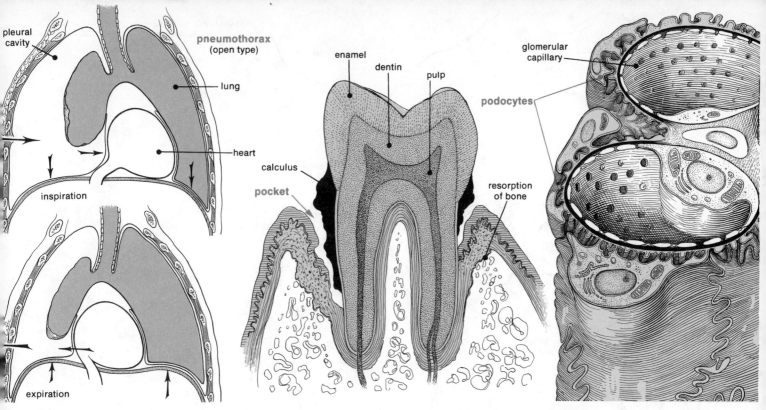

nal fluid of the subarachnoid space with a gas.

pneu′mogram. 1. Tracing made by a pneumograph. **2.** Roentgenogram following injection of air or gas into a bodily space.

pneu′mograph. An instrument for recording the movements of respiration; also called pneumonograph and pneumatograph.

pneumog′raphy. Roentgenography of any air- or gas-filled bodily space.

   retroperitoneal p., roentgenography following the injection of gas into the retroperitoneal space to increase the contrast between organs (adrenal gland, kidney, etc.) and the surrounding tissues.

pneumohemopericar′dium. See hemopneumopericardium.

pneumohemotho′rax. The presence of gas or air and blood in the thoracic cavity.

pneumohydrome′tra. The presence of gas and fluid in the uterine cavity.

pneumohydrotho′rax. See hydropneumothorax.

pneu′molith. A calculus or concretion present in the lung.

pneumol′ogy. Study of the lungs.

pneumolys′ia, pneumol′ysis. Surgical separation of the pleura from the chest wall in order to allow the lung to collapse.

pneumomediasti′num. The presence of free air in the mediastinum (the central space of the chest containing all the thoracic organs except the lungs).

pneumomyco′sis. Any disease of the lungs caused by fungi or bacteria; also called pneumonomycosis.

pneumon-. See pneumo-.

pneumonec′tomy. Surgical removal of a lung or a portion of it; also called pneumectomy and pulmonectomy.

pneumo′nia. Inflammation of the lungs, caused by viruses, bacteria, or chemical and physical agents.

   acute p., lobar pneumonia.

   aspiration p., pneumonia resulting from aspiration of food particles, vomit, water, or infected material from the upper respiratory tract.

   bacterial p., disease of sudden onset caused by a variety of bacterial agents (pneumococcus being the most common); high fever, chills, stabbing chest pains, cough, and rusty sputum are typical findings.

   bronchial p., see bronchopneumonia.

   chemical p., pneumonia caused by inhalation of extremely poisonous gas such as phosgene; characterized by edematous and hemorrhagic lungs.

   desquamative interstitial p., diffuse proliferation of alveolar lining cells, which desquamate into the air sacs, producing gradual onset of dyspnea and nonproductive cough, with roentgenographic changes.

   double p., lobar pneumonia involving both lungs.

   Eaton agent p., see mycoplasmal pneumonia.

   Friedländer's p., a severe form of lobar pneumonia caused by infection with *Klebsiella pneumoniae* (Friedländer's bacillus); marked by much swelling of the affected pulmonary lobe.

   hypostatic p., pulmonary congestion occurring in the aged or in ill individuals who lie in the same position for long periods of time.

   lipid p., lipoid p., condition caused by aspiration of oily or fatty substances; also called oil pneumonia.

   lobar p., acute pneumonia usually caused by a type of pneumococcus bacteria; marked by fever, chest pains, cough, and blood-stained sputum, with inflammation and consolidation of one or more lobes of the lungs.

   Löffler's p., Löffler's syndrome.

   mycoplasmal p., a severe form of insidious onset caused by infiltration of the lungs with *Mycoplasma pneumoniae* (Eaton agent); marked predominantly by severe cough, tracheal tenderness, pharyngitis with ear involvement, and occasionally blood-specked sputum; also called primary atypical or Eaton agent pneumonia.

   pneumococcal p., acute lobar pneumonia caused by the pneumococcus organism.

   primary atypical p., see mycoplasmal pneumonia.

   secondary p., inflammation of the lungs occurring as a complication of another disease.

   viral p., acute systemic disease, caused by a variety of viruses (e.g., myxoviruses, adenoviruses), with involvement of the lungs.

pneumon′ic. 1. Of or relating to the lungs. **2.** Relating to pneumonia.

pneumoni′tis. Inflammation of the lungs.

pneumono-. See pneumo-.

pneu′monocele. See pneumatocele (3).

pneumon′ocyte. See pneumocyte.

pneumonomyco′sis. See pneumomycosis.

pneumonot′omy. Incision into the lung; also called pneumotomy.

pneumopericar′dium. The presence of air in the sac encasing the heart.

pneumoperitone′um. The presence of air or gas in the peritoneal cavity from perforation of a viscus or therapeutic installation.

pneumoperitoni′tis. Inflammation of the peritoneum with accumulation of air or gas in the peritoneal cavity.

pneumopyotho′rax. See pyopneumothorax.

pneumoroentgenog′raphy. X-ray examination of a bodily part into which air or gas has been injected to provide additional outlines.

pneumor′rhachis. The presence of gas in the spinal canal.

pneumorrha′gia. Bleeding from or into the lung.

pneumotho′rax. The presence of air or gas in the pleural cavity.

pneumot′omy. See pneumonotomy.

PNS. Abbreviation for peripheral nervous system.

p.o. Abbreviation of the Latin *per os*.

Po. Chemical symbol of the element polonium.

P$_{O_2}$. Symbol for partial pressure of oxygen; also written pO$_2$.

pock. A pustule caused by an eruptive disease, especially smallpox.

pock′et. 1. A saclike cavity. **2.** A space between a tooth and the inflamed gum. **3.** To enclose the pedicle of a tumor (after its removal) within the edges of the wound. **4.** A collection of pus.

pock′mark. The scar left on the skin after the healing of a smallpox pustule.

pod-. See podo-.

podag′ra. Gout of the metatarsophalangeal joint of the big toe.

pod′agral, podag′ric, pod′agrous. Relating to or suffering from gout.

podal′gia. Pain in the foot.

podal′ic. Relating to feet.

podarthri′tis. Inflammation of the foot joints.

podi′atrist. A specialist in podiatry; also called chiropodist.

podi′atry. The study and treatment of foot diseases, injuries, and defects; also called chiropody.

podi′tis. An inflammatory disorder of the foot.

podo-, pod-. Combining forms indicating a relationship to the foot.

podobromidro′sis. Perspiration or sweating of the feet with a strong, offensive odor.

pod′ocyte. An epithelial cell of the renal glomerulus which squats upon the glomerular basement membrane, spreading thin cytoplasmic projections over the membrane; the outer surface of the engorged cell projects into the glomerular (Bowman's) space, where it is bathed by the glomerular ultrafiltrate.

pododynamom′eter. Device for measuring the strength of the foot or leg muscles.

podophyl′lin. Podophyllum resin; see under resin.

podophyllotox′in. The active principle of podophyllum resin; it has laxative properties.

podophyl′lum. The rhizome of the mayapple (*Podophyllum peltatum*), used as a bulk-forming laxative.

   p. resin, see under resin.

pogo′nion. The most anterior midpoint of the

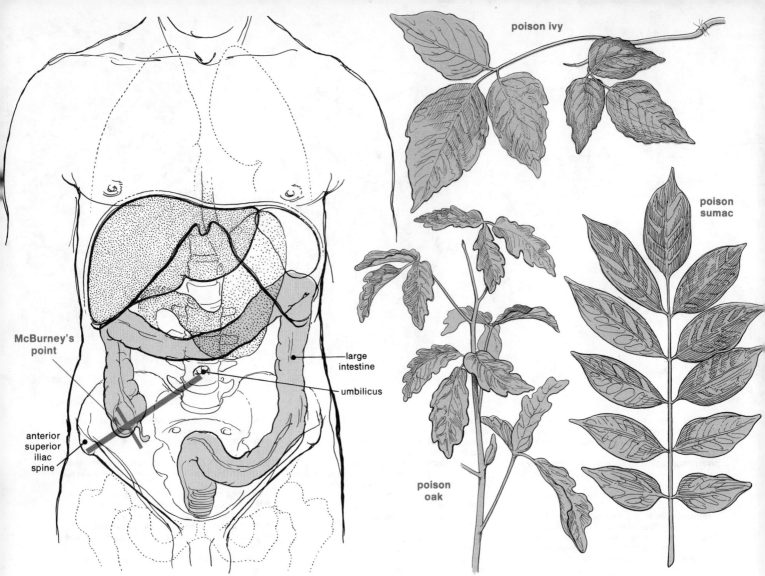

poison ivy

poison sumac

poison oak

McBurney's point

anterior superior iliac spine

large intestine

umbilicus

---

mandible or chin.

-poiesis, -poesis. Combining forms meaning production.

poikilo-. Combining form meaning varied or irregular.

poikil′ocyte. A red blood cell assuming an abnormal and often bizarre shape; it could be pear-shaped, racquet-shaped, or pessary-shaped; characteristically found in severe hemolytic anemias.

poikilocyto′sis. The presence in the blood of abnormally shaped red blood cells (poikilocytes); also called poikilocythemia.

poikiloder′ma. An atrophic skin condition that has streaks, marks, or patches of a different color or colors.

poikil′otherm. An animal having a temperature that varies with the environment.

point. 1. A minute spot or area. **2.** The sharp or tapered end of an object. **3.** A specific condition or degree.

  alveolar p., see prosthion.

  boiling p., the temperature at which a liquid boils, i.e., at which the vapor pressure of a liquid is equal to the atmospheric pressure.

  contact p., the small area of the proximal surface of a tooth that touches the adjacent tooth; also called contact area.

  craniometric p., any one of many fixed points on the skull used as landmarks in craniometry.

  dew p., temperature at which the moisture of the air condenses.

  end p., in volumetric analysis of a solution, the point at which a reaction is completed.

  freezing p., the temperature at which a liquid changes to a solid state.

  isoelectric p. (pl), the pH at which an amphoteric electrolyte, such as an amino acid or protein, is electrically neutral owing to equality of ionization; above or below this pH, it acts as an acid or base, respectively.

  J p., J junction; the junction between the QRS complex and the ST segment in the electrocardiogram.

  jugal p., the point where the zygomatic arch meets with the frontal process of the zygomatic bone.

  McBurney's p., the point located on a line between the anterior superior spine of the right ilium and the umbilicus, about one-third of that distance from this spine; the especially tender point in acute appendicitis.

  melting p., the temperature at which a solid changes into a liquid state.

  mid-inguinal p., the point on the inguinal ligament halfway between the pubic symphysis and the anterior superior iliac spine.

  p. of fixation, the retinal point on which an image is formed; in normal vision it is the fovea.

  p. source, in photometry, the source of light from which light radiates in straight lines in all directions.

  pressure p., (1) a point at which pressure can be exerted to control hemorrhage from an arterial injury; (2) a point on the skin surface which is extremely sensitive to pressure.

point′ing. The process of reaching a point.

  p. of an abscess, an abscess or boil that is about to open spontaneously.

  past p., incoordination of voluntary movements characterized by inability to place a finger on some designated site (the finger moves past the site).

poise. The unit of dynamic viscosity of a liquid equal to one dyne-second per square centimeter.

poi′son. Any substance that is injurious to health or causes death, either taken internally or applied externally.

  p. ivy, (1) *Rhus radicans;* a shrub or vine which grows abundantly throughout the United States and parts of sourthern Canada and has smooth, glossy leaflets of three with margins varying from crenate or serrate to deeply lobate; it causes a rash on contact; (2) the acute, intensely itchy vesicular skin eruption caused by the toxic material (oleoresin) in the sap of the poison ivy plant; the blisters are usually grouped; also called ivy dermatitis.

  p. oak, *Rhus diversilobum;* A North American shrub having varied leaflets, often with three to seven subacute lobes resembling the leaves of some common oak; it causes a rash on contact.

  p. sumac, a swamp shrub, *Rhus vernix,* that grows in marshy areas of eastern North America and has compound leaves with branches of seven to 13 elongated leaflets; it produces an acutely irritating oil that causes a rash on contact; also called poison ash, poison dogwood, and poison elder.

  "purse" p., medication carried in the purse for personal use that results in poisoning of the curious child who seeks candy or gum and finds attractive multicolored pills and tablets.

poi′soning. The condition produced by a poison.

  arsenic p., poisoning caused by ingestion of arsenic-containing compounds, usually insecticides or rodenticides; arsenic reacts with sulfhydryl groups to disrupt vital enzyme systems; symptoms of chronic poisoning include skin changes and peripheral neuropathy; headache and confusion may be seen in both acute and chronic forms.

  blood p., a vague colloquial term; see septicemia and bacteremia.

  carbon monoxide p., acute, potentially fatal poisoning with various degrees of severity, caused by inhalation of carbon monoxide; severe headache is usually an early symptom; subquently, nausea, weakness, and exertional dyspnea develop, and collapse and coma may supervene.

  carbon tetrachloride p., poisoning due to ingestion, inhalation, or absorption of carbon tetrachloride, an industrial solvent; causes hepatic and renal necrosis.

  cyanide p., poisoning caused by inhalation or ingestion of compounds of cyanide; death may occur in minutes; cyanides combine with iron-con-

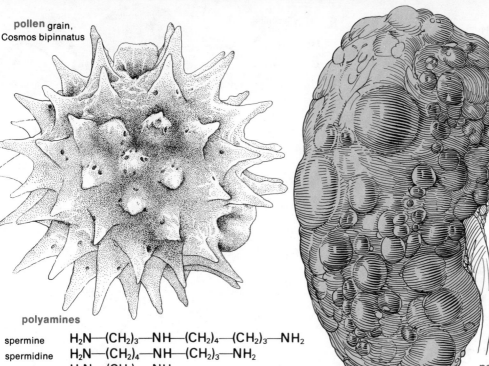

pollen grain,
Cosmos bipinnatus

polyamines

spermine	$H_2N—(CH_2)_3—NH—(CH_2)_4—(CH_2)_3—NH_2$
spermidine	$H_2N—(CH_2)_4—NH—(CH_2)_3—NH_2$
cadaverine	$H_2N—(CH_2)_5—NH_2$
putrescine	$H_2N—(CH_2)_4—NH_2$

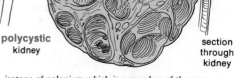

cyst cavities

renal pelvis

polycystic kidney

section through kidney

taining enzymes such as cytochromes and catalase to block energy-releasing metabolism and cause tissue asphyxia; most common sources are fungicides and insecticides.

food p., poisoning causing acute gastrointestinal illness, or neurologic manifestations accompanied by intestinal complaints; resulting from ingestion of foods that (a) have become contaminated with microorganisms, (b) may themselves be poisonous, or (c) may contain harmful chemicals.

heavy metal p., poisoning caused by such metals as antimony, arsenic, bismuth, cadmium, copper, gold, lead, mercury, silver, and thallium; BAL and EDTA are used to treat many of these disorders.

lead p., acute or chronic intoxication with lead or its salts, causing gastrointestinal and mental disturbances, anemia, basophilic stippling of red blood cells, and a bluish "lead line" on the gums; most commonly seen in young children who eat paint scales; other sources include lead toys, motor fuel, and lead water pipes; also called plumbism.

mercury p., poisoning caused by ingestion of soluble mercury salts such as mercuric chloride ($HgCl_2$), producing corrosive damage to the gastrointestinal tract and destruction of the kidney tubules; repeated inhalation of mercury vapor or ingestion of small amounts of mercury salts may lead to chronic mercury poisoning, characterized by mental symptoms, renal damage, and stomatitis.

po'lar. 1. Relating to poles. **2.** Having poles; said of certain nerve cells.

polarim'eter. Instrument used to determine the amount of polarization of light or the rotation of the plane of polarization.

polarim'etry. The process of using the polarimeter.

polar'iscope. Instrument used to study the properties of polarized light.

polar'ity. 1. Having two opposite poles. **2.** Manifesting two opposite tendencies or attributes.

polariza'tion. 1. In optics, the process of altering the transverse wave motion of a light ray, whereby the vibrations of the wave occur in one plane only. **2.** In electricity, the deposition of gas in one or both electrodes of an electric cell, whereby the action of the battery is impeded. **3.** The development of ions of opposite charges (i.e., differences in potential) in two points of living tissue, as on both sides of a cell membrane.

po'larize. To induce polarization.

po'larizer. The part of a polarimeter or polariscope that receives and polarizes the light.

polarog'raphy. In qualitative or quantitative microanalysis, the recording of the relationship between an increasing current flowing through a solution being analyzed and the increasing voltage used to produce the current.

pole. 1. Either end of an axis. **2.** Either of two points having opposite physical properties; e.g., terminals of an electric cell or battery.

animal p., the site in the early ovum near the nucleus where most of the protoplasm is concentrated, and from which the polar bodies are pinched off; also called germinal pole.

germinal p., see animal pole.

negative p., cathode.

positive p., anode.

vegetal p., vegetative p., the pole of an ovum where the bulk of the yolk is located, opposite to the germinal disk; also called vitelline pole and antigerminal pole.

vitelline p., see vegetal pole.

polio-. Combining form indicating a relationship to the gray matter of the nervous system.

polio. Colloquial term for poliomyelitis.

poliodys'trophy. Wasting of the gray substance of the nervous system.

polioencephali'tis. Inflammation of the gray substance of the brain.

poliomyeli'tis. A highly contagious, infectious disease caused by a filterable virus and occurring most commonly in children; in its acute form it involves the spinal cord, causing paralysis, atrophy, and permanent deformity of one or more muscular groups; also called polio and infantile paralysis.

poliomyelop'athy. Any disease principally affecting the gray matter of the spinal cord and medulla oblongata.

pol'len. The powder-like microspores (male fertilizing elements) produced by the anthers of flowering plants which are carried by wind or insects and play a major role in the etiology of hay fever and some cases of asthma.

polleno'sis, pollino'sis. Hay fever excited by certain airborne pollens.

pol'lex. The thumb.

pollino'sis. See pollenosis.

pollut'ant. A substance that contaminates; especially one that contaminates the air, water, or food.

pollute'. To make impure; to dirty; to contaminate.

pollu'tion. The act or process of contaminating, as the discharge of noxious substances into the atmosphere or into a body of water.

polo'nium. A radioactive metallic element; symbol Po, atomic number 84, atomic weight 210; one of the rarest naturally occurring elements, a product of radium disintegration; discovered by Pierre and Marie Curie and named after Mme. Curie's native land, Poland.

polo'nium-210 (^{210}Po). A 138.4-day α-emitter isotope of polonium which is a member of the uranium natural radioactive decay series.

po'lus, *pl.* **po'li.** Latin for pole.

poly-. Prefix denoting (a) many, often, multiplicity, or much; e.g., polyarteritis; (b) excessive; e.g., polydipsia; (c) polymer of; e.g., polypeptide.

polyac'id. An acid that yields more than one hydrogen ion per molecule.

polyadeni'tis. Inflammation of several lymph nodes.

polya'mine. Any of a group of substances, widely distributed in small quantities among living forms, which are essential growth factors for a number of microorganisms such as *Hemophilus parainfluenzae*; they serve as agents which stabilize membranous structures; putrescine, cadaverine, spermidine, and spermine are polyamines.

polyarteri'tis. Simultaneous inflammation of several arteries.

p. nodosa, polyarteritis with formation of numerous nodules within the walls of the arteries; a collagen vascular disease which may involve a variety of different organ systems, producing renal, gastrointestinal, or nervous system findings; also called periarteritis nodosa.

polyarthri'tis. Inflammation of several joints.

polyba'sic. An acid that has more than one replaceable hydrogen atom.

polycho'lia. Excessive production and flow of bile.

polychondri'tis. A rare syndrome marked by a widespread inflammatory and degenerative process in cartilaginous structures, such as those in the nose, ear, joints, and tracheobronchial tree; destruction of cartilage leaves deformities, such as saddle nose or floppy ear; death may occur from suffocation due to loss of stability in the tracheobronchial tree.

polychroma'sia, polychroma'tia. Polychromatophilia.

polychromat'ic. Multicolored; exhibiting many colors.

polychro'matophil, polychro'matophile. 1. A cell or other element that stains readily with both acidic and basic dyes, especially certain red blood cells. **2.** A young or degenerating red blood cell which manifests acidic and basic staining affinities.

polychromatophil'ia. 1. Tendency to stain with basic and acid stains. **2.** Condition marked by the presence of an excessive number of red blood cells that stain with basic, acid, and neutral dyes.

polyclin'ic. A clinic, dispensary, or hospital that treats any disease or injury.

polycys'tic. Made up of several cysts.

polycystic disease of kidney. An inherited kidney disease marked by formation of multiple cysts of varying sizes, resulting in renal parenchymal

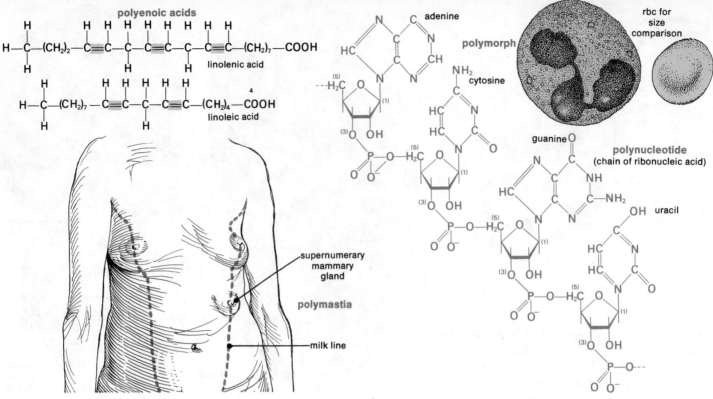

polyenoic acids

linolenic acid

linoleic acid

adenine

cytosine

guanine

uracil

polymorph

rbc for size comparison

polynucleotide
(chain of ribonucleic acid)

supernumerary mammary gland

polymastia

milk line

degeneration and gradual loss of renal function; the adult form of the disease shows autosomal dominant inheritance; uremia results usually in early or middle adult life; bilateral polycystic kidney disease of infants and children often causes stillbirths or deaths within the first few months of life, is frequently associated with cysts in other organs, and does not follow an autosomal dominant inheritance.

polycystic ovary syndrome. Condition of unknown cause characterized by bilaterally enlarged polycystic ovaries, small uterus, menstrual abnormalities, anovulatory infertility (i.e., failure to produce ova), and hirsutism; also called Stein-Leventhal syndrome.

polycythe′mia. The presence of an abnormally large number of red corpuscles in the blood.

p. hypertonica, polycythemia associated with hypertension, in the absence of splenic enlargement.

p. vera, a disease of unknown cause characterized by hyperplasia of all the cellular elements of the bone marrow and manifested by an increase in the total number of red blood cells in the body, usually accompanied by leukocytosis and thrombocytosis; also called primary polycythemia and erythremia.

primary p., see polycythemia vera.

relative p., an increase in the number of red blood cells per unit volume of blood due to a decrease in the total plasma of the body.

secondary p., an increase in the total number of red blood cells in the body due to another condition; e.g., the chronic tissue hypoxia of advanced pulmonary disease, high altitude, or the secretion of erythropoietins by certain tumors.

polydac′tyly. Congenital abnormality marked by the presence of more than ten fingers or toes; also called polydactylia and polydactylism.

polydip′sia. Insatiable thirst.

polydyspla′sia. Condition marked by multiple developmental abnormalities of tissues, organs, or systems.

poly′ene. A chemical compound containing many conjugated (alternating) double bonds; e.g., carotenoids.

polyeno′ic acid. A polyunsaturated fatty acid, essential in the diet, with more than one double bond in the carbon chain; e.g., linoleic acid (two double bonds) and linolenic acid (three double bonds).

polyeth′ylene. A resin, $(CH_2CH_2)_n$, produced by the polymerization of ethylene under high pressure; a straight-chain paraffin hydrocarbon of high molecular weight.

p. glycol 300, a condensation product of ethylene oxide and water; $HOCH_2 (CH_2OCH_2)_nCH_2OH$, with n varying from five to six; used in nitrofurazone

ointment and solution.

p. glycol 400, a condensation product of ethylene oxide and water; $H(OCH_2CH_2)_nOH$, with n varying from eight to 10; used in ointments.

p. glycol 1540, Carbowax compound 1540, a condensation product of ethylene oxide and water; $HOCH_2(CH_2OCH_2)_nCH_2OH$, with n varying from 28 to 36; a soft petrolatum-like semisolid used in nitrofurazone ointment and solution.

p. glycol 4000, Carbowax compound 4000, a condensation product of ethylene oxide and water; $H(OCH_2CH_2)_nOH$ with n varying from 70 to 85; solid component of so-called greaseless polyethylene glycol ointment.

pol′ygen. A chemical element with two or more valences.

pol′ygene. One of a group of genes that, acting together, control a quantitative character such as height.

polygen′ic. Relating to a quantitative character (e.g., height) dependent on the action of several genes.

polygland′ular. See pluriglandular.

pol′ygraph. An instrument for simultaneously recording changes in such physiologic processes as blood pressure, respiratory motion, and galvanic skin resistance; sometimes used to study emotional reactions, as in lie detection; also called lie detector.

polyhe′dral. Having many faces.

polyhydram′nios. An excess volume of amniotic fluid in pregnancy, usually greater than 2000 ml.

polyhy′dric. Containing more than one hydroxyl group.

polyhypermenorrhe′a. Frequent menstruation accompanied by excessive flow.

polyhypomenorrhe′a. Frequent menstruation accompanied by a scanty flow.

polylep′tic. Having many relapsing phases; said of a disease.

polylo′gia. Garrulity or talkativeness (often incoherent) caused by a mental disorder.

polymas′tia. The presence of more than two breasts in the human; also called multimammae.

pol′ymer. A complex compound of high molecular weight formed by a chain of simpler molecules; e.g., the combining of many ethylene molecules to form polyethylene.

addition p., a large molecule formed by a chain of smaller molecules (monomers) without the formation of any other product.

condensation p., a large molecule formed by a chain of smaller molecules, involving the elimination of water or some other simple compound.

polymerase. Any enzyme that promotes polymerization.

polymeriza′tion. The chemical joining of similar monomers to form a compound of a high molecular weight.

polymethylmethac′rylate. The principal base resin employed in making dentures; it is transparent and can be tinted to any shade of translucence; also used as bone cement.

polymicrolipomato′sis. A morbid condition marked by the presence of a number of small, nodular, fairly discrete masses of lipid (lipomata) in the subcutaneous connective tissue.

pol′ymorph. Shortened version of polymorphonuclear leukocyte (PMN).

polymor′phic, polymor′phous. Occurring in many morphologic forms.

polymor′phism. The occurrence of two or more genetically different classes in the same population; e.g., Rh-positive and Rh-negative humans.

polymorphonu′clear. Having nuclei of varied shapes, or so deeply lobulated that they appear to be multiple; said of a variety of leukocytes (PMNs).

polymyal′gia. Persistent pain in several muscles.

p. rheumatica, a syndrome of muscular rheumatism in old people, more frequent in men than women, characterized by a markedly elevated erythrocyte sedimentation rate; often associated with cranial arteritis.

polymyosi′tis. A painful inflammation of the muscles which may also involve skin and subcutaneous tissue; the muscles most affected are those of the pelvic and shoulder girdles and pharynx; when skin changes are prominent the disorder is often called dermatomyositis; in 15 to 20 per cent of cases there is an associated neoplasm.

polymyx′in. Any of a group of antibiotic substances derived from strains of the soil bacterium *Bacillus polymixa;* they are polypeptides containing various amino acids and a branched fatty acid, (+)-6-methyloctanoic acid; there are five different types, designated A, B, C, D, and E.

polyneuri′tis. Inflammation of several peripheral nerves at the same time, characterized by widespread sensory and motor disturbances; also called multiple neuritis.

polyneurop′athy. A disease in which several peripheral nerves are affected at the same time.

polyneu′roradiculi′tis. Inflammation involving nerve roots and peripheral nerves.

polynu′clear. Multinuclear; containing more than one nucleus.

polynucleo′tidase. A class of enzymes which help to hydrolyze or split up nucleic acids of high molecular weight into their constituent mononucleotide units.

polynu′cleotide. Compound containing several

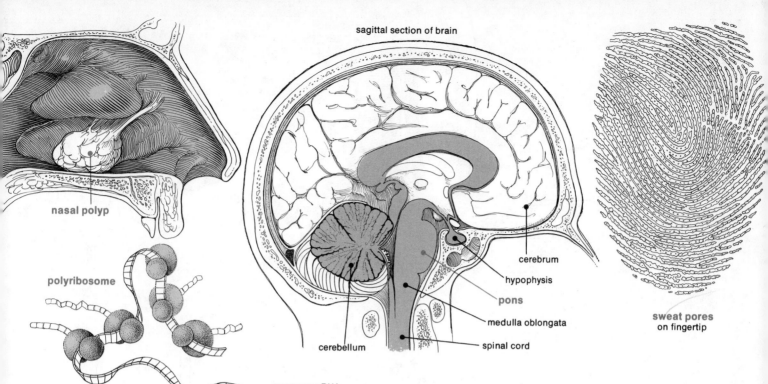

sagittal section of brain

nasal polyp

polyribosome

messenger RNA

cerebrum
hypophysis
pons
medulla oblongata
spinal cord
cerebellum

sweat pores
on fingertip

or many nucleotides; a nucleic acid.

polyol. General term for an alcohol that contains more than one hydroxyl group in the molecule.

polyo'pia. A condition in which a person perceives more than one image of the same object; multiple vision; also called polyopsia and polyopy.

  p. monophthalmica, condition in which only one eye is affected.

polyor'chidism, polyor'chism. The presence of more than two testes.

pol'yp. A general term denoting a growth or mass of tissue that protrudes from a mucous membrane, commonly found in the nose, uterus, rectum, and bladder.

  pedunculated p., one that is attached to the mucosa by a slender stalk or pedicle.

  sessile p., one that has a broad base.

polypec'tomy. Surgical removal of a polyp.

polypep'tide. A compound containing two or more amino acids united by peptide linkage; the ribosome is the site of polypeptide synthesis in the cytoplasm.

polypeptide'mia. The presence of polypeptides in the blood.

polypha'gia. Morbid or pathological overeating.

polyphen'ic. See pleiotrophic.

pol'yplast. Derived from several structures.

polyplas'tic. Capable of taking many forms.

polyple'gia. Paralysis of several muscles.

pol'yploidy. The state of having a chromosome number that is a multiple of the normal diploid number, resulting from the replication of chromosome sets without subsequent division of the nucleus; e.g., tetraploid = 92 chromosomes, triploid = 69 chromosomes, etc.

pol'yploid. Having the outward appearance of a polyp.

polypo'sis. The presence of numerous polyps.

pol'ypotome. A cutting instrument for excising polyps.

pol'ypous. Relating to or characterized by the presence of polyps.

polyri'bosome. A multiple structure composed of two or more ribosomes held together by a molecule of messenger RNA; also called polysome and ergosome.

polys. A colloquial term for polymorphonuclear leukocytes.

polysacch'aride. A carbohydrate containing a large number of saccharide units, such as starch and glycogen.

polyserosi'tis. Inflammation of several serous membranes; also called multiple serositis.

polyso'me. See polyribosome.

polyso'my. The state of a cell nucleus in which

some but not all of the chromosomes of a set are reduplicated beyond the normal diploid number.

polysor'bate 80. Polyoxethylene sorbitan monooleate; a yellow, bitter oil, used as an emulsifier in the preparation of ointments; Tween 80®.

polysper'mia. Excessive secretion of semen.

polysper'my. The entry of more than one sperm into an ovum during fertilization.

polytetrafluoroeth'ylene. A waxy synthetic fabric, used for surgical implantation, which resists the clotting of blood upon its surface; Teflon®.

polythe'lia. The presence of more than two nipples.

polytrich'ia. The presence of excessive hair.

polyunsaturated. Having two or more unsaturated (double) bonds; said of certain long-chain carbon compounds, especially fats and oils.

polyu'ria. Passage of abnormally large quantity of urine.

polyv'alent. See multivalent.

polyvin'ylpyrrol'idone (PVP). A synthetic polymer used as a dispersing and suspending medium; also called povidone.

Pompe's disease. Type 2 glycogenosis; see under glycogenosis.

pom'pholyx. Dyshidrosis (2); a deep eruption of blisters occurring primarily on the hands and feet, accompanied by intense itching.

pom'phus. A blister or a wheal.

POMR. Abbreviation for problem-oriented medical record.

pons. 1. The part of the brain located between the cerebral peduncle above and the medulla oblongata below. **2.** Any bridgelike structure connecting two parts of an organ.

pon'tic. An artificial tooth on a fixed partial denture which replaces the missing natural tooth.

pon'tile, pon'tine. Relating to a pons, especially of the brain (pons varolii).

pool. A collection of blood in a part.

pop'les. The back of the knee.

poplit'eal. Relating to the back of the knee.

por'celain. A fine ceramic powder (composed of clay, quartz, and flux) mixed with water to form a paste; used in the manufacture of artificial teeth, inlays, jacket crowns, and dentures.

por'cine. Relating to pigs.

pore. A minute opening on a surface, as of a sweat gland on the skin.

  gustatory p., a minute surface opening of a taste bud.

  slit p., the linear ultraminute space between the footlike processes (pedicles) of the podocytes that cover the outside of the capillary of the renal corpuscle.

sweat p., the surface opening of a sweat gland.

porenceph'aly. Congenital malformation of the brain characterized by a cystic outpouching of the ventricular system.

porokerato'sis. A rare skin disease marked by cornification around pores and progressive centrifugal atrophy.

por'phin. $C_{20}H_{14}N_4$; a fundamental substance which contains four pyrrole-like rings linked by four CH groups or methene bridges in a ring system; the unsubstituted tetrapyrrole nucleus of the porphyrins.

porphobilin'ogen. Organic compound present in large quantities in the urine of individuals with acute or congenital porphyria.

porphy'ria. A disorder of blood pigment metabolism in which there is a marked increase in the formation and excretion of porphyrins.

por'phyrin. Any of various organic compounds present in protoplasm, forming the foundation structure for hemoglobin, chlorophyll, and other respiratory pigments; they are capable of combining with metals such as iron, magnesium, copper, etc. (metalloporphyrins), and with nitrogenous substances.

porphyrinu'ria, porphyru'ria. Presence of porphyrin in the urine in excess of the normal amount.

porri'go. Any disease of the scalp.

por'ta. The point at which vessels, nerves, and excretory ducts enter and leave an organ.

  p. hepatis, the fissure on the under surface of the liver through which the portal vein, the hepatic artery, and the hepatic ducts pass.

portaca'val. Relating to the portal vein and the inferior vena cava.

por'tal. Relating to any entrance; specifically, to the porta hepatis.

por'tio, pl. portio'nes. Latin for part.

por'togram. An x-ray film of the portal vein.

portog'raphy. Splenic photography, a roentgenographic technique in which the splenic and portal veins and their tributaries are visualized after injection with a radiopaque material; widely used as a diagnostic and prognostic tool in cirrhosis.

po'rus, pl. po'ri. Latin for pore; an orifice.

position. 1. The placement of the body in a special way to facilitate specific diagnostic or therapeutic procedures. **2.** The particular arrangement of bodily parts. **3.** In obstetrics, the relationship of a designated point on the presenting part of the fetus to a designated point in the maternal pelvis. **4.** The place occupied. **5.** To place the body in a particular way.

  anatomic p., one in which the body is erect with the arms and hands turned forward.

  centric p., the position of the mandible in its most

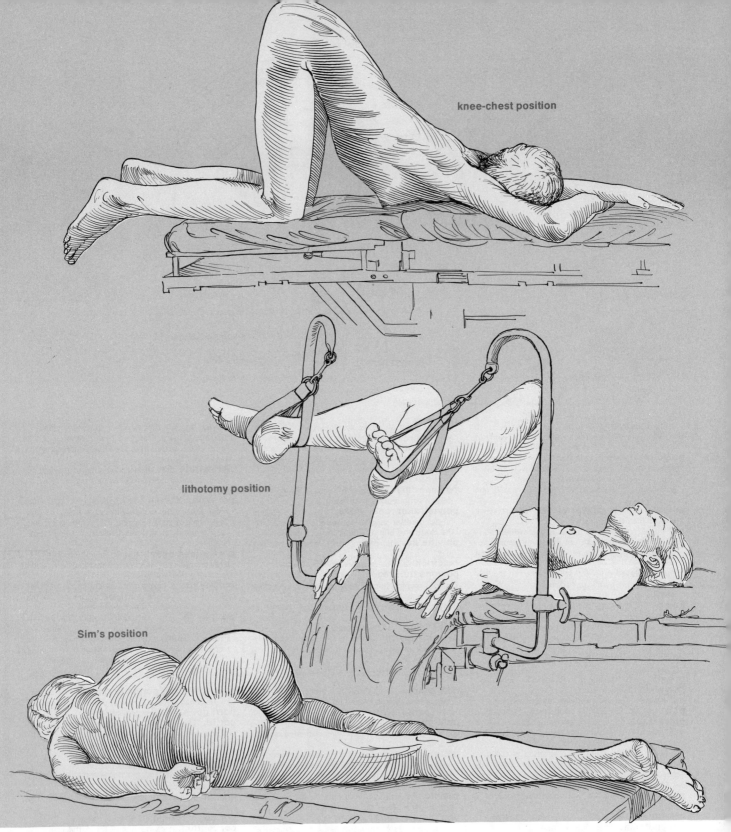

knee-chest position

lithotomy position

Sim's position

retruded relation to the maxilla; the position in which an individual normally closes his jaws.

eccentric p., any position of the mandible other than the centric position.

Fowler's p., an inclined position obtained by raising the head of the bed about 20 inches.

frog leg p., lying on the back with both thighs acutely extended and knees flexed, as seen in infants with scurvy; also called pithed frog position.

genupectoral p., knee-chest position.

jackknife p., one in which the individual is on his back with shoulders elevated and thighs at right angles to the abdomen; used to facilitate urethral instrumentation.

knee-chest p., a prone posture resting on the knees and chest with forearms supporting the head;

assumed for rectal examinations.

left lateral recumbent p., one in which the individual lies on the left side with the right thigh and knee drawn upward; assumed by parturient women; also called obstetric position.

lithotomy p., the individual lies on his back with buttocks at the end of the examining or operating table, the hips and knees being fully flexed with feet supported by slings or mechanical braces.

obstetric p., see left lateral recumbent position.

occlusal p., the relation of the mandible to the maxilla when the jaws are closed and the teeth are in contact.

orthopneic p., a sitting position with the individual's head and arms resting on an overbed table or on the arms of a chair.

prone p., lying face down.

recumbent p., a restful position in which the individual is on his back with legs slightly extended and flexed.

Sim's p., one in which the individual lies on the left side with the right thigh acutely flexed and the left thigh slightly flexed; the left arm is behind the body; used to facilitate vaginal and rectal examinations, curettement of uterus, intrauterine irrigation after labor, tamponade of vagina, etc.

supine p., lying on the back.

Trendelenburg's p., one in which the individual lies on his back on an operating table, inclined at an angle of 45 degrees with the head lower than the rest of the body; the legs and feet hang over the end of the table.

position | **position**

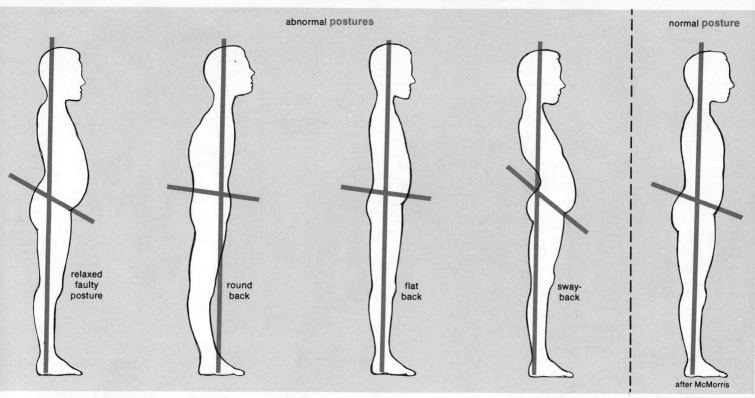

abnormal **postures**　　　　normal **posture**

relaxed
faulty
posture

round
back

flat
back

sway-
back

after McMorris

pos'itive. 1. Definite; reactive; affirmative; not negative. **2.** Denoting the presence of a particular disorder upon examination. **3.** Having a quantity greater than zero. **4.** Irrefutable.

pos'itron. A subatomic particle of the same mass as the electron and of equal but opposite (positive) charge.

Posner-Schlossman syndrome. Recurrent episodes of unilateral noncongestive glaucoma characterized by an open angle and pigmented precipitates on the posterior surface of the cornea.

post-. Prefix denoting behind, posterior to, or subsequent to.

postcardiotomy syndrome. See postpericardiotomy syndrome.

postcholecystectomy syndrome. A group of symptoms suggestive of biliary disease, such as right upper quadrant pain, indigestion, and food intolerance, which continue to persist after cholecystectomy.

postci'bal. After meals; after eating.

post cibum (p.c.). Latin for after meals.

postclavic'ular. Situated in back of the clavicle (collarbone).

postclimac'teric. Following the termination of the reproductive period.

postco'itus. The time immediately or soon after coitus (sexual intercourse).

postcom'missure. Posterior commissure of the brain; see under commissure.

postcommissurotomy syndrome. Fever, chest pains, and inflammation of the pericardium and pleura, occurring suddenly, within a few weeks, in patients who have undergone surgery of the heart valves.

postencephalit'ic. Occurring after encephalitis.

poste'rior. 1. Located behind a structure. **2.** Relating to the back or dorsal side of the human body.

posterior inferior cerebellar artery occlusion syndrome. Syndrome occurring in occlusion of the posterior inferior cerebellar artery; symptoms include muscular weakness and loss of pain and temperature senses of the face, soft palate, pharynx, and larynx on the same side as the lesion, associated with loss of pain and temperature sensations of the extremities and trunk on the side opposite the lesion; also called Wallenberg's syndrome.

posteroante'rior. From the back to the front.

posterolat'eral. Behind and to one side.

posterome'dial. Behind and to the inner side.

postganglion'ic. Situated behind or distal to a ganglion.

postgastrectomy syndrome. See dumping syndrome.

pos'thioplasty. Plastic surgery of the prepuce.

posthi'tis. Inflammation of the prepuce; also called acrobystitis.

postic'tal. Following a convulsion.

postmatu'rity. Condition in which the fetus remains in the uterus in excess of three weeks after the calculated date of birth.

postmenopau'sal. Relating to the period after the menopause.

postmor'tem. Pertaining to or occurring after death.

postmyocardial infarction syndrome. Fever and pericarditis often accompanied by pleuritis occurring a week or more after a myocardial infarction.

postna'sal. Behind the nasal cavity.

postna'tal. After birth.

postop'erative. Occurring after a surgical operation.

postpar'tum. Pertaining to or occurring after childbirth.

postpericardiot'omy. Occurring after surgery that involved cutting through the pericardium (two-layer membrane enveloping the heart).

postpericardiotomy syndrome. An unusual complication of heart surgery in which there is a delayed pericardial or pleural reaction characterized by fever, pleuropericarditis, chest pain, and raised erthrocyte sedimentation; also called postcardiotiomy syndrome.

postphlebitic syndrome. Chronic swelling of the leg, pain, and dermatitis secondary to stagnation of blood in the veins.

postpran'dial. After a meal.

postpu'bertal. Of or occurring during the period immediately after puberty.

postsynap'tic. 1. The time immediately following the transmission of an impulse from one neuron to another; occurring right after the crossing of a synapse. **2.** Situated distal to a synapse.

post-traumat'ic. Occurring after an injury or resulting from it.

pos'tulate. An unproved assertion.

 Koch's p.'s., to prove that a microorganism is the cause of a specific disease, it must be present in all cases of the disease, inoculations of its pure culture most produce the same disease in animals, and from these it must be obtained in pure cultures and propagated.

pos'ture. Way of bearing one's body.

postvac'cinal. After vaccination.

pot. A shortened version of the Mexican Indian word *potaguaya* meaning marijuana.

po'table. Fit to drink; drinkable.

potas'sium. A soft alkaline metallic element; symbol K (kalium), atomic number 19, atomic weight 39.10; it plays an important physiologic role in muscular contraction, conduction of nerve impulses, enzyme action, and cell membrane function; normal potassium concentration of extracellular fluid is between 3.5 and 5 mEq/liter.

 p. chloride, a colorless crystalline solid or powder, KCl; used in the treatment of potassium deficiency.

 p. iodide, a crystalline powder, KI; soluble in water and used medicinally as a source of iodine.

 p. nitrate, KNO_3; a translucent, crystalline compound; also called niter and saltpeter.

 p. permanaganate, a dark purple crystalline compound, $KMnO_4$; used as an antiseptic and deodorizing agent; also called purple salt.

potas'sium-42 (^{42}K). An artificial isotope used as a tracer in studies of potassium distribution in body fluid compartments.

po'tency. 1. The quality of being potent; strength. **2.** The comparative expression of drug activity relating to the dose required to produce a specific effect of given intensity as compared to a standard of reference. **3.** Inherent ability for growth and development.

 sexual p., ability of a male to perform sexually.

po'tent. 1. Powerful. **2.** Capable of producing a particular physiologic or chemical effect of strong intensity. **3.** Possessing sexual potency.

poten'tia. Latin for potency.

poten'tial. 1. Capable of doing or being, but not yet realized. **2.** The force necessary to drive a unit positive charge from one point in an electrical field to another; the electromotive force which drives a current from one point to another.

 action p., the electric current developed in a nerve, muscle, or other excitable tissue during its activity.

 dark p. of the eye, see resting potential of the eye.

 demarcation p., see injury potential.

 excitatory postsynaptic p. (EPSP), the change in potential seen in the postsynaptic membrane when an impulse which has an excitatory influence arrives at the synapse; a local change in the direction of depolarization.

 inhibitory postsynaptic p. (IPSP), the change in potential seen in the postsynaptic membrane when an impulse which has an inhibitory influence arrives at the synapse; a local change in the direction of hyperpolarizaton.

 injury p., the potential developed between the injured and uninjured parts of a nerve, due to the exposure of the negatively charged inner surface of the polarized membrane at the site of injury; also called demarcation potential.

 membrane p., the difference in potential between

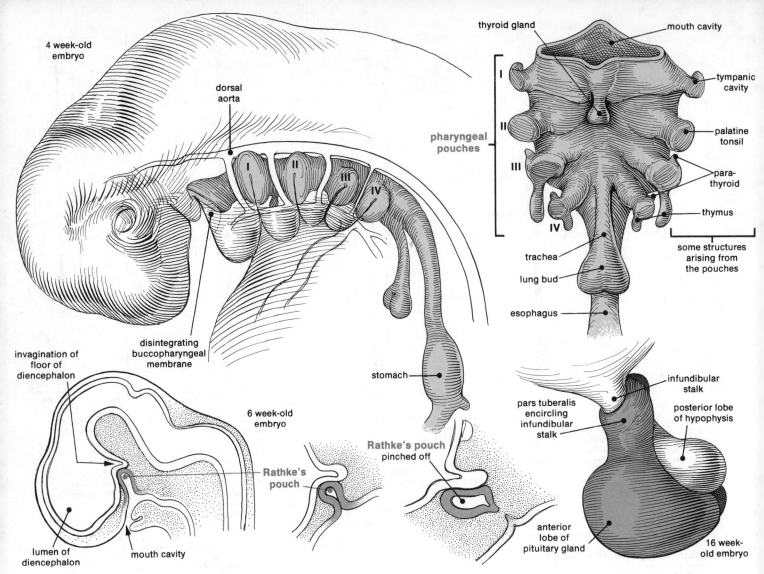

4 week-old embryo

dorsal aorta

pharyngeal pouches

thyroid gland

mouth cavity

tympanic cavity

palatine tonsil

para-thyroid

thymus

some structures arising from the pouches

trachea

lung bud

esophagus

disintegrating buccopharyngeal membrane

stomach

6 week-old embryo

invagination of floor of diencephalon

Rathke's pouch

Rathke's pouch pinched off

infundibular stalk

posterior lobe of hypophysis

pars tuberalis encircling infundibular stalk

anterior lobe of pituitary gland

16 week-old embryo

lumen of diencephalon

mouth cavity

the two sides of a cell membrane, especially of nerve or muscle fibers; the outside is positive in contrast to the inside.

oxidation-reduction p., the relative potential, in volts, exerted by an inert (nonreacting) metallic electrode in a solution, as measured against that exerted by a normal hydrogen electrode at absolute temperature; the potential difference between an inert electrode and a reversible oxidation-reduction system in which it is submerged; also called redox potential.

redox p., see oxidation-reduction potential.

resting p. of the eye, the direct current potential difference between the anterior pole of the eye (cornea) and the posterior one (retina); usually expressed in millivolts; also called dark potential of the eye.

visual evoked p., the potential as measured from electroencephalographic recordings taken from the occipital scalp area as the subject fixates a light flashing at 1/4-second intervals; the computer averages the response of 100 consecutive flashes.

potentia'tion. The increase in the power of an activity, such as in the force of the contraction of a muscle; the term is frequently used improperly in reference to drug interaction as a synonym of synergism.

potentiom'eter. Instrument for measuring precisely electromotive forces.

po'tion. A large liquid dose, especially of medicine.

Pott's disease. Tuberculous spondylitis; see under spondylitis.

pouch. A sac or pocket-like space.

Douglas' p., rectouterine pouch.

Hartmann's p., a dilatation at the neck of the gallbladder.

Heidenhain p., one made for the experimental study of gastric secretions; an isolated part of the stomach, with the nervous supply interrupted, is opened to the outside through the abdominal wall.

Pavlov p., one made for the study of gastric secretions; an isolated part of the stomach, with the nervous supply left intact, is opened to the outside through an opening in the abdominal wall.

pharyngeal p.'s, paired lateral pouches of the embryonic pharynx; each pouch is in close relationship to an aortic arch and is situated opposite a branchial cleft.

Rathke's p., in embryology, the outpocketing of the stomodeum (embryonic mouth) occurring when the embryo is about three weeks old and subsequently forming the anterior (glandular) lobe of the hypophysis; also called craniobuccal or neurobuccal pouch.

rectouterine p., the pocket-like space between the uterus and the rectum; also called Douglas' pouch.

rectovesical p., the pouch between the rectum and the bladder in the male.

uterovesical p., the pouch between the bladder and the uterus.

poul'tice. A hot, moist, soft mass of bread meal, linseed, or any other cohesive substance, applied to the skin between two pieces of muslin to soothe, relax, or stimulate an aching or inflamed part of the body.

pound. A unit of weight equal to 16 ounces (avoirdupois weight) or 12 ounces (apothecaries' weight).

po'vidone. See polyvinylpyrrolidone.

pow'der. 1. In pharmaceutics, a mixture of dry, fine particles. **2.** A single dose of such a powder, enclosed in paper.

Seidlitz p.'s, a mild laxative composed of sodium bicarbonate, tartaric acid, and potassium sodium tartrate.

talcum p., a fine, soft toilet powder of perfumed talc.

pow'er. 1. The ability or capacity to produce effectively. **2.** In optics, the refractive vergence of a lens. **3.** Might.

back vertex p., the vergence power of a lens as measured from surface toward eye; standard for measurement of ophthalmic lenses.

focal p., see vergence power.

refractive p., the vergence power of a refracting optical system.

resolving p., a measure of the ability of a lens to image closely spaced objects so that they are recognized as separate objects; calculated by dividing the wavelength of the light used by twice the numerical aperture of the objective.

vergence p., the capability of an optical system to change the vergence of a cylinder of rays; also called focal power.

pox. 1. Any disease characterized by purulent eruptions on the skin. **2.** A colloquial term for syphilis.

poxvi'ruses. The largest and most complex of all DNA viruses infecting man; they multiply in the cytoplasm of cells (unlike other DNA viruses) and cause smallpox, alastrim, and molluscum contagiosum.

PP. Abbreviation for pyrophosphate.

ppa. Abbreviation for Latin *phiala prius agitate*.

PPD. Abbreviation for purified protein derivation.

P-Pf. Abbreviation for pellagra-preventing factor.

PPLO. Abbreviation for pleuropneumonia-like organisms.

ppm. Abbreviation for parts per million.

ppt. Abbreviation for precipitate.

P-pulmonale. In electrocardiography, the P-wave pattern characteristic of cor pulmonale; a tall peaked P wave, usually seen in leads II, III, and AVF.

Pr. 1. Abbreviation for presbyopia. **2.** Chemical symbol of the element praseodymium.

p.r. Abbreviation for per rectum.

prac'tice. 1. The exercise of a profession or occupation. **2.** To engage in, especially as a profession. **3.** Collective term for the patients of a physician.

practitioner. One who exercises a profession.

pragmatagno'sia. Loss of the power of recogniz-

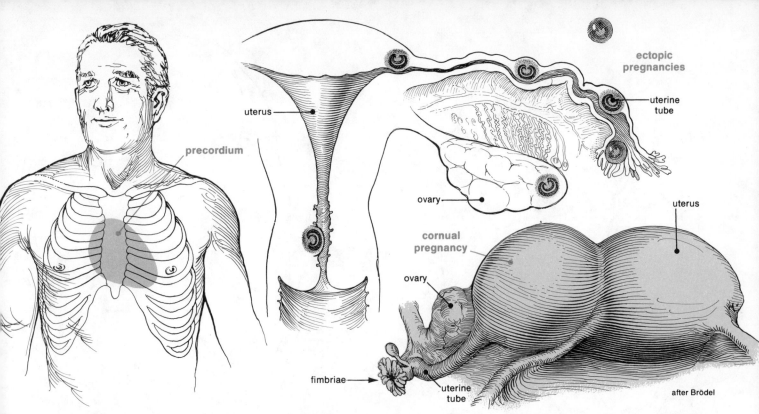

precordium

uterus

ectopic pregnancies

uterine tube

ovary

cornual pregnancy

ovary

uterus

fimbriae

uterine tube

after Brödel

ing objects formerly known to the individual.

praseodym'ium. A soft, silvery, rare-earth element; symbol Pr, atomic number 59, atomic weight 140.907.

praxiol'ogy. The study of behavior or conduct.

pre-. Prefix denoting before, in time or space.

preag'onal, preagon'ic. Preceding the act of dying.

prealbu'min. A protein constituent of plasma, so named because its mobility is greater than that of albumin (at the alkaline pH values used for electrophoresis).

 thyroxine-binding p., one of the three carrier proteins of thyroxine in plasma.

prea'nal. In front of the anus.

preanesthet'ic. Before anesthesia; a medication administered to facilitate the subsequent induction of general anesthesia.

preauric'ular. Situated in front of the auricle of the ear.

precan'cerous. Subject to malignancy; said of a tumor.

precip'itant. Anything that causes the chemical separation of a solid from a solution.

precip'itate. 1. To cause a substance in solution to separate and form a solid deposit. **2.** The solid deposit thus formed. **3.** Occurring abnormally quickly, as a precipitate labor.

precipita'tion. 1. The act of separating a solid held in suspension or solution. **2.** The clumping of protein in serum caused by the action of a specific precipitin.

precip'itin. An antibody that reacts specifically with a soluble antigen to cause a precipitate.

preclin'ical. 1. Occurring before the onset of disease; referring to the stage of a disorder before clinical symptoms can be recognized and diagnosed. **2.** Occurring before clinical work; referring to medical training that usually takes place during the first two years.

preco'cious. Characterized by unusually early physical or mental maturity.

preco'city. Unusually early development, physical or mental.

 sexual p., a complex condition characterized by premature development and maturation of genital organs and secondary sexual characteristics.

precogni'tion. Extrasensory perception of an event not yet experienced.

precon'scious. In psychoanalysis, thoughts and ideas that can be recalled by conscious effort.

preconvul'sive. Preceding a convulsion.

precor'dial. Relating to the area of the chest over the heart.

precor'dium. Antecardium; the area of the chest

wall which corresponds to the location of the heart.

precos'tal. In front of the ribs.

precu'neus. A lobule on the mesial surface of each cerebral hemisphere located between the cuneus and paracentral lobules.

precur'sor. Anything in the course of a process that is the forerunner or precedes a later stage, as a premalignant lesion, or as a physiologically inactive substance that is converted to an active substance such as a hormone or enzyme.

prediabe'tes. An early stage in the course of diabetes before there is any recognizable impairment of carbohydrate metabolism.

predias'tole. The interval in the cardiac rhythm cycle just preceding the diastole; also called late systole.

prediges'tion. Artificial initiation of the digestive process in protein and starch before they are used therapeutically as food.

predispose'. To render susceptible or liable.

predisposi'tion. The state of being predisposed or susceptible to a disease; a special tendency or inclination toward a disease.

prednis'olone. A synthetic glucocorticoid; white bitter crystals, soluble in water; used as a cortisone substitute.

pred'nisone. A synthetic glucocorticoid; white bitter crystals, insoluble in water; used as a cortisone substitute, as it produces less water retention.

predor'mitum, predormi'tion. The state of waning consciousness which precedes sound sleep.

preeclamp'sia. Toxemia of pregnancy in which convulsions have not occurred. See also toxemia.

preemy. Informal term for premature infant.

preexcita'tion. Premature activation of the ventricular myocardium by a supraventricular impulse which bypasses the normal A-V conduction pathway; an intrinsic part of the Wolff-Parkinson-White syndrome.

preexcitation syndrome. See Wolff-Parkinson-White syndrome.

prefron'tal. Located in the anterior part of the frontal lobe or region of the brain.

preganglion'ic. Situated before or proximal to a ganglion.

preg'nancy. The period of time between conception and birth of the child; the normal duration of pregnancy is about 280 days or nine calendar months; also called gestation.

 abdominal p., development of the impregnated ovum in the abdominal cavity resulting from an early rupture of a tubal pregnancy.

 cervical p., a rare form of ectopic pregnancy resulting from implantation of the fertilized ovum in the lining of the cervix.

 cornual p., rare ectopic pregnancy, usually occurring in women with a double uterus, in which the fertilized ovum implants in a (usually rudimentary) uterine horn.

 ectopic p., one resulting from implantation of the fertilized ovum in a site other than the normal one in the uterine cavity, i.e., the interstitial portion of the uterine tube and the cervix as well as the ovary, the uterine tube, and the abdominal cavity.

 extrauterine p., one occurring outside the cavity of the uterus.

 false p., a spurious pregnancy.

 interstitial p., one resulting from implantation of the fertilized ovum in the portion of the uterine tube which pierces the wall of the uterus.

 multiple p., the simultaneous presence of two or more developing fetuses.

 ovarian p., a rare form of ectopic pregnancy in which the impregnated ovum develops in the ovary; also called oothecocyesis.

 spurious p., the presence of symptoms of pregnancy without the occurrence of conception, usually occurring in women nearing menopause or in young women with an intense desire to be pregnant; also called pseudocyesis and false or phantom pregnancy.

 tubal p., implantation and development of the fertilized ovum in a uterine tube.

preg'nane. A saturated steroid hydrocarbon, derivative of cholane; a precursor of progesterone and several adrenocortical hormones.

pregnan'ediol. $C_{21}H_{36}O_2$; the main metabolic end product of progesterone; its concentration in the urine is an indicator of corpus luteum function.

pregnan'etriol. A precursor in the biosynthesis of cortisol.

preg'nant. Carrying a developing offspring within the body; also called gravid.

preg'nene. An unsaturated steroid derivative of pregnane.

prehen'sile. Adapted for grasping.

prehor'mone. An inactive glandular secretion capable of being converted into an active hormone.

preic'tal. Before a convulsion or stroke.

preinfarction syndrome. The sudden onset or worsening of angina pectoris prior to myocardial infarction.

preleuke'mia. A defect of cellular differentiation and maturation that precedes the onset of diagnosable acute leukemia as a primary maturational disturbance.

pre'load. The stretch imposed on the heart muscle due to the ventricular and diastolic volume; also called venous return.

preluxa'tion. Forward dislocation.

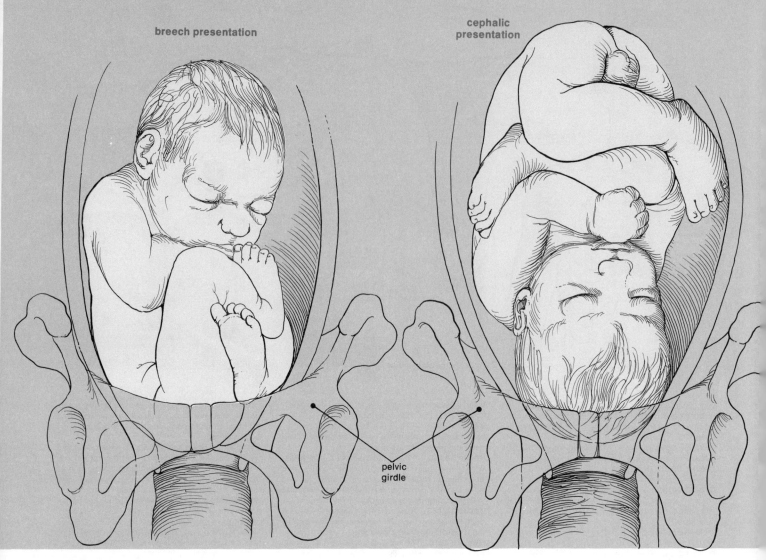

breech presentation

cephalic presentation

pelvic girdle

premalig'nant. Preceding malignancy; also called precancerous.

premature'. Occurring prior to correct or expected time.

premature infant. See infant, premature.

prematu'rity. The state of being premature.

pre'med. An abbreviated version for premedical, or premedical student.

premedica'tion. A drug or drugs administered prior to a general anesthetic to allay apprehension and produce sedation.

premel'anosome. All particulate stages in the maturation of melanosomes.

premenar'chal. Taking place or existing prior to the onset of menstruation.

premen'strual. Denoting the time of month prior to the menstrual flow.

premenstrual syndrome. The occurrence of all or some of the following symptoms two or three days before the menstrual flow: lumbar and low abdominal pain, nervous irritability, headache, tenderness of the breasts, and pelvic congestion.

premo'lar. A bicuspid tooth.

premuni'tion. Immunity established against a particular microorganism by infection (in a chronic form) with another related organism.

prena'ris, *pl.* **prena'res.** Nostril.

prena'tal. Prior to birth.

preop'erative. Prior to an operation.

prepal'lium. The cerebral cortex in front of the central sulcus (fissure of Rolando).

prepara'tion. 1. Readiness. **2.** A substance, such as medicine, prepared for a particular purpose. **3.** The reduction of a natural tooth in order to be able to receive a prosthesis, such as a crown.

  cavity p., the removal of caries from a tooth and the establishment of a cavity that is able to receive and retain a restoration.

  depot p., a drug whose physical state is altered so that it can be absorbed over an extended period of time; e.g., special microcrystalline suspensions of penicillin.

prepatel'lar. In front of the kneecap (patella).

prepu'berty. The phase immediately preceding puberty.

pre'puce. The loose fold of skin that partly or completely covers the glans penis; it is this tissue which is removed by circumcision; also called foreskin.

  p. of clitoris, a fold of the labia minora that forms a cap over the clitoris.

preputiot'omy. Surgical incision of the prepuce (foreskin) of the penis, usually to relieve tightness (phimosis).

prere'nal. Located in front of a kidney.

prerenal azothemia. See azothemia, prerenal.

presbycu'sis. Progressive loss of hearing occurring in old age.

presbyo'pia. Diminution of accommodation power in the eyes due to advancing age; commonly known as old sight.

prescribe'. To recommend a remedy in the treatment of a disorder.

prescrip'tion. A written instruction by a licensed health science practitioner for the preparation and administration of any remedy, such as medication or corrective lenses.

  shotgun p., a drug prescription containing many ingredients, given with the hope that one or more of them may be effective; also called blunderbuss prescription.

presenil'ity. 1. Premature old age. **2.** Period immediately preceding old age.

present'. To appear first; said of the part of the fetus that is felt by the examining finger.

presenta'tion. The position of the fetus in the uterus during labor with respect to the birth canal.

  breech p., presentation of the pelvic extremity, known as (1) frank breech presentation when the legs of the fetus extend over the anterior surface of its body, (2) full breech presentation when the fetal thighs and legs are flexed, and (3) foot or footling presentation when one or both feet are the presenting parts.

  cephalic p., one in which the head is the presenting part, known as (1) vertex presentation when the fetal head is flexed with its chin and thorax in contact, (2) sincipital presentation when the large fontanel is the presenting part, (3) brow presentation when the fetal brow is the presenting part, and (4) face presentation when the face is the presenting part; also called head presentation.

  head p., see cephalic presentation.

  placental p., see placenta previa.

  shoulder p., presentation in which the long axis of the fetus lies transversely with the maternal long axis and a shoulder is the presenting part.

preser'vative. 1. A substance added to food products, such as fatty acids, for inhibiting the growth of food-spoiling bacteria. **2.** Capable of preserving.

preso'mite. In embryology, before the appearance of somites.

pres'sor. Causing constriction of blood vessels and a rise in blood pressure; said of certain substances and nerve fibers.

pressorecep'tor. See baroreceptor.

pres'sure. A force applied or acting against resistance.

  atmospheric p., the pressure exerted by the atmosphere; approximately 15 pounds per square inch at sea level, capable of supporting a column of mercury 760 millimeters high; also called standard pressure.

  back p., pressure exerted in the circulatory system resulting from obstruction to flow.

  blood p., the pressure of the circulating blood on the walls of the arteries, primarily maintained by the contraction of the left ventricle, the resistance of the arterioles and capillaries, the elasticity of the arte-

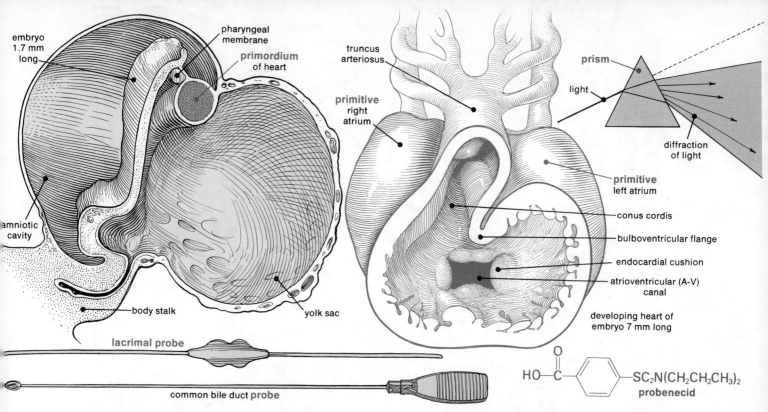

embryo 1.7 mm long

pharyngeal membrane

primordium of heart

amniotic cavity

body stalk

yolk sac

truncus arteriosus

primitive right atrium

primitive left atrium

conus cordis

bulboventricular flange

endocardial cushion

atrioventricular (A-V) canal

developing heart of embryo 7 mm long

prism

light

diffraction of light

lacrimal probe

common bile duct probe

$$HO-\overset{\overset{\displaystyle O}{\|}}{C}-\!\!\!\!\!\bigcirc\!\!\!\!\!-SC_2N(CH_2CH_2CH_3)_2$$

probenecid

rial walls, and the volume and viscosity of the blood; the maximum or systolic blood pressure occurs at the moment of systole of the left ventricle of the heart; the minimum or diastolic blood pressure occurs during diastole of the ventricle; the upper limits of normal in adults are generally set at 140/90 mm Hg.

cerebrospinal p., tension of the cerebrospinal fluid, normally 100 to 150 millimeters of water (with individual lying on one side).

critical p., the pressure required to condense or liquefy a gas at the critical temperature.

diastolic p., arterial pressure during diastole; see blood pressure.

effective osmotic p., the portion of the total osmotic pressure of a solution that regulates the tendency of its solvent to pass through a boundary, such as a semipermeable membrane.

hyperbaric p., pressure higher than normal atmospheric pressure; used in therapy for shock, carbon dioxide poisoning, clostridial infections, and for some operations.

intracranial p., (ICP), pressure within the skull.

intraocular p., the pressure of the fluid within the eye; (measured by a tonometer, usually in millimeters of mercury).

intrapulmonic p., the pressure of air within the lungs.

negative p., a pressure lower than that of ambient atmosphere.

occlusal p., any force exerted upon the occlusal surfaces of teeth.

oncotic p., osmotic pressure exerted by colloids in solution.

osmotic p., pressure or stress exerted by dissolved substances on a semipermeable membrane which separates a solution from the pure solvent.

partial p., the portion of the total pressure exerted by each component of a gas mixture, expressed in millimeters of mercury (mmHg).

pulse p., the difference between the systolic (maximum) and diastolic (minimum) blood pressures within an artery during the cardiac cycle; it normally varies between 30 and 50 mmHg.

systolic p., arterial pressure during systole; see blood pressure.

vapor p., the pressure exerted by the molecules of a vapor in equilibrium with its solid or liquid phase.

wedge p., intravascular pressure determined by positioning a catheter in branches of the pulmonary or hepatic venous system; the pressure thus obtained is felt to be a close reflection of pressure at the other end of the capillary bed and helps define the site of increased pressures across either of the two organs.

presynap'tic. 1. Existing or taking place before the synapse is crossed. **2.** Situated proximal to a synapse.

presys'tole. The interval immediately preceding the systole.

presystol'ic. Occurring immediately before the systole.

pretib'ial. Pertaining to the front of the leg, especially that portion in front of the tibia.

prev'alence. The number of people with a specific condition in a given population.

preven'tive. Acting to ward off or hinder the occurrence of something such as a disease.

prever'tebral. In front of a vertebra or of the vertebral column.

preves'ical. In front of the bladder.

pre'vius. Latin for in the way; usually applied to anything that obstructs the birth canal during childbirth. See also placenta previa.

pri'apism. A continuous and pathologic erection of the penis without sexual desire; usually associated with general disorders, especially sickle cell anemia.

priapi'tis. Inflammation of the penis.

pri'macy. The state of being first in importance or in a sequence.

pri'ma fa'cie. Latin for on first appearance.

primaquine phosphate. Bitter, orange crystals, soluble in water; used in the treatment of malaria.

pri'mary. 1. Being first in a sequence or importance. **2.** The simplest or most primitive form.

primary aldosteronism. See aldosteronism, primary.

pri'mate. A member of the order Primates.

Prima'tes. The highest order of mammals, including man and those animals, such as apes, monkeys, and lemurs, nearest him in physical characteristics; from Latin *primus,* meaning first.

primigrav'ida. A woman in her first pregnancy; also called unigravida.

primip'ara. A woman who has completed one pregnancy to the stage of viability, regardless of whether it was a single or multiple birth, or whether the fetus was live or stillborn.

prim'itive. Primary, embryonic.

primor'dial. 1. Relating to the embryonic group of cells that develops into an organ or structure. **2.** Formed during the early stage of development.

primor'dium. 1. The earliest cells forming an organ in the embryo. **2.** Anlage.

prin'ceps. Latin for chief, principal; applied to certain arteries.

prin'ciple. 1. A fundamental concept. **2.** The essential ingredient characteristic of a drug or chemical compound.

active p., the constituent of a drug to which its

physiologic effect is due.

antianemic p., substance (chiefly found in liver) that stimulates remission of symptoms in pernicious anemia.

Fick p., principle utilized in measurement of cardiac output and blood flow to some organs.

hematinic p., vitamin B_{12}.

pleasure p., in psychoanalytic theory, the concept that man instinctively tries to avoid pain and discomfort, and endeavors to obtain gratification and pleasure.

reality p., in psychoanalytic theory, the concept that the pleasure principle is normally modified in personality development by the demands of the external world; e.g., postponement of gratification to a more appropriate time.

Starling p., the principle that the exchange of fluids across capillary membranes is governed by the net difference between the hydrostatic and osmotic pressures.

prism. A transparent body, usually made of optical glass or crystalline material, with at least two polished plane faces inclined toward each other from which light is reflected or through which light is refracted.

p.r.n. Abbreviation for Latin *pro re nata*.

pro-. Prefix meaning before.

Pro. Symbol for the amino acid proline or its radical forms.

proaccel'erin. See factor V.

probabil'ity. Likelihood; the ratio of the likelihood of occurrence of a specific event to total events.

probacter'iophage. See prophage.

pro'band. See propositus.

pro'bang. A long, slender, flexible rod with a tuft of sponge or some other soft material at the end; used chiefly in removing obstructions from the esophagus or larynx.

probe. A slender metal rod with a blunt tip, used to explore bodily cavities or wounds.

lacrimal p., a probe, usually made of silver, that can be passed into the upper and lower puncta of the eyelids, through the upper and lower canaliculi, and down the nasolacrimal duct into the nose.

proben'ecid. An agent that enhances the excretion of uric acid by inhibiting its reabsorption by the kidney; also inhibits excretion of penicillin by the kidney; Benemid®.

prob'lem. 1. Any situation that presents difficulty or uncertainty. **2.** In psychiatry, term often used to denote a person whose behavior deviates from the norm; e.g., problem child; sometimes used in preference to the terms behavior disorder or mental disorder.

pressure | problem

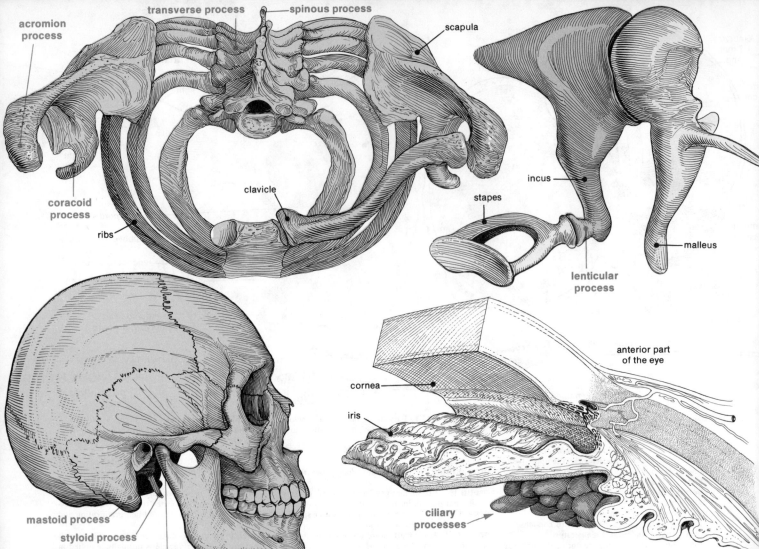

acromion process

transverse process — spinous process

scapula

coracoid process

ribs

clavicle

incus

stapes

malleus

lenticular process

mastoid process

styloid process

condylar process of mandible

anterior part of the eye

cornea

iris

ciliary processes

probos′cis, pl. **probos′cises.** A tubular structure located near the oral cavity of certain insects and worms, often associated with feeding and used as a means of attachment.

procainamide hydrochloride. White crystals, soluble in water; a cardiac depressant used in treating ventricular arrhythmias.

procaine hydrochloride. A frequently used local anesthetic, $C_{13}H_{20}O_2N_2 \cdot HCl$; Novocaine®.

procar′yote. Any simple unicellular organism that does not have a nuclear membrane, membrane-bound organelles, and characteristic ribosomes; e.g., bacteria and blue-green algae.

proce′dure. A manner of effecting something.

cataract operative p., any of several operations to remove a cataractous lens.

procer′coid. The larval stage of certain tapeworms, occurring in the intermediate host.

process. 1. A marked prominence extending from an anatomic structure, usually for the attachment of muscles and ligaments. 2. A series of actions that attain a result.

acromion p., the outer end of the spine of the scapula overhanging the glenoid fossa.

articular p. of vertebra, one of the small projections on the upper and lower surfaces of the vertebra, forming the vertebral joint; the surface is coated with hyaline cartilage.

ciliary p.'s, radiating pigmented ridges (from 60 to 80) on the inner surface of the ciliary body of the eye; formed by the inward folding of the various layers of the choroid.

clinoid p., one of three pairs of extensions from the sphenoid bone of the skull.

condylar p. of the mandible, the articular process of the ramus of the mandible and the constricted portion (neck) that supports it.

coracoid p., a thick, curved bony projection from the scapula (shoulder blade) overhanging the glenoid fossa; it provides attachment for muscles and ligaments.

dendritic p., see dendrite.

hamulus p., hamulus.

lenticular p., a right angle extension of the long limb of the incus bone of the middle ear; it articulates with the stapes.

mastoid p., a conical downward projection of the mastoid part of the temporal bone of the skull; situated behind the ear with the apex on a level with the lobe of the auricle; it serves for the attachment of the sternocleidomastoid muscle, the splenius muscle of the head, and the longissimus muscle of the head.

odontoid p., a toothlike process of the second cervical vertebra (axis) that articulates with the first cervical vertebra (atlas).

primary p., a type of thinking characterized by the lack of any sense of time, and the use of allusion, analogy, and symbolic representation; also called nonlogical thinking.

pterygoid p., a long process extending downward from the junction of the body and great wing of the sphenoid bone on either side; it consists of a medial and lateral plate, the upper parts of which are fused together.

secondary p., a type of thinking controlled by the laws that govern conscious (or preconscious) mental activity.

spinous p., the dorsal projection of the vertebra from the junction of the laminae, forming, with those of other vertebrae, the spine.

styloid p., a slender, pointed projection extending downward and slightly forward from the petrous portion of the temporal bone; it gives attachment to the styloglossus, stylohyoid, and stylopharyngeus muscles, and the stylohoid and stylomandibular ligaments.

transverse p., a lateral projection present on each side of a vertebra.

trochlear p., a projection from the lateral side of

the calcaneus bone of the foot between the tendons of the long and short peroneal muscles.

xiphoid p., xiphoid cartilage at the lower end of the sternum (breastbone).

zygomatic p. of maxillary bone, a rough triangular eminence from the maxilla that articulates with the zygomatic bone.

zygomatic p. of temporal bone, a long arch projecting from the temporal bone that articulates with the temporal process of the zygomatic bone to form the zygomatic arch.

prochlorper′azine. Phenothiazine compound used as a tranquilizer and to relieve nausea and vomiting; Compazine®.

prochon′dral. Relating to the stage preceding the development of cartilage.

prochor′dal. Anterior to the notochord.

prociden′tia. Complete prolapse of an organ.

procol′lagen. A precursor of collagen.

proconver′tin. See factor VII.

pro′create. To produce offspring.

proct-. See procto-.

proctal′gia, proctag′ra. Pain in the rectum or in and around the anus; also called proctodynia.

p. fuga, acute spasmodic pain of only a few minutes' duration in the rectum; occurring in young men usually at night.

proctatre′sia. Imperforation of the anus.

protecta′sia. Dilatation of the anus or rectum.

proctec′tomy. Removal of the rectum.

proctenclei′sis, proctencli′sia. Stricture of the anus or rectum.

procti′tis. Inflammation of the rectum.

procto-, proct-. Combining forms indicating a relationship to the anus or, more frequently, the rectum.

proc′tocele. See rectocele.

proctoc′lysis, proctoc′lysia. Continuous, slow infusion of saline solution into the rectum and colon.

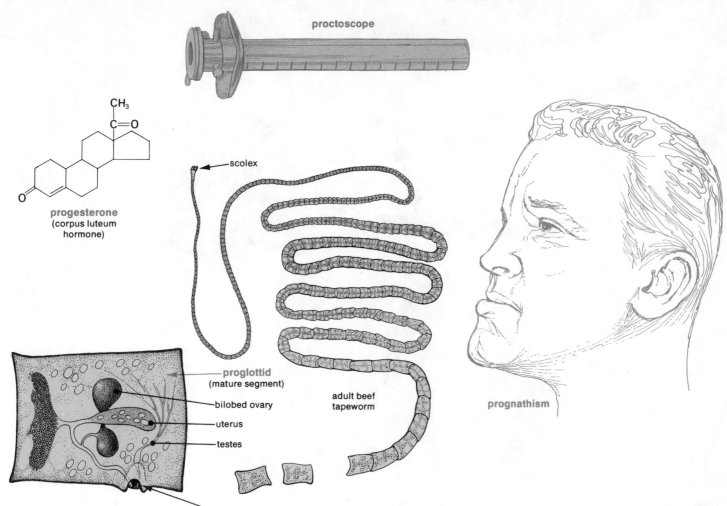

proctoscope

progesterone
(corpus luteum
hormone)

scolex

proglottid
(mature segment)

bilobed ovary

uterus

testes

adult beef
tapeworm

prognathism

common genital pore

proctocoli′tis. See coloproctitis.

proctocolonos′copy. Examination of the rectum and colon.

proctocolpoplas′ty. Surgical closure of a rectovaginal fistula.

proctocys′tocele. Bulging of the bladder into the rectum.

proctocystot′omy. The incising of the bladder from the rectum.

proctode′um. The hollowed ectodermal surface located beneath the tail of the fetus; it rapidly depresses toward the cloaca and comes in contact with the outer surface of the cloacal wall.

proctodyn′ia. See proctalgia.

proctolog′ic. Of or relating to proctology.

proctol′ogist. A specialist in proctology.

proctol′ogy. The branch of medicine concerned with the study of the rectum and anus and the treatment of their diseases.

proctome′nia. Vicarious menstruation involving the rectum.

proctoparal′ysis. Paralysis of the anus, resulting in fecal incontinence.

proctoperine′oplasty. Plastic surgery of the anus and perineum; also called rectoperineorrhaphy.

proc′topexy. Surgical fixation of a prolapsed rectum by suturing to another part; also called rectopexy.

proc′toplasty. Plastic surgery of the anus or rectum; also called rectoplasty.

proctople′gia. Paralysis of the muscles of the rectum and anus.

proctopto′sia, proctopto′sis. Prolapse of the rectum and anus.

proctorrha′gia. Bloody discharge from the rectum.

proctor′rhaphy. Suturing of a lacerated rectum or anus.

proctorrhe′a. Mucous discharge from the rectum.

proc′toscope. Instrument used for inspecting the rectum; a speculum; also called rectoscope.

proctos′copy. Examination of the rectum with a proctoscope.

proctosigmoidec′tomy. Surgical removal of the rectum and sigmoid colon.

proctosigmoidi′tis. Inflammation of the rectum and sigmoid colon.

proctosigmoidos′copy. Examination of the interior of the rectum and sigmoid by means of a sigmoidoscope.

proc′tospasm. Spasmodic contraction of the rectum or anus.

proc′tostat. A tube containing radium for insertion through the anus in the treatment of cancer of the rectum.

proctosteno′sis. Abnormal narrowing of the rectum or anus; also called rectostenosis.

proctos′tomy. The establishment of a permanent opening into the rectum.

proctot′omy. Surgical incision of the anus or rectum.

proctovalvot′omy. Incision of rectal valves.

procum′bent. Lying face down.

pro′dromal. Relating to prodrome.

pro′drome. An early symptom of a disease, as one seen before the rash of a communicable disease.

prod′uct. Any substance produced, naturally or artificially.

   cleavage p., substance resulting from the splitting of large molecules into simpler ones.

   fission p., atomic species resulting from the splitting of large atoms.

produc′tive. Denoting an inflammatory condition leading to the formation of new tissue.

proenceph′alon. See prosencephalon.

proen′zyme. The inactive precursor of an enzyme that requires some change to render it active; e.g., profibrolysin; also called zymogen.

proeryth′roblast. The earliest red blood cell pre-

cursor, generally 12 to 19 μ in diameter; characterized by scanty, basophilic cytoplasm without hemoglobin, and a nucleus having fine chromatin; also called pronormoblast and rubriblast.

proery′throcyte. The precursor of a red blood cell; an immature erythrocyte with a nucleus.

profun′dus, pl. **profun′da.** Latin for deep; applied to certain anatomic structures.

progen′ital. On the exposed surface of the external genitalia.

proge′ria. Premature senility or old age.

progesta′tional. 1. Conducive to pregnancy. **2.** Referring to progesterone.

proges′terone. A hormone produced in the ovary by the corpus luteum; it stimulates changes in the wall of the uterus in preparation for implantation of the fertilized ovum.

proges′tin. 1. A hormone of the corpus luteum that acts on the lining of the uterus (endometrium). **2.** General term for any synthetic drug providing such action.

proges′togen. An agent that produces effects similar to those of progesterone.

proglos′sis. The tip of the tongue.

proglot′tid. One of the segments of the tapeworm which contains both male and female reproductive organs; in a mature proglottid, ovules are produced and fertilized hermaphroditically.

prognath′ic. See prognathous.

prog′nathism. Abnormal forward projection of the lower jaw.

prog′nathous. Having a projecting lower jaw; also called prognathic.

prognose′. To predict the probable course and outcome of a disease; also called prognosticate.

progno′sis. A prediction of the outcome of a disease.

prognos′ticate. Prognose; to give a prognosis.

program, quality assurance. A program designed to insure the quality of patient care within a

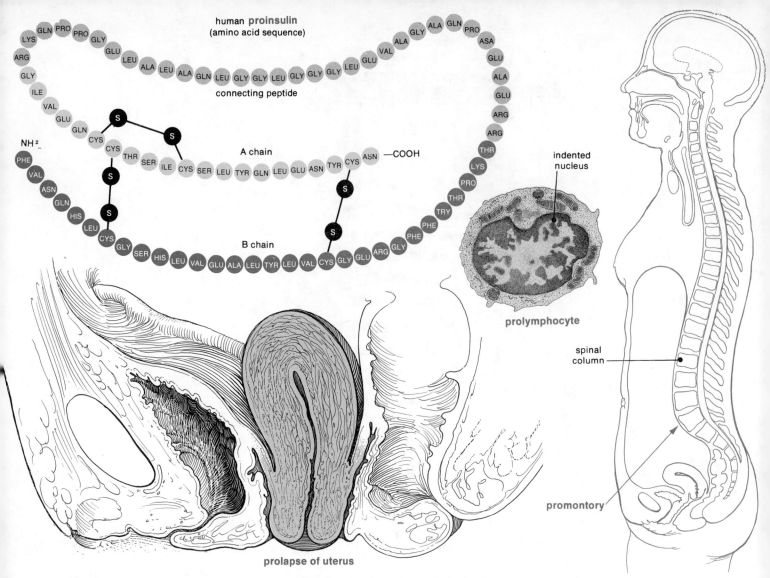

human **proinsulin**
(amino acid sequence)

connecting peptide

A chain

B chain

NH²

—COOH

indented
nucleus

prolymphocyte

spinal
column

promontory

prolapse of uterus

health facility; peer groups monitor the care given to a patient; necessary changes are brought about through continuing education.

progran'ulocyte. See promyelocyte.

progres'sive. Advancing; usually denoting the unfavorable course of a disease, as from bad to worse.

prohor'mone. Any precursor of a hormone; e.g., proinsulin.

proin'sulin. A single chain precursor of insulin; formed in the endoplasmic reticulum of the cell and transferred to the Golgi apparatus where the connecting peptide (C-peptide) is removed enzymatically, resulting in the formation of insulin.

projec'tion. 1. A prominence. **2.** The referring of sensations from the sense organs to the source of the stimulus. **3.** The referring to another of one's own unacceptable, repressed attributes. **4.** The application of x rays to a bodily part in a particular direction as it relates to the x-ray tube, e.g., anteroposterior (AP), posteroanterior (PA), right anterior oblique (RAO), right posterior oblique (RPO), etc.

prokaryo'sis. A state in which the nuclear substance of a primitive cell is mixed or is in direct contact with the rest of the protoplasm, due to not having a nuclear envelope.

prola'bium. The full thickness of the prominent central part of the upper lip.

prolac'tin. A hormone produced by the anterior lobe of the pituitary gland that stimulates milk secretion.

prolapse'. 1. To fall down or slip down. **2.** The slipping down of an organ or part from its normal position.

  p. of rectum, protrusion of the inner surface of the rectum through the anus.

  p. of uterus, falling of the uterus into the vagina due to stretching and laxity of its supporting structures.

prolifera'tion. Multiplication of similar cells.

prolif'ic. 1. Copiously productive. **2.** Fertile; bearing offspring in great abundance.

pro'line. A naturally occurring amino acid; unlike other amino acids, it is readily soluble in alcohol.

prolym'phocyte. A cell midway in maturity between the lymphoblast and the lymphocyte; it has the capacity to divide, and may serve as a reservoir of immunologically uncommitted cells.

promas'tigote. The flagellate stage of a trypanosomatid microorganism; formerly called leptomonad and leptomonad stage.

promazine hydrochloride. Phenothiazine compound used as a tranquilizer and antiemetic; Sparine®.

promeg'aloblast. A large nucleated red blood cell; an early stage in the maturation of the megaloblast.

promet'aphase. A stage of mitosis, between prophase and metaphase, marked by the disintegration of the nuclear membrane and formation of the spindle.

promethazine hydrochloride. An antihistaminic compound used also as an adjuvant with narcotics; Phenergan®.

prome'thium. A radioactive rare-earth element; symbol Pm; atomic number 61; atomic weight 147 (best-known isotope); half-life 2.6 years; used as a source of β-rays.

prom'inence. A projection.

  laryngeal p., the projection in front of the neck produced by the thyroid cartilage; also called Adam's apple.

prom'ontory. A projection or elevation.

promo'tor. 1. A substance that increases the activity of a catalyst. **2.** The area on DNA in which RNA polymerase binds and initiates transcription.

promy'elocyte. The developmental stage of a granular leukocyte, between a myeloblast and myelocyte, containing a variable number of large ovoid or irregularly spherical granules; nucleoli are often

present; also called progranulocyte.

pro'nate. To assume, or to be placed in, a prone or face-down position.

prona'tion. The act of lying face downward or of rotating the forearm so that the palm of the hand is turned backward or downward.

prone. Lying with the face downward.

proneph'ros, *pl.* **proneph'roi.** The primitive excretory organ of the embryo, consisting of a series of rudimentary tubules; it is replaced by the transitory mesonephros which forms caudally to it.

pro'nograde. The horizontal position of the body of a quadruped; opposed to orthograde.

pronom'eter. An instrument for determining the degree of pronation or supination of the forearm.

pronor'moblast. The earliest red blood cell precursor, generally 12 to 19 μ in diameter; characterized by scanty, basophilic cytoplasm without hemoglobin, and a nucleus having fine chromatin; also called proerythroblast and rubriblast.

pronu'cleus. One of two nuclei, or haploid nuclei, undergoing fusion, as of an egg or sperm at the time of fertilization.

proof spirit. A mixture of alcohol and water or a beverage containing 50 per cent (100 proof) of ethyl alcohol by volume at 60°F.

propaga'tion. 1. Reproduction. **2.** The continuance of an impulse along a nerve fiber.

propantheline bromide. An anticholinergic agent used in treatment of gastrointestinal disorders; Pro-Banthine®.

proparacaine hydrochloride. An effective surface anesthetic derived from aminobenzoic acid; used principally in ophthalmology; Ophthaine®.

pro'penyl. Glyceryl; the trivalent radical, $C_3H_5O_3$, of glycerol.

proper'din. A natural euglobulin protein in human blood serum with molecular weight approximately eight times that of γ-globulins; it acts in conjunction with complement and magnesium ions and plays a

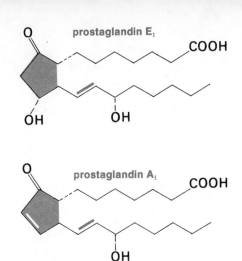

prostaglandin E₁

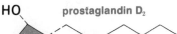

prostaglandin E₂

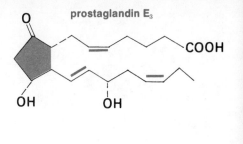

prostaglandin E₃

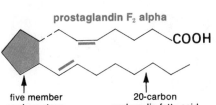

prostaglandin A₁

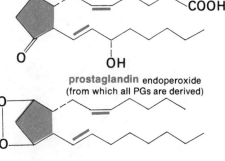

prostaglandin D₂

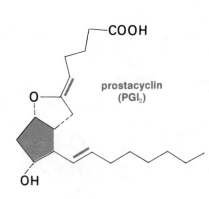

prostaglandin endoperoxide
(from which all PGs are derived)

prostacyclin
(PGI₂)

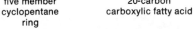

prostaglandin F₂ alpha

five member
cyclopentane
ring

20-carbon
carboxylic fatty acid

role in providing immunity from infectious diseases, and possibly in initiating other immune processes.

properitone'al. Situated in front of the peritoneum, i.e., between the parietal peritoneum and the abdominal wall.

pro'phage. In lysogenic bacteria, the structure that conveys genetic coding for the creation of a given type of phage and bestows specific hereditary traits on the host; also called probacteriophage.

pro'phase. The first stage of cell division by mitosis, during which chromatin collects into a chromosomal thread which breaks up into pairs of rod-shaped chromosomes; each chromosome then splits longitudinally into chromatids.

prophylac'tic. 1. Relating to the prevention of disease. **2.** An agent that wards off disease. **3.** Common name for a condom.

prophylax'is. 1. Precautions taken to prevent a disease; preventive treatment. **2.** In dentistry, cleaning of the teeth.

propos'itus, *pl.* **propos'iti,** *female* **propos'ita.** The member of a family in which a particular trait is first observed and through whom the rest of the family is brought under observation for the study of the hereditary characteristics of the trait; also called proband and index case.

propoxyphene hydrochloride. A mild analgesic; Darvon®.

propranolol hydrochloride. An adrenergic β-receptor blocking agent which diminishes the rate and contractile force of the heart, causing a fall in cardiac output, arterial pressure, and arterial blood flow.

propriocep'tor. A sensory nerve ending, primarily located within the muscles and tendons, which receives stimuli pertaining to movements and position of the body.

  muscle p., neuromuscular spindle; see under spindle.

proptom'eter. See exophthalmometer.

propto'sis. Bulging or protrusion of an organ, as of the eyeball.

propul'sion. Displacement of the center of gravity producing a tendency to lean forward, seen in persons suffering from paralysis agitans (Parkinson's disease).

pro'pyl. The radical of propyl alcohol or propane.

propyl alcohol. A clear colorless fluid, $CH_3CH_2CH_2OH$, more toxic than ethyl alcohol and widely used as a solvent.

prop'ylene. A flammable colorless gas soluble in water; $CH_2 = CHCH_3$.

propylpar'aben. Any of several compounds used as preservatives in a number of pharmaceutical preparations; known to cause contact dermatitis

when used in skin creams, lotions, etc.

propylthiou'racil. Compound used in the treatment of hyperthyroidism.

pro re nata (p.r.n.). Latin for when necessary; used in prescription writing.

proru'bricyte. Basophilic normoblast; see under normoblast.

prosec'tion. An anatomic dissection made specifically for demonstration or for exhibition.

prosec'tor. One who prepares or dissects anatomic structures for demonstration.

prosecto'rium. A dissecting room for preparing prosections; also called anatomy laboratory.

prosenceph'alon. The part of the embryonic brain developed from the most anterior portion of the embryonic neural tube; later it forms the telencephalon and the diencephalon; also called forebrain and proencephalon.

prosodem'ic. Denoting a disease that is spread from one individual to another; an outbreak of a disease arising in this manner, in contrast to an epidemic.

pros'ody. The variations in the stress and intonation patterns of speech by which different shades of meaning are communicated.

prosopagno'sia. A form of visual agnosia in which the individual is unable to recognize, or has great difficulty recognizing, familiar faces.

pros'opople'gia. Facial palsy; see under palsy.

prosopoto'cia. Face presentation in childbirth.

prostacy'clin. See prostaglandin.

prostaglan'din (PG). One of a family of hormone-like, lipid-soluble, acidic compounds derived from long-chain polyunsaturated fatty acids; occurring in nearly all tissues (including cerebrospinal fluid), and possessing an intricate array of physiologic actions (e.g., suppression of gastric acid secretions, peripheral vasodilation, increased renal blood flow, and bronchodilation); used for inducing labor and treating peptic ulcers; other potential uses are in hypertension and asthma; aspirin, indomethacin, phenylbutazone, and other nonsteroidal antiinflammatory agents prevent prostaglandin synthesis; first found in semen and believed to originate from the prostate, thus the name prostaglandin. PGs are classified by chemical structure, using letters (e.g., PGA, PGB) to designate ring substitution and numerical subscripts (e.g., PGA₁) to denote number of unsaturated bonds. Prostacyclin or PGI₂, a powerful inhibitor of platelet aggregation, is found in endometrium; it appears of importance in maintaining the integrity of blood vessel walls.

prostat-, prostato-. Combining forms denoting the prostate gland.

prostatal'gia. Pain in the prostate gland.

pros'tate. A chestnut-shaped body in the male

consisting of glandular and muscular tissue that surrounds the urethra immediately below the bladder; it secretes a milky fluid that is discharged by excretory ducts into the urethra at the time of ejaculation.

prostatec'tomy. Surgical removal of the prostate, or a portion of it.

prostat'ic. Relating to the prostate.

pros'tatism. Any condition caused by hypertrophy or other disease of the prostate; usually refers to symptoms of obstructive uropathy caused by prostatic hypertrophy.

prostati'tis. Inflammation of the prostate.

prostatocysti'tis. Inflammation of the prostate and the bladder.

prostatocystot'omy. Incision through the prostate and bladder wall.

prostat'olith. A stone of the prostate.

prostat'olithot'omy. Incision of prostate for removal of a calculus.

prostatomeg'aly. Marked enlargement of the prostate.

prostatomyomec'tomy. Surgical removal of a myomatous or hypertrophied prostate.

prostatorrhe'a. Abnormal discharge from the prostate.

prostatot'omy. Incision of the prostate.

pros'tatovesiculec'tomy. Surgical removal of the prostate and the seminal vesicles.

pros'tatovesiculi'tis. Inflammation of the prostate and the seminal vesicles.

prosthe'sis. An artificial device used to replace a missing part of the body.

  cleft palate p., appliance used to correct a congenital structural deficiency in the roof of the mouth.

  dental p., artificial replacement of one or more teeth and/or related structures.

  discoid valve p., an artificial heart valve consisting of a free disc in an open cage.

  ocular p., an artificial eye.

  trileaflet aortic valve p., a one-piece trileaflet artificial heart valve which permits a full central flow pattern similar to that of the normal valve.

prosthet'ic. Relating to an artificial part of the body.

prosthet'ics. The making and adjusting of artificial parts of the body.

  dental p., see prosthodontics.

pros'thion. A craniometric point situated on the maxillary alveolar process that projects most anteriorly in the midline; used in measuring facial depth; also called alveolar point.

prosthodon'tics. The branch of dentistry pertaining to the restoration and maintainance of oral func-

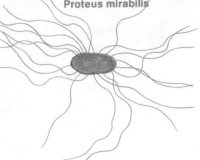

Proteus mirabilis

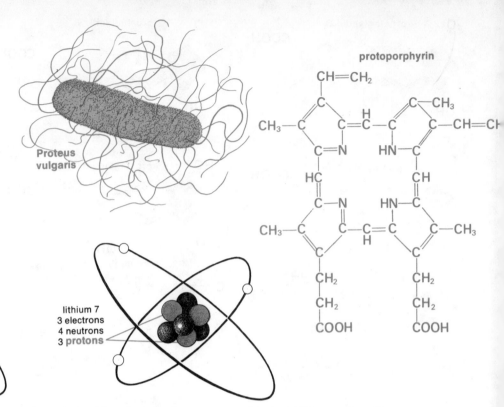

Proteus vulgaris

protoporphyrin

lithium 6
3 electrons
3 neutrons
3 protons

electron

lithium 7
3 electrons
4 neutrons
3 protons

tion by the replacement of missing teeth and associated structures by artificial appliances; also called dental prosthetics.

prosthodon′tist. A specialist in prosthodontics.

pros′thoker′atoplas′ty. Reparative surgery of the eye by means of which excised corneal tissue is replaced by a transparent prosthetic implant.

prostra′tion. A state of extreme exhaustion.

prot-. See proto-.

protactin′ium. A rare radioactive element, symbol Pa, atomic number 91, atomic weight 231; similar to uranium.

protam′inase. An enzyme of the proteinase class which normally splits up protamines to peptides in the intestine; also called carboxypeptidase B.

protam′ine. Any of a group of simple, highly basic proteins, rich in arginine and soluble in water; they neutralize the anticoagulant action of heparin.

　p. sulfate, a heparin antagonist used to neutralize excess amounts of heparin.

protano′pia. Inability to differentiate red, orange, yellow, and green; also called red blindness and anerythropsia.

pro′tean. Changeable in form; having the capacity to readily assume different shapes or forms; variable.

pro′tease. Any enzyme that acts upon the peptide bonds of proteins and peptides; a protein-splitting or hydrolyzing enzyme; also called proteolytic enzyme.

protection, personal injury. In automobile insurance, first party no-fault coverage under which an insurance firm pays, within specified limits, medical, hospital, or funeral costs of the insured, others in his vehicle, or pedestrians hit by him.

protec′tive. 1. Providing immunity. **2.** Agent applied to a part to afford protection.

pro′tein. Any of a group of complex nitrogenous substances of high molecular weight that contain amino acids as their fundamental structural units, are present in the cells of all animals and plants, and function in all phases of chemical and physical activity of the cells.

　Bence Jones p., a protein found in the urine of individuals with multiple myeloma; when the urine is heated, a precipitate forms at 50 to 60°C which dissolves when the temperature is raised to near boiling point; also called Bence Jones albumin.

　conjugated p., compound formed by the combination of a protein with a nonprotein (prosthetic) group.

　C-reactive p., abnormal protein found in the blood serum of persons in acute stages of inflammatory diseases such as rheumatic fever.

　denatured p., one that has undergone a change,

so that its characteristic properties are lost.

　foreign p., one that differs from those normally found in the blood, lymph, or bodily tissues.

　immune p., antitoxin.

　native p., one in its natural state.

　plasma p.'s, proteins present in blood plasma; e.g., albumin, globulins, fibrinogen, etc.

　plasma p. fraction, selected proteins from blood plasma of adult human donors, used as a blood volume supporter.

　p. hydrolysate (intravenous), a product of protein hydrolysis used after surgery of the intestinal tract and certain severe illnesses; also called casein hydrolysate 5%; Amigen®.

　simple p., one that yields only amino acids upon hydrolysis.

pro′teinase. Any enzyme that hydrolyzes native protein or polypeptides; e.g., pepsin.

proteino′sis. Condition marked by an increase in proteins in the tissues, especially abnormal proteins.

　pulmonary alveolar p., a chronic progressive disease of the lungs, marked by accumulation of a homogeneous granular substance in the alveoli (air sacs); it affects adults and its cause is unknown.

proteinu′ria. Excretion of protein in the urine in excess of the normal daily amount; an average-size healthy individual normally excretes up to 100 mg of protein per day.

　continuous p., persistent p., urinary excretion of protein at an abnormally high rate which is not intermittent or related to position of the body; usually associated with primary renal disorders producing vascular and parenchymal changes in the kidney.

　febrile p., proteinuria occurring with fever.

　heavy p., excretion of more than four grams of protein daily, usually caused by renal disorders that greatly increase glomerular permeability.

　orthostatic p., see postural proteinuria.

　persistent p., see continuous proteinuria.

　postural p., orthostatic p., excessive excretion of protein in the urine, usually mild, in healthy adolescents and young adults, occurring when the individual is upright, and disappearing during recumbency.

　transient p., proteinuria that may occur with febrile disorders, abdominal crises, heart disease, severe anemia, and emotional stress; also called intermittent or functional proteinuria.

proteol′ysis. The breaking down (hydrolysis) of proteins into simpler, soluble forms by the action of enzymes, as in digestion.

proteolyt′ic. Causing proteolysis.

pro′teose. One of the intermediate products of protein digestion, between a protein and a peptone.

Pro′teus. A genus of gram-negative bacteria, mo-

tile only at 25°C; most commonly associated with urinary tract and wound infections; may also be seen in diarrhea and gastroenteritis.

　P. mirabilis, a species found in putrid meat, effusions, and abscesses; thought to be a cause of gastroenteritis.

　P. morganii, species that is a common inhabitant of the gastrointestinal tract; seen in normal and diarrheal stools.

　P. vulgaris, species found in putrefying tissues and abscesses; certain strains are agglutinated by typhus serum and therefore are used in diagnosing the disease (Weil-Felix reaction).

prothrom′bin. Factor II; a plasma protein that is converted into thrombin during the second stage of blood coagulation; an enzymically inactive precursor of thrombin; formerly called thrombinogen.

Protis′ta. A third kingdom or division of living things comprised of unicellular organisms such as bacteria, protozoa, and many fungi and algae.

pro′tium. See hydrogen-1.

proto-, prot-. Combining forms meaning the first in a series.

protodiastol′ic. Relating to the initial one-third of a cardiac diastole or the period immediately following the second heart sound.

pro′ton. The unit of positive electricity; the nucleus of the hydrogen atom; a particle of all other atomic nuclei having a mass of 1.0073 units and a positive charge equal numerically to the negative charge of an electron.

pro′toplasm. Living matter; the essential substance of which all living cells, vegetable and animal, are made.

pro′toplast. A spherical, osmotically fragile wall-defective microbial form with external surface free of cell wall components.

protoporphy′ria. Condition marked by high concentrations of protoporphyrin in red blood cells, plasma, and feces.

protopor′phyrin. A porphyrin which, linked with iron, forms the heme of hemoglobin and the prosthetic groups of myoglobin, catalase, cytochromes, etc.

pro′totroph. The nutritionally independent, wild-type strain of any organism. Cf. auxotroph.

pro′totype. The primitive or ancestral species from which others develop or to which they conform.

protover′atrines A and B. A mixture of two alkaloids isolated from *Veratrum album*; formerly used as antihypertensive agents; the antihypertensive action is obtained by sensitization of the carotid sinus baroreceptors.

protox′ide. The oxide of a metal exclusive of suboxides containing the lowest proportion of oxygen.

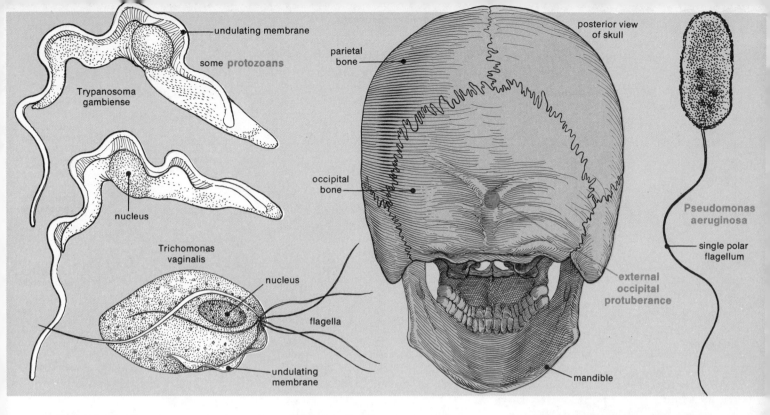

some protozoans

Trypanosoma gambiense — undulating membrane — nucleus

Trichomonas vaginalis — nucleus — flagella — undulating membrane

posterior view of skull — parietal bone — occipital bone — external occipital protuberance — mandible

Pseudomonas aeruginosa — single polar flagellum

Protozo´a. A phylum of the animal kingdom which includes all unicellular organisms.

protozo´an. A unicellular organism, member of the phylum Protozoa; also called protozoon.

protozoi´asis. Infestations with protozoans.

protozool´ogy. The biological study of the simplest or most primitive forms of animal life (protozoa).

protozo´on. See protozoan.

protozo´ophage. A cell that ingests protozoa.

protrac´tion. In dentistry, condition in which teeth or other maxillary or mandibular structures are located anterior to their normal position.

protrac´tor. 1. An instrument for extracting a foreign object, such as a bullet, from a deep wound. **2.** A muscle that extends a limb; an extensor muscle.

protru´sion. In dentistry, position of the mandible forward or laterally forward from the centric position.

protu´berance. An eminence, projection, or bulge.

external occipital p., a prominence at the center of the outer surface of the occipital bone.

internal occipital p., a prominence at the midpoint of the inner surface of the occipital bone.

mental p., a triangular elevation on the lower portion of the outer surface of the mandible, at the midline, that helps to form the chin.

provi´rus. A virus that has become an integral part of the host cell chromosome and is transmitted from one cell generation to another.

provi´tamin. A substance in certain foods which may be converted into a vitamin; a precursor of a vitamin such as carotene; also called previtamin.

prox´imal. 1. Nearest the center, midline, point of attachment, or point of origin; opposite of distal. **2.** In dentistry, the surface of a tooth, either mesial or distal, which is nearest an adjacent tooth.

prox´imate. Nearest, next; approximate; immediate.

prox´imoatax´ia. Lack of muscular coordination of the proximal portions of the extremities.

prune. The partially dried fruit of the common plum *Prunus domestica*; used as a mild laxative.

prur´ient. Denoting morbid interest in aberrant matter, especially of a sexual nature.

prurig´inous. Relating to prurigo.

pruri´go. An itchy skin eruption of papules.

prurit´ic. Itchy.

pruri´tus. Itching.

p. ani, intense itching at the anus; may be caused by infections, hemorrhoids, or allergy; also, fecal soiling of the perianal skin may play an important role, inducing a chemical dermatosis.

prus´siate. 1. A salt of hydrocyanic acid; a cyanide. **2.** A ferricyanide or ferrocyanide.

prus´sic acid. See hydrocyanic acid.

psammo´ma. A type of meningioma; a benign calcified tumor derived from a connective tissue and occurring along the blood vessels of dura and skull; characterized by the formation of multiple, discrete, concentrically laminated, calcareous bodies (psammoma bodies).

pseud-. See pseudo-.

pseudarthro´sis. A false joint formed on the shaft of a long bone, at the site of a fracture that failed to fuse; also called neoarthrosis.

pseudesthe´sia, pseudoesthe´sia. 1. Subjective sensation without an external stimulus. **2.** Sensation referred to an absent limb after an amputation.

pseudo-, pseud-. Combining forms meaning false; deceptive resemblance.

pseudoaliele´. A gene that behaves as an allele, but occupies a different, closely linked position on a chromosome; it can be separated by crossing over.

pseudoan´eurysm. Dilatation of an artery resembling an aneurysm.

pseudocoarcta´tion. An elongated and tortuous condition of the aortic arch in the area of the ligamentum arteriosum without occlusion of the vessel.

pseudocroup´. See laryngismus stridulus.

pseudocryp´torchism. Condition in which the testes occasionally move high into the inguinal canal.

pseudocye´sis. Spurious pregnancy; pseudopregnancy; condition in which several signs of pregnancy occur without conception.

pseu´docyst. 1. Accumulation of fluid without an enclosing membrane. **2.** An aggregation of *Toxoplasma* parasites within a host cell.

pseudoesthe´sia. See pseudesthesia.

pseudofrac´ture. Condition in which new bone tissue and thickening of periosteum is formed at the site of an injury.

pseudogan´glion. A localized thickening of a nerve trunk simulating a ganglion.

pseudoglauco´ma. An abnormality of the optic disk resembling glaucoma, due to conditions other than pressure within the eyeball.

pseu´dogout. A disease characterized by calcified deposits in articular cartilage which are free of urate and consist of calcium pyrophosphate crystals; a form of chondrocalcinosis; it leads to goutlike attacks of pain, swelling, stiffness, local warmth, and joint tenderness; the knee is the joint predominantly affected.

pseudohe´mophil´ia. An acquired condition resembling hemophilia but caused by another disorder.

pseudohemop´tysis. Spitting of blood from a source other than the lungs or bronchi.

pseudohermaph´roditism. Condition in which a person is distinctly of one sex but has superficial characteristics of the opposite sex; commonly, and wrongly, called hermaphroditism.

male p., condition in which a person has testes but secondary sexual characteristics of both sexes.

female p., condition in which a person has ovaries but secondary sexual characteristics of both sexes.

pseudoher´nia. A swelling resembling a hernia, caused by inflammation of an inguinal gland or scrotal tissue.

pseudohy´pha. A structure of many fungi which is formed by budding, is composed of a chain of cells, and resembles a hypha.

pseudohy´poparathy´roidism. A genetic disorder resembling hypoparathyroidism in which the primary defect is renal unresponsiveness to parathyroid hormone; usually characterized by short stature, round face, and ectopic calcifications and associated with hyperphosphatemia and hypocalcemia; transmitted as an X-linked dominant trait.

pseudomem´brane. See membrane, false.

Pseudomo´nas. A genus of gram-negative motile bacteria with polar flagella, occurring in soil, water, sewage, and air.

P. aeruginosa, a species found in human feces and skin; it causes blue pus infections of wounds and burns, and may cause infections in other parts of the body through the use of instruments, as in the urinary tract, or in the subarachnoid space through lumbar puncture; some strains produce a blue compound soluble in chloroform (pyocyanin); others produce a greenish compound soluble in water (fluorescin).

P. mallei, a species causing glanders in horses, sheep, goats, and man; also called glanders bacillus; formerly called *Actinobacillus mallei*.

P. pseudomallei, the species causing melioidosis; formerly called *Malleomyces pseudomallei*.

pseudomu´cin. A gelatinous substance similar to mucin.

pseudomyce´lium. A group of pseudohyphae.

pseudomyo´pia. Eye condition resulting from spasm of the ciliary muscle, causing the same focusing defect as myopia.

pseudomyxo´ma. A gelatinous tumor or tumorlike condition resembling a myxoma but composed of epithelial mucus.

pseudone´oplasm. An aggregation of nonneoplastic material that clinically resembles a true neoplasm.

pseudoparal´ysis. Apparent loss of power of voluntary movement.

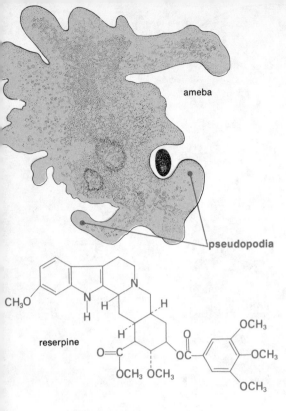

ameba

pseudopodia

reserpine

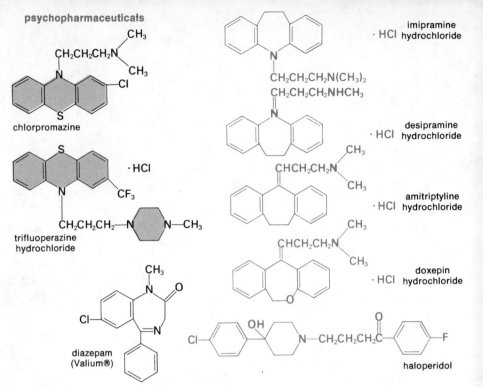

chlorpromazine

trifluoperazine
hydrochloride

diazepam
(Valium®)

imipramine
· HCl hydrochloride

desipramine
· HCl hydrochloride

amitriptyline
· HCl hydrochloride

doxepin
· HCl hydrochloride

haloperidol

pseudoparaple´gia. Apparent loss of power of voluntary movement of the lower extremities.

pseudopo´dium, *pl.* **pseudopo´dia. 1.** A cytoplasmic process used by certain protozoa (e.g., amebae) for locomotion and feeding. **2.** A small cytoplasmic extension from a cell.

pseudopol´yp. A protruding mass in the colon, composed of edematous mucosa, granulation tissue, or inflamed epithelium; commonly associated with ulcerative colitis.

pseudopreg´nancy. See pregnancy, spurious.

pseudo-pseudohy´poparathy´roidism. Heritable disorder which has the constitutional features of pseudohypoparathyroidism (round face, short stature, obesity, abnormally short hands and feet) but lacks the chemical findings.

pseudopteryg´ium. A superficial adhesion of the cornea to the conjunctiva, resulting from injury; also called scar pterygium.

pseudosmia. A sensation of an odor that is not present.

pseudotu´bercle. A nodule resembling a tuberculous granuloma, but not caused by the tubercle bacillus.

pseudotu´mor. The occurrence of symptoms and signs indicating the presence of a tumor in the absence of one, with subsequent spontaneous recovery.

p. cerebri, a condition producing signs of increased intracranial pressure suggesting the presence of an intracranial tumor in the absence of any neoplasm; also called benign intracranial hypertension.

pseudoxanthoma elasticum. A condition marked by slightly elevated papules or plaques on the skin that, as yellowish aggregates, resemble but are not xanthomas; the lesions generally appear on the neck, axillae, abdomen, and thighs, and are due to degenerated elastic tissue; so-called angioid streaks occur in the retina; premature arterial degeneration is common and internal hemorrhage occurs in 10 per cent of cases.

psi. Abbreviation for pounds per square inch.

Psilocybe mexicana. A species of mushrooms (family Agaricaceae) containing the hallucinogenic substance psilocybin; commonly known as the Mexican magic mushroom.

psilocy´bin. Hallucinogenic substance obtained from *Psilocybe mexicana.*

psilo´sis. Falling or loss of hair.

psittaco´sis. A viral disease of birds, transmitted to man by parrots or parakeets through inhalation of infective material; in humans, the disease is characterized by fever, chills, headache, sore throat, and cough. See also ornithosis.

pso´as. See table of muscles.

psorias´iform. Resembling psoriasis.

psori´asis. A chronic skin disease characterized by reddish patches covered with silvery scales, occurring mostly on the knees, elbows, scalp, and trunk.

psoriat´ic. Relating to psoriasis.

PSP. Abbreviation for phenolsulfonphthalein.

psych-. See psycho-.

psychasthe´nia. Term formerly used for a neurosis characterized by marked anxiety, obsessions, compulsions, phobias, and feelings of inadequacy.

psy´che. The mind as distinguished from the body.

psychedel´ic. Relating to drugs that cause hallucinations, distortions of perception, and, sometimes, conditions resembling psychosis.

psychiat´ric. Relating to psychiatry.

psychi´atrist. A specialist in psychiatry.

psychi´atry. The branch of medicine concerned with the study, diagnosis, and treatment of mental diseases.

psy´chic. 1. Relating to the mind. **2.** Relating to extraordinary mental or spiritual processes, such as mental telepathy or extrasensory perception.

psycho-, psych-. Combining forms denoting the mind or mental processes.

psy´cho. Street term for a psychopath.

psychoanal´ysis. A method of psychotherapy in which a patient is made to recall past experiences, through free association, in order to bring into consciousness repressed experiences causing the emotional problems; originated by Sigmund Freud.

psychoan´alyst. A psychiatrist trained in the techniques of psychoanalytic therapy; also called analyst.

psychobiol´ogy. The study of the biology of the mind based on the concept of the individual as a biologic unit whose personality development is dependent on its environmental setting; especially the theory of Adolph Meyer.

psychodiagno´sis. The use of psychological tests to determine the causes of abnormal behavior.

psychodram´a. A method of group psychotherapy in which patients dramatize their emotional problems.

psychodynam´ics. The science of human behavior and its unconscious motivation.

psychodyslep´tic. Any agent which has the capability or producing abnormal mental phenomena, particularly in the perceptual and cognitive spheres.

psychogalvan´ic. Relating to electrical changes in the skin induced by mental processes.

psychogen´esis. 1. Development of mental faculties. **2.** Production of symptoms by mental factors.

psychogen´ic, psychogenet´ic. Originating in the mind.

psychogeriat´rics. The study of old age as it relates to psychological problems and mental illnesses.

psychogno´sis. Diagnosis of mental disorders or psychiatric states.

psy´chogram. A chart depicting the personality traits of an individual; also called psychograph.

psychokine´sis (PK). In parapsychology, the influence on motion, especially of distant inanimate objects, through concentrated directed thought.

psycholag´ny. Sexual excitement and satisfaction from mental imagery.

psycholog´ic. Relating to mental processes and behavior.

psychol´ogist. One who is trained to perform psychological evaluation, therapy, or research.

psychol´ogy. The science concerned with the study of the mind in all its aspects, especially as they are manifested in behavior.

psychom´etry. The measuring of mental efficiency, functioning, and potential.

psychomo´tor. Relating to the mental origin of muscular activity, as compulsive movements.

psychoneuro´sis. Emotional and behavioral disorder manifested by anxiety and symptoms such as depression, phobias, compulsions, or obsessions without gross distortion of reality orientation; commonly called neurosis.

psychoneurot´ic. Relating to or suffering from a psychoneurosis.

psy´chopath. An individual with a personality disorder, manifested by asocial behavior without accompanying guilt.

psychopath´ic. Relating to mental disease or psychopathy.

psychopathol´ogy. The pathology of mental disorders; the nature or study of mental disease.

psychop´athy. Any mental disorder.

psychopharmaceut´icals. Any of several drugs used in the treatment of emotional disorders.

psychopharmacol´ogy. The study of the action of drugs on the mind and emotions.

psychophys´ical. Relating to physical stimuli and mental responses.

psychophys´ics. The branch of psychology concerned with the relationships between physical stimuli and sensory responses.

psychophysiolog´ic. 1. Relating to psychophysiology. **2.** Denoting a disease with primarily physical manifestations but emotional causes.

psychophysiol´ogy. The study of the interaction of psychologic and physiologic processes.

psychople´gia. A form of dementia or mental weakness characterized by sudden onset.

psychople´gic. 1. Relating to psychoplegia. **2.**

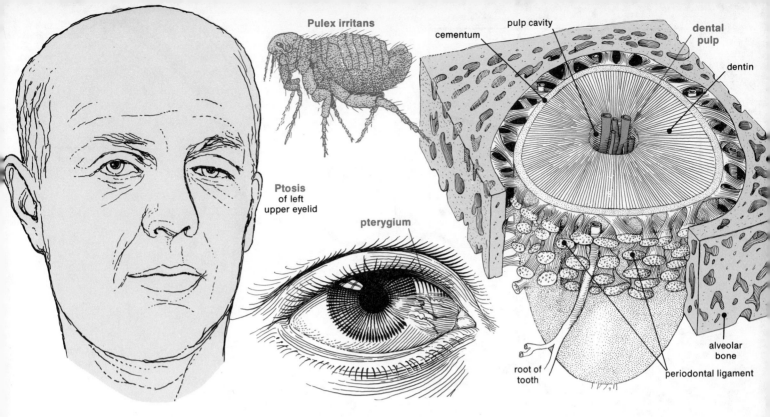

Pulex irritans

Ptosis of left upper eyelid

pterygium

cementum
pulp cavity
dental pulp
dentin
root of tooth
periodontal ligament
alveolar bone

An agent that dulls mental activity.

psychosen′sory. Of or relating to the perception and interpretation of sensory stimuli.

psychosex′ual. Relating to the mental or emotional aspects of sex.

psycho′sis. A severe mental illness of organic and/or emotional origin, marked by loss of contact with reality and frequently by regressive behavior, delusions, or hallucinations; see also insanity.

 Korsakoff's p., see Korsakoff's syndrome.

 manic-depressive p., conspicuous mood swings from elation to depression.

psychoso′cial. Involving psychological and social factors.

psychosomat′ic. Referring to the influence of the mind over the body; specifically, physical symptoms that have an emotional or mental origin.

psychosomimet′ic. See psychotomimetic.

psychostim′ulant. Any agent that has the capability of increasing the level of an individual's alertness and/or motivation.

psychosur′gery. Brain surgery for the treatment of mental disorders; e.g., lobotomy.

psychother′apy. Treatment of emotional disorders conducted primarily by means of psychologic methods such as suggestion, persuasion, psychoanalysis, and reeducation.

psychot′ic. Relating to, afflicted with, or caused by a psychosis.

psychot′ogen. An agent that produces psychotic symptoms.

psychotogen′ic. Producing psychosis; said of certain drugs like LSD.

psychotomimet′ic. Producing symptoms that resemble those of a psychosis; said of certain drugs; also called psychosomimetic.

psychotrop′ic. Denoting drugs that affect the mind.

psychro-. Combining form meaning cold.

psychrom′eter. Device used to calculate the relative humidity of the atmosphere; it consists of two thermometers, one with a bulb that is kept wet to cause evaporation and the other with a dry bulb.

psychrom′etry. 1. The science of the physical laws that control air and water mixture. **2.** Estimation of the relative humidity of the air by means of the psychrometer.

psychrophil′ic. Thriving in cold temperature; said of some bacteria.

psychropho′bia. 1. Abnormal fear of cold temperatures. **2.** Extreme sensitiveness to cold.

psyl′lium. 1. A plant of the genus *Plantago.* **2.** Plantago seed; see under seed.

P.T. Abbreviation for physical therapy.

Pt. Chemical symbol of the element platinum.

pt. Abbreviation for (a) pint; (b) patient.

PTA. Abbreviation for plasma thromboplastin antecedent (factor XI).

ptar′mic. An agent that causes sneezing.

PTC. Abbreviation for plasma thromboplastin component (factor IX).

pter′idine. A diaminopyrimidine derivative; a two-ring heterocyclic compound found as a component of pteroic acid and the pteroylglutamic acids.

pte′rion. A craniometric point on either side of the skull at the junction of the frontal, sphenoid, parietal, and temporal bones.

pteroylglutam′ic acid. See folic acid.

pteryg′ium. A horizontal, triangular growth of the bulbar conjunctiva, extending usually from the inner canthus to the border of the cornea or beyond; a slowly advancing lesion, believed to be caused by ultraviolet radiation.

pter′ygoid. Wing-shaped.

pterygopal′atine. Relating to the pterygoid process of the sphenoid bone and the bony palate.

PTH. Abbreviation for parathyroid hormone.

ptilo′sis. Loss of eyelashes.

pto′maine. Vague term denoting a poisonous substance.

 p. poisoning, poisoning attributed to toxic decomposition of ingested food; most of these cases are probably caused by viral or bacterial infection.

ptosed. Prolapsed.

-ptosis. Combining form denoting a downward displacement.

pto′sis. 1. A prolapse or sinking down of an organ. **2.** Drooping of an upper eyelid when the eyes are open.

ptot′ic. Relating to ptosis or prolapse.

PTT. Abbreviation for partial thromboplastin time.

ptyal-, ptyalo-. Combining forms denoting saliva.

pty′alin. An enzyme present in the saliva, which changes starch into dextrin, maltose, and glucose.

pty′alolith. See sialolith.

ptyalolithi′asis. See sialolithiasis.

ptyalolithot′omy. See sialolithotomy.

Pu. Chemical symbol of the element plutonium.

pubar′che. The beginning of puberty.

pu′beral, pu′bertal. Relating to the beginning of sexual maturity.

puber′tas. Puberty.

 p. precox, early arrival of sexual maturity.

pu′berty. The stage of development in which an individual is first capable of reproduction, usually between the ages of 13 and 16 in boys and 12 and 14 in girls.

pubes′cence. The beginning of sexual maturity.

pubes′cent. One who is reaching the age of sexual maturity.

pu′bic. Relating to the pubic bone or area.

pu′bis, *pl.* **pu′bes. 1.** The pubic bone. **2.** The region over the pubic bone. **3.** The hair of the pubic region.

pubomade′sis. Loss or absence of pubic hair.

puboves′ical. Relating to the pubic bone and the bladder.

pubovesicocer′vical. Relating to the pubic symphysis, bladder, and uterine cervix.

puden′dal. Relating to the genitals.

puden′dum, *pl.* **puden′da.** External genitals, especially the female genitals; the vulva.

puer′iculture. The care of the unborn child through attention to the health of the pregnant woman.

pu′erile. 1. Relating to childhood. **2.** Childish.

pu′erilism. Second childhood.

puer′pera. A woman who had just given birth.

puer′peral. Relating to the first few weeks following childbirth.

puer′peralism. Any disease state consequent upon childbirth.

puerpe′rium. The period from the end of labor to the return of uterus to normal size, usually from three to six weeks.

Pu′lex. A genus of fleas.

 P. cheopis, former name for the Oriental rat flea species, *Xenopsylla cheopis.*

 P. irritans, the species of flea that commonly infects and parasitizes man and various animals; its bite produces itching.

pulicide, pulicicide. Any agent which destroys fleas.

pullula′tion. Sprouting; budding.

pul′mo, *pl.* **pulmo′nes.** Latin for lung.

pul′monary. Relating to the lungs.

pulmonec′tomy. See pneumonectomy.

pulmon′ic. Pulmonary.

pul′motor. Apparatus used to induce artificial respiration by introducing oxygen into the lungs.

pulp. Any soft, moist tissue.

 dental p., the vascular and innervated connective tissue contained in the pulp cavity of the tooth.

pul′pal. Relating to the pulp or to the pulp cavity of a tooth.

pulpec′tomy. Removal of the pulp tissue from the entire tooth, including the pulp in the root canals.

pulpefac′tion, pulpifac′tion. The act of reducing to pulp.

pulpi′tis. Inflammation of the pulp of a tooth; also called odontitis.

pulp′less. Having a nonfunctioning or dead pulp or one that has been replaced with an inert substance; said of a tooth.

pulpot′omy. Surgical removal of a portion of the

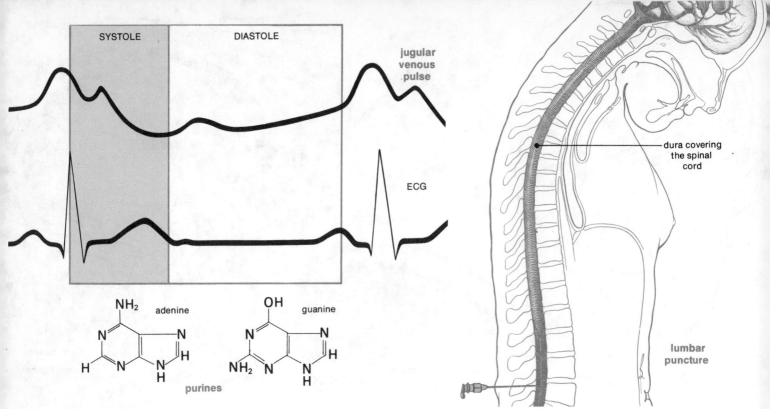

SYSTOLE | DIASTOLE

jugular venous pulse

ECG

NH₂ adenine

OH guanine

purines

dura covering the spinal cord

lumbar puncture

---

pulp from a tooth, usually the coronal portion.

pul′py. The condition of a solid when it is soft and moist.

pul′sate. To expand and contract, or beat, rhythmically, as the heart.

pul′satile. Throbbing; pulsating.

pulsa′tion. 1. The act of pulsating. **2.** A single throb, as of the heart.

pulse. The rhythmic increase in pressure within a blood vessel produced by the increased volume of blood forced through the vessel with each contraction of the heart.

  alternating p., one with alternating weak and strong beats; also called pulsus alternans.

  anacrotic p., a pulse (usually palpable in the carotid arteries) in which the ascending limb of the pulse wave has a secondary notch.

  bigeminal p., a pulse in which two beats occur in rapid succession followed by a longer pause; usually produced by a small premature ectopic beat after a normally conducted beat.

  capillary p., see Quincke's pulse.

  Corrigan's p., one characterized by an abrupt rise with rapid collapse; also called water-hammer pulse.

  coupled p., twice-beating p., a pulse in which two waves are palpated during each cardiac cycle; also called double beat.

  jugular venous p., jugular p. (JVP), pulsation observed in a jugular vein.

  paradoxical p., a reduction in the amplitude of the pulse during inspiration; also called pulsus paradoxus.

  plateau p., one with a slowly rising pressure and sustained peak.

  p. deficit, the difference between the number of heart beats (greater) and the number of beats counted at the wrist (less) due to failure of a very early ventricular contraction to propel sufficient blood to produce a palpable pulse.

  Quincke's p., alternate pallor and reddening of capillary areas, such as the nail bed; seen in aortic insufficiency; also called capillary pulse.

  thready p., a small fine pulse.

  trigeminal p., one occurring in groups of three.

  twice-beating p., see coupled pulse.

  venous p., one occurring in the veins.

  water-hammer p., see Corrigan's pulse.

pulseless disease. Progressive inflammation and obliteration of the brachiocephalic trunk, left subclavian, and left common carotid arteries, leading to loss of pulse in the arms and neck among other symptoms; also called Takayashu's syndrome. See also aortic arch syndrome.

pulsim′eter. Instrument used to measure the force

and frequency of the pulse.

pul′sion. A swelling.

pul′sus. Latin for pulse.

  p. alternans, see pulse, alternating.

  p. paradoxus, see pulse, paradoxical.

  p. parvus, a small pulse.

  p. tardus, a pulse with a delayed rise and fall, as seen in aortic stenosis.

pul′verize. To reduce to a powder.

pulvi′nar. The angular prominence constituting the posteromedial portion of the thalamus.

pul′vinate. Having the shape of a cushion.

pul′vis, *pl.* **pul′veres.** Latin for powder.

pum′ice. A porous volcanic substance; in dentistry, used in powdered form to polish teeth and dentures.

pump. An apparatus for transferring a liquid or gas through tubes from or to any part.

  Alvegniat's p., a mercurial vacuum pump for determining the amount of free gaseous constituents of the blood.

  breast p., a suction pump for withdrawing milk from the breast.

  Carrel-Lindbergh p., a perfusion pump by means of which an organ taken out of the body may be kept functioning; also called Lindbergh pump.

  coronary-sucker p., a pump for aspirating the small quantity of blood that enters the heart while the heart-lung machine is used during open-heart surgery.

  electrolyte p., a process which derives its energy from the metabolic activities of the cell and which can cause a solute to move from an area of relatively low to one of higher chemical potential; e.g., a sodium pump located in renal tubular cells.

  p.-oxygenator, a mechanical apparatus that facilitates open heart surgery by temporarily substituting for both the heart (pump) and the lungs (oxygenator).

  sodium p., electrolyte p.

  stomach p., a suction pump with a flexible tube for removing the contents of the stomach in an emergency, as in a case of poisoning.

punch-drunk. Suffering from brain dysfunction caused by repeated concussions; characterized by slow body movements, unsteady gait, hesitant speech, and slow intellect; condition seen in some professional boxers.

punc′tate. 1. Marked with minute dots. **2.** Material withdrawn by means of a puncture.

punc′tiform. Of the size and shape of a very small point, usually having a diameter of less than one millimeter; used principally to describe minute colonies of bacteria.

punc′tum, *pl.* **punc′ta.** A point or a spot.

  lacrimal p., the minute opening of the lacrimal

duct on the margin of each eyelid at the inner canthus.

punc′ture. 1. To pierce with a pointed instrument. **2.** A small hole made with a needle.

  lumbar p., puncture made into the subarachnoid space between two of the lower lumbar vertebrae to remove cerebrospinal fluid for diagnostic purposes, or to inject an anesthetic solution; also called spinal puncture and spinal tap.

  spinal p., see lumbar puncture.

PUE. Abbreviation for pyrexia of unknown etiology. See also FUO and PUO.

PUO. Abbreviation for pyrexia of unknown origin. See also FUO and PUE.

pu′pil. The circular opening in the center of the iris, through which light enters the eye.

  Argyll-Robertson p., a pupil characterized by the loss of response to light, with retention of a normal response to convergence accommodation.

  fixed p., one that is unresponsive to all stimuli.

pu′pillary. Relating to the pupil.

pupillog′raphy. The recording of pupillary reactions to light stimuli.

pupillom′eter. Coreometer; an instrument used to measure the diameter of the pupil.

pupillom′etry. Coreometry; measurement of the pupil of the eye.

pupillomo′tor. Relating to motor activity affecting the size of the pupil; specifically, denoting the motor nerve fibers supplying the iris.

pupillople′gia. Slow or absent response of the pupil to a light stimulus.

pupillostatom′eter. Instrument used to measure the distance between the pupils of the eyes.

pure. 1. In genetics, denoting (a) an inherited trait that is transmitted without a break in several generations; (b) an individual who is not a hybrid. **2.** Free from contamination.

pure′bred. An animal derived from a line subjected to inbreeding.

purga′tion. Catharsis; vigorous evacuation of the bowels effected by a cathartic medicine (purgative).

pur′gative. See cathartic.

purge. 1. To induce evacuation of the bowels. **2.** Any agent having such properties.

pu′rine. The base of a group of organic compounds (uric acid compounds), known as purines or purine bases; when synthetically produced, it is a colorless crystalline compound; it is not known to exist as such in nature.

pur′pura. Condition in which spontaneous bleeding occurs in the subcutaneous tissues, causing the appearance of purple patches on the skin.

  anaphylactoid p., see Henoch-Schönlein purpura.

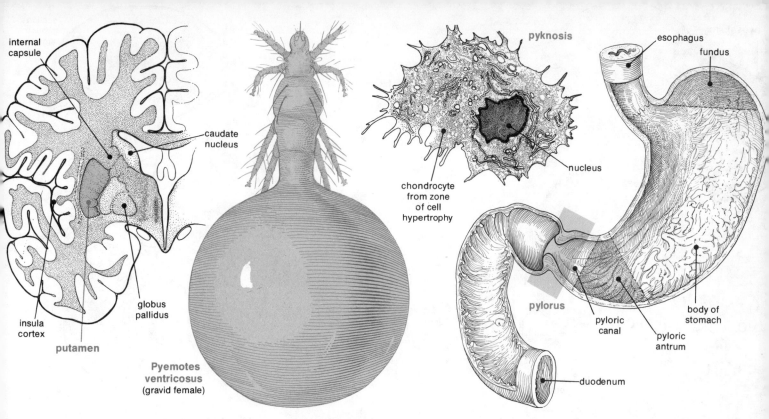

internal capsule

caudate nucleus

pyknosis

esophagus

fundus

nucleus

chondrocyte from zone of cell hypertrophy

globus pallidus

insula cortex

putamen

Pyemotes ventricosus
(gravid female)

pylorus

pyloric canal

pyloric antrum

body of stomach

pyloric

duodenum

annular telangiectatic p., a form characterized by lesions (usually limited to the lower extremities) appearing as circular pigmented areas with a yellow-ish necrosed center; also called Majocchi's disease.

Henoch-Schönlein p., purpura, seen especially in children and young adults, associated with gastrointestinal symptoms, joint pains, and hematuria; the appearance of cutaneous lesions (most common on the extremities) is preceded by a pinprick itchy sensation; also called Schönlein's disease and anaphylactoid purpura.

rheumatic p., purpura associated with acute rheumatic arthritis.

thrombocytopenic p., a form associated with deficiency in platelet count.

thrombotic thrombocytopenic p., a severe and frequently fatal form characterized by a low platelet count in the blood and thrombosis in the terminal arterioles and capillaries of many organs; findings may include azotemia, hemolytic anemia, hypertension, and central nervous system symptoms.

purpu′ric. Relating to or afflicted with purpura.

purpurif′erous. Forming the visual purple or rhodopsin.

pu′rulence, pu′rulency. The condition of containing or producing pus.

pu′rulent. Containing or producing pus.

pus. A thick, viscous, yellowish fluid, product of inflammation, composed chiefly of dead white blood cells (leukocytes) and a thin liquid (liquor puris), and often the microbiologic agent responsible for the inflammation.

pus′tular. Characterized by pustules.

pustula′tion. The formation or development of pustules.

pus′tule. A small elevation of the skin containing pus.

pus′tuliform. Resembling a pustule.

puta′men. A thick, convex, dark gray mass in the brain between the insular cortex laterally and the globus pallidus and the internal capsule medially.

putrefac′tion. 1. Decomposition of organic matter, especially proteins, by the action of bacteria, resulting in the formation of foul-smelling compounds. **2.** Decomposed matter.

putrefac′tive. Relating to or causing the decomposition of organic matter.

pu′trefy. To decompose or decay.

putres′cence. Rottenness.

pu′trid. Decayed; rotten.

PVP. Abbreviation for polyvinylpyrrolidone.

pyarthro′sis. The presence of pus in a joint cavity.

pycni′dium, *pl.* **pycni′dia.** A flask-shaped or round spore fruit of various imperfect fungi; it contains conidia.

pyel-, pyelo-. Combining forms denoting relationship to the renal pelvis.

pyelecta′sia. Dilatation of the renal pelvis.

pyelec′tomy. Surgical removal of the redundant portion of a greatly distended kidney pelvis.

pyeli′tis. See pyelonephritis.

pyelocysti′tis. Inflammation of the kidney pelvis and the bladder.

py′elogram. A roentgenogram of the kidney pelvis and the ureter.

pyelog′raphy. The making of roentgenograms of the ureter and the kidney pelvis.

pyelolithot′omy. Surgical removal of a stone from the pelvis of the kidney.

pyeloneos′tomy. The division and reimplantation of a ureter for the improvement of kidney drainage.

pyelonephri′tis. Inflammation of the kidney, especially the renal pelvis; also called pyelitis. •

　acute p., active pyogenic infection of the kidney.

　chronic p., disease of the kidney thought to result from scarring from previous bacterial infections.

　xanthogranulomatous p., a rare form of chronic pyelonephritis in which the kidney shows xanthogranulomas with lipid-containing foam cells, multinucleated giant cells, lymphocytes, and plasma cells.

pyeloneph′rolithot′omy. Removal of kidney stones by combining an incision in the kidney pelvis with one in the cortex.

pyeloplas′ty. Plastic operation on the kidney pelvis either for the purpose of improving drainage or to reduce its size.

pyeloplica′tion. Operation to reduce the size of the kidney pelvis when abnormally dilated.

pyelos′copy. Fluoroscopic examination of the kidney pelvis after introduction of a radiopaque solution through the ureter or intravenously.

pyelos′tomy. Surgical formation of an opening into the pelvis of the kidney.

pyelot′omy. Incision into the pelvis of the kidney.

pyeloureterec′tasis. Dilatation of kidney pelvis and ureter.

pyem′esis. The vomiting of purulent material.

pye′mia. A form of septicemia in which there is a general secondary infection with formation of multiple abscesses in several areas of the body; also called metastatic infection.

pye′mic. Afflicted with pyemia.

Pyemotes ventricosus. A small parasite of insect larvae (esp. the grain moth and the wheat grain worm); the young female has an elongated body which becomes greatly distended when gravid; the fertilized eggs are retained in her abdomen where they hatch and become mature mites before they

are discharged; the mites may burrow in the epidermis of individuals in contact with grains, straw or hay, causing a skin eruption; also called hay or grain itch mite.

pye′sis. Suppuration.

pyg′myism. Primordial dwarfism; see under dwarfism.

pyk′nic. Having a short, stocky, well rounded body build with ample body cavities.

pyknomor′phous. Having the stainable elements closely packed; said of a cell.

pykno′sis. Condensation and shrinking of a cell nucleus; e.g., during maturation of a red blood cell prior to ejection of the nucleus from the cell.

py′la. The opening between the third ventricle of the brain and the cerebral aqueduct (aqueduct of Sylvius).

pylemphrax′is. Obstruction of the portal vein.

phylephlebecta′sia. Dilatation of the portal vein.

pylephlebi′tis. Inflammation of the portal vein or its branches.

pylethrombophlebi′tis. Inflammation and thrombosis of the portal vein.

pylethrombo′sis. Thrombosis of the portal vein or its branches.

py′lic. Referring to the portal vein.

py′lon. A temporary artificial leg.

pyloral′gia. Pain in the pyloric area of the stomach.

pylorec′tomy. Surgical removal of the pylorus.

pylor′ic. Of or relating to the pylorus.

pyloric-channel syndrome. A syndrome characterized by inflammation of the pylorus and the prepyloric region with muscle hypertrophy and narrowing of the pyloric canal, resulting in pyloric obstruction.

pyloristeno′sis. Stricture of the pylorus.

pylori′tis. Inflammation of the pyloric area of the stomach.

pylorogastrec′tomy. Surgical removal of the pyloric portion of the stomach.

pyloromyot′omy. Operative technique for the treatment of congenital pyloric stenosis; also called Fredet-Ramstedt operation.

pylo′roplasty. Plastic operation of the pylorus, especially one to enlarge a constricted pylorus; performed sometimes in the treatment of peptic ulcers.

pylo′rospasm. Spasm of the pylorus or the pyloric area of the stomach; in adults, usually associated with nearby duodenal or gastric ulcer or severe gastritis.

pylorot′omy. Surgical incision of the pylorus.

pylo′rus. The opening between the stomach and duodenum.

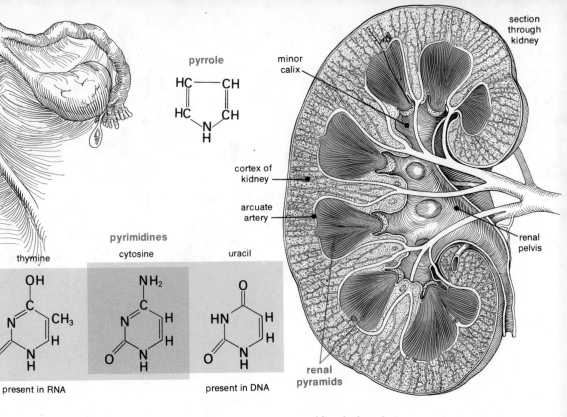

pyosalpinx

pyrrole

section through kidney

minor calix

cortex of kidney

arcuate artery

renal pelvis

pyrimidines

thymine
cytosine
uracil

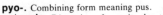
pyridoxal phosphate

present in RNA

present in DNA

renal pyramids

pyo-. Combining form meaning pus.

py'ocele. Distention of a cavity due to accumulation of pus.

pyoceph'alus. The presence of a purulent fluid within the skull.

pyoche'zia. The discharge of pus with the stools.

pyococ'cus. A pus-producing microorganism, as *Streptococcus pyogenes.*

pyocol'pos. Accumulation of pus in the vagina.

pyocyan'ic. Relating to blue pus or to the bacillus that produces it (*Pseudomonas aeruginosa*).

pyocy'anin. An antibiotic substance obtained from the bacillus *Pseudomonas aeruginosa.*

py'ocyst. A pus-containing cyst.

pyoder'ma, pyoder'mia. Any pus-producing disease of the skin.

   p. gangrenosum, an eruption of chronic pustules associated with ulcerative colitis.

py'ogen. Anything that causes pus formation.

pyogen'esis. The formation of pus; also called pyopoiesis.

pyogen'ic. Producing pus.

pyohemotho'rax. The presence of pus and blood in the pleural cavity.

py'oid. Resembling pus; also called puriform.

pyolabyrinthi'tis. Suppurative inflammation of the labyrinth of the internal ear.

pyome'tra. Accumulation of pus in the uterus.

pyometri'tis. Inflammation of the wall of the uterus with accumulation of pus in its cavity.

pyomyosi'tis. Condition marked by the formation of single or multiple deep-seated abscesses in voluntary muscles; caused by *Staphylococcus aureus;* also called tropical pyomyositis.

pyonephrolithi'asis. The presence of pus and stones in the kidney.

pyonephro'sis. Distention of the calices and pelvis of the kidney with pus.

pyoova'rium. Pus in the ovary; also called ovarian abscess.

pyopericardi'tis. Suppurative inflammation of the pericardium.

pyopericar'dium. Accumulation of pus in the sac enveloping the heart (pericardium).

pyoperitoni'tis. Suppurative inflammation of the peritoneum.

pyophthal'mia, pyophthalmi'tis. Suppurative inflammation of the eye, especially the conjunctiva.

pyophysome'tra. An accumulation of gas and pus in the uterine cavity.

pyopneu'mocholecysti'tis. Distention of an inflamed gallbladder with gas and pus; caused by gas-producing organisms or by the entry of air from the intestine through the biliary tree.

pyopneumopericar'dium. A condition marked by the presence of pus and gas in the membranous sac surrounding the heart (pericardium).

pyopneumoperitone'um. A condition marked by the presence of pus and gas in the peritoneal cavity.

pyopneumothor'ax. The presence of pus and air in the pleural cavity; also called pneumopyothorax.

pyopoie'sis. Pyogenesis; the formation of pus.

pyopoiet'ic. Pus-producing.

pyop'tysis. Spitting of pus.

pyorrhe'a. See periodontitis.

pyosalpingi'tis. Suppurative inflammation of the uterine tube.

pyosalpingo-oophori'tis. Suppurative inflammation of the uterine tube and the ovary.

pyosal'pinx. Accumulation of pus in the uterine tube.

pyo'sis. Suppuration.

pyostat'ic. Denoting an agent that arrests the formation of pus.

pyoure'ter. Pus in a ureter.

pyr'amid. Any of numerous anatomic structures that are pyramidal or cone-shaped.

   cerebellar p., the pyramid of the vermis; the central portion of the inferior vermis of the cerebellum between the uvula and tuber.

   malpighian p., see renal pyramid.

   p. of light, a triangular area on the anterior inferior surface of the tympanic membrane which reflects light brightly; it extends from the umbo to the periphery; also called cone of light.

   p.'s of the medulla, two anterior and two posterior longitudinal fiber bundles within the medulla oblongata that resemble narrow elongated pyramids.

   p. of thyroid gland, pyramidal lobe of thyroid gland; see under lobe.

   renal p., one of a number of pyramidal masses formed by the medullary substance of the kidney, containing part of the secreting and collecting tubules; the apex projects into the minor calix; also called malpighian pyramid.

pyram'idal. Relating to or having the shape of a pyramid; said of certain anatomic structures.

pyret'ic. Feverish.

pyretogen'esis. The causation of fever.

pyretogenet'ic. Relating to pyretogenesis.

pyretother'apy. 1. Treatment of disease by intermittent raising of body temperature. **2.** Treatment of fever.

pyrex'ia. A fever; elevation of body temperature above normal.

pyr'idine. A colorless, flammable liquid, C_5H_5N, used in the preparation of vitamins and drugs, as a solvent, and as a denaturant of alcohol.

pyridoxal phosphate. A vitamin derivative or coenzyme essential to many reactions of amino acid metabolism, as transamination, decarboxylation, and racemization.

pyridox'ine. Common name for a group of water-soluble substances of the vitamin B complex, essential in protein metabolism; also called vitamin B$_6$.

pyrimeth'amine. An antimalarial agent.

pyrim'idine. The fundamental substance of several organic bases, some of which are components of nucleic acid.

pyro-. Combining form meaning fire.

pyrogal'lol. Pyrogallic acid, $C_6H_3(OH)_3$; used in the treatment of skin disorders, as psoriasis and ringworm.

py'rogen. A fever-producing agent.

pyrogen'ic. 1. Producing or caused by fever. **2.** Produced by or generating heat.

pyrolig'enous. Relating to or obtained from the destructive distillation of wood.

pyrol'ysis. Chemical change produced by heat.

pyroma'nia. A morbid desire to set things on fire.

pyrom'eter. An electric thermometer for measuring extremely high temperatures.

py'ronin. A basic red dye used in histologic stains.

pyropho'bia. Abnormal fear of fire.

pyrophos'phatase. Any enzyme that splits a pyrophosphate.

pyrophos'phate. A salt of pyrophosphoric acid.

pyrophosphoric acid. A water-soluble, crystalline substance, $H_4P_2O_7$, obtained by heating phosphoric acid.

pyro'sis. Heartburn; a burning sensation in the esophagus caused by the rising of small amounts of acid liquid or gas from the stomach. See also water brash.

pyrot'ic. 1. Relating to heartburn. **2.** Caustic.

pyr'role. A toxic heterocyclic compound possessing an odor suggestive of chloroform; the parent of many biologically important natural compounds such as bile pigments, porphyrins, chlorophyll, etc; also called azole.

py'ruvate. A salt or ester of pyruvic acid.

   p. kinase, enzyme that promotes the transfer of phosphate from phosphoenolpyruvate to ADP, forming ATP and pyruvate; deficiency of pyruvate kinase in red blood cells is the cause of an autosomal recessive hemolytic anemia; also called phosphoenolpyruvate kinase.

pyruvic acid. A colorless liquid, $CH_3COCOOH$, with an odor similar to that of acetic acid; an intermediate product in the metabolism of carbohydrate.

pyrvinium pamoate. A deep red, crystalline substance; used in the eradication in pinworms.

pyu'ria. The presence of pus in the urine.

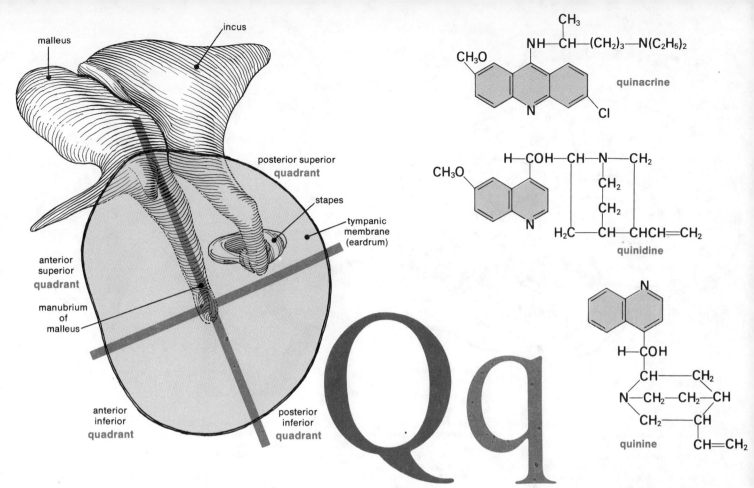

malleus · incus · posterior superior **quadrant** · stapes · tympanic membrane (eardrum) · anterior superior **quadrant** · manubrium of malleus · anterior inferior **quadrant** · posterior inferior **quadrant**

quinacrine

quinidine

quinine

Qq

Q. 1. Abbreviation for (a) coulomb (unit of quantity of electricity); (b) quadrant. **2.** Symbol for (a) the first downward deflection of the QRS complex of the electrocardiogram; (b) the seventh in a series, e.g., the seventh orbit of electrons in the atom.

Q_{10}. Symbol for the increase in rate of a process as a result of raising the temperature 10°C.

QCO_2. Symbol for the carbon dioxide given off (in microliters) per milligram of tissue per hour at standard pressure and temperature.

QO_2. Symbol for oxygen consumption (in microliters) per milligram of tissue per hour at standard pressure and temperature.

q.d. Abbreviation for Latin *quaque die*.

q.h. Abbreviation for Latin *quaque hora*.

q.i.d. Abbreviation for Latin *quater in die*.

q.l. Abbreviation for Latin *quantum libet*.

q.q.h. Abbreviation for Latin *quaque quarta hora*.

q.s. Abbreviation for Latin *quantum sufficit*.

qt. Abbreviation for quart.

quack. One who fraudulently misrepresents his medical or dental capability to diagnose and treat disease and who generally makes extravagant claims as to the effects achieved by the treatment he offers.

quack'ery. A false claim to medical knowledge and experience in treating the sick.

quadr-. See quadri-.

quad'rant. 1. One-quarter of a circle. **2.** In anatomy, one of the four sections into which roughly circular areas of the body are divided for descriptive purposes; e.g., the tympanic membrane, the fundus of the eye, the abdomen.

quadrantanop'sia. Blindness in approximately a quarter of the visual field; also called quadrantic hemianopsia.

quad'rate. Having equal sides; square-shaped; four-sided.

quadra'tus. Denoting certain muscles which have a seemingly square shape.

quadri-, quadr-. Combining forms indicating four; e.g., quadripara.

quadriba'sic. Referring to an acid that has four replaceable hydrogen atoms.

quad'riceps. Having four heads, as some muscles.

quadrigem'inal. Occurring in a group of four; four-fold, having four parts.

quadrip'ara. A woman who has given birth to four children.

quadriple'gia. Paralysis of all four extremities; also called tetraplegia.

quadripleg'ic. One whose four limbs are paralyzed.

quad'risect. To divide or cut into four parts.

quadriv'alent. Having the combining ability of four hydrogen atoms; also called tetravalent.

quad'ruplet. One of four offspring born at one birth.

quan'ta. Plural of quantum.

quan'tum, *pl.* **quan'ta. 1.** A unit of radiant energy. **2.** A specified amount.

   q. libet (q.l.), Latin for as much as desired.

   q. sufficit (q.s.), Latin for sufficient amount or as much as suffices.

   q.vis (q.v.), Latin for as much as you want; used in prescription writing.

quaque die (q.d.). Latin for every day.

quaque hora (q.h.). Latin for every hour; used in prescription writing.

quaque quarta hora (q.q.h.). Latin for every four hours.

quar'antine. 1. The restriction of freedom of movement of persons who have been exposed to a communicable disease; originally the period of restriction was 40 days. **2.** The isolation of a person afflicted with a communicable disease.

quart. 1. A measure of fluid capacity equal to two pints; one-fourth of a gallon; 32 ounces; 0.9468 liter; 57.75 cubic inches. **2.** A unit of volume in dry measure equal to 67.2 cubic inches.

   imperial q., a British unit of volume or capacity equal to 1.201 liquid quarts.

quar'tan. Recurring every four days, as a malarial fever; actually, the attack occurs on day one and day four, so that there is really only an interval of two days.

quartz. A form of silica, used in dentistry as one of three main ingredients of dental porcelain.

qua'ter in di'e (q.i.d.). Latin for four times a day.

quater'nary. 1. The member of a series which is fourth in order. **2.** A chemical compound containing four different elements; e.g., $NaHSO_4$.

Queckenstedt's sign. Absence of variation in pressure of the cerebrospinal fluid when the veins of the neck are compressed; indicative of a block in the vertebral canal.

quick. A sensitive part, painful to the touch.

quick'ening. The sensation caused by the movement of the fetus within the uterus, felt by the mother for the first time about the fourth or fifth month of pregnancy.

quick'silver. See mercury.

quin'acrine. A bright yellow antimalarial drug with a biologic half-life of 10 days; Atabrine®.

Quincke's disease. Angioneurotic edema; see under edema.

Quincke's sign. Quincke's pulse; see under pulse.

quinhy'drone. A compound of equimolecular quantities of quinone and hydroquinone; $C_6H_4O_2 \cdot C_6H_4(OH)_2$; used in pH determinations.

quin'idine. An alkaloid from cinchona bark; used to control cardiac arrhythmias.

quin'ine. A white, crystalline, bitter powder, obtained from the bark of the cinchona tree; used in the treatment of malaria; also called quinina and Jesuit's or Cardinal's bark.

quin'inism. See cinchonism.

quin'one. Any of a group of aromatic crystalline compounds used in making dyes.

quinquagenar'ian. An individual in his fifties.

quinqui'na. Cinchona bark from which quinine is extracted.

quin'sy. Acute suppurative inflammation of the tonsils and surrounding tissue.

quintip'ara. A woman who has given birth to five children.

quintup'let. One of five children born of a single birth.

quod vi'de (q.v.). Latin for which see; usually placed in parentheses after a cross-reference.

quotid'ian. Recurring every day, as a fever.

quo'tient. The number of times a quantity is contained in another.

   blood q., color index, see under index.

   intelligence q. (IQ), the ratio of a person's mental age, determined by the Binet-Simon scale, to his actual age, multiplied by 100.

   respiratory q., the ratio between the volume of carbon dioxide expired and the volume of oxygen consumed; it varies with the diet, but normally is about 0.82.

q.v. Abbreviation for (a) Latin *quantum vis*; (b) Latin *quod vide*.

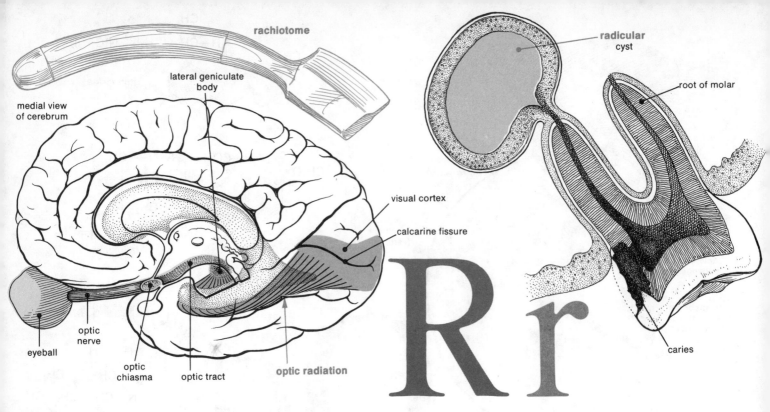

medial view of cerebrum

rachiotome

lateral geniculate body

eyeball

optic nerve

optic chiasma

optic tract

optic radiation

visual cortex

calcarine fissure

radicular cyst

root of molar

caries

Rr

R. 1. Abbreviation for respiration. **2.** Symbol for (a) electrical resistance; (b) gas constant; (c) registered trademark (often enclosed in a circle, ®); (d) organic radical; (e) roentgen.

r. 1. Abbreviation for (a) radius; (b) ratio; (c) refraction. **2.** Symbol for (a) oxidation-reduction potential; (b) radius.

RA. Abbreviation for (a) rheumatoid arthritis; (b) right atrium.

Ra. Chemical symbol of the element radium.

rab′id. Afflicted with rabies.

ra′bies. A viral encephalitis transmitted through saliva of an infected animal; the incubation period varies from 10 days to several months; invariably fatal in man unless preventive treatment is administered; also called hydrophobia.

race. A class of individuals having common genetically transmitted physical characteristics.

race′mic. 1. Composed of clustered parts; said of glands. **2.** Denoting a chemical compound composed of equal parts of dextrorotatory and levorotatory substances, therefore incapable of rotating the plane of polarized light.

racemiza′tion. The chemical conversion of an optically active substance into another that is relatively, or completely, inactive.

race′mose. Resembling a bunch of grapes.

rachi-, rachio-. Combining forms meaning spine.

ra′chial. Spinal.

rachial′gia. Pain in the spine (vertebral column); also called spondylalgia.

rachicente′sis. Lumbar puncture.

rachid′ian. Spinal.

rachiocamp′sis. Spinal curvature.

rachiocente′sis. Spinal puncture.

rachiodyn′ia. Pain in the spinal muscles.

rachiop′athy. Any disease of the spinal cord; also called spondylopathy.

ra′chiotome. A surgical bone-cutting instrument for dividing the vertebral laminae; also called rachitome.

rachiot′omy. The operative procedure of cutting into the vertebral column.

ra′chis. The vertebral column.

rachis′chisis. Myelocele; developmental defect in which the vertebral arches are absent.

rachit′ic. Relating to or affected with rickets.

rachi′tis. Rickets; a disease of infants and children caused by deficiency of vitamin D.

rachitogen′ic. Producing or causing rickets, as a vitamin D-deficient diet.

ra′chitome. See rachiotome.

rad. A unit of radiation exposure expressing the absorbed dose; one rad represents absorption of 100 ergs of energy per gram, and is roughly equiva-

lent to a roentgen.

radarkymog′raphy. Videotaping of heart motions during fluoroscopy with the aid of an image intensifier; it enables the movements to be calibrated through graphic tracings.

radec′tomy. Removal of a portion or the whole of the root of a tooth.

radiabil′ity. The property of being permeable by x rays.

ra′dial. 1. Relating to a bone in the forearm (radius) or to any radius. **2.** Diverging in various directions from a central point.

ra′dial-immunodiffu′sion. A method of quantifying immunoglobulins; plates of agar impregnated with various antisera to specific immunoglobulins are used as receptacles for the plasma to be tested; as the test sample immunoglobulin diffuses into the agar, a circle of precipitation forms, the diameter of which is proportional to the amount of immunoglobulin in the test sample.

ra′diant. 1. Emitting heat or light rays. **2.** A central point from which rays diverge. **3.** Emitted as radiation.

ra′diate. 1. To expose to radiation. **2.** To emit radiation. **3.** To diverage in all directions from a center.

radia′tion. 1. The emission and projection of energy (waves or particles) through space. **2.** A bundle of white fibers in the brain.

  background r., the measured radioactivity in a given location, in the absence of a sample.

  "hard" r., short wavelength radiation having high energy and the ability to penetrate deeply.

  optic r., a band of fibers in the brain passing from the lateral geniculate body of the thalamus to the cortex of the occipital lobe.

  scattered r., the change in direction of the x-ray photon as a result of collision with matter.

  "soft" r., long wavelength radiation of low penetrability.

rad′ical. 1. A group of atoms that can pass from one compound to another without changing, and which forms one of the basic parts of a molecule; in chemical formulas it is enclosed in parentheses. **2.** Carried to the farthest limit in dealing with the root or cause of a disease.

  acid r., a radical formed by an acid by loss of one or more hydrogen ions.

  free r., chemical group that has unshared electrons available for reaction; e.g., as CH_3.

rad′icle. A small rootlike structure; a rootlet.

radicot′omy. See rhizotomy.

radicul′gia. Neuralgia of the sensory root of a spinal nerve, usually due to an irritation.

radic′ular. Relating to a root, especially a nerve or

a tooth root.

radiculec′tomy. Resection of a spinal nerve root.

radiculi′tis. Inflammation of the portion of a spinal nerve root within the dura mater.

radic′ulomyelop′athy. Disease of the spinal cord and nerve roots.

radic′uloneurop′athy. Disease of the spinal nerve roots and nerves.

radic′ulop′athy. Disease of the spinal nerve roots.

radio-. Combining form denoting radiation.

radioac′tive. Relating to or possessing radioactivity.

radioactiv′ity. The property, possessed by certain elements of high atomic weight, of emitting rays and subatomic particles, either through unstable atomic nuclei or as a result of nuclear reaction.

radioau′tograph. See autoradiograph.

radiobiol′ogy. The branch of science concerned with the effects of radiation on living tissues and with the use of radioactive isotopes.

radiocal′cium (^{45}Ca). Radioisotope of calcium, usually used in bone tumor localization and bone metabolism studies.

radiocar′bon (^{14}C). Radioactive isotope of carbon.

radiocar′pal. Relating to the radius and the carpal bones, especially the joint between the radius and the proximal row of carpal bones.

radiochem′istry. The study of chemical reactions of radioactive elements.

radiocinematog′raphy. The technique of making motion pictures of the passage of a radiopaque substance through the internal organs as seen on x-ray examination.

radiocur′able. Susceptible to cure by irradiation; said of some cancer cells.

radiodermati′tis. Inflammation of the skin caused by excessive exposure to x or γ rays.

radiodon′tics. The branch of dentistry that specializes in the taking and interpreting or roentgenograms of teeth and related structures.

radioelec′trophysiol′ograph. Apparatus by means of which changes in the electrical potential of brain or heart are radiotransmitted and recorded at some other site; the apparatus is carried by the person, who is unrestricted in his movements.

radioel′ement. Any radioactive element.

radioepidermi′tis. Inflammation of the skin caused by exposure to ionizing radiation; also called radiodermatitis.

radiofre′quency. A frequency of electromagnetic radiation in the range between audio frequencies and infrared frequencies.

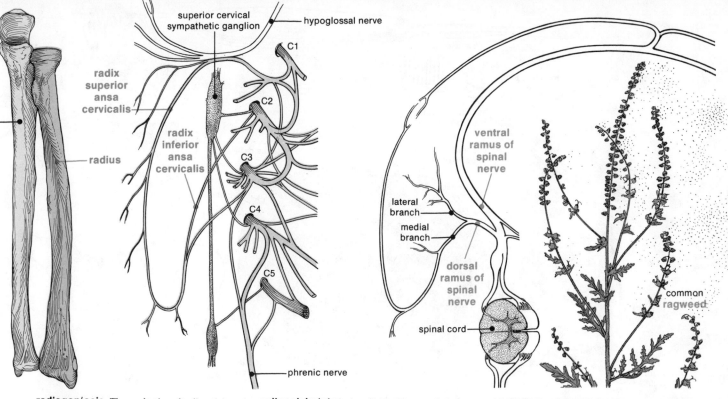

Labels on illustrations: ulna · radix superior ansa cervicalis · radius · radix inferior ansa cervicalis · superior cervical sympathetic ganglion · hypoglossal nerve · C1 · C2 · C3 · C4 · C5 · phrenic nerve · ventral ramus of spinal nerve · lateral branch · medial branch · dorsal ramus of spinal nerve · spinal cord · common ragweed

radiogen′esis. The production of radioactivity.

radiogen′ic. 1. Producing rays. **2.** Produced by radioactivity.

ra′diogram. Term sometimes used instead of the preferred terms roentgenogram and radiograph.

ra′diograph. The processed photographic film produced in radiography.

radiog′raphy. The development of an image of a bodily part by transmitting radioactive energy (x or γ rays) through it onto a sensitized film.

radiohu′meral. Relating to the radius and the humerus.

ra′dioimmu′noassay. A method of analysis, such as determination of the concentration of substances in blood plasma, through the use of radioactive antibodies.

ra′dioimmu′nodiffu′sion. The study of antigen-antibody reactions by gel diffusion using radioisotope-labeled antigen or antibody.

ra′dioimmu′noelec′trophore′sis. Immunoelectrophoresis using radioisotope-labeled antigen or antibody.

radioi′odinated. Combined or treated with radio-iodine.

radioi′odine. A radioactive isotope of iodine; about two dozen are known, the most commonly used at present being ^{131}I and ^{125}I.

radioi′sotope. An isotope of an element which is naturally or artificially radioactive.

radiolog′ic. Relating to radiology.

radiol′ogist. A physician with specific training in radiology.

radiol′ogy. The science that deals with radiant energy (x rays, radium, and radioactive isotopes) and its use for the diagnosis and treatment of disease. Cf roentgenology.

radiolu′cency. The state of being moderately transparent to x rays or other forms of radiation.

radiomimet′ic. Denoting a chemical that has a destructive effect on tissues which is similar to that of high energy radiation; e.g., sulfur mustards, nitrogen mustards.

radionecro′sis. Destruction of tissues due to radiation.

radionu′clide. A radioactive nuclide; a species of nuclide with an unstable nucleus; found in a natural state or a chemical element made radioactive through bombardment by neutrons in a cyclotron or atomic pile.

radiopa′city. The state of being impenetrable by any form of radiation.

radiopaque′. Impenetrable by x rays or any form of radiation.

radiopathol′ogy. The study and treatment of conditions caused by radiation.

radiopelvim′etry. A radiographic procedure for determining the size and shape of the maternal pelvis, the fetus, and its presenting part.

radiopharmaceut′ical. A radioactive pharmaceutical preparation used for diagnostic or therapeutic purposes.

radio-phar′macist. A pharmacist specializing in the preparation and dispensing of radioactive drugs.

radio-phar′macy. The branch of pharmacy dealing with the preparation and dispensing of radioactive drugs utilizing short-lived radioisotopes.

radioreac′tion. A bodily reaction to radiation, especially of the skin.

radiorecep′tor. A receptor capable of responding to radiant energy, such as light or heat.

radioresis′tance. The relative resistance of cells or organisms to the injurious action of radiation.

radios′copy. Roentgenoscopy; examination of internal structures of the body by x rays.

radiosen′sitive. Affected by radiation.

radiosensitiv′ity. Relative susceptibility of biologic tissues or substances to the action of radiation; also called radiosensitiveness.

radiosur′gery. Use of radioactive objects such as radium needles or radon seeds in surgical treatment.

radiother′apist. A physician who specializes in radiotherapy.

radiother′apy. The treatment of disease by any radioactive substance or radiant energy.

radiotoxe′mia. Radiation sickness.

radiotranspar′ent. Allowing the passage of radiant energy.

radioul′nar. Relating to the radius and the ulna.

ra′dium. A radioactive metallic element which emits α-, β-, and γ-radiation and a radioactive gas called radon; it has a half-life of 1,590 years; symbol Ra, atomic number 88, atomic weight 226.05; in medicine, it is used in the treatment of some malignancies.

ra′dius, *pl.* **ra′dii. 1.** The smaller of the two bones of the forearm, on the side of the thumb. **2.** A straight line extending from the center to the periphery of a circle.

ra′dix, *pl.* **rad′ices.** Latin for root; the beginning or primary portion of a structure, as a nerve at its origin from the spinal cord.

　r. inferior ansa cervicalis, fibers from the second and third cervical nerves that form the inferior root of the cervical loop (ansa cervicalis).

　r. linguae, root of the tongue; the posterior attached part of the tongue.

　r. superior ansa cervicalis, fibers from the first and second cervical nerves that form the superior root of the cervical loop (ansa cervicalis).

ra′don. A colorless gas emanating from radium,

with a half-life of about four days; it is a natural isotope produced during the radioactive decay of radium; symbol Rn, atomic number 86, atomic weight 222; also called radium emanation.

raf′finose. $C_{18}H_{3}O_{16} \cdot 5H_2O$; a sugar occurring in cottonseed meal and in sugar beets, composed of D-galactose, D-glucose, and D-fructose; also called melitose.

rage. Intense, violent anger.

　sham r., an outburst of motor activity in an animal whose cerebral hemispheres have been removed, characterized by manifestations of fear and anger on slight provocation and accompanied by struggling, piloerection, dilatation of pupils, and increase in blood pressure.

rag′weed. A weed of the genus *Ambrosia*, especially the species *Ambrosia artemisiifolia* (comon ragweed), *Ambrosia trifida* (giant ragweed) or *Ambrosia psilostachya* (Western ragweed), whose abundant pollen is a hazard to many hay fever sufferers; sometimes called bitterweed.

rale. Abnormal sound heard on auscultation of the chest, originating in the pulmonary airway, and usually indicating disease of the bronchi or lungs.

　coarse r., see rhonchus.

　fine r., short, high-pitched sound originating in the alveoli and terminal bronchi; the sound is simulated by rubbing hair between one's fingers close to the ear.

　medium r., one having a pitch that is lower than that of a fine rale.

rami. Plural of ramus (branch).

ram′ify. To branch.

ra′mose, ra′mous. Branching.

ram′ulus. A minute terminal branch.

ra′mus, *pl.* **ra′mi.** A branchlike part of a nerve, artery, or vein, especially a primary division.

　dorsal r. of spinal nerve, a bundle of nerve fibers given off by a spinal nerve immediately after the union of its dorsal and ventral roots; it innervates the structures of the back.

　r. communicans, a bundle of nerve fibers connecting two nerves or a nerve to a ganglion.

　ventral r. of spinal nerve, the continuation of a spinal nerve soon after it emerges from the intervertebral foramen, dividing ultimately into the lateral and anterior divisions; it innervates the limbs and the anterolateral parts of the body wall; the major plexuses (cervical, brachial, and lumbosacral) are formed by the ventral rami of spinal nerves.

ran′ine. Pertaining to the undersurface of the tongue.

ran′ula. A cystic tumor occurring on the floor of the mouth or the undersurface of the tongue; also called sublingual cyst.

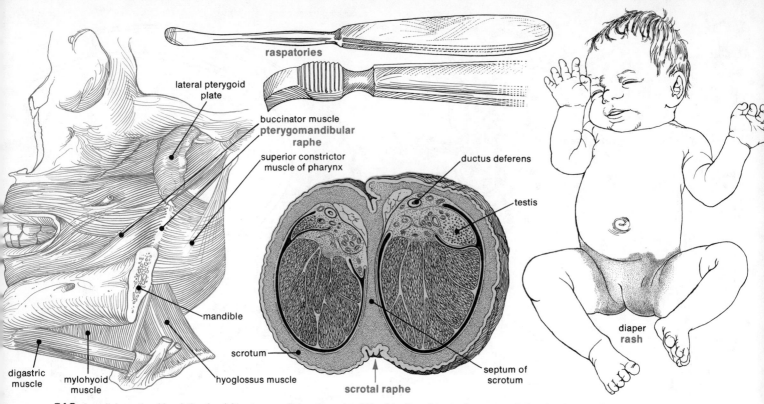

raspatories

lateral pterygoid plate

buccinator muscle
pterygomandibular raphe

superior constrictor muscle of pharynx

ductus deferens

testis

mandible

scrotum

septum of scrotum

digastric muscle

mylohyoid muscle

hyoglossus muscle

scrotal raphe

diaper **rash**

RAO. In radiology, the abbreviation for right anterior-oblique projection.

rape. The criminal act in which an individual forces another individual to submit to sexual intercourse; also called rape of the first degree.

 statutory r., sexual intercourse with a female under the legal age of consent; also called rape of the second degree.

ra′phe. A ridge or line marking the union of two similar structures.

 scrotal r., one extending from the anus to the base of the penis; it marks the attachment of the scrotal septum which separates the testes.

rapport. Relationship, especially one of mutual understanding; also called accord.

rap′tus. Any sudden seizure.

rarefac′tion. The process of becoming less dense.

rar′efy. To make light, less dense, or less compact.

RAS. Abbreviation for reticular activating system.

rash. Any eruption of the skin.

 heat r., see heat, prickly.

 morbilliform r., condition of the skin resembling the eruption of measles.

 nettle r., urticaria.

ras′patory. Instrument for scraping bone.

rat. Any of various long-tailed rodents of the genus *Rattus;* vectors of human disease.

 albino r., white rat used extensively in laboratory experiments.

 black r., English black rat, *Rattus rattus*, that harbors the flea, *Zenopsylla cheopis*, responsible for transmitting plague to humans.

 brown r., large brownish-gray rat, *Rattus norvegicus*, with short ears and a smaller than usual tail.

 spontaneously hypertensive r. (SHR), A strain of rats prone to develop hypertension without recourse to special diets or hormones; originally developed in Japan; a useful animal in research in hypertension.

 Sprague-Dawley r., genetically similar, inbred strain of rats developed by the Sprague-Dawley Company.

 Wistar r., a white rat extensively used in experimental biology and medicine; strain developed at the Wistar Institute.

rate. A quantitative measurement of an event or process in terms of its relationship to some fixed standard; a measured quantity expressed as the ratio of one quantity to another.

 basal metabolic r. (BMR), see metabolism, basal.

 case r., see morbidity rate.

 death r., see mortality rate.

 erythrocyte sedimentation r. (ESR), the rate (in millimeters per hour) of settling of red blood cells

when anticoagulated blood is allowed to stand under standard conditions in a vertical glass column; the two standard methods commonly used are those of Wintrobe and Westergren (see under method); also called sedimentation rate.

 fetal heart r. (FHR), the number of fetal heart beats per minute, normally ranging from 120 to 140.

 glomerular filtration r. (GFR), the volume of plasma filtered through the glomerular capillary membranes of the kidney in one minute; determined by the rate of glomerular perfusion, the permeability of the capillary wall, the plasma oncotic pressure, and the intracapillary hydrostatic pressure; measured indirectly by determining the rate of removal or clearance from plasma to urine of a measurable substance (usually inulin) which is freely filtered at the glomerulus and neither reabsorbed from nor secreted into the tubule; the normal GFR is generally around 120 milliliters per minute per 1.73 square meters.

 growth r., absolute or relative growth increase, expressed in units of time.

 morbidity r., the number of cases of a particular disease occurring in a year per given unit of the total population; also called case rate.

 mortality r., the ratio between the number of registered deaths in a specified area and the total population during a given period, usually one year; also called death rate.

 pulse r., the number of beats per minute of a peripheral arterial pulse.

 respiration r., the rate of breathing; the number of inspirations (breaths) per minute.

 sedimentation r., erythrocyte sedimentation rate.

ra′tio. Proportion; the relation that one thing bears to another in respect to magnitude or quantity; also called rate.

 body-weight r., body weight in grams divided by the height in centimeters.

 cardiothoracic r., the ratio of the transverse diameter of the heart to the internal diameter of the thoracic cage at its widest point.

 extraction r., the fraction of a substance removed from the blood by an organ; $A - V/A$ (A and V being the concentration of the substance in arterial and venous renal plasma, respectively).

 mendelian r., the ratio in which the offspring, or later generations, show the characteristics of their parents, in accordance with genetic principles.

 nucleocytoplasmic r., the ratio of the volumes of nucleus and cytoplasm within a given cell; the ratio is generally constant for a particular cell type, and is usually increased in malignant neoplasms; also

called nucleoplasmic ratio.

 nucleoplasmic r., see nucleocytoplasmic ratio.

 segregation r., ratio of the various segregating genotypes among offspring.

 therapeutic r., the ratio of the maximally tolerated dose of a drug to the minimal effective dose; the higher the ratio the safer the drug.

rational. 1. In possession of reasoning qualities; not delirious. **2.** Based on reason.

rationaliza′tion. The provision of an explanation to justify an act which is governed by factors other than reason.

rat′tlesnake. Any of numerous poisonous snakes (genera *Crotalus* and *Sistrurus*) that have a series of horny segments loosely interlocking at the end of the tail which make a rattling sound when vibrated.

rauwol′fia. An alkaloid derived from a number of tropical trees and shrubs of the genus *Rauwolfia*.

 r. serpentina., the dried root of *Rauwolfia serpentina* which is the source of tranquilizing alkaloid drugs such as reserpine.

ray. 1. A straight-line, narrow beam of electromagnetic radiation such as light, heat, or other form of radiation. **2.** A linear anatomic structure.

 actinic r., a light ray toward and beyond the violet end of the spectrum, capable of producing chemical changes; photochemically active radiation.

 α-r.'s, fast moving streams of minute alpha particles of matter composed of positively charged composite particles, indistinguishable from helium atom nuclei; derived from radioactive substances.

 Becquerel r.'s, α-, β-, and γ-rays emitted from uranium, radium, and other radioactive substances.

 β-r.'s, fast moving streams of negatively charged beta particles of matter, especially of electrons, that have greater penetrative power than the α-rays; derived from radioactive substances.

 borderline r.'s, grenz rays.

 cathode r.'s, a stream of electrons emitted by the negative electrode (cathode) in a vacuum tube (Crookes' tube); their bombardment against the glass wall of the tube or against the anode gives rise to the x rays (roentgen rays).

 cosmic r.'s, high energy particles that bombard the earth from outer space.

 γ-r., electromagnetic radiation emitted from the nucleus of an atom during the radioactive decay process; analogous to the x ray but of shorter wave length.

 grenz r.'s, very soft x rays, greater in length than one Å; closely allied to the ultraviolet rays in their wavelength and in their biologic action upon tissue; used in x-raying soft tissues; also called borderline rays.

 hard r., x ray of short wavelength and great pene-

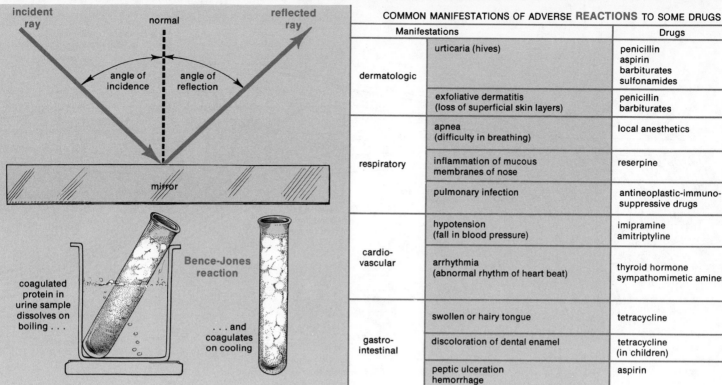

COMMON MANIFESTATIONS OF ADVERSE REACTIONS TO SOME DRUGS

Manifestations		Drugs
dermatologic	urticaria (hives)	penicillin aspirin barbiturates sulfonamides
	exfoliative dermatitis (loss of superficial skin layers)	penicillin barbiturates
respiratory	apnea (difficulty in breathing)	local anesthetics
	inflammation of mucous membranes of nose	reserpine
	pulmonary infection	antineoplastic-immuno- suppressive drugs
cardio- vascular	hypotension (fall in blood pressure)	imipramine amitriptyline
	arrhythmia (abnormal rhythm of heart beat)	thyroid hormone sympathomimetic amines
gastro- intestinal	swollen or hairy tongue	tetracycline
	discoloration of dental enamel	tetracycline (in children)
	peptic ulceration hemorrhage	aspirin

Bence-Jones reaction

coagulated protein in urine sample dissolves on boiling . . .

. . . and coagulates on cooling

---

trability; produced by a high-voltage tube.

Hertzian r.'s, radio waves; see under wave.

incident r., a ray that strikes the surface before reflection.

infrared r.'s, rays having wavelengths greater than 7700 Å, beyond the red end of the spectrum.

medullary r., the center of the renal lobe, which has the shape of a small steep pyramid, consisting of straight ascending or descending limbs of the nephronic loop or collecting tubules; also called pars radiata lobuli corticalis renis.

reflected r., a ray of radiant energy thrown back from a nonabsorbent surface.

roentgen r., see x ray (1).

soft r., one of long wavelength and slight penetrability.

ultraviolet r.'s, rays having wavelenghs between 4000 and 40 Å, between the violet end of the visible spectrum and the x-ray region of the electromagnetic spectrum.

vital ultraviolet r.'s, rays of wavelengths between 3200 and 2900 Å which are necessary for normal growth; they promote calcium metabolism.

x r., (1) an electromagnetic radiation (high energy photon) with a very short wavelength (0.05 to 100 Å), generated at the point of impact of a stream of high-speed cathode electrons on the target of an x-ray tube; x rays, because of their penetrating power, are used to record on film shadows of the varying densities within a portion of the body; also called roentgen ray; (2) a photograph taken with x rays, properly termed roentgenogram.

Raynaud's disease. Bilateral cyanosis of the fingers due to spasmodic contraction of the peripheral arteries, usually precipitated by cold or by emotion.

Rb. Chemical symbol of the element rubidium.

RBBB. Abbreviation for right bundle-branch block.

RBC. Abbreviation for red blood cell.

RBE. Abbreviation for relative biologic effectiveness.

RBF. Abbreviation for renal blood flow.

RDA. Abbreviation for recommended dietary allowance.

RDS. Abbreviation for respiratory distress syndrome.

R.E. Abbreviation for right eye.

re-. Prefix meaning again, back, against, and behind.

Re. Chemical symbol of the element rhenium.

reabsorp′tion. The process of reabsorbing or the state of being reabsorbed.

active r., one requiring the expenditure of energy.

passive r., one requiring no energy expenditure; the substances are reabsorbed along a concentration gradient.

tubular r., selective reabsorption of extracellular fluid in the tubules of the kidney; it helps restore essential components to the body.

react′. To participate in a chemical reaction or undergo chemical change.

reac′tance. Opposition to the flow of an alternating electric current, by passage through a coil of wire or a condenser.

reac′tant. Any substance that takes part in a chemical reaction.

reac′tion. 1. A force produced by and opposing an acting force. **2.** Any response to a stimulus. **3.** The transformation of molecules into others. **4.** The observable color change in, or produced by, indicators or reagents in chemical analysis.

acid r., a positive test indicating the presence of hydrogen ions in a solution; e.g., the reddening of blue litmus.

alarm r. (AR), the body's response to a sudden exposure to a violent or stressful stimulus.

alkaline r., a positive test indicating the presence of hydroxyl ions in a solution; e.g., the bluing of red litmus.

allergic r., one stimulated by exposure to a substance (allergen) to which the individual has become sensitized.

amphoteric r., the reaction of a substance that is capable of reacting chemically both as an acid and as a base.

anamnestic r., the increased and more rapid production of antibodies upon a second exposure to antigens; also called secondary response.

antigen-antibody r., the specific binding of antibody with the same type of antigen that activated the formation of the antibody, resulting in precipitation, agglutination, or neutralization of exotoxin.

anxiety r., an uncontrollable apprehension out of proportion to any apparent external cause.

arousal r., change in the brain wave pattern of an individual when suddenly awakened.

Arthus r., a severe local sensitivity reaction produced at the site of injection of antigen into an animal possessing specific precipitating serum antibodies.

Bence-Jones r., the coagulation of Bence-Jones protein when a urine sample from a patient with Bence-Jones proteinuria is heated, followed by its redissolving on boiling, and coagulation again on cooling.

biuret r., a chemical test used to detect and to quantitate protein.

chain r., a series of chemical reactions, each one initiated by the one preceding.

complement fixation r., reaction occurring when antibody-coated erythrocytes are added to a mixture of a test antigen and a patient's heated serum in the presence of a measured amount of complement; if the patient's serum contains antibody, an antigen-antibody reaction takes place and complement is consumed (fixed); no free complement is left to lyse the sensitized erythrocytes; the reaction is the basis for many serologic tests for infections (e. g., syphilis).

consensual r., constriction of the pupil of one eye when a light is flashed into the other eye; also called pupillary reflex and indirect light reflex.

conversion r., process through which unacceptable unconscious impulses or repressed ideas are converted into bodily symptoms; also called somatic conversion.

cross r., one occurring between an antibody and an antigen of a type different but related to the one that stimulated the production of the antibody.

delayed r., a late response of the body to an agent to which it is hypersensitive.

dissociative r., one marked by dissociated behavior, such as amnesia, sleepwalking, dream states, etc.

drug r., an adverse reaction arising during the therapeutic administration of a drug; may be immediate (within minutes), accelerated (from one to 72 hours), or late (after three days).

endergonic r., one requiring the expenditure of energy; e.g., certain biologic syntheses.

endothermal r., endothermic r., chemical reaction in which heat is absorbed.

exergonic r., one that liberates energy, as in certain catabolic processes.

exothermal r., exothermic r., one in which heat is liberated.

false-negative r., an erroneous negative reaction; a negative reaction occurring in the presence of the condition being tested for.

false-positive r., an erroneus positive reaction; a positive reaction occurring in the absence of the condition being tested for.

first-order r., one in which the rate is proportional to the concentration of the substance undergoing chemical change.

Herxheimer's r., see Jarisch-Herxheimer reaction.

id r., a skin eruption occurring in an area of the body other than that of the infection, e.g., on the hands during acute tinea infection of the feet; most commonly follows fungus infections of the feet or the scalp, severe contact dermatitis of the hands, and varicose ulcers; considered to be an allergic reaction.

immune r., (1) the response activated in the lym-

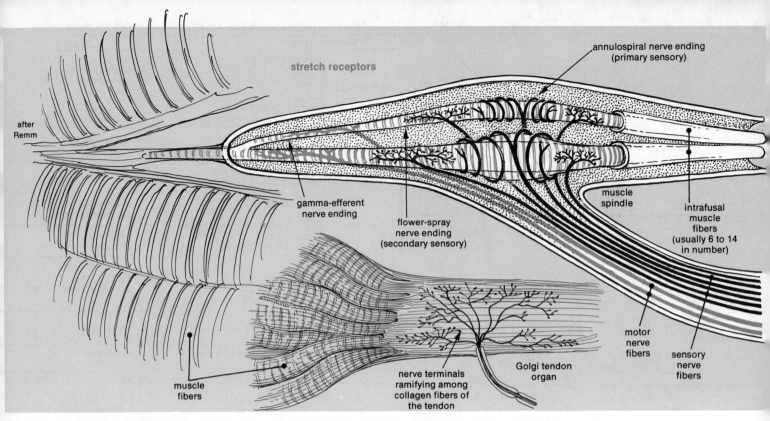

stretch receptors

annulospiral nerve ending (primary sensory)

after Remm

gamma-efferent nerve ending

flower-spray nerve ending (secondary sensory)

muscle spindle

intrafusal muscle fibers (usually 6 to 14 in number)

muscle fibers

nerve terminals ramifying among collagen fibers of the tendon

Golgi tendon organ

motor nerve fibers

sensory nerve fibers

phoreticular system of vertebrates by the presence of a foreign substance (antigen); the response may be a direct functioning of the cells (e.g., phagocytosis), or the elaboration of a cell product (antibody); (2) the formation of a slight papule without vesicle formation following smallpox vaccination of an immune person.

IMViC r., the four tests used in classifying coliform bacteria; indol, methyl red, Voges-Proskauer, and citrate (the lower case *i* is added to the term for euphony).

Jarisch-Herxheimer r., an inflammatory reaction sometimes induced by arsphenamine, mercury, or antibiotics in the treatment of syphilis; believed to be due to rapid release of treponemal antigen; aslo called Herxheimer's reaction.

leukemoid r., condition marked by the presence of increased white blood cells in the blood; similar to, but not associated with, leukemia and occurring in certain conditions, such as infectious diseases and some malignant tumors.

ninhydrin r., the production of violet color by proteins, peptones, peptides, and amino acids having a free carboxyl and an α-amino group, when boiled with ninhydrin.

normal lymphocyte transfer r. (NLT reaction), reaction resulting from the injection of allogeneic lymphocytes into the skin.

nuclear r., one in which an atomic nucleus changes its atomic number (number of protons) or its mass number (number of nucleons), as a result of natural or artificial radioactivity, or through direct nuclear bombardment.

Pandy's r., a qualitative and quantitative test to detect the presence of proteins in the spinal fluid; also called Pandy's test.

Prausnitz-Kustner r., reaction occurring when blood serum from an allergic person is injected into the skin of a nonallergic individual, followed (48 hours later) by injection of antigens to which the donor is allergic; a wheal appears at the site of injection; also called Prausnitz-Kustner or P-K test.

quellung r., Neufeld capsular swelling; see under swelling.

Schultz-Charlton r., blanching of scarlatinal rash at site of intracutaneous injection of scarlatina antiserum; also called Schultz-Charlton phenomenon.

Schultz-Dale r., smooth muscle contraction produced in vitro when antigen is applied to the excised muscle of a sensitive animal.

transfusion r., general term for a variety of nonimmune (e.g., hepatitis) and immune complications occurring during or after transfusion of whole blood or blood products; the immune transfusion reaction may be caused by the destruction of the recipient's

red blood cells by antibodies present in the blood of either the donor or the recipient or by a reaction to infused white blood cells.

Voges-Proskauer r., a chemical reaction used to determine the presence of acetyl-methyl carbinol, produced by certain bacteria.

Wassermann r., see test, Wassermann.

Weil-Felix r., the agglutination of *Proteus* X bacteria with blood serum of persons with typhus fever.

wheal-flare, r., a skin sensitivity reaction due to histamine, characterized by an edematous elevation and erythematous flare.

white-graft r., a reaction to a tissue graft in which the graft fails to vascularize and is quickly rejected.

Widal's r., agglutination reaction used in the diagnosis of typhoid.

zero-order r., a reaction that, regardless of the concentration of the reactants, proceeds at a definite rate.

reac'tivate. To restore activity, as in an inactivated immune serum to which normal serum is added.

reactiv'ity. The ability to react.

reading mistake. The wrong placement of an amino acid residue in a polypeptide chain during the synthesis of protein.

rea'gent. Any substance, added to a solution, that participates in a chemical reaction, especially one employed in chemical analysis for the detection of biologic constituents.

Benedict-Hopkins-Cole r., magnesium glyoxalate, made by adding a saturated solution of oxalic acid to powdered magnesium; used for testing proteins for the presence of tryptophan.

biuret r., an alkaline solution of copper sulfate.

diazo r., a reagent consisting of two solutions, sodium nitrite and acidified sulfanilic acid; used to bring about diazotization.

Esbach's r., a reagent consisting of a one per cent aqueous solution of picric acid mixed with a two per cent solution of citric acid; used in estimating quantity of albumin in urine.

Fehling's r., see solution, Fehling's.

Lloyd's r., precipitated aluminum silicate; used in absorbing alkaloids from solutions.

Nessler's r., one used in determining the level of urea nitrogen in the blood and in the urine.

Sulkowitch's r., a reagent consisting of oxalic acid, ammonium oxalate, glacial acetic acid, and distilled water; used in detection of calcium in the urine.

re'agin. An antibody that has an affinity for cells; also homocytotropic antibody in the human primarily associated with IgE globulins.

real'ity. The sum of all things that have an objective

existence.

r. principle, see under principle.

ream'er. A dental instrument used to enlarge root canals.

rebase'. To replace or add to the base material of a denture without changing the occlusal relations of the teeth.

re'bound. 1. In anesthesia, new reflex activity following the withdrawal of a stimulus. **2.** Reappearance of a phenomenon, often with greater force than originally, after the effect of a therapeutic agent has worn off; e.g., when the effect of a vasoconstrictor (e.g., nosedrops) wears off and there is subsequently increased vasocongestion.

recall'. 1. The process of summoning back a memory into consciousness; to bring back to awareness; to remember. **2.** In psychiatry, the term refers to the recollection of events in the immediate past.

recan'aliza'tion. The process of recanalizing; e.g., the restoration of a lumen in a blood vessel following thrombotic occlusion.

receiver. 1. An electronic device capable of receiving incoming electromagnetic signals and converting them to perceptible forms. **2.** In chemistry, a vessel attached to a condenser in which the products of distillation are collected.

receptac'ulum. A pouchlike structure.

r. chyli, see cisterna chyli.

recep'tor. 1. The sensory end-organ; the small structure in which a sensory nerve fiber terminates; it receives stimuli and converts them into nervous impulses. **2.** In pharmacology, a constituent in a cell that combines with a specific drug, resulting in a change of the cell's function.

adrenergic r.'s, constituents of effector tissues innervated by adrenergic postganglionic fibers of the sympathetic nervous system.

α-adrenergic r.'s, adrenergic receptors that are blocked by the action of compounds such as phenoxybenzamine and phentolamine.

β-adrenergic r.'s, adrenergic receptors that are blocked by action of such compounds as propranolol.

stretch r., one whose function is to detect elongation; e.g., the muscle spindle and the Golgi tendon organ.

re'cess. A shallow cavity.

piriform r., a recess in the pharynx on each side of the opening of the larynx.

reces'sion. The process of withdrawing.

gingival r., displacement of gingiva with resulting added exposure of tooth surface.

tendon r., posterior surgical displacement of the insertion of an eye muscle.

reces'sive. 1. Latent; not dominant. **2.** In ge-

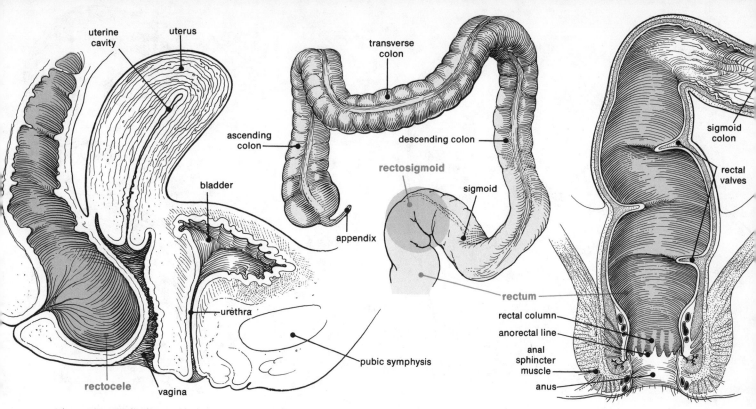

Labels on illustration: uterine cavity, uterus, transverse colon, ascending colon, descending colon, sigmoid colon, rectosigmoid, bladder, sigmoid, rectal valves, appendix, rectum, urethra, rectal column, anorectal line, anal sphincter muscle, pubic symphysis, anus, rectocele, vagina

netics, not expressed unless present in both sets of chromosomes (homozygous).

reces′sus, *pl.* **reces′sus.** Latin for recess.

recidiva′tion. Reappearance of a disease or symptom.

recid′ivism. The tendency of an individual to relapse into a previous mode of behavior, especially a tendency to return to criminal or delinquent habits.

recid′ivist. A person who tends to relapse into a previous pattern of bad behavior after rehabilitation; e.g., a habitual criminal.

recipe. Latin for take, usually represented by the symbol R_x. **1.** The heading or superscription of a physician's presescription. **2.** The prescription itself.

recip′iomo′tor. The recipient of a motor stimulus.

Recklinghausen's disease. See neurofibromatosis.

Recklinghausen's disease of bone. Osteitis fibrosa cystica.

recombina′tion. The formation of gene combinations in the offspring that were not present in either parent, caused by the exchange of genes between homologous chromsomes (crossing over).

re′con. In genetics, the smallest unit of a single DNA nucleotide capable of recombination.

reconduc′tion. Retrograde conduction; see under conduction.

reconstitu′tion. 1. Restoration to original form, as of a substance previously altered for preservation. **2.** Regeneration of a lost bodily part.

rec′ord. Information preserved in an enduring form.

   interocclusal r., a record of the positional relations of teeth or jaws to each other.

   maxillomandibular r., maxillomandibular registration, a record of any positional relations of the maxilla to the mandible.

   problem oriented medical r. (POMR), a system of recording medical information about a patient, characterized by a defined universe of information for the data base, a complete up-to-date problem list, and numbered and titled plans and progress notes that preserve the course of action of the physicians and other medical personnel; it is adaptable for the computer.

   r. base, see baseplate.

   source oriented medical r., the traditional method of recording medical information about a patient as it happens.

record′ing. Preserving, in writing or any other permanent form, the results of a study.

rec′rement. 1. Any secretion, such as saliva or bile, that is reabsorbed after having performed its function. **2.** Waste matter.

recrudes′cence. A return of a morbid process after a dormant or inactive period.

recruit′ment. 1. In the testing of hearing, the abnormally rapid increase in loudness experienced by the patient when the sound stimulus is gradually increased. **2.** A gradual increase in response to a stimulus which has a constant intensity but prolonged duration.

rec′tal. Relating to the rectum.

rectal′gia. Proctalgia.

rec′tify. 1. To purify a liquid through redistillation. **2.** To transform an alternating current into a direct one. **3.** To correct.

recto-. Combining form meaning rectum.

rectoabdom′inal. Relating to both the rectum and abdomen, especially a method of examination in which one hand is placed on the abdomen, and one or more fingers of the other hand are inserted into the rectum.

rec′tocele. Prolapse of the rectum into the perineum; also called proctocele.

rectocoli′tis. See coloproctitis.

rectoperineor′rhaphy. See proctoperineoplasty.

rec′topexy. See proctopexy.

rec′toplasty. See proctoplasty.

rec′toscope. See proctoscope.

rectosig′moid. The portion of the intestinal tract adjacent to the junction of the rectum and the sigmoid colon, on both sides.

rectosteno′sis. See proctostenosis.

rectoure′thral. Relating to both the rectum and the urethra.

rectou′terine. Relating to both the rectum and the uterus.

rectovag′inal. Relating to both the rectum and the vagina.

rectoves′ical. Relating to both the rectum and the bladder.

rec′tum. The terminal portion of the intestinal tract extending from the sigmoid colon to the anus.

rec′tus. Straight; describes some muscles which run a straight course, such as the abdominal rectus muscle.

recum′bent. Lying down; leaning or reclining.

recu′perate. To recover.

recur′rence. 1. A return of symptoms, a natural characteristic of certain diseases, e.g., yellow fever. **2.** The return of a morbid state after a period of improvement.

recur′rent. Returning after abatement or disappearance.

recurva′tion. A backward bending or curving.

red. A bloodlike hue; one of the primary colors emanating from the long-wave end of the spectrum, evoked by radiant energy of wavelengths from 620

to 770 nm.

   carmine r., a specific stain for glycogen and mucus in which the active ingredient is carminic acid; also used for staining embryos, small animals, and large blocks of tissue.

   congo r., a red azo dye, used in biologic stains and as an indicator (red in alkaline solutions and blue in acid solutions).

   methyl r., a red compound, $C_{15}H_{15}O_2N_3$, soluble in alcohol; used as an indicator with a pH range of 4.4 to 6 (red at 4.4, yellow at 6).

   neutral r., a dye used as an indicator with a pH range of 6.8 to 8 (red at 6.8, yellow at 8).

   oil r. 0, see stain, oil red 0.

   phenol r., see phenolsulfonphthalein.

Red Cross. 1. Red Cross Society; an international organization established for the purpose of caring for the injured and homeless during wartime and natural disasters. **2.** The emblem of the Red Cross Society, a red Geneva cross or red Greek cross on a white background; a sign of neutrality.

re′dia, *pl.* **re′diae.** The larval stage in the life cycle of a trematode.

red′ox. In chemistry, a coined term meaning a reduction-oxidation reaction or state.

re′duce. 1. To return a part to its normal position; e.g., the ends of a fractured bone. **2.** To decrease the valence number of an atom by adding electrons.

redu′cible. Capable of being reduced.

reduc′tant. The donor of electrons in an oxidation-reduction reaction.

reduc′tase. The reducing enzyme in an oxidation-reduction reaction.

reduc′tion. 1. The correction, through surgical or manipulative methods, of a hernia, a fracture, or a dislocation. **2.** In chemistry, the removal of oxygen from a substance or the addition of hydrogen; the reverse of oxidation.

reduplica′tion. A doubling.

reen′try. The return of an impulse to an area of heart muscle which it has recently stimulated, as occurs in reciprocal heart rhythms.

REF. Abbreviation for renal erythropoietic factor (erythrogenin).

refine. To purify.

reflect′. 1. To bend back from a surface, as light or heat rays. **2.** To meditate.

reflec′tion. 1. The return of light from an optical surface to the same medium from which it came. **2.** A bending back. **3.** Meditation.

reflec′tor. A surface that reflects light, heat, or sound waves.

re′flex. 1. An involuntary and immediate response to a stimulus. **2.** Turned backward; reflected.

   abdominal r., contraction of the muscles of the

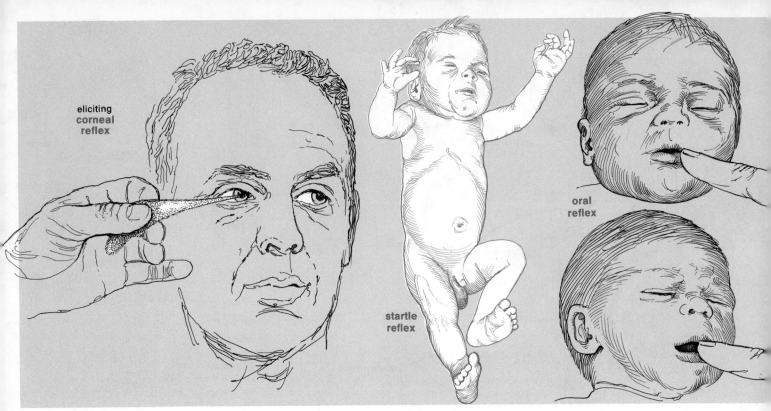

eliciting corneal reflex

startle reflex

oral reflex

abdominal wall upon stroking of the overlying skin.

accommodation r., the increase in convexity of the crystalline lens when the eyes are directed from a distant to a near object, in order to bring the image into focus; initiated by an out-of-focus image on the retina.

Achilles tendon r., calcaneal tendon reflex.

acquired r., conditioned reflex.

anal r., contraction of the anal sphincter muscle upon irritation of the perianal area, or upon insertion of a finger into the rectum.

ankle r., calcaneal tendon reflex.

attitudinal r., see statotonic reflex.

Babinski's r., Babinski's sign; extension of the large toe with fanning of the small toes upon scratching the sole of the foot.

Bainbridge r., acceleration of the heart beat caused by a rise in pressure in the great veins at the entrance to the right atrium.

biceps r., flexion of the forearm when the tendon of the biceps is struck.

brachioradial r., flexion of the forearm upon tapping of the brachioradial muscle at its attachment to the lower end of the radius.

calcaneal tendon r., contraction of the calf muscles with resulting plantar flexion of the foot on striking of the calcaneal (Achilles) tendon; also called Achilles tendon reflex, ankle jerk, and ankle reflex.

carotid sinus r., see carotid sinus syndrome.

ciliary r., contraction of the pupils when the gaze is directed from a distant to a near object.

ciliospinal r., see pupillary-skin reflex.

conditioned r., one that is developed through association with, and repetition of, a stimulus; also called trained reflex.

conjunctival r., closure of the eyelids upon touching of the conjunctiva with a fine wisp of cotton.

coordinated r., one in which several muscles take part.

corneal r., blinking induced by touching of the cornea with a fine wisp of cotton while the patient looks in the direction opposite to the approaching cotton.

cremasteric r., retraction of the testicle upon gently scratching the inner aspect of the upper thigh of the same side.

crossed r., one that causes movement on one side of the body when the opposite side is stimulated.

crossed adductor r., inward rotation of the leg upon tapping of the sole.

crossed extension r., response elicited from a newborn infant indicating spinal cord integrity; placing the child in the supine position, the examiner extends and presses down on one of the child's legs and stimulates the sole of the foot; this causes the free leg to flex, adduct, and then extend.

deep r., deep tendon r., tendon r., contraction of a muscle upon tapping of its tendon.

elbow r., see triceps reflex.

fundus r., the red glow seen in the pupil during inspection of the interior of the eyeball, produced by reflection of light from the choroid.

gag r., gagging initiated by introduction of a foreign body into the pharynx; also called pharyngeal reflex.

gastrocolic r., the wavelike contraction of the colon, propelling its contents onward, initiated by introduction of food into the empty stomach.

Gordon r., extension of the big toe upon firm squeezing of the calf.

grasp r., the immediate grasping of an object placed in the hand; occurring normally only in infants.

Hering-Breuer r., the effects of afferent impulses from the pulmonary vagi in the control of respiration; e.g., deflation of the lungs brings on inspiration.

Hoffmann's r., flexion of the thumb and fingers when the last joint of the middle finger is quickly flexed and extended.

hung-up r., prolonged relaxation time of the deep tendon reflexes (particularly the ankle jerks in hypothyroidism).

knee-jerk r., patellar reflex.

light r., constriction of the pupil upon light stimulation of the retina.

magnet r., normal response elicited from a newborn infant; with the baby in the supine position with legs semiflexed, the examiner presses his thumbs against the soles of the child's feet; this causes the child to extend his legs.

micturition r., any of the reflexes controlling effortless urination and the subconscious ability to retain urine within the bladder; also called bladder or urinary reflex.

milk-ejection r., the release of milk from the breast upon stimulation of the nipple.

Moro's r., see startle reflex.

myotatic r., contraction of a muscle in response to a passive stretching force; also called stretch reflex.

Oppenheim's r., extension of the toes elicited by pressing down firmly on the shin from the knee to the ankle.

oral r., nomal reflex elicited from a newborn infant; when one corner of his mouth is touched, the bottom lip lowers on the same side and the tongue moves forward and toward the examiner's finger.

orbicularis pupillary r., unilateral contraction of the pupil while trying to close the eyelids which are forcibly held open; also called Westphal's pupillary reflex.

palmomental r., unilateral twitching of the chin upon scratching of the palm of the hand of the same side; also called palm-chin reflex.

patellar r., extension of the leg upon tapping of the patellar tendon while the leg hangs loosely at right angles to the thigh.

patellar-tendon r., patellar reflex.

pharyngeal r., see gag reflex.

pilomotor r., formation of goose flesh on lightly touching the skin, or on exposure to cold or emotional stimuli.

plantar r., flexion of the toes on scratching of the sole of the foot; also called sole reflex.

primitive r's., the reflexes occurring naturally in the newborn infant; they are an indication of normal neuromuscular development.

proprioceptive r., any of various reflexes brought about by stimulation of proprioceptors (labyrinth, carotid sinus, etc.).

papillary r., any alteration in the diameter of the pupil.

pupillary-skin r., dilatation of the pupil upon scratching of the neck; also called ciliospinal reflex.

quadriceps r., patellar reflex.

radial r., flexion of the forearm upon tapping of the end of the radius.

rectal r., desire to defecate stimulated by accumulation of feces in the rectum.

righting r.'s, reflexes that cause the head and body to resume their normal position in space; initiated by displacement of the body from its normal position.

rooting r., response elicited from a newborn infant; when the cheek is lightly touched, the infant's head turns in the direction of the touch and his lips purse in preparation for sucking.

startle r., Moro's r., response of the newborn to loud noises or sudden changes in position; characterized by tensing of muscles, a wide embracing motion of the arms, and extension of the thighs, legs, and fingers, except the thumb and index, which remain in a "C" position.

statotonic r., attitudinal r., any of several reflexes stimulated by changes of position of the body in space.

superficial r., any reflex elicited by stimulation of the skin or mucous membranes.

tendon r., see deep reflex.

trained r., see conditioned reflex.

triceps r., a sudden extension of the forearm on tapping of the triceps tendon at the elbow while the forearm hangs loosely at a right angle to the arm; also called elbow reflex and or jerk.

reflex | reflex

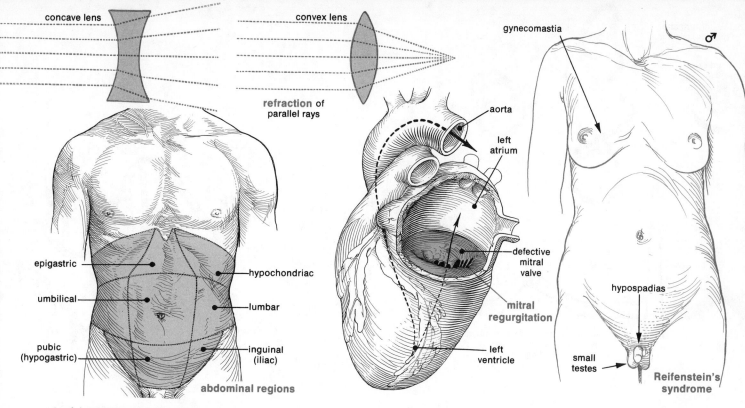

concave lens

convex lens

refraction of parallel rays

gynecomastia ♂

aorta

left atrium

defective mitral valve

mitral regurgitation

left ventricle

epigastric

hypochondriac

umbilical

lumbar

pubic (hypogastric)

inguinal (iliac)

abdominal regions

hypospadias

small testes

Reifenstein's syndrome

---

trunk-incurvation r., reflex occurring in a newborn infant with normal spinal cord; while the baby is in the prone position, the examiner runs his finger along one side of the spine, causing the child's body to curve in the direction of the stimulus.

tympanic r., percussion sound heard over a hollow structure.

vagovagal r., a cardiac reflex elicited by irritation of the respiratory tract.

vesical r., the desire to urinate in response to pressure within the bladder when full.

Westphal's pupillary r., see orbicularis pupillary reflex.

reflex'ograph. An apparatus for graphically recording a reflex.

re'flux. Backward flow.

refract'. 1. To change the direction of a propagating wave, as of light. 2. To measure the refractive and muscular state of the eyes.

refrac'tion. 1. The clinical measurement and/or correction of refractive errors of the eye. 2. The deflection of a ray of light as a result of passing obliquely from one medium to another of different optical density.

refrac'tive. Relating to refraction.

refractom'eter. An instrument that measures indices of refraction in translucent substances.

refrac'tory. 1. Not responsive or readily yielding to treatment. 2. Not responsive to stimulation, said of a muscle or nerve; immediately after responding to an initial stimulation, it enters a period of functional inactivity during which it does not respond to a second stimulation. 3. Resisting the action of heat; difficult to melt or work.

refrac'ture. The breaking again of a bone that was improperly set.

refrig'erant. An agent that produces a sensation of coolness.

Refsum's syndrome. A rare recessive hereditary disorder marked by cerebellar ataxia, chronic polyneuritis, pigmentary degeneration of the retina, and night blindness; death is commonly due to degenerative heart disease at an early age; also called heredopathia atactica polyneuritiformis.

refu'sion. The return of the circulation of blood after its temporary removal from the same individual.

regenera'tion. 1. The replacement of a lost or damaged part by the growth of new tissue. 2. A form of asexual reproduction.

reg'imen. A systematic procedure or regulation of an activity (exercise, diet) designed to achieve certain ends, usually hygienic or therapeutic in nature.

re'gio, *pl.* **regio'nes.** Latin for region.

re'gion. 1. Any large segment of a bodily surface

with more or less definite boundaries. 2. A bodily part having a special nervous or vascular supply. 3. A portion of an organ having a special function, as the motor region of the brain.

abdominal r.'s, the nine areas into which the abdomen is divided by four imaginary planes.

registra'tion. In dentistry, a record of jaw relations.

regres'sion. 1. Abatement of symptoms. 2. Relapse. 3. Return to a more primitive or infantile pattern of behavior due to inability to function at a logical adult level (psychological or atavistic regression).

regula'tion. 1. A law or rule designed to control details of procedure. 2. In experimental embryology, the power of a very young embryo to regenerate and continue its development in spite of experimental interference.

regurgita'tion. A backward flow, as the return of stomach contents.

mitral r., the back flow of blood from the left ventricle to the left atrium due to a malfunctioning mitral valve (left atrioventricular valve).

rehabilita'tion. 1. Restoration of form and function following illness or injury. 2. Restoration of an individual's capability to achieve the fullest possible life compatible with his abilities and disabilities.

oral r., the restoration of all lost tooth structure.

physical r., see physiatrics.

rehala'tion. Rebreathing; procedure sometimes used in anesthesia.

Reifenstein's syndrome. Familial male pseudohermaphrodism associated with hypospadias, small testes and sterility, absence of beard, short stature, and often gynecomastia; inherited as an X-linked recessive or an autosomal dominant male-limited trait; also called hereditary familial hypogonadism.

reimplanta'tion. Replantation; replacement of a bodily structure to its natural position, as a tooth to the socket from which it was previously removed.

reinfec'tion. A second infection by the same agent following recovery or during the course of the primary infection.

reinforce'ment. Added force or strength, such as (a) the increased reflex response when the person performs some mental or physical work while the reflex is being elicited; (b) a structural addition to strengthen a denture.

reinnerva'tion. The restoration of a damaged nerve either by grafting of a live nerve or by spontaneous regrowth of nerve fibers.

reintegra'tion. In psychiatry, the resumption of normal functioning after a mental disorder.

Reiter's syndrome (RS). A symptom complex

consisting of urethritis, conjunctivitis, arthritis, and mucocutaneous lesions; recurrences or chronicity occur in more than one-half of the patients; etiology remains unknown.

rejec'tion. 1. The term applied to the immunologic response to an incompatible transplanted organ which prevents the graft from being accepted. 2. Something rejected.

second-set graft r., accelerated rejection of a second graft due to immunity developed to a primary graft.

re'lapse. The return of a disease after apparent recovery or improvement.

rela'tion. The way in which one object stands when considered in association with another.

centric r., the most posterior position of the mandible from which lateral jaw movements can be made at any given degree of jaw separation.

eccentric r., any deviation from the centric relation.

rest r., the relation of the mandible to the maxilla when the person is resting in an upright position and the jaws are not in contact.

rela'tionship. An association; a kinship.

coefficient of r., see under coefficient.

object r., in psychiatry, the emotional bonds existing between one individual and another.

relative biologic effectiveness (RBE). A measure of the capacity of absorbed doses of various types of radiation (x ray, neutrons, alpha particles, etc.) to produce a specific biologic effect; it may vary with the kind and degree of biologic effect considered, the duration of the exposure, and other factors.

relax'. 1. To loosen or slacken; to make lax or less tense. 2. To relieve from tension, effort, or strain.

relax'ant. 1. A drug or therapeutic treatment that produces relaxation by relieving muscular or nervous tension. 2. Tending to reduce tension or to relax.

relaxa'tion. 1. Loosening. 2. The lengthening of muscle fibers.

relax'in. A polypeptide ovarian hormone secreted by the corpus luteum of pregnancy; it relaxes the pubic symphysis and dilates the cervix of some animals during labor; in humans it is thought to inhibit premature contraction of the uterus during pregnancy and to dilate the cervix, thus facilitating delivery of the fetus.

relief'. 1. The lessening of pain or distress, physical or mental; ease from discomfort. 2. In dentistry, the removal of pressure from a specific area under a denture base.

relieve'. 1. To free wholly or partly from pain, discomfort, anxiety, fear, or the like. 2. To elimi-

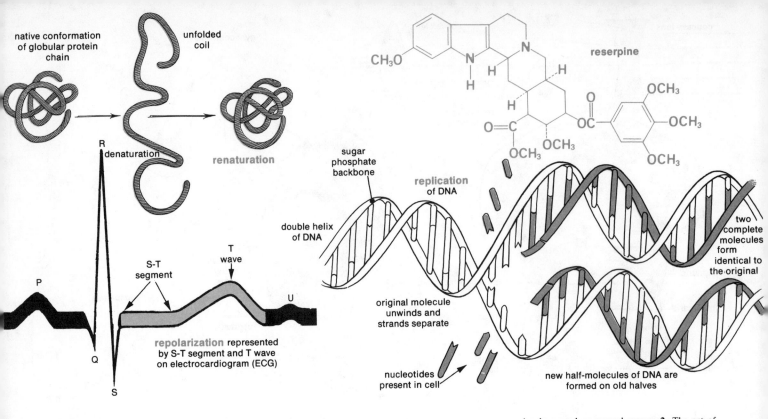

native conformation of globular protein chain

unfolded coil

denaturation

renaturation

R

P

S-T segment

T wave

Q

S

U

repolarization represented by S-T segment and T wave on electrocardiogram (ECG)

reserpine

replication of DNA

sugar phosphate backbone

double helix of DNA

two complete molecules form identical to the original

original molecule unwinds and strands separate

nucleotides present in cell

new half-molecules of DNA are formed on old halves

nate bodily waste.

reline'. To resurface the tissue side of a denture with new base material in order to make it fit better.

REM. Abbreviation for rapid eye movements (a phase of sleep); see under movement and sleep.

rem. Acronym for roentgen-equivalent-man; the amount of ionizing radiation, absorbed by man, that is required to produce a biologic effect equivalent to the absorption of one roentgen of x or γ rays.

reme'diable. Capable of being cured or remedied; also called curable.

reme'dial. Able to correct a deficiency, especially a reading deficiency.

rem'edy. 1. Something, such as a drug or therapy, that cures, palliates, or prevents disease, or corrects a disorder. **2.** To effect a cure.

remem'bering. The neural mechanism involved in the retrieval of stored information; the "read out phase" of learning; the mental faculty of reviving an impression or idea of which the mind has once been conscious.

remineraliza'tion. Restoration of mineral elements to the body, especially of calcium salts to bone.

remis'sion. A diminution of the severity of a disease or abatement of its symptoms.

remit'. To temporarily abate in severity without absolutely ceasing; to diminish.

remit'tent. Characterized by alternating periods of abatement and returning of symptoms.

re'nal. Relating to the kidneys; also called nephric.

renatura'tion. The return of normal characteristic biologic activity to denatured protein, accompanied by the return of its native form; also called refolding and annealing.

Rendu-Osler-Weber syndrome. Hereditary hemorrhagic telangiectasia; see under telangiectasia.

ren'iform. Kidney-shaped.

re'nin. An enzyme formed by the kidney and released into the blood stream; it has an important role in the formation of angiotensin, a potent pressor agent.

ren'net. A dry extract containing rennin, obtained from the lining of the fourth stomach of the calf; used in curdling milk.

ren'nin. A milk-curdling enzyme obtained from rennet, used in making cheese; also called chymosin.

reno-. Combining form denoting a relationship to the kidney. See also nephro-.

renogram, radioactive. A graphic record produced by the continuous recording of radioactivity of the kidney after injection of a radiopharmaceutical; an aid in the clinical evaluation of kidney function.

renog'raphy. Roentgenography of the kidney.

renomeg'aly. Abnormal enlargement of the kidney.

renopriv'al. Resulting from removal of kidneys or absence of kidney function.

renotroph'ic. Affecting the growth of the kidney; also called nephrotropic.

renotro'phin. An agent that affects the growth of the kidney.

renovas'cular. Referring to the blood vessels of the kidneys.

reovi'ruses. An RNA group of viruses replicating in the cytoplasm; found in the respiratory and intestinal tracts of man but not yet associated with any disease.

rep. Abbreviation for roentgen-equivalent-physical; see under roentgen.

repel'lent. 1. Capable of repelling; tending to repel. **2.** Any agent that repels something, especially one that repels insect pests.

repetition compulsion. In psychoanalysis, the impulse to reenact earlier experiences.

replanta'tion. Replacement of a bodily part to its natural position, as the reinsertion of a dislodged tooth into its original socket; for the soft interior pulp to survive, the tooth should be replanted within about a half-hour; the outer periodontal tissues may survive and reattach after periods of up to six hours; also called reimplantation.

replica'tion. The process of duplicating something; e.g., the repeated formation of the same molecule, as of DNA; also called autoreproduction.

repolariza'tion. A process, immediately following depolarization of the cell, in which the surface of the cell membrane is polarized again by the gradual restoration of the positive charges on the outer and negative charges on the inner surface; for cardiac muscle, graphically shown on the electrocardiogram by the S-T segment and T wave.

repos'itor. An instrument used to replace a prolapsed or dislocated organ, especially the uterus.

repositioning. Reduction (1); the return of a part to its normal position.

repres'sion. 1. A defense mechanism by which painful experiences are forced into the unconscious sphere; repression effected unconsciously. **2.** The prevention of the formation of an enzyme as programmed by a structural gene in the presence of a small corepressor molecule.

repres'sor. The product of a regulatory gene, capable of combining with a corepressor to form an active complex, or with an inducer to form an inactive complex.

reproduc'tion. 1. The process of producing offspring by sexual or asexual means. **2.** The act of bringing to mind again a past experience, as a memory.

   asexual r., reproduction without the union of male and female sex cells.

   sexual r., reproduction by the union of male and female sex cells.

   somatic r., reproduction by splitting or budding of cells other than sex cells.

Reptil'ia. A class of cold-blooded, usually egg-laying vertebrates that includes snakes, lizards, turtles, and crocodiles.

repul'sion. 1. The act of repelling, or the condition of being repelled. **2.** Extreme dislike.

reradia'tion. Radiation emanating from a substance as a result of its absorbing radiation.

RES. Abbreviation for reticuloendothelial system.

research'. Investigation or experimentation.

resect'. To cut off.

resec'table. Amenable to surgical removal; capable of being cut off.

resec'tion. The surgical removal of a portion of any part.

resec'toscope. An instrument for removing prostate gland tissue through the urethra.

reser'pine. An alkaloid, $C_{33}H_{40}N_2O_9$, isolated from the roots of certain species of *Rauwolfia*; used to reduce blood pressure in hypertension and as a tranquilizer.

reserve'. Something available, but stored for future use or a special purpose.

   cardiac r., the work which the heart is capable of performing beyond ordinary requirements.

reset'. To set again, as a broken bone.

res'ident. An individual who is in graduate training to qualify as a specialist in a field of medicine or dentistry.

resid'ual. Relating to the quantity remaining or left behind at the end of a process; left over.

res'idue. Material remaining after the completion of an abstractive physical or chemical process; also called residuum.

resid'uum. 1. Residue. **2.** That which remains after removal of a part.

   gastric r., the stomach contents during the interdigestive period.

   sporal r., the residual substance after sporulation.

resil'ience. Elasticity.

res'in. 1. Any of various viscous substances of plant origin, such as amber and rosin, that are usually transparent or translucent; used in synthetic plastics, adhesives, and pharmaceuticals. **2.** Any of various polymerized synthetics as polyethylene, epoxies, and silicones, that are used with other components to form plastics. **3.** In dentistry, a plastic

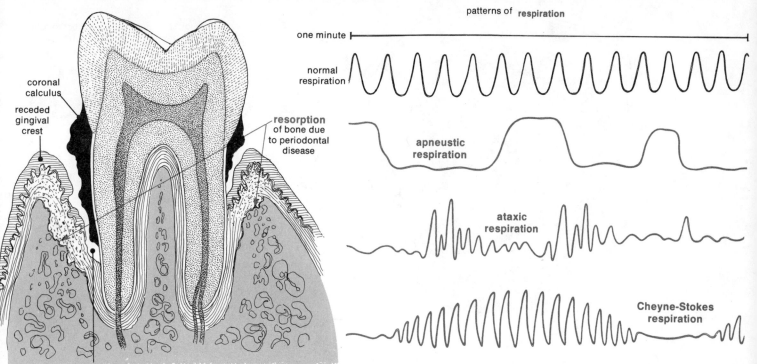

coronal calculus

receded gingival crest

resorption of bone due to periodontal disease

periodontal pocket

patterns of **respiration**

one minute

normal respiration

apneustic respiration

ataxic respiration

Cheyne-Stokes respiration

filling material having good esthetic appearance.

acrylic r., a thermoplastic resinous material of the various esters of acrylic acid; the principal ingredient of many plastics used in dentistry.

autopolymer r., a resin which can be polymerized by an activator and a catalyst rather than by the application of heat; it sets at room or body temperature; also called cold-curing, quick-curing, or self-curing resin.

cold-curing r., see autopolymer resin.

cholestyramine r., an insoluble chloride salt of a basic anion exchange resin that binds bile acids in the intestine and prevents their reabsorption; the reduced levels of bile acids increase the rate of conversion of cholesterol to bile acids in the liver; used in treatment of hyperlipoproteinemia; Cuemid®; Questran®.

dental r., a synthetic acrylic resin widely used in dentistry.

epoxy r., any thermosetting resin that is a condensation polymer of epichlorohydrin and bisphenol and forms a tight cross-linked structure that exhibits strong adhesion and chemical resistance; used in surface coatings, adhesives, and as embedding medium for electron microscopy.

ion-exchange r., an insoluble, porous solid material of high molecular weight containing an active electrolyte; it contains either acidic groups (cation-active) or basic groups (anion-active); used for lowering the potassium content of the body in the treatment of hyperkalemia.

methyl methacrylate r., a stable, transparent resin of remarkable clarity that is liquid at room temperature and is polymerized by the use of a chemical initiator; widely used in medical and dental appliances.

podophyllum r., a bitter-tasting resin derived from the dried rhizome and root of the May apple (*Podophyllum peltatum*); used as a cathartic and topical caustic.

quick-curing r., see autopolymer resin.

quinine carbacrylic r., a quinine salt of a resin containing about two per cent of quininium ion; used in testing deficiency of acids in the gastric juice, especially of hydrochloric acid.

self-curing r., see autopolymer resin.

thermoplastic r., a synthetic resin that becomes soft when heated and hard when cooled.

res′inous. Relating to a resin.

resis′tance. 1. Any force that opposes and/or retards motion. **2.** In electricity, the opposition to the passage of electric current. **3.** In psychiatry, an individual's psychologic defense against recalling repressed or unpleasant experiences.

drug r., a state of decreased response to drugs that ordinarily inhibit cell growth or cause cell death.

expiratory r., resistance in the air passages to the flow of air out of the lungs.

peripheral r., see total peripheral resistance.

total peripheral r., the sum of resistance to the flow of blood through the blood vessels; also called peripheral resistance.

resolu′tion. The termination of a morbid condition such as inflammation or the disappearance of a swelling.

visual r., the ability to perceive two separate adjacent objects as two.

resolve′. To return to normal after an inflammatory process.

resol′vent. 1. Causing or capable of causing resolution of a tumor or swelling. **2.** Any substance that promotes the dissipation of a pathologic growth or reduces an inflammation. **3.** Promoting the separation into constituents.

res′onance. 1. The sound heard on percussion. **2.** In chemistry, the property of a substance whereby two or more structural forms of the substance are simultaneously present.

amphoric r., sound resembling that produced by blowing over the mouth of an empty bottle.

electron spin r. (ESR), in spectrometry, resonance arising from electron spin, related to the extent of activity of free radicals in an organic reaction.

nuclear magnetic r. (NMR), a measure of the magnetic dipole moment of atomic nuclei (ratio of the maximum torque applied to the nuclei in a magnetic field to the magnetic induction of the field); used to determine the particular characteristics of covalent bonds involved in an organic reaction.

tympanic r., percussion sound heard over a hollow structure.

vesicular r., sound heard on percussion of normal lungs.

vocal r., voice sounds heard on auscultation of the chest.

res′ona′tor. An apparatus designed to create an electric current of very high potential and small volume.

resor′cinol. A keratolytic compound, $C_6H_4(OH)_2$; in concentrations of two per cent to 10 per cent, it is used in treating acne by causing a mild irritation that produces some peeling.

resorp′tion. 1. The assimilation of excreted material. **2.** The dissolution of tissue by physiologic or pathologic means, as of the gums or of the bones surrounding the teeth.

res′pirable. Fit for breathing.

respira′tion. 1. The physical and chemical processes through which an organism acquires oxygen and releases carbon dioxide. **2.** The act of breath-

ing.

abdominal r., respiration effected mainly by the abdominal muscles; also called diaphragmatic respiration.

aerobic r., one effected in the presence of air through the consumption of free oxygen.

anaerobic r., one that is carried on in the absence, or near absence, of air, without involving free oxygen.

apneustic r., breathing characterized by inspiratory spasms of varying duration, often lasting several seconds; seen in persons with lesions of the lower pons.

artificial r., the maintenance of respiratory movements through artificial means.

assisted r., in anesthesia, one in which the patient's own respiratory effort initiates the cycle but the volume of air is increased by mechanical means; also called augmented respiration and assisted breathing.

ataxic r., gasping, irregular (in rate and depth) breathing; seen in individuals with medullary lesions; also called Biot's breathing.

Cheyne-Stokes r., a rhythmic increase and decrease in the depth of respiration.

controlled r., in anesthesiology, artificial respiration requiring no effort by the patient; each inspiration is initiated by a timing mechanism of the respirator; also called controlled ventilation.

diffusion r., introduction of oxygen into the lungs through a catheter; also called apneic oxygenation.

external r., the interchange of gases in the lungs; also called pulmonary respiration.

forced r., voluntary increase in the rate and depth of breathing.

internal r., tissue respiration.

Kussmaul r., respiration marked by deep sighing; characteristic of diabetic acidosis.

mouth-to-mouth r., see under resuscitation.

tissue r., the exchange of gases between tissue cells and blood.

res′pirator. 1. An apparatus used to administer artificial respiration. **2.** A screenlike device fitted over the nose and mouth to protect the respiratory passages.

Drinker r., an airtight metal tank designed to enclose the body (except the head) and provide artificial respiration by exerting intermittent negative air pressure on the chest; commonly known as iron lung.

res′piratory. Of or relating to respiration.

respiratory distress syndrome of newborn. (RDS), A disease of unknown cause characterized by acute difficulty in breathing, cyanosis, easy collapsibility of alveoli, and loss of pulmonary

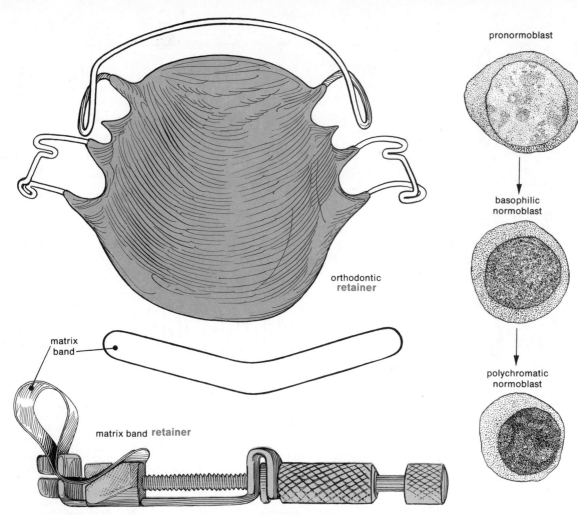

orthodontic **retainer**

matrix
band

matrix band **retainer**

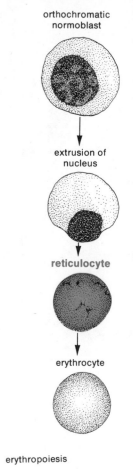

pronormoblast

orthochromatic
normoblast

basophilic
normoblast

extrusion of
nucleus

polychromatic
normoblast

reticulocyte

erythrocyte

erythropoiesis

surfactant; seen most frequently in premature infants, and those born of diabetic mothers or delivered by cesarean section.

respire′. To breathe.

respirom′eter. Spirometer.

response′. A reaction to a specific stimulus.

   autoimmune r., an immune response in which the action of an autoantibody is directed to a "self" antigen; distinguished from autoimmune disease, with which it may or may not be associated.

   evoked r., a change in the electrical activity of the nervous system resulting from an incoming sensory stimulus.

   galvanic skin r., the change in skin resistance in response to a stimulus.

   immune r., a specific response resulting in immunity, which includes an afferent phase during which responsive cells are primed by antigen, a central reponse during which antibodies are formed, and an efferent response in which immunity is effected by antibodies.

   triple r., the three degrees of reaction of the skin to injury; i.e., a red line, a flare around the red line, and a wheal surrounded by a flare.

rest. 1. Repose. **2.** To cease temporarily from any activity. **3.** A portion of displaced embryonic tissue that becomes embedded in other structures. **4.** In dentistry, an extension from a prosthesis that aids in supporting a restoration.

   adrenal r., an accessory adrenal gland.

resteno′sis. Recurrence of stenosis, especially of a heart valve after corrective surgery of the primary condition.

res′tiform. Shaped like a rope, as the ropelike restiform body (inferior peduncle) connecting the cerebellum to the medulla oblongata.

restitution, external rotation. In obstetrics, the return of the rotated head of the fetus to its natural relation with the shoulders after its complete emergence from the vulva.

restless legs syndrome. A feeling of creepiness, twitching, and restlessness deep in the legs, usually occurring in older individuals after lying down; the cause is unknown.

restora′tion. 1. The process of returning to a healthy state. **2.** In dentistry, a prosthetic device or appliance designed to replace lost teeth or oral tissues.

restor′ative. Tending to renew health.

restraint′. In psychiatry, the act of controlling by physical means an excited or violent patient.

resus′citate. To restore to life after apparent death.

resuscita′tion. The return to life or consciousness of one who is apparently dead.

   cardiopulmonary r. (CPR), restoration of respiration and cardiac contraction by means of external assistance (e.g., mouth-to-mouth breathing and external cardiac compression).

   mouth-to-mouth r., artificial respiration in which the operator places his mouth over the patient's mouth (and nose, if the patient is a small child) and blows rhythmically at a rate of about 20 cycles per minute.

resus′citator. An apparatus that forces gas, usually oxygen, into the lungs to initiate respiration as in asphyxia.

retain′er. 1. An appliance or device used to maintain teeth in the proper position after orthodontic treatment. **2.** The part of a fixed denture (dental bridge) which attaches the prosthesis to the abutment tooth; it may be an inlay, partial-veneer, or a complete crown. **3.** Any form of device, such as a clasp, used for the stabilization of a prosthesis.

   continuous bar r., a metal bar placed in contact with the lingual surfaces of teeth to aid in stabilizing the teeth or in retaining a partial denture.

   direct r., a clasp or attachment placed on a supporting tooth for the purpose of maintaining a removable appliance in position.

   indirect r., an attachment of a removable partial denture which assists the direct retainers in preventing displacement of free end denture bases.

retar′date. A mentally retarded individual.

retarda′tion. Slowing down of mental and physical processes, seen in certain forms of severe depression.

   mental r., subnormal intellectual functioning,

originating during the individual's developmental period, and associated with impairment of either adjustment (social and learning) or maturation, or both; it may be borderline (I.Q. 68–83), mild (I.Q. 52–67), moderate (I.Q. 36–51), severe (I.Q. 20–35), or profound (I.Q. below 20).

retch′ing. Involuntary but ineffectual effort to vomit.

re′te, pl. **re′tia.** A network, as of nerve fibers or minute blood vessels.

reten′tion. 1. The act of holding food and drink in the stomach. **2.** The holding back of body wastes. **3.** The ability to remember. **4.** Maintaining in position.

   denture r., the means by which a denture is maintained in proper position in the mouth.

   direct r., retention of a removable partial denture by means of clasps attached to the anchoring teeth.

   indirect r., retention of a removable partial denture by means of an attachment used in conjunction with a direct retainer.

   r. lug, a metal attachment soldered either to an orthodontic band or an artificial crown to insure stabilization of a dental prosthesis.

retic′ular. Netlike; pertaining to a reticulum.

retic′ulin. A scleroprotein present in the connective fibers of reticular or lymphatic tissues.

retic′ulocyte. The youngest red blood cell in the circulating blood; when it is supravitally stained with cresyl blue the scattered ribosomes clump together, giving the cell a reticulated appearance; it constitutes one per cent of the red blood cell population in the circulating blood.

reticulocytope′nia. Diminution of reticulocytes in the blood.

reticulocyto′sis. The abnormal increase in the percentage of reticulocytes in the blood.

retic′uloendothe′lial. Relating to the reticuloendothelium, i.e., to tissues having both reticular and endothelial properties.

retic′uloendothelio′ma. A localized neoplasm derived from reticuloendothelial tissue; e.g., malignant lymphoma.

retic′uloendothelio′sis. Abnormal conditions, especially hyperplasia, of the reticuloendothelium

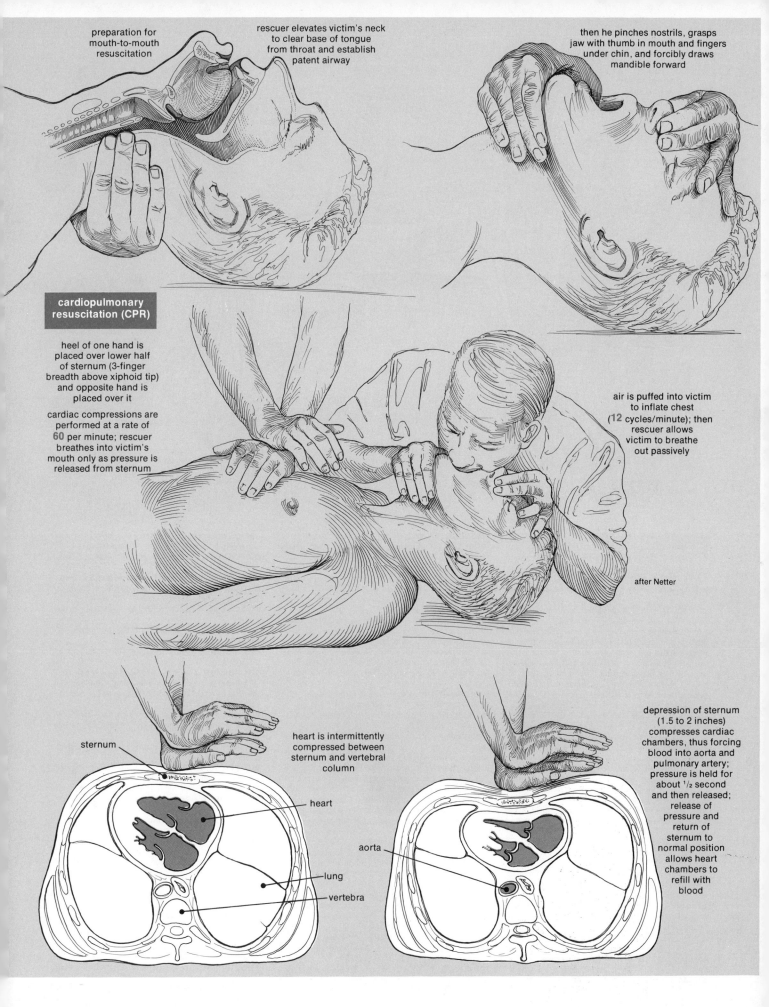

preparation for mouth-to-mouth resuscitation

rescuer elevates victim's neck to clear base of tongue from throat and establish patent airway

then he pinches nostrils, grasps jaw with thumb in mouth and fingers under chin, and forcibly draws mandible forward

cardiopulmonary resuscitation (CPR)

heel of one hand is placed over lower half of sternum (3-finger breadth above xiphoid tip) and opposite hand is placed over it

cardiac compressions are performed at a rate of **60** per minute; rescuer breathes into victim's mouth only as pressure is released from sternum

air is puffed into victim to inflate chest (**12** cycles/minute); then rescuer allows victim to breathe out passively

after Netter

heart is intermittently compressed between sternum and vertebral column

depression of sternum (1.5 to 2 inches) compresses cardiac chambers, thus forcing blood into aorta and pulmonary artery; pressure is held for about ¹/₂ second and then released; release of pressure and return of sternum to normal position allows heart chambers to refill with blood

sternum

heart

lung

vertebra

aorta

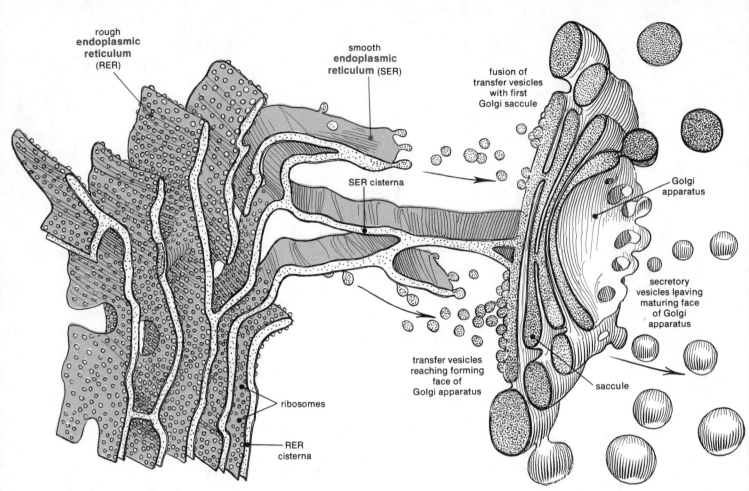

rough **endoplasmic reticulum (RER)**

smooth **endoplasmic reticulum (SER)**

fusion of transfer vesicles with first Golgi saccule

SER cisterna

Golgi apparatus

secretory vesicles leaving maturing face of Golgi apparatus

transfer vesicles reaching forming face of Golgi apparatus

saccule

ribosomes

RER cisterna

in any of the organs or tissues.

retic′uloendothe′lium. A widely dispersed bodily system of morphologically varied cells concerned with phagocytosis; present in the thymus gland, spleen, lymph nodes, etc.

reticulo′sis. A brief term for reticuloendotheliosis.

retic′ulum. A fine network, especially one formed of protoplasmic material within a cell.

 endoplasmic r., an extensive network of fine parallel membranes interspersed throughout the cytoplasm of the cell; it is continuous with the outer portion of the nuclear membrane and with the Golgi apparatus. One possessing ribosomes on its cytoplasmic surface is known as granular or rough endoplasmic reticulum; it receives synthesized material from the ribosomes and isolates it from the rest of the cytoplasm while channeling it to the Golgi apparatus for packaging; differentiated cells engaged in synthesis of protein contain an abundant amount of rough endoplasmic reticulum. One whose surface is free of ribosomes is known as agranular or smooth endoplasmic reticulum; depending on the cell type in which it resides, it can play a role in detoxification of certain drugs, lipid and cholestrol metabolism, production of steroid hormones, etc.

ret′ina. The innermost of the three tunics of the eyeball, consisting of an outer pigmented layer and an inner nervous stratum or retina proper which, in turn, is composed of eight microscopic layers, named from within outward as follows: (1) nerve fiber layer, (2) ganglionic layer, (3) inner plexiform layer, (4) inner nuclear layer, (5) outer plexiform layer, (6) outer nuclear layer, (7) layer of rods and cones, (8) pigment layer.

ret′inal. 1. Pertaining to the retina. **2.** The aldehyde of retinol present in the visual pigments of the retina; one isomere (11-*cis*-retinal) occurs in rhodopsin in combinaton with the protein group opsin; another (all-*trans*-retinal) is the yellow pigment resulting from the bleaching of rhodopsin by light; formerly called retinene and vitamin A_1 aldehyde.

retinac′ulum, *pl.* **retinac′ula.** A retaining bandlike ligament, as seen in the wrist and ankle.

ret′inene. See retinal.

retini′tis. Inflammation of the retina (the innermost layer of the eyeball).

 r. pigmentosa, hereditary degeneration and atrophy of the retina, usual!y with migration of pigment, causing gradual reduction of peripheral vision; its first symptom, night blindness, is usually seen in children and adolescents.

retinoblasto′ma. A congenital malignant tumor of the retina, composed of embryonic retinal cells; usually observed before the age of four.

retinochoroidi′tis. Chorioretinitis; inflammation of the choroidal and retinal layers of the eye.

ret′inol. A 20-carbon alcohol; also called vitamin A_1.

retinomala′cia. Degeneration of the retina.

retinopapilli′tis. See papilloretinitis.

retinop′athy. Any degenerative noninflammatory disease of the retina.

 diabetic r., progressive disease of the blood vessels in the retina, occurring as a complication of diabetes; it may lead to severe visual disability.

 hypertensive r., disease of the blood vessels in the retina occurring as a complication of hypertension; the initial change is narrowing of the arterioles caused by spasm; in later stages hemorrhages and exudates are seen; papilledema may appear in extreme cases associated with hypertensive encephalopathy.

 macular r., see maculopathy.

retinopie′sis. The pressing of a detached retina back into its normal position, as by air, intravitreal silicone, saline, etc.

ret′inoscope. An optical instrument for examining the refractive state of the eye.

retinos′copy. Ophthalmologic examination with a retinoscope to determine the objective measurements of the refractive properties of the eyes; also called shadow test, skiametry, and skiascopy.

retort′. A closed, long-necked laboratory vessel resembling a flask, used in distillation.

retract′. 1. To shrink back. **2.** To pull back.

retrac′tile. Capable of being drawn back.

retrac′tion. 1. Drawing back. **2.** A shrinking.

 gingival r., retraction of the gums from the tooth surface due to an underlying inflammation.

retrac′tor. A surgical instrument used to draw apart the edges of a wound.

retro-. Prefix meaning backward or situated behind.

retrobul′bar. 1. Located behind the eyeball. **2.** Located posterior to the medulla oblongata.

retroce′cal. Situated behind or posterior to the cecum.

retrocer′vical. Located behind the uterine cervix.

retrocol′ic. Behind the colon.

retrodisplace′ment. Backward displacement of an organ.

retroflex′ion. The backward bending of an organ.

 r. of uterus, the backward bending of the body of the uterus while the cervix remains in its normal position.

retrogna′thia. Condition characterized by a retruded position of the lower jaw without diminution of its size.

ret′rograde. Moving backward; retracing original course.

retrogre′ssion. 1. A return to an earlier or more primitive condition. **2.** Degeneration, especially of tissues.

retroillumina′tion. The technique of examining transparent or semitransparent tissues, as the cornea, by reflecting light from posteriorly located tissues.

retrolen′tal. Located behind the lens of the eye.

retromandib′ular. Located behind the lower jaw.

retroperitone′al. Located behind the peritoneum.

retroperitone′um. The retroperitoneal space between the parietal peritoneum and the posterior bodily wall.

retropharyn′geal. Located behind the pharynx.

retropla′sia. The state of decreased or retrogressive activity in a tissue.

retroposi′tion. Backward displacement of an organ without retroflexion or retroversion.

retropul′sion. An involuntary walking or falling backward.

ret′rospon′dylolisthe′sis. Posterior displace-

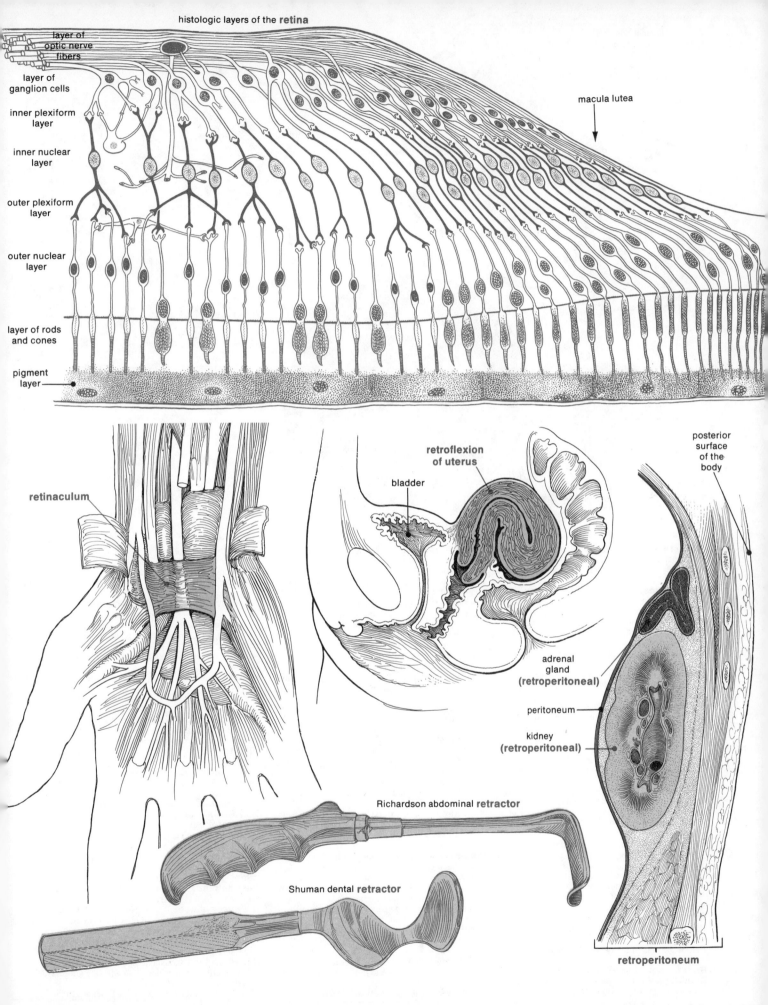

histologic layers of the retina

layer of optic nerve fibers

layer of ganglion cells

inner plexiform layer

inner nuclear layer

outer plexiform layer

outer nuclear layer

layer of rods and cones

pigment layer

macula lutea

retinaculum

bladder

retroflexion of uterus

posterior surface of the body

adrenal gland (**retroperitoneal**)

peritoneum

kidney (**retroperitoneal**)

Richardson abdominal **retractor**

Shuman dental **retractor**

retroperitoneum

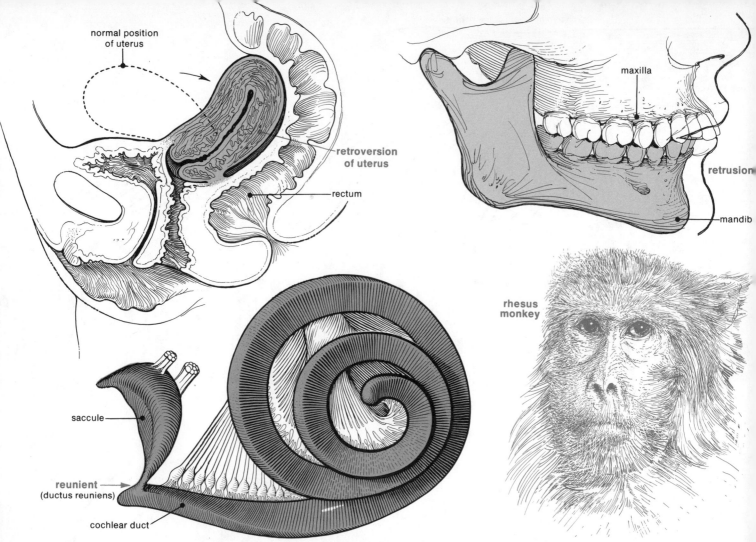

normal position of uterus

retroversion of uterus

rectum

maxilla

retrusion

mandib

rhesus monkey

saccule

reunient (ductus reuniens)

cochlear duct

ment of a vertebra, bringing it out of alignment with the other vertebrae.

retroster′nal. Situated behind the sternum (breast bone).

retrou′terine. Situated behind the uterus.

retrover′sion. The backward tilting of an entire organ.

  r. of uterus, the leaning backward of the uterus with the cervix pointing forward.

retrover′ted. Inclined backward.

retru′sion. The backward displacement of the lower jaw.

reu′nient. Connecting; denoting the ductus reuniens which connects the saccule to the cochlear duct in the internal ear.

revasculariza′tion. The reestablishment of blood supply to a part of the body by blood vessel grafting, or by development of collateral channels.

rever′sal. A turning in the opposite direction.

  sex r., the apparent change to the opposite sex, as in certain pseudohermaphroditic individuals.

rever′sible. Capable of returning to the original form or state.

rever′sion. 1. Reverse mutation; the restoration in a mutant gene of its ability to produce a functional protein. **2.** The appearance in an individual of a characteristic that has been absent for several generations.

Reye's syndrome. An acute and frequently fatal childhood syndrome marked by encephalopathy, hepatitis, and fatty accumulations in the viscera; usually starts as a mild illness with respiratory and gastrointestinal symptoms of a few days' duration, terminating in rapid brain swelling, hepatomegaly, convulsions, and coma.

Rf. Chemical symbol of the element rutherfordium.

RF. Abbreviation for (a) rheumatoid factor; (b) releasing factor.

RH. Abbreviation for (a) relative humidity; (b) releasing hormone.

Rh. Chemical symbol of the element rhodium.

Rhabdi′tis. A genus of small phasmid nematode worms; some are parasitic in man.

rhabdo-, rhabd-. Combining forms meaning (a) rod-shaped; (b) striated.

rhab′doid. Rod-shaped.

rhab′domyol′ysis. An acute, fulminating, potentially fatal disease of skeletal muscle, characterized by disintegration of skeletal muscle accompanied by excretion of myoglobulin in the urine; also called paroxysmal idiopathic myoglobulinuria.

rhabdomyo′ma. A benign tumor or neoplasm of striated muscle elements.

rhab′domy′osarco′ma. A malignant tumor derived from skeletal muscle.

rhab′dovi′ruses. A group of relatively large, bullet-shaped RNA viruses; one of its members causes rabies.

rhag′ades. Cracks or fissures in the skin, especially around bodily openings; seen in congenital syphilis and in vitamin deficiencies.

rhagad′iform. Denoting the shape of a fissure.

-rhagia, -rhage. Combining forms meaning a profuse flow from a burst vessel; usually denoting bleeding from a part.

RHD. Abbreviation for rheumatic heart disease.

rhe. The absolute unit of fluidity; the reciprocal of the unit of viscosity.

rhe′nium. A rare, silvery-white metallic element with a melting point exceeded only by tungsten and carbon; symbol Re, atomic number 75, atomic weight 186.2.

rheo-. A combining form denoting a flow or current; e.g., rheology.

rhe′obase. The minimal strength of an electric stimulus required to excite a tissue if allowed to flow through it for an adequate time.

rhe′oencephalog′raphy. The measurement of blood flow in the brain.

rheol′ogy. The study of the deformation and flow of liquids and semisolids; e.g., the flow of blood through the heart.

rheom′eter. 1. A device for measuring the velocity of viscous liquids, such as blood. **2.** A galvanometer.

rheom′etry. The measurement of blood flow.

rhe′ostat. An appliance for regulating the current entering an electric circuit; it basically consists of a continuously variable electrical resistor.

rheotax′is. The movement of an organism in response to the direction of fluid flow.

  negative r., rheotaxis in which the organism moves in the same direction as that of fluid flow.

  positive r., rheotaxis in which the organism moves in the opposite direction from that of fluid flow.

rhesus monkey. A light brownish monkey, *Macaca mulata,* of India and China; used in medical research.

rheum. Any watery discharge from the nose or eyes.

rheumat′ic. Relating to or afflicted with rheumatism.

rheumatic heart disease. A manifestation of rheumatic fever consisting of inflammatory changes (carditis) and/or damaged heart valves.

rheu′matid. An eruption sometimes accompanying rheumatism.

rheu′matism. A general term applied to various diseases that cause pain in the muscles, joints, and fibrous tissues.

rheu′matoid. 1. Resembling rheumatism. **2.** Associated with rheumatoid arthritis.

rheumatol′ogy. The study of the diagnosis and treatment of rheumatic conditions.

rhex′is. The rupture of a vessel or an organ.

rhin-, rhino-. Combining forms meaning nose.

rhi′nal. Relating to the nose.

rhinal′gia. Pain in the nose.

rhinede′ma. Edema or swelling of the nasal mucous membrane.

rhinenceph′alon. The region of the forebrain involved with the function of olfaction (smell), consisting of the olfactory bulb and peduncle, parolfactory area, subcallosal gyrus, and anterior perforated substance.

rhineuryn′ter. A dilatable bag which is inflated after insertion into a nostril to arrest a profuse nosebleed (epistaxis).

rhin′ion. A craniometric point; the lower end of the

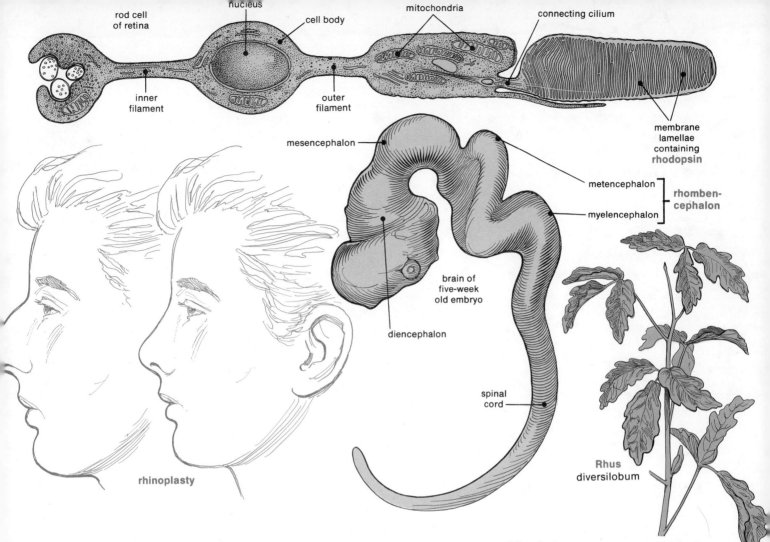

rod cell of retina / nucleus / cell body / mitochondria / connecting cilium

inner filament / outer filament

membrane lamellae containing rhodopsin

metencephalon / rhomben-cephalon / myelencephalon

mesencephalon

brain of five-week old embryo

diencephalon

spinal cord

rhinoplasty

Rhus diversilobum

suture between the nasal bones.

rhini'tis. Inflammation of the mucous membrane of the nose accompanied by excessive mucus discharge.

   acute r., cold in the head.

   allergic r., pale boggy swelling of nasal mucosa associated with sneezing and watery discharge due to hypersensitivity to foreign substances such as pollens, dust, etc.

   atrophic r., chronic rhinitis causing thinning of the mucous membrane; often associated with crusts and foul-smelling discharge.

   hypertrophic r., chronic rhinitis causing permanent thickening of the mucous membrane.

   vasomotor r., rhinitis without infection.

rhinoantri'tis. Inflammation of the mucous membrane of the nasal cavity and maxillary sinuses.

rhinocanthec'tomy. Surgical incision of the inner canthus of the eye; also called rhinommectomy.

rhinochi'loplasty. Reparative surgery of the nose and lip.

rhinoclei'sis. Nasal passageway obstruction.

rhinodac'ryolith. A concretion in the nasolacrimal duct.

rhinog'enous. Originating in the nose.

rhinokypho'sis. A deformity of the nose characterized by an abnormal hump in the ridge.

rhinola'lia. Nasal speech due to disease or defect of the nasal passages.

rhi'nolith. A stone in the nasal cavity formed in layers, usually around a foreign body.

rhinolithi'asis. The presence of calculi in the nose.

rhinol'ogy. The study of the nose and its diseases.

rhinomanom'eter. Instrument for determining the amount of nasal obstruction.

rhinom'eter. Instrument for measuring the nasal passages.

rhinomyco'sis. Fungus infection of the mucous membrane of the nose.

rhinop'athy. Disease of the nose.

rhinopharyngi'tis. Inflammation of the mucous

membrane of the nasopharynx.

   r. mutilans, see gangosa.

rhinophar'ynx. See nasopharynx.

rhinophy'ma. Acne rosacea of the nose, causing the skin to become coarsened, purplish, and thickened with nodulation and pitted scars.

rhi'noplasty. 1. Plastic surgery of the nose. **2.** Surgical reconstruction of the nose with tissue taken from another site.

rhinorrha'gia. Nosebleed.

rhinorr'haphy. Operation for the relief of epicanthus, in which a piece of skin is removed from the bridge of the nose and the edges of the wound are sutured together.

rhinorrhe'a. A profuse, watery nasal discharge.

rhi'nosal'pingi'tis. Inflammation of the nasal mucosa and the lining of the auditory (eustachian) tube.

rhi'nosclero'ma. Chronic disease involving the nose and upper respiratory tract, marked by the formation of hard nodules, sometimes leading to deformity.

rhi'noscope. An instrument for inspection of the nasal cavity; a speculum; also called nasoscope.

rhinos'copy. Visual examination of the nasal cavity with a rhinoscope.

   median r., inspection of the nasal cavity and the openings of the ethmoid cells and sphenoidal sinus with a long nasal speculum.

rhinosteno'sis. Abnormal narrowing of the nasal passage; nasal obstruction.

rhinot'omy. Operative incision of the nose.

rhinovi'ruses. A subgroup of RNA viruses, the major cause of the common cold; they belong to the picornavirus group.

rhi'zome. A horizontal rootlike stem, growing under or along the ground, which gives off roots from its lower side and leafy shoots or buds from its upper side.

rhizomeningomyeli'tis. Inflammation of the nerve roots, the meninges, and the spinal cord; also called radiculomeningomyelitis.

rhi'zoplast. A fine fibril connecting the flagellum to the nucleus of certain flagellate organisms.

Rhizopo'da. A subclass of protozoa of the class Sarcodina characterized by having rootlike pseudopodia.

rhizot'omy. Surgical division of a posterior spinal nerve root for the relief of pain; also called radicotomy and radiculotomy.

rho'dium. A hard metallic element of the platinum group, symbol Rh, atomic number 45, atomic weight 102.91.

rhodo-, rhod-. Combining forms denoting a reddish-rose color.

rhodop'sin. A purplish red, light-sensitive pigment found in the membrane of the outer segments of the rod-shaped photoreceptor cells of the retina; composed of a vitamin A derivative (11-*cis*-retinal) and a protein group (opsin); when light is absorbed by rhodopsin, it is transformed and separated into all-*trans*-retinal and opsin, but regenerates in the dark (the all-*trans*-retinal reverts back to 11-*cis*-retinal, which combines with opsin to form rhodopsin); this unique property makes possible the transformation of light energy into visual perception; also called visual purple.

rhombenceph'alon. The embryonic hindbrain; the third cephalic dilatation of the neural tube which divides into the metencephalon (anterior portion), which later forms the pons and cerebellum, and the myelencephalon (posterior portion), which develops into the medulla oblongata.

rhom'bocele. Rhomboidal sinus; the terminal expansion of the central canal of the spinal cord in the lumbar region.

rhom'boid. Resembling a rhomb or parallelogram with unequal adjacent sides; somewhat kite-shaped.

rhon'chus, *pl.* **rhon'chi.** A loud rale or snoring sound produced in the bronchial tubes or the trachea; also called coarse rale.

Rhus. A genus of plants (family Anacardiaceae) various species of which produce pruritic skin lesions on contact in sensitized individuals; the irritat-

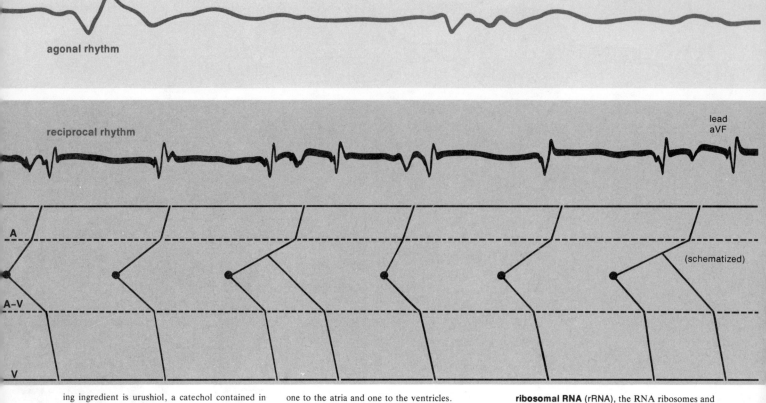

agonal rhythm

reciprocal rhythm

lead aVF

A

A–V

V

(schematized)

ing ingredient is urushiol, a catechol contained in the sap.

R. radicans, see poison ivy (1).

R. diversiloba, see poison oak.

R. vernix, see poison sumac.

rhythm. The pattern of recurrence of a biologic cycle; e.g., the heart beat and sexual cycle.

agonal r., one appearing in the electrocardiogram as wide disorted ventricular complexes, often seen in dying patients.

alpha r., see wave, alpha.

A-V nodal r., a heart rhythm originating in the atrioventricular (A-V) node; resulting from anything that suppresses sinus node activity, or from anything that enhances A-V node automaticity; also called nodal rhythm and junctional rhythm.

beta r., see wave, beta.

bigeminal r., heart rhythm in which every beat is followed by a weak premature beat and then a pause, so that the beats appear coupled; also called coupling.

cantering r., see gallop.

circus r., see movement, circus.

coronary nodal r., term, not uniformly accepted, for rhythm appearing in the electrocardiogram with normal upright P waves in leads I and II with a short P-R interval; occasionally called short P-R interval.

coronary sinus r., one appearing in the electrocardiogram with inverted P waves in inferior leads with a normal P-R interval; thought to originate in the coronary sinus.

delta r., see wave, delta (1).

ectopic r., heart rhythm originating from any focus other than the sinus node.

gallop r., see gallop.

idionodal r., a slow independent heart rhythm arising in the atrioventricular (A-V) junction and controlling only the ventricles.

idioventricular r., a slow independent heart rhythm arising in an ectopic center in the ventricles and controlling only the ventricles.

junctional r., see A-V nodal rhythm.

r. method, see under method.

nodal r., see A-V nodal rhythm.

quadruple r., a quadruple cadence of the heart sounds, not heard in normal hearts.

reciprocal r., phenomenon in which the impulse arises in the A-V junction and travels both downward to the ventricles and upward to the atria; before reaching the atria, it is reflected and descends to reactivate the ventricles; also called reciprocal beating.

reciprocating r., a variation of the reciprocal rhythm in which the impulse circulates around the A-V junction and gives off two daughter impulses,

one to the atria and one to the ventricles.

sinus r., the normal heart rhythm originating in the sinoatrial node.

theta r., see wave, theta.

trigeminal r., trigeminy; one in which the heart beats are grouped in three; either two premature beats follow each normal beat, or two normal beats are followed by a premature beat.

triple r., a triple cadence to the heart sounds, generally caused by the presence of a third (diastolic) or fourth (presystolic) heart sound or gallop in addition to the usual first and second heart sounds.

rhytidec'tomy. see rhytidoplasty.

rhytidoplas'ty. A face lift; surgical elimination of wrinkles from the face; the excess skin is removed so that the remaining skin may be tightened, thus smoothing out the wrinkles; also called rhytidectomy.

rhytido'sis. 1. Premature wrinkling of the face. **2.** Wrinkling of the cornea.

rib. One of a series of long, thin, rather elastic, curved bones which articulates posteriorly with a thoracic vertebra and extends anteriorly toward the sternum; normally there are 12 on each side.

cervical r., an extra rib similar to, but independent of, the first dorsal rib; usually attached to the seventh cervical vertebra.

false r., one of the five lower pairs of ribs that is not directly connected in front, through the costal cartilage, to the sternum; also called vertebrochondral rib.

floating r., one of the two lower pairs of false ribs that is free at the anterior end; also called vertebral rib.

true r., one of the seven upper pairs of ribs that is connected in front, through the costal cartilage, to the sternum.

ribofla'vin. A yellow, crystalline pigment present in milk, egg yolk, and fresh meat, and produced synthetically; it acts as coenzyme for hydrogen transfer in reactions catalyzed by flavoproteins; also called vitamin B_2; formerly called vitamin G.

ribonu'clease. An enzyme responsible for the breakdown of ribonucleic acid.

ribonucleic acid (RNA). Any of a family of polynucleotides, component of all living cells, especially the cytoplasm and nucleolus, which are characterized by their constituent sugar (*d*-ribose) and singlestranded molecules.

messenger RNA (mRNA), an RNA fraction with a base ratio that corresponds to the DNA of the same organism; it carries information from DNA to the protein-forming areas of the cell; also called template RNA.

ribosomal RNA (rRNA), the RNA ribosomes and polysomes.

soluble RNA (sRNA), transfer RNA.

template RNA, see messenger RNA.

transfer RNA (tRNA), an RNA molecule that transfers an amino acid to a growing polypeptide chain; the smallest biologically active nucleic acid known, present in cells in at least 20 varieties; also called soluble RNA.

ri'bonucleopro'tein (RNP) A complex macromolecule containing ribonucleic acid (RNA) and protein.

ribonu'cleoside. A nucleoside in which the sugar component is ribose; e.g., adenosine, cytidine, guanosine, and uridine.

ribonu'cleotide. A compound consisting of a purine or pyrimidine base bonded to the sugar component ribose, which in turn is esterified with a phosphate group; the most common ribonucleotides are adenylic, guanylic, cytidylic, and uridylic acids.

ri'bose. A five-carbon sugar present in ribonucleic acid (RNA); an aldopentose.

ri'boside. A glycoside that, on hydrolysis, yields ribose.

ri'bosome. One of the minute granules free in the cytoplasm or attached to the endoplasmic reticulum of a cell, containing a high concentration of RNA; it plays an important role in protein synthesis and ranges in size from 100 to 150 Å in diameter; it is assembled from two subunits produced in the nucleolus; also called microsome.

ribosu'ria. The excessive excretion of ribose in the urine; seen in muscular dystrophy.

ri'bosyl. The radical formed from ribose, $C_5H_9O_4$.

ribovi'ruses. RNA viruses; see under virus.

rib-spreader. A surgical instrument for widening and maintaining space between ribs, facilitating intrathoracic operations.

ri'cin. A highly toxic protein occurring in the castoroil bean; used as a biochemical reagent.

rick'ets. A disease of infants and young children caused by deficiency of vitamin D, resulting in defective bone growth; also called rachitis.

renal r., a form of rickets occurring in children due to chronic disease of the kidneys.

vitamin D-resistant r., a severe form of rickets which is not relieved by the administration of vitamin D; it is caused by a congenital defect of the kidneys; the disease is seen most frequently in males.

Ricket'tsia. A genus of gram-negative, pathogenic, intracellular parasitic bacteria which are transmitted to humans through the bites of infected fleas, ticks, mites, and lice.

R. akari, a species which is the causative agent of

Rhus | **Rickettsia**

418

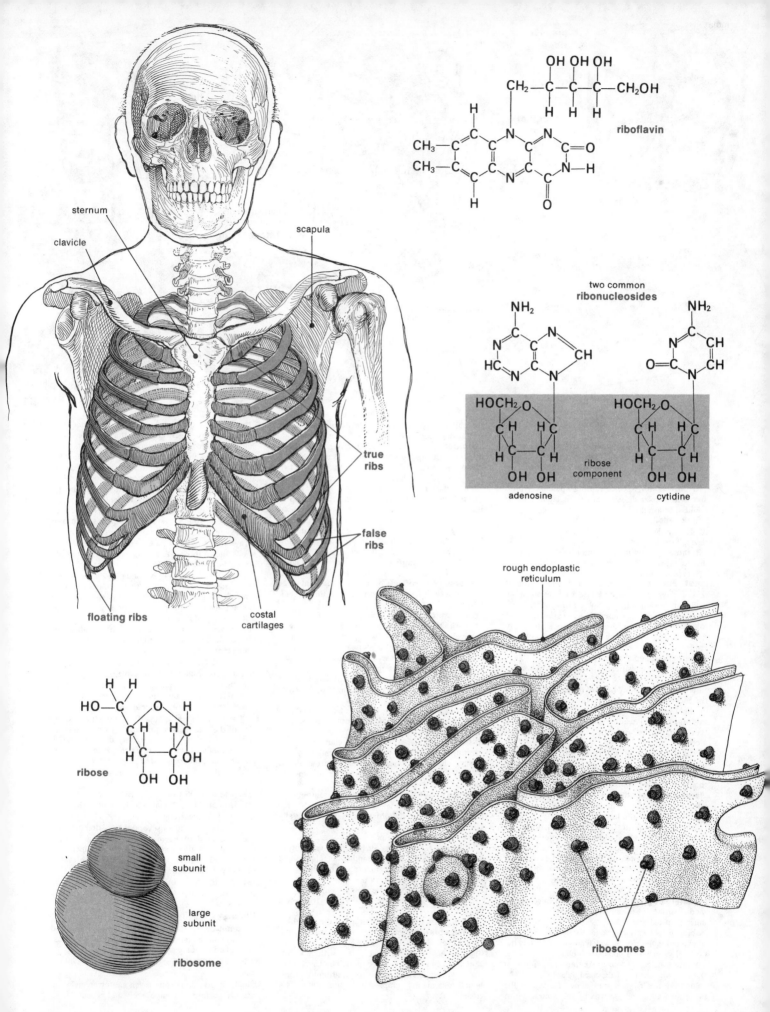

sternum

clavicle

scapula

true ribs

false ribs

floating ribs

costal cartilages

riboflavin

two common ribonucleosides

ribose component

adenosine

cytidine

ribose

small subunit

large subunit

ribosome

rough endoplastic reticulum

ribosomes

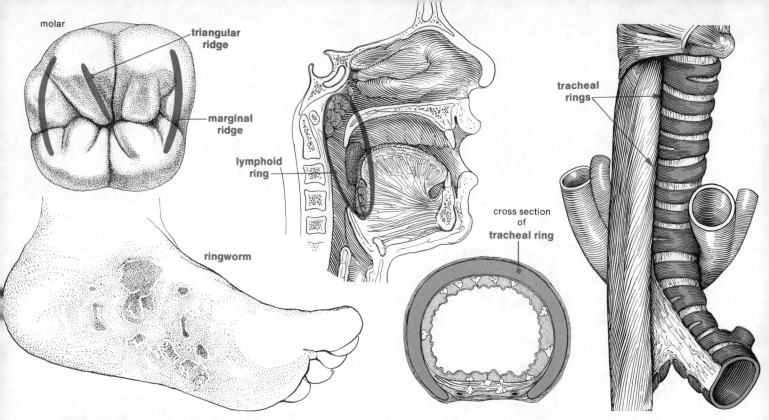

molar

triangular ridge

marginal ridge

lymphoid ring

tracheal rings

cross section of tracheal ring

ringworm

rickettsialpox; transmitted to humans by a mite that infests mice.

R. mooseri, a species which is the causative agent of murine (endemic or flea-borne) typhus; transmitted to man by the rat flea; also called *Rickettsia typhi.*

R. prowazekii, species causing epidemic typhus and Brill-Zinsser disease (carrier or latent type of typhus); transmitted by lice.

R. rickettsii, a species which is the causative agent of Rocky Mountain spotted fever; transmitted through the bites of infected ticks.

R. tsutsugamushi, species causing tsutsugamushi disease (scrub typhus); transmitted by mites.

R. typhi, see *Rickettsia mooseri.*

rickett′sialpox. An acute, mite-borne disease of several days' duration, characterized by an initial cutaneous lesion followed by a rash, fever, backache, and headache; caused by *Rickettsia akari.*

rickettsio′sis. Any disease due to a species of *Rickettsia,* such as Rocky Mountain spotted fever, epidemic typhus, endemic typhus, scrub typhus, rickettsialpox, and Q fever.

ridge. A linear elevation or projection on a bone or a tooth.

alveolar r., the bony ridge of the jaw that contains the sockets (alveoli) in which the roots of the teeth are held.

dental r., any linear elevation on the surface of a tooth forming the border of a cusp or the margin of a crown.

incisal r., the cutting portion of the crown of an anterior tooth.

labial r., one of three smooth, vertical ridges on the labial surface of an anterior tooth.

lateral supracondylar r., a curved ridge on the lateral surface of the humerus to which two of the dorsal muscles of the forearm attach.

lingual r., a vertical ridge extending from the cingulum on the lingual surface of an anterior tooth; on the cuspid it may be confluent with the cusp tip.

marginal r., the rounded border of the enamel of a tooth which forms the proximal margin of the occlusal surface of a posterior tooth and of the lingual surface of an anterior tooth.

medial supracondylar r., a curved ridge on the medial surface of the humerus to which two of the muscles of the arm attach.

oblique r., a variable ridge, formed by the union of two triangular ridges, which crosses obliquely the occlusal surface of a maxillary molar.

palatine r., one of four or six transverse ridges on the anterior portion of the hard palate.

Passavant's r., the prominence formed in the posterior wall of the pharynx by the contraction of

the superior constrictor muscle during the act of swallowing; also called Passavant's cushion or bar.

supraorbital r., the curved elevation of the frontal bone forming the upper border of the orbit.

transverse r., a ridge, formed by the union of two triangular ridges, which crosses transversely the occlusal surface of a posterior tooth.

triangular r., the ridge that runs from the tip of the cusp toward the central part of the occlusal surface of a posterior tooth.

rigid′ity. 1. Stiffness; immobility; the quality of being rigid or inflexible. **2.** In psychiatry, an individual's excessive resistance to change.

anatomic r., rigidity of the uterine cervix in labor without any pathologic infiltration.

cerebellar r., stiffness of the body and limbs due to an injury or lesion of the vermis of the cerebellum.

clasp-knife r., see spasticity, clasp-knife.

cogwheel r., rigidity of a muscle which, when passively stretched, gives way to a series of small jerks, as seen in Parkinson's disease.

lead-pipe r., the diffuse tonic contraction of muscles as seen in paralysis agitans.

mydriatic r., a tonic pupil, usually large, which responds very slowly, if at all, to light and accommodation.

pathologic r., rigidity of the uterine cervix in labor, due to fibrosis, cancer, or other diseases.

postmortem r., rigor mortis.

rig′or. 1. Rigidity; stiffness. **2.** A chill.

r. mortis, stiffness of the body occurring from one to seven hours after death and lasting from one to six days; caused by coagulation of the muscle plasma.

Riley-Day syndrome. Familial dysautonomia; see under dysautonomia.

rim. The outer edge, border, or margin, generally circular in form.

bite r., see occlusion rim.

occlusion r., occluding surface built on denture bases for recording maxillomandibular relation and for arranging teeth; also called record or bite rim.

record r., see occlusion rim.

ri′ma. A slit or elongated opening.

r. glottidis, the opening between the true vocal cords.

r. oris, the longitudinal aperture of the mouth.

r. palpebrarum, the slit between the lids of the closed eye.

ring. 1. A circular or oval object with a vacant center. **2.** In anatomy, any circular band surrounding an opening. **3.** In chemistry, a group of atoms bound in a manner graphically representable as a circle.

benzene r., the hexagonal ring arrangement of carbon and hydrogen atoms in the benzene molecule; also called benzene nucleus.

casting r., a metal ring or tube in which a mold is made for casting metal tooth restorations or dental appliances; also called refractory flask.

inguinal r., one of two (superficial or subcutaneous and deep or abdominal) openings of the inguinal canal through which pass the spermatic cord in males or round ligament in females. See also anulus inguinalis, superficialis and profundus.

Kayser-Fleischer r., a brownish pigmented ring, about one to three millimeters wide, in the periphery of the cornea; seen in Wilson's disease.

lymphoid r., a mass of lymphoid tissue, encircling the entrance to the pharynx, that includes the palatine, pharyngeal, and lingual tonsils and the small lymph follicles on the posterior oropharyngeal wall; also called Waldeyer's ring.

teething r., a ring, usually of hard rubber or plastic, designed for a teething baby to bite on.

tonsillar r., lymphoid ring.

tracheal r., one of the cartilages forming the trachea; also called tracheal cartilage.

umbilical r., the opening in the linea alba of the fetus through which the umbilical vessels pass.

Waldeyer's r., see lymphoid ring.

ring′worm. Tinea; a superficial infectious condition of the skin marked primarily by ring-shaped or oval itchy lesions; caused by any of a number of fungi, chiefly of the genera *Trichophyton, Microsporum,* and *Epidermophyton.*

RISA. Abbreviation for radioiodinated serum albumin.

risk. The possibility of harm; also called hazard.

risk factor. An element that influences the likelihood of an occurrence.

coronary r. f., any of several factors that increase the likelihood of having a greater than average chance of suffering a coronary occlusion, including high blood pressure, diabetes mellitus, elevated blood lipids, smoking, and heredity.

ristoce′tin. Antibiotic produced by *Nocardia lurida;* used against staphylococcic and enterococcic infections.

ri′sus. A laugh.

r. caninus, r. sardonicus, a peculiar grin caused by spasm of the facial muscles, occurring in tetanus; also called sardonic grin.

Ritter's disease. See dermatitis exfoliativa infantum.

ritual. In psychiatry, any psychomotor behavior or activity performed compulsively and repeatedly to

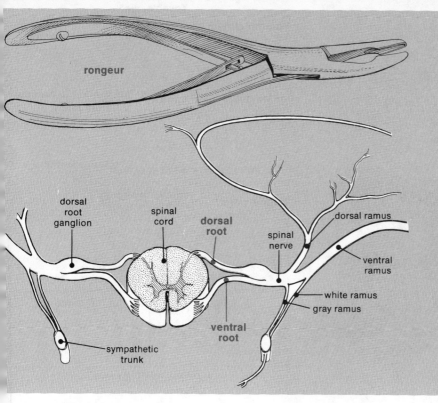

rongeur

dorsal root ganglion — spinal cord — **dorsal root** — dorsal ramus — spinal nerve — ventral ramus — white ramus — gray ramus — **ventral root** — sympathetic trunk

MANDIBULAR TEETH	LENGTH OF **ROOT OF TOOTH**	LENGTH OF CROWN OF TOOTH
central incisor	12.5 mm	9.0 mm
lateral incisor	13.0 mm	9.5 mm
cuspid	16.0 mm	11.0 mm
first bicuspid	14.0 mm	8.5 mm
second bicuspid	14.5 mm	8.5 mm
first molar	14.0 mm	8.0 mm
second molar	13.0 mm	7.5 mm
third molar	11.5 mm	7.0 mm
MAXILLARY TEETH		
central incisor	13.0 mm	10.5 mm
lateral incisor	12.0 mm	9.0 mm
cuspid	17.0 mm	10.0 mm
first bicuspid	14.0 mm	8.5 mm
second bicuspid	14.0 mm	8.5 mm
first molar	12.5 mm	7.5 mm
second molar	11.5 mm	7.0 mm
third molar	10.5 mm	6.5 mm

relieve or forestall anxiety; seen in obsessive-compulsive neurosis.

riz′iform. Resembling rice grains.

R.N. Abbreviation for registered nurse.

Rn. Chemical symbol of the element radon.

RNA. Abbreviation for ribonucleic acid.

RNase, RNAase. Abbreviations for ribonuclease.

RNP. Abbreviation for ribonucleoprotein.

Robin syndrome. See Pierre Robin syndrome.

Rocher's sign. See drawer sign.

rod. 1. Any slender, cylindrical structure or formation. **2.** One of the cells forming, with the cones, the layer of rods and cones of the retina.

rodent′icide. An agent lethal to rodents.

roent′gen (r). The primary unit of x-ray dosage, equal to the quantity of ionizing radiation that can produce one electrostatic unit of electricity in one cubic centimeter of dry air at 0°C and standard atmospheric pressure.

r.-equivalent-man (rem), the amount of ionizing radiation absorbed by man that is required to produce a biologic effect equivalent to the absorption of one roentgen of x or γ rays; the dose is determined by multiplying the dose in rads (units of radiation exposure expressing the absorbed dose) by the appropriate RBE (relative biologic effectiveness); maximum permissible doses (MPD) used as a guideline for occupational exposure are as follows: gonads, red bone marrow, and whole body, five rems in a year; skin, thyroid, and bone, 30 rems in a year; hands and forearms, 75 rems in a year; all other organs, 15 rems in a year.

r.-equivalent-physical (rep), the amount of ionizing radiation which, upon absorption by living tissue, produces an energy gain per gram of tissue equivalent to that produced by one roentgen of x rays or γ rays.

roent′genism. 1. The use of x rays in the treatment of disease. **2.** Any disorder caused by x-ray radiation.

roentgenky′mograph. Apparatus for graphically recording the movements of the heart and great vessels on a single x-ray film.

roent′genogram. A processed photographic film on which an image is produced by x rays striking a sensitized film after their passage through a portion of the body; loosely called an x ray.

roentgenog′raphy. Radiography with the use of x rays.

body section r., tomography; sectional roentgenography in which a single layer of a part of the body is put into focus.

roentgenol′ogist. A specialist in the use of x rays in the diagnosis and treatment of disease. Cf radiol-ogist.

roentgenol′ogy. The study of x rays as applied to diagnosis and treatment of disease. Cf radiology.

roentgenom′etry. Measurement of (a) the therapeutic dosage of x rays; (b) the penetrating power of x rays.

roentgenos′copy. Examination of any bodily part by visualization of shadows cast upon a roentgenoscope, fluoroscope, or fluorescent screen by a beam of x rays, following introduction of a radiopaque material; also called radioscopy.

Roger's disease. Congenital heart anomaly consisting of a small defect of the interventricular septum; also called maladie de Roger.

role. 1. The pattern of social behavior which an individual develops, influenced by what others expect or demand of him. **2.** A part played by an individual in relation to a group.

role-playing. A method of treating emotional conflicts by having the subject assume various roles.

Romberg's disease. Facial hemiatrophy; see under hemiatrophy.

Romberg's sign. Swaying and loss of balance when standing with feet together and eyes closed; it indicates a loss of proprioceptive control; occurring in disease of the posterior columns of the spinal cord.

Romberg's syndrome. Facial hemiatrophy; see under hemiatrophy.

rongeur′. Instrument used to cut bone.

roof. A top covering structure.

r. of fourth ventricle, the upper structure of the fourth ventricle of the brain; formed by the superior and inferior medullary vela and by the epithelial lining, the tela choroidea; also called tegmen ventriculi quarti.

r. of mouth, the palate; the bony and muscular partition between the nasal and oral cavities.

room. An area in a building surrounded by walls.

delivery r., a hospital room to which women in labor are taken for delivery.

emergency r. (ER), an area in a hospital where immediate attention is given by trained personnel to individuals brought in who have developed sudden and unexpected medical problems, such as acute illness, trauma, etc; also called accident ward.

operating r. (OR), a hospital facility in which surgical procedures are performed.

recovery r. (RR), a hospital room provided for the immediate care of postoperative patients.

root. 1. The embedded part of a structure, as of a tooth, hair, or nail. **2.** The origin of a structure; e.g., the proximal end of a nerve.

anatomic r., the root of a tooth extending from the cervical line to its apical extremity and con-tained in the bony socket of the jaw.

anterior r.'s, see ventral roots.

clinical r., the portion of the tooth below the gingival crevice.

dorsal r.'s, the nerve roots which carry impulses from bodily parts to the back of the spinal cord; they are attached along the dorsal lateral sulcus of the cord by six to eight rootlets; also called sensory or posterior roots.

motor r.'s, see ventral roots.

posterior r.'s, see dorsal roots.

r. of aorta, the origin of the ascending aorta from the left ventricle.

r. of hair, the part of hair embedded in the hair follicle.

r. of lung, all the structures entering or emerging at the hilus of the lung, forming a pedicle.

r. of nail, the proximal end of the nail, embedded under a fold of skin.

r. of penis, the proximal attached part of the penis, including the two crura of the corpora cavernosa and the bulb.

r. of tooth, the part of the tooth below the neck which is normally embedded in the alveolar process and covered with cementum.

sensory r.'s, see dorsal roots.

ventral r.'s, the nerve roots whch carry impulses from the anterior part of the spinal cord out to muscles and other structures; they are attached along the ventral lateral sulcus in two or three irregular rows of rootlets; also called motor or anterior roots.

rosa′cea. chronic inflammatory disorder superficially resembling acne; occurring most often in middle-aged individuals; characterized by papules, pustules, and dilation of capillaries on the cheeks and nose and sometimes the forehead and chin; also called acne rosacea.

rosan′ilin. Red needles, soluble in water; a component of the stain fuchsin.

ro′sary. An arrangement resembling a string of beads.

rachitic r., a row of nodules at the junction of the ribs with their cartilages, sometimes seen in rachitic children; also called rachitic beads.

Rosenbach's sign. 1. Fine tremor of gently closed eyelids, occurring in exophthalmic goiter. **2.** Loss of abdominal reflexes seen in cases of acute inflammation of the abdominal organs.

roseo′la. A reddish rash.

r. infantum, exanthem subitum.

rosette. A spherical group of fine red vacuoles surrounding the cytocentrum of a monocyte.

ros′in. The solid resin of Pinus palustris; used in the preparation of plasters and ointments.

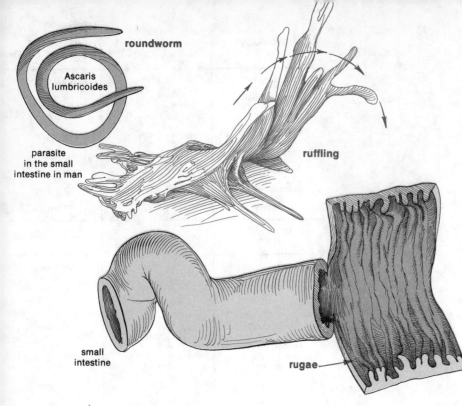

roundworm

Ascaris lumbricoides

parasite in the small intestine in man

ruffling

small intestine

rugae

Young's rule

$$\text{dose for child} = \text{adult dose} \times \frac{\text{age} + 12}{\text{age of child (in years)}}$$

Clark's rule

$$\text{dose for child} = \text{adult dose} \times \frac{\text{weight of child (in pounds)}}{150 \text{ pounds}}$$

Fried's rule

$$\text{dose for infant} = \text{adult dose} \times \frac{\text{age (in months)}}{150}$$

Nägele's rule

estimated day of birth (of the following year)

	May								June					
		1	2	3	4	5						1	2
6	7	8	9	10	11	12	3	4	5	6	7	8	9
13	14	15	16	17	18	19	10	11	12	13	14	15	16
20	21	22	23	24	25	26	17	18	19	20	21	22	23
27	28	29	30	31			24	25	26	27	28	29	30

	July								August					
1	2	3	4	5	6	7				1	2	3	4
8	9	10	11	12	13	14	5	6	7	8	9	10	11
15	16	17	18	19	20	21	12	13	14	15	16	17	18
22	23	24	25	26	27	28	19	20	21	22	23	24	25
29	30	31					26	27	28	29	30	31	

day of last menstrual period

---

rostel′lum. The anterior, hook-bearing portion of a tapeworm.

ros′tral, ros′trad. 1. Directed toward the front end of the body. **2.** Relating to any beaklike structure.

ros′trum. Any beak-shaped structure.

rot. 1. To decay. **2.** The process of decomposition.

rotam′eter. A flow-rate meter used to measure gases during administration of anesthesia.

rota′tion. 1. Motion around an internal axis. **2.** In obstetrics, the turning of the fetal head or any presenting part, whereby it is accommodated to the birth canal.

rota′tor. A muscle that rotates a part, as one of several muscles that rotate the vertebral column.

ro′tenone. The insecticidal component of derris root and other roots; used as an insecticide in the treatment of scabies and in veterinary medicine.

Rothmund′s syndrome. A hereditary syndrome, probably transmitted as an autosomal recessive trait, characterized by juvenile cataracts, saddle nose, premature graying and loss of hair, and wasting of muscles; also called Rothmund-Thomson or congenital poikiloderma-juvenile cataract syndrome.

rouge. A fine red powder of iron oxide; used as a final polishing agent for dental restorations made of gold and precious metal alloys.

rough. Denoting the granular surface of certain bacterial colonies.

rough′age. Indigestible material in the diet (coarse vegetable fibers and cellulose) that serves to stimulate peristalsis.

round′worm. A member of the phylum Nemathelminthes.

RPF. Abbreviation for renal plasma flow.

r.p.m. Abbreviation for revolutions per minute.

r.p.s. Abbreviation for revolutions per second.

R.Q. Abbreviation for respiratory quotient.

RR. Abbreviation for recovery room.

-rrhaphy. Combining form denoting a joining by sutures; e.g., herniorrhaphy.

-rrhea, -rrhoea. Combining form denoting a discharge; e.g., menorrhea.

-rrhexis. Combining form meaning rupture; e.g., erythrocytorrhexis.

rRNA. Abbreviation for ribosomal ribonucleic acid.

RSV. Abbreviation for Rous sarcoma virus (leukovirus).

RS virus. Abbreviation for respiratory syncytial virus.

R.U. Abbreviation for rat unit.

Ru. Chemical symbol of the element ruthenium.

rub. 1. To apply pressure and friction on a surface. **2.** Friction encountered in moving a structure against another.

friction r., the auscultatory sound produced by the rubbing together of two serous surfaces roughened by an inflammatory exudate; also called friction sound.

pericardial r., a friction or scraping sound produced by the rubbing together of inflamed pericardial surfaces during each heart beat.

pleuritic r., a grating sound produced by the rubbing together of the inflamed surfaces of the costal and visceral pleurae.

rubber-dam. See dam.

rube′do. Temporary redness of the skin.

rubefa′cient. Causing redness and irritation of the skin.

rubel′la. A contagious exanthematous disease of short duration, caused by a virus and capable of causing congenital defects in infants born of mothers who acquire the disease during the first three months of pregnancy; the incubation period is usually two to three weeks; also called German measles.

rube′ola. See measles.

rubeo′sis. Redness.

r. iridis, the formation of numerous new blood vessels on the anterior surface of the iris; most frequently associated with diabetes; occasionally seen in other conditions.

rubes′cent. Reddening.

rubid′ium. Chemical element; symbol Rb, atomic number 37, atomic weight 85.48.

ru′bor. Latin for redness.

ru′briblast. See pronormoblast.

ru′bricyte. Polychromatic normoblast; see under normoblast.

rubrospi′nal. Relating to the red nucleus and the spinal cord.

ru′diment. An incompletely developed structure.

rudimen′tary. Incompletely developed.

Ruffini′s cor′puscle. Ruffini's nerve ending; see under ending.

ruf′fling. The method by which a cell moves (perambulates) across a surface; characterized by the extension of thin, veil-like folds (ruffles) sprouting upward, extending out like an arm, and then dropping to the surface; when this "arm" adheres to the surface the cell flows into it as if it were pulling itself along.

ru′ga, *pl.* **ru′gae.** A fold or wrinkle.

gastric r., one of the folds in the lining of the stomach.

r. palatina, one of several transverse ridges on the anterior portion of the palate.

r. of vagina, one of several transverse folds of the vaginal mucosa.

ru′gal. Wrinkled; creased; corrugated.

ru′gitus. Intestinal rumbling.

ru′gose. Marked by rugae or ridges; wrinkled.

rugos′ity. 1. The state of having folds or ridges. **2.** A fold or ridge (ruga).

rule. A guide.

American Law Institute r., a 1962 American rule stating, ". . . a person is not responsible for criminal conduct if at the time of such conduct as a result of mental disease or defect he lacks substantial capacity either to appreciate the wrongfulness of his conduct or to conform his conduct to the requirements of law."

Durham r., a 1954 American test of criminal responsibility stating, ". . . an accused is not criminally responsible if his unlawful act was the product of mental disease or mental defect." This test was repudiated in 1966 (Brawner vs. U.S.) by the court that originated it; now it is a law only in Maine.

M′Naghten r., McNaughton r., a British test of criminal responsibility stating, ". . . it must be shown that, at the time of committing the act, the accused was acting under such defect of reason from a diseased mind as not to know the nature and quality of the act or if he knew this, that he did not know that what he was doing was wrong."

Nägele′s r., estimation of the day of birth by counting back three months from the first day of the last menstrual period and adding seven days.

Young′s r., a rule to determine the dose of a drug for a child; the adult dose is divided by a calculated number (the child's age plus 12, divided by the age); e.g., for a child of 3 years: $3 + 12 = 15$; $15 \div 3 = 5$; the adult dose divided by five is the proper dose for the child.

ru′minant. Any of various hoofed, usually horned, animals (cattle, goats, etc.) that have a stomach with four compartments and that regurgitate and chew partially digested food (cud).

rumina′tion. 1. The process of chewing cud. **2.** The recurring of thoughts.

rump. Buttocks or gluteal region.

rup′ture. 1. Hernia. **2.** The bursting or tearing of a part.

rut. A period of sexual desire in the males of certain species of mammals; it corresponds to heat or estrus in the female.

ruthe′nium. A rare, brittle, metallic element; symbol Ru, atomic number 44, atomic weight 101.1.

ruth′erford. Unit of radioactivity, equal to the amount of radioactive material that undergoes one million disintegrations per second.

RV. Abbreviation for (a) right ventricle; (b) residual volume.

rypopho′bia. A morbid fear of dirt.

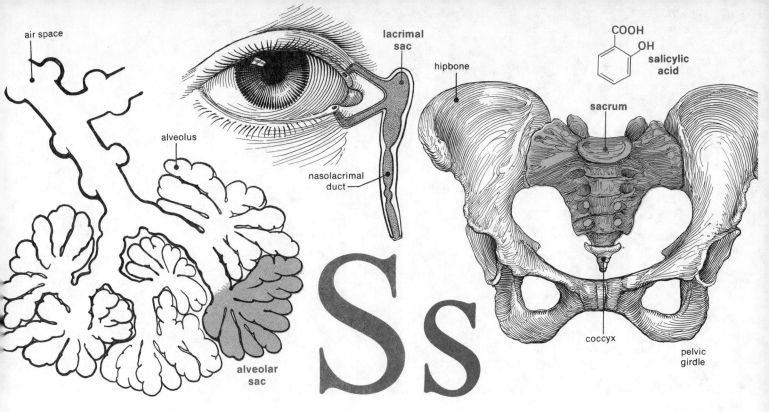

air space

alveolus

lacrimal sac

hipbone

nasolacrimal duct

salicylic acid

sacrum

coccyx

pelvic girdle

alveolar sac

S s

S. 1. Abbreviation for the Latin *signa* (in prescription writing, mark or signature). **2.** Symbol for sulfur.

s. Abbreviation for the Latin *sinister* (left).

Sa. Chemical symbol of the element samarium.

S-A. Abbreviation for sinoauricular or sinoatrial.

sab′ulous. Sandy; gritty.

sac. A bag or pouchlike anatomic structure.

abdominal s., the part of the embryonic coelom that develops into the abdominal cavity.

air s., see alveolar sac.

allantoic s., the dilated distal part of the allantois.

alveolar s., a cluster of alveoli in the lungs sharing a common central air space; also called air sac.

aneurysmal s., the dilated wall of an artery in a saccular aneurysm.

dental s., the fibrous layer of mesenchyme surrounding a developing tooth.

endolymphatic s., the blind extremity of the endolymphatic duct of the inner ear.

greater s. of peritoneum, the main part of the peritoneal cavity; it extends across the whole breadth of the abdomen, and from the diaphragm to the pelvis.

heart s., pericardium.

hernial s., the peritoneal envelope of a hernia.

lacrimal s., the slightly dilated upper part of the nasolacrimal duct situated in the lacrimal fossa; also called tear sac.

lesser s. of the peritoneum, the smaller part of the peritoneal cavity; a diverticulum of the greater sac of the peritoneum, situated behind the lesser omentum; it extends upward as far as the diaphragm and downward between the layers of the greater omentum; it opens through the epiploic foramen; also called omental bursa.

omental s., a recess of the lesser sac of the peritoneum situated between the layers of the greater omentum.

pleural s., a closed sac enveloping each lung, composed of a double-layered membrane (pleura).

synovial s., a closed sac formed by the synovial membrane; it contains a thick, viscous, lubricating fluid (similar to the white of an egg) that facilitates movement of joints.

tear s., see lacrimal sac.

vitelline s., see yolk-sac.

saccad′ic. Quick; jerky; sudden; said of certain movements of the eye.

sac′cate. Pouched.

sacch′arate. A salt of saccharic acid.

sacch′arated. Sweetened; sugary.

sacch′aric. Relating to sugar.

s. acid, a white crystalline compound; obtained by oxidation of glucose or its derivatives.

sacch′aride. Any of a series of compounds containing carbon, hydrogen, and oxygen in which the ratio of hydrogen to oxygen is 2:1; a sucrate.

saccharif′erous. Containing or producing sugar.

saccharim′eter. A device for measuring the amount of sugar in a solution.

sacch′arin. A white crystalline powder, $C_6H_4COSO_2NH$; used as a sugar substitute.

sacch′arine. Sweet.

sacch′arometab′olism. Utilization of sugar by the tissues.

Saccharomy′ces. A genus of yeast fungi, some species of which ferment sugar.

S. cerevisiae, the beer, wine, and bread yeast; also called brewer's, baker's, or wine yeast.

sacch′arose. See sucrose.

sacch′arum. Latin for sucrose.

saccharu′ria. Glycosuria.

sac′ciform. Baglike.

sac′cular. Resembling a bag.

sac′culated. Formed of or divided into a series of pouches.

saccula′tion. The presence or the formation of sacs.

sac′cule, sac′culus. 1. A small sac. **2.** The smaller of the two sacs of the membranous labyrinth in the vestibule of the internal ear.

sac′cus, *pl.* **sac′ci.** Latin for sac.

sacr-, sacro-. Combining forms relating to the sacrum.

sacrad. Toward the sacrum.

sa′cral. Relating to the sacrum.

sacral′gia. Pain in the sacral area; also called sacrodynia.

sacraliza′tion. A bony anomaly in which one or both (usually both) transverse processes of the fifth lumbar vertebra are wing-shaped and long, and articulate with the sacrum or ilium, or both.

sacrec′tomy. Surgical removal of a portion of the sacrum.

sacrococcyg′eal. Relating to both the sacrum and coccyx.

sacroil′iac. Relating to the sacrum and the ilium, as the sacroiliac joint.

sacroscia′tic. Relating to the sacrum and ischium.

sacrospi′nal. Relating to the sacrum and spine.

sacroverte′bral. Relating to the sacrum and the vertebrae.

sa′crum. A slightly curved, triangular bone made up of five fused vertebrae, wedged dorsally between the two hip bones, and forming the posterior section of the pelvis.

sad′dle. Denture base; see under base.

sa′dism. The existence of destructive-aggressive

attitudes in an individual; i.e., the person derives pleasure from inflicting physical or psychological pain on others, in both social and sexual relationships.

sa′dist. One who practices sadism.

sadomas′ochism. The simultaneous existence of destructive-aggressive and self-destructive-passive attitudes in an individual, in both social and sexual relationships.

saf′flower. A plant having seeds from which safflower oil is extracted.

saf′ranin O. A red basic dye used in biologic stains.

safranophile. Staining readily with safranin.

sag′ittal. In an anteroposterior direction.

sal, *pl.* **sal′es.** Latin for salt.

sal′icin. A glucoside obtained from the bark of willow and poplar trees; used as a bitter tonic.

salicylam′ide. A white, crystalline compound having analgesic properties.

salic′ylate. A salt of salicylic acid.

methyl s., oil of wintergreen.

salicylaz′osulfapyr′idine. A sulfonamide used in the treatment of ulcerative colitis.

salicylic acid. A white crystalline powder, $C_7H_6O_3$, derived from phenol; used externally for the local treatment of corns and warts.

sal′icylism. Poisoning by salicylic acid or its salts.

salicyluric acid. $C_9H_9NO_4$; an acid found in the urine after administration of salicylic acid or some of its derivatives.

sa′lient. Projecting; protruding.

salifi′able. Capable of combining with acids to form salts; said of certain bases.

sal′ify. To convert into a salt.

salim′eter. Instrument used to determine the concentration of saline solutions.

sa′line. Relating to or containing salt.

sali′va. The fluid mixture of secretions from the parotid, sublingual, and submandibular glands and the mucous glands of the oral cavity; it contains an enzyme (ptyalin) which partially digests carbohydrates.

sal′ivant. 1. Increasing the flow of saliva. **2.** An agent having such an effect.

sal′ivary. Relating to saliva.

salivary gland virus disease. See cytomegalic inclusion disease.

sal′ivate. To produce excessive secretion of saliva.

saliva′tion. 1. The secretion of saliva. **2.** Sialorrhea; excessive flow of saliva.

Salmonel′la. A genus of gram-negative, rod-shaped, motile bacteria, some species of which cause acute intestinal inflammation.

S. typhi, species that is the causative agent of

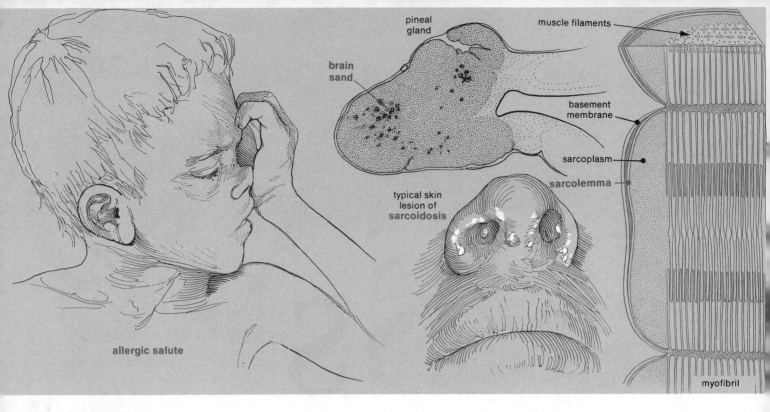

allergic salute

pineal gland

brain sand

muscle filaments

basement membrane

sarcoplasm

sarcolemma

typical skin lesion of **sarcoidosis**

myofibril

---

typhoid fever; formerly called *Salmonella typhosa*; also called typhoid bacillus.

S. typhimurium, species causing food poisoning in man.

S. typhosa, former name for *Salmonella typhi*.

salmonello′sis. Infection with bacteria of the genus *Salmonella*, usually marked by severe diarrhea.

salping-, salpingo-. Combining forms denoting a tube.

salpingec′tomy. Surgical removal of a uterine tube; also called tubectomy.

salpingemphrax′is. Obstruction of a uterine or an auditory tube.

salpin′gian. Relating to the uterine (fallopian) or to the auditory (eustachian) tubes.

salpingi′tis. Inflammation of the uterine tube.

salpin′gocele. Hernia of a uterine (fallopian) tube.

salpingocye′sis. Tubal pregnancy; see under pregnancy.

salpingog′raphy. Radiography of a uterine tube after the injection of a radiopaque compound.

salpingol′ysis. The release of adhesions about a uterine (fallopian) tube or its fringed end.

salpingo-oophrec′tomy. Surgical removal of an ovary and its corresponding uterine (fallopian) tube.

salpingo-oophori′tis. Inflammation of a uterine tube and ovary; also called salpingo-oothecitis.

salpingo-oothec i′tis. See salpingo-oophoritis.

salpingoperitoni′tis. Inflammation of a uterine (fallopian) tube and adjacent peritoneum.

salpingopharyn′geal. Relating to the auditory tube and the pharynx.

salpingoplas′ty. Reparative operation on a uterine tube.

salpingor′rhaphy. Stitching of a uterine (fallopian) tube.

salpingos′tomy. The making of an artificial opening in a uterine tube when the fringed end of the tube is occluded; an operative treatment for sterility.

salpingot′omy. Surgical inclusion into a uterine tube.

sal′pinx. A tube; denoting the uterine (fallopian) tube or the auditory (eustachian) tube.

salt. 1. Compound produced by the reaction between an acid and a base in which all or part of the hydrogen ions of the acid are replaced by one or more radicals of the base. **2.** Table salt (sodium chloride).

acid s., one containing unreplaced hydrogen atoms from the acid; e.g., NaHSO₄.

basic s., one containing unreplaced hydroxyl radicals from the base; e.g., Bi(OH)Cl₂.

binary s., one containing only two elements.

effervescent s., one of several preparations containing sodium bicarbonate, tartaric and citric acids, and an active salt; when it is mixed with water the acids break up the sodium bicarbonate, releasing the carbonic acid gas.

Epsom s., see magnesium sulfate.

iodized s., table salt containing one part sodium or potassium iodide to 10,000 parts sodium chloride.

smelling s., a preparation of ammonium carbonate with any of several aromatic oils, sniffed as a restorative.

salta′tion. Leaping, as in certain nervous disorders.

sal′ting out. The separation of a protein from its solution by the addition of a neutral salt such as sodium chloride.

saltpe′ter. See potassium nitrate.

salu′brious. Healthful.

salure′sis. Excretion of sodium in the urine.

saluret′ic. Promoting excretion of sodium.

sal′utary. Healthful.

salute′, aller′gic. Rubbing of the tip of the nose in a characteristic transverse or upward motion, commonly seen in children afflicted with allergic rhinitis.

salve. 1. An ointment. **2.** Anything that soothes or heals. **3.** To dress with salve; to soothe.

sama′rium. Metallic element of the rare earth group; symbol Sm, atomic number 62, atomic weight 150.35.

sam′ple. 1. A representative segment of the whole. **2.** In biostatistics, the portion of the population being studied. **3.** A specimen.

san′ative. Curative.

sanato′rium. An institution for the treatment of long term illnesses, as tuberculosis, mental disorders, etc.; often confused with sanitarium.

san′atory. Curative.

sand. Granules of disintegrated rock.

brain s., minute crystals, mainly composed of calcium carbonate, present in the pineal body; also called acervulus.

sane. Relating to sanity or to one who is of sound mind.

sanguif′erous. Conveying blood.

sanguin′eous. Relating to or containing blood.

sanguin′olent. Blood-tinged.

sanguinopur′ulent. Denoting a discharge or matter containing blood and pus.

san′guis. Latin for blood.

sanguiv′orous. Blood-sucking, as certain animals.

sa′nies. A watery discharge containing blood and pus.

saniopu′rulent. Denoting a blood-tinged discharge with pus.

saniose′rous. Denoting a blood-tinged serum.

sanita′rium. A health resort. Cf sanatorium.

san′itary. Relating to or conducive to health.

sanita′tion. Application of measures to create environmental conditions conducive to health.

san′ity. Soundness of mind; in a legal sense, the state of a person's mind whereby he is legally responsible for his actions and their consequences.

san′tonin. The bitter principle of santonica (dried flower heads of the plant *Artemicia cina*); sometimes used to effect expulsion of roundworms.

saphenec′tomy. Surgical removal of a saphenous vein.

saph′enous. 1. Relating to either of two large superficial veins of the leg (saphena) that carry blood from the toes upward. **2.** Denoting various structures in the leg.

sapona′ceous. Soapy; resembling soap.

saponifica′tion. The formation of a soap by the hydrolytic action of an alkali upon fat.

sapon′ify. To convert fat into soap.

sap′onin. Any of a group of vegetable substances possessing the property of making suds.

sapph′ism. Lesbianism.

sap′rogen. An organism that causes decay of organic matter.

saprogen′ic. Causing decay.

saprog′enous. Resulting from decay.

saproph′ilous. Thriving on decaying matter.

sap′rophyte. A plant, such as a bacterium or fungus, that lives on dead or decaying organic matter; also called necroparasite.

saprophyt′ic. Relating to a saprophyte; deriving nourishment from dead organic matter.

saprozo′ic. Thriving in decaying organic material; said of certain protozoa.

sarco-. A combining form meaning flesh.

sar′cocele. A fleshy tumor of the testis.

sar′coid. 1. Sarcoidosis. **2.** Resembling flesh.

sarcoido′sis. Multiple benign nodular lesions involving any tissue of the body, especially the lungs; a systemic granulomatous disease of undetermined etiology; also called Boeck's sarcoid.

sarcolem′ma. The delicate plasma membrane that invests every striated muscle fiber.

sarco′ma. A malignant tumor composed of connective tissue.

Ewing's s., a rapidly growing malignant tumor arising from medullary tissue within a single bone, usually the long bones; occurring most frequently in individuals between the ages of 10 and 25 years; symptoms include fever, pain, and leukocytosis;

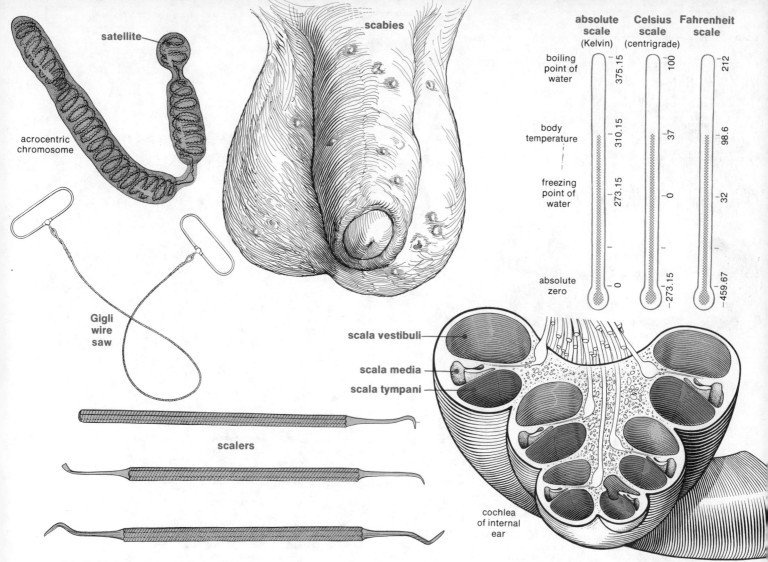

satellite

acrocentric chromosome

scabies

Gigli wire saw

scalers

	absolute scale (Kelvin)	Celsius scale (centigrade)	Fahrenheit scale
boiling point of water	375.15	100	212
body temperature	310.15	37	98.6
freezing point of water	273.15	0	32
absolute zero	0	−273.15	−459.67

scala vestibuli
scala media
scala tympani

cochlea of internal ear

---

also called Ewing's tumor and diffuse endothelioma of bone.

   Rous s., a sarcoma-like growth of fowl; shown in 1910 by Peyton Rous to be caused by a virus.

sarco′matoid. Resembling a sarcoma.

sarco′matous. Pertaining to or of the nature of sarcoma.

sar′comere. One of a series of repeated segments of a muscle fibril that comprises the fundamental units of contraction; the area between two Z′lines, composed of overlapping thick and thin myofilaments.

sar′coplasm. The interfibrillary cytoplasm of a muscle fiber; the substance in which the muscle fibrils are embedded.

sarcopoiet′ic. Forming muscle.

Sarcoptes scabiei. The species of itch mite that causes the parasitic skin disorder scabies; the fertilized female tunnels intradermally and deposits eggs and excreta; the male mites generally do not burrow, but remain on the surface of the skin searching for unfertilized females.

sar′cosome. A mitochondrion of muscle; in cardiac muscle, sarcosomes are large, numerous, and usually aligned in columns between the myofibrils.

sarcosto′sis. Ossification of muscle tissue.

sarcotu′bules. A system of membranous tubules surrounding each fibril of striated muscle.

sardon′ic grin. See risus caninus.

sat. Abbreviation for saturated.

sat′ellite. In genetics, a small globoid chromatin mass attached to the end of the chromosome by a slender secondary constriction; in man, usually associated with the short arm of an acrocentric chromosome.

satellito′sis. Phenomenon in which interstitial brain cells of a certain type (oligodendroglia), normally found as satellites about nerve cells, increase in number about a damaged nerve cell.

sat′urate. 1. To impregnate completely. **2.** To neutralize.

sat′urated. Denoting a solution in which the addition of any more of a solute will cause precipitation.

sat′urnine. Relating to lead.

sat′urnism. Lead poisoning.

satyri′asis. Excessive sexual desire in the male.

sauri′asis. Severe ichthyosis; also called lizard skin.

saw. A cutting instrument with a serrated edge, used to cut bone.

   Gigli wire s., a wire with saw teeth.

Sb. Chemical symbol of the element antimony (stibium).

SBE. Abbreviation for subacute bacterial endocarditis.

Sc. Chemical symbol of the element scandium.

scab. 1. The crust formed on the surface of an ulcer or a superficial wound, composed of dried pus, lymph, or blood. **2.** To develop a scab.

sca′bicide. An agent destructive to itch mites.

sca′bies. A contagious, parasitic skin disorder caused by the mite *Sarcoptes scabiei*; the female mite excavates tunnels in the superficial layers of the skin and deposits eggs and irritating excreta, causing red lesions, itching, and swelling of the skin surface along the elevated tracts; the most common sites of entry are between the fingers, the hands, and wrists; the infection can persist for months or years in untreated individuals, hence the colloquial term seven-year itch; also called sarcoptic acariasis.

scabrit′es. Rough, scaly skin.

sca′la. One of the spiral canals of the cochlea.

   s. media, cochlear duct; see under duct.

   s. tympani, the spiral canal of the cochlea located below the spiral lamina; also called tympanic canal.

   s. vestibuli, the spiral canal of the cochlea located above the spiral lamina; also called vestibular canal.

scald. 1. To burn with a hot liquid or vapor. **2.** The lesion produced in such a manner. **3.** Any crusty lesion of the scalp.

scale. 1. A small thin piece of epithelium shed from the skin. **2.** To shed such material. **3.** In dentistry, to scrape tartar off the teeth. **4.** A system of marks at regular intervals serving as a standard of measurement. **5.** An instrument having such marks.

   absolute s., a temperature scale with its zero point at absolute zero (approximately −273.16°C); also called Kelvin scale.

   Celsius s., a temperature scale in which 0° represents the freezing point of water and 100° its boiling point, at sea level; the normal human body temperature is recorded at 37°; named after Anders Celsius, the Swedish astronomer who invented it; also called centigrade scale.

   centigrade s., one having 100 equal units between two standard points; e.g., the Celsius scale.

   Fahrenheit s., temperature scale that records the freezing point of water at 32°, the boiling point of water at 212°, and the normal heat of the human body at 98.6° under standard atmospheric pressure; named after the German physicist Gabriel D. Fahrenheit.

   Kelvin s., see absolute scale.

scalen′e. Having sides of unequal length; said of a triangle or a muscle of such proportions.

scalenec′tomy. Surgical removal of a scalene muscle, or a portion of it.

scalenus-anticus syndrome. Pain in the shoulder, often radiating to the arm and back of the neck, caused by compression of nerves and vessels between the first thoracic rib and a hypertonic anterior scalene (scalene anticus) muscle.

sca′ler. An instrument designed to be used in removing deposits, especially tartar, from the teeth.

scal′ing. Removal of calculus from the exposed surfaces of the teeth and the area under the margin of the gums by use of special instruments called scalers.

scalp. The skin covering the cranium.

scal′pel. A thin surgical knife, usually with a re-

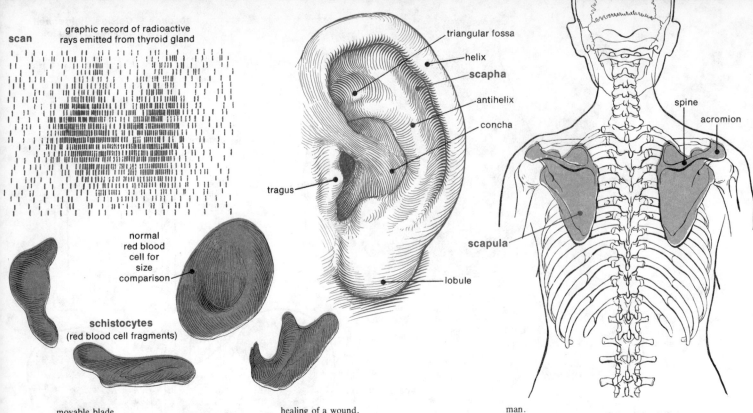

scan. graphic record of radioactive rays emitted from thyroid gland

normal red blood cell for size comparison

schistocytes (red blood cell fragments)

triangular fossa
helix
scapha
antihelix
concha
tragus
lobule

spine
acromion
scapula

movable blade.

scal′priform. Resembling a chisel.

scaly. 1. Flaking. **2.** Covered with scales or flakes.

scan. 1. A graphic record of the distribution of a specific radioactive element within an organ. **2.** To obtain a record of the distribution of radioactivity within an organ.

scan′dium. A light, silvery-white metallic element that reacts rapidly with acids; symbol Sc, atomic number 21, atomic weight 44.956; present in the earth's crust in a concentration of about five parts per million.

scan′ner. 1. Apparatus used to determine radioactivity distribution within an organ; it consists of a sensitive, collimated detector which is mechanically coupled to a recorder. **2.** Any device that scans a region point by point in a continuous systematic manner.

    ACTA s., a CAT scanner capable of doing whole body as well as head scans.

    CAT s., a machine for performing computerized axial tomography; also called CT scanner.

    EMI s., a CAT scanner developed by the EMI company.

scan′ning. The procedure of making a radioactivity scan.

    bone s., a sensitive technique of scanning bone for detecting lesions; a valuable aid in the diagnosis, treatment, and prognosis of a variety of benign and malignant skeletal disorders.

    brain s., one of the essential methods of cerebrospinal diagnosis; it entails injection or inhalation of radioisotopes and production of pictures by radiation detectors; also called radioisotopic brain scanning.

    radioisotopic brain s., see brain scanning.

sca′pha. The long longitudinal depression or furrow between the helix and the antihelix of the auricle.

scaphocephal′ic. Characterized by scaphocephalism.

scaphoceph′alism. A deformity in which the skull is abnormally long and narrow (high vertex, bulging forehead, lateral flattening, and increased anteroposterior diameter), due to the premature closure of the sagittal suture.

scaphoceph′aly. Scaphocephalism.

scaph′oid. Boat-shaped; sunken; hollowed.

scap′ula. Either of two large, flat, triangular bones overlying the upper portion of the ribs, and forming the back of the shoulder; articulates with the clavicle and the humerus; also called shoulder blade.

scap′ular. Of or relating to the scapula (shoulder blade).

scar. Cicatrix; the fibrous tissue formed during the healing of a wound.

scarifica′tion. The making of several superficial scratches on the skin, as when vaccinating.

scarlati′na. Scarlet fever; an acute infectious disease caused by a β-hemolytic streptococcus.

scarlatin′iform. Resembling scarlatina; said of a rash.

scato-, scat-. Combining forms meaning feces or excrement.

scatol′ogy. 1. The scientific study and analysis of the feces. **2.** In psychiatry, the study relating to disorder manifestations connected with excrement.

scato′ma. An inspissated fecal mass in the colon or rectum resembling, on palpation, an abdominal tumor.

scatoph′agy. Eating of feces or filth; also called rhypophagy.

scatos′copy. Examination or inspection of the feces for diagnostic purposes.

scat′tering. The change in direction or dispersal of a beam of particles or radiation as a result of physical interaction, as the dispersal of electrons by the specimen in the electron microscope.

Sc.D. Abbreviation for Doctor of Science.

Schamberg's disease. Progressive pigmentary dermatosis, a benign chronic disorder marked by repeated crops of petechiae on feet and legs, especially in men; associated microscopically with capillary dilatation, diapedesis, and hemosiderosis.

sche′ma. An arrangement or plan.

Schilder's disease. See encephalitis periaxialis diffusa.

Schilling's hemogram. A differential blood count in which the polymorphonuclear leukocytes are separated into four groups according to the number and arrangement of nuclear segments in the cells; also called Schilling's blood count and Schilling's index.

schisto-, schist-. Combining forms meaning split, division, cleft, or fissure.

schistoce′lia. Congenital furrow of the abdominal wall.

schistocys′tis. Fissure or exstrophy of the bladder; a congenital gap in the anterior wall of the bladder and the abdominal wall in front of it, with the posterior wall of the bladder presenting through the opening.

schis′tocyte, schiz′ocyte. A fragment of a red blood cell; it can assume a variety of sizes and shapes.

schistocyto′sis. The occurrence of many red blood fragments (schistocytes) in the blood.

schistoglos′sia. Congenital cleft of the tongue.

Schistoso′ma. A genus of blood flukes (class Trematoda), some species of which are parasitic in man.

schis′tosome. A member of the genus Schistosoma.

schistosomi′asis. Infestation with schistosomes (blood flukes); involves mainly the intestinal tract, liver, or bladder; also called bilharziasis and bilharziosis.

schizo-, schiz-. Combining forms meaning split, division, cleft, or cleavage.

schizog′ony. A stage in the asexual cycle of the malarial parasite occurring in the red blood cells of man; also called multiple fission.

schi′zoid. See under personality.

Schizomyce′tes. A class of microorganisms containing all bacteria.

schiz′ont. The adult asexual form of the malarial parasite in man, following the trophozoite, with two or more divisions of its nucleus; it eventually divides, producing merozoites.

schizopha′sia. The disordered, incomprehensible speech of the schizophrenic individual; also referred to as "water-salad" speech.

schizophre′nia. A category of severe emotional disorders marked by disturbances of thinking including misinterpretation of reality and sometimes delusions and hallucinations; there are associated changes in mood and behavior, particularly withdrawal from people; formerly called dementia precox.

schizophren′ic. Relating to or afflicted with schizophrenia.

schizotrich′ia. A splitting of hairs at their ends; also called scissura pilorum.

Schlemm's canal. Scleral venous sinus; see under sinus.

Schmidt's syndrome. 1. Primary hypothyroidism and adrenal insufficiency; organ-specific antibodies against the adrenal gland and thyroid gland may be present; diabetes mellitus may also be present. **2.** Unilateral paralysis of a vocal cord, the palate, and the trapezius and sternocleidomastoid muscles.

Schönlein's disease. Henoch-Schönlein purpura; see under purpura.

Schüffner's dots. The dots or stipples appearing in red blood cells infected with malarial parasites (especially Plasmodium vivax), due to accumulation of granules; also called Schüffner's granules.

Schüller disease. See Hand-Schüller-Christian syndrome.

schwanno′ma. See neurilemoma.

    granular cell s., see tumor, granular cell.

Schwann's sheath. See neurilemma.

sciage′. The back and forth sawing movement of the hand in massage.

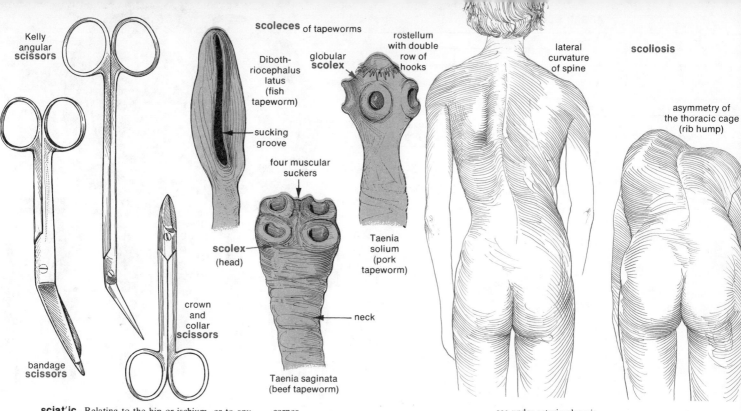

Kelly
angular
scissors

bandage
scissors

crown
and
collar
scissors

scoleces of tapeworms

Diboth-
riocephalus
latus
(fish
tapeworm)

—sucking
groove

globular
scolex

rostellum
with double
row of
hooks

four muscular
suckers

scolex
(head)

Taenia
solium
(pork
tapeworm)

—neck

Taenia saginata
(beef tapeworm)

lateral
curvature
of spine

scoliosis

asymmetry of
the thoracic cage
(rib hump)

sciat'ic. Relating to the hip or ischium, or to any structure in its vicinity, as the sciatic nerve.

sciat'ica. Any condition characterized by pain along the course of the sciatic nerve; usually a neuritis and generally caused by mechanical compression or irritation of the 5th lumbar spinal root.

scinticisternog'raphy. A test for diagnosing hydrocephalus, and for studying the dynamics of cerebrospinal fluid movement, by use of a radioactive tracer.

scin'tigram. A Scintiscan.

scintilla'tion. A flash of light produced in a chemical crystal by absorption of an ionizing photon; the minuscule flash of light seen on a fluorescent screen results from the spontaneous emission of charged alpha particles across the sensitized surface.

scin'tillator. Scintillation counter; see under counter.

scin'tiscan. A graphic pattern recorded on paper of pulses derived from a radioactive isotope, revealing its concentration in a specific organ or tissue; it serves to outline the tissue or organ or its actively metabolizing portion.

scin'tiscan'ner. A directional scintillation counter which automatically scans a region of the body to record the concentration of a γ-ray-emitting isotope in tissue.

scirrho-, scirrh-. Combining forms meaning hard.

scir'rhoid. Resembling a scirrhus (hard fibrous cancer).

scir'rhous. Relating to a scirrhus; hard.

scir'rhus. A hard cancerous tumor composed chiefly of fibrous connective tissue.

scissors. A double-bladed cutting instrument.

scler-. See sclero-.

scler'a. The tough, white, membranous tunic, outermost of three, which covers all of the eyeball except the anterior portion, which is occupied by the cornea.

scleradeni'tis. Inflammatory hardening of a gland.

scle'ral. Of or pertaining to the sclera.

sclerecta'sia. Bulging of the sclera.

sclerec'tomy. Surgical removal of a small portion of the sclera, as for the treatment of glaucoma.

sclerede'ma. Disease of unknown cause marked by induration and swelling of the skin and subcutaneous tissues.

sclere'ma. Hardening of the skin and underlying tissues.

scleri'tis. Inflammation of the sclera.

annular s., anterior scleritis which extends around the limbus of the cornea (ring-shaped).

anterior s., scleritis of the anterior part of the eyeball where the sclera adjoins the limbus of the cornea.

brawny s., annular scleritis involving the episcleral tissue of the peripheral part of the cornea.

herpetic s., herpes zoster involving the sclera.

posterior s., inflammation of the posterior sclera and Tenon's capsule; may also involve the underlying choroid and retina.

pyogenic s., scleritis caused by a bacterial embolus lodged in a scleral vessel, resulting in an abscess.

sclero-, scler-. Combining forms meaning hard, or indicating a relationship to the sclera, the tough outer coat of the eyeball.

sclerochoroi'dal. Relating to both the sclera and choroid, the outer and middle layers of the eyeball.

scleroconjunc'tival. Relating to the sclera and the conjunctiva.

sclerocor'nea. The sclera and cornea considered as a unit.

sclerodac'tyly. Scleroderma affecting the fingers or toes.

scleroder'ma. Progressive thickening and hardening of the skin.

sclerodermati'tis, sclerodermi'tis. Inflammation, thickening, and hardening of the skin.

sclerog'enous. Producing a hard tissue or substance; causing sclerosis; also called sclerogenic.

scleroiri'tis. Inflammation of the sclera and iris.

sclero'ma. A circumscribed area of hard or granulation tissue in the skin or mucous membrane.

scleromala'cia. Extreme thinning of the sclera, occurring in patients with rheumatoid arthritis.

scleronych'ia. Excessively hardened and thickened condition of the nails.

sclero-oophori'tis. Inflammatory hardening of the ovary; also called sclero-oothecitis.

sclero-oothecи'tis. See sclero-oophoritis.

sclerophthal'mia. Rare congenital condition in which scleral tissue encroaches on the cornea, with only a small central area remaining clear.

scleroplas'ty. Reparative surgery of the sclera.

scleropro'tein. A hard fibrous protein resembling albumin; also called albuminoid.

sclerose'. To harden or to become sclerotic.

sclero'sis. Hardening of tissues due to proliferation of connective tissue, usually originating in chronic inflammation.

amyotrophic lateral s., a disease characterized by degeneration of the lateral motor tracts of the spinal cord, causing progressive muscular atrophy and exaggerated reflexes.

arterial s., see arteriosclerosis.

endocardial s., endomyocardial fibroelastosis; see under fibroelastosis.

medial calcific s., Mönckeberg's arteriosclerosis;

see under arteriosclerosis.

multiple s., (MS), disease of the brain and spinal cord affecting mostly young adults and characterized by loss of the fatty sheaths (myelin) that surround nerve fibers; its name is derived from the plaques or patches of scarred (sclerosed) nervous fibers that dot the central nervous system; symptoms vary with distribution of the sclerotic patches, but the most frequently seen are weakness, incoordination, scanning (halting, monosyllabic) speech, involuntary oscillation of the eyeballs (nystagmus), and coarse tremors.

tuberous s., a familial disease marked by progressive mental deterioration, epileptic convulsions, and sometimes sebaceous adenomas of the skin.

scleros'tomy. The operative creation of a fistulous opening in the sclera, as for the relief of glaucoma.

sclerother'apy. Injection of a chemical into a vein to obliterate its lumen; a method of treating varicose veins.

sclerot'ic. 1. Relating to or characterized by sclerosis. **2.** Of or relating to the sclera or outer layer of the eyeball.

scle'rotome. In embryology, the cells that break off from the somite, surround the notochord and spinal cord, later differentiate into cartilage, and eventually form the vertebrae.

sclerot'omy. Surgical incision of the sclera.

scle'rous. Hardened; indurated; calloused; leather-like; scarred.

SCM. Abbreviation for state certified midwife.

sco'leces. Plural of scolex.

scolecol'ogy. See helminthology.

sco'lex, *pl.* **sco'leces.** The head of a tapeworm by which it attaches to the mucosa of the small intestine; it is connected by a short and narrow neck to a large number of proglottids (segments).

scolio'sis. A rotary lateral curvature of the spine.

congenital s., scoliosis resulting from malformation of the spine or chest.

idiopathic s., lateral spinal curvature in which the cause is unknown; constitutes 80 per cent of all cases of scoliosis.

myopathic s., scoliosis due to weakness of the spinal muscles.

osteopathic s., lateral curvature resulting from pathologic conditions of the vertebrae, such as tuberculosis, rickets, osteomalacia, and tumors.

static s., scoliosis due to difference in the length of the legs.

scoliot'ic. Relating to or afflicted with scoliosis.

-scope. A combining form indicating an instrument for inspection.

scopo'lamine. A nonbarbiturate hypnotic alka-

sciatic | **scopolamine**

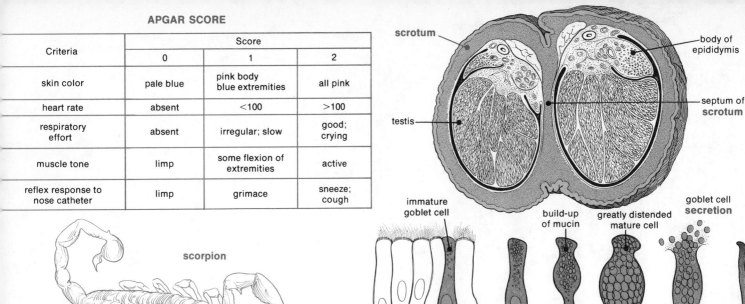

APGAR SCORE

Criteria	Score		
	0	1	2
skin color	pale blue	pink body blue extremities	all pink
heart rate	absent	<100	>100
respiratory effort	absent	irregular; slow	good; crying
muscle tone	limp	some flexion of extremities	active
reflex response to nose catheter	limp	grimace	sneeze; cough

scorpion

scrotum
body of epididymis
septum of scrotum
testis

immature goblet cell
epithelial cells
build-up of mucin
greatly distended mature cell
goblet cell secretion

loid found in the leaves and seeds of *Hyoscyamus niger* (henbane), *Scopola carniolica, Atropa belladonna,* and other solanaceous plants; in toxic doses, it can cause excitation, hallucinations, delirium, and other peculiar mental effects; because of its amnestic qualities, it is used with morphine to produce "twilight sleep"; formerly used extensively in obstetrics.

scorbu′tus. See scurvy.

score. An evaluative record, usually expressed numerically.

  Apgar s., evaluation of the general condition of a newborn soon after birth; numerical values are assigned to the status of skin color, heart rate, respiratory effort, muscle tone, and reflex irritability; a score of ten denotes a newborn in excellent condition.

scor′pion. A member of the order Scorpionida having a segmented body and an erectile tail which possesses a venomous sting.

scoto-. A combining form denoting a relationship to darkness.

scotochrom′ogens. Group II mycobacteria that produce a yellow pigment when grown in the dark and an orange pigment in the presence of light.

scoto′ma. 1. An abnormal blind spot; an area in the visual field in which vision is absent or greatly diminished. **2.** In psychiatry, a figurative blind spot in an individual's psychologic awareness characterized by an absence of insight into or inability to grasp a mental problem.

scotom′atous. Relating to an area of absent or depressed vision (scotoma) in the visual field.

scotom′eter. Instrument used to plot and measure an isolated area of absent or depressed vision (scotoma) in the visual field.

scotopho′bia. Abnormal fear of the dark.

scoto′pia. See vision, scotopic.

scotop′ic. 1. Relating to vision that is adapted to low levels of illumination. **2.** Denoting the low levels of illumination to which the eye's sensitivity to light becomes greatly increased when it is dark-adapted.

scra′pie. 1. A disease-causing viroid that may represent a missing link between viruses and genes, and may be an agent of extrachromosomal inheritance. **2.** A contagious disease of sheep and goats, manifested by various nervous symptoms and usually leading to death.

screen. 1. A thin sheet of any material used as a shield. **2.** To make a fluoroscopic examination.

  fluorescent s., one coated with calcium tungstate crystals, used in the fluoroscope.

  tangent s., a large, usually black screen used in the clinical measurement of the central field of vi-

sion.

screening. 1. The process of examining large groups of people for a given disease. **2.** Survey of a specimen for a variety of substances; e.g., a narcotic screen of a urine sample.

scrof′ula. Tuberculous inflammation of lymph nodes of the neck in children, caused by *Mycobacterium bovis;* relatively rare in the United States as a result of elimination of tuberculous cattle and pasteurization of milk; also called cervical adenitis.

scrofuloder′ma. Tuberculosis of the skin.

scro′tal. Of or relating to the scrotum.

scrotec′tomy. Surgical removal of part of the scrotum.

scroti′tis. Inflammation of the scrotum.

scro′tocele. A complete inguinal hernia which rests in the scrotum; also called scrotal hernia.

scro′toplasty. See oscheoplasty.

scro′tum. The two-layered sac enclosing the testes and lower part of spermatic cords; composed of skin, muscles, and fascia, and divided on its surface into two portions by a ridge (raphe).

scruff. Nape.

scru′ple. A unit of apothecary weight equal to 20 grains or one-third of a dram.

scur′vy. A nutritional deficiency disease resulting from a lack of vitamin C (ascorbic acid), characterized by spongy, swollen, and bleeding gums, hemorrhages, and extreme weakness; also called scorbutus.

scute. A thin lamina or plate, as the thin bony plate separating the upper part of the middle ear from the mastoid cells.

scyb′alum. An abnormally hard mass of feces in the intestine.

scyphozo′an. An animal of the class Scyphozoa.

Scyphozo′a. A class of marine animals (phylum Coelenterata) which includes the jellyfishes.

S.D. Abbreviation for (a) standard deviation, (b) skin dose.

S.E. Abbreviation for standard error.

Se. Chemical symbol of the element selenium.

seal. 1. To effect an airtight closure. **2.** Any agent used to prevent seepage of air or moisture.

sea nettle. A stinging jellyfish.

sea′sickness. Nausea, pallor, sweating, and vomiting provoked by the motion of a vessel at sea.

seba′ceous. Relating to or secreting fatty material (sebum).

seborrhe′a. See dermatitis, seborrheic.

se′bum. The secretion of a sebaceous gland.

secobarb′ital. A short-acting, fast-onset sedative and hypnotic; Seconal®.

sec′ondary. 1. Sequential to something considered primary; e.g., secondary syphilis, a stage of

syphilis that must be preceded by the primary stage. **2.** Sequential to anything; not primary; e.g., secondary infection, an infection which is superimposed upon an existing condition.

secondary aldosteronism. See aldosteronism, secondary.

secre′ta. Secretions.

secre′tagogue, secre′togogue. 1. A substance that promotes secretion, as of the stomach. **2.** Stimulating secretion.

secrete′. To produce cell products and deliver them into the blood or bodily cavity either through a duct or by direct diffusion.

secre′tin. An intestinal hormone released primarily by the mucosa of the duodenum during digestion; it stimulates the secretion of water and bicarbonate by the pancreas.

secre′tion. 1. The production of a substance by a cell or a gland. **2.** The substance produced.

secre′togogue. See secretagogue.

secretomo′tor, secre′tomo′tory. Stimulating secretion; said of certain nerves.

secre′tor. A person whose saliva and other body fluids contain water-soluble forms of the ABO blood group antigens.

secre′tory. Relating to secretion.

sec′tile. Capable of being cut.

sec′tion. 1. The act of cutting. **2.** One of several component segments of a structure. **3.** A thin slice of tissue suitable for examination under the microscope. **4.** A cut surface.

  cesarean s., incision through the walls of the abdomen and uterus for delivery of the fetus.

  coronal s., a section parallel to the coronal suture of the skull, at right angles to the saggital section.

  cross s., a section at right angles to the long axis.

  saggital s., an anteroposterior section which divides the body in more or less equal right and left parts.

  serial s., one of several consecutive histologic sections of a structure (e.g., spinal cord) for the purpose of microscopic examination.

secundigrav′ida. A woman who has been pregnant twice.

sec′undines. The placenta, umbilical cord, and membranes expelled from the uterus after the birth of the child; also called the afterbirth.

secun′dipara. A woman who has given birth twice; also called bipara.

sedate′. 1. To bring under the influence of a sedative. **2.** To administer a sedative to an individual.

seda′tion. The reduction of anxiety or stress by the administration of a sedative drug.

sed′ative. Any agent that slows down nervous activity.

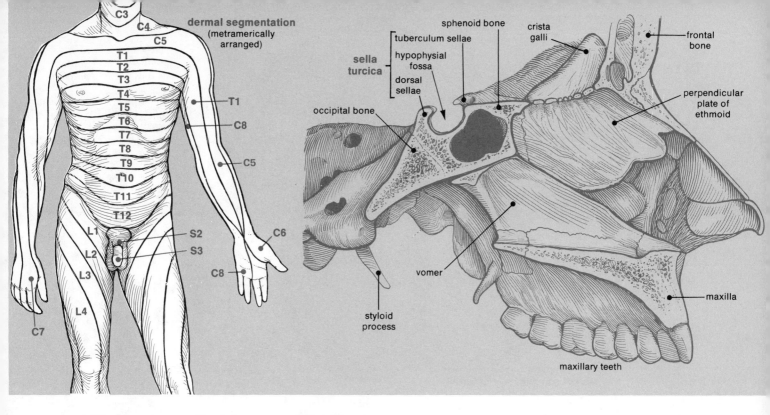

dermal segmentation (metramerically arranged)

sella turcica { tuberculum sellae, hypophysial fossa, dorsal sellae }

sphenoid bone · crista galli · frontal bone

occipital bone · perpendicular plate of ethmoid

vomer · maxilla

styloid process

maxillary teeth

anxiolytic s., any minor tranquilizer that acts on the central nervous system and has the capability of reducing pathologic anxiety, tension, and agitation without side effects of delusions and hallucinations; e.g., diazepam (Valium®).

sed'iment. The insoluble material that settles to the bottom of a liquid; also called hypostasis (that which rises to the surface is called epistasis).

urinary s., the solid matter that sinks to the bottom after the urine has been allowed to stand for some time or has been centrifuged; microscopic examination of the urine is usually performed on sediment resuspended in a few drops of the supernatant urine.

sedimenta'tion. The formation of a deposit of insoluble materials at the bottom of a liquid.

sedimenta'tor. Centrifuge.

seed. The fertilized ovule of a plant.

plantago s.'s, the seeds of the herb *Plantago psyllium,* which, when moist, swell and become gelatinous; used as a mild laxative (cathartic) in the treatment of simple constipation and as a demulcent in intestinal irritation; also called plantain or psyllium seeds, and psyllium.

seg'ment. 1. One of the parts into which a structure can be divided. **2.** A differentiated subdivision of an organism or part, as a metamere.

segmenta'tion. 1. The process of becoming divided into similar parts. **2.** Cleavage, as of the fertilized ovum.

cutaneous s., see dermal segmentation.

dermal s., cutaneous s., the division of the skin into segments (dermatomes) according to the different nervous innervation of each segment.

segrega'tion. In meiosis, the separating of two alleles of a pair of allelic genes so that they can pass to different gametes.

seizure. An attack; the sudden onset of a disease or symptoms, especially of epilepsy.

jacksonian s., a form of epilepsy with involuntary clonic motion or sensation.

selectiv'ity. In pharmacology, a comparative measure of the tendency of one drug to produce several effects; the relationship between the desired and undesired effects of a drug. Cf potency.

sele'nium. A poisonous element; symbol Se, atomic number 34, atomic weight 78.96; it resembles sulfur.

self. A person's awareness of his own being.

self-abuse'. Masturbation.

self-accusa'tion. Condemning oneself to misery, often because of some trivial error; a psychiatric symptom seen frequently in the depressive phase of manic-depressive psychosis.

self-anal'ysis. See autoanalysis

self-diges'tion. See autodigestion.

self-hypno'sis. See autohypnosis.

self-infec'tion. See autoinfection.

self-lim'ited. Denoting a disease which runs a definite course in a specific time, limited by its own characteristics rather than external factors.

self-poi'soning. 1. Autointoxication. **2.** The intentional or accidental taking of a substance that causes illness or death, especially by chemical means.

sella tur'cica. A depression with two prominences (anterior and posterior) on the upper surface of the sphenoid bone at the base of the skull, resembling a Turkish saddle and housing the pituitary gland.

SEM. Abbreviation for scanning electron microscope; see under microscope.

S.E.M. Abbreviation for standard error of the mean.

semeiog'raphy. See semiography.

semeiol'ogy. See semiology.

semelin'cident. Occurring only once; said of certain diseases.

se'men. A viscous whitish secretion of the male reproductive organs; composed chiefly of sperm, fructose-rich secretions from the seminal vesicles, and secretion from the prostrate gland (sperm usually comprises about 10 per cent of the semen); also called seminal fluid.

semenu'ria. The discharge of seminal fluid with the passage of urine; also called seminuria and spermaturia.

semi-. Prefix meaning half or partly.

semico'ma. A state of unconsciousness from which one can be aroused.

semico'matose. In a state of unconsciousness or stupor from which one can be aroused.

semicon'scious. Partly conscious; half-conscious.

semiflex'ion. The position of an extremity midway between extension and flexion.

semilu'nar. Shaped like a half-moon; also called crescentic.

semimem'branous. Consisting partly of membrane or fascia.

sem'inal. Of or relating to the semen.

semina'tion. Insemination.

seminif'erous. Conveying semen.

semino'ma. A malignant testicular neoplasm made up of large cells resembling spermatogonia; they usually metastasize to paraortic lymph nodes; also called dysgerminoma of the testis.

ovarian s., see dysgerminoma.

seminor'mal (0.5 N, N/2). Half normal; denoting a solution which contains one-half the strength

of a normal solution or one-half of an equivalent weight of the active reagent.

seminu'ria. See semenuria.

semiog'raphy, semeiog'raphy. A description of the symptoms of a disease.

semiol'ogy, semeiol'ogy. See symptomatology (1).

semipen'niform. Shaped like a feather on only one side; said of certain muscles.

semiper'meable. Of or relating to a membrane that allows some molecules in a solution to pass through but not others.

semiprone'. About three-quarters prone, between the midposition and pronation.

se'mis (ss, s). Latin for half; in prescriptions, it follows the sign indicating the measure.

semisul'cus. A slight groove on the edge of a structure which, when united with a similar groove of an adjoining structure, forms a complete sulcus.

semisupina'tion. A position midway between supination and pronation.

semisupine'. Lying in semisupination.

semisynthet'ic. Made from chemical reactions in which a naturally occurring substance was used as a starting material.

semiten'dinous. Partly tendinous, as the semitendinous muscle.

Senear-Usher disease, Senear-Usher syndrome. An eruption of scaling macules and blisters resembling both lupus erythematosus and pemphigus vulgaris; occurs on the scalp, face, and trunk; also called pemphigus erythematosus.

senes'cence. The process of aging or growing old.

senes'cent. Aging; growing old.

se'nile. 1. Characteristic of or resulting from old age. **2.** Exhibiting mental deterioration with old age.

se'nilism. Premature old age or senility, as in progeria.

senil'ity. 1. The condition of being senile. **2.** The physical and mental changes associated with old age.

sen'na. The dried leaves of the plants *Cassia acutifolia* or *Cassia angustifolia;* a laxative.

seno'pia. The unaided improvement of near vision in the aged; usually a sign of incipient cataract; also called second sight and gerontopia.

sensa'tion. The conscious perception of a stimulus acting on any of the organs of sense.

sense. 1. The power of perceiving any stimulus. **2.** Any of the special functions of sight, hearing, touch, taste, or smell.

sensibil'ity. The capability of perceiving sensations.

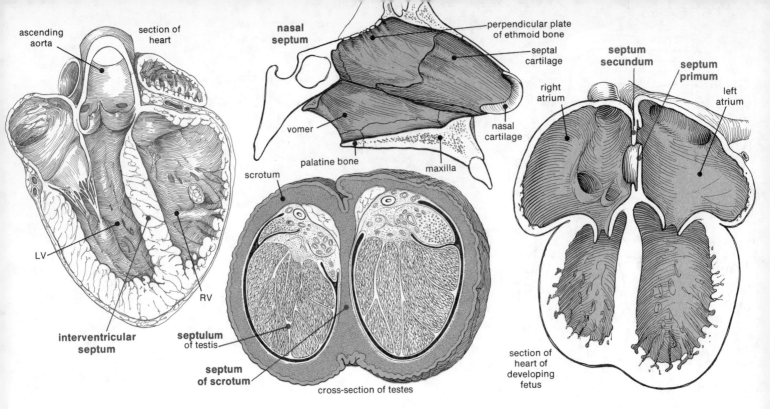

ascending aorta

section of heart

nasal septum

perpendicular plate of ethmoid bone

septal cartilage

septum secundum

septum primum

right atrium

left atrium

vomer

nasal cartilage

palatine bone

maxilla

LV

RV

scrotum

interventricular septum

septulum of testis

septum of scrotum

cross-section of testes

section of heart of developing fetus

sen'sible. 1. Perceptible by the senses. **2.** Able to feel.

sensim'eter. An instrument for measuring degrees of cutaneous sensation, as in anesthetized areas.

sen'sitive. 1. A state of increased capacity to respond specifically to an antigen or hapten. **2.** Responsive to external stimulation. **3.** Easily irritated or altered by the action of some agents.

sensitiv'ity. The state of being sensitive.

   disk s., a measurement of the susceptibility of a bacterial species to a variety of antibiotics placed on the culture medium in the form of disks; the sensitivity is measured by the area of inhibition of growth produced by the antibiotic disk.

sensitiza'tion. The process of increasing the reactivity of a subject, usually to specific antibodies or immune cells.

sen'sitize. To render sensitive; to increase the specific reactivity of a subject to an agent.

sensorimo'tor. Both sensory and motor; said of certain nerves.

senso'rium. In psychiatry, the state of mental clarity and consciousness at a given time.

sen'sory. Relating to sensation; said of a nerve.

sen'timent. 1. An attitude, thought, or judgment based on feeling instead of reason. **2.** Feeling or emotion regarding a specific matter. **3.** Susceptibility to a nostalgic feeling, verging on sentimentality.

sep'arator. 1. Instrument used to separate two teeth, so as to gain access to adjacent surfaces. **2.** A substance applied to a surface that prevents other material from adhering to that surface.

sep'sis. Presence in the blood of pus-forming microorganisms or their toxins.

sep'ta. Plural of septum.

sep'tal. Of or relating to a septum.

sep'tate. Divided into compartments by a septum.

septa'tion. The formation of thin dividing walls or septa.

septec'tomy. Surgical removal of part of the nasal septum.

sep'tic. Relating to sepsis.

septice'mia. Systemic disease caused by the presence of pathogenic microorganisms in the body.

septiv'alent. Having a valency of seven.

septomar'ginal. Relating to the margin of a partition or septum.

septona'sal. Relating to the nasal septum.

sep'totome. An instrument for incising the nasal septum.

septot'omy. Surgical incision of a septum.

sep'tulum, *pl.* **sep'tula.** Latin for a minute partition or septum.

sep'tum, *pl.* **sep'ta.** A thin wall dividing two bodily cavities or masses of soft tissue.

   interalveolar s., one of the bony partitions between the tooth sockets.

   interatrial s., the partition between the atria of the heart.

   interventricular s., the musculomembranous wall dividing the ventricles of the heart; also called ventricular septum.

   nasal s., the thin wall dividing the nasal cavities, composed posteriorly of bone and anteriorly of cartilage.

   s. lucidum, see septum pellucidum.

   s. pellucidum, a thin triangular partition between the anterior portions of the lateral ventricles of the brain; it is composed of the two laminae and is attached to the undersurface and reflected portion of the corpus callosum and to the fornix; also called septum lucidum.

   s. primum, in embryology, the sickle-shaped partition that initiates the division of the single atrial cavity of the embryonic heart into right and left chambers.

   rectovaginal s., the thin layer of fascia separating the vagina from the anterior wall of the rectum.

   s. of scrotum, the layer of fascia dividing the scrotum into two completely separate sacs, each containing a testis.

   s. secundum, the sickle-shaped partition apearing on the roof of the right atrium of the embryonic heart, adjacent to the septum primum; it never closes completely; its unclosed area forms the foramen ovale.

se'quel, sequel'a, *pl.* **se'quels, seque'lae.** Any abnormal condition following and caused by another disease.

sequencer, protein. An instrument that sequentially removes amino acids from the parent protein chain in order to determine the composition and structure of the protein.

seques'ter. 1. To undergo sequestration. **2.** To detach, separate, or isolate.

sequestra'tion. 1. The formation of a sequestrum. **2.** The isolation of a person with a contagious disease. **3.** An increase in the quantity of blood within the blood vessels, occurring physiologically or produced artificially.

   bronchopulmonary s., congenital anomaly marked by the presence of an independent mass of lung tissue having its own bronchial branch and artery (a branch from the thoracic aorta).

sequestrec'tomy. The surgical removal of a dead bone fragment that has become separated from the surrounding healthy bone.

seques'trum. A piece of dead bone that has become separated from the surrounding healthy bone tissue.

Ser. Symbol for the amino acid serine, and its aminoacyl (seryl) form.

se'ra. Plural of serum.

ser'ies. A group of related events, objects, or compounds, arranged systematically.

   aromatic s., compounds derived from benzene.

   erythrocytic s., the group of cells in various stages of development that ultimately form red blood cells.

   fatty s., the series of saturated open-chain hydrocarbons, denoted by the suffix -ane (methane, ethane, propane, etc.); also called methane series and paraffin series.

   granulocytic s., the cells in various stages of development, culminating in the formation of granulocytes.

   homologous s., a succession of organic compounds, each one differing from the preceding one by a radical or atomic group such as CH_2.

   lymphocytic s., cells in different stages of development leading to the formation of mature lymphocytes.

se'rine. A nonessential amino acid; one of the hydrolysis products of proteins.

se'riograph. Instrument for taking a series of six to eight radiographic exposures; used in radiography of the cerebral blood vessels.

seriscis'sion. Division of soft tissue, as the pedicle of a tumor, by a silk ligature.

sero-, ser-. Combining forms indicating serum or serous; e.g., serology.

seroconver'sion. A change in immunologic reactivity of the serum from negative to positive for a particular antibody; most commonly refers to one of the serologic tests for syphilis.

serocys'tic. Composed of or relating to cysts containing serous fluid.

serodiagno'sis. Diagnosis by means of reactions tested in the blood stream; also called orthodiagnosis.

seroenteri'tis. Inflammation of the serous or peritoneal coat of the intestine.

serofi'brinous. Containing serum and fibrin; said of a discharge or exudate.

serofi'brous. Relating to both a serous membrane and a fibrous tissue.

seroimmu'nity. Passive immunity; see under immunity.

serolog'ic. Relating to serology.

serol'ogy. 1. The study of serum, especially with respect to immunity phenomena. **2.** Commonly used to refer to a serologic test for syphilis.

sero'ma. A tumor-like mass formed by the collection of serum in the tissues, usually in a wound site.

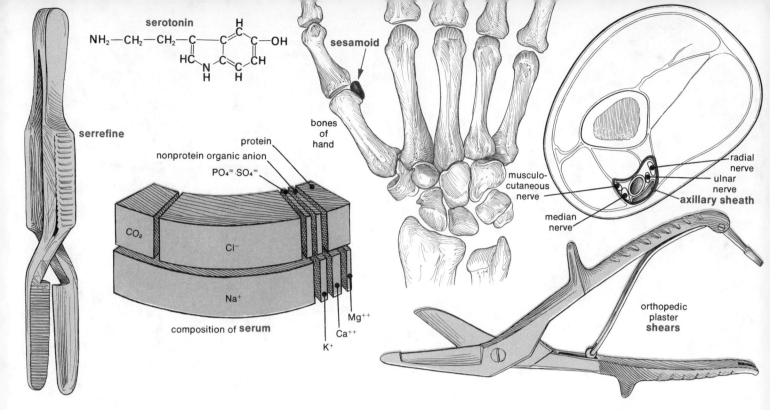

serotonin

serrefine

sesamoid

bones
of
hand

protein
nonprotein organic anion
$PO_4^=$ $SO_4^=$
CO_2
Cl^-
Na^+
Mg^{++}
Ca^{++}
K^+

composition of **serum**

musculo-cutaneous nerve
median nerve
radial nerve
ulnar nerve
axillary sheath

orthopedic
plaster
shears

---

seromem'branous. Relating to a serous membrane.

seromu'cous. Composed of serum and a mucinous material.

seropu'rulent. Containing serum and pus; said of a discharge.

se'ropus. Serum mixed with pus.

sero'sa. Any smooth membrane, such as that covering the intestines, composed of a mesothelial layer and a layer of connective tissue.

serosan'guinous. Containing serum and blood; said of an exudate or discharge.

serose'rous. Relating to two or more serous membranes.

serosi'tis. Inflammation of a serous membrane.
  multiple s., see polyserositis.

serosynovi'tis. Inflammation of the synovial membrane of a joint with effusion of serum.

seroto'nin. 5-Hydroxytryptamine; $C_{10}H_{12}N_2O$; a stimulant of smooth muscle contraction; occurs predominantly in the gastrointestinal mucosa, in small amounts in blood platelets, and in the brain; also found in carcinoid tumors.

se'rotype. A taxonomic subdivision of bacteria based on the antigenic characteristics of the microorganisms.

se'rous. Relating to, resembling, secreting, or containing serum.

serovaccina'tion. Combination of injection of serum to produce passive immunity and vaccination to produce active immunity.

serpig'inous. Creeping; denoting an ulcer or skin lesion that heals at one margin while spreading on the opposite side.

serpi'go. 1. Ringworm. **2.** Herpes. **3.** Any creeping eruption.

ser'rate, ser'rated. Notched.

serra'tion. 1. The state of having a sawlike edge. **2.** A series of toothlike projections.

serrefine'. A fine clamp; a small surgical spring forceps, usually used for clamping blood vessels.

ser'rulate, ser'rulated. Having small notches.

se'rum, *pl.* **se'rums** *or* **se'ra. 1.** The clear fluid of blood, devoid of fibrinogen and cells. **2.** Loosely used term denoting serum that contains antitoxins, used for therapeutic or laboratory diagnostic purposes.
  anticomplementary s., one that destroys complement.
  antilymphocyte s. (ALS), one used to inhibit rejection of grafts of organ transplants.
  antitoxic s., one containing antibodies to the toxins of a disease-causing microorganism.
  blood s., the clear, fluid portion of blood that is left after fibrinogen (a protein) and the cellular

elements of blood are removed by coagulation; distinguished from plasma, which is the cell-free liquid portion of uncoagulated blood.
  convalescent s., blood serum from a person recovering from an infectious disease.
  immune s. globulin, γ-globulin; see under globulin.
  polyvalent s., one containing antibodies against more than one strain of a microorganism.
  s. sickness, generalized allergic reaction to a foreign serum or to a drug; characterized by fever, skin rash, enlarged lymph nodes, and painful joints.
  truth s., a name for certain chemicals (sodium amobarbital and sodium thiopental) administered intravenously to facilitate questioning of an individual who is unwilling or unable to answer queries; it is in fact a misnomer since the subject's revelations elicited under the influence of the drug are not necessarily factually true.

servomech'anism. 1. An automatic control device used to maintain the operation of a mechanical system. **2.** A self-regulatory biologic process.

ses'amoid. Resembling a grain of sesame; denoting a small bone that is embedded in a tendon or in a joint capsule; it is found mainly in the hands and feet; the patella (kneecap) is the largest such bone in the body.

ses'sile. Attached by a broad base rather than by a peduncle; applied to certain cysts.

set. 1. To put into a position that will restore function; said of a fractured bone. **2.** Denoting plastic material after it has hardened or jelled.

se'ta. A short bristle-like hair or structure.

seta'ceous. 1. Having bristles or setae. **2.** Resembling a bristle.

set'ting. Hardening, as of plaster of Paris.

set'up. The arrangement of artificial teeth on a trial denture base, preliminary to construction of an appliance.

sex. The classification of organisms as male or female by means of their reproductive characteristics.
  chromosomal s., an individual's sex determined by the presence or absence of the Y chromosome in the spermatozoon at the time of its union with the ovum.
  genetic s., chromosomal sex.
  morphologic s., sex determined by the morphology of the external genitalia.
  s. influence, the occurrence of autosomal traits predominantly in one sex, either male or female.
  s. limitation, the occurrence of autosomal traits in one sex only, either male or female.
  s. linkage, see under linkage.

sexiv'alent. Having the combining power of six hydrogen atoms.

sex-linked. X-linked; determined by a gene which is carried on the X chromosome; said of a trait; often used synonymously with X-linked, but as a Y-linked trait is also sex-linked, the preferred term is X-linked.

sexol'ogy. The study of the sexes and their relationship.

sexop'athy. Sexual perversion.

sex'tan. Denoting a malarial paroxysm recurring every sixth day.

sex'ual. 1. Relating to or endowed with sex. **2.** Causing erotic desires.

sexual'ity. The state of having sexual characteristics, experiences, and behaviors.
  infantile s., in psychoanalysis, the capacity of the infant and child to have experiences of a sexual nature.

Sézary syndrome. Exfoliative dermatitis with intense pruritus, associated with highly distinctive monocytoid cells in the peripheral blood.

s.g. Abbreviation for specific gravity.

SGOT. Abbreviation for serum glutamic oxaloacetic transaminase; see under transaminase.

SGPT. Abbreviation for serum glutamic pyruvic transaminase; see under transaminase.

SH. Abbreviation for serum hepatitis.

shadow-casting. A method of increasing the visibility of ultramicroscopic specimens under the microscope by coating them with a film of carbon, platinum, or chromium.

shakes. 1. Severe chills, especially those of malarial fever. **2.** A popular name for the tremor associated with withdrawal from acute alcoholism.

shank. The leg; the part of the human leg from the knee to the ankle.

shears. Large double-bladed cutting instrument, similar to a pair of scissors.

sheath. An enveloping structure.
  axillary s., a tubular, fibrous membrane encasing the large vessels and nerves of the arm (axillary artery and vein and brachial plexus); located between the clavicle (collarbone) and the first rib.
  carotid s., a tubular sheath enclosing the carotid artery, internal jugular vein, and vagus nerve; extends from the base of the skull to the first rib and sternum (breastbone).
  femoral s., a funnel-shaped sheath located in the groin below the inguinal ligament and divided into three compartments by two vertical partitions; the lateral compartment contains the femoral artery, the middle one contains the femoral vein, and the medial one (femoral canal) contains lymphatic vessels and a lymph node; also called crural sheath.
  Henle's s., see endoneurium.
  medullary s., myelin sheath.

seromembranous | **sheath**

cross section of axon of nerve cell

myelin sheath (jelly-roll configuration)

Schwann cell

nucleus

nipple shield

breast shield

superior vena cava

right atrium

septal defect

right ventricle

left atrium

section of heart

left-to-right shunt

---

myelin s., the multiple-layered covering of many of the axons of both central and peripheral nerves; composed of lipid and protein molecules and serving mainly to increase the velocity of conduction of nerve impulses.

s.'s of optic nerve, the three sheaths (dura, arachnoid, and pia) surrounding the optic nerve; continuous with the membranes of the brain.

s. of Schwann, see neurilemma.

synovial tendon s., a double-layered sheath forming a closed sac; one layer surrounds the tunnel through which the tendon passes, the other covers the surface of the tendon; serves to facilitate the gliding of tendons through fibrous and bony tunnels.

Sheehan's disease, Sheehan's syndrome. Hypopituitarism due to postpartum pituitary necrosis, usually following hemorrhage and shock during delivery; results in failure to lactate, absence of menstrual function, loss of hair, cold intolerance, atrophy of sex organs, and wrinkling of the skin; a specific form of Simmond's disease.

sheet, draw. A folded sheet placed under the buttocks of a bedridden patient, with its long axis across the bed, to facilitate its removal without lifting the patient.

shelf. A structure in the body resembling a shelf.

rectal s., one occurring in the rectum due to infiltration by neoplasm or inflammation; also called Blumer's shelf.

shield. 1. A means of protection, such as a lead rubber apron or sheet used to protect an individual from radiation. **2.** A dense substance that encloses radioisotopes in order to reduce the amount of radiation that escapes into the area. **3.** To protect from radiation or other toxic agents.

breast s., a rubber cap or dome, used to protect inflamed or irritated nipples from contact with clothing.

Buller's s., a watchglass in a frame of adhesive tape secured over the unaffected eye to protect it from the other infected eye.

embryonic s., a swelling of the embryonic blastoderm within which the primitive streak appears.

eye s., a protective covering for the eye.

nipple s., a round glass or plastic plate with a short central projecting tube to which a rubber nipple is attached; used over sore nipples during nursing so that the pressure from the infant's mouth is attenuated by the resistance of the rubber nipple.

shift. A change.

axis s., see deviation, axis.

Doppler s., the magnitude of the frequency change with the velocity of motion in the Doppler effect.

s. to the left, increased percentage of young neutrophils in the blood.

threshold s., a deviation in decibels from an individual's previous audiogram, indicating loss of hearing.

Shigel′la. A genus of nonmotile, gram-negative bacteria (family Enterobacteriaceae) which is the principal cause of human dysentery; divided into four major groups (A, B, C, and D) and subdivided serologically into different types.

S. dysenteriae, group A species, a particularly virulent form that causes dysentery in man; found in the excreta of infected individuals or convalescent carriers.

S. flexneri, group B species, one of the commonest causes of dysentery epidemics and sometimes of infantile gastroenteritis.

S. sonnei, group D species, it causes mild dysentery in man and summer diarrheal disorders in children.

shigello′sis. Acute infection of the bowel caused by *Shigella* organisms often occurring in epidemic patterns; characterized by frequent passage of stools containing blood, pus, and mucus and accompanied by cramps, tenesmus, and fever.

shin. The anterior portion of the leg below the knee.

shin splints. Irritation or inflammation of the extensor muscles of the lower lateral area of the legs caused by an unusually great adduction of the legs and aggravated by overexercise.

shinbone. See tibia.

shingles. See herpes zoster.

shiv′er. To shudder or shake, especially from a chill produced by fever-induced decreased skin temperature.

shock. A severe physiologic reaction to bodily trauma characterized by pale clammy skin, diminished blood pressure, weak rapid pulse, and sometimes unconsciousness.

anaphylactic s., violent reactions, sometimes accompanied by a rash, following injection of a foreign protein to which the individual has been previously sensitized.

cardiogenic s., shock due to the sudden reduction of the cardiac output, as in mycocardial infarction.

deferred s., delayed s., shock occurring a number of hours after the injury.

electric s., the effects of the passage of an electric current through any part of the body.

histamine s., shock produced by the injection of histamine.

hypovolemic s., one produced by reduction of blood volume, as in hemorrhage.

insulin s., shock resulting from a sudden reduction of blood sugar caused by an overdose of insulin.

irreversible s., shock that does not respond to any form of treatment.

neurogenic s., shock due to the action of the nervous system immediately after injury.

primary s., one appearing immediately after a severe injury, mainly due to anxiety, pain, etc.

septic s., shock due to severe infection, particularly with gram-negative bacilli.

spinal s., loss of spinal reflexes after injury to the spinal cord, manifested in the muscles innervated by the nerves situated below the injury.

shoe. An outer covering for the human foot having a durable sole and heel.

Scarpa's s., a metal brace that prevents plantar extension of the foot beyond a right angle; used in treating talipes equinus.

short bowel syndrome. Condition which occurs following removal of an extensive segment of small intestine, characterized by intractable diarrhea with impaired absorption of fats, vitamins, and other nutrients; ultimately leads to malnutrition, anemia, and continued weight loss.

shortsight′edness. See myopia.

sho′shin. The acute fulminating form of cardiovascular beriberi. See also beriberi.

shoul′der. The bodily part between the neck and upper arm where the scapula joins with the clavicle and humerus.

s. girdle, see under girdle.

s. blade, see scapula.

shoulder-hand syndrome. Pain and stiffness of the shoulder and hand, sometimes with late atrophy of hand muscles; usually associated with neck or upper arm injuries or with myocardial infarction; thought to be a reflex sympathetic dystrophy.

show. The discharge from the vagina of blood-stained mucus indicating the onset of labor; it is caused by the expulsion of the mucus plug that has filled the cervical canal during pregnancy.

SHR. Abbreviation for spontaneously hypertensive rat.

shu′mac. See sumac.

shunt. 1. To bypass or divert. **2.** A passage between two natural channels; may be congenital, as a defect between the two atria of the heart, or a surgical anastomosis to divert blood from one part of the body to another or to divert intestinal contents from one portion of the intestinal tract to another.

left-to-right s., diversion of blood from the left to the right side of the heart (through a septal defect) or from the systemic to the pulmonary circulation (through a patent ductus arteriosus).

metabolic s., catabolism of a substance by an

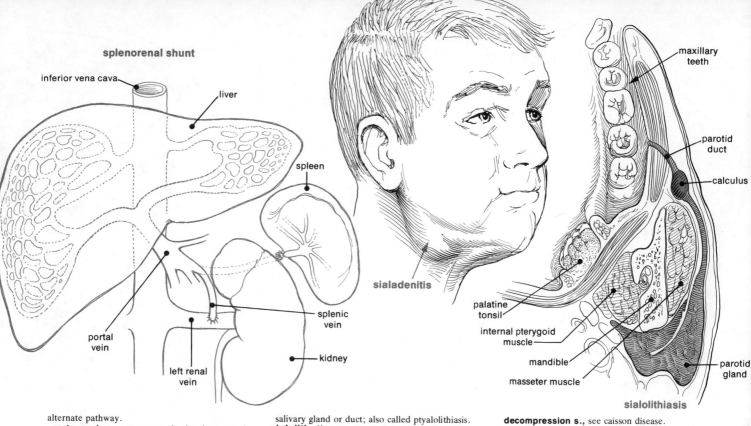

splenorenal shunt

inferior vena cava · liver · spleen · splenic vein · portal vein · left renal vein · kidney

sialadenitis

maxillary teeth · parotid duct · calculus · palatine tonsil · internal pterygoid muscle · mandible · masseter muscle · parotid gland

sialolithiasis

alternate pathway.

  portacaval s., any communication between the portal vein and the systemic veins; surgical anastomosis between the portal and caval veins.

  splenorenal s., surgical anastomosis between the splenic vein and the left renal vein.

Shy-Drager syndrome. A rare condition, resembling parkinsonism, characterized by tremors, muscular wasting, atrophy of the iris, ocular palsies, and ortho- static hypotension.

SI. Abbreviation for International System of Units; from the French equivalent, Système International d'Unités. See under system.

Si. Chemical symbol of the element silicon.

sialadeni'tis. Inflammation of a salivary gland.

sialadenotrop'ic. Influencing the activity of salivary glands.

sialapo'ria. Deficient secretion of saliva.

sialecta'sis. Dilatation of a salivary duct.

sial'ic. Salivary.

sialic acids. A group of naturally occurring derivatives of a 9-carbon, 3-deoxy-5-amino sugar acid; present in bacteria and in animal tissue as constituents of lipids, polysaccharides, and mucoproteins.

si'alism, sialis'mus. Sialorrhea.

sialo-, sial-. Combining forms indicating a relationship to saliva or the salivary glands.

sialoadenec'tomy. Surgical removal of a salivary gland.

sialoadeni'tis. Sialadenitis.

sialoadenot'omy. Incision of a salivary gland.

sialoangiec'tasis. 1. Condition in which a salivary duct is vastly dilated by stagnated saliva, usually resulting from an obstructive stone or ductal constriction. **2.** Dilatation of salivary ducts, usually by means of bougies.

sialoangii'tis. Inflammation of a salivary duct.

sialodochi'tis. Inflammation of the duct of a salivary gland.

sialodochoplas'ty. Repair of a salivary duct.

sialog'enous. Producing saliva.

sial'ogogue. An agent that promotes the secretion of saliva.

sial'ogram. A roentgenogram of one or more salivary ducts, produced by sialography; also called sialograph.

sial'ograph. See sialogram.

sialog'raphy. Roentgenographic examination of the salivary glands and ducts after the injection of radiopaque material into the ducts; an invaluable technique for determining the presence and location of an obstruction in the salivary ducts and the condition of the salivary acini.

sial'olith. Salivary calculus; also called ptyalolith.

sialolithi'asis. The presence of a calculus in the

salivary gland or duct; also called ptyalolithiasis.

sialolithot'omy. Surgical incision of a salivary duct or gland for the removal of a calculus; also called ptyalolithotomy.

sialorrhe'a. An excessive flow of saliva for any reason, including teething, mental retardation, ill-fitting dental appliances, mercurialism, periodontic disease, and acute inflammation of the mouth; also called salivation.

sialos'chesis. Suppression of the secretion of saliva; also called dry mouth.

sialo'sis. Salivation (1).

sialosteno'sis. Stricture or stenosis of a salivary duct.

sialosy'rinx. 1. A salivary fistula. **2.** A syringe for cleansing the salivary ducts. **3.** A salivary duct drainage tube.

sib. Abbreviation for sibling.

sib'ilant. Hissing or whistling; said of a rale.

sib'ilus. A hissing or whistling sound heard on auscultation.

sib'ling. One of two or more children having one, but especially both, parents in common.

sib'ship. Relationship between children of the same parents; occasionally used to denote all blood relatives.

sic'cant. Drying.

sicca syndrome. See Sjögren's syndrome.

siccolab'ile. Destroyed by drying.

siccosta'bile. Not destroyed by drying.

sic'cus. Latin for dry.

sick. 1. Ill. **2.** Nauseated. **3.** Mentally disturbed.

sickle cell C disease. Hemolytic anemia present in patients who are heterozygous for hemoglobin S and C.

sickle form. See crescent, malarial.

sickle'mia. Outmoded term, formerly used to denote any sickle cell disorder.

sickling. The production of sickle-shaped blood cells.

sick'ness. Disease.

  African sleeping s., African trypanosomiasis; disease of the central nervous system caused by protozoans of the genus *Trypanosoma*, transmitted by several species of tsetse flies (genus *Glossina*).

  air s., motion sickness occurring during travel in aircraft flying at low altitude where the atmosphere is most turbulent.

  altitude s., giddiness, headache, difficult rapid breathing on exertion, insomnia, and nausea are symptoms experienced by some unacclimatized individuals within a few hours after exposure to high altitude; also called mountain sickness.

  car s., motion sickness brought about by riding in an automobile or on a train.

  decompression s., see caisson disease.

  morning s., nausea and/or vomiting sometimes occurring during early pregnancy.

  motion s., a group of symptoms such as pallor, sweating, excessive salivation, nausea, and frequently vomiting, occurring in persons riding in airplanes, automobiles, ships, or trains and occasionally in children riding in playground equipment; caused by stimulation of the semicircular canals and/or certain psychic factors.

  mountain s., see altitude sickness.

  radiation s., illness caused by excessive exposure to ionizing radiation; massive exposure usually causes symptoms occurring in four stages: (1) nausea, vomiting, and sometimes diarrhea and weakness; (2) a period of relative well being; (3) fever, loss of appetite, nausea, abdominal distention, bloody diarrhea, and nausea (death usually occurs during this stage); (4) those who survive experience temporary sterility and eventually develop cataracts.

  sea s., seasickness.

  serum s., an immune response following injection of a foreign serum, marked by fever, skin eruptions, edema, and painful joints.

  sleeping s., African sleeping sickness.

sick-sinus syndrome (SSS). A syndrome caused by failure of the sinus node to maintain normal rhythmicity; characterized by chaotic atrial activity with continual changes in P wave contour, bradycardia interspersed with multiple and recurring ectopic beats, and by runs of atrial or nodal tachycardia; also called sick sinus node.

side effect. See under effect.

sidero-. Combining form meaning iron.

sid'eroblast. An immature red blood cell containing granules of iron.

sid'erocyte. A red blood cell having iron-containing granules.

sideroder'ma. Brownish discoloration of the skin of the legs caused by accumulation of hemosiderin deposits.

siderofibro'sis. Abnormal formation of fibrous tissue associated with multiple small deposits of iron.

side'rope'nia. Iron deficiency, especially in the blood and bone marrow.

sid'erophil. A cell or tissue that has an affinity for iron.

si'derophilin. See transferrin.

sidero'sis. 1. Pneumoconiosis due to inhalation of iron dust. **2.** Deposit of iron dust or particles in a tissue.

  s. bulbi, rusty discoloration of the eyeball caused by the prolonged presence of an iron foreign body in

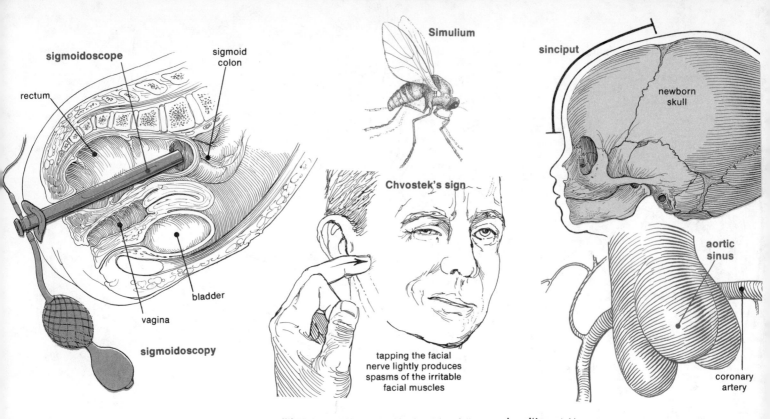

sigmoidoscope · **sigmoid colon**

rectum

sigmoidoscopy

bladder

vagina

Simulium

Chvostek's sign

tapping the facial
nerve lightly produces
spasms of the irritable
facial muscles

sinciput

newborn
skull

**aortic
sinus**

coronary
artery

the eye.

SIDS. Abbreviation for sudden infant death syndrome.

Sig. Abbreviation for Latin *signa*.

sigh. 1. A deep audible inspiration and expiration made involuntarily under the influence of some emotion or an anesthetic. **2.** To emit such a sound.

sight. The ability to see.
 day s., see nyctalopia.
 far s., see hyperopia.
 near s., see myopia.
 night s., see hemeralopia.
 old s., see presbyopia.
 second s., see senopia.

sig′matism. Inability to pronounce sibilant (s, sh) sounds correctly.

sig′moid. Having the shape of the letter S.

sigmoidec′tomy. Surgical removal of part of the sigmoid colon; excision of the sigmoid flexure.

sigmoi′dopexy. Suturing of the sigmoid colon to the abdominal wall for the correction of a prolapsed rectum.

sigmoi′doscope. An instrument for inspecting the interior of the sigmoid colon.

sigmoidos′copy. Inspection of the interior of the sigmoid colon by means of an instrument (sigmoidoscope).

sigmoidot′omy. Surgical incision of the sigmoid colon.

sign. 1. Any objective evidence indicative of disease, perceptible to the examiner, as compared to subjective sensations (symptoms) of the patient. For individual signs, see specific names. **2.** An indication of continued existence.
 vital s.'s, breathing, heart beat, and blood pressure; the signs of life.

sig′na (Sig. or S.). Latin for write, or set a mark upon; used in prescriptions to introduce the signature.

sig′nature. The part of a pharmaceutical prescription containing instruction to the patient for the use of the medication; also called transcription. See also superscription, inscription, and subscription.

signif′icant. In statistics, anything that is probably not the result of chance.

sil′ica. Silicon dioxide, SiO_2; a white or colorless crystalline compound; one of the three major ingredients of dental porcelain.

sil′icate. A salt of silicic acid.

silicic acid. Generally, any acid containing silicon.

silicious. Resembling, relating to, or containing silica.

sil′icon. A nonmetallic element abundantly present in the earth's crust in silica and silicates; symbol Si, atomic number 14, atomic weight 28.09.

sil′icone. Any of a group of semiorganic polymers marked by physiochemical inertness and a high degree of water repellence and lubricity; used in prosthetic replacement of bodily parts, protective coatings, and adhesives.

silico′sis. Fibrosis of the lungs caused by prolonged inhalation of silica dust (stone dust, SiO_2); a pneumoconiosis; also called stone mason's disease and potters' phthisis.

silicotuberculo′sis. Silicosis associated with tuberculosis.

silk. The fine lustrous fiber produced by the silkworm to make its cocoon.
 surgical s., thread made from the cocoon fiber of the mulberry silkworm; used as suture material in surgical operations.

sil′ver. A lustrous white, malleable, ductile metallic element; symbol Ag (from the Latin *argentum*), atomic number 47, atomic weight 107.87.
 s. nitrate, a caustic colorless crystalline compound, $AgNO_3$, which becomes grayish black when exposed to light; used in solution as an antiseptic in the eyes of the newborn.

Simmond's disease. See panhypopituitarism.

simula′tion. 1. Imitation; said of a disease or symptom that resembles or mimics another. **2.** A feigning or pretending; also called malingering.

sim′ulator. A device designed to produced effects simulating or approximating actual conditions.
 patient s., a functional replica of a bodily part.
 space s., a hermetically sealed chamber with human or animal subjects at ground level, used to study some of the physiologic effects of space traveling.

Simu′lium. a genus of biting black gnats (family Simuliidae), some species of which transmit onchocerciasis.

sincip′ital. Relating to the forehead and upper part of the head.

sin′ciput. 1. The upper anterior part of the head from the forehead to the crown. **2.** Bregma; the top of the skull where the sagittal and coronal sutures meet.

sin′e (s, ś). Latin for without; used in prescription writing.

sine (sin). A trigonometric ratio between parts of a triangle; in a right triangle, it is the side opposite an acute angle divided by the side opposite the right angle (hypotenuse); graphed with two coordinates, the values produce a sinusoid or sine curve with the equation $y = \sin x$.

sin′ew. A tendon.

singlet. A single member, as a single microtubule in the middle of a cilium.

singulta′tion. Hiccupping.

singul′tus. A hiccup.

sinis′ter(s). Latin for left.

sinis′tral. 1. Of or relating to the left side. **2.** Left-handed.

sinistral′ity. Left-handedness.

sinistrocar′dia. Displacement of the heart toward the left, beyond its normal position.

sinistrocer′ebral. Relating to the left hemisphere of the brain.

sinistroc′ular. 1. Having better vision in the left eye. **2.** Relating to dominance of the left eye.

sinistrop′edal. Using the left foot in preference to the right.

sinistrotor′sion. A turning or rotating to the left, especially of the eye.

sinoa′trial, sinoauric′ular. Relating to the sinus venosus and the right atrium of the heart; especially the sinus (S-A) node.

si′nus. 1. A mucus-lined, air-filled cavity in one of the cranial bones which communicates with the nasal cavity. **2.** A dilated channel for the passage of blood or lymph, which lacks the coats of an ordinary vessel; applied especially to those of the dura; e.g., cavernous sinus. **3.** An abnormal fistula or tract.
 aortic s., any of the three slight dilatations of the aorta between each semilunar valve and the wall of the aorta; also called sinus of Valsalva.
 carotid s., a slight dilatation of the most proximal part of the internal carotid artery containing in its wall pressoreceptors which, when stimulated by changes in blood pressure, cause slowing of the heart, vasodilation, and a fall in blood pressure; also called carotid bulb.
 cavernous s., a paired, irregularly shaped venous sinus in the dura mater on each side of the body of the sphenoid bone in the middle cranial fossa; it drains the superior ophthalmic vein, superficial middle cerebral vein, and sphenoparietal sinus; it empties by way of the petrosal sinuses into the transverse sinus and internal jugular vein.
 cerebral s.'s., see dura mater sinuses.
 circular s., (1) a venous ring around the hypophysis (pituitary gland) formed by the anterior and posterior intercavernous sinuses communicating with the cavernous sinus; also called Ridley's sinus; (2) the venous sinus at the periphery of the placenta; (3) the scleral venous sinus of the eye.
 coronary s., the short venous sinus receiving most of the veins of the heart, situated in the posterior part of the coronary sulcus between the left atrium and the ventricle; it opens into the right atrium between the inferior vena cava and the atrioventricular orifice.
 dermal s., a congenital sinus tract lined with skin and usually extending from the skin to the spinal

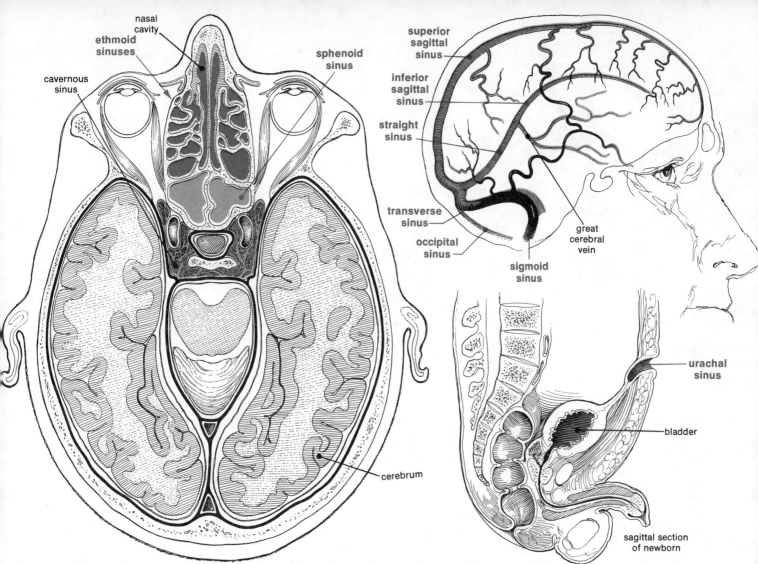

nasal cavity

ethmoid sinuses

cavernous sinus

sphenoid sinus

superior sagittal sinus

inferior sagittal sinus

straight sinus

transverse sinus

occipital sinus

great cerebral vein

sigmoid sinus

cerebrum

urachal sinus

bladder

sagittal section of newborn

---

canal.

dura mater s.'s, the venous sinuses in the dura mater; e.g., cavernous, superior sagittal, and transverse; also called cerebral sinuses.

epididymal s., a narrow slitlike recess between the upper part of the testis and the overlying epididymis; formed by the invagination of the tunica vaginalis.

ethmoid s., any of the air cells of the ethmoid bone.

frontal s., one of the paired sinuses in the lower part of the frontal bone; it communicates by way of the nasofrontal duct (infundibulum) with the nasal cavity of the same side.

jugular s.'s, two slight dilatations of the internal jugular vein; a superior one located at its origin near the base of the skull and an inferior one near its termination, just before it unites with the subclavian vein.

lactiferous duct s., the spindle-shaped dilated portion of the lactiferous duct of the mammary gland, just before it enters the nipple.

lymphatic s., irregular, tortuous channels of a lymph node through which a continuous flow of lymph passes on its way to the efferent lymphatic vessels.

marginal s. of placenta, a discontinous, circumferential venous sinus at the margin of the placenta.

maxillary s., a mucus-lined air cavity in the body of the maxilla on either side, communicating with the middle meatus of the nasal cavity.

occipital s., the smallest of the sinuses of the dura mater, usually unpaired, that drains the area of the foramen magnum, ascends along the attached margin of the falx cerebelli, and terminates in the confluence of the sinuses near the internal occipital protuberance.

omphalomesenteric duct s., a sinus caused by persistent patency of the distal part of the embryonic omphalomesenteric (vitelline) duct.

paranasal s., any of the mucus-lined air sinuses (frontal, ethmoid, sphenoid, maxillary) in the bones of the face which open into the nasal cavity.

petrosal s., inferior, a paired venous sinus passing along in the groove of the petro-occipital fissure connecting the cavernous sinus with the beginning of the internal jugular vein.

petrosal s., superior, a paired venous sinus passing along the attached margin of the tentorium cerebelli connecting the cavernous sinus with the transverse sinus.

pilonidal s., a congenital sinus in the sacral region, leading to the exterior; often containing a tuft of hair and prone to suppuration.

piriform s., piriform recess; see under recess.

prostatic s., the sinus or recess on either side of the urethral crest in the prostatic part of the urethra.

rhomboidal s., a dilatation of the central canal of the spinal cord in the lumbar region; also called rhombocele.

Rokitansky-Aschoff s., one of a number of small evaginations of the gallbladder extending through the lamina propria and muscular layer; may be seen in chronic cholecystitis.

sagittal s., superior, an unpaired venous sinus in the sagittal groove of the cranium, beginning near the crista galli and extending backward to empty into the confluence of the sinuses near the internal occipital protuberance; it is invaginated by arachnoid granulations.

sagittal s., inferior, an unpaired venous sinus in the lower margin of the cerebral falx, running parallel to the superior sagittal sinus and emptying into the upper end of the straight sinus.

scleral venous s., the ringlike sinus in the corneoscleral junction of the eye; it serves as a flow drainage for the excess aqueous humor of the anterior chamber of the eye; also called venous sinus of the sclera and Schlemm's canal.

sigmoid s., the S-shaped continuation of the

transverse sinus on either side, situated along the posterior surface of the petrous portion of the temporal bone to the jugular foramen where it joins the jugular vein.

s. rectus, straight sinus.

s. of Valsalva, see aortic sinus.

s. venosus, the common venous chamber of the embryonic heart into which the cardinal, vitelline, and umbilical veins drain.

sphenoid s., one of the paired, asymmetrical, mucus-lined sinuses situated in the body of the sphenoid bone; it opens into the nasal cavity, of which it forms part of the roof.

sphenoparietal s., a small dural venous sinus along the lesser wing of the sphenoid bone; it empties into the cavernous sinus.

splenic s.'s, dilated venous sinusoids, lined with reticuloendothelial cells, that connect splenic capillaries with collecting venules and serve to convey blood through the spleen.

straight s., a triangular venous sinus formed by the union of the great cerebral vein and the inferior sagittal sinus; it receives the cerebellar veins before draining into the transverse sinus.

tonsillar s., tonsillar fossa; see under fossa.

transverse s., either of two (right and left) large venous sinuses of the dura mater lying along the attached margin of the tentorium cerebelli; the right one is frequently the direct continuation of the superior sagittal sinus, the left, of the straight sinus; at their origin in the confluence, they communicate with each other; they drain via the sigmoid sinuses to the internal jugular veins.

urachal s., congenital abnormality which occurs when the lumen of either end of the embryonic allantois (which extends from the navel to the bladder) fails to close.

urogenital s., in embryology, an elongated sac formed by the division of the cloaca below the entrance of the genital ducts; it develops into the

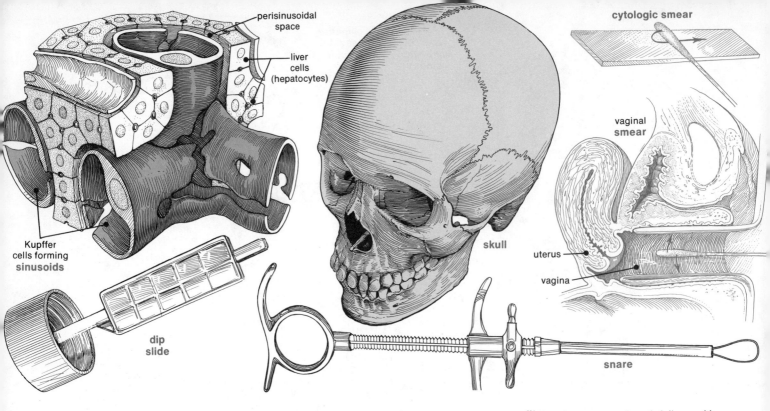

perisinusoidal space

liver cells (hepatocytes)

Kupffer cells forming sinusoids

dip slide

skull

cytologic smear

vaginal smear

uterus

vagina

snare

lower part of the bladder in both sexes, the vestibule in the female, and most of the urethra in the male.
venous s. of sclera, see scleral venous sinus.
sinusi′tis. Inflammation of the mucous membrane of a sinus, especially of a paranasal sinus.
   frontal s., infection in the frontal sinuses.
si′nusoid. 1. Like a sinus. **2.** An irregular blood channel formed by anastomosing blood vessels; present in certain organs, such as the liver and spleen.
si o′pus sit. (S.O.S.). Latin for if there is need.
si′phon. 1. A U-shaped tube, used to transfer liquids or in draining wounds. **2.** The act of transferring a fluid by means of a siphon.
   carotid s., the U-shaped bend of the intracranial portion of the internal carotid artery alongside the sella turcica.
Sipple syndrome. A familial syndrome consisting of pheochromocytoma and medullary thyroid carcinoma with occasional parathyroid carcinoma.
site. A location.
   active s., the area of an enzyme molecule that binds the substrate (substance that undergoes chemical change) and activates the reaction.
   allosteric s., the part of an enzyme molecule that binds an effector (substance that does not undergo chemical change but either inhibits or accelerates the enzymatic reaction); also called regulatory site.
sitos′terol. Any of several widely occurring plant sterols, or a mixture of such sterols.
si′tus. Position or location; especially normal location.
   s. inversus, congenital anomaly in which internal organs are located on the side of the body opposite to their normal location.
Sjögren′s syndrome. Disorder of unknown cause marked chiefly by atrophic changes of the lacrimal and salivary glands, leading to scanty lacrimal and salivary secretions with dryness of the eyes and mouth (keratoconjunctivitis sicca and xerostomia), and rheumatoid arthritis; rheumatoid factor is usually present and other abnormal antibodies are common in the patient's serum; also called sicca syndrome.
ska′tole. A crystalline compound formed in the intestine as a result of protein decomposition.
skein. A length of coiled thread; said mainly of the coiled chromatin seen in the prophase stage of mitosis.
skel′etal. Relating to the skeleton.
skeletog′enous. Giving rise to bone formation.
skel′eton. The internal framework of vertebrates, composed of bones and cartilages and supporting the soft tissues.
skenei′tis, skeni′tis. Inflammation of Skene's

glands of the female urethra.
skeocyto′sis. See neocytosis.
skin. The membranous covering of the body; the human skin is an integument composed of a thin outer layer (epidermis) and a thicker, deeper, connective tissue layer (dermis).
skin pop′ping. Slang expression denoting the injection of a narcotic drug intradermally; often results in ulcerations.
skull. The framework of the head composed of the bones encasing the brain and the bones of the face; also called cranium.
SLE. Abbreviation for systemic lupus erythematosus.
sleep. A natural, periodically recurring state of rest in which consciousness is temporarily interrupted.
   paroxysmal s., see narcolepsy.
   rapid eye movement s., REM s., phenomenon occurring at regular intervals during the dreaming phase of sleep, in which both eyes move rapidly and in unison under the closed eyelids; thought to represent the activated state of sleep, in which activity levels of many functions approach those occurring during wakefulness.
   REM s., see rapid eye movement sleep.
   twilight s., state in which, although pain is felt, the memory of it is abolished, induced by injection of a mixture of morphine and scopolamine.
sleep′lessness. Insomnia.
sleep′talking. Somniloquism; talking while asleep or while in a condition resembling sleep.
sleep′walking. Somnambulism; walking while asleep.
slide. A glass plate for mounting specimens to be examined under the microscope.
   dip s., a special plastic slide capable of holding an even thickness of culture medium on a molded grid; used to quantify the bacterial population of urine.
sling. A band suspended from the neck, serving as a supporting bandage for an injured arm or hand.
slit. A long, narrow opening, entrance, or cleft.
   vulvar s., the cleft between the labia majora.
slit′lamp. An instrument that projects obliquely a thin beam of intense light for illuminating any reasonably transparent structure, such as the cornea, by sections; usually used in examination of the eye through a magnifying apparatus.
slough′. A mass of dead tissue which has separated from, or is partially attached to, a living structure.
sludge. A muddy sediment.
sluggish sinus node syndrome. A syndrome of reduced sinoatrial (S-A) nodal automaticity; it often precedes the development of the sick-sinus syndrome.
Sm. Chemical symbol of the element samarium.

small′pox. A severe contagious viral disease with an incubation period of 12 days; at the onset symptoms are headache, fever, abdominal and muscular pain, and vomiting; after three or four days, symptoms lessen and the eruptive stage occurs, with papules developing into vesicles and pustules throughout the body, especially on the face, hands, and feet; the trunk and legs are last affected; the lesions in any area are all in the same stage of development; after about three weeks, scabs form and upon falling leave permanent markings on the skin (pock marks); also called variola.
smear. A substance or preparation spread thinly on a slide for microscopic examination.
   buccal s., a smear obtained by scraping the inside of the cheek.
   cervical s., one obtained from the uterine cervix.
   cytologic s., cytosmear: one made by spreading the specimen onto a glass slide, then fixing it and staining it.
smeg′ma. The material that collects under the foreskin of the penis, consisting of sebaceous secretions of preputial glands mixed with desquamated epithelial cells.
smell. 1. To perceive the scent of a substance by means of the olfactory apparatus. **2.** To emit an odor.
smog. A fog made heavier and darker by industrial gases, motor vehicle exhaust fumes, or smoke.
Sn. Chemical symbol of the element tin; from Latin *stannum*.
snap. A sharp sound.
   closing s., the accentuated first sound of the heart occurring during closure of the abnormal mitral valve in mitral stenosis.
   opening s., a highpitched click heard during diastole; caused by opening of the abnormal mitral valve in mitral stenosis.
snare. A surgical instrument with a wire loop which is tightened about the pedicle of a tumor, polyp, etc., in order to sever it; also used to remove an intrauterine device.
sneeze. The forceful, involuntary expulsion of air through the nose and mouth.
snore. 1. To breathe through the mouth and nose with a rattling noise produced by vibration of the soft palate. **2.** The noise produced while snoring.
snort′ing. Slang expression denoting the inhalation of a narcotic drug, especially heroin or cocaine.
snuff. 1. To inhale forcibly through the nose; to sniff. **2.** Finely pulverized tobacco which is inhaled through the nostrils or applied to the gums. **3.** Any medicated powdery substance which is inhaled through the nose.
snuf′fles. Noisy breathing due to obstructed nasal

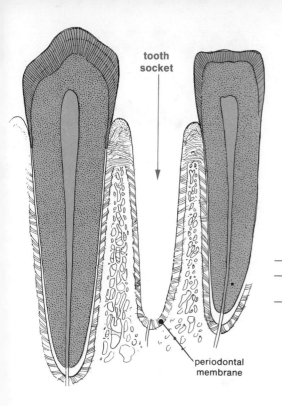

tooth socket

periodontal membrane

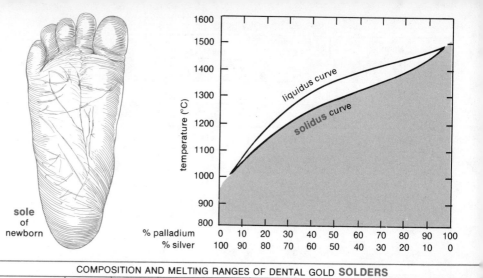

sole of newborn

% palladium / % silver

Solder no.	Gold %	Silver %	Copper %	Zinc %	Tin %	Melting range °F	°C
A	65.4	15.4	12.4	3.9	3.1	1375–1445	745–785
B	66.1	12.4	16.4	3.4	2.0	1385–1480	750–805
C	65.0	16.3	13.1	3.9	1.7	1410–1470	765–800
D	72.9	12.1	10.0	3.0	2.0	1390–1535	755–835
E	80.9	8.1	6.8	2.1	2.0	1375–1595	745–870

COMPOSITION AND MELTING RANGES OF DENTAL GOLD SOLDERS

passages; when occurring in the newborn, it is usually caused by congenital syphilis.

soap. A cleansing agent; a salt formed by fatty acids with potassium or sodium.

insoluble s., a salt formed by fatty acids and metals other than sodium or potassium; insoluble in water and without detergent properties.

soap'stone. A relatively soft stone having a soapy feel and composed mainly of talc and chlorite.

social psychiatry. The application of psychiatric principles to the solutions of social problems and issues.

socioacu'sis. Denoting a hearing loss caused by a noisy environment.

sociomed'ical. Pertaining to the interrelations of the practice of medicine and social welfare.

so'ciopath. An individual with a behavior disorder marked by disregard for societal rules, immaturity, difficulty in postponing gratification, poor impulse control, and little ability to consider the consequences of his actions.

sock'et. A cavity into which another part fits, as the socket of the eye or of a joint.

dry s., a condition sometimes occurring after extraction of a tooth in which the blood clot in the socket disintegrates, leading to exposure of the bone and secondary infection.

eye s., see orbit.

tooth s., the cavity in the jaw in which a tooth is embedded; also called alveolus.

so'da. General term commonly used to designate sodium bicarbonate, sodium carbonate, and sodium hydroxide.

so'dium. A soft, silvery-white metallic element; symbol Na, atomic number 11, atomic weight 22.99.

s. benzoate, a white, crystalline, odorless powder, C_6H_5COONa; used as a food preservative and in the manufacture of pharmaceuticals; also called benzoate of soda.

s. bicarbonate, a white crystalline compound with a slight alkaline taste, $NaHCO_3$; used medicinally as a gastric antacid; also called baking soda and bicarbonate of soda.

s. biphosphate, a colorless, water-soluble, crystalline powder, $NaH_2PO_4 \cdot H_2O$; used to increase acidity of the urine.

s. bisulfite, white, water-soluble crystals, $NaHSO_3$; used as a preservative, a disinfectant, and an antioxidant in certain injections.

s. borate, a colorless crystalline compound, $Na_2B_4O_7 \cdot 10 H_2O$; used in dentistry as a retardant and in the manufacture of pharmaceuticals and detergents; also called borax.

s. carbonate, (1) a white powdery compound, Na_2CO_3; used as a reagent and in water treatment; (2) any of several hydrated forms, such as $Na_2CO_3 \cdot 10H_2O$ (washing or sal soda).

s. chloride, a crystalline compound, NaCl; used medicinally in solution; also called table or common salt.

s. citrate, a white, water-soluble, granular powder, $Na_3C_6H_5O_7 \cdot 2 H_2O$; used as a blood anticoagulant.

s. cyclamate, a water-soluble powder, used as an artificial sweetener.

s. diatrizoate, a radiopaque, water-soluble powder; an organic compound of iodine, $C_{11}I_8O_4 \cdot N_2I_3Na \cdot 4 H_2O$; used in excretory radiography of the urinary tract.

s. glutamate, a white crystalline compound with a meatlike taste; used in cooking; also called monosodium glutamate.

s. group, the alkali metals, lithium, sodium, potassium, rubidium, and cesium.

s. hydroxide, alkaline, water-soluble compound, NaOH; used in the chemical and pharmaceutical industries; also called caustic soda and lye.

s. iodide, white crystalline powder, NaI; used as a source of iodine.

s. levothyroxine, the sodium salt of the natural isomer of thyroxin; used in the treatment of thyroid deficiency conditions.

s. liothyronine, the sodium salt of L-triiodothyronine; used in the treatment of thyroid deficiency.

s. nitrate, white crystalline compound, $NaNO_3$; formerly used to treat dysentery; also called Chile saltpeter and soda niter.

s. pentothal, see thiopental sodium.

s. perborate, a white odorless compound, $NaBO_2H_2O_2 \cdot 3H_2O$; used as an antiseptic.

s. peroxide, a white or yellowish powder, Na_2O_2; used in the manufacture of pharmaceuticals.

s. phosphate, a crystalline, water-soluble sodium salt of phosphoric acid, $Na_2HPO_4 \cdot H_2O$; used as a laxative.

s. salicylate, white scales, soluble in water; formerly used in the treatment of rheumatic fever.

s. thiosulfate, a crystalline compound, $Na_2S_2O_3 \cdot 5H_2O$; used as an antidote in cyanide poisoning, to prevent ringworm infection, and as a photographic fixing agent; also called hypo and hyposulfite.

sodo'ku. Rat-bite fever; see under fever.

sod'omy. Sexual practice in which the penis is introduced into the anus or mouth of another person.

sof'tening. The process of becoming soft; also called malacia.

gray s., a stage in softening of the brain in which absorption of fat occurs, following yellow softening.

hemorrhagic s., red softening.

red s., softening of the brain with bleeding into the necrotic tissue.

white s., softening of the brain caused by obstruction of blood supply.

yellow s., late stage in softening of the brain in which fatty degeneration takes place.

sol. 1. A colloidal dispersion of a solid in a liquid. **2.** Abbreviation for solution.

Solana'ceae. A family of herbs, shrubs, and trees, including several poisonous species and some that are used medicinally.

solana'ceous. Relating to the family Solanaceae.

sola'tion. In chemistry, the conversion of a gel into a sol, as the melting of gelatin.

sold'er. A fusible alloy of metals used to join metallic parts when applied in the melted state to the solid metal.

sold'ering. The joining of metals by the fusion of intermediate alloys which are of a lower melting point than that of the components to be connected.

sole. The plantar surface (undersurface) of the foot.

sol'id. 1. Of definite shape; not liquid or gaseous. **2.** Compact; firm; without gaps.

sol'idus. The temperature line on a constitution diagram below which the indicated metal element or alloy is in a solid state.

solubil'ity. 1. The property of being soluble. **2.** The degree to which a substance possesses the property of being soluble.

sol'uble. Capable of being dissolved.

solut'e. The substance dissolved in a solution.

solu'tion (sol). **1.** A homogeneous substance formed by the mixture of a gaseous, liquid, or solid substance (solute) with a liquid or a noncrystalline solid (solvent), and from which the dissolved substance can be recovered. **2.** The process of making such a mixture.

alcoholic s., one in which alcohol is used as the solvent.

Benedict's s., a water solution of sodium citrate, sodium carbonate, and copper sulfate; used to detect the presence of reducing substances in the urine.

Burrow's s., a solution of aluminum acetate.

Dakin's s., mixture of hypochlorite and perborate of sodium with hypochlorous and boric acids; an antiseptic; also called Dakin's modified solution.

Fehling's s., a mixture of two aqueous solutions (1) copper sulfate and (2) potassium sodium tartrate (Rochelle salt) with sodium hydroxide (caustic soda); used for detection of reducing sugars.

gram-molecular s., molar solutions.

hyperbaric s., a solution possessing a higher

SELECTED SOLVENTS

Name	Molecular weight	Melting point °C	Boiling point °C
water	18.02	0.0	100.0
methanol	32.04	−97.7	64.7
acetaldehyde	44.05	−123.0	20.4
ethanol	46.07	−114.1	78.3
acetone	58.05	−94.7	56.3
acetic acid	60.05	16.7	117.9
cyclopentane	70.13	−93.8	49.3
benzene	78.12	5.5	80.1
hexane	86.17	−95.3	68.7
pyruvic acid	88.06	13.6	165.0
toluene	92.14	−94.9	110.6
phenol	94.12	40.9	181.8
caprylic acid	144.22	16.5	239.9
engenol	164.20	9.2	255.0
oleic acid	282.47	13.4	360.0

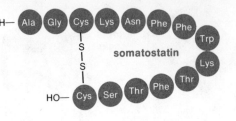

somatostatin

MOLECULAR WEIGHT OF SOME PROTEINS

ribonuclease	14,000
somatotropin (growth hormone)	21,500
carboxypeptidase	34,000
pepsin	35,500
serum albumin	66,500
catalase	250,000
fibrinogen	330,000
urease	480,000
thyroglobulin	660,000

specific gravity than a standard of reference; e.g., in spinal anesthesia, one having a specific gravity higher than that of the cerebrospinal fluid (CSF), thereby producing anesthesia below the level of injection due to its downward migration.

hypertonic s., a solution possessing a higher osmotic pressure than a standard of reference; e.g., a solution of sodium chloride having a higher osmotic pressure than that of blood; often denoting a solution which, when surrounding a cell, causes a flow of water to leave the cell through the semipermeable cell membrane.

hypobaric s., a solution possessing a lower specific gravity than a standard of reference; e.g., in spinal anesthesia, one having a specific gravity lower than that of the cerebrospinal fluid (CSF), thereby producing anesthesia above the level of injection due to its upward migration.

hypotonic salt s., a solution possessing a lower specific gravity than a standard of reference; e.g., a solution of sodium chloride having a lower osmotic pressure than that of blood; often denoting a solution which, when surrounding a cell, causes a flow of water to enter the cell through the semipermeable cell membrane.

iodine s., a solution containing approximately two per cent iodine and two and one half per cent sodium iodide in water; generally applied to superficial lacerations to prevent bacterial infections.

iodine s., strong, one containing iodine 5 g, potassium iodide 10 g, and enough distilled water to make 100 ml; used as a source of iodine; also called Lugol's solution.

isotonic sodium chloride s., solution of sodium chloride with the same osmotic pressure as plasma; 0.9 per cent sodium chloride; also called physiologic salt solution.

lactated Ringer's s., one containing sodium chloride 600 mg, sodium lactate 310 mg, calcium chloride 20 mg, and potassium chloride 30 mg in 100 ml of boiled distilled water; the ionic concentration of the solution is 130 mEq sodium, 4 mEq potassium, 4 mEq calcium, 111 mEq chloride, and 27 mEq lactate.

Locke-Ringer s., one containing sodium chloride 9 g, calcium chloride 0.24 g, potassium chloride 0.42 g, and magnesium chloride 0.2 g, with sodium bicarbonate 0.5 g, glucose 0.5 g, and water to make one liter; used for physiologic and pharmacologic experiments.

Locke's s., one consisting of sodium chloride 0.9 g, calcium chloride 0.024 g, potassium chloride 0.042 g, with sodium bicarbonate 0.01 to 0.03 g, glucose 0.1 g, and distilled water to make 100 ml; used for irrigation of tissues during laboratory experiments.

Lugol's s., see iodine solution, strong.

molal s., one in which one-gram molecular weight of the solute is dissolved in enough solvent to make one liter.

molar s., one in which one-gram molecular weight of the solute is dissolved in one liter of the solvent.

normal s., one that contains one gram equivalent weight of the dissolved substance in each liter of solution.

ophthalmic s., a sterile solution for application into the eye, containing a preservative and having an osmotic pressure and pH similar to that of normal tears.

ophthalmic irrigating s., see eyewash.

phsyiologic salt s., isotonic sodium chloride solution.

pickling s., an acid solution used to remove oxide and other impurities from dental casts; commonly made from one part of concentrated hydrochloric acid and one part water.

Ringer's s., one containing sodium chloride 8.6 g, potassium chloride 0.3 g, and calcium chloride 0.33 g in one liter of boiled distilled water; the ionic concentration of the solution is 147 mEq sodium, 4 mEq potassium, 5 mEq calcium and 156 mEq chloride; used locally for burns and wounds; also called Ringer's mixture.

saline s., a solution of any salt, especially of sodium chloride; commonly known as saline.

saturated s., one containing the maximum amount of solute that a given amount of solvent can dissolve.

sclerosing s., one that causes formations of fibrous tissue; used in oral surgery to arrest bleeding, cauterize ulcers, etc.

Shohl's s., one containing citric acid 140 g, sodium citrate 90 g, and enough water to make one liter.

standard s., one of known concentration, used as a basis of comparison.

supersaturated s., one containing a greater amount of the solute than a given amount of solvent would dissolve at ordinary temperatures.

test s., standard solution of specific substances, used in analysis.

Tyrode's s., one containing sodium chloride 8 g, potassium chloride 0.2 g, calcium chloride 0.2 g, and magnesium chloride 0.1 g, with sodium biphosphate 0.05 g, sodium bicarbonate 1 g, glucose 1 g, and water to make one liter; used in irrigation of the peritoneal cavity and in laboratory work.

volumetric s. (vs), a standard solution containing a specific quantity of a substance (usually 1, ¹/₂, or ¹/₁₀ mole) dissolved in one liter of water.

Ziehl's s., a staining solution for microorganisms such as the tubercle bacillus; containing basic fuchsin, ethyl alcohol, phenol, and distilled water; also called carbolfuchsin.

solv. Abbreviation for Latin *solve.*

sol'vate. A compound formed by the loose combination of a solvent (the dissolving substance) and a solute (the substance dissolved).

sol've (solv). Latin for dissolve.

sol'vent. Capable of dissolving another substance; also called dissolvent.

so'ma. 1. An organism as a whole, exclusive of its germ cells. **2.** The body, distinguished from the mind.

somatesthe'sia. Bodily awareness; also called somesthesia.

somat'ic. 1. Of or pertaining to the body. **2.** Parietal; relating to the wall of the body cavity.

somato-, somat-, somatico-. Combining forms indicating body; e.g., somatology.

somatogen'ic. Of bodily origin; originating in the body cells.

somatol'ogy. The study of the human body in relation to form and function.

somatomammatropin. See lactogen, human placental.

so'matome. Somite.

somatom'etry. Measurement of the body.

somatop'athy. Disease of the body.

somat'oplasm. The totality of protoplasm of all cells (except germ cells) that make up the body.

somatopsy'chic. Relating to the relationship of the body and mind; denoting the effects of the body on the mind.

somatopsycho'sis. An emotional disorder associated with visceral disease.

somatosex'ual. Relating to both physical and sexual characteristics; usually refers to physical manifestations of sexual development.

somatosta'tin. A peptide found in the central nervous system, stomach, small intestine, and islets of Langerhans; it inhibits the release of growth hormone, insulin, and glucagon; it may act as a neurotransmitter in the central nervous system; also called somatotropin release-inhibiting factor.

somatother'apy. Treatment directed toward physical ailments, as opposed to psychiatric treatments.

somatoto'nia. Personality type marked by dominance of vigorous muscular activity and assertiveness.

somatotrop'ic, somatotro'phic. Having a stimulating effect on body growth or an influence on the body.

somatotro'pin. Growth hormone; a hormone se-

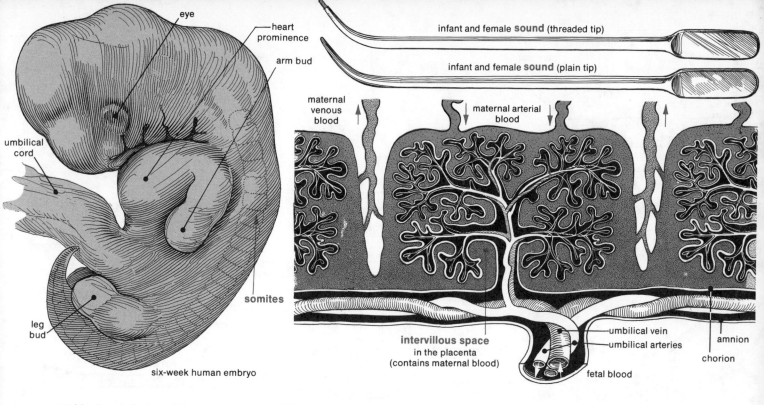

eye

heart prominence

arm bud

infant and female **sound** (threaded tip)

infant and female **sound** (plain tip)

maternal venous blood

maternal arterial blood

umbilical cord

somites

leg bud

six-week human embryo

intervillous space
in the placenta
(contains maternal blood)

umbilical vein

umbilical arteries

amnion

chorion

fetal blood

creted by the anterior lobe of the pituitary gland which affects the rate of skeletal growth and gain in body weight.

somat'otype. A classification of individuals based on physical characteristics of the body; also called biotype, physique and body build.

somesthe'sia. See somatesthesia.

so'mite. One of paired, segmented blocks of epithelioid cells on either side of the neural tube of the embryo, which in later stages of development give rise to connective tissue, bone, muscle, and the dermis and subcutaneous tissue of the skin; the size of the embryo may be expressed in the number of somites; usually 42 to 44 develop in man.

somnam'bulism. Walking while asleep without any recollection upon awakening; applied also to some states of hypnosis; also called sleepwalking and noctambulism.

somnam'bulist. One who walks in his sleep.

somnil'oquism, somnil'oquence. Talking while asleep or in a condition resembling sleep; also called sleeptalking.

somnil'oquist. A person who talks in his sleep.

som'nolence, som'nolency. Drowsiness; sleepiness.

som'nolent. 1. Drowsy. **2.** Soporific; producing sleep.

som'nus. Latin for sleep.

sone. A subjective unit of loudness; the intensity of sound of a pure tone of 1000 cycles per second at 40 decibels above an individual's threshold of audibility.

son'ic. 1. Of or pertaining to audible sound. **2.** Relating to the speed of sound in air (approximately 740 miles per hour at sea level).

sonography. A diagnostic aid in which high-frequency sound waves are used to detect the presence of pregnancy and pelvic tumors, to locate the placenta, and to measure the fetal biparietal diameter.

so'por. Stupor; unusually profound sleep.

soporif'ic. Producing sleep; also called somnolent.

so'porose, so'porous. Comatose.

sorbefa'cient. Facilitating absorption.

sor'bitan. A general term for esters of sorbitol.

sorbitan polyoxyalkalene. A compound from which the nonionic emulsifying compounds with the trademark Tween are derived.

sor'bitol. A sweet crystalline substance occurring in mountain ash fruits and made synthetically by reduction of glucose; used in the preparation of ascorbic acid and as a laxative, working by an osmotic effect; also called D-glucitol.

sor'des. Foul brown or blackish crust formed about the lips and teeth of patients with some forms of prolonged low grade fever.

sore. Any open skin lesion.

bed s., decubitus ulcer; see under ulcer.

canker s., aphthous stomatitis; see under stomatitis.

cold s., a lesion occurring singly or in clusters, usually on the lips, caused by the virus herpes simplex; it often accompanies a fever, common cold, or exposure to the sun; also called fever blister. See also herpes simplex.

hard s., see chancre.

oriental s., cutaneous leishmaniasis; see under leishmaniasis.

pressure s., decubitus ulcer; see under ulcer.

soft s., see chancroid.

S.O.S. Abbreviation for Latin *si opus sit.*

souf'fle. A soft blowing sound heard on auscultation.

fetal s., a blowing, whistling sound synchronous with the fetal heart beat, heard during late pregnancy; caused by blood rushing through the umbilical arteries when the umbilical cord is subject to torsion, tension, or pressure; also called funic or umbilical souffle.

mammary s., a blowing murmur heard at the medial border of the breast during late pregnancy and lactation; attributed to a change of dynamics in blood flow through the internal thoracic (mammary) artery.

placental s., uterine souffle.

splenic s., a soft blowing sound heard over the spleen in malaria.

umbilical s., fetal souffle.

uterine s., a soft, blowing sound synchronous with the maternal heart beat, heard during late pregnancy; caused by blood flowing through engorged uterine vessels; also may be heard in nonpregnant women with large myomatous tumors of the uterus or enlarged ovaries.

sound. 1. Noise. **2.** A cylindrical, usually curved metal instrument used for exploring bodily cavities or for dilating a canal such as the urethra. **3.** Healthy.

heart s.'s, normal sounds heard on auscultation over the area of the heart: first heart sound is caused by closure of the atrioventricular valves (mitral and tricuspid); second heart sound results from closure of the semilunar valves (aortic and pulmonary); third sound is audible sometimes during rapid filling of the ventricles; fourth sound coincides with atrial contraction and is normally inaudible, but frequently recorded by phonocardiography; also called cardiac sounds.

friction s., friction rub; a grating sound heard on auscultation, produced by the rubbing of two inflamed surfaces.

soy'a. The seed of the soybean plant.

soy'bean. 1. A leguminous, climbing Asiatic plant, *Glycine soya* or *Glycine hispida.* **2.** The seed of this plant, rich in protein and low in starch content; given to individuals who are allergic to cow's milk.

space. Any bodily area or volume between specified boundaries; a delimited three-dimensional area.

antecubital s., cubital fossa; see under fossa.

arachnoid s., subarachnoid space.

Bowman's s., the space or sac between the parietal and visceral epithelial of the renal corpuscle; it receives the filtrate of the blood from the glomerular vessels; also called glomerular or urinary space.

corneal s.'s, the interlamellar spaces of the cornea; very small spaces between the lamellae of the corneal stroma; they contain tissue fluid.

dead s., (1) a space or cavity left after improper closure of a surgical or other wound; (2) the portion of the respiratory tract from the nostrils to the terminal bronchioles where no gaseous interchange can take place; also called anatomic dead space.

epidural s., the space between the spinal dura mater and the periosteum of the vertebrae; it contains loose areolar tissue and a plexus of veins.

epitympanic s., the upper portion of the middle ear cavity above the tympanic membrane; it contains the head of the malleus and the body of the incus.

free-way s., interocclusal distance; see under distance.

glomerular s., see Bowman's space.

intercostal s., the space or interval between two adjacent ribs; the breadth is greater between the upper ribs and ventrally.

interpleural s., the space in the middle of the chest between the two pleurae.

interproximal s., the space between adjacent teeth in a dental arch.

interradicular s., the space between the roots of a multirooted tooth, occupied by bony septum and the periodontal membrane.

intervillous s., the space in the placenta in which maternal blood bathes chorionic villi, thus allowing exchange of materials between the fetal and maternal circulation; it is bounded by the chorion on the fetal side and the decidua basalis on the maternal side.

medullary s., the central cavity and the cellular intervals between the trabeculae of marrow-containing bone.

palmar s., a large fascial space in the hand, divided by a fibrous septum into the middle palmar space (toward the little finger) and the thenar space

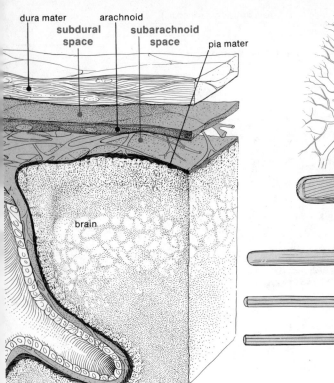

dura mater   arachnoid

subdural space   **subarachnoid space**   pia mater

brain

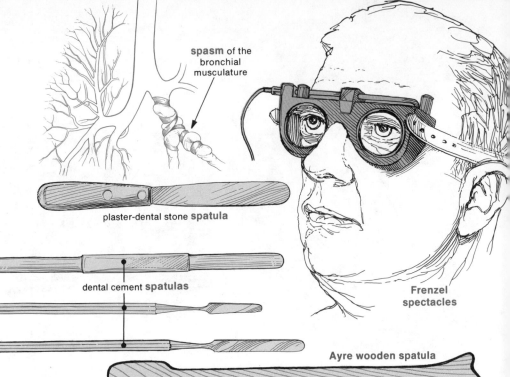

spasm of the bronchial musculature

plaster-dental stone **spatula**

dental cement **spatulas**

Frenzel spectacles

Ayre wooden spatula

(toward the thumb).

pharyngeal s., the area within the pharynx.

physiologic dead s., the portion of the respiratory passage at the end of inspiration, which is filled with air that has not mixed with alveolar air.

pleural s., the potential space between the parietal and visceral layers of the pleura; also called cavum pleurae.

retroperitoneal s., the space between the parietal peritoneum and the structures of the posterior abdominal wall.

retropubic s., the extraperitoneal area of loose connective tissue separating the bladder from the pubis and anterior abdominal wall; also called Retzius' space.

Retzius' s., see retropubic space.

s.'s of Fontana, the spaces of the trabecular tissue that connect the anterior chamber of the eye to the venous sinus of the sclera (Schlemm's canal); involved with drainage of the aqueous humor.

subarachnoid s., the space or interval between the arachnoid and the pia mater; it is filled with a delicate meshwork of fibrous trabeculae and contains cerebrospinal fluid.

subdural s., the narrow space between the dura mater and the arachnoid; it contains only a small amount of fluid sufficient to moisten the opposing surfaces of the two membranes.

subphrenic s., the space between the diaphragm and the organs immediately below it.

subpodocytic s.'s, spaces beneath the cell body of the podocyte and its trabeculae; they contain numerous fine foot processes (pedicels) which support the trabeculae on the basement membrane of glomerular capillaries.

Traube's s., a semilunar space on the left side of the chest about three inches wide, bounded on the right by the sternum, above by an oblique line from the cartilage of the sixth rib to the ninth rib, and below by the inferior border of the rib cage (costal margin).

urinary s., see Bowman's space.

Zang's s., lesser supraclavicular fossa; see under fossa.

zonular s., the circumlental space between the equator of the lens of the eye and the ciliary processes; it contains aqueous humor.

space maintainer. A dental appliance, either fixed or removable, used to preserve the space created by the premature loss of a tooth.

space obtainer. An orthodontic appliance that slowly increases space between teeth.

Spanish fly. See cantharis.

spargano′sis. Infection with spargana.

spar′ganum. The intramuscular parasitic larva of tapeworms of the genus *Spirometra*.

spargo′sis. Excessive distention, especially of the breasts with milk.

spas′m. An involuntary, sudden, violent contraction of a muscle or a group of muscles.

carpopedal s., spasm of the feet and hands occurring in tetany and other disorders.

clonic s., one characterized by alternate rigidity and relaxation of the muscles.

intention s., one occurring when voluntary movements are attempted.

nictitating s., involuntary winking.

tailor's s., see cramp, tailor's.

tonic s., a spasm in which the muscular contraction is persistent.

spasmod′ic. Relating to or characterized by spasm.

spasmogen′ic. Causing spasms.

spasmol′ysis. The arrest or elimination of spasm.

spasmolyt′ic. Antispasmodic; a drug that reduces spasm.

spast′ic. Convulsive.

spastic′ity. Increased tone or rigidity of a muscle.

clasp-knife s., spasticity of the extensor muscles induced by passive flexion of a joint which suddenly gives way on exertion of further pressure, allowing the joint to be easily flexed; the rigidity is due to an exaggeration of the stretch reflex; also called clasp-knife rigidity.

spat′ula. 1. A thin, flat, blunt, blade-shaped instrument used especially for spreading or mixing substances such as dental impression materials. **2.** A device used for scraping tissue for biopsy.

Ayre wooden s., a spatula generally used for taking a smear from the cervix or fornix of the uterus.

Roux s., a small steel spatula for transferring bits of infected material to culture tubes.

spat′ulate. 1. Shaped like a spatula, or having a flat blunt end. **2.** To mix substances by forced compression with a spatula.

spatula′tion. The manipulation of two or more substances with a spatula in order to mix them into a homogeneous mass; usually done by repeatedly and forcefully smoothing out the mass on the side of a mixing bowl or on a flat surface.

spay. To remove the ovaries of an animal.

SPCA. Abbreviation for serum prothrombin conversion accelerator (factor VII).

specialist. One who confines his interest to one branch of knowledge, as a physician who confines his practice to the treatment of a specific group of patients (e.g., children) or of diseases (e.g., urogenital).

specialize. To channel one's training or practice to a specific branch of health science.

specialty. The branch of health science to which one devotes oneself.

spe′cies. 1. A toxonomic classification of organisms, ranking after a genus and before a variety, which bear a close resemblance to one another and are capable of interbreeding; a subdivision of a genus. **2.** A variety or type of pharmaceutical preparation consisting of a mixture of crushed, but not pulverized, dried leaves used in making decoctions. **3.** Latin for tea.

specif′ic. 1. Relating to a species. **2.** Relating to one disease only. **3.** A remedy intended for one particular disease.

specific′ity. The state of having a fixed relationship to a particular cause, or to a definite result, as the discriminatory relation of an antigen to its specific antibody or vice versa.

spec′imen. A small part or sample of any substance, as tissue, blood, or urine, obtained for analysis and diagnosis.

spec′tacles. A pair of lenses set in a frame that holds them in front of the eyes; also called eyeglasses and glasses.

crutch s., spectacles with a ptosis crutch attachment (little offsets of smooth metal which engage below the upper eyelid to keep it raised above the pupil); also called Masselon's spectacles.

Frenzel s., plano spectacles with built-in illumination and 20-diopter lenses for the purpose of dazzling the eyes and preventing their fixation on an external object; used in a darkened room to observe and record nystagmus.

half-glass s., see pantoscopic spectacles.

Masselon's, see crutch spectacles.

pantoscopic s., eyeglasses used for reading in which the top halves of the lenses are removed so as not to affect distant vision; also called clerical or half-glass spectacles.

stenopaic s., spectacles having, in place of lenses, opaque disks with narrow slits or circular perforations allowing a minimum amount of light to enter.

spec′trin. Term denoting the two heaviest polypeptide components with molecular weights of 255,000 and 220,000; accounts for approximately 30 per cent of all protein in the membrane of red blood cells.

spectrochem′istry. The study and analysis of chemical substances by the use of light waves (spectroscopy); the study of the spectra of substances.

spec′trocolorim′eter. A form of spectroscope (colorimeter) using a light source from a selected wavelength (spectral light source) for detecting perception of one color.

spec′trogram. 1. A machine that translates

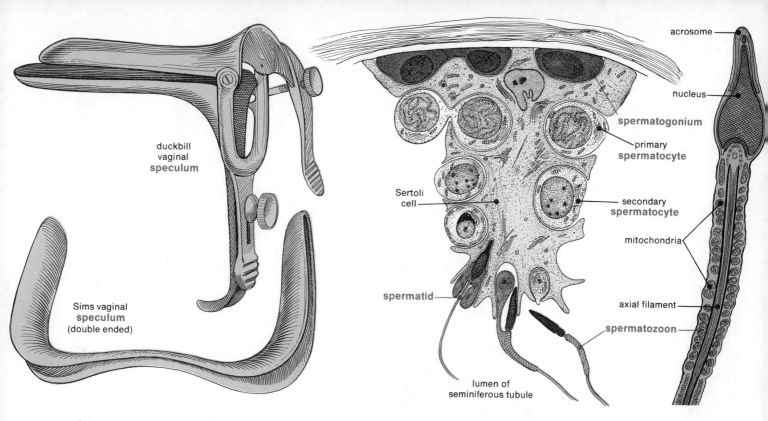

duckbill vaginal **speculum**

Sims vaginal **speculum** (double ended)

acrosome

nucleus

spermatogonium

primary **spermatocyte**

Sertoli cell

secondary **spermatocyte**

mitochondria

spermatid

axial filament

spermatozoon

lumen of seminiferous tubule

---

sounds into a pattern on paper. **2.** A photograph, graph, or map of a spectrum.

spec′trograph. A spectroscope specifically designed for photographic recording of a spectrum.

spectrom′eter. An instrument designed to break up light from a source into its constituent wavelengths and to indicate wavelength on its calibrated scale.

  nuclear magnetic resonance s., one that makes it possible to observe the magnetic properties of atoms in a molecule and provide information which describes their spatial relationships and movements.

spectrom′etry. Measuring of the wavelengths of rays of a spectrum with the spectrometer.

spec′tropho′tofluorim′etry. The photometric measurement and analysis of the intensity and quality of fluorescence spectra.

spec′trophotom′eter. An optical instrument for measuring photometrically the intensity of any particular wavelength range absorbed by a colored solution.

spec′tropolarim′eter. An instrument for measuring optical rotation of different wavelengths of light passing through a solution or translucent solid; a combined spectroscope and polariscope.

spec′troscope. Any one of several forms of optical instruments used for dispersion of light and visual observation of the resulting spectrum.

spectros′copy. The experimental observation and study of optical spectra.

spec′trum. 1. An orderly distribution of radiant energy presented when white light is dispersed into its constituent colors by passing through a prism or a diffraction grating; the colors, arranged according to the increasing frequency of molecular vibration or decreasing wavelength, are red, orange, yellow, green, blue, indigo, and violet. **2.** A range of activity of pathogenic microorganisms affected by an antibiotic or antibacterial agent.

  antibacterial s., spectrum (2).

  s. of disease, the complete range of manifestations of a disease.

spec′ulum. An instrument used to dilate and hold open the orifice of a body cavity or canal to facilitate the inspection of its interior.

speech. The production of articulate sounds to convey ideas.

  esophageal s., speech produced by swallowing air and regurgitating it; used by an individual who has had his larynx removed.

  scanning s., slow speech with pauses between syllables.

  staccato s., jerky, abrupt speech in which each syllable is pronounced separately.

  telegraphic s., a sparse speech usually consisting mainly of nouns, important adjectives, and transitive verbs, omitting articles, prepositions, and conjunctions; seen in certain types of aphasia.

speed. Slang name for methamphetamine hydrochloride.

sperm. 1. Spermatozoon; a mature reproductive cell of the male. **2.** Semen.

spermat′ic. Relating to the sperm.

sper′matid. One of the four cells resulting from the division of a spermatocyte; it develops into a spermatozoon without further division.

spermato-, spermat-. Combining forms indicating a relationship to semen or spermatozoa.

sper′matoblast. See spermatogonium.

sper′matocele. An intrascrotal, painless cyst containing sperm, usually less than one centimeter in diameter and occurring just above and posterior to the testis; caused by obstruction of the sperm-transporting tubules; also called spermatocyst.

sper′matocide. Any agent that destroys spermatozoa; also called spermicide.

sper′matocyst. 1. Seminal vesicle; see under vesicle. **2.** See spermatocele.

spermatocystec′tomy. Removal of the seminal vesicles.

sper′matocyte. A cell originating from the division of a spermatogonium which in turn divides into four spermatids.

spermatogen′esis. The formation of spermatozoa.

spermatogenet′ic. Relating to spermatogenesis.

spermatogen′ic, spermatog′enous. Producing sperm.

sper′matogo′nium, sper′matogone. An undifferentiated young cell located close to the basement membrane of the seminiferous tubules which either gives rise to new spermatogonia (type A) or differentiates to a more developed primary spermatocyte (type B), which eventually becomes a sperm; also called spermatoblast.

sper′matoid. Resembling semen.

spermatol′ysin. A specific lysin of spermatozoa formed in the female body following exposure to spermatozoa.

spermatol′ysis. Destruction with dissolution of the spermatozoa.

spermatorrhe′a. Abnormal involuntary discharge of semen without orgasm.

spermatos′chesis. Suppression of seminal discharge; nonsecretion of semen.

spermatox′in. Spermotoxin.

spermatozo′a. Plural of spermatozoon.

spermatozo′on, pl. **spermatozo′a.** The male sexual cell produced in the testes; a nucleated cell with a thin motile tail by means of which it migrates up the female reproductive passages where fertilization takes place.

spermatu′ria. See semenuria.

spermia′tion. The release of spermatozoa from the seminiferous epithelium.

spermio-, spermo-. Combining forms indicating a relationship to semen or spermatozoa.

spermiogen′esis. The phase of spermatogenesis in which spermatids develop into spermatozoa.

sper′molith. A stone in the deferent (spermatic) duct.

spermotox′in. A cytotoxic antibody destructive to spermatozoa; produced by injecting an animal with spermatozoa; also called spermatotoxin.

sp. gr. Abbreviation for specific gravity; less common form is s. g.

sphacelate. To become gangrenous.

sphaceloder′ma. Gangrene of the skin.

sphe′nion. A craniometric point located at the tip of the sphenoid angle of the parietal bone.

spheno-. Combining form meaning wedge-shaped.

sphen′oid. Wedge-shaped; denoting a large wedge-shaped bone at the base of the skull.

sphenoidi′tis. Inflammation of the sphenoid sinus.

sphenoidos′tomy. Removal of a portion of the anterior wall of the sphenoid sinus.

sphenoidot′omy. Incision into the sphenoid sinus.

sphenopal′atine. Relating to the sphenoid and palatine bones.

sphenor′bital. Relating to the sphenoid bone and the orbit.

sphenosquamo′sal. Relating to the sphenoid bone and the thin portion of the temporal bone.

sphere. A ball-shaped structure; a globular body.

  attraction s., see astrosphere.

  Morgagni's s.'s, Morgagni's globules; see under globule.

sphe′rocyte. A red blood cell which appears spherical in the living state and has a diameter of less than six microns; it has a greater than normal density of hemoglobin and a decreased surface-to-volume ratio; characteristic of hereditary spherocytosis and certain other hemolytic anemias.

spherocyto′sis. The presence of red blood cells which are more spherical than biconcave, as in hemolytic anemia; also called congenital spherocytic anemia.

spher′ule. 1. A small sphere. **2.** A minute, thick-walled, spherical structure containing many fungal spores; characteristic of the parasitic phase of *Coccidioides immitis.*

  rod s., the miniature terminal part of the retinal rod cell that forms synaptic relationships with the

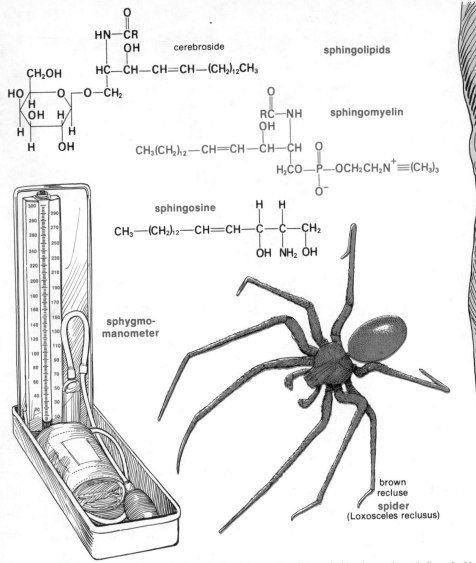

cerebroside

sphingolipids

sphingomyelin

sphingosine

sphygmo-manometer

brown recluse
spider
(Loxosceles reclusus)

spina
bifida

processes of bipolar cells and horizontal cells of the retina.

sphinc'ter. 1. Any circular muscle which, when contracted, closes a natural body opening. **2.** A portion of a tubular structure that functions as a sphincter.

external anal s., a two-layered flat band of muscular fibers, elliptical in shape, surrounding the anal orifice.

ileocecal s., ileocecal valve; see under valve.

internal anal s., a muscular ring surrounding about 2.5 cm of the anal canal; in contact with, but separate from, the external anal sphincter.

lower esophageal s. (LES), a high pressure zone in the distal portion of the esophagus where resting pressure is usually higher than pressure in the fundus of the stomach; acts as a barrier preventing the reflux of gastric contents; cannot be identified anatomically but its pressure can be measured and demonstrated; normally it straddles the diaphragm, extending 1–3 cm below to 1–2 cm above the diaphragmatic hiatus.

pupillary s., a narrow circular band of muscle fibers, about one millimeter in width, in the pupillary margin of the iris.

vesicular s., a thickening of the middle circular layer of the muscular fibers of the bladder, surrounding the internal urethral opening.

sphincteral'gia. Pain in a sphincter muscle, especially of the anus.

sphincteri'tis. Inflammation of a sphincter, particularly the sphincter of the hepatopancreatic duct.

sphincterot'omy. Surgical division of a sphincter muscle.

sphingolip'id. A group of lipids containing in their structure a long-chain, aliphatic base; e.g., ceramide, cerebroside, sphingomyelin, ganglioside; found primarily in tissues of the central nervous system.

sphingolipido'sis. General term for a number of

disorders marked by abnormal metabolism of sphingolipids.

cerebral s., any of a group of inherited diseases caused by a disturbance of metabolism resulting in increased lipids in the brain and characterized by progressive decrease in vision leading to complete blindness (usually within two years), severe mental deterioration, retinal atrophy, convulsions, and paralysis; there are four types of the disorder: infantile (Tay-Sachs disease), early juvenile (Jansky-Bielschowsky disease), late juvenile (Spielmeyer-Vogt or Batten-Mayou disease), and adult (Kufs' disease); also called cerebromacular degeneration; formerly called amaurotic familial idiocy.

sphingomy'elin. One of a group of phospholipids present in large quantities in brain and nerve tissue; on hydrolysis, it yields a fatty acid, phosphoric acid, choline, and the amino alcohol sphingosine.

sphing'osine. A complex amino alcohol; a constituent of cerebrosides.

sphygm-, sphygmo-. Combining forms meaning pulse.

sphyg'mic. Relating to the pulse.

sphyg'mogram. A curve representing the arterial pulse, made with a sphygmograph.

sphyg'mograph. Instrument used to make a graphic representation (curve) of the arterial pulse.

sphygmog'raphy. 1. The graphic recording of the arterial pulse by means of the sphygmograph. **2.** A treatise on the pulse.

sphyg'moid. Resembling the pulse.

sphygmomanom'eter. An instrument for measuring arterial blood pressure.

sphygmom'eter. Sphygmomanometer.

sphygmopalpa'tion. Feeling or "taking" the pulse; palpation of the pulse.

sphyg'mophone. An instrument for rendering audible the vibrations of each individual beat of the pulse.

sphyg'moscope. Instrument used to render the

pulse beat visible.

spi'ca. A plaster cast resembling a figure 8, used to immobilize the trunk and an extremity; e.g., shoulder spica; its name is derived from the overlapping turns that give it the appearance of an ear of barley.

spic'ule. A small needle-shaped structure.

spi'der. 1. Any of numerous arachnids having four pairs of legs, usually eight eyes, a body divided into a cephalothorax and an abdomen, and a complex of web-spinning spinnerets that produce silk; some venomous spiders are the black widow (*Latrodectus mactans*), brown recluse (*Loxosceles reclusus*), Chilean brown (*Loxosceles laeta*), and red-legged widow (*Latrodectus bishopi*). **2.** Exhibiting a pattern suggestive of a spider or a spider's web.

arterial s., a dilated arteriole in the skin with radiating capillary branches resembling the legs of a spider; characteristic of parenchymatous liver disorder, but also seen in pregnancy and at times in normal individuals; also called spider nevus, spider hemangioma, and nevus arachnoideus.

Spielmeyer-Vogt disease. Cerebral sphingolipidosis; see under sphingolipidosis.

spike. A brief electrical cerebral activity of three to 25 milliseconds' duration that is recorded on the electroencephalogram as a rising and falling vertical line.

spill'way. The labial, buccal, and lingual embrasures or passageways through which food escapes from the occlusal surfaces of teeth during chewing.

spi'na, *pl.* **spi'nae. 1.** The spine. **2.** Any sharp projection.

s. bifida, congenital defect in which part of the vertebral column is absent; it allows the spinal membranes and sometimes the spinal cord to protrude.

s. bifida occulta, spina bifida without protrusion of the spinal cord or its membranes; also called cryptomerorachischisis.

spi'nal. 1. Relating to a spine. **2.** Relating to the vertebral column.

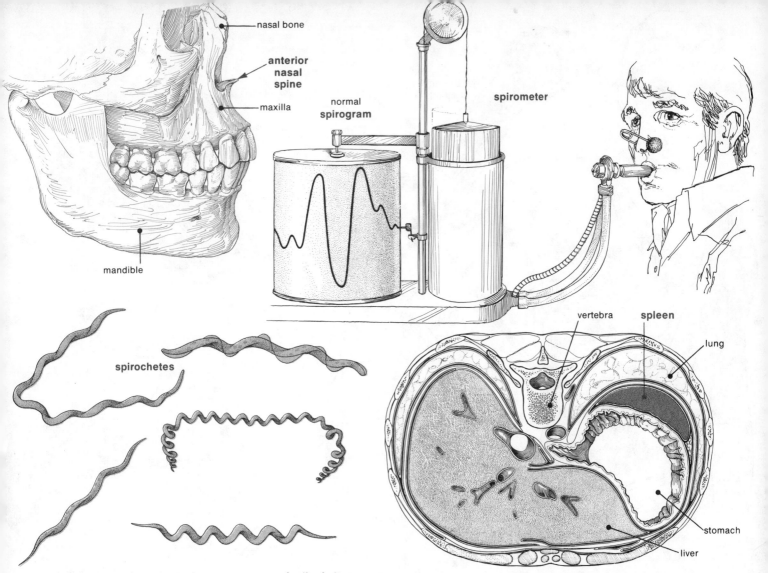

normal spirogram

spirometer

spirochetes

vertebra   **spleen**

lung

stomach

liver

s. column, see column, vertebral.

s. cord, see cord, spinal.

s. curvature, deviation of the vertebral column.

spin'dle. Any spindle-shaped or fusiform anatomic structure.

  mitotic s., the fusiform figure characteristic of a dividing cell formed by protoplasmic fibers extending between the two asters, along which the chromosomes are distributed.

  muscle s., neuromuscular spindle.

  neuromuscular s., small bundle of delicate muscular fibers (intrafusal fibers) invested by a capsule within which the sensory nerve fibers terminate; they vary in length from 0.8 to 5 mm and have a fusiform appearance; also called muscle proprioceptor.

  neurotendinous s., Golgi tendon organ; an enclosed capsule containing a number of enlarged tendon fasciculi (intrafusal fasciculi) around which the sensory nerve fibers terminate; chiefly found near the junctions of tendons and muscles.

spine. 1. A short projection of bone. **2.** Vertebral column; see under column.

  anterior nasal s., the anterior projection of the anterior crest of the maxilla.

  cervical s., the seven cervical vertebrae considered as a whole.

  iliac s., one of the four spines of the ilium.

  ischial s., a spine situated on the posterior aspect of the ischium near the posteroinferior border of the acetabulum.

  lumbar s., the five lumbar vertebrae considered as a whole.

  mental s., one of two spines located on the internal surface of the mandible, near the lower part of the midline.

  neural s., the middle spinous process of a typical vertebra.

  thoracic s., the twelve thoracic vertebrae considered as a whole.

spinn'barkeit. The ability to form a thread; designates the stringy cervical mucus of decreased or low viscosity which, when smeared on a slide, dries in a fernlike pattern and is indicative of ovulation in some women; also called spinnbarkheit.

spinobul'bar. Relating to the spine and the medulla oblongata.

spiradeno'ma. A benign tumor or overdevelopment of sweat glands.

spi'ral. Circling around a fixed center; coiled.

  Curschmann's s.'s, coiled masses of mucus sometimes found in the sputum in bronchial asthma.

spirillo'sis. Any disease caused by bacteria of the family Spirillaceae.

Spiril'lum. A genus (family Spirillaceae) of flagellated spiral or corkscrew-shaped bacteria which are found in water and putrid infusions.

spir'it. 1. An alcohol solution of a volatile substance. **2.** Archaic term denoting any liquid produced by distillation. **3.** Used in the plural, an alcoholic beverage.

  pyroxylic s., methyl alcohol; see under alcohol.

spiro-. Combining form denoting (a) spiral or coil-shaped; e.g., spirochete; (b) a relationship to breathing; e.g., spirograph.

Spirochae'ta. A genus of nonflagellated microorganisms with a slender wavy shape; found in sewage and stagnant water.

spi'rochete. Any organism of the genus *Spirochaeta.*

spirocheto'sis. Any infection caused by a spirochete, such as syphilis.

spi'rogram. The tracing made by a spirometer.

spi'rograph. A device for graphically recording the depth and rapidity of respiratory movements.

spirom'eter. Device for measuring the rate and volume of breathing; it records the volume of air and the time used to complete both inspiration and expiration.

spironolac'tone. A drug that acts directly on the renal tubules (blocks the action of aldosterone), producing sodium loss with potassium retention; used to minimize the hypokalemia induced by the thiazides or other potassium-losing diuretics; Aldactone®.

spis'sated. Thickened by evaporation or absorption of fluid.

spit. 1. To expectorate. **2.** Saliva.

spit'tle. Saliva.

splanch-. See splanchno-.

splanchnecto'pia. Malposition of any of the abdominal organs.

splanch'nic. Pertaining to the viscera.

splanchnicec'tomy. Surgical resection of a portion of the greater splanchnic nerve, usually performed along with a sympathectomy for treating essential hypertension.

splanchnicot'omy. Surgical transection of a splanchnic nerve or nerves; a surgical procedure tried in the treatment of arterial hypertension.

splanchno-, splanch-. Combining forms denoting a relationship to the viscera.

splanch'nocele. 1. Hernia of an abdominal organ. **2.** The embryonic body cavity.

splanchnomeg'aly. Abnormal largeness of abdominal organs.

splay'foot. See flatfoot.

spleen. A large vascular lymphatic organ situated in the abdominal cavity on the left side below the diaphragm; it is the sole lymphatic tissue specialized to filter blood; it removes effete or worn out cells from the circulatory system, converts hemoglobin to bilirubin, and releases iron into the blood for reuse; also called lein.

  accessory s., a mass of splenic tissue sometimes present in one of the peritoneal folds.

  sago s., deposits of amyloid in the spleen.

splen-. See spleno-.

splenec'tomy. Surgical removal of the spleen.

splene'olus. Accessory spleen.

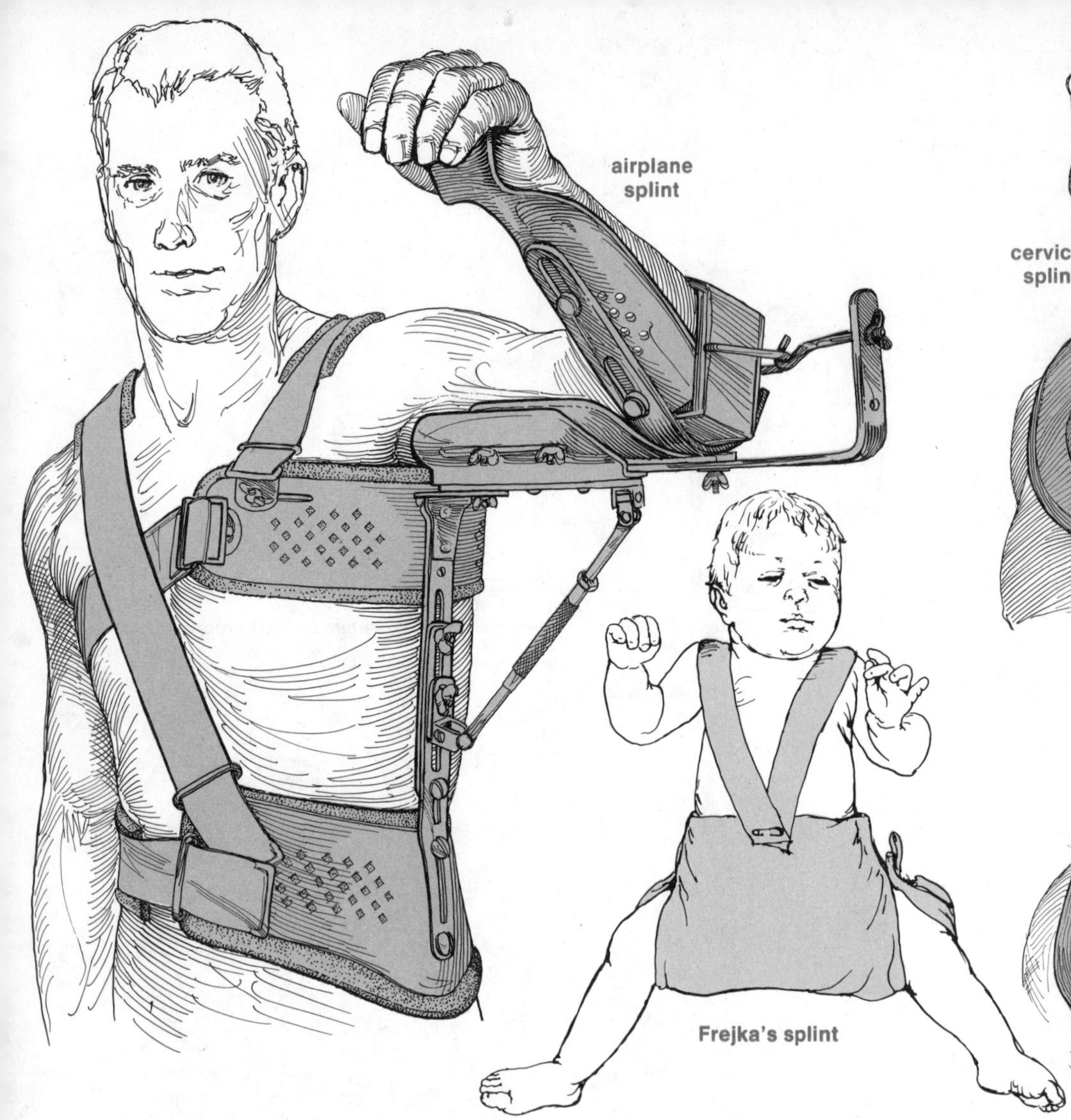

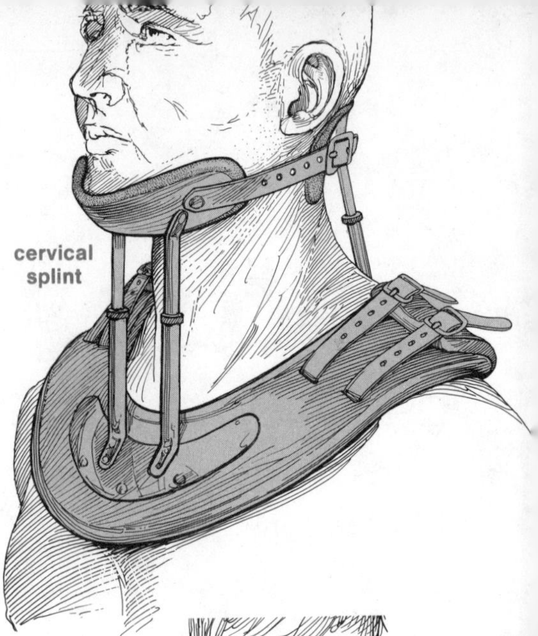

airplane
splint

cervical
splint

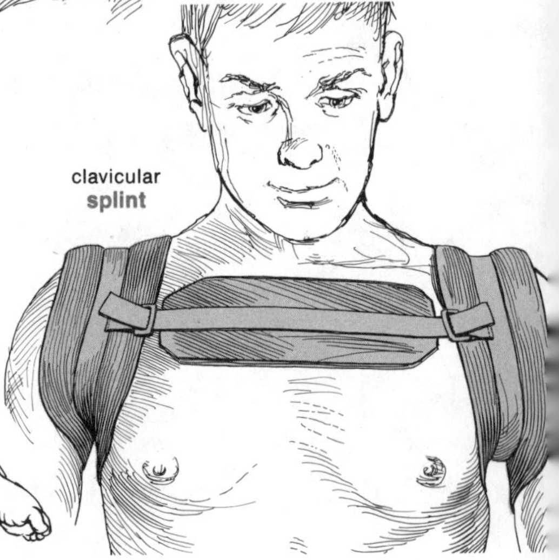

clavicular
splint

Frejka's splint

splen′ic. Relating to the spleen.

splenic flexure syndrome. Painful discomfort in the upper left abdomen which may radiate to the area over the heart and to the left shoulder; believed to be due to distention or spasmodic contraction of the colon.

spleni′tis. Inflammation of the spleen.

sple′nium. A bodily structure resembling a bandaged part.

s. of corpus callosum, the round, thick, posterior part of the corpus callosum of the brain.

spleno-, splen-. Combining forms denoting a relationship to the spleen.

sple′nocele. 1. Hernial protrusion of the spleen. **2.** A splenic tumor.

splenocol′ic. Relating or belonging to the spleen and colon, as the peritoneal fold connecting the organs.

sple′nocyte. A large mononuclear white blood cell of the spleen which is phagocytic; a splenic macrophage.

sple′nogram. A roentgenogram of the spleen.

splenogranulomato′osis. A granulomatous condition of the spleen with enlargement of the organ and thickening of the capsule.

splenog′raphy. Roentgenography of the spleen following injection of radiopaque material into it.

splenohepatomeg′aly. Abnormal enlargement of the spleen and the liver.

splenol′ysis. Destruction (lysis) of the spleen tissue.

splenomala′cia. Pathologic softening of the spleen.

splenomeg′aly. Enlargement of the spleen; also called splenomegalia and megalosplenia.

chronic congestive s., disorder usually following hypertension of the portal vein, marked by splenic enlargement, anemia, and occasional gastrointestinal bleeding; leukopenia and thrombocytopenia may develop in some cases; also called Banti's syn-

drome and splenic anemia.

tropical s., visceral leishmaniasis; see under leishmaniasis.

splenoneph′ric. See splenorenal.

splenopancreat′ic. Relating or belonging to the spleen and the pancreas.

splenop′athy. Any disease or disorder of the spleen.

splenophren′ic. Relating to the spleen and the diaphragm.

splenopor′togram. X-ray picture of the splenic and portal veins obtained after injection of radiopaque material into the spleen.

splenopto′sis. Abnormal mobility of the spleen resulting in downward displacement.

splenore′nal. Relating to the spleen and the kidney; also called splenonephric.

splenorrha′gia. Bleeding from a ruptured spleen.

spleno′sis. The presence of numerous nodules composed of splenic tissue throughout the peritoneal cavity.

splenot′omy. Incision into the spleen.

splenotox′in. A cytotoxin that has a particular affinity for the cells of the spleen.

splint. A device used to immobilize, support, and correct injured, displaced, or deformed structures.

acrylic s., one covering only the labial and lingual (outside and inside) surfaces of teeth and connected around the last molar by continuous acrylic material or a wire; used only to anchor fractured jaws of children with deciduous teeth.

acrylic resin bite-guard s., one used to eliminate movement of teeth.

airplane s., one designed to hold the arm in abduction at shoulder level.

Balkan s., see frame, Balkan.

cast cap s., a one-piece metal appliance, cemented over the crowns of teeth to immobilize the fragments of a fractured jaw.

cervical s., a splint for supporting the head, thus

taking some pressure off the cervical area.

Cramer's s., a flexible splint resembling a ladder, consisting of two parallel wires connected with a series of fine wires.

Denis Browne s., one used to correct clubfoot, consisting of two padded metal plates which are securely fastened to the infant's feet and connected by a metal crossbar.

Frejka's s., a pillow splint used to correct dislocations of the hip in infants under the age of 12 months.

Hodgen's s., one designed for a fractured femur, essentially used to apply balanced traction.

Thomas' s., one used to immobilize the leg, consisting of an iron ring that fits on the upper thigh (near the groin) connected to a continuous iron bar which has a W shape at the opposite end.

splint′ing. 1. The application of a rigid device to a limb to prevent motion of a dislocated joint or the ends of a fractured bone. **2.** In dentistry, the linking of two or more teeth with a fixed restoration. **3.** Protection against pain by reducing motion of the painful part; e.g., the shallow breathing and fixed position assumed by a patient to reduce pain in his chest.

split′ting. In chemistry, the conversion of a complex substance into two or more simpler products.

spodo-. Combining form denoting waste material.

spodog′enous. Resulting from accumulation of waste material in an organ.

spodoph′agous. Denoting one who eats body wastes.

spondyl-. See spondylo-.

spondylarthri′tis. Inflammation of one or more intervertebral articulations.

spondyli′tis. Inflammation of one or more vertebrae.

ankylosing s., ossification of the ligaments of the spine with involvement of the hips and shoulders; also called Strümpell-Marie arthritis, Marie-Strüm-

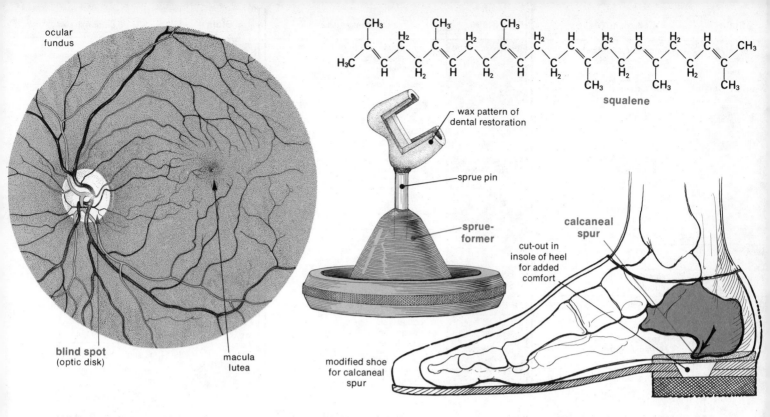

ocular
fundus

blind spot
(optic disk)

macula
lutea

squalene

wax pattern of
dental restoration

sprue pin

sprue-
former

calcaneal
spur

cut-out in
insole of heel
for added
comfort

modified shoe
for calcaneal
spur

---

pell disease, and rheumatoid spondylitis.

tuberculous s., tuberculosis of the spine; also called Pott's disease.

spondylo-, spondyl-. Combining forms relating to the vertebrae or vertebral column.

spondyloisthe′sis. Forward slippage of one vertebra over another, usually of a lumbar vertebra on the vertebra below it, or upon the sacrum; also called spondyloptosis.

spondylol′ysis. Breaking down or destruction of a vertebra.

spondylop′athy. Rachiopathy; any disorder of the vertebrae.

spondylopto′sis. See spondylolisthesis.

spondylopyo′sis. Suppurative inflammation of the body of a vertebra.

spondylos′chisis. Myelocele; congenital fissure of the vertebral column.

spondylo′sis. Abnormal immobility and fixation of a vertebral joint.

sponge. 1. The light fibrous skeleton of certain aquatic animals used as an absorbent. **2.** A folded piece of gauze or cotton.

absorbable gelatin s., a sterile, absorbable, water-insoluble gelatine-based sponge, used in surgery to control bleeding.

spon′giform. Resembling a sponge.

spon′gioblast. An embryonic cell of the supportive (non-neuronal) component of the central nervous system.

spongioblasto′ma. Tumor composed mainly of spongioblasts.

spon′giocyte. 1. A cell of the supportive tissue of the central nervous system. **2.** One of the vacuolated cells situated in the cortex of the adrenal gland.

spongiosi′tis. Inflammation of the corpus spongiosum of the penis.

sponta′neous. Arising without apparent cause.

spoon. 1. An implement consisting of a small, shallow, oval bowl on a handle. **2.** A slang expression for a measure of pure heroin, about $^1/_{16}$ ounce.

cataract s., one used for removing a cataractous lens from the eye.

sharp s., a sharp-edged spoon used for scraping away granulations, carious bone, or other diseased tissue.

sporad′ic. 1. Occurring infrequently or at irregular intervals. **2.** Not widespread.

sporan′gia. Plural of sporangium.

sporan′giophore. A fungal structure that bears one or more sporangia.

sporan′gium, *pl.* **sporan′gia.** A capsule or encystment within a plant in which spores are produced.

spore. A primitive, thick walled, usually unicellular reproductive cell that is capable of giving rise to a new plant.

spor′icide. A substance that destroys spores.

sporid′ium. The spore stage of a protozoan organism.

sporo-, spor-. Combining forms indicating spore; e.g., sporogenesis.

spor′oblast. An early stage in the development of a sporocyst, from which sporozoites later develop.

spo′rocyst. A stage in the life cycle of many protozoa in which two or more parasites are enclosed within a common wall.

sporogen′esis. The production of spores.

sporog′ony. A sexual cycle of certain protozoans in which spores are produced as a result of sexual fusion of gametes prior to multiple fission.

spor′ont. A sexually mature protozoan parasite.

sporotricho′sis. A fungal disease usually affecting cutaneous, subcutaneous, and lymphatic tissues; caused by *Sporotrichum schenkii.*

Sporot′richum. A genus of cigar-shaped parasitic fungi.

S. schenkii, the cause of sporotrichosis in man and animals.

Sporozo′a. A class of the phylum Protozoa which includes parastic organisms that reproduce by spores.

sporozo′an. A member of the class Sporozoa.

sporozo′ite. The infectious stage in the life cycle of sporozoan organisms; one of the minute elongated bodies formed by division of the encysted zygote (oocyst); in malaria, forms of the plasmodium organism are concentrated in the salivary glands of mosquitoes and transferred to man in the act of feeding.

sporozo′on. Sporozoan.

spor′ulate. To produce spores.

sporula′tion. Reproduction by spores.

spor′ule. A minute spore.

spot. 1. A small area of discoloration. **2.** To discharge a small amount of blood from the vagina.

blind s., optic disk; the area in the eye where the optic nerve enters the retina which is insensitive to light.

cafe au lait s.'s, hyperpigmented light brown patches on the skin as seen in neurofibromatosis.

Koplik's s.'s, one of the signs of measles; minute bluish white lesions surrounded by a bright ring on the mucous membrane of the cheeks, occurring about two days before the appearance of the skin rash.

liver s.'s, see chloasma.

rose s.'s, pinkish spots on the abdomen, seen in the early stages of typhoid fever.

Roth's s.'s, round white spots sometimes seen in the retina of patients with bacterial endocarditis.

soft s., see fontanel.

Tay's cherry red s., the cherry red spot in the macular area of the retina, seen in patients with Tay-Sachs disease.

yellow s., see macula retinae.

sprain. Injury to a joint in which only the soft tissues are affected.

spray. 1. A jet of liquid droplets. **2.** To sprinkle.

sprue. 1. A malabsorptive disorder; see celiac disease. **2.** In dentistry, the wax or metal used to form the opening through which a material such as gold or resin is poured into a mold to make a casting; also the waste piece of material that fills the opening.

nontropical s., see celiac disease.

tropical s., disease occurring in certain tropical areas, characterized by abnormal small bowel structure and malabsorption; unlike celiac disease, it is not associated with gluten intolerance but is caused by vitamin deficiencies and/or bacterial contamination of the intestines; it responds to treatment with folic acid, sometimes supplemented by antibiotics. Cf celiac disease.

sprue-former. In dentistry, the cone-shaped base to which the sprue pin is anchored while the wax pattern is being invested.

spur. A spinelike projection from a bone or a horny outgrowth from the skin.

calcaneal s., a bony outgrowth from the plantar surface of the calcaneous (heel bone), which often causes pain when walking; also called heel spur.

heel s., see calcaneal spur.

spu′tum, *pl.* **spu′ta.** Expectorated matter from the air passages; also called expectoration.

squal′ene. An unsaturated terpene hydrocarbon found in shark liver oil and an intermediate in the biosynthesis of cholesterol; present in small amounts in blood plasma.

squa′ma, *pl.* **squa′mae. 1.** A thin plate of bone. **2.** A scalelike structure.

squamomas′toid. Relating to the squamous and mastoid portions of the temporal bone.

squamopetro′sal. Relating to the squamous and petrous parts of the temporal bone.

squamo′sa. The scalelike portion (squama) of the temporal bone.

squa′mous. 1. Scaly; covered with scales. **2.** Resembling scales.

squint. Strabismus.

Sr. Chemical symbol of the element strontium.

SRF. Abbreviation for somatotropin-releasing factor (growth hormone-releasing factor).

sRNA. Abbreviation for soluble ribonucleic acid (transfer ribonucleic acid).

Stain	demonstrates	Stain	demonstrates	Stain	demonstrates
acid stain acid-fast stain	pancreatic alpha cells acid-free bacteria	hematoxylin and eosin stain	cytoplasm and nuclei of cells muscle fibers collagen	silver and gold impregnation stain	reticular fibers collagenous connective tissue Golgi apparatus neurofibrils
alcian blue stain	mucoproteins	Janus-green stain	mitochondria	Sudan stain	lipids myelin
aldehyde fuchsin	elastic fibers basement membranes beta cells of islets of Langerhans neuro secretion mast cell granules thyrotrophs	Mallory's stain	collagen reticular fibers elastic fibers nuclei neuroglia	Toluidine blue stain	nucleic and cytoplasmic ribonucleic acid cartilage matrix mast cell granules basophilic granules Nissl bodies
azan stain	nuclei of cells muscle fibers collagen	Nissl stain	cell bodies of neuron dendrites of neuron	van Gieson's stain	connective tissue
basic stain	nuclei of cells	Oil red O stain	lipids	von Kossa's stain	calcium salts in bone
Best's carmine stain	glycogen	orcein stain	elastic fibers	Weigert's stain	elastic fibers nerve fibers
brilliant cresyl blue stain	platelets reticulocytes	osmic acid stain	lipids myelin Golgi apparatus	Wright's stain	bone marrow erythrocytes eosinophils basophils neutrophils malarial parasites
Feulgen nuclear reaction stain	chromatin	periodic acid Schiff test	glycoproteins glycogen basement membranes granules in some pituitary cells	Ziehl-Neelsen stain	tubercle bacilli
Giemsa stain	blood, spleen, and bone marrow certain protozoan parasites	picric acid and carmine stain	collagenous fibers epithelium muscle fibers		
Golgi stain	nerve tissue	potassium dichromate stain	catecholamine granules of the adrenal medulla and paraganglionic cells		

SRS, SRS-A. Abbreviation for slow-reacting substance (slow-reacting substance of anaphylaxis); see under substance.

ss. Abbreviation for the Latin *semis*.

SSS. Abbreviations for (a) specific soluble substance; (b) sick-sinus syndrome.

S₁S₂S₃ syndrome. Prominent S waves in the three standard limb leads with a small R′ deflection in V_1 and a normal QRS interval; most commonly seen in young adults without heart disease, but it may also be seen in right ventricular hypertrophy, and occasionally with acute myocardial infarction.

stab. To pierce or wound with a pointed instrument or weapon.

sta′bile.1. Stable; unchangeable; fixed; immobile; unaffected, as certain constituents of serum which are unaffected by ordinary degrees of heat, etc. **2.** Resistant to chemical change.

stabil′ity. 1. The condition of being resistant to change in the presence of forces. **2.** The ability of a denture to resist displacement by functional forces.

   dimensional s., the property of a material to retain its shape.

   emotional s., character of a person not given to marked mood swings or labile emotions.

sta′bilizer. 1. An instrument employed in an x-ray unit to render constant the milliamperage output of the x ray. **2.** Any substance used to maintain the equilibrium or velocity of a chemical reaction.

stable. Denoting a balanced condition, resisting alteration.

staff. 1. The personnel who have a specific responsibility and authority in a hospital. **2.** A grooved probe or sound used for guiding the scalpel, as in a lithotomy; also called guide. **3.** A pole, rod, or stick, especially when used as a symbol.

   house s., the resident or junior physicians and surgeons of a hospital.

   s. of Aesculapius, see under Aesculapius.

stage. 1. A phase in the course of a disease or the life cycle of an organism. **2.** The platform of a microscope on which the slide is placed for viewing.

   anal s., stage in infantile psychosexual development during which interest is focused on elimination and retention of feces; also called anal phase.

   Arneth s.'s, classification of polymorphonuclear neutrophils according to the number of lobes in their nuclei.

   exoerythrocytic s., stage in the life cycle of the malarial parasite (*Plasmodium*) outside of the red blood cells of the host.

   genital s., stage in psychosexual development (usually between the ages of three and six) during which the child becomes aware of his/her genitals and the pleasure derived from their stimulation;

also called phallic stage (regardless of sex) and genital phase.

   incubation s., stage in the course of a disease prior to the appearance of symptoms.

   mechanical s., device attached to, or built into, the stage of a microscope which permits moving of the specimen slide while holding it in the plane of focus.

   Oedipal s., stage in psychosexual development in which the child has an erotic attachment to the parent of the opposite sex; also called Oedipal phase.

   oral s., stage of infantile psychosexual development (from birth to approximately 12 months); divided into oral erotic, associated with the pleasurable sensation of sucking, and oral sadistic, related to aggressive biting; also called oral phase.

   phallic s., see genital stage.

   prodromal s., incubation stage.

   psychosexual s.'s, stages of development of infantile sexuality, especially in psychoanalytic theory (oral, anal, phallic).

   resting s., a misnomer for the period in the life of a cell when no mitotic changes occur, but when the cell is actively synthesizing DNA; more properly called the interphase.

   s.'s of labor, see under labor.

stag′ger. To walk or stand unsteadily.

stagna′tion. The condition of not flowing, occurring in any body fluid that normally should circulate.

stain. 1. Any dye used to render cells and tissues visible for microscopic study. **2.** To impart color to cells and tissues for microscopic examination. **3.** A superficial discoloration of the skin.

   acid s., a dye salt whose acid radical combines with the basic components of cells; it stains mainly the protoplasm.

   acid-fast s., procedure for staining acid-free bacteria (those retaining Ziehl's solution even when decolorized with acid alcohol); after decolorization, a contrasting second stain (counterstain) is applied; the acid-fast cells remain red; others take the color of the counterstain.

   aldehyde fuchsin s., one containing potassium permanganate, sulfuric acid, sodium bisulfate, fuchsin, and paraldehyde; used to demonstrate elastic fibers, β-cells of islets of Langerhans, and basement membranes.

   basic s., a dye salt whose basic radical combines with the acidic components of cells; it stains mainly the nuclei.

   contrast s., one used to stain a portion of tissue which is unaffected by a previously used dye of another color.

   differential s., one used to differentiate between kinds of bacteria that are morphologically indistinguishable although of different species.

   Giemsa s., one consisting of azur II eosin, azur II, glycerin, and methanol; used for blood cells, Negri bodies, and certain protozoan parasites.

   Golgi s., a heavy metal stain used to enhance the cytoarchitectural appearance of nervous tissue; usually the metal (silver or gold) becomes impregnated along the membranes or within neurons or neuroglia.

   Gram's s., method used to classify bacteria, based on the ability of the organisms to retain a basic dye (crystal violet); those retaining the violet stain are gram positive and those that do not retain it are gram negative.

   H & E s., hematoxylin and eosin stain.

   hematoxylin and eosin s., method of tissue staining employed in numerous variations; consists mainly of the use of a water solution of hematoxylin and eosin; it stains cytoplasm pink and nuclei blue.

   Janus-green B s., a supravital stain used to demonstrate mitochondria.

   Mallory's aniline blue s., one suitable for demonstrating connective tissue and secretion granules.

   metachromatic s., one that stains different cell elements a different color from that of the dye employed.

   Nissl s., a method for staining neuronal cell bodies and proximal dendrites; based on the ability of the cell to take up basic aniline dyes, such as cresyl-fast violet, thionine, or toluidine blue.

   oil red O s., oil red O in isopropyl alcohol; it stains lipid a cherry red color.

   orcein s., a natural dye used to demonstrate elastic fibers and membranes.

   osmic acid s., aqueous solution of osmic acid (OsO₄) used in electron microscopy as a fixative and stain.

   Papanicolaou s., one employed on smears of body secretions to detect the presence of malignancy; consists generally of aqueous hematoxylin with multiple counterstaining dyes in ethyl alcohol.

   periodic acid-Schiff' s. (PAS), a tissue stain for demonstration of polysaccharides and mucopolysaccharides of epithelial mucins, basement membranes, and connective tissue.

   port-wine s., port-wine hemangioma; a capillary hemangioma varying in color from pink to purple.

   potassium dichromate s., one used to demonstrate catecholamine granules of the adrenal medulla and paraganglionic cells.

   silver and gold impregnation s., solutions of silver and gold compounds used to demonstrate reticular fibers, collagenous connective tissue, Golgi

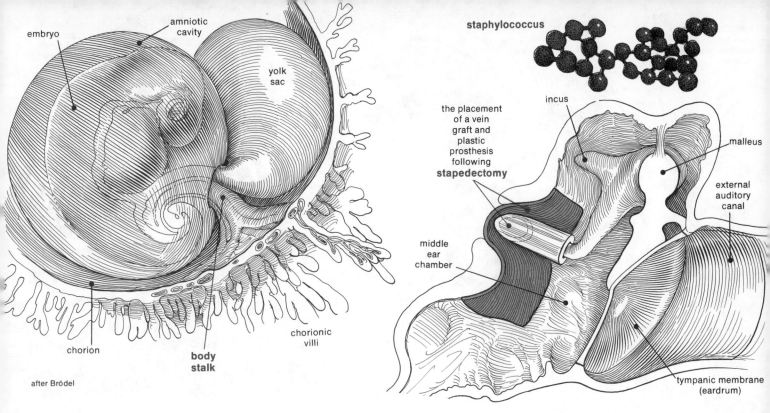

embryo

amniotic cavity

yolk sac

staphylococcus

the placement of a vein graft and plastic prosthesis following **stapedectomy**

incus

malleus

external auditory canal

middle ear chamber

chorionic villi

body stalk

chorion

tympanic membrane (eardrum)

after Brödel

apparatus, and neurofibrils.

Sudan s.'s, oil-soluble compounds used for demonstrating lipids.

supravital s., a relatively nontoxic dye such as neutral red; used to study living cells.

tumor s., in radioscopy, a dense area in an x-ray film indicating accumulation of contrast material in abnormal distorted blood vessels, thought to represent a tumor.

vital s., a dye introduced into a living organism.

von Kossa's s., a silver nitrate stain for calcium salts in bone.

Weigert s., one that stains nerve fiber tracts blue to black.

Wright's s., a stain commonly used for the demonstration of blood cells that consists of both acid (eosin) and basic (methylene blue, methylene azure, and methylene violet) dyes; also used to stain malarial parasites.

Ziehl-Neelsen s., stain used in the identification of tubercle bacilli.

stain'ing. 1. The coloration of a microscopic specimen with a dye to improve the visibility of certain parts. **2.** In dentistry, modification of the color of teeth.

negative s., process of suspending bacteria in an opaque medium (e.g., India ink) which fails to penetrate the organism, thus providing contrast.

simple s., staining with one dye only.

stalagmom'eter. Device used to obtain and measure drops from a liquid at definite intervals with a view to calculating the surface tension of the liquid.

stalk. A slender or elongated connection with a structure or organ.

allantoic s., a narrow connection between the urogenital sinus and the allantoic sac.

body s., a bridge of mesenchymal mass connecting the caudal end of the young embryo to the inner face of the chorionic vesicle.

optic s., a slender structure connecting the optic vesicle to the forebrain in the early embryo.

yolk s., omphalomesenteric duct; see under duct.

stam'mering. A faltering manner of speaking marked by involuntary pauses and syllabic repetitions; distinguished from stuttering.

stanch, staunch. To arrest bleeding.

stan'dard. An established rule of comparison for qualitative or quantitative value.

standardiza'tion. 1. The formulation of standards for any preparation or procedure. **2.** Making anything fit a standard.

stan'nic. Relating to or containing tin with valence four.

stan'nous. Relating to or containing tin with valence two.

stan'num. Latin for tin.

stapedec'tomy. Surgical removal of the stapes from the middle ear chamber.

stape'dial. Relating to the stapes of the middle ear.

stapediotenot'omy. Surgical division of the stapedius muscle of the middle ear.

stapediovestib'ular. Relating to both the stapes and the vestibule of the ear.

stape'dius. A minute muscle in the middle ear. See table of muscles.

sta'pes. The smallest and innermost of the three ossicles of the middle ear; it articulates by its head with the incus, and its base (footplate) is inserted and attached to the margin of the oval window; the smallest bone of the human body; also called stirrup.

staphyl-. Combining form denoting the uvula.

staphylec'tomy. Surgical removal of the uvula.

staph'yline. Resembling a bunch of grapes.

staphyl'ion. A craniometric landmark; the midpoint of the posterior edge of the hard palate.

staphylococ'cal. Relating to or caused by staphylococci.

staphylococce'mia. The presence of staphylococci in the blood.

staphylococ'cus, *pl.* **staphylococ'ci.** Any organism of the genus *Staphylococcus.*

Staphylococ'cus. A genus (family Micrococcaceae) of gram-positive, nonmotile, usually pathogenic bacteria which tend to aggregate in irregular grapelike clusters.

S. aureus, a species containing the pigmented, coagulase-positive variety which causes boils, carbuncles, abscesses, and other suppurative inflammations.

S. epidermidis, a species containing the nonpigmented, mannitol- and coagulase-negative nonpathogenic variety which causes stitch abscesses; normally present on skin.

staphyloder'ma. Pus-forming skin disorder caused by staphylococci.

staphylol'ysin. 1. A substance elaborated by a staphylococcus that causes destruction of red blood cells and liberation of hemoglobin. **2.** An antibody causing dissolution of staphylococci.

staphylo'ma. Protrusion of the cornea or sclera, usually lined with uveal tissue.

staph'yloplasty. Surgical repair of the uvula and/or the soft palate.

staphylopto'sia, staphylopto'sis. Relaxation or lengthening of the uvula.

starch. 1. A carbohydrate with the general formula $(C_6H_{10}O_5)_n$; exists abundantly in the vegetable kingdom and is converted into dextrins and glucose

by amylase enzyme action in saliva and pancreatic juice. **2.** A substance consisting of granules separated from the mature grain of *Zea mays* (Indian corn), used in pharmaceuticals and as a dusting powder.

stare. To look intently with a steady, often wide-eyed, unblinking gaze.

postbasic s., an odd expression of the eyes marked by downward rolling of the eyeballs and retraction of the upper eyelids; seen in persons with posterior basic meningitis.

starva'tion. The condition of suffering from prolonged lack of food.

sta'sis. Stoppage of the flow of a fluid, especially of the blood.

stat. Abbreviation for Latin *statim.*

state. Condition.

anxiety s., anxiety neurosis; see under neurosis.

carrier s., the condition of harboring pathogenic microorganisms without being affected by them.

central excitatory s., a condition of hyperexcitability of nerve cells produced by the storing up of subthreshold stimuli in a reflex center of the spinal cord.

convulsive s., spasmodic jerking of the extremities and trunk with varying degrees of unconsciousness.

dreamy s., a semiconscious condition associated with an attack of epilepsy.

paranoid s., psychotic disorder in which the primary abnormality consists of a delusion, usually of persecution or grandeur.

refractory s., the reduced excitability of a nerve following a response to previous stimulation.

standard s., the pure and stable form of an element at 1.0 pressure and 25°C temperature.

steady s., dynamic equilibrium.

twilight s., condition of impaired consciousness in which a person may perform elaborate purposeful acts and have no recollection of them afterward.

sta'tim (stat). Latin for at once, immediately; used in prescription writing.

statis'tics. A collection of organized numerical data.

vital s., a collection of data pertaining to human birth, health, disease, and death.

statoco'nia. See otoconia.

stat'ure. The natural height of a person.

sta'tus. State; condition.

s. choleraicus, the stage of shock and collapse in cholera, marked by cold skin, weak pulse, and lethargy.

s. epilepticus, a series of epileptic attacks in rapid succession.

s. thymicolymphaticus, enlargement of the thy-

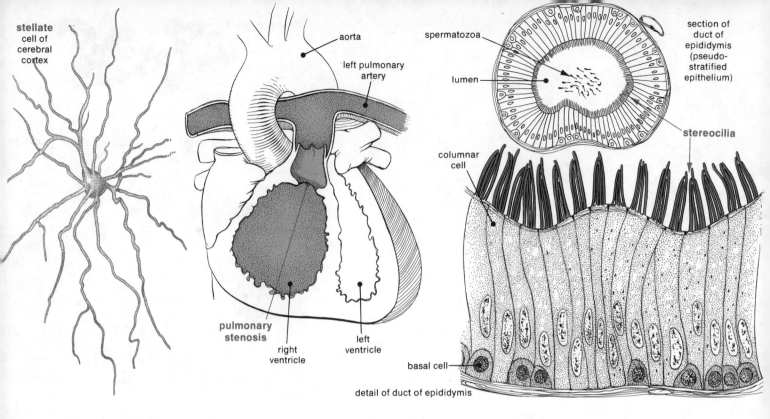

stellate
cell of
cerebral
cortex

aorta

left pulmonary
artery

pulmonary
stenosis

right
ventricle

left
ventricle

spermatozoa

lumen

columnar
cell

basal cell

section of
duct of
epididymis
(pseudo-
stratified
epithelium)

stereocilia

detail of duct of epididymis

---

mus and lymph nodes; formerly believed to cause crib death of infants.

staunch. See stanch.

steap'sin. A fat-splitting enzyme in pancreatic juice; also called pancreatic lipase.

ste'arate. A salt of stearic acid.

stearic acid. A common fatty acid made by the hydrolysis of fats; used in pharmaceutical preparations; also called octodecanoic acid.

ste'arin. The triglyceride of stearic acid; a solid fat that melts at 71°C; also called glyceryl stearate.

stearo-. Combining form meaning fat.

steati'tis. Inflammation of fatty tissue.

steato-, steat-. Combining forms denoting a relationship to fat or tallow; e.g., steatorrhea.

steatocrypto'sis. Dysfunction of sebaceous glands.

steatocysto'ma. A sebaceous cyst.

s. multiplex, see steatomatosis.

steatog'enous. 1. Causing fat degeneration. **2.** Producing any disease of the sebaceous glands.

steatol'ysis. The hydrolysis or emulsion of fat preparatory to absorption.

steato'ma. 1. A tumor composed chiefly of fatty tissue. **2.** A sebaceous cyst.

steatomato'sis. A condition characterized by the presence of numerous sebaceous cysts, often widespread; also called steatocystoma multiplex.

steatonecro'sis. A histologic abnormality seen almost exclusively in the liver of an alcoholic patient; marked by the presence of Mallory bodies (coagulated, hyalinized cytoplasm that forms a coarse, acidophilic network around the nucleus of liver cells), usually in association with fatty changes.

steatop'athy. Disorder of the sebaceous glands.

steatopy'gia, steatopy'ga. Excessively fat buttocks.

steatorrhe'a. Excessive amount of fat in the feces, a manifestation of the malabsorption syndrome.

steato'sis. 1. Fatty degeneration. **2.** Any disease of the sebaceous glands.

stegno'sis. 1. Stoppage of secretions or excretions. **2.** Constriction.

Stein-Leventhal syndrome. Polycystic ovary syndrome; condition characterized primarily by menstrual abnormalities, enlarged cystic ovaries, and infertility.

stel'late. Having the shape of a star.

stellec'tomy. Excision of the stellate ganglion; usually performed for the relief of intractable pain; also called stellate ganglionectomy.

Stellwag's sign. Infrequent and incomplete blinking; seen in exophthalmic goiter.

stem cell renewal. A residual population of cells that retain the ability to divide.

sten'ion. The craniometric point located at each end of the shortest transverse diameter of the skull in the temporal region.

steno-. A combining form indicating narrowness or constriction.

stenocho'ria. Constriction of a duct or orifice.

stenope'ic. Having a narrow opening.

stenosed'. Constricted.

steno'sis. Abnormal constriction of a channel or orifice.

aortic s., pathologic constriction of the orifice between the aorta and the left ventricle of the heart.

congenital pyloric s., see hypertrophic pyloric stenosis.

hypertrophic pyloric s., overdevelopment of the pyloric sphincter muscle causing narrowing of the pyloric orifice and projectile vomiting, occurring in the second or third week of life; also called congenital pyloric stenosis.

hypertrophic subaortic s., functional constriction during systole of the left ventricular opening into the aorta in the presence of normal aortic valves; thought to be due to abnormal hypertrophy of tissue in the outflow tract.

infundibular pulmonic s., obstruction of the infundibulum (outflow tract) of the right ventricle of the heart, usually caused by either or both of two conditions: (1) a fibrous ring just below the pulmonic valve; (2) hypertrophy of heart muscle surrounding the infundibulum.

mitral s., narrowing of the opening between the left atrium and the left ventricle.

pulmonary s., constriction of the orifice between the pulmonary artery and the right ventricle.

pyloric s., constriction of the pyloric orifice of the stomach.

subaortic s., subvalvular s., obstruction of the outflow tract of the left ventricle of the heart; caused by either a fibrous band or muscular hypertrophy just below the aortic valve.

tricuspid s., narrowing of the tricuspid orifice of the heart.

stenosteno'sis. Constriction of the parotid duct.

stenosto'mia. A narrow state of the oral cavity.

stenother'mal. Capable of withstanding only slight changes in temperature.

stenotho'rax. An abnormally narrow chest.

stenot'ic. Narrowed abnormally; affected with stenosis.

step'page. High steppage gait; see under gait.

stercobil'in. A brown pigment present in the feces, derived from bile.

ster'colith. A fecal concretion.

stercora'ceous. Fecal; relating to feces.

ste're. A metric unit of volume equal to one kiloliter or 1,000 liters (nearly one cubic meter).

stereo-. A combining form denoting a solid or three-dimensionality.

stereoanesthe'sia. See astereognosis.

stereoarthrol'ysis. Surgical creation of a movable joint.

stereocampim'eter. Instrument used to examine the central visual field of each eye separately while both eyes fixate similar targets.

stereochem'istry. The branch of chemistry concerned with the spatial arrangement of atoms in a compound.

stereocil'ia. Unusually long, slender, nonmotile microvilli, found primarily in parts of the male reproductive tract; thought to aid in secretion and absorption.

stereocinefluorog'raphy. Motion picture photography of x-ray images obtained by stereoscopic fluoroscopy, producing three-dimensional visualization.

stereogno'sis. The recognition of objects through the sense of touch.

stereoi'somer. One of two compounds which contain the same number and kind of atoms and the same chemical structure but which have different optical properties because the atoms in each have different spatial positions.

stereoisom'erism. Isomerism in which two compounds have the same structural formula but the atoms are linked in a different order.

stereol'ogy. A study of the three-dimensional aspects of morphology, especially ultrastructure.

stereo-orthopter. A visual training instrument used to correct strabismus.

stereop'sis. Visual depth perception produced by slight disparateness of images, i.e., when images fall on slightly disparate points of the retina.

stereoroentgenog'raphy. The taking of an x-ray picture from two slightly different positions to produce a three-dimensional effect.

ster'eoscope. Instrument that permits two different portions of the same picture (or two photographs of different views of the same object) to be viewed by the two eyes at the same time, resulting in a three-dimensional perception.

stereospecif'ic. Denoting enzymes or synthetic organic reactions that act only with a given molecule or with a limited class of molecules.

stereotax'is. 1. The localization of the three-dimensional arrangement of body structures by means of coordinate landmarks. **2.** The movement of an organism toward, or away from, a rigid surface with which it comes in contact; applied to the organism as a whole.

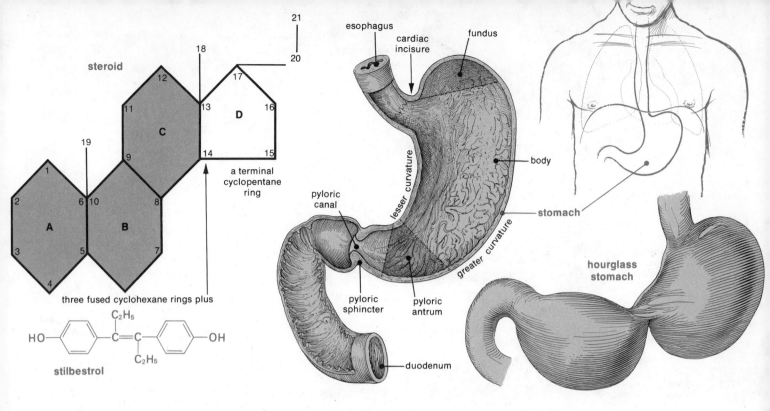

steroid

three fused cyclohexane rings plus

a terminal cyclopentane ring

stilbestrol

esophagus — cardiac incisure — fundus — body — stomach — hourglass stomach — lesser curvature — greater curvature — pyloric canal — pyloric sphincter — pyloric antrum — duodenum

stereotax'y. A method of inserting an electrode into a specific area of the brain by means of a stereotaxic apparatus; used to destroy nuclear masses and fiber tracts within the brain.

stereot'ropism. The movement of parts of an organism toward (positive stereotropism) or away from (negative stereotropism) a solid body with which it comes in contact.

ste'reotypy. The persistent mechanical repetition of certain movements or speech; common in schizophrenia.

oral s., see verbigeration.

ste'ric. Relating to stereochemistry.

ster'ile. 1. Incapable of reproducing. **2.** Free from bacteria or other microorganisms; also called aseptic.

steril'ity. Absence or nonfunctioning of the organs of reproduction.

steriliza'tion. 1. A treatment that deprives living organisms of the ability to reproduce. **2.** The process of destroying or removing all living microorganisms.

ster'ilizer. An apparatus for rendering anything germ-free.

ster'nal. Of or relating to the sternum (breastbone).

sternal'gia. 1. Pain in the sternum or sternal area; also called sternodynia. **2.** Angina pectoris.

sterno-. Combining form denoting sternum.

sternoclavic'ular. Relating to the sternum and the clavicle.

sternoclei'dal. Relating to the sternum and the clavicle.

sternocleidomas'toid. Relating to the sternum, clavicle, and mastoid process; denoting the muscle that has its origin and insertion on these structures.

sternocos'tal. Relating to the sternum and the ribs.

sternodyn'ia. See sternalgia.

sternot'omy. Cutting through the sternum.

ster'num. A long, flat bone forming the middle part of the anterior wall of the thoracic cage, articulating with the clavicles and the costal cartilages of the first seven pairs of ribs; also called breastbone.

ste'roid. 1. One of a family of chemical substances characterized by four interlocking rings of carbon atoms; included are the adrenal steroids, corticosteroids, the male and female sex hormones, and the D vitamins; cholesterol is one of the main building blocks for the other steroids; examples include aldosterone, androsterone, cholecalciferol, cholesterol, cortisol, cortisone, estradiol, estriol, progesterone, and testosterone. **2.** A shortened form for an adrenal corticosteroid or a synthetic compound with similar actions.

steroidogen'esis. The natural production of steroids.

steroid withdrawal syndrome. Weakness, nausea, fever, malaise, and slight hypotension experienced by persons upon withdrawal of steroid therapy to which they have been subjected for prolonged periods.

ster'ol. One of a group of unsaturated solid alcohols, a subdivision of the steroids, present in all animal and plant tissue except bacteria; the best known member of the group is cholesterol.

ster'tor. A snoring sound produced in breathing.

ster'torous. Characterized by snoring.

steth-, stetho-. Combining forms denoting chest.

stethal'gia. Pain in the chest.

steth'ograph. Apparatus used for recording the respiratory movements of the chest.

steth'oscope. An instrument used for listening to sounds produced within the body, especially respiratory and vascular sounds; originally designed by René Laënnec.

Stevens-Johnson syndrome. Erythema multiforme exudativum; see under erythema.

STH. Abbreviation for somatotropin (growth hormone).

sthenom'etry. The measurement of bodily or muscular strength.

stib'ialism. Poisoning with antimony.

stib'ium. Latin for antimony.

stiff-man syndrome. A chronic disorder of unknown cause marked by fluctuating muscular rigidity and spasm which progresses to generalized stiffness involving the extremities, neck, and trunk; associated with severe muscle pains and disability, dysphagia, and weight loss; also called Moersch-Woltmann syndrome.

stig'ma, *pl.* **stig'mata. 1.** Visible evidence characteristic of a disease (spot, blemish, symptom, sign, etc.). **2.** The pigmented eyespot of certain protozoa.

stilbes'trol. A colorless crystalline compound derived from stilbene; formerly used as an estrogen in humans and as a fattener for livestock; now thought to have carcinogenic properties; also called diethylstilbestrol.

still'birth. Death of the fetus while in the uterus.

still'born. Born dead.

sti'lus. A pencil-shaped medicinal preparation for external application.

stim'ulant. Anything that accelerates organic activity.

stimula'tion. 1. The process of exciting the body, or a part, to increased functional activity. **2.** The state of being stimulated.

photic s., the use of a flickering light to alter the pattern of the electroencephalogram.

stim'ulator. An agent that increases functional activity.

cerebellar electrical s., brain pacemaker; see under pacemaker.

long-acting thyroid s. (LATS), substance found in the blood of hyperthyroid patients, not elaborated in the pituitary gland, and having a prolonged stimulatory action on the thyroid gland.

stim'ulus, *pl.* **stim'uli. 1.** Anything causing a response. **2.** A stimulant; an agent or action that elicits a physiologic or psychologic activity.

conditioned s., a stimulus which prior to the procedure does not evoke the specific reflex or response under study.

unconditioned s., a stimulus which normally evokes the particular response under study.

sting. 1. To pierce the skin with a sharp-pointed organ or part, such as the ovipositor of a wasp, and deposit venom. **2.** The sharp transitory pain produced by stinging.

stip'pling. In histology, the staining of basophilic granules in a cell protoplasm when exposed to the action of a basic stain.

Ziemann's s., fine spots sometimes seen in red blood cells of persons with quartan malaria.

stir'rup. See stapes.

stitch. 1. A suture. **2.** A sudden, short sharp pain. **3.** The act of suturing.

stoichiom'etry. The study of the combining proportions (by weight and volume) of elements participating in a chemical reaction.

Stokes-Adams syndrome. See Adams-Stokes syndrome.

sto'ma. 1. Any small opening. **2.** The mouth or an artificial opening between two cavities or channels or between any cavity or tube and the exterior.

stom'ach. The enlarged, saclike portion of the digestive tract, between the esophagus and the small intestine, in which ingested food is acted on by the enzymes and hydrochloric acid of gastric juice, and then released spasmodically into the duodenum by gastric peristalsis; the stomach is entirely covered with peritoneum and normally has a capacity of about one quart.

hourglass s., one with a stricture at the midpoint.

leather-bottle s., see linitis plastica.

stom'achache. Pain in the stomach or abdomen.

sto'mal. Pertaining to a stoma or small aperture.

stomatal'gia. Pain in the mouth, occurring in varying degrees of severity as a result of injury or disease; also called stomatodynia.

stomat'ic. Relating to (a) the mouth; (b) an artificial opening.

stomati'tis. Inflammation of the mucous mem-

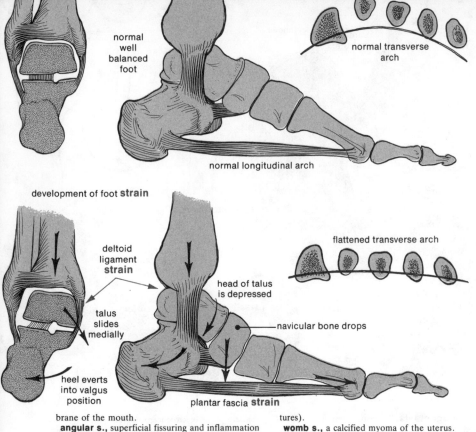

normal
well
balanced
foot

normal transverse arch

normal longitudinal arch

development of foot **strain**

deltoid
ligament
strain

talus
slides
medially

heel everts
into valgus
position

flattened transverse arch

head of talus
is depressed

navicular bone drops

plantar fascia **strain**

**divergent
strabismus**

brane of the mouth.

angular s., superficial fissuring and inflammation at the angles of the mouth.

aphthous s., ulcerative s., a chronically recurrent disease marked by the appearance of small, painful, single or multiple ulcers on the mucous membrane of the mouth; also called canker and canker sore.

gangrenous s., see noma.

herpetic s., a recurrent infection of the oral mucosa, caused by the herpes simplex virus, with painful vesicle and ulcer formation.

ulcerative s., see aphthous sore.

Vincent's s., necrotizing ulcerative gingivitis; see under gingivitis.

stomato-, stoma-. Combining forms relating to the mouth or an opening.

stomat'ocyte. Red blood cell in which the central area appears as a slit rather than a biconcave circular area.

stomatodyn'ia. See stomatalgia.

stomatol'ogy. The study of the structures, functions, and diseases of the mouth.

stomatomala'cia. Abnormal softening of structures in the mouth.

stomatomyco'sis. Fungal disease of the mouth.

stomatop'athy. Any disorder of the oral cavity.

stomatorrha'gia. Bleeding from any structure in the mouth.

stomode'um. A midline invagination or depression of the ectoderm of the embryo between the maxillary and mandibular processes which later develops into the mouth cavity.

-stomy. Combining form meaning surgical opening.

stone. An abnormal concretion usually composed of mineral salts and formed most frequently in the cavities of the body which serve as reservoirs for fluids; also called calculus.

bladder s., one lodged in the bladder; it may be either formed in the bladder or passed from the kidney or ureter; also called vesical calculus.

chalk s., see tophus.

dental s., α-hemihydrate; gypsum that has been calcined under steam pressure to 130°C; used for making casts and models of the oral cavity.

gallbladder s., gallstone.

kidney s., stone in the kidney, most commonly made up of uric acid, calcium oxalate, or calcium phosphate; also called renal calculus.

pulp s., the collection of calcified material in the pulp chamber of a tooth or a projection into the chamber from the cavity wall; also called pulp nodule and denticle.

tear s., dacryolith; one located in the lacrimal apparatus (tear-forming and tear-conducting structures).

womb s., a calcified myoma of the uterus.

stool. 1. A bowel movement. **2.** Feces.

tarry s., bloody stool, especially one in which blood can be grossly recognized.

stop'cock. A valve that stops or regulates the flow of a liquid through a tube or pipe.

storm, thyroid. Thyrotoxic crisis; see under crisis.

strabis'mal, strabis'mic. Relating to or afflicted with strabismus.

strabismom'eter. Instrument used to measure the angle of strabismus.

strabis'mus. A visual disorder in which one eye cannot focus with the other; also called heterotropia.

convergent s., one in which the eye deviates inward, toward the nose; also called cross-eye, internal strabismus, and esotropia.

divergent s., one in which the eye deviates outward; also called wall-eye, external strabismus, and exotropia.

strabot'omy. Division of one or more of the ocular muscles or their tendons in treatment of strabismus.

straight back syndrome. Loss of the physiologic dorsal kyphosis of the thoracic spine; this may result in the leftward shift of the heart or a "pancake" appearance; the close proximity of the outflow structures to the anterior chest wall results in an easily heard innocent systolic murmur.

strain. 1. To injure a part by misuse or excessive effort. **2.** The injury resulting from such activity. **3.** A group or stock of microorganisms, such as bacteria, made up of descendants of a single isolation in pure culture. **4.** An inherited trait.

S s., the strain of pneumococcus that has a slime capsule and causes pneumonia.

strait. A narrow space or passageway.

inferior pelvic s., pelvic plane of outlet; see under plane.

superior pelvic s., pelvic plane of inlet; see under plane.

strait jacket. See under jacket.

stramo'nium. 1. The dried leaves of jimsonweed (*Datura stramonium*), used in the treatment of asthma. **2.** Jimsonweed.

strang'le. To suffocate by compressing the trachea so as to prevent respiration; to choke.

strangula'tion. 1. Constriction of the air passages that interferes with or terminates normal breathing. **2.** Compression that cuts off the blood supply to a part, specifically to a loop of intestine.

stran'ury. Difficult, slow, painful urination.

strap. 1. A strip of adhesive plaster. **2.** To bind with adhesive plaster.

strat'ified. Arranged in layers.

strat'iform. Arranged in a series of superimposed layers.

stra'tum, *pl.* **stra'ta.** A layer, especially of differentiated tissue comprising one of several associated layers.

horizontal strata, portion of dorsal horn of gray matter of spinal cord; formerly called zona spongiosa.

malpighian s., stratum germinativum.

s. bacillare retinae, the neuroepithelial layer of rods and cones of the retina.

s. basale, the deepest (basal) layer of the endometrium (mucosa of the uterus) which undergoes only minimal changes during the menstrual cycle; the portion of the endometrium which is not sloughed off during menstruation; it contains the narrow terminal portion of the uterine glands.

s. basale epidermidis, the deepest (basal) layer of the epidermis consisting of columnar or high cuboidal cells arranged in a single row and resting on a thin basement membrane; usually contains granules of melanin pigment.

s. compactum, the innermost layer of the endometrium (mucosa of the uterus) containing the necks of the uterine glands and a rather compact layer of interglandular tissue.

s. corneum, the outermost horny keratinized layer of the epidermis, composed of flattened, dehydrated, nonnucleated epithelial cells; it is very thick in the palms and soles; also called corneum.

s. cylindricum, stratum basale epidermidis.

s. functionale, the thick part of the lining of the uterus (endometrium) which is sloughed off during menstruation; it consists of a compact layer and a spongy layer.

s. germinativum, the growing part of the epidermis containing several rows of cells undergoing mitosis; composed of a basal layer (stratum basale) and a spiny layer (stratum spinosum); also called malpighian layer.

s. granulosum epidermidis, the layer of epidermis between the stratum spinosum and the stratum lucidum composed of a few rows of flattened rhombic cells with their long axis parallel with the skin; thought to represent the transitional stage in the formation of soft keratin; the cells contain conspicuous granules of keratohyalin.

s. granulosum ovarii, the epithelial layer of granulosa (follicular) cells in the developing ovarian follicle, located between the zona pellucida surrounding the ovum and the glassy membrane.

s. lucidum, a narrow homogeneous layer of the epidermis between the stratum corneum and the stratum granulosum; it consists of a few rows of

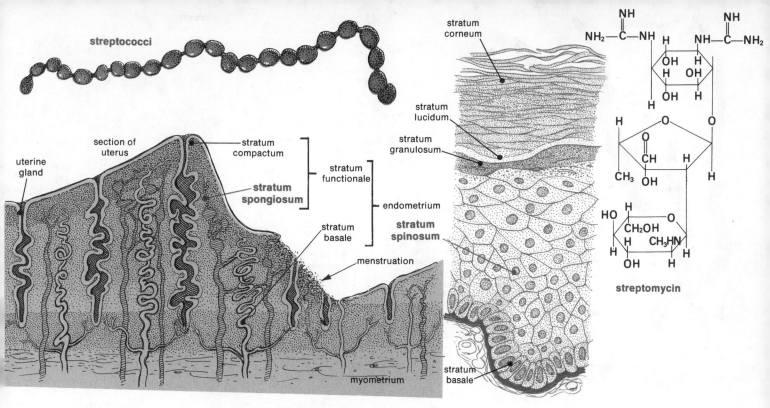

streptococci

stratum corneum

stratum lucidum

stratum granulosum

stratum spinosum

stratum basale

section of uterus

stratum compactum

stratum functionale

stratum **spongiosum**

endometrium

stratum basale

menstruation

uterine gland

myometrium

streptomycin

flattened clear cells containing a refractile substance (eleidin); nuclei and cell boundaries are not visible.

s. pigmenti retinae, the outer pigmented layer of the retina.

s. spinosum, the thick layer of the epidermis between the stratum basale and stratum granulosum, composed of irregular polyhedral cells with short cytoplasmic spines which may contain melanin; mitosis is frequent in this layer; also called prickle-cell layer.

s. spongiosum, the middle of three layers of the lining of the uterus (endometrium) containing the tortuous and dilated glands and a small amount of interglandular tissue; the layer is discharged at each menstrual flow and at the termination of pregnancy.

streak. A striation, line, or furrow.

angioid s.'s, brownish-red pigmented lines in the fundus of the eye, radiating from the disk and situated beneath the retinal vessels, due to degeneration of the lamina vitrea of the choroid; may be seen in pseudoxanthoma elasticum, osteitis deformans, and sickle-cell anemia.

germinal s., primitive streak.

Knapp's s.'s, pigmented streaks resembling blood vessels, seen occasionally in the retina following hemorrhage; also called Knapp's striae.

medullary s., the embryonic neural groove, the closure of which forms the primordium of the brain and spinal cord.

meningeal s., a congested streak, sometimes with petechial hemorrhage, occurring when the skin is scratched; may be seen in meningitis, when skin capillaries generally become unduly irritable; also called tache cérébrale.

primitive s., a midline narrow groove, with slightly bulging regions on either side, situated on the caudal end of the embryonic disk; site from which the mesodermal cells migrate from the surface to form the middle germ layer; clearly visible in a 15- to 16-day embryo and provides the earliest evidence of the cephalocaudal axis.

strephosymbo'lia. A perception disorder, occurring mainly in children, in which certain letters or words are seen reversed, as if in a mirror.

strep'itus. A sound heard on auscultation.

strepto-. Combining form meaning twisted, curved, or flexible.

Streptobacil'lus. A genus (family Bacteriodiaceae) of bacteria containing gram-negative rods; some species are pathogenic.

streptococ'cal. Relating to or caused by streptococcus.

streptococcem'ia. The presence of streptococci in the blood.

streptococ'ci. Plural of streptococcus.

streptococco'sis. Any infection with streptococci.

Streptococ'cus. A genus of gram-positive, round or ovoid bacteria (family Lactobacillaceae), pathogenic and/or nonpathogenic in man, occurring in pairs or chains; medically classified according to their hemolytic activity on blood agar as α-hemolytic streptococci, which produce a zone of incomplete hemolysis and green discoloration adjacent to the colony, β-hemolytic streptococci, which produce a clear zone of hemolysis around the colony, and γ-streptococci, which produce no hemolysis.

S. cremoris, nonpathogenic species isolated from raw milk and milk products; used as commercial starter in the manufacture of butter and cheese.

S. fecalis, an enterococcus normally found in the intestinal tract; a cause of subacute bacterial endocarditis.

S. lactis, a species which is the most common cause of the souring of milk.

S. pneumoniae, a rarely spherical species which causes lobar pneumonia and other acute pus-forming conditions such as middle ear infections and meningitis; formerly called *Diplococcus pneumoniae.*

S. pyogenes, a species which is the cause of several acute pyogenic (pus-forming) infections in man, such as scarlet fever, erysipelas, and sore throat.

S. salivarius, species found in saliva and throughout the intestinal tract; generally nonpathogenic but has been implicated in contributing to the formation of dental caries.

streptococ'cus, *pl.* **streptococ'ci.** Any member of the genus *Streptococcus.*

streptodermati'tis. Inflammation of the skin caused by streptococci.

streptodor'nase. Enzyme produced by hemolytic streptococci, capable of causing liquefaction of purulent exudates.

streptokin'ase. Enzyme present in hemolytic streptococci, capable of dissolving fibrin; used to dissolve blood clots and fibrinous adhesions.

streptol'ysin. A hemolysin produced by streptococci.

Streptomy'ces. A genus of bacteria (family Streptomycetacea) present in the soil; antibiotics have been obtained from cultures of some species.

S. antibioticus, species that yields actinomycin.

S. fradiae, species that yields neomycin.

S. griseus, species that yields streptomycin.

S. rimosus, species that yields oxytetracycline.

streptomy'cete. A member of the genus *Streptomyces.*

streptomy'cin. An antibiotic obtained from cultures of *Streptomyces griseus;* white granules or powder soluble in water, acid alcohol, and methyl alcohol; active against the tubercle bacillus, many gram-negative bacteria, and some gram-positive bacteria; excessive dosage leads to damage to the eighth cranial nerve, usually affecting the vestibular part first.

streptotricho'sis. Infection with bacteria of the genus formerly called *Streptothrix* but now classified in other genera, e.g., *Actinomyces, Nocardia, Streptobacillus.*

stress. 1. The internal force of a body generated to resist an external force that tends to deform it. **2.** In dentistry, pressure against the teeth and their attachments exceeding that produced by normal function. **3.** Abnormal conditions that tend to disrupt normal functions of the body or mind. **4.** An emotionally disrupting influence.

stress'breaker. An attachment in a removable partial denture that relieves the anchoring teeth of all or part of the pressure during mastication.

stretch'er. A canvas stretched over a frame, used to transport disabled or dead persons; also called litter.

stri'a, *pl.* **stri'ae.** A thin stripe or band, especially one of several that are more or less parallel.

s. atrophica, one of several glistening white bands in the skin of the abdomen, breasts, buttocks, and thighs, caused by overstretching and weakening of the elastic tissues; associated with pregnancy, obesity, rapid growth during puberty, Cushing's syndrome, and other conditions.

stri'ate, stri'ated. Marked by striae; striped.

stria'tion. 1. A stria. **2.** The state of having stria.

stric'ture. An abnormal narrowing of a tubular structure.

strid'ent. Harsh, shrill, or grating, as certain sounds heard on auscultation.

stri'dor. A harsh, shrill respiratory sound, as in acute laryngeal obstruction.

strid'ulous. Having a harsh, shrill sound.

strip. A streak.

Mees' s.'s., white strips on fingernails occurring in arsenic poisoning.

strip'ping. 1. Excision of a varicose vein of the leg. **2.** Milking; the removal of the contents of a tubular structure by gentle pressure.

strobi'la, *pl.* **strobi'lae. 1.** The linear collection of segments comprising the body of a tapeworm. **2.** The larva of a scyphozoan comprised of a series of individuals produced by transverse fission.

strob'iloid. Resembling the segmented body of a tapeworm.

strobolaryn'goscope. A type of stroboscope used to observe in detail the vibratory motion of the

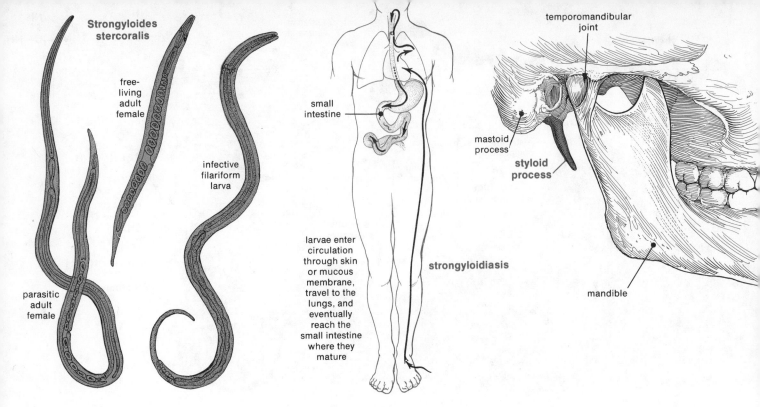

Strongyloides stercoralis

free-living adult female

infective filariform larva

parasitic adult female

small intestine

larvae enter circulation through skin or mucous membrane, travel to the lungs, and eventually reach the small intestine where they mature

strongyloidiasis

temporomandibular joint

mastoid process

styloid process

mandible

---

vocal cords.

stro′boscope. 1. An instrument used to observe moving objects by making them appear stationary through intermittently interrupted illumination. **2.** An electronic instrument that produces brief pulses of light at controllable frequency, used to alter electrical activity of the cerebral cortex.

stroke. Any sudden, severe attack or seizure.

  apoplectic s., see apoplexy.

  heat s., condition caused by excessive exposure to high temperatures, marked by high fever, dry skin, and in severe cases, coma.

  paralytic s., sudden paralysis caused by injury to the brain.

stro′muhr. Instrument used to measure the amount of blood flowing per unit of time through a blood vessel.

Strongyloi′des. A genus (class Nematoda) of intestinal parasites of herbivorous animals and man.

  S. stercoralis, a species which is the causative agent of strongyloidiasis of man.

strongyloidi′asis, strongyloido′sis. Parasitic infection caused by a nematode, *Stronglyloides stercoralis;* the threadlike worms enter the body through the skin or mucous membrane of the mouth, travel to the lungs, and eventually reach the small intestine where the female lays her eggs.

stro′ma. The framework of an organ, usually composed of connective tissue, which supports the functional elements or cells.

stron′tium. A soft, easily oxidized metallic element similar to calcium in chemical properties; symbol Sr, atomic number 38, atomic weight 87.62.

  s. 90, a radioactive isotope which emits a high energy beta particle and has a half-life of 28 years; a product of atom bomb blasts that constitutes an important fallout hazard, since it is incorporated into bone tissue upon absorption.

strophan′thin. A poisonous glycoside or mixture of glycosides resembling digitalis; used as a cardiac tonic.

Strophan′thus. A genus of African vines of the family Apocynaceae.

  S. gratus, species containing ouabain, a cardiac glycoside.

  S. kombe, species containing strophanthin, a cardiac glycoside.

struc′ture. The configuration of the component parts of an entity.

  brush heap s., the fibrils in a gel or hydrocolloid impression material.

  denture-supporting s., the tissues, teeth, and/or residual ridges that serve as support for removable dentures (partial or complete).

  fine s., see ultrastructure.

stru′ma. Goiter.

  Hashimoto's s., lymphocytic thyroiditis; see under thyroiditis.

  s. lymphomatosa, lymphocytic thyroiditis; see under thyroiditis.

  Riedel's s., see thyroiditis, Riedel's.

strumi′tis. Inflammation of the thyroid gland accompanied by swelling.

strych′nine. An extremely poisonous alkaloid, derived from seeds of *Strychnos nux-vomica* and possessing an intensely bitter taste; occasionally used as a stimulant for the central nervous system.

strych′ninism. A toxic condition resulting from excessive use of strychnine; also called chronic strychnine poisoning.

Strych′nos. A genus of tropical trees or shrubs (family Loganiaceae) that yield the alkaloids strychnine, curare, ignatia, and brucine.

STS. Abbreviation for serologic test for syphilis.

study. The pursuit and acquisition of information.

  bioavailability s., see bioequivalence study.

  bioequivalence s., the comparison of two or more different formulations of the same parent drug, one of which is an acceptable standard; also called bioavailability study.

  blind s., a study in which the patient is not aware of the type of medication being administered.

  double blind s., a study in which neither the patient nor the individual in contact with the patient is cognizant of the type of medication being administered in order to obviate bias of observation.

  longitudinal s., a study of a defined cohort (group of individuals having a statistical factor in common) over a protracted period of time, in contrast to a cross-sectional study examining a cohort at a particular time.

stump. 1. The extremity of a limb left after amputation. **2.** The pedicle remaining after removal of the tumor which was attached to it.

stun. To daze, stupefy, or render senseless, as by a blow or other force.

stupe. A hot compress applied externally as a counterirritant; prepared by wringing out a cloth of hot water; a medicament is usually added to the water or directly to the cloth.

stupefa′cient. 1. Causing stupor. **2.** Any agent that causes stupor, as a narcotic.

stupefac′tion. The act of inducing stupor or narcosis.

stu′pefy. To make senseless; to induce a stupor.

stu′por. A state of semiconsciousness.

stu′porous. In a semiconscious state.

Sturge-Weber syndrome. An uncommon congenital condition marked by localized atrophy and calcification of the cerebral cortex and an ipsilateral port-wine hemangioma on the face; often associated with mental retardation; attributed to faulty development of certain mesodermal and ectodermal elements.

stut′tering. A speech disorder characterized by involuntary spasmodic hesitation and repetition of sounds.

St. Vitus' dance. Acute chorea; see under chorea.

stye, sty. See hordeolum.

sty′let, sty′lette, style. A wire inserted into the lumen of a flexible catheter in order to stiffen it during passage.

sty′liform. Styloid; having the shape of a peg.

stylo-. Combining form meaning a point.

styloglos′sus. Relating to the styloid process of the temporal bone and the tongue; the term is given to certain structures, as a muscle extending between the tongue and the process.

sty′loid. Shaped like a peg; denoting certain bony processes; also called styliform.

stylomas′toid. Relating to the styloid and mastoid processes of the temporal bone.

stylostix′is. Acupuncture.

sty′lus. A sharply pointed instrument used in drawing or as the marking instrument on certain recorders.

stype. A tampon; a plug or pledget of absorbent material.

styp′sis. 1. The action of an astringent or hemostatic agent. **2.** The application of an astringent.

styp′tic. An agent that contracts the tissues; an astringent.

sub-. Prefix meaning under or less than.

subacro′mial. Situated beneath the acromion process.

subacute′. Denoting the intensity of a disease, somewhat between acute and chronic.

subalimenta′tion. Insufficient nourishment.

subarach′noid. Beneath the arachnoid membrane of the brain or spinal cord.

subar′cuate. Slightly bowed.

subare′olar. Beneath the areola, particularly of the nipple.

subatom′ic. Relating to the components of the atom.

subau′ral. Below the ear.

subcap′sular. Situated beneath a capsule.

subcar′bonate. Any basic carbonate such as bismuth subcarbonate; a complex of a base and its carbonate.

subcartilag′inous. 1. Beneath a cartilage. **2.** Partly cartilaginous.

subchon′dral. Beneath or just under the cartilages of the ribs.

subcla′vian. 1. Situated beneath the clavicle. **2.**

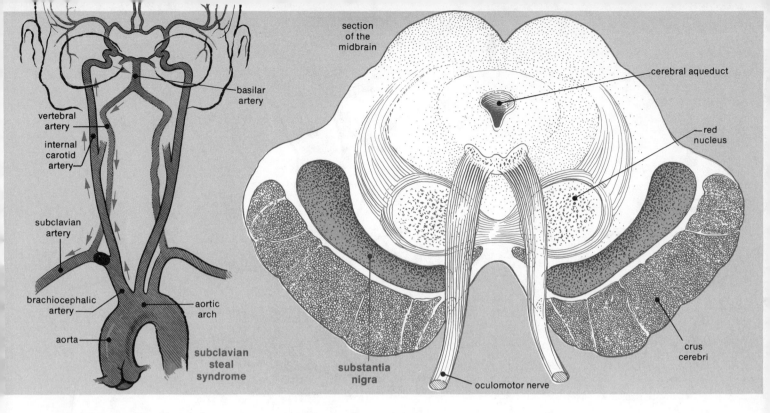

section of the midbrain

cerebral aqueduct

red nucleus

basilar artery

vertebral artery

internal carotid artery

subclavian artery

brachiocephalic artery

aorta

aortic arch

subclavian steal syndrome

crus cerebri

substantia nigra

oculomotor nerve

Relating to the subclavian artery.

subclavian steal syndrome. Reduced blood supply of the brain stem caused by obstruction of the subclavian artery proximal to the origin of the vertebral artery; blood flow through the vertebral artery is reversed and diverted from the brainstem to the arm; thus the subclavian "steals" cerebral blood.

subclavic′ular. Situated beneath the clavicle (collarbone).

subclin′ical. Denoting the phase of a disease prior to the manifestation of symptoms.

subconjuncti′val. Under the conjunctiva of the eye.

subcon′scious. 1. Less than fully conscious. **2.** In psychology, not fully in conscious awareness but easily accessible; distinguished from unconscious, which implies inaccessibility to awareness.

subcor′neal. Beneath or just under the stratum corneum of the skin.

subcor′tex. The portion of an organ immediately below the cortex, especially below the cerebral cortex.

subcos′tal. Beneath the ribs.

subcra′nial. Below the skull.

sub′culture. A secondary culture of microorganisms, derived by inoculation from the primary culture.

subcuta′neous. Located beneath the skin; also called hypodermic.

subcutic′ular. Below the epidermis.

subcu′tis. The loose fibrous tissue directly below the skin; also called tela subcutanea.

subder′mic. Subcutaneous.

subdiaphragmat′ic. Located beneath the diaphragm; also called subphrenic.

subdu′ral. Located beneath the dura mater.

subendocar′dial. Under the endocardium.

subfam′ily. A taxonomic category between a family and a tribe.

subfertil′ity. Less than normal ability, in either the male or the female, to accomplish fertilization.

subge′nus. A taxonomic classification ranking between a genus and a species.

subgin′gival. At a level below the gingival margin.

subglot′tic. Situated or occurring beneath the glottic opening between the vocal cords.

subhepat′ic. Situated below the liver.

subin′timal. Under the intima (of a vessel).

subinvolu′tion. Failure of an organ to return to its normal size, as when the uterus remains abnormally large after childbirth.

subja′cent. Situated beneath or below.

sub′ject. 1. A person or animal under treatment or

experimentation. **2.** A cadaver used for dissection.

subjec′tive. Perceived by the patient only and not by the examiner; e.g., the symptom of pain or a sense of fatigue or malaise.

subla′tion. Detachment of a bodily part.

suble′thal. Slightly less than lethal.

sub′limate. 1. To convert a solid into a gas and back into a solid without passing through the liquid stage. **2.** A substance that has been subjected to sublimation. **3.** In psychoanalysis, to divert consciously unacceptable, instinctive drives into personally and socially acceptable channels; an unconscious process.

sublima′tion. 1. The conversion of a solid directly into vapor and then back into the solid state without passing through the intermediate liquid stage. **2.** The unconscious process of changing instinctive impulses which may be socially unacceptable into personally and socially acceptable channels.

sublim′inal. Below the level of sensory perception.

subli′mis. Latin for superficial.

sublin′gual. Located beneath the tongue.

subluxa′tion. Partial dislocation.

s. of lens, incomplete dislocation of the lens of the eye.

submandib′ular. Situated below the lower jaw.

submax′illary. Located beneath the upper jaw.

submen′tal. Situated beneath the chin.

submicroscop′ic. Too small to be seen through an ordinary light microscope.

submuco′sa. The layer of tissue located beneath the mucous membrane.

subnor′mal. Less than normal.

suboccip′ital. Situated below the occipital bone or the back of the head (occiput).

subor′bital. Located beneath the orbit.

sub′order. A taxonomic classification ranking between an order and a family.

subox′ide. An oxide of an element (e.g., carbon suboxide) containing the smallest proportion of oxygen. Cf protoxide.

sub′phylum. A taxonomic classification ranking between a phylum and a class.

subscap′ular. Located beneath or below the scapula (shoulder blade).

subscle′ral. Beneath the sclera.

subscrip′tion. The part of a pharmaceutical prescription that contains directions to the pharmacist for the compounding of ingredients, or dispensing of medication, in a form suitable for use by the patient; it indicates the class of preparation (e.g., capsules) and the number of doses (e.g., 20). See also superscription, inscription, and signature.

subse′rous. Located beneath a serous membrane.

sub′stage. An attachment to a microscope, situated beneath the stage, by means of which accessories (mirror, diaphragm, condenser, or prism) are held in place.

sub′stance. Matter; material.

gray s., the gray portion of the brain and spinal cord composed of cell bodies; also called substantia grisea and gray matter.

reticular s., (1) a mass of filaments seen in immature red blood cells after vital staining; also called alpha substance and filar mass; (2) see formation, reticular.

Rolando's s., substantia gelatinosa of Rolando.

slow-reacting s. (SRS SRS-A), substance released in anaphylactic shock, formed through the interaction of antigen with sensitized cells; produces a slow prolonged contraction of smooth muscle.

specific capsular s., a polysaccharide present in the capsule of many bacteria, believed to have a role in the transport of nutrients and protection against noxious agents; also called specific soluble substance.

specific soluble s., see specific capsular substance.

white s., the white portion of the brain and spinal cord consisting of nerve fibers; also called substantia alba and white matter.

substan′tia. Latin for substance.

s. adamantina, tooth enamel.

s. alba, see substance, white.

s. eburnea, the dentine of teeth.

s. gelatinosa of Rolando, a mass of translucent gelatinous tissue, containing small nerve cells, on the posterior gray column of the spinal cord; appearing in cross-section as a crescentic cap over the horn.

s. grisea, see substance, gray.

s. nigra, a layer of gray substance in the cerebral peduncles containing deeply pigmented nerve cells; it extends from the upper border of the pons into the subthalamic region; on cross-section it appears crescentic; also called black substance and intercalatum.

subster′nal. Situated beneath the sternum (breastbone).

substitu′tion. 1. In chemistry, the replacement of one or more atoms of one element by those of another. **2.** An unconscious mechanism by which an unacceptable goal or emotion is replaced by a more acceptable one.

sub′strate. Any substance upon which an enzyme or ferment acts.

substra′tum. Any layer of tissue located beneath.

sub′structure. A structure or a dental appliance

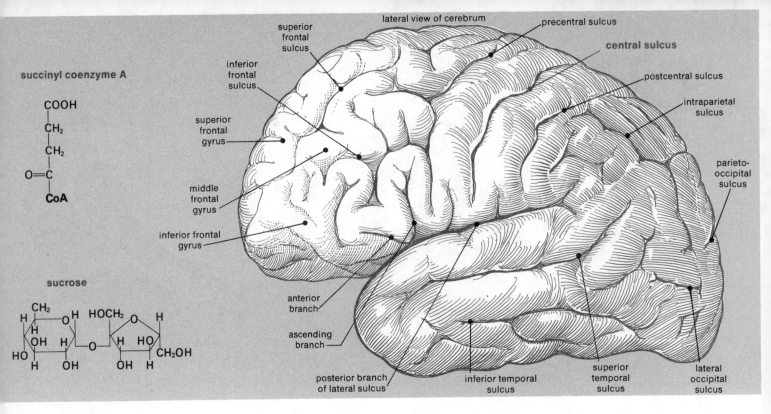

succinyl coenzyme A

COOH
|
CH$_2$
|
CH$_2$
|
O=C
|
CoA

sucrose

lateral view of cerebrum

superior frontal sulcus — precentral sulcus — **central sulcus** — postcentral sulcus — intraparietal sulcus — parieto-occipital sulcus — inferior frontal sulcus — superior frontal gyrus — middle frontal gyrus — inferior frontal gyrus — anterior branch — ascending branch — posterior branch of lateral sulcus — inferior temporal sulcus — superior temporal sulcus — lateral occipital sulcus

---

which is partly beneath the surface.

subthalam′ic. 1. Situated beneath the thalamus. **2.** Relating to the subthalamus.

subthal′amus. The portion of the diencephalon lying immediately beneath the thalamus, between the tegmentum of the midbrain and the dorsal thalamus.

subun′gual. Beneath the nail of a toe or finger; also called hyponychial.

sub′unit. A secondary unit or part of a more comprehensive unit.

subure′thral. Located beneath the urethra.

subvir′ile. Characterized by deficient potency or masculine vigor; lacking in virility.

subvit′rinal. Beneath the vitreous body.

subvolu′tion. The operative procedure of turning over a flap of mucous membrane to prevent adhesion.

suc′cagogue. 1. Stimulating glandular secretion. **2.** An agent having such property.

succeda′neum. A substitute, as the permanent teeth that replace the deciduous teeth, or a drug with properties similar to those of another.

succentu′riate. Supplemental; accessory.

suc′cinate. A salt of succinic acid.

succinic acid. An intermediate in the metabolism of tricarboxylic acid.

succinylcholine chloride. Choline chloride succinate, a muscle-relaxant drug used as an anesthetic.

succinyl coenzyme A (succinyl-CoA). The condensation product of succinic acid and coenzyme A.

succorrhe′a. An excessive flow of a digestive fluid, such as saliva or gastric juice.

suc′cus, *pl.* **suc′ci. 1.** Juice. **2.** The fluid component of tissues. **3.** A fluid secretion, especially of the digestive tract.

s. entericus, intestinal juice.

succus′sion. The act of shaking the body as a diagnostic procedure; a splashing sound is produced in the presence of fluid and air in a body cavity.

suck. 1. To draw fluid into the mouth. **2.** To draw fluid into a tube by establishing a partial vacuum.

su′crase. See invertase.

su′crose. A disaccharide, C$_{12}$H$_{22}$O$_{11}$, which on hydrolysis yields glucose and fructose (monosaccharides); obtained chiefly from sugar cane, sugar beet, and maple; used as a sweetener and preservative; also called cane sugar and saccharose.

suc′tion. The process of aspirating or sucking.

suda′men, *pl.* **sudam′ina.** A minute vesicle formed by retention of sweat.

Sudan. Name given to a series of histologic dyes; see under stain.

sudanophil′ia. Affinity for Sudan stain.

suda′tion. Sweating.

sudden infant death syndrome (SIDS). The sudden death of a baby caused by a disease which can be neither predicted nor prevented and that displays no specific symptoms; it is a major cause of death in infants after the first month of life; also called crib death.

Sudeck's atrophy. See Sudeck's syndrome.

Sudeck's syndrome. Bone atrophy usually of the hands, wrists, or feet following minor injuries; associated with painful swelling of the overlying soft tissue; thought to be due to abnormal vasomotor regulation; also called Sudeck's atrophy.

sudomo′tor. Stimulating sweat glands.

su′dor. Perspiration.

sud′oral. Relating to perspiration.

sudore′sis. Profuse perspiration.

sudorif′erous. Producing or carrying perspiration.

sudorif′ic. Causing perspiration; also called diaphoretic and sudoriferous.

sudorip′arous. Producing perspiration.

su′et. The fat within the abdomen or around the kidneys of sheep and cattle.

prepared s., purified suet from sheep, used in pharmaceutical ointments.

suf′focate. To impede respiration; to choke.

suffu′sion. 1. Pouring of a fluid over the body. **2.** Flushing of the skin. **3.** Extravasation or spreading of a bodily fluid, such as blood, into surrounding tissues.

sugar. A type of carbohydrate having a sweet taste.

amino s., hexosamine; sugar containing an amino group; e.g., glucosamine.

blood s., glucose.

cane s., see sucrose.

deoxy s., a sugar that contains fewer atoms of oxygen than of carbon; e.g., deoxyribose.

fruit s., see fructose.

grape s., glucose.

hexose s., a simple sugar having six carbon atoms per molecule.

invert s., a mixture of equal parts of glucose and fructose, used in solution as a parenteral nutrient; also called invertose.

malt s., see maltose.

milk s., see lactose.

pentose s., one having five carbon atoms per molecule.

sugges′tion. 1. In psychiatry, the technique by which a therapist induces an idea or attitude which is adopted by the patient without questioning. **2.** Any idea or attitude so induced.

su′icide. 1. The act of taking one's own life voluntarily and intentionally. **2.** One who commits such an act.

suicidol′ogy. The study of the nature, causes, and control of suicide.

suigen′derism. The natural nonerotic relationship between members of the same sex, as in a child's interest in associating with others of his own gender.

suit. An outer garment designed to be worn under particular environmental conditions.

antiblackout s., anti-G suit.

anti-G s., a flight garment worn by pilots to increase their ability to withstand the effects of high acceleration (gravitational force or G) by exerting pressure on parts of the body below the chest; bladders (balloons) in the suit expand to apply external pressure to the abdomen and lower extremities during positive G maneuvers in flight, thereby preventing the pooling of blood in those areas.

G-suit, anti-G suit.

sul′cate, sul′cated. Furrowed.

sul′culus, *pl.* **sul′culi.** A small groove.

sul′cus. A groove or furrow.

alveololabial s., the oral sulcus between the anterior alveolar bone and the lips.

alveololingual s., the sulcus at the floor of the mouth between the mandibular alveolar bone and the tongue.

arterial sulci, grooves on the interior surface of the skull which house the meningeal arteries; also called arterial grooves.

calcarine s., a deep arched fissure on the medial surface of the occipital lobe; it divides the cuneus from the lingual gyrus; also called calcarine fissure.

central s., central fissure; a deep sulcus between the parietal and frontal lobes of the brain.

cingulate s., a sulcus on the medial surface of each cerebral hemisphere from the front of the corpus callosum to a point just behind the central sulcus.

collateral s., a long sagittal sulcus on the inferior surface of each cerebral hemisphere; it separates the fusiform gyrus from the hippocampal and lingual gyri.

coronary s., a sulcus encircling the external surface of the heart between the atria and ventricles, and occupied by arterial and venous vessels; also called atrioventricular groove.

dorsal lateral s., a shallow longitudinal sulcus on either side of the dorsal median sulcus of the spinal cord; it marks the line of entrance of the posterior nerve roots.

dorsal median s., a shallow sulcus in the median line of the posterior surface of the spinal cord.

gingival s., the shallow space or groove between

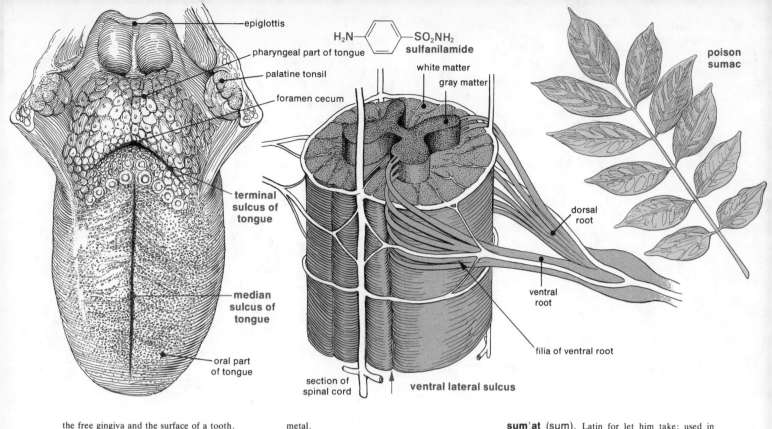

epiglottis
pharyngeal part of tongue
palatine tonsil
foramen cecum
terminal sulcus of tongue
median sulcus of tongue
oral part of tongue

H₂N— —SO₂NH₂
sulfanilamide

white matter
gray matter
dorsal root
ventral root
filia of ventral root
section of spinal cord
ventral lateral sulcus

poison sumac

---

the free gingiva and the surface of a tooth.

horizontal s. of cerebellum, horizontal fissure of cerebellum; see under fissure.

median s. of tongue, a slight, median, longitudinal depression running forward on the dorsal surface of the tongue from the foramen cecum; it divides the tongue into symmetrical halves.

occlusal s., a sulcus on the occlusal surface of a tooth.

parietooccipital s., a sulcus on the medial surface of the occipital region of each cerebral hemisphere extending upward from the calcarine sulcus; it separates the occipital lobe from the parietal lobe.

postcentral s., a sulcus on the lateral surface of the parietal lobe of the cerebrum; it separates the postcentral gyrus from the remainder of the parietal lobe.

precentral s., an interrupted sulcus on the lateral surface of the frontal lobe, anterior and somewhat parallel to the central sulcus.

terminal s. of tongue, a shallow V-shaped groove on the tongue running laterally and forward from the foramen cecum; it marks the separation between the oral and pharyngeal parts of the tongue; also called sulcus terminalis.

ventral lateral s., an indistinct sulcus on either side of the ventral median fissure of the spinal cord, marking the line of exit of the ventral nerve roots.

sulf-. see sulfo-.

sul'fa. Denoting any of the sulfa drugs chemically similar to sulfonamide, such as sulfisoxazole and sulfadiazine.

sulfadi'azine. One of a group of antibacterial compounds commonly known as sulfa drugs (sulfonamides); occurs as a white or yellowish odorless powder soluble in water.

sulfamer'azine. An antibacterial compound of the sulfonamide group (sulfa drugs); commonly used in mixtures with two other sulfonamides.

sulfameth'azine. An antibacterial drug of the sulfonamide group, usually given in combination with sulfadiazine and sulfamerazine.

sulfanil'amide. A potent antibacterial crystalline compound, $C_6H_8N_2SO_2$; first of the sulfonamides discovered and used in the treatment of bacterial infections.

sul'fate. A salt of sulfuric acid; a compound containing the group SO_4.

sulfhemoglo'bin. A compound derived from the action of hydrogen sulfide on hemoglobin; also called sulfmethemoglobin.

sulfhemoglobine'mia. Condition marked by persistent cyanosis, caused by the presence of sulfhemoglobin in the blood.

sul'fide. A compound of bivalent sulfur with a metal.

sulfisox'azole. A sulfonamide (sulfa drug) used chiefly in the treatment of bacterial infections of the urinary tract; Gantrisin®.

sul'fite. A salt of sulfurous acid.

sulfmethemoglo'bin. Compound formed by the combination of sulfide with the ferric ion of methemoglobin.

sulfo-, sulf-. Combining forms indicating the presence of a sulfur atom in the compound. The spelling sulph- is no longer used.

sulfobromophthalein sodium (BSP). A crystalline powder, soluble in water and used in testing liver function; Bromsulphalein®.

sulfon'amides. General term for a group of antibacterial drugs containing the sulfanilamide group; commonly known as sulfa drugs.

sul'fonate. 1. A salt of sulfonic acid. **2.** To treat with sulfonic acid.

sul'fone. Any of various compounds containing the radical SO_2 and carbon.

sulfon'ic acid. Any of various acids containing one or more sulfonic groups ($-SO_3H$).

sulfonylurea compounds. Derivative compounds of isopropylthiodiazylsulfanilamide; because of their hypoglycemic action, they are used in the treatment of certain cases of diabetes mellitus; also called sulfonylureas.

sulfosalicylic acid. A soluble solid, $C_6H_3(OH)\cdot(COOH)\cdot SO_3H$, used as a reagent for albumin and ferric ion.

sul'fur. A pale yellow nonmetallic element, symbol S, atomic number 16, atomic weight 32.06; used in the preparation of pharmaceuticals and insecticides.

sulfur-35 (^{35}S). A radioactive sulfur isotope; a β-emitter with a half-life of 87.1 days; used as a tracer in studying protein systems, since it can be taken up by proteins by way of the sulfur-containing amino acids.

sulfur'ic. Containing sulfur, especially with valence 6.

sulfuric acid. A heavy, oily, highly corrosive liquid, H_2SO_4; also called oil of vitriol.

sul'furize. To combine with sulfur.

sul'furous. 1. Containing or derived from sulfur; denoting compounds of sulfur with a low valence (+4). **2.** Having the characteristics of sulfur.

sulfurous acid. A solution of sulfur dioxide, H_2SO_3; used as a disinfectant and bleaching agent.

sum. Abbreviation for the Latin terms *sumat, sumendum.*

su'mac, shu'mac. Any of various plant species of the genus *Rhus;* some cause an acute itching lesion shortly after contact.

swamp s., poison sumac.

sum'at (sum). Latin for let him take; used in prescription writing.

sumen'dum (sum). Latin for to be taken; used in prescription writing.

summa'tion. 1. Totality. **2.** The quality of two or more drugs whereby their combined effects are equal to the sum of their individual effects.

s. of stimuli, muscular or neural effects produced by the frequent repetition of slight stimuli, one of which alone might not excite a response.

sun'burn. an inflammation or blistering of the skin caused by excessive exposure to ultraviolet rays of the sun.

sun'stroke. A state of extreme prostration and collapse caused by prolonged exposure to intense sunlight.

super-. Prefix indicating (a) a placement above or superior; (b) excess.

superacid'ity. An excess of acid beyond the normal; particularly increased acidity of the gastric juice; also called hyperacidity.

superacute'. Extremely acute; said of a disease.

superalimenta'tion. The therapeutic administration of nutrients in excess of the patient's nutritional requirements for the treatment of certain wasting diseases.

superalkalin'ity. Excessive alkalinity beyond the normal; also called hyperalkalescence.

supercil'iary. Relating to or located in the area of the eyebrow.

supercil'ium. The eyebrow.

supere'go. In psychoanalytical theory, the part of the personality structure associated with ethics and standards formed during the individual's early life through identification with important persons, particularly his parents; the conscience.

superexcita'tion. Excessive stimulation.

superfam'ily. A taxonomic category between an order and a family.

superfat'ted. Containing additional fat; said of certain soaps.

superfecunda'tion. The impregnation of two or more ova, liberated at the same ovulation, by successive coital acts.

superfe'male. Nonscientific term for metafemale.

superficial. 1. On, near, or affecting the surface, as a wound. **2.** Shallow, not thorough.

superinfec'tion. Appearance of a new infectious agent complicating an infection already under treatment.

supe'rior. The upper surface of an organ; located higher; toward the head; also called cephalic.

superior cerebellar artery syndrome. Syndrome occurring in occlusion of the superior cere-

sulcus | superior cerebellar artery syndrome

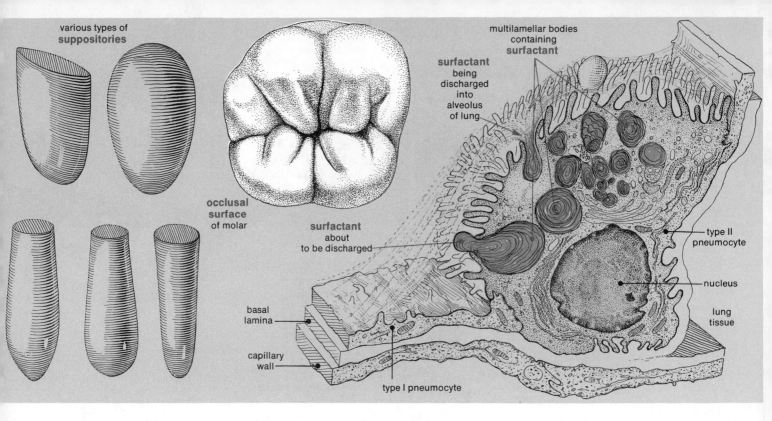

various types of
suppositories

**occlusal
surface** of molar

multilamellar bodies
containing
surfactant

surfactant
being
discharged
into
alveolus
of lung

surfactant
about
to be discharged

type II
pneumocyte

nucleus

lung
tissue

basal
lamina

capillary
wall

type I pneumocyte

---

bellar artery; consists of loss of pain and temperature sensations on the side of the face and body opposite to that of the lesion, with incoordination in executing skilled movements.

superior pulmonary sulcus syndrome. See Pancoast's syndrome.

superior vena cava syndrome. Edema of the face, neck, and/or upper arms caused by obstruction of the superior vena cava, usually by lung cancer or lymphoma invading the mediastinum.

su´permale. Nonscientific term for metamale.

superna´tant. Floating on a surface; denoting the liquid floating above a precipitate.

su´pernate. Colloquial term for supernatant fluid.

supernu´merary. 1. Accessory. **2.** Exceeding a normal or fixed number.

supersat´urate. To add a substance beyond saturation.

superscrip´tion. The part of the pharmaceutical prescription that directs the pharmacist to take the drugs listed to prepare the medication; indicated by the symbol R_x (derived from the Latin term *recipe*, take). See also inscription, subscription, and signature.

superson´ic. 1. Having a frequency above the level of audibility of the human ear. **2.** Of or relating to speeds greater than the speed of sound in air.

supervol´tage. A very high electromotive force, from 10 to 50 million electron volts; used in radiotherapy.

supina´tion. 1. The act of lying on the back. **2.** Rotation of the forearm so that the palm of the hand is turned forward or upward.

su´pinator. A muscle that supinates the forearm.

supin´e. Lying on the back.

support´. A device for holding a part in position.

suppos´itory. A solid medication designed for introduction into and melting within a body cavity other than the mouth.

suppres´sion. 1. In psychoanalysis, the conscious exclusion from awareness of painful memories or feelings, as distinguished from repression, which is unconscious. **2.** The cessation of a secretion; contrasted with retention, in which secretion occurs without discharge from the body.

suppura´tion. The production and discharge of pus.

sup´purative. Pus-forming.

supra-. Prefix meaning above.

supra-a´nal. Situated above the anus.

suprabuc´cal. Above the cheek.

supracho´roid. The outer layer of the vascular (choroid) coat of the eye, consisting chiefly of pigmented, loose, connective tissue.

supraclavic´ular. Located above a clavicle (col-

larbone).

supracon´dylar, supracon´dyloid. Situated above a condyle.

supracos´tal. Located above or over the ribs.

supradiaphragmat´ic. Located above the diaphragm.

supraduc´tion. In vertical divergence testing, upward movement of one eye when an ophthalmic prism is placed base down before it.

suprahepat´ic. Located above the liver.

suprahy´oid. Located above the hyoid bone.

suprain´guinal. Located above the groin.

supralim´inal. Above the threshold of sensory perception.

supralum´bar. Located above the lumbar region.

supramandib´ular. Located above the mandible (lower jaw).

supramen´tal. Above the chin.

supranu´clear. Situated above a nucleus.

supraor´bital. Located above the orbit.

suprapub´ic. Located above the pubic arch.

supraren´al. 1. Situated above or over the kidney. **2.** Pertaining to the adrenal (suprarenal) gland.

suprascap´ular. Situated above or in the upper part of the scapula (shoulder blade).

suprasel´lar. Above the sella turcica of the sphenoid bone.

supraspi´nal. Located above or over a spine or spinal column.

supraspinatus syndrome. Pain and tenderness over the supraspinatus tendon upon abduction of the arm.

supraspi´nous. Situated above a spine, especially those of the vertebrae.

supraster´nal. Located above the sternum (breastbone).

supratympan´ic. Above the middle ear.

supraventric´ular. Above the ventricles.

supraver´gence. The upward movement of one eye while the other remains stationary; also called sursumvergence.

supraver´sion. 1. Condition in which a tooth is abnormally elongated. **2.** The upward movement of both eyes; also called sursumversion.

su´ra. Latin for the calf of the leg.

sur´face. The outer boundary of an object.

buccal s., the surface of premolars and molars facing the cheek.

distal s., (1) the surface of a structure which is farther from a point of reference; (2) the surface of a tooth most distant from the median line.

dorsal s., (1) the surface of a structure that is directed toward the back of the human body; (2) the back of the human body.

facial s., the combined buccal and labial surfaces

of anterior teeth.

incisal s., the cutting surface of incisors and cuspids.

labial s., the surface of incisors and cuspids facing the lips.

lingual s., the surface of a tooth facing the tongue.

mesial s., the proximal surface of a tooth facing the median line.

occlusal s., the grinding surface of a posterior tooth which comes in contact with one in the opposite jaw during occlusion.

proximal s., (1) one that is nearer to a point of reference; (2) the surface of a tooth that faces an adjoining tooth in the same dental arch.

ventral s., (1) the anterior or abdominal surface of the human body; (2) the surface of a structure that is directed toward the anterior side of the human body.

surface-active. Altering the surface of a liquid, usually by reducing the surface tension.

surfac´tant. A surface-active lipoprotein that normally serves to decrease the surface tension of fluids within the alveoli of the lungs, thus permitting the pulmonary tissues to expand during inspiration.

sur´geon. A health practitioner who specializes in surgery.

dental s., a dentist.

house s., a resident training in surgery in a hospital who acts under the orders of the attending surgeon.

oral s., a dental specialist who deals with the diagnosis and the surgical and adjunctive treatment of diseases, injuries, and defects of the jaws and associated structures.

Surgeon General. The chief medical officer in the United States Army, Air Force, or Public Health Service; although the chief medical officer in the Navy is referred to as the Surgeon General, he is more properly called the Chief of the Bureau of Medicine and Surgery.

sur´gery. The treatment of disease, injury, or deformity by means of manual and instrumental operations.

dental s., dentistry.

open heart s., surgical correction of defects of the heart's interior through direct visualization.

oral s., the branch of dentistry dealing with the surgical treatment of disorders of the oral cavity.

orthopedic s., the branch of surgery specializing in the treatment of injuries and deformities of bones and chronic joint diseases.

plastic s., surgery for the repair of physical defects or for the replacement of tissues lost through injury.

sur´rogate. 1. A person who substitutes for an-

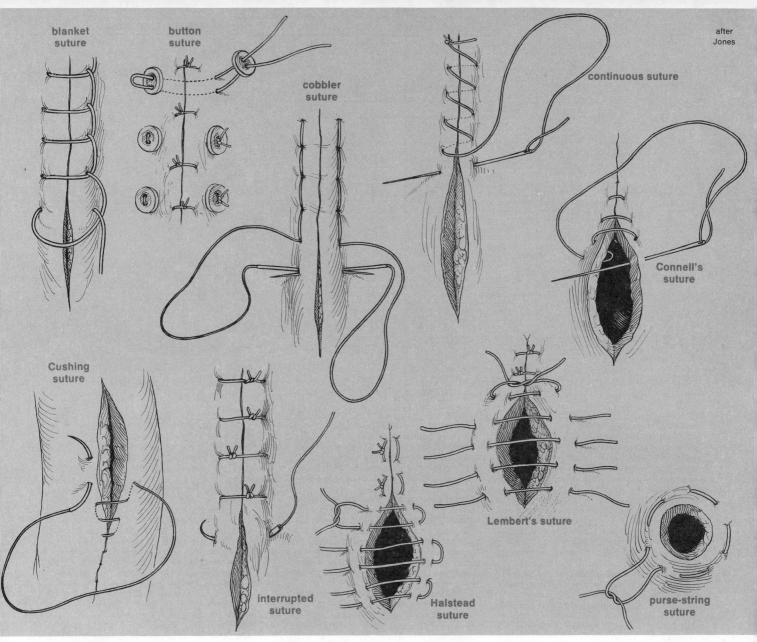

blanket suture

button suture

cobbler suture

continuous suture

after Jones

Connell's suture

Cushing suture

interrupted suture

Halstead suture

Lembert's suture

purse-string suture

other. **2.** In psychiatry, usually refers to a person who replaces a parent in the feelings of the patient; e.g., father-surrogate.

survey'ing. In dentistry, studying the relative position of teeth and associated structures before designing a removable partial denture, in order to select a path of insertion and removal that will encounter the least interference.

susceptibil'ity. 1. The condition or quality of being sensitive or predisposed, as to a familial disease. **2.** The state of lacking bodily resistance to disease.

suscep'tible. 1. Capable of being influenced or affected. **2.** Unresistant or not immune to an infectious disease.

sus'citate. To stimulate; to excite; to arouse to increased activity.

suspen'sion. 1. The lifting of a bodily part from a support from which it is allowed to hang in order to subject it to traction. **2.** A noncolloidal dispersion of solid particles in a liquid.

suspen'sory. 1. A structure, such as a ligament or muscle, that aids in keeping an organ or part in place. **2.** A support for a dependent bodily part, such as a pouch attached to a body belt that provides support for the scrotum (used to relieve discomfort from such conditions as orchitis, varicocele, or epididymitis, or from scrotal surgery).

sustentac'ular. Supporting.

sustentac'ulum. A supporting structure.

  s. lienis, the phrenicocolic ligament which supports the left flexure of the colon, and upon which rests the base of the spleen (lien).

  s. tali, a process which projects medially from the

anterior end of the calcaneus and which serves to support the head of the talus bone of the foot.

Sutton-Rendu-Osler-Weber syndrome. See telangiectasia, hereditary hemorrhagic.

sutu'ra. A type of immovable fibrous articulation occurring only between the bones of the skull; a cranial suture.

su'ture. 1. Stitch or stitches used in surgery to unite two surfaces. **2.** To apply a surgical stitch. **3.** The material used. **4.** Sutura; an immovable joint uniting the bones of the skull.

  absorbable s., a sterile strand obtained from tissues of healthy animals that is capable of being gradually absorbed by living tissue; it may be treated to alter its absorbability, may be impregnated with antimicrobial substances, and may be treated with coloring materials.

  blanket s., a continuous self-locking stitch; also called lock-stitch suture.

  button s., one in which the ends of the strand are passed through the eyes of a button and then tied.

  catgut s., an absorbable type obtained from the small intestine of sheep.

  cobbler s., one made with a needle at each end of the strand.

  continuous s., one running the length of the wound with only two anchoring knots, at the beginning and at the end.

  Connell's s., continuous suture in which the apposing edges are inverted.

  cranial s., sutura; a junction between the bones of the skull.

  Cushing s., a continuous inverting suture passed through the seromuscular layers of the gastrointestinal tract.

  Halstead s., interrupted inverting stitch, parallel to the wound and tied on one side.

  interrupted s., a single stitch inverted and tied separately.

  inverting s., one that turns in the apposing surfaces.

  Lembert s., an inverting suture, either continuous or interrupted, used to join two segments of intestine without entering the lumen.

  lock-stitch s., see blanket suture.

  mattress s., one that may be parallel to the wound (interrupted and continuous) or at right angles (interrupted on-end or vertical) and is inserted deep into the tissues.

  nonabsorbable s., one that is not absorbed by living tissues, i.e., silk, cotton, plastic, and alloy steel wire.

  purse-string s., a continuous, circular inverting suture.

  subcuticular s., continuous suture inserted so as to approximate the tissues immediately under the skin, without penetrating the skin.

  tension s., large simple or mattress interrupted stitch used to prevent undue stress.

  uninterrupted s., continuous suture.

Svedberg (S). Unit of sedimentation, proportional to the rate of sedimentation of a molecule in a given centrifugal field; a sedimentation constant of 1×10^{-13} sec.

swab. A small ball of cotton or gauze wrapped around the end of a stick or wire; used for cleansing, for applying medication, or for obtaining samples of material for bacteriologic examination.

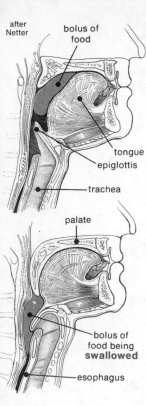

after Netter

bolus of food

tongue
epiglottis

trachea

palate

bolus of food being **swallowed**

esophagus

Sb	antimony	N	nitrogen
As	arsenic	Os	osmium
Ba	barium	O	oxygen
Bi	bismuth	Pb	palladium
Br	bromine	P	phosphorus
Cd	cadmium	Pt	platinum
Ca	calcium	Pu	plutonium
C	carbon	K	potassium
Cl	chlorine	Ra	radium
Cr	chromium	Rn	radon
Co	cobalt	Se	selenium
Cu	copper	Si	silicone
F	fluorine	Ag	silver
Au	gold	Na	sodium
He	helium	Sr	strontium
H	hydrogen	S	sulfur
I	iodine	Sn	tin
Fe	iron	W	tungsten
Pb	lead	U	uranium
Mg	magnesium	Xe	xenon
Mn	manganese	Y	yttrium
Hg	mercury	Zn	zinc

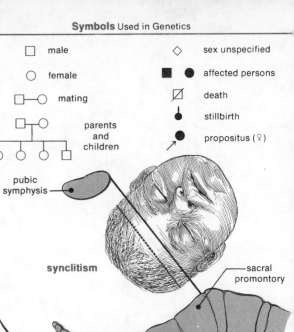

male sex unspecified
female affected persons
mating death
parents and children stillbirth
  propositus (♀)

pubic symphysis

synclitism

sacral promontory

swal′low. To pass a substance from the mouth via the throat and the esophagus into the stomach; to perform deglutition.

swarm′ing. Denoting the progressive spreading of motile bacteria, especially *Proteus* species, over the surface of the colony or solid culture medium.

sway-back. See lordosis.

sweat. 1. Perspiration. **2.** To perspire.

sweet′bread. The thymus gland or pancreas of a calf used for food.

swel′ling. An enlargement that may be inflammatory or noninflammatory; like fever, it is not a disease in itself, but rather a sign of an underlying disorder.

　Neufeld capsular s., swelling and opacity of the capsule of pneumococci when exposed to specific immune serum; also called quellung reaction.

syco′ma. 1. A pendulous growth. **2.** A large soft wart.

syco′siform. Latin for resembling the form of a fig; resembling sycosis.

syco′sis. Disease involving the hair follicles of the beard, marked by pustules and crusting of the skin.

sym′biont. One of the organisms associated with another in a symbiotic relationship; also called symbiote and symbion.

symbio′sis. 1. The living together in intimate association of two dissimilar organisms. **2.** In psychiatry, the relationship of two disturbed individuals who become dependent on each other.

sym′biote. See symbiont.

symbleph′aron. Adhesion of the eyelid to the eyeball.

symbleph′aropteryg′ium. Adhesion of the eyelid to the eyeball through a cicatricial band resembling a pterygium.

sym′bol. 1. A mark or character representing a substance, quality, quantity, or relation. **2.** Something that represents something else.

　chemical s., a symbol (letter or combination of letters) representing an atom or molecule of an element.

　phallic s., in psychoanalysis, any slender, upright, pointed object representing, in disguise, a penis (phallus).

symboliza′tion. An unconscious mental process whereby one object or idea stands for another through some aspect that both have in common.

sym′metry. Exact correspondence of constituent parts on opposite sides of a dividing plane or about an axis.

sympath-, sympatheto-, sympathico-, sympatho-. Combining forms indicating the sympathetic (autonomic) nervous system.

sympathec′tomy, sympathec′tomy. Surgical removal of a portion of a sympathetic nerve or of a sympathetic ganglion.

　chemical s., interruption of a sympathetic nervous pathway by means of a chemical.

sympathet′ic. 1. Denoting the thoracolumbar autonomic nervous system. **2.** Of or expressing sympathy.

sympath′icotrip′sy. Crushing of a ganglion of the sympathetic nervous system.

sympath′icotrop′ic. Having an influence upon the sympathetic nervous system.

sym′pathin. A name originally used to describe the substance produced at post-ganglionic sympathetic nerve endings upon stimulation of sympathetic nerve fibers; now known to be norepinephrine.

sym′pathoadre′nal. Relating to the sympathetic nervous system and the hormones of the medulla of the adrenal gland, epinephrine and norepinephrine, which produce effects similar to those produced by sympathetic stimulation.

sym′pathoblast. One of the primitive undifferentiated cells that migrate from the embryonic neural crest and give rise to sympathetic ganglion cells and to the adrenal medulla.

sym′pathoblasto′ma. See neuroblastoma.

sympathogo′nia. The primitive ectodermal stem cells that migrate down from the neural crest to form the medulla of the adrenal (suprarenal) glands during embryologic development.

sym′pathogonio′ma. See neuroblastoma.

sympatholyt′ic. Inhibiting the activity of the sympathetic nervous system; also called sympathoparalytic.

sympathomimet′ic. Producing effects similar to those caused by stimulation of the sympathetic nervous system.

sympathoparalyt′ic. See sympatholytic.

sym′pathy. 1. Expression of compassion or sorrow for another's grief. **2.** The capacity for understanding the feelings of another person.

symphys′eal. Relating to a symphysis.

symphysior′rhaphy. Fastening of a divided symphysis.

symphysiot′omy, symphyseot′omy. Division of the pubic symphysis, by means of a wire saw, to facilitate delivery.

sym′physis. 1. A type of articulation in which two bones are united by fibrocartilage, as the pubis. **2.** In pathology, the abnormal fusion of two surfaces.

symp′tom. Any manifestation of illness experienced by an individual. For individual symptoms, see specific names.

symptomat′ic. Relating to a symptom.

symptomatol′ogy. 1. The group of symptoms of a disease. **2.** The study of the symptoms of a disease, their causes, and the information they furnish; also called semiology and semeiology.

syn-. Prefix meaning together or joined.

synal′gia. Pain felt in an area other than the site of its origin.

syn′apse. The junction between nerve cells; a synaptic gap, about a millionth of a inch wide, exists through which a nerve impulse must pass to be transmitted from one nerve cell to another; this is accomplished by release of a transmitter substance.

　axodendritic s., the junction of the axon of a nerve cell with a dendrite of another nerve cell.

　axosomatic s., the junction of the axon of a nerve cell with the cell body of another.

synap′sis. Process during the prophase stage of meiosis in which homologous chromosomes pair off and unite.

synap′tic. Relating to a synapse.

synarthro′sis. Synarthrodial joint; one in which two bones are united by fibrous tissue permitting little or no movement between the bones.

syncan′thus. Adhesion of the eyeball to orbital structures.

synchondro′sis. The union of two bones by cartilage, in some instances replaced by bone before adulthood, as in the skull of the newborn or the union of the manubrium with the body of the sternum (breastbone).

synchro′nia. 1. Synchronism. **2.** The formation and development of tissues at the normal time.

syn′chronism. The simultaneous occurrence of two or more events.

syn′chrotron. An accelerator for generating high speed electrons or protons around a fixed circular path by a radio-frequency potential.

syn′chysis. Condition of the eye marked by liquefaction of the vitreous body.

　s. scintillans, the presence of numerous minute, glistening particles floating in a liquefied vitreous body, occurring secondarily to degenerative disease of the eye.

syn′clitism. A condition in which the planes of the fetal head and the maternal pelvis are parallel; the fetal head presents into the pelvis with the sagittal sutures midway between the maternal pubic symphysis and sacral promontory; also called parallelism.

syn′copal. Relating to fainting.

syn′cope. A brief loss of consciousness; a faint.

syncytiotro′phoblast. The outer layer of cells covering each chorionic villus of the placenta and in contact with maternal blood or decidua; also called syntrophoblast and syncytial trophoblast.

syncy′tium. A mass of protoplasm with many nu-

swallow | **syncytium**

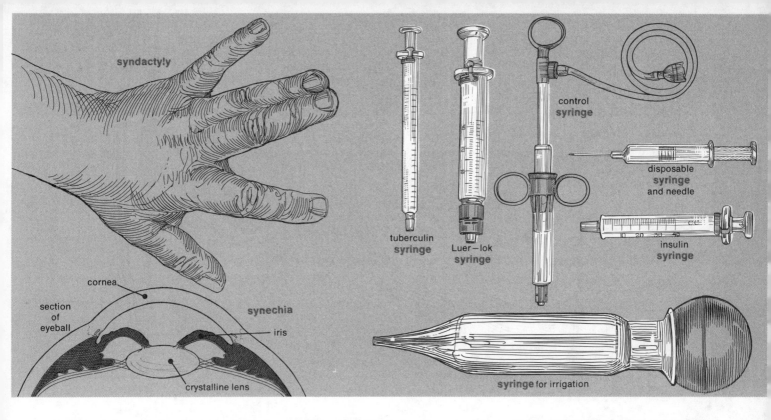

syndactyly

section of eyeball

cornea

synechia

iris

crystalline lens

tuberculin **syringe**

Luer–lok **syringe**

control **syringe**

disposable **syringe** and needle

insulin **syringe**

syringe for irrigation

clei, seemingly resulting from the merging of several cells.

syndac'tyly, syndactyl'ia, syndac'tilism. The partial or total webbing or fusion of two or more fingers or toes.

syndesmec'tomy. The excision of a section of a ligament.

syndesmi'tis. 1. Inflammation of a ligament. **2.** Conjunctivitis.

syndesmol'ogy. The anatomic study of ligaments and related joints.

syndes'mopexy. The operative fixation of a dislocation by reconstruction of the ligaments of the joint.

syndes'moplas'ty. Reparative surgery of a ligament.

syndesmor'rhaphy. Surgical suture or repair of a ligament.

syndesmo'sis. A type of fibrous articulation in which the fibrous tissue between the bones forms a membrane or ligament, as the tibiofibular articulation or the union of the footplate of the stapes to the oval window of the internal ear.

syndesmot'omy. The surgical incision or division of a ligament.

syn'drome. A set of signs and symptoms that appear together with reasonable consistency. For individual syndromes, see specific names.

synech'ia, *pl.* **synech'iae.** Any adhesions; especially adhesion of the iris to the cornea or to the crystalline lens.

synechiot'omy. Division of the adhesions in synechia.

synectenterot'omy. The separation of intestinal adhesions.

syner'esis. The shrinking or contraction of gels upon prolonged standing, causing the solid components to become more concentrated and droplets of the liquid medium to form on the surface; e.g., the shrinkage of blood clots, agar culture media, custards, etc.

syn'ergism, syn'ergy. 1. Cooperation in action, as the coordinated action of two or more substances or organs to produce an effect of which each is individually incapable. **2.** In pharmacology, the quality of two drugs whereby their combined effects are greater than the algebraic sum of their individual effects.

syn'ergist. Anything, such as a drug or muscle, that acts in conjunction with another toward a common purpose.

synesthe'sia. Condition in which, in addition to the normal sensation, a stimulus produces another unrelated sensation.

synesthesial'gia. Condition in which a stimulus,

in addition to exciting the normal sensation, produces pain somewhere else.

syn'gamy. Conjugation or union of the nuclei of two gametes in fertilization to produce a zygote nucleus.

syngene'ic. Relating to genetically identical (isogenic) or near-identical mammals (identical twins or highly inbred animals).

syn'graft. Isograft.

synkar'yon. The nucleus formed when the nuclei of two cells fuse during fertilization.

synkine'sis. Involuntary motion of one part when another part is moved.

synop'tophore. A modified stereoscope used in training individuals afflicted with ocular muscle imbalance.

synor'chidism, syn'orchism. Congenital fusion of the testes.

synosto'sis. The fusion of adjacent bones, normally separate, by means of osseous tissue.

synovec'tomy. Surgical removal of a portion or all of a diseased synovial membrane of a joint.

syno'via. The clear, thick, lubricating fluid in a joint, bursa, or tendon sheath; it is secreted by the membrane lining the cavity or tendon sheath (synovial membrane).

syno'vial. Relating to, containing, or secreting synovia.

synovianal'ysis. The microscopic examination, crystal identification, and cell count of joint fluid (synovia); five categories can be distinguished: (1) normal, (2) noninflammatory, (3) inflammatory, (4) purulent, and (5) hemorrhagic.

syno'vin. Mucinous substance found in synovia (joint fluid).

synovi'tis. Inflammation of the membranes lining a joint (synovial membranes).

synther'mal. Of the same temperature.

syn'thesis. A building up; especially the formation of a compound by the combination of simpler compounds or elements.

syn'thesize. To combine so as to produce a complex compound from simpler compounds; to form by synthesis.

syn'thetase. Trivial name for a ligase.

synthet'ic. Made by synthesis.

synton'ic. In balance.

syn'trophism. Enhanced growth of a strain of bacteria resulting from admixture with or nearness of another strain.

syntroph'oblast. See syncytiotrophoblast.

syn'trophus. Any congenital disease.

syph'ilid. Any of the skin lesions of syphilis; also called syphiloderma.

syph'ilis. An infectious venereal disease caused by

Treponema pallidum, transmitted through sexual intercourse or any direct contact; the first symptoms develop after an incubation period of 12 to 20 days.

congenital s., syphilis present at birth.

late latent s., a form of the disease in which there is serologic or historic evidence of syphilis of more than four years' duration; it is not detectable by physical examination, by examination of the cerebrospinal fluid, or by roentgenographic examination of the heart and aorta.

latent s., a phase of syphilis following the primary infection in which the organisms disappear from the skin and blood, and the foci of infection are beyond diagnostic reach; if evidence of infection is present in the cerebrospinal fluid the stage is designated as asymptomatic neurosyphilis.

primary s., the first stage of the disease, beginning with the appearance on the genitalia, and sometimes the oral cavity, of a small ulcer which develops into a chancre.

secondary s., the second stage of syphilis, beginning after healing of the initial chancre (between six and 12 weeks after its appearance) and lasting indefinitely; it is marked by infectious, copper-colored skin eruptions, mucous patches, fever, and other constitutional symptoms.

tertiary s., the final, noninfectious stage of the disease, beginning after a lapse of several months or years; marked by the development throughout the body of masses of granulomatous tissue (gummas); serious disorders of the nervous and vascular systems may occur.

syphilit'ic. Relating to or suffering from syphilis.

syph'ilize. To infect with syphilis, especially in an attempt to immunize against syphilis by inoculation with *Treponema pallidum*.

syphilogen'esis. Origin of syphilis.

syph'iloid. Resembling or characteristic of syphilis.

syphilol'ogy. The medical study pertaining to the nature and treatment of syphilis.

syphilo'ma. A gumma; a syphilitic tumor.

syphilopho'bia. An unwarranted fear of acquiring syphilis.

syphilophy'ma. Syphilitic growth; a gumma.

syr. Abbreviation of Latin *syrupus*.

syring-. See syringo-.

syringadeno'ma. A benign sweat gland tumor; also called syringoadenoma.

syringadeno'sus. Relating to sweat glands.

syringe'. A device used for injecting or withdrawing fluids.

fountain s., an apparatus consisting of a reservoir for holding water or special solutions, to the bottom of which is attached a tube with a nozzle at the end;

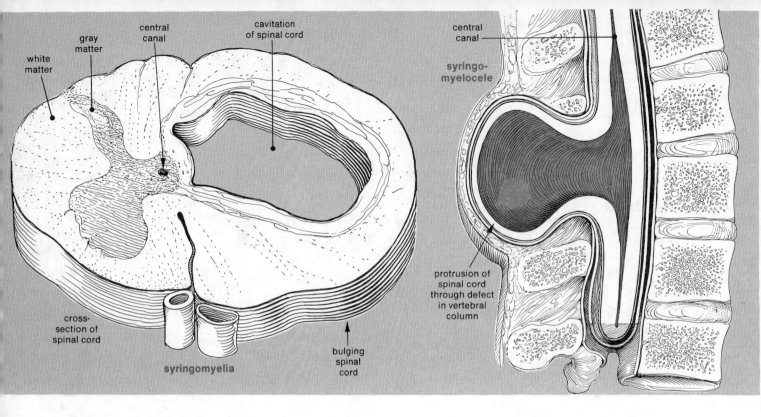

white matter · gray matter · central canal · cavitation of spinal cord

cross-section of spinal cord

syringomyelia

bulging spinal cord

central canal

syringo-myelocele

protrusion of spinal cord through defect in vertebral column

used for enemas and vaginal irrigations (douches).

hypodermic s., a syringe for the introduction of liquid remedies through a hypodermic needle into subcutaneous tissues.

syringi'tis. Inflammation of a bodily tube, such as the uterine tube.

syringo-, syring-. Combining forms denoting a relationship to a tube; e.g., syringitis.

syringoadeno'ma. See syringadenoma.

syringobul'bia. The presence of abnormal cavities in the brain stem.

syringocysto'ma. Cystic tumor of a hair follicle.

syringo'ma. A benign neoplasm of the tubular portion of a sweat gland.

syringomye'lia. A disease marked by the presence of cavities in the gray matter adjacent to the central canal of the spinal cord, causing loss of the senses of pain and temperature with retention of the sense of touch; in advanced cases, it often causes paralysis of the extremities and scoliosis of the lumbar spine.

syring'omyeli'tis. Inflammation of the spinal cord with formation of cavities in its substance.

syring'omy'elocele. Protrusion of the spinal cord, with the central canal greatly distended with cerebrospinal fluid, through an abnormal gap in the vertebral column.

syrin'gotomy. See fistulotomy.

syr'inx. A cavity in the brain or spinal cord caused by disease.

syr'up. In pharmacy, a solution of sugar in water used as a vehicle for active ingredients.

syssarco'sis. A muscular articulation; the union of bones by muscular tissue, as in the connection between the hyoid bone and the mandible (lower jaw).

sys'tem. 1. A functionally related group of parts or organs. **2.** An organized set of interrelated ideas, procedures, techniques, etc.

ascending reticular activating s., the upward neural projections of the reticular formation and thalamus which are responsible for normal wakefulness and alertness.

autonomic nervous s., the division of the nervous system that innervates the striated muscles of the heart and the smooth muscles and glands of the body; it is divided into the sympathetic (thoracolumbar) system and the parasympathetic (craniosacral) system.

cardiovascular s. (CVS), the heart and blood vessels.

centimeter-gram-second s., a system of metric units in which the basic units of length, mass, and time are the centimeter, gram, and second.

central nervous s. (CNS), the brain and spinal cord.

digestive s., the alimentary canal from the mouth to the anus and the associated glands.

endocrine s., collectively, all the ductless glands.

extrapyramidal s., a functional system of tracts in the brain which controls and coordinates motor activities, especially postural, static, and supportive.

female reproductive s., the genital organs in the female, consisting of the ovaries, uterine tubes, uterus, vagina, and external genitalia.

genitourinary s., the reproductive organs, kidneys, and urinary tract considered as a whole; also called urogenital system.

haversian s., see osteon.

hematopoietic s., the blood-producing organs.

heterogeneous s., a combination of matter containing two or more distinct components that have definite boundaries; e.g., a suspension or an emulsion.

International s. of units, a system of units for the basic quantities of length; mass; time; electric current; temperature; luminous intensity; and amount of substance; the corresponding units are: meter; kilogram; second; ampere; kelvin; candela; and mole. In all languages it is abbreviated SI. See page 462.

limbic s., term loosely applied to the part of the nervous system that controls autonomic functions and the emotions.

lymphatic s., the lymphatic vessels, nodes, tonsils, spleen, thymus, and lymphoid or adenoid tissue.

lymphoreticular s., in immunology, a collection of cellular elements strategically distributed throughout the body; they can be activated by a variety of influences which are recognized as foreign by the host.

male reproductive s., the genital organs in the male, consisting of the testes, excretory ducts, seminal vesicles, prostate gland, and penis.

metric s., a system of measures and weights based upon the meter and the gram, respectively.

muscular s., the muscles of the body collectively.

nervous s., the brain and spinal cord (central nervous system), the cranial and spinal nerves (peripheral nervous system), and the autonomic nervous system.

neuromuscular s., the nerves and the muscles which the nerves supply.

oculomotor s., the part of the nervous system that controls eye movements.

oxidation-reduction s., one in which the reversible oxidation-reduction reaction can take place; e.g., the enzyme systems of living cells.

parasympathetic nervous s., a division of the autonomic nervous system.

peripheral nervous s. (PNS), the nervous system which connects the central nervous system (CNS) to the rest of the body.

portal s., the arrangement of vessels and capillaries in the liver; the portal vein and its branches.

Purkinje s., the system of modified muscle fibers in the heart concerned with conduction of impulses.

respiratory s., the air passages, lungs, and the muscles of respiration.

reticular activating s., a portion of the central cephalic brain stem which controls wakefulness, arousal from sleep, and focusing of attention.

reticuloendothelial s. (RES), the phagocytic cells present in the bone marrow, spleen, and liver, where they free the blood or lymph of foreign matter.

sympathetic nervous s., a division of the autonomic nervous system.

triaxial reference s., in electrocardiography, the figure resulting from rearranging the sides of the Einthoven triangle (which represent the three standard limb leads) so that they bisect one another.

urogenital s., see genitourinary system.

vascular s., the blood vessels.

systemat'ic. Relating to a system or arranged in accordance with a system.

systematiza'tion. Formulation or arrangement of ideas in orderly sequence, according to a system.

sys'tematized. Denotes widespread pathology that has a significant pattern rather than haphazard distribution.

system'ic. Relating to or affecting the entire body.

sys'tole. The rhythmic and synchronous contraction of the muscles of the heart chambers.

atrial s., auricular s., atrial contraction giving impetus to the blood flowing from the atria into the ventricles; it has a duration of about 0.1 sec.

ventricular s., ventricular contraction immediately following atrial systole; it is divided into two phases: (a) isometric contraction, which occurs when the ventricular pressure firmly closes the atrioventricular valves, and (b) the period of ejection, occurring when the pressure in the ventricles overcomes the diastolic pressure of the aorta and pulmonary arteries and the aortic and pulmonic valves open, forcefully ejecting the ventricular blood; in an individual with a heart rate of 70 beats per minute, the ejection period lasts 0.3 sec.

systol'ic. Relating to or resulting from ventricular systole.

systrem'ma. A cramp in the muscles of the leg, chiefly of the bellies of the gastrocnemius and soleus muscles; may be associated with swimmer's cramp or a charleyhorse.

syringe | **systremma**

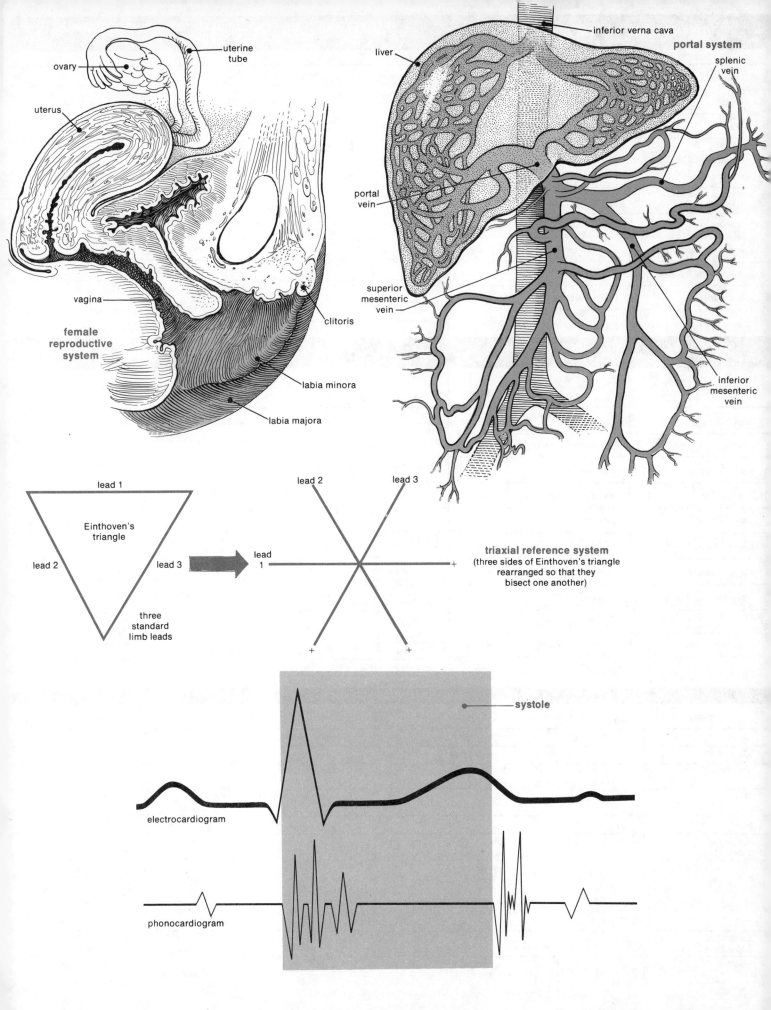

female reproductive system

ovary

uterine tube

uterus

vagina

clitoris

labia minora

labia majora

portal system

liver

inferior verna cava

splenic vein

portal vein

superior mesenteric vein

inferior mesenteric vein

lead 1

Einthoven's triangle

lead 2

lead 3

three standard limb leads

lead 1

lead 2

lead 3

triaxial reference system
(three sides of Einthoven's triangle rearranged so that they bisect one another)

systole

electrocardiogram

phonocardiogram

INTERNATIONAL SYSTEM OF UNITS (SI)

Quantity	Name	Symbol
SI base units:		
length	meter	m
mass	kilogram	kg
time	second	s
electric current	ampere	A
thermodynamic temperature	kelvin	K
amount of substance	mole	mol
luminous intensity	candela	cd
SI supplementary units:		
plane angle	radian	rad
solid angle	steradian	sr

PREFIXES AND THEIR SYMBOLS USED TO DESIGNATE DECIMAL MULTIPLES AND SUBMULTIPLES

Prefix	Symbol	Factor	
tera	T	10^{12} =	
giga	G	10^9 =	1 000 000 000
mega	M	10^6 =	1 000 000
kilo	k	10^3 =	1 000
hecto	h	10^2 =	100
deka	da	10^1 =	10
deci	d	10^{-1} = 0.1	
centi	c	10^{-2} = 0.01	
milli	m	10^{-3} = 0.001	
micro	μ	10^{-6} = 0.000 001	
nano	n	10^{-9} = 0.000 000 001	
pico	p	10^{-12} = 0.000 000 000 001	
femto	f	10^{-15} = 0.000 000 000 000 001	
atto	a	10^{-18} = 0.000 000 000 000 000 001	

EXAMPLES OF SI DERIVED UNITS EXPRESSED IN TERMS OF BASE UNITS

Quantity	SI unit	Unit Symbol
area	square meter	m^2
volume	cubic meter	m^3
speed, velocity	meter per second	m/s
acceleration	meter per second squared	m/s^2
wave number	1 per meter	m^{-1}
density, mass density	kilogram per cubic meter	kg/m^3
current density	ampere per square meter	A/m^2
magnetic field strength	ampere per meter	A/m
concentration (of amount of substance)	mole per cubic meter	mol/m^3
specific volume	cubic meter per kilogram	m^3/kg
luminance	candela per square meter	cd/m^2

SI DERIVED UNITS WITH SPECIAL NAMES

Quantity	Name	Symbol	Expression in terms of other units
frequency	hertz	Hz	s^{-1}
force	newton	N	$kg \cdot m/s^2$
pressure, stress	pascal	Pa	N/m^2
energy, work, quantity of heat	joule	J	$N \cdot m$
power, radiant flux	watt	W	J/s
quantity of electricity, electric charge	coulomb	C	$A \cdot s$
electric potential, potential difference, electromotive force	volt	V	W/A
capacitance	farad	F	C/V
electric resistance	ohm	Ω	V/A
conductance	siemens	S	A/V
magnetic flux	weber	Wb	$V \cdot$
magnetic flux density	tesla	T	Wb/m^2
inductance	henry	H	Wb/A
luminous flux	lumen	lm	$cd \cdot sr$
illuminance	lux	lx	lm/m^2
activity (of a radionuclide)	becquerel	Bq	s^{-1}
absorbed dose	gray	Gy	J/kg

RECOMMENDED UNITS

Quantity	Symbol	Dimension	Unit	Unit symbol	Recommended sub-units	Not recommended units
Length	l	L	meter	m	$mm, \mu m, nm$	$cm, \mu, u, m\mu, mu, A$
Area	A	L^2	square meter	m^2	$mm^2, \mu m^2$	cm^2, μ^2
Volume	V	L^3	cubic meter / liter	m^3 / l	$dm^3, cm^3, mm^3, \mu m^3$ / $ml, \mu l, nl, pl, fl$	cc, ccm, μ^3, u^3 / $L, \lambda, ul, \mu\mu l, uul$
Mass	m	M	kilogram	kg	$g, mg, \mu g, ng, pg$	$Kg, gr, \gamma, ug, m\mu g, mug, \gamma\gamma, \mu\mu g, uug$
Number	N	I	one	1	$10^9, 10^6, 10^3, 10^{-3}$	all other factors
Amount of substance	n	N	mole	mol	$mmol, \mu mol, nmol$	$M, eq, val, g\text{-}mol, mM, meq, mval, \mu M \mu eq, \mu val, nM, neq, nval$
Mass concentration		$L^{-3} m$	kilogram per liter	kg/l	$g/l, mg/l, \mu g/l, ng/l$	$g/ml, \%, g\%, \% (w/v), g/100\ ml, g/dl, ^0/_{00}, ^0/_{00}, ^0/_{00} (w/v), mg\%, mg\% (w/v), mg/100\ ml, mg/dl, ppm, ppm (w/v), \mu g\%, \mu g\% (w/v), \mu g/100\ ml, \mu/dl, \gamma\%, ppb, ppb (w/v), \mu\mu g/ml, uug/ml$
Substance concentration	c	$L^{-3} N$	mole per liter	mol/l	$mmol/l, \mu mol/l, nmol/l$	$M, eq/l, val/l, N, n, mM, meq/l, mval/l, \mu M, uM, \mu eq/l, nM, neq/l$
Molality	m	$M^{-1} N$	mole per kilogram	mol/kg	$mmol/kg, \mu mol/kg$	$m, mmol/g, \mu mol/mg, mm, \mu m, mm$

Periodic Table

Group	I	II												III	IV	V	VI	VII	O

Tt

METALS   periodic table   NONMETALS

Period

| Period 1: H 1 | | | | | | | | | | | | | | | | | | He 2 |

Period 2: Li 3, Be 4 — B 5, C 6, N 7, O 8, F 9, Ne 10

Period 3: Na 11, Mg 12 — Al 13, Si 14, P 15, S 16, Cl 17, Ar 18

Period 4: K 19, Ca 20, Sc 21, Ti 22, V 23, Cr 24, Mn 25, Fe 26, Co 27, Ni 28, Cu 29, Zn 30, Ga 31, Ge 32, As 33, Se 34, Br 35, Kr 36

Period 5: Rb 37, Sr 38, Y 39, Zr 40, Nb 41, Mo 42, Tc 43, Ru 44, Rh 45, Pd 46, Ag 47, Cd 48, In 49, Sn 50, Sb 51, Te 52, I 53, Xe 54

Period 6: Cs 55, Ba 56, *57-71, Hf 72, Ta 73, W 74, Re 75, Os 76, Ir 77, Pt 78, Au 79, Hg 80, Ti 81, Pb 82, Bi 83, Po 84, At 85, Rn 86

Period 7: Fr 87, Ra 88, **89-103, Rf 104, Ha 105

* lanthanide elements (rare earth): La 57, Ce 58, Pr 59, Nd 60, Pm 61, Sm 62, Eu 63, Gd 64, Tb 65, Dy 66, Ho 67, Er 68, Tm 69, Yb 70, Lu 71

** actinide elements: Ac 89, Th 90, Pa 91, U 92, Np 93, Pu 94, Am 95, Cm 96, Bk 97, Cf 98, Es 99, Fm 100, Md 101, No 102, Lw 103

T. 1. Abbreviation for tension. **2.** Symbol for absolute temperature.

t. Abbreviation for (a) temperature; (b) Latin *ter*.

t₁/₂. Abbreviation for (a) biologic half-life, the time it takes for the body to eliminate 50 per cent of a drug; (b) half-life, the time required for one-half of a given number of radioactive atoms to disintegrate.

T₂. Abbreviation for diiodotyrosine.

T₃. Abbreviation for the thyroid hormone triiodothyronine.

T₄. Abbreviation for the thyroid hormone tetraiodothyronine (thyroxin).

T-1824. Evans blue; see under blue.

Ta. Chemical symbol of the element tantalum.

Taba'nus. A genus of biting flies, some species of which transmit anthrax, infectious equine anemia, and other diseases; commonly called horseflies, gadflies, and breezeflies.

tabefac'tion. Atrophy or wasting of the body.

ta'bes. Progressive wasting away.

   t. dorsalis, a late manifestation of syphilis characterized by sclerosis of the sensory nerve roots and the posterior columns of the spinal cord; the usual symptoms are: shooting pains, muscular incoordination and atrophy, and functional disturbance of certain organs; also called locomotor ataxia.

tabes'cent. Wasting away progressively.

tabet'ic. Afflicted with tabes.

tabet'iform. Resembling tabes dorsalis.

table. 1. An orderly arrangement of written, typed, or printed data. **2.** A flat layer, as one of the two laminae, separated by the diploë, into which the cranial bones are divided. **3.** An article of furniture having a flat horizontal surface.

   Aub-DuBois t., table of rates of basal metabolism in calories per square meter of body surface per hour for all age groups.

   examining t., one on which the patient lies during a medical examination.

   operating t., one on which a patient is placed during a surgical procedure.

   periodic t., an arrangement of chemical elements listed according to their atomic number; it demonstrates the recurrence of similar properties after certain intervals.

   tilt t., one with a top that tilts so that the patient lying on it can be brought into a semierect position.

   Reuss' color t.'s, diagrams in which colored letters are superimposed on colored backgrounds as a test for colorblindness.

   vitreous t., the inner table of the cranial bones; it is denser than the outer table.

ta'blespoon (tbsp). A large spoon used as a measure in the dosage of liquid medicines; equivalent to 15 milliliters, four liquid drams, one-half fluid ounce, or three teaspoons.

tab'let. A small disc containing measured amounts of medicinal substances.

   buccal t., one placed between the cheek and the gum where it dissolves quickly, permitting the medicinal substance to be absorbed through the mucosa.

   compressed t., one prepared by compressing granulated medicinal substances under several hundred kilograms of pressure per square centimeter.

   enteric coated t., one coated with material that does not disintegrate in stomach fluids; the medication is released in the intestines.

   hypodermic t., a small water-soluble tablet, intended to be dissolved in the barrel of a hypodermic syringe prior to injection.

   sublingual t., one placed under the tongue to permit absorption of the medicinal ingredients through the mucosa.

tabopar'esis. Condition marked by symptoms of tabes dorsalis and general partial paralysis.

tab'ular. 1. Arranged as a table or list. **2.** Having a flat surface.

tache. A minute spot or blemish.

   t. cérébrale, meningeal streak; see under streak.

   t. noir, the crust-covered lesion produced by the bite of a tick.

tach'istesthe'sia. Perception of a flicker of light.

tachis'toscope. Instrument that projects a slide for a brief period of time; used in experimental optics to measure the speed of conscious visual perception.

tach'ogram. The graphic record made by tachography.

tachog'raphy. The recording of the rate of arterial blood flow.

tachy-. Combining form meaning rapid or accelerated; e.g., tachycardia.

tachyarrhyth'mia. Heart rhythm with over 100 beats per minute.

tachycar'dia. An abnormally fast heart beat; also called tachyrhythmia.

   paroxysmal atrial t. (PAT), sudden onset of rapid heart action originating in the atria.

   paroxysmal atrial t. with block, PAT with a block in transmission of all the beats from the atria to the ventricles so that the ventricular rate is less than the atrial.

tachycar'diac. Relating to or afflicted with tachychardia.

tachycrot'ic. Relating to a rapid pulse.

tachyla'lia. Tachylogia.

tachylo'gia. Rapid speech.

tachym'eter. Instrument for measuring speed of motion.

tachypha'gia. Abnormally rapid eating; bolting of food.

tachyphra'sia. Tachylogia.

tachyphylax'is. Rapid production of immune tolerance, as by repeated injections of small doses of a substance.

tachypne'a. Abnormally rapid, shallow breathing.

tachyrhyth'mia. See tachycardia.

tachys'terol. A sterol produced by ultraviolet irradiation of ergosterol.

tachysys'tole. Tachycardia.

tac'tile. Relating to the sense of touch.

tac'tion. 1. An act of touching; a contact. **2.** The sense of touch.

tactom'eter. Instrument used to determine the condition of the sense of touch.

tac'tor. A sensory (tactile) end-organ.

tac'tal. Of, derived from, or relating to the sense of touch.

tac'tus. Latin for touch; the sense of touch.

Tae'nia. A genus of tapeworms (family Taeniidae).

   T. echinococcus, *Echinococcus granulosus.*

   T. saginata, the common tapeworm transmitted

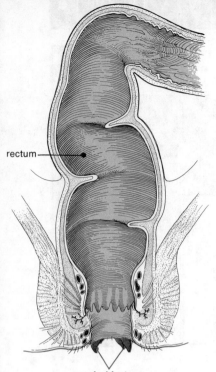

rectum

anal skin tags

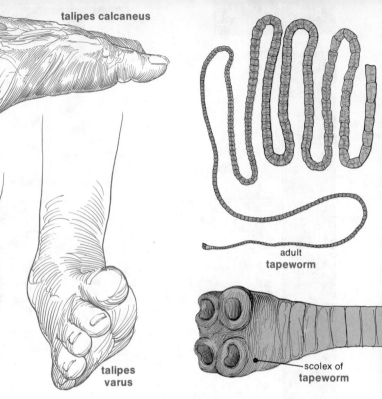

talipes calcaneus

talipes valgus

talipes varus

adult tapeworm

scolex of tapeworm

to man by the ingestion of infected beef; the larvae exist in the muscles and organs of cattle; the adults, measuring from 5 to 10 meters in length, are found in the human small intestine, attached to the mucosa by means of muscular suckers on the scolex (head); also called beef tapeworm.

T. solium, a species whose larval state exists in the muscles of the hog; the adult forms are found in the human intestine, to which they gain access by the ingestion of insufficiently cooked infested pork; also called pork tapeworm and armed tapeworm because of the double row of hooks present on its head.

TAF. Abbreviation for tumor angiogenesis factor.

tag. 1. To introduce a radioactive isotope to a substance. **2.** The radioactive material so used. **3.** A small outgrowth of flaplike appendage.

  anal skin t., a polypoid projection in the anus.

  skin t., a small flesh-colored to brown polypoid growth; also called fibroepithelial papilloma.

tagged. Labeled; said of a compound to which a radioactive isotope has been added.

Takayashu's syndrome. Pulseless disease occurring mostly in young females. See also pulseless disease and aortic arch syndrome.

take. A successful grafting procedure.

talal'gia. Discomfort or pain in the heel or ankle.

talc, tal'cum. A fine-grained hydrous magnesium silicate, having a soft texture; used in face and talcum powder, and in cosmetic and pharmaceutical preparations.

talco'sis. Disorder of the lungs produced by inhalation of talc.

tal'iped. 1. A person who is afflictd with a clubfoot. **2.** Clubfooted.

tal'ipes. General term that denotes a deformity involving the ankle and foot.

  t. calcaneovalgus, a relatively common congenital disorder in which the ankle joint is dorsiflexed and the foot is everted; believed to be caused by the position of the fetus in the uterus; the opposite of clubfoot (talipes equinovarus).

  t. calcaneus, fixed dorsiflexion of the foot, causing the weight of the body to rest on the heel.

  t. equinovarus, see clubfoot.

  t. equinus, fixed plantar extension of the foot, causing the weight of the body to rest on the ball of the foot; the ankle joint is plantar flexed.

  t. valgus, outward turning of the foot, causing only the inner side of the sole to touch the ground; accompanied by flattening of the longitudinal arch.

  t. varus, deformity considered to be an incomplete form of clubfoot (talipes equinovarus); characterized by a turning inward of the foot, causing only the outer part of the sole to touch the ground; accompanied by increased height of the longitudinal arch.

talocalca'neal. Pertaining to the talus and calcaneus bones of the foot; denoting the joint between those bones and the ligaments attaching them.

talocru'ral. Relating to the ankle joint.

talonavic'ular. Relating to the talus and the navicular bone.

ta'lus. The large bone articulating with the tibia and fibula to form the ankle joint; also called astralagus and ankle bone.

tambour'. A drum-shaped apparatus used to transmit and register slight movements.

tam'pon. A plug of any absorbent material placed in a canal or cavity to control hemorrhage or absorb secretions.

tamponad'e, tam'ponage. The use of a tampon as a surgical aid.

  cardiac t., compression of the heart due to accumulation of blood in the pericardium, as in rupture of the heart or after penetrating wounds.

T and A. Abbreviation for tonsillectomy and adenoidectomy.

Tangier disease. An inherited disorder of lipid metabolism marked by deficiency of high density lipoproteins, deposition of cholesterol esters in foam cells, enlargement of liver, spleen, and lymph nodes, enlarged orange-colored tonsils, and corneal opacity; the disease was named after Tangier Island, a geographically isolated community located in the Virginia part of the Chesapeake Bay, where the disease was first discovered.

tann'ate. A salt of tannic acid.

tan'nic acid. A lustrous brownish-yellow amorphous, powdered, or spongy mass, $C_{76}H_{52}O_{46}$, extracted from the bark and fruit of various plants; used as an astringent and styptic, and occasionally in treating diarrhea; toxic to the liver; also called tannin.

tan'nin. See tannic acid.

tan'talum. A metallic noncorrosive element; symbol Ta, atomic number 73, atomic weight 180.95; used in surgery as a skull plate, a wire mesh in the abdominal wall, etc.

tan'trum. Unprovoked fit of bad temper; unreasoning anger that may be accompanied by violent acts or gestures.

tap. 1. To deliver a quick, gentle blow or blows, as when eliciting a tendon reflex. **2.** To strike lightly but audibly. **3.** To withdraw fluid from a bodily cavity.

  spinal t., lumbar puncture; see under puncture.

tape'tum. 1. The portions of the corpus callosum that border the posterior horns (laterally) of the lateral ventricles of the brain. **2.** The outer and posterior part of the choroid (the vascular layer of the eyeball).

tape'worm. Any of several ribbonlike worms (class Cestoda) that infest the intestines of vertebrates, including man; its body consists of a head or scolex with hooks for attachment to the intestinal wall and a series of segments or proglottids (from four to several thousand) containing the reproductive organs.

  beef t., see *Taenia saginata.*

  fish t., see *Diphyllobothrium latum.*

  dwarf t., dwarf mouse t., see *Hymenolepis nana.*

  pork t., see *Taenia solium.*

taphopho'bia. A morbid fear of being buried alive.

tapinocephal'ic. Characterized by a flattened skull.

tapinoceph'aly. Deformity in which the skull is flattened.

tapotement'. Tapping with the side of the hand; a massage movement.

tar. A dark, semisolid substance obtained from the destructive distillation of various organic materials, as wood or coal.

  coal t., tar obtained from bituminous coal; used in the preparation of certain drugs and dyes.

  pine t., a dark, viscous syrup produced by the destructive distillation of pine wood; it contains resins, turpentine, and oils and is used as a disinfectant and antiseptic in the treatment of skin disorders such as eczema; also called wood tar and liquid pitch.

taran'tula. Any of several large, hairy, dark spiders (family Theraphosidae) capable of inflicting a painful but not significantly poisonous bite.

  black t., *Sericopelma communis,* a large black tarantula of Panama, whose bite is poisonous although the effect is localized.

tar'dive. Late; tardy; applied to the characteristic lesion of a disease that is late in appearing.

tare. In chemistry, (a) the weight of an empty container; (b) a weight used to counterbalance the weight of the container holding the substance being weighed.

tar'get. An object of fixation or observation used in vision training or testing.

tarsadeni'tis. Inflammation of the borders of the eyelids and of the meibomian glands.

tar'sal. 1. Relating to the small bones forming the instep of the foot. **2.** Relating to the border of an eyelid.

tarsec'tomy. 1. Surgical removal of the tarsus of the foot, or part of it. **2.** Surgical removal of the margin of an eyelid, or part of it.

tarsi'tis. 1. Inflammation of the margin of the eyelid; also called marginal blepharitis. **2.** Inflamma-

Taenia | **tarsitis**

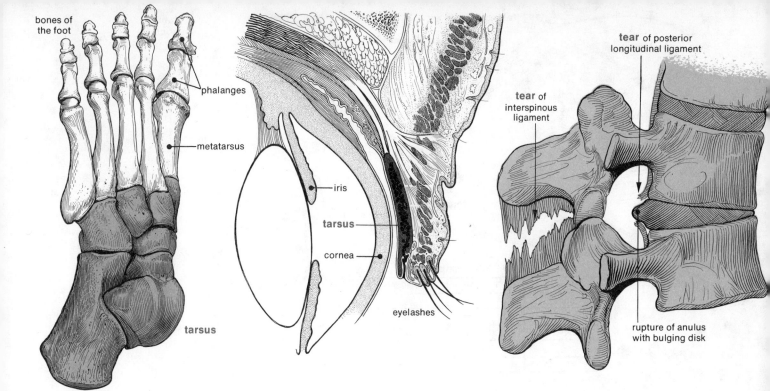

bones of the foot

phalanges

metatarsus

tarsus

iris

tarsus

cornea

eyelashes

tear of posterior longitudinal ligament

tear of interspinous ligament

rupture of anulus with bulging disk

tion of the tarsus of the foot.

tarsocla′sia, tarsoc′lasis. Surgical fracture of the tarsus, as for the correction of clubfoot.

tarsomala′cia. Softening of the tarsal cartilage of an eyelid.

tarsometatar′sal. Relating to the tarsus and metatarsus.

tarsophy′ma. A tarsal tumor.

tar′soplasty. Plastic surgery of the eyelid; also called blepharoplasty.

tarsor′rhaphy. A surgical procedure to close or to reduce the length of the palpebral fissure by suturing the upper and lower eyelids.

tarsot′omy. Surgical incision of the eyelid.

tar′sus, *pl.* **tar′si. 1.** The part of the foot between the leg and the metatarsus formed by seven small bones. **2.** The fibrous tissue that strengthens and shapes the edge of the eyelid.

tar′tar. Dental calculus; a hard yellow to brown deposit on the teeth, usually most heavily accumulated on the teeth nearest the salivary duct openings.

tartaric acid. A soluble white powder, a laxative and refrigerant, used in preparing Seidlitz powders and effervescing tablets.

tar′trate. A salt of tartaric acid.

tar′trated. Containing tartar or tartaric acid.

taste. 1. The special sense that distinguishes the different flavors of substances that come in contact with the taste buds in the mouth. **2.** To perceive such sensations.

tatoo′. A permanent design made on the skin by ingraining an indelible pigment through punctures.

tau′rine. Water-soluble, colorless crystals produced by the decomposition of taurocholic acid.

taurocho′late. A salt of taurocholic acid.

taurocholic acid. A bile acid; a compound of cholic acid and taurine; also cholytaurine.

Taussig-Bing syndrome. Congenital malformation of the heart in which the aorta arises from the right ventricle (instead of the left) and the pulmonary artery arises from both ventricles, anteriorly to the aorta; a ventricular septal defect is also present.

tautom′erism. Phenomenon in which a chemical compound exists in a state of equilibrium between two isomeric forms and is able to react according to either; also called dynamic allotropy.

tax′is. 1. Correction of a dislocation or reduction of a hernia by gentle pressure. **2.** The reaction of certain organisms to a stimulus, i.e., motion away from or toward the stimulus, or arrangement in a particular position relating to the stimulus; used with a prefix indicating the type of stimulus; e.g., chemotaxis, electrotaxis, etc.

tax′on, *pl.* **tax′a.** A category in a systematic classification; e.g., genus, species.

taxon′omy. The classification of living organisms into categories (taxa).

Tay-Sachs disease. Cerebral sphingolipidosis; see under sphingolipidosis.

Tb. Chemical symbol of the element terbium.

tb. Abbreviation for tuberculosis.

t.b. Abbreviation for tubercle bacillus.

TBG. Abbreviation for thyroxin-binding globulin.

TBPA. Abbreviation for thyroxin-binding prealbumin.

tbsp. Abbreviation for tablespoon.

TBW. Abbreviation for total body water.

Tc. Chemical symbol of the element technetium.

t.d.s. Abbreviation of Latin *ter die sumendum*.

Te. Chemical symbol of the element tellurium.

tear. 1. The clear saline liquid secreted by the lacrimal gland, serving to keep the cornea and conjunctiva moist and to facilitate movement of the eyelid. **2.** The act of secreting tears.

tear. 1. To pull apart or divide forcefully. **2.** To wound by lacerating.

tease. To separate gently with a fine instrument, as the minute components of a tissue.

tea′spoon (tsp). A small spoon used as a measure in the dosage of fluid medicines, equivalent to 5 milliliters.

teat. A nipple or breast.

techne′tium. A radioactive element; symbol Tc, atomic number 43, atomic weight 99; employed in clinical medicine because of its readily detected 140-kev γ-rays, absence of β-radiation, and a half-life of six hours; used to determine the blood flow pattern and location of tumors in a number of different areas by scintillation scanning.

tech′nical. 1. Relating to technique. **2.** Specialized.

technician. A person who has a high school diploma or an Associate Degree and who has been trained in the performance of special technical procedures.

dental laboratory t., a person trained in the making of dental appliances, such as dentures, crown and bridge work, restorations, and orthodontic appliances.

histologic t., one trained in processing body tissues that have been removed from the body for microscopic examination (such as fixing, embedding, sectioning, mounting, and staining).

medical laboratory t., a person who has an Associate Degree with special training in medical laboratory techniques (such as physical, chemical, and microscopic analysis of body fluids and tissues) and who works under appropriate supervision, such as

that of a certified medical technologist. Cf medical technologist.

radiation therapy t., one who assists the radiologist in treatment of disease by exposing specific areas of the patient's body to prescribed doses of x-ray or other forms of ionizing radiation.

x-ray t., a person trained to make x-ray films of a bodily part; also called radiologic technologist.

technique. The systematic procedure by which a surgical operation, scientific experiment, or any complex act is accomplished.

hydro-flow t., in dentistry, a method of cavity preparation in which the tooth being prepared is kept under a stream of water.

flush t., one used to determine the systolic blood pressure in infants.

Ouchterlony t., a double diffusion method for performing a precipitin test.

Shouldice t., a technique for repairing direct and indirect inguinal hernias.

technol′ogist. An individual who is a graduate of a four-year college with special training in a particular field and who is certified in that field.

medical t., one who performs or supervises test procedures in the clinical laboratory, including the fields of serology, immunology, chemistry, blood typing, hematology, parasitology, microbiology, urinalysis, and histochemistry. Cf medical technician.

nuclear medicine t., a certified medical technologist or a registered nurse who has been trained in the use of radioactive materials for diagnostic purposes.

pharmaceutical laboratory t., certified medical technologist in industry who analyzes and tests medications for strength and purity.

tecton′ic. Relating to plastic surgery or grafting.

tecto′rial. Relating to or forming a cover or roof.

tecto′rium. Any rooflike structure.

tec′tum. Any anatomic covering or roofing structure, especially the roofplate of the midbrain; it is dorsal to the cerebral aqueduct and includes the superior and inferior colliculi, their brachii, and the tectal lamina.

teeth′ing. The eruption of the primary or baby teeth into the oral cavity.

teg′men. A structure that covers or roofs over a part.

t. tympani, roof of the middle ear chamber formed by the thin plate of the petrous part of the temporal bone; it separates the middle ear chamber from the middle cranial fossa.

t. ventriculi quarti, roof of fourth ventricle; see under roof.

tegmen′tum. The larger dorsal portion of the

telangiectasia
dilatation of small blood vessels

tenaculum

tenia mesocolica
meso-colon
tenia omentalis
tenia liberia
colon

NORMAL RECTAL BODY temperatures

Species	°F (±1°F)	°C (±0.5°C)
mouse	97	36
man	98.6	37.0
cat	101.5	38.5
dog	102	39
chicken	106.2	41.5

brain stem.

teg′ument. See integument.

te′la, *pl.* **te′lae.** A thin, delicate, weblike membrane.

telangiecta′sia, telangiec′tasis. Dilatation of a group of capillaries.

　hereditary hemorrhagic t., telangiectasia in the skin and mucous membranes, usually appearing after puberty; transmitted as a simple dominant trait; also called Rendu-Osler-Weber disease and Sutton-Rendu-Osler-Weber syndrome.

telangiectat′ic. Afflicted with telangiectasia.

telangio′ma. A tumor made up of dilated capillaries or arterioles.

tele-, tel-. Combining forms denoting distance; e.g., telediagnosis.

telecar′diophone. An instrument through which heart sounds can be heard by listeners at some distance from the patient.

telediagno′sis. Diagnosis of disease in a patient located at some distance from the physician by evaluation of data transmitted to a receiving station.

telelec′trocar′diogram. An electrocardiogram recorded at some distance from the patient; also called telecardiogram.

telelec′trocar′diograph. An apparatus for the transmission and remote reception of electrocardiograph signals; also called telecardiograph.

telem′etry. The science and technology of remote sensing for monitoring living systems by use of radio transmitters placed in or on animal or human subjects; such parameters as blood pressure, heart rate, etc., may be monitored in this way.

telenceph′alon. The portion of the embryonic brain from which develop the cerebral hemispheres, the lateral ventricles, the anterior part of the third ventricle, and the olfactory lobes; together with the diencephalon it makes up the prosencephalon.

teleneu′ron. A nerve ending.

teleol′ogy. Doctrine according to which all biologic events are directed toward some final purpose.

telep′athy. The phenomenon of communication of thought from one individual to another without the aid of physical means; since the means of extrasensory thought transference is unknown, it is generally not accepted as scientifically valid.

telerecep′tor. An organ that perceives sense stimuli from a distance; e.g., the eye.

telether′apy. Radiotherapeutic treatment with an external radiation source many centimeters from the patient.

tellu′rium. A lustrous semimetallic element; symbol Te, atomic number 52, atomic weight 127.6.

telo-, tel-. Combining forms denoting (a) a final form or phase; e.g., telophase; (b) a relationship to

an end; e.g., telangectasia.

telocen′tric. Denoting a chromosome with its centromere at the end.

teloden′dron. The terminal branching of an axon.

tel′ogen. The resting or final phase of a hair cycle; the period of time before a hair is shed.

tel′omere. One of the two ends of a chromosome.

te′lophase. The last stage of cell division by mitosis, beginning when the chromatids reach the poles of the cell and the nuclear membranes enclose each new set of chromosomes to complete the separation of two daughter cells.

TEM. Abbreviations for triethylenemelamine.

tem′perament. The unique natural predispositions of an individual that influence his manner of thinking, behaving, and reacting.

tem′perature. 1. Intensity of heat as measured in any of several arbitrary scales. **2.** A feverish condition.

　absolute t. (T), temperature measured on an absolute scale.

　critical t., temperature above which a gas cannot be reduced to liquid form.

　effective t., a comfort index that takes into consideration the temperature, movement, and moisture content of the air.

　normal t., the temperature of a normal person at rest (usually about 98.6°F or 37°C oral).

temperature coefficient. See under coefficient.

temper-tantrum. A habit disorder, seen principally among emotionally immature children, characterized by screaming and kicking.

tem′plate. 1. The macromolecular mold for the synthesis of another macromolecule. **2.** In dentistry, a curved or flat plate used as an aid in setting teeth; a pattern.

　wax t., a wax impression of the occlusion of the teeth.

tem′ple. The lateral region on either side of the forehead above the zygomatic arch.

tempola′bile. Unstable over a period of time or changed or destroyed by time; said of a serum.

tem′poral. Relating to the side of the head or temple.

temporomandib′ular. Relating to the temporal bone and mandible, as the articulation of the lower jaw (TMJ).

temporo-occip′ital. Relating to the temporal and occipital bones of the skull.

temposta′bile, temposta′ble. Not altered by the passage of time; said of certain chemicals.

tena′cious. Sticky; adhesive.

tenac′ity. The state of being adhesive or cohesive.

tenac′ulum. A hooked surgical instrument for grasping and holding parts, such as the divided end

of a blood vessel during an operation.

tenal′gia. Pain in a tendon; also called tenontodynia and tenodynia.

ten′der. Painful on pressure; sensitive.

ten′derness. Abnormal sensitivity to pressure or contact.

　rebound t., pain felt when pressure is released suddenly; in the abdomen it is characteristic of peritonitis.

tendini′tis. Inflammation of a tendon; also called tenontitis, tenonitis, and tendonitis.

tendinoplas′ty. See tenoplasty.

ten′dinous. Relating to or of the nature of a tendon.

tendol′ysis. The removal of adhesions from a tendon; also called tenolysis.

ten′don. A fibrous band that attaches a muscle to a bone.

　Achilles t., see calcaneal tendon.

　calcaneal t., the large common tendon that attaches the gastrocnemius and soleus muscles to the calcaneus (heel bone); also called Achilles tendon and tendo calcaneus.

　conjoined t., the fused tendons of the transversus abdominis and internal oblique muscles; it inserts onto the crest of the pubic bone and the pectineal line; also called inguinal falx and conjoint tendon.

tendoni′tis. See tendinitis.

ten′doplasty. See tenoplasty.

tendot′omy. See tenotomy.

tenec′tomy. Surgical removal of part of a tendon.

tenes′mic. Relating to or afflicted with tenesmus.

tenes′mus. A painful, ineffectual straining to defecate or urinate.

te′nia, *pl.* **te′niae. 1.** Any narrow bandlike anatomic structure. **2.** The line of attachment of a choroid plexus. **3.** Any flatworm of the genus *Taenia*.

　t. coli, any of three thickened bands of longitudinal muscular fibers about six millimeters broad, on the wall of the colon.

　t. libera, the tenia coli almost midway between the tenia mesocolica and tenia omentalis; also called free band.

　t. mesocolica, the tenia coli situated along the attachment of the mesocolon to the colon.

　t. omentalis, the tenia coli of the transverse colon situated along the site of attachment of the greater omentum.

　t. thalami, the tenia, or line of attachment, of the choroid plexus that runs along the dorsomedial border of the thalamus; the lateral ventricles lie above it and the third ventricle lies below it; also called tenia of the thalamus and tenia of the third ventricle.

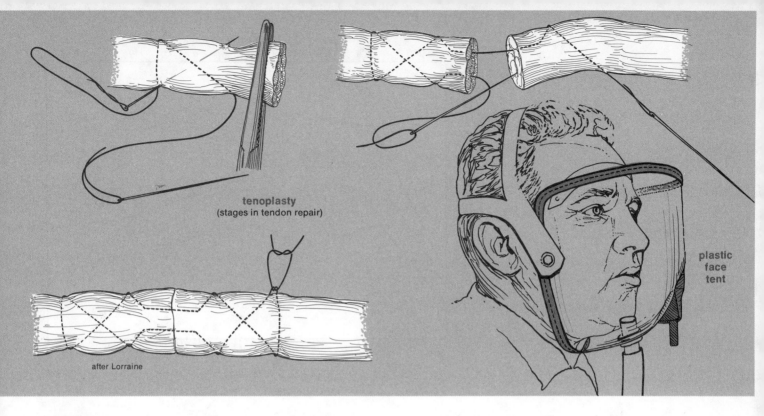

tenoplasty
(stages in tendon repair)

after Lorraine

plastic
face
tent

te'niacide. Any agent that destroys tapeworms.

teniafuge. An agent for expelling tapeworms.

te'nial. 1. Relating to a tapeworm. **2.** Relating to a band of tissue (tenia).

teni'asis. Infestation with tapeworms in the intestine.

te'nioid. 1. Resembling a ribbon. **2.** Resembling a tapeworm.

teno-, tenon-. Combining forms denoting tendon; e.g., tenotomy.

tenod'esis. The transferring of the proximal end of a tendon to another site.

tenol'ysis. See tendolysis.

tenonec'tomy. Surgical procedure for shortening a tendon in which a segment of the tendon is removed and the two remaining ends are joined.

Tenon's capsule. Bulbar fascia; see under fascia.

tenonti'tis. See tendinitis.

ten'ophyte. A growth of cartilaginous or bony tissue attached to a tendon.

ten'oplasty. Reparative surgery of the tendons; also called tendinoplasty, tendoplasty, and tenontoplasty.

tenorrh'aphy. The suturing of a divided tendon.

tenosynovec'tomy. Surgical removal of a tendon sheath.

tenosynovi'tis. Inflammation of a tendon sheath; also called tenovaginitis.

tenot'omy. The cutting of a tendon for corrective measures, as for clubfoot or strabismus; also called tendotomy.

tenovagini'tis. See tenosynovitis.

ten'sion. 1. The act of stretching or the condition of being taut or strained. **2.** A force tending to produce extension or expansion, as of a liquid or gas, when a confining force is removed. **3.** Emotional or mental strain.

  arterial t., the pressure produced on the wall of an artery by the blood current at the peak of a pulse wave.

  interfacial surface t., the resistance to separation offered by the film of liquid between two well adapted surfaces, as that of the thin film of saliva between a denture base and the tissues.

  intraocular t., pressure within the eyeball.

  premenstrual t., temporary condition marked by irritability, nervousness, and/or headache, occurring during the week prior to menstruation and disappearing after the onset of the menstrual flow.

  surface t., the force that tends to pull together the molecules of a liquid surface when in contact with another substance.

ten'sor. A muscle that makes a part tense or firm.

tent. 1. A covering of canvas or plastic placed over a patient's bed for the administration of inhaled medications or oxygen. **2.** An expandable plug placed in an orifice to keep it open.

  oxygen t., one placed over a patient's bed into which oxygen is conducted.

  plastic face t., one placed over a patient's face to facilitate the administration of gaseous medications.

  steam t., one in which steam is provided.

tento'rial. Of or relating to the tentorium.

tento'rium. A membranous partition.

  t. cerebelli, a fold of dura mater separating the cerebellum and the posterior part of the cerebrum.

tephromala'cia. Condition marked by softening of the gray substance of the brain and spinal cord.

ter. Latin for three times.

  t. die sumendum (t.d.s.), Latin for to be taken three times a day; used in prescription writing.

  t. in die (t.i.d.), three times a day; used in prescription writing.

tera-. Combining form used in the metric system to indicate a trillion (10^{12}); e.g., teraohm.

teras. A greatly deformed fetus.

terato-. Combining form denoting a relationship to a greatly deformed fetus.

ter'atocarcino'ma. 1. A malignant tumor composed of several types of tissues, usually occurring in the testis. **2.** A malignant epithelial tumor originating in a teratoma.

ter'atogen. A chemical that induces abnormal fetal development when administered during pregnancy.

teratogen'esis, teratog'eny. The origin of congenital malformations.

ter'atoid. Resembling a malformed fetus.

teratol'ogy. The subspecialty of developmental anatomy that deals with abnormal development; also called desmorphology.

terato'ma. A tumor composed of multiple tissues, including tissues not normally found in the organ in which it arises; occurs most frequently in the ovary, where it is usually benign and forms dermoid cysts; also occurs in the testis, where it is usually malignant, and, uncommonly, in other sites.

terato'matous. Relating to or having the characteristics of a teratoma.

teratopho'bia. Morbid fear of giving birth to a grossly deformed baby.

terato'sis. A gross anomaly; also called teratism.

ter'bium. A metallic element; symbol Tb, atomic number 65, atomic weight 158.93.

te'res. Round and elongated, such as certain ligaments and muscles.

term. 1. A definite or limited period of time. **2.** A point of time starting or ending a period.

  at t., at the normal time; at the end of a normal pregnancy or gestation period.

ter'minal. 1. Relating to the end. **2.** Relating to, situated at, or forming the extremity of any structure. **3.** The part of an electric circuit at which an electric connection is generally made.

  computer t., a machine resembling a typewriter, sometimes equipped with a television-like cathode ray screen, which is directly connected to a computer for the purpose of entering and retrieving information; also called interactive or on-line terminal.

  interactive t., see computer terminal.

  on-line t., see computer terminal.

terms. The menses.

ter'nary. Composed of three, as a molecule containing three different types of atoms.

ter'ra. Earth; soil.

  t. alba, (1) a finely pulverized powder, barium sulfate, which because of its radiopaque properties is used to outline structures during roentgenography of the digestive tract; (2) a clay, kaolin.

ter'tian. Recurring every third day, as a type of malarial fever; the attack actually occurs on day one and day three, so that there is really only an interval of one day.

ter'tiarism, tertiaris'mus. The combined symptoms of the third stage of syphilis.

ter'tigrav'ida. A woman who has been pregnant three times.

tertip'ara. A person who has borne three children.

test. 1. An examination. **2.** A means to determine the presence and quantity of a substance. **3.** To perform such functions. **4.** A substance used in a test.

  acetone t., one used to detect the presence of acetone in the urine; a few drops of sodium nitroprusside are added to the urine sample and shaken; strong ammonia water is then poured over the mixture; if acetone is present, a magenta ring forms at the line of contact.

  acoustic impedance t., a test that assesses the integrity and function of the middle ear, especially transmission characteristics, by measuring the reflected sound waves (acoustic impedance) at the tympanic membrane.

  Adson's t., one for the detection of thoracic outlet syndrome; the patient sits with the palm of the hands on his knees, chin held high, head turned toward the side to be examined; if on deep inspiration the radial pulse disappears, it indicates temporary occlusion of the subclavian artery.

  alkali denaturation t., test to determine the concentration of fetal hemoglobin.

  antiglobulin t., see Coombs' test.

  Aschheim-Zondek t., a test for the determination

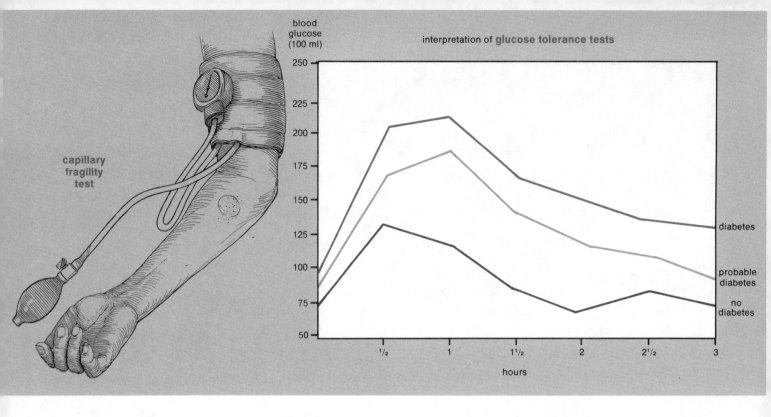

blood glucose (100 ml)

interpretation of **glucose tolerance tests**

diabetes

probable diabetes

no diabetes

hours

capillary fragility test

---

of pregnancy; small quantities of first morning urine are injected subcutaneously into four immature female mice; if the woman is pregnant, the ovaries of the mice become swollen, hyperemic, and hemorrhagic, and may also exhibit premature maturation of the ovarian follicles.

association t., a method for examining the content of the mind, whereby the subject is required to respond as quickly as possible to a given stimulus word with the first word that comes to mind; also called word association test.

balloon t. for cervical incompetency, Mann test.

Bender-Gestalt t., a test of visual motor function in which the subject is asked to copy nine standard designs; its chief application is to determine organic brain dysfunction in both children and adults and level of development of visual motor function in children; secondarily used to assess personality variables; also called Bender visual-motor Gestalt test.

Benedict's t., a test for detecting glucose in urine; the urine sample is mixed with the reagent (copper sulfate, sodium citrate, and sodium carbonate) and placed in a boiling water bath for five minutes; a green, yellow, or orange-red precipitate forms in the presence of glucose.

benzidine t., test to detect the presence of blood; a portion of the suspected sample is added to benzidine reagent (benzidine, glacial acetic acid, and hydrogen peroxide); a blue color develops in the presence of blood.

Binet t., Stanford-Binet t., one used to determine the mental age of a child; it consists of a series of questions standardized according to the mental capacity of normal children at different ages.

biuret t., test used to determine the presence of proteins in body fluids; the sample is mixed with alkaline copper sulfate; a violet-pinkish color indicates a positive result.

blood urea clearance t., see urea clearance test.

Brodie-Trendelenburg t., test for determining the presence of incompetent valves in the communicating veins between the superficial and deep vessels in patients with varicose veins; tourniquet is applied around the thigh with the individual in the recumbent position; if the valves are incompetent, they allow the varicosities to fill rapidly when the person assumes an erect position.

bromsulfalein (BSP) t., a sensitive test for determining hepatic function; bromsulfalein is injected intravenously; within the liver cell it becomes conjugated with glutathione and then excreted; the rate of excretion is indicative of the state of hepatic function; normal value is less than five per cent remaining in serum 45 minutes after injection of 5 mg per kg of body weight; also called sulfobromophthalein test.

capillary fragility t., a tourniquet test to determine weakness of the capillary walls; a circle 2.5 cm in diameter is drawn on the inner aspect of the forearm 4 cm below the crease of the elbow, and a blood pressure cuff is inflated above the elbow (not to exceed 100 mm Hg) for five minutes; the petechiae (minute hemorrhagic spots) formed within the circle are counted; a number over 20 is abnormal; also called Rumpel-Leede test.

cephalin-cholesterol flocculation t., obsolete test to distinguish between obstructive and hepatogenous jaundice.

complement-fixation t., a widely used test to detect the presence of antibodies in serum; based on the fact that antibodies, when combined with their specific antigens, are able to fix or remove complement (thus making it undetectable in a subsequent test).

Coombs' t. (CT), an agglutination test designed to detect the presence on cells of serum proteins (commonly functionally univalent antibodies) not usually identifiable by simple in vitro agglutination techniques; two methods may be combined: direct (test for antibody on cells) or indirect (test for antibody in serum); also called antiglobulin test. See also direct and indirect Coombs' tests.

cross-agglutination t., one of several tests used in blood typing; red blood cells from a donor of an unknown blood type are mixed with sera of known blood types.

cytotoxicity t., cytoxicity t., one used in testing for compatibility for organ transplant; living cells are mixed with antibody and complement; if antibody to a cell-bound antigen is present, cell death will occur in the presence of complement.

Dick t., intracutaneous test to detect susceptibility to scarlet fever.

direct Coombs' t., test for detecting sensitized red blood cells in erythroblastosis fetalis and acquired hemolytic anemia; a sample of the patient's red blood cells is washed with saline and mixed with Coombs' antihuman globulin, then centrifuged; agglutination indicates a positive test.

double-blind t., one in which neither the person giving the test nor the one receiving it knows whether the drug used is active or inert.

draw-a-person t., in psychology, (a) a method of determining a child's level of intellectual development based upon the complexity of the subject's "best" drawing of a human figure; also called Goodenough test; (b) a projective personality test requiring the subject to draw a person; also called Machover test.

Ellsworth-Howard t., The measuring of urinary phosphate after intravenous administration of parathyroid extract for the diagnosis of pseudohypoparathyroidism; an increase in urinary phosphate is seen in hypoparathyroidism but not in pseudohypoparathyroidism (however, exceptions may occur).

ether t., one used to estimate arm-to-lung circulation time; diluted ether is injected intravenously into the arm; the time elapsed is recorded when the subject coughs, grimaces, or tastes or smells ether; normal arm to lung time is four to eight seconds; a prolonged time is found in congestive heart failure, particularly when the right ventricle is involved.

FIGlu t., a test to determine a deficiency in folic acid based upon the excretion of formiminoglutamic acid (FIGlu) in the urine; after ingestion of histidine, urine is collected over a period from three to eight hours; FIGlu is then separated from it by electrophoresis and measured by converting to glutamic acid with ammonia.

fluorescent treponemal antibody-absorption t. (FTA-ABS t.), a specific test for syphilis using a suspension of *Treponema pallidum* (Nichols strain).

fragility t., one that measures the osmotic fragility of red blood cells; cells are placed in a series of test tubes with saline of decreasing concentrations ranging from 0.85 to 0.10 per cent; the red cells absorb water, swell to a spheroid shape, and rupture; in normal cells hemolysis begins at concentrations of 0.45 to 0.39 per cent, and complete hemolysis occurs at 0.33 to 0.30 per cent.

Frei t., test for detection of lymphogranuloma venereum; if the person has the disease, a red papule forms when antigen (prepared from pus obtained from a lesion) is injected intracutaneously.

galactose tolerance t., a liver function test that measures the ability of the liver to convert galactose to glycogen; after ingestion of 40 grams of galactose, excretion of not more than three grams in urine after five hours is considered normal.

glucose tolerance t. (GTT), test for diabetes based on the response to a glucose load; in the oral glucose tolerance test (OGTT), 100 grams of glucose are ingested after an overnight fast; normally, blood sugar rises quickly, then falls to normal within two hours; in diabetes mellitus, the increase is greater and the return to normal is abnormally prolonged; additional information can be obtained if plasma insulin levels are measured simultaneously; in patients with gastrointestinal disease a smaller dose of glucose (usually 25 grams) may be given intravenously to avoid difficulty in interpretation due to abnormal absorption.

histamine t., (1) a test for determining the absence of gastric acidity; histamine phosphate is in-

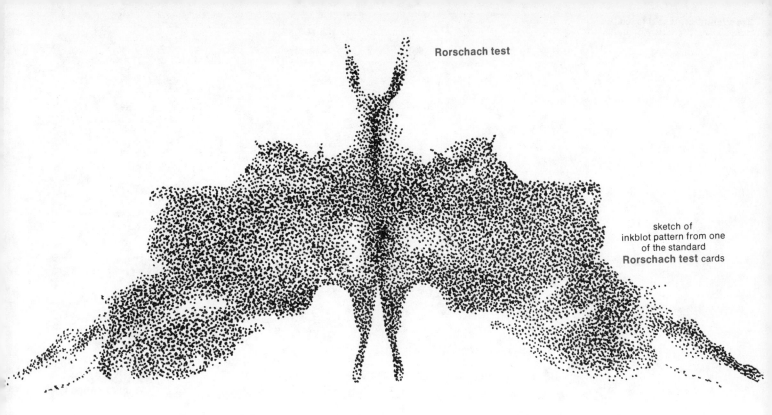

sketch of
inkblot pattern from one
of the standard
Rorschach test cards

jected subcutaneously to stimulate secretion of gastric juice; (2) a provocative test for pheochromocytoma; histamine phosphate is injected intravenously; normally there is a prompt, slight fall in blood pressure, but if a lesion is present, a marked rise in blood pressure follows immediately after the fall.

Howard t., a test used to determine functional disparities between two kidneys in the diagnosis of renovascular hypertension; bilateral ureteral catheterization is performed and urine from each side is obtained for measurement of flow rate, sodium concentration, and creatine concentration; a reduction of urine flow of 40 per cent or more and reduction in urinary sodium concentration of 15 per cent or more, or increase in creatinine concentration of 50 per cent or more, suggests that a particular kidney may be responsible for the individual's hypertension; also called split-function test. See also Ellsworth-Howard test.

immunologic pregnancy t., test utilizing latex particles coated with human chorionic gonadotropin (HCG) as antigen, anti-HCG serum, and urine to be tested; if the latex particles do not clump, the woman is pregnant; also called agglutination inhibition test for pregnancy.

indirect Coombs' t., test used in crossmatching of blood and transfusion reaction studies; the patient's serum is incubated with a suspension of donor red blood cells; after a washing with saline, Coombs' serum is added; clumping indicates that the cells had been coated or sensitized by antibodies present in the patient's serum.

intelligence t., any test designed to measure the mental capacity of the subject.

Ishihara t., a test for detection of color blindness, based on the ability to see patterns in a series of multicolored plates or cards (Ishihara plates).

Kolmer's t., (1) a complement-fixation test for certain bacterial diseases; (2) a modified Wassermann test for syphilis.

Kveim t., test for detection of sarcoidosis; a dose of ground sarcoid lymph nodes, tested for sterility and preserved in phenol, is injected intradermally; a papule appears; biopsy of the papule in a positive test shows giant cell formation.

latex t., one for rheumatoid arthritis; minute spherical particles of latex in suspension are coated with antigen and incubated with the patient's serum; when rheumatoid factor is present in the serum, clumping of the latex particles occurs; also called latex agglutination or latex fixation test.

Liebermann-Burchard t., a test for cholesterol; the suspected substance is mixed with acetic anhydride and sulfuric acid in chloroform; a blue-green color develops when cholesterol is present.

Mann t., the insertion of a special rubber balloon filled with an opaque substance into the uterus to check the competency of the cervix.

Mantoux t., a tuberculin test in which a derivative of tuberculin, such as purified protein derivative (PPD), is injected intracutaneously; considered positive if redness and induration of 10 mm diameter occur.

Master's t., Master's two-step exercise t., two-step exercise test.

oyster ciliary t., the sera from individuals with cystic fibrosis inhibit ciliary activity in preparations of oyster gills.

Pap t., Papanicolaou t., microscopic examination of secretion (especially from the female genital tract) for the detection of cancer and for evaluation of the hormonal state.

partial thromboplastin time t., a one-stage clotting test for detection of plasma factor deficiencies.

patch t., a test for allergic sensitivity made by placing filter paper or gauze saturated with a suspected allergen against the skin (usually of the forearm) under a small patch; on removal of the patch the reaction of the skin is observed; a positive reaction is indicated by reddening at the site; also used for tuberculin testing.

paternity t., a medicolegal test based upon genetic interpretation of blood groups of mother, child, and alleged father for the purpose of excluding the possibility of paternity.

Paul-Bunnell t., a test to determine the presence of heterophil antibodies in the circulating blood; an elevated titer is found in infectious mononucleosis.

Phalen's t., a test for determining median nerve compression in the carpal tunnel of the wrist; the wrists are placed in a flexed position; if there is median nerve compression, paresthesias of the fingers usually occur after several seconds; most normal individuals develop paresthesias after a few minutes of acute wrist flexion.

phenolsulfonphthalein t. (PSP test), a test for renal function; thirty minutes after an individual drinks two or three glasses of water, one millimeter of phenolsulfonphthalein (PSP) is administered intravenously; urine specimens are obtained 15, 30, 60, and 120 minutes later to determine the rate of dye excretion; normal values are 25 per cent or more in 15 minutes and 40 per cent or more in 30 minutes; delayed excretion of the dye (low PSP test) indicates a renal disorder such as a general loss of nephron function.

phentolamine t., test for pheochromocytoma in patients with sustained hypertension; administration of phentolamine produces a sustained fall in blood pressure in the presence of pheochromocytoma.

postprandial blood sugar t., a test utilizing a sample of blood drawn, usually two hours after the ingestion of a 100-gram carbohydrate meal for the diagnosis of diabetes mellitus.

precipitin t., any test in which a positive result is indicated by the formation of a precipitate; also called precipitation test.

pregnancy t., any test for pregnancy (e.g., Aschheim-Zondek test, immunologic pregnancy test).

protein-bound iodine t., PBI t., a common test for thyroid function; it reflects the rate at which the gland secretes thyroxin into the circulation by measuring the amount of protein-bound iodine in the blood; more specific tests for circulating thyroid hormone are now generally used.

prothrombin t., one that determines the amount of thrombin present in plasma, based on the clotting time of blood; used to measure blood coagulability and as a guide to anticoagulation with coumarin and related drugs.

provocative t., a test for pheochromocytoma performed on patients with normal blood pressure; the presence of pheochromocytoma causes a sudden rise in blood pressure immediately following the administration of histamine, tyramine, or glucagon.

psychological t., any test dealing with mental phenomena.

pulp t., see vitality test.

pyrogen t., test to detect the presence of pyrogens (fever-causing substances) in a fluid to be given to a patient intravenously; the material to be tested is injected into a rabbit, whose temperature is taken 15 minutes before and every hour (for three hours) after the injection.

Queckenstedt-Stookey t., when the jugular vein is compressed in a healthy person, there is a rapid increase in the pressure of the cerebrospinal fluid (CSF), and an equally rapid return to normal when pressure is released; when there is a block in the vertebral canal, compression of the jugular vein causes little or no increase in pressure.

Rinne's t., hearing test that compares bone conduction with air conduction by alternately holding a vibrating tuning fork in contact with the skull and in the air near the auditory orifice; in normal hearing the vibrations are heard twice as long by air as by bone conduction; in conductive hearing loss the ratio varies in favor of bone conduction.

Rorschach t., projective psychological test for evaluating conscious and unconscious personality traits and emotional conflicts through the individual's associations to a set of inkblot patterns.

test | **test**

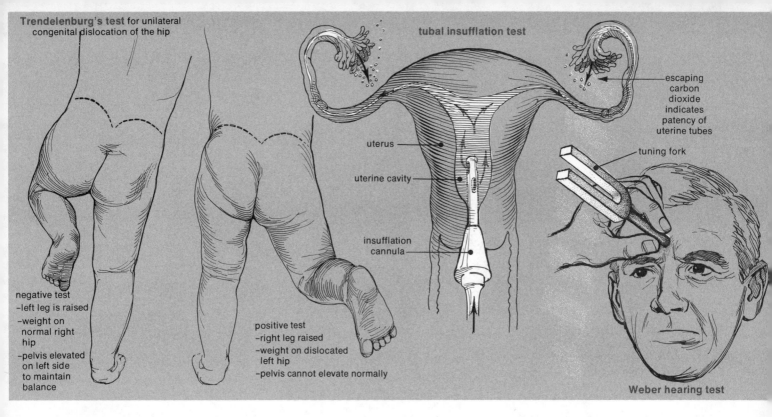

Trendelenburg's test for unilateral congenital dislocation of the hip

tubal insufflation test

escaping carbon dioxide indicates patency of uterine tubes

uterus

uterine cavity

tuning fork

insufflation cannula

negative test
–left leg is raised
–weight on normal right hip
–pelvis elevated on left side to maintain balance

positive test
–right leg raised
–weight on dislocated left hip
–pelvis cannot elevate normally

Weber hearing test

Rumpel-Leede t., capillary fragility test.

Sabin-Feldman dye t., one used to diagnose toxoplasmosis; heat-inactivated serum from the patient (in the presence of a nonspecific serum factor) kills *Toxoplasma* organisms; methylene blue fails to stain damaged organisms.

Schick t., a test to measure immunity to diphtheria; diphtheria toxin (one-fiftieth of a guinea pig median lethal dose) is injected intracutaneously; if the person does not have sufficient antitoxin to neutralize the dose of toxin, an inflammation appears at the site of injection, usually within 48 hours.

Schiller's t., a test for early squamous cell carcinoma of the cervix; the cervix is coated with an aqueous iodine solution; a normal cervix turns brown; a cancerous cervix turns yellowish-white.

Schirmer's t., test to measure the production of tears with a strip of filter paper.

scratch t., see skin test.

screening t., one devised to separate individuals or objects according to a fixed characteristic or property.

secretin t., test for excretory function of the pancreas; secretion of pancreatic enzymes is stimulated for analysis by intravenous injection of the hormone secretin.

serologic t., any test using serum.

sickle cell t., when blood is mixed with sodium bisulfite, red blood cells containing the abnormal sickle hemoglobin (Hb S) assume a crescentic or elongated shape.

skin t., any test for allergy or infectious disease in which the allergen or an extract of a disease-causing organism is injected intracutaneously or applied to the skin by means of a patch; also called scratch test.

skinfold t., measurement of skinfolds with special constant tension calipers to determine the degree of obesity.

Stanford-Binet t., see Binet test.

string t., any of various tests to determine the approximate site of bleeding from the upper gastrointestinal tract, using a white string which is passed into the duodenum or beyond; the string is removed and checked along its length for blood; the blood-stained portion indicates the site of hemorrhage.

sweat t., one for diagnosis of cystic fibrosis of the pancreas; high concentration of sodium chloride in the sweat is suggestive of the disease.

thematic apperception t. (TAT), psychological test in which the subject is asked to tell stories about ambiguous pictures that may be interpreted in different ways, according to the individual's personality.

three-glass t., one devised to locate the site of inflammation of the male urinary tract in which the patient urinates into three glass containers; the contents of each container reveal the approximate site; the urine in the first container has washings from the anterior urethra, that in the second from the bladder, and that in the third from the posterior urethra, prostate, and seminal vesicles.

thromboplastin generation t. (TGT), a coagulation test based on the principle of mixing reagents; if thromboplastin formation is deficient, recombination of reagents determines which of the ingredients is defective.

tilt t., (1) test for pheochromocytoma; excretion of urinary epinephrine and norepinephrine is measured during consecutive three-hour intervals with the patient first in a horizontal and then in a nearly vertical position; a marked increase in the second period indicates a positive test; (2) a rise in pulse or drop in blood pressure as a patient is moved from the supine toward the upright position, indicating a loss of extracellular fluid, as during hemorrhage or dehydration.

tine t., test for skin sensitivity performed by pressing tines previously impregnated with antigens into the skin; used for tuberculin testing.

Töpfer's t., quantitative test for free hydrochloric acid in the gastric contents, by means of the indicator *p*-dimethylaminoazobenzene (0.5 per cent alcoholic solution).

Trendelenburg's t., test for unilateral congenital dislocation of the hip; when weight is borne on the normal side of the hip, the opposite side of the pelvis is elevated to maintain balance (negative test); when weight is borne on the dislocated side, the opposite side of the pelvis cannot be elevated normally (positive test).

treponemal immobilization t. (TPI), test for syphilis; serum from a syphilitic patient (in the presence of complement) immobilizes the actively motile *Treponema pallidum* obtained from testes of a syphilitic rabbit (antigen).

triiodothyronine uptake t. (T_3 t.), an in vitro measurement using the patient's serum and radioactive triiodothyronine to determine the concentration of thyroxin-binding globulin present.

tubal insufflation t., insufflation of the uterus with carbon dioxide to determine patency of the uterine (fallopian) tubes; if patent, the escape of gas into the abdominal cavity is heard over the lower abdomen; also called Rubin test.

tuberculin t., any test for tuberculosis in which tuberculin or its protein derivative is introduced into the skin by means of a patch (patch test), multiple punctures (tine test), or injection (Mantoux test).

two-step exercise t., test for coronary insufficiency in which the person makes two steps nine inches high repeatedly for 1½ minutes; a depression of the ST segment of the electrocardiogram indicates coronary insufficiency; also called Master's test.

urea clearance t., a renal function test based on the volume of blood which is cleared of its urea per minute; urea clearance is related in part to urine flow; maximum clearance is obtained at flow rates over two milliliters per minute; standard clearance is generally 40 to 65 ml/min; maximum clearance, 60 to 100 ml/min; also called blood urea clearance test.

van den Bergh's t., a test used to determine bilirubin in body fluids.

VDRL t., flocculation test for syphilis developed by the Venereal Disease Research Laboratory of the United States Public Health Service.

vitality t., a test that measures the response of the dental pulp to various stimuli (thermal, electrical, or mechanical); it determines whether a pulp is alive, diseased, or dead; also called pulp test.

vitamin A absorption t., a gastrointestinal absorption test; after a fasting blood specimen is obtained, the subject ingests 200,000 units of vitamin A in oil; serum vitamin A level normally should rise to twice fasting level in three to five hours.

Wassermann t., a complement-fixation test used in the diagnosis of syphilis; the antigen is a cardiolipin diphosphatidylglycerol; also called Wassermann reaction.

Weber hearing t., the application of a vibrating tuning fork to the midline of the forehead, bridge of the nose, and against the chin, for audiologic assessment; if the individual hears the tone in the middle of his head, he may have either normal hearing or deafness equal on both sides; if there is nerve deafness on one side, the tone will be heard better on the other side; when asymmetric conductive deafness is present, the tone is heard better in the poor ear.

d-**xylose absorption t.,** a test of gastrointestinal absorption; after fasting for eight hours, an individual drinks 10 milliliters per kilogram body weight of a five per cent solution of *d*-xylose and then abstains from eating or drinking until the test is completed; all urine voided during the following five hours is pooled; blood samples are taken just prior to ingestion of the solution and at one and two hours later; normally, 16 to 33 per cent of the ingested xylose is excreted within five hours; the serum xylose reaches a level between 25 and 40 mg/100 ml after one hour and is maintained at this level for another 60 minutes.

test | **test**

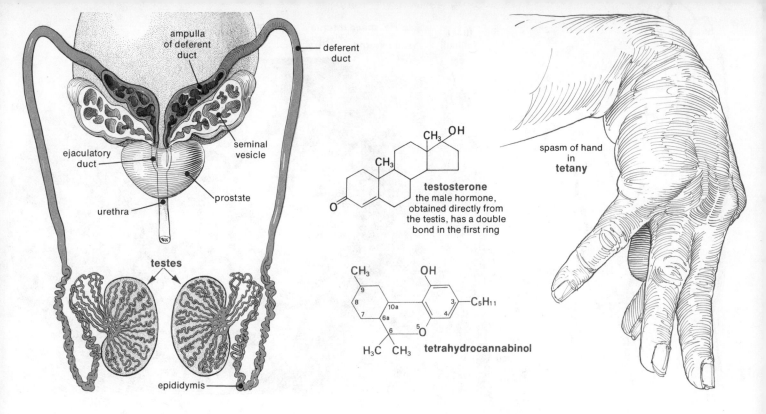

ampulla of deferent duct

deferent duct

ejaculatory duct

seminal vesicle

prostate

urethra

testes

epididymis

testosterone
the male hormone, obtained directly from the testis, has a double bond in the first ring

tetrahydrocannabinol

spasm of hand in tetany

tes'ta. An outer shell.

testal'gia. Orchialgia; testicular pain.

test'cross. A way of determining an unknown genotype by crossing it with a homozygous recessive.

tes'tes. Plural of testis.

tes'ticle. See testis.

testic'ular. Of or relating to the testes.

testicular feminization syndrome. Familial male pseudohermaphroditism marked by female external genitalia with a short vaginal pouch and absent uterus, undescended or labial testes, and absent or sparse pubic and axillary hair; the karyotype is XY, but there is a lack of end organ response to testosterone.

tes'tis, *pl.* **tes'tes.** One of the two egg-shaped glands which produce spermatozoa, normally situated in the scrotum; also called testicle.

   descent of the t., the gradual change of location of the testis, in the fetus and infant, from the abdominal cavity to the scrotum.

   undescended t., retained t., a testis that fails to descend into the scrotum, but remains in the abdominal cavity or inguinal canal.

testi'tis. See orchitis.

testos'terone. A hormone produced by the testes, responsible for the development and maintenance of secondary sexual characteristics; the most potent of the naturally produced androgens, it is produced in the Leydig's cells under control of luteinizing (interstitial cell-stimulating) hormone.

test types. Letters or figures printed on a card, used to test vision.

   Jaeger's t. t., words and phrases printed in ordinary printer's type of varying sizes, used to test near vision.

   Snellen's t. t., block letters of varying sizes printed on a white card; used to test visual acuity.

tetan'ic. Relating to tetanus or tetany.

tetan'iform. Resembling tetanus.

tet'anize. To produce a sustained contraction of a muscle by the application of numerous stimuli in rapid succession.

tet'anode. The quiet period between the muscle spasms in tetanus.

tet'anoid. 1. Resembling tetanus. **2.** Resembling tetany.

tetanol'ysin. A hemolysin produced by the tetanus bacillus (*Clostridium tetani*).

tet'anospas'min. The neurotoxin produced by *Clostridium tetani*, the causative agent of tetanus; it interferes with neuromuscular transmission by inhibiting the release of acetylcholine from nerve terminals in muscles; sites of action include: the motor end plates in skeletal muscles, spinal cord, brain,

and sympathetic nervous system.

tetanotox'in. A filtrate of a culture of *Clostridium tetani* (the tetanus bacillus) containing the toxins tetanospasmin and tetanolysin.

tet'anus. 1. An acute infectious disease caused by the toxin of *Clostridium tetani*, which affects the central nervous system, and marked by painful muscular contraction, most commonly beginning in the jaws (trismus) and neck muscles; it results from deposition of spores of *Clostridium tetani* in an area of injury, often minor, where the devitalized tissue permits growth; its incubation period is from three days to four weeks or longer; in generalized tetanus, the mobility rate approximates 50 per cent; severity is related to the rapidity of onset of symptoms; also called lockjaw. **2.** Sustained or prolonged contraction of a muscle.

   local t., one which affects only the muscles of the immediate area of the wound.

   t. neonatorum, a form of tetanus affecting newborn infants due to infection through the open end of the umbilical cord.

tet'any. A disorder marked by intermittent muscle spasms, usually beginning with sharp flexion of the wrists and ankles, and progressing to involve other muscles and produce convulsions; it occurs as a result of hypocalcemia, alkalosis, or hypokalemia.

   hyperventilation t., tetany caused by reduction of carbon dioxide in the blood, as in prolonged forced breathing.

   latent t., tetany which is made apparent only by certain stimulating procedures.

   neonatal t., a relatively continuous hypertonicity of muscles in newborn infants.

tetartanop'sia. Loss of vision in homonymous quadrants of the visual fields of both eyes; e.g., the lower nasal quadrant of one eye and lower temporal quadrant of the other eye.

tetra-, tetr-. Combining forms denoting four; e.g., tetrachloride.

tet'racaine hydrochlo'ride. A white crystalline compound used as a local or spinal anesthetic.

tetrachlor'ide. A compound possessing four atoms of chlorine per molecule.

tetrachlormeth'ane. See carbon tetrachloride.

tetracyc'line. A yellow crystalline compound produced synthetically or from certain species of *Streptomyces;* a broad spectrum antibiotic.

tet'rad. 1. A set of four related things. **2.** In chemistry, an element that has the combining power of four. **3.** A group of four chromatids (chromosomal elements) that were formed during meiosis.

tetradac'tyl. Having only four fingers or toes.

tetraethylammonium chloride. Compound of ammonium having a ganglionic blocking action of

short duration.

tetrahydrocannab'inol (THC). The chief active ingredient in marijuana; it has no accepted medical use.

3,5,3',5'-tetraiodothy'ronine (T$_4$). See thyroxin.

tetral'ogy. Any series of four related elements, such as four concurrent defects.

   t. of Fallot, a form of cyanotic congenital heart disease; the four abnormalities which constitute the deformity are pulmonic stenosis (usually infundibular), right ventricular hypertrophy, ventricular septal defect, and overriding of the aorta; thought to be due to a single embryologic error whereby the conus septum is located in an abnormally anterior position.

tetraple'gia. Quadriplegia; paralysis of the four extremities.

tet'raploid. A cell with four haploid sets of chromosomes in its nucleus.

tetrav'alent. See quadrivalent.

tet'rose. A four-carbon sugar; a monosaccharide containing four carbon atoms; e.g., threose and erythrose.

TG. Abbreviation for triglyceride.

Th. Chemical symbol of the element thorium.

thalam'ic. Relating to the thalamus.

thalamic syndrome. Hemianesthesia, hemichorea, central pain, and hemiparesis caused by arterial occlusion; also called Dejerine-Roussy syndrome.

thalamocor'tical. Relating to the thalamus and the cerebral cortex.

thalamolentic'ular. Relating to the thalamus and the lentiform nucleus of the brain.

thalamomam'millary. Relating to the thalamus and the mammillary bodies of the brain.

thalamotegmen'tal. Relating to the tegmentum of the brain stem and the thalamus.

thalamot'omy. Operative destruction of a portion of the thalamus.

thal'amus, *pl.* **thal'ami.** An ovoid gray mass about four cm in length, located on either side of the third ventricle of the cerebrum, which primarily serves as a relay center for sensory impulses in the cerebral cortex; it is also an important structure for the perception of some types of sensation.

thalasse'mia. A genetically transmitted type of hemolytic anemia; caused by a decreased rate of synthesis of one of the polypeptide chains in the globin portion of hemoglobin; the different forms are classified according to the polypeptide chain involved, i.e., α, β, or γ; in the presence of one normal gene and one thalassemia gene (the heterozygote state), clinical findings are generally mild and the condition is termed thalassemia trait or

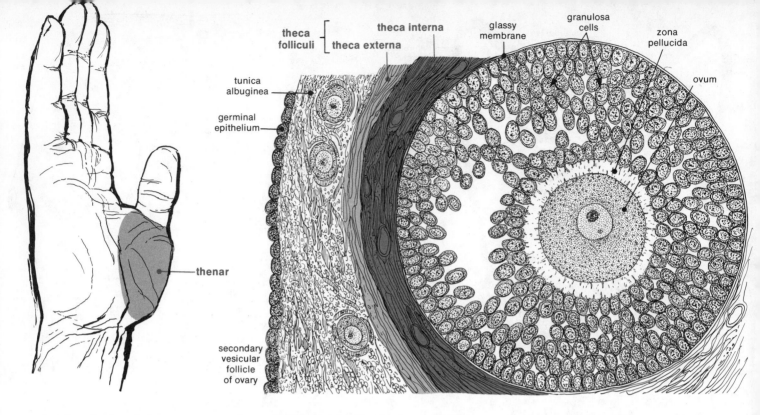

thenar

tunica albuginea

germinal epithelium

secondary vesicular follicle of ovary

theca folliculi { theca interna / theca externa }

theca interna

glassy membrane

granulosa cells

zona pellucida

ovum

thalassemia minor; the homozygous state produces thalassemia major, generally a severe illness characterized by the appearance, in early childhood, of anemia, hepatosplenomegaly, jaundice, and growth retardation.

A₂ t., β thalassemia.

β t., thalassemia characterized by a decrease in the rate of synthesis of the β polypeptide chain of hemoglobin; if the defect is only in the β chain, levels of hemoglobin A₂ are increased even in the heterozygous form; also called Cooley's or Mediterranean anemia.

F t., a form of thalassemia in which heterozygotes show high levels of fetal hemoglobin and normal levels of A₂ hemoglobin; both β and γ polypeptide chains are affected.

α t., a form in which there is a decrease in the rate of synthesis of the α polypeptide chain of hemoglobin; the homozygous form is incompatible with life.

thalassopho'bia. A morbid fear of the sea.

thalid'omide. A sedative and hypnotic drug, $C_{13}H_{10}N_2O_4$; when taken by pregnant women, it has been associated with abnormalities of the fetus' limbs.

thal'lium. A rare metallic element, symbol Tl, atomic number 81, atomic weight 204.37; the lightest known element with naturally radioactive isotopes; used in scintillation scanning.

thal'lospore. An organ of reproduction derived directly from the thallus or vegetative portion of certain fungi and algae.

thallotoxico'sis. Poisoning resulting from the intake (accidental or purposeful) of thallium salts (widely used as pesticides); clinical features include ptosis, ataxia, tremors, paresthesias, and a toxic encephalopathy.

thal'lus. The vegetative plant body of certain fungi and algae, which is not differentiated into root, stem, and leaf.

than'atoid. 1. Resembling death. **2.** Deadly.

thanatol'ogy. The science of death in all its aspects.

thanatopho'bia. Extreme fear of death.

thanatop'sia, than'atopsy. Autopsy.

THC. Abbreviation for tetrahydrocannabinol.

the'ca, *pl.* **the'cae.** A sheath, such as the one covering a tendon or a vesicular ovarian follicle.

t. externa, the outer fibrous part of the theca folliculi; it is poorly vascularized.

t. folliculi, an envelope of concentrically arranged hypertrophied stromal cells surrounding the vesicular ovarian follicle.

t. interna, the inner secretory part of the theca folliculi; it is permeated by a rich capillary network.

theci'tis. Inflammation of a tendon sheath.

theco'ma. A functional ovarian neoplasm, composed of spindle-shaped cells (predominantly theca lutein cells with bands of collagen), that produces considerable quantities of feminizing endocrine substances; it generally causes irregularities in the menstrual cycle, breast enlargement, and occassionally increased libido; also called theca lutein cell or theca cell tumor.

thelar'che. The beginning of breast development at puberty.

the'leplasty. Reparative surgery of the nipple.

theler'ethism. Erection of the nipple.

theli'tis. Inflammation of the nipple.

thelorrha'gia. Hemorrhage or bleeding from the nipple.

the'nar. 1. The fleshy mass of the palm on the thumb side. **2.** Denoting any structure situated on or associated with this area.

theoph'ylline. An alkaloid present in tea leaves; a smooth muscle relaxant, heart stimulant, and vasodilator; used in the treatment of bronchial asthma and to stimulate the heart muscle.

the'orem. A proven proposition.

the'ory. A hypothetical concept given credibility by working experimentation but lacking absolute proof.

atomic t., one stating that the molecules of a substance are made up of smaller particles in definite proportions.

Bohr's t., one in which the atom is conceived as a positively charged nucleus around which electrons revolve.

clonal selection t., theory according to which certain predestined antibody-producing cells, when exposed to the host's own tissues during fetal life, were deleted or destroyed; thus there would be no "antiself" clones or colonies of cells to react against one's own tissues.

germ t., the theory, now a doctrine, that all infectious diseases are caused by microorganisms.

germ layer t., the concept that the embryo develops three primary germ layers (ectoderm, mesoderm, and endoderm) and that each layer gives rise to specific tissues and organs.

gestalt t., theory claiming that mental phenomena are total configurations and cannot be analyzed into their component parts.

Lamarckian t., the theory that acquired characteristics may be transmitted.

Planck's t., see quantum theory.

quantum t., theory that atoms emit and absorb energy discontinuously, in finite discrete amounts (quanta) in individual acts of emission and absorption, rather than in a continuous fashion; also called Planck's theory.

reentry t., theory that extrasystoles are caused by reentry of the sinus impulse into the ectopic focus.

van't Hoff's t., substances in dilute solutions obey the gas laws.

Young-Helmholtz t., the theory that the perception of colors depends on three sets of receptors in the retina: for red, green, and violet.

therapeu'tic. Curative or healing.

t. blood level, see under level.

therapeu'tics. The aspect of medicine concerned with the treatment of disease.

ther'apist. A specialist in the conduction of therapy, as in speech therapy, physical therapy, etc.

radio t., see radiotherapist.

rehabilitation t., a member of the health-care team (i.e., physical, occupational, and recreational therapists) engaged in restoring the injured, the disabled, and the physically or mentally sick to their rightful place in society.

ther'apy. The treatment of disease or disability.

anticoagulant t., the use of drugs that prevent or arrest formation of blood clots in the cardiovascular system.

collapse t., an obsolete treatment of pulmonary tuberculosis by collapsing or reducing the volume of the diseased lung.

electroshock t. (EST), **electroconvulsive t.** (ECT), a form of shock treatment for mental illness (especially depressive reactions) in which an electric current is used to produce unconsciousness and/or convulsions.

fever t., treatment of disease by artificially increasing body temperature.

gestalt t., a type of psychotherapy concerned with treatment of the person as a whole: his physical make-up and functioning, his perceptual configuration, and his relationship with his environment; the person's sensory awareness of his immediate experience is emphasized rather than his recollection of past experiences.

hyperbaric oxygen t., the use of oxygen in a compression chamber at a prevailing pressure greater than one atmosphere.

inhalation t., administration of gases, steam, or vaporized medications through inhalation.

occupational t., an adjunctive method of treatment for the sick or injured through purposeful and healthy activity.

oxygen t., treatment with oxygen inhalation.

parenteral t., administration of medications through routes other than the alimentary canal, i.e., intramuscular or intravenous.

physical t., the use of physical agents (heat, massage, electricity, and exercise) to restore bodily functions; also called physiotherapy.

thalassemia | therapy

472

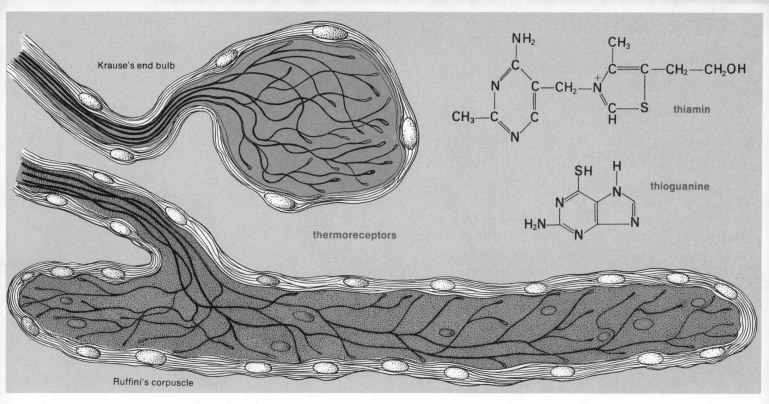

Krause's end bulb

thermoreceptors

Ruffini's corpuscle

thiamin

thioguanine

radium t., radiotherapy.

replacement t., administration of natural body products, or synthetic substitutes, to compensate for a deficiency.

roentgen t., treatment with x rays.

shock t., see treatment, shook.

specific t., administration of medication that has a selective action upon the cause of a disease.

speech t., the application of special techniques to correct speech disabilities.

therm-, thermo-. Combining forms meaning heat.

therm. Any of the following units of quantity of heat: a small calorie; a large calorie; 1000 large calories; 100,000 British thermal units.

ther'mal. Relating to heat.

thermalge'sia. Extreme sensitivity to heat.

thermanalge'sia. See thermoanesthesia.

thermatol'ogy. The study of heat as applied to the treatment of disease.

thermelom'eter. An electric thermometer.

thermo-. See therm-.

thermoanesthe'sia. Inability to distinguish between heat and cold or to feel variations in temperature; also called ardanesthesia and thermalgesia.

thermocau'tery. The destruction of tissue (cauterization) by means of a heated wire; also called thermoelectric cautery.

thermochem'istry. The branch of chemistry concerned with the relationship of heat and chemical reactions.

ther'mochrose. The property of heat rays which enables them to be reflected, refracted, and absorbed.

thermocoagula'tion. Coagulation effected by the application of heat.

ther'mocouple. Device used to measure slight variations in temperature; also called thermopile.

thermodiffu'sion. Diffusion of a gas or a liquid through heat; the rise in temperature increases the molecular motion.

thermodilu'tion. Reduction in temperature of a liquid occurring when it is added to a colder liquid; the volume of the latter liquid can be calculated from the degree of rise in its temperature; the principle is employed to measure the volume or the rate of flow through a chamber; e.g., ventricular volume, cardiac output, or renal blood flow.

thermodynam'ics. The branch of physics concerned with heat and its conversion to other forms of energy.

thermoesthe'sia. The ability to perceive changes in temperature; also called thermesthesia.

thermogen'esis. The production of heat in the body; a physiologic process.

ther'mogram. A colored photograph displaying the surface temperatures of the body; produced by infrared sensing devices.

ther'mograph. A thermometer that records variations in temperature.

thermog'raphy. A process for measuring temperature by photographically recording infrared radiations emanating from the body's surface; it can aid in diagnosing underlying pathology by indicating thermal variations.

thermohy'peresthe'sia. Extreme sensitivity to variations in temperature.

thermohy'pesthe'sia. Diminished sensitivity to temperature fluctuations; also called thermohypoesthesia.

thermoinhib'itory. Preventing or arresting the production of heat.

thermola'bile. Susceptible to alteration or destruction by heat.

thermol'ysis. 1. The loss of body heat. **2.** The chemical decomposition of compounds by heat.

thermomassag'e. The use of heat and massage in physical therapy.

thermom'eter. A device for measuring temperature, usually consisting of a graduated, sealed, glass vacuum tube with a bulb at its lower extremity and containing a liquid, generally mercury (sometimes alcohol), that rises in the tube when expanded by increase in temperature.

digital t., an electronic thermometer that reads and/or numerically prints out the temperature.

electronic t., one that measures and/or electronically records temperature.

thermom'etry. Measurement of temperature by direct contact.

ther'mophile, ther'mophil. An organism which grows best at warm temperatures, usually from 40° to 70°C.

ther'mophore. An appliance for (1) applying heat to a bodily part; (2) maintaining the temperature of the mask during ether inhalation.

thermoplacento'graphy. Determination of the placental location by recording the increased temperature (due to large amounts of blood) with the thermograph.

thermoplas'tic. A type of material which can be made soft by heating and which rehardens upon cooling (without chemical change).

thermople'gia. Heat stroke.

thermorecep'tor. A special nerve-ending (receptor) that is sensitive to change in temperature.

thermoregula'tion. The regulation of heat; also called temperature control.

ther'moset. A material which becomes rigid or hardened by a chemical reaction involving heat.

thermosta'ble, thermosta'bile. Not changed or destroyed by moderate heat.

thermotax'is. 1. Movement of an organism toward (positive thermotaxis) or away from (negative thermotaxis) a heat source. **2.** The adjustment of the body to temperature changes.

thermother'apy. The use of heat as an aid in the treatment of disease.

thesauro'sis, thesaurismo'sis. Abnormal or excessive storage in the body, or in particular organs, of phosphatides, fats, heavy metals, or other material.

the'sis. An essay containing results of original research written by a candidate for an academic degree.

thi-. See thio-.

thiam'inase. A thiamine-splitting enzyme.

thi'amine, thi'amin. A vitamin of the B-complex, present in yeast, meat, and the bran coat of grains; essential in carbohydrate metabolism; lack of thiamine causes beriberi; also called vitamin B_1.

t. pyrophosphate (TPP), the diphosphoric ester of thiamine; a coenzyme which is a cofactor in decarboxylation; also called cocarboxylase.

thi'azides. A shortened term for the class of diuretics called benzothiadiazides; widely used in treating both edema and hypertension.

thigh. The portion of the upper leg between the knee and the hip.

driver's t., inflammation of the sciatic nerve due to prolonged pressure on the nerve, as from the continued use of the accelerator pedal in long distance driving of an automobile.

thigh'bone. The femur; see table of bones.

thig'mesthe'sia. Sensitiveness to touch; also called tactile sensibility.

thigmotax'is. The reaction of an organism that comes in contact with a solid body.

thio-, thi-. A combining form denoting the replacement of oxygen by sulfur in the compound to the name of which it is attached.

thioal'cohol. See mercaptan.

thiobarbit'urates. One of a series of hypnotic compounds obtained by the condensation of thiourea and malonic acid.

thiogua'nine. An antineoplastic agent used in the treatment of some types of leukemia.

thi'ol. 1. The univalent radical —SH. **2.** Mercaptan; any substance containing the radical —SH bound to carbon.

-thi'ol. Combining form indicating the presence of a thiol (—SH) group.

thi'onine. A greenish-black powder giving a violet color in solution; often used to stain the Nissl substance of nerve cells; also called Lauth's violet.

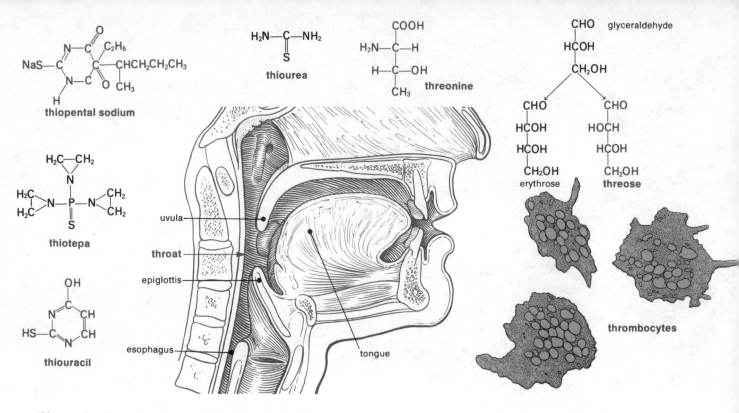

thiopental sodium

thiotepa

thiouracil

thiourea

threonine

glyceraldehyde

erythrose threose

uvula

throat

epiglottis

esophagus

tongue

thrombocytes

---

thiopental sodium. A rapid-acting, potent barbiturate capable of inducing anesthesia within 30 to 60 seconds after being administered intravenously or rectally; also called sodium pentothal; Pentothal Sodium®.

thi'osemicar'bazone. One of several compounds containing the radical =N—NH—C(S)—NH₂, having an inhibitory effect on tuberculous infections.

thiosul'fate. A salt of thiosulfuric acid.

thiosulfuric acid. A highly unstable acid, $H_2S_2O_3$, which decomposes readily to sulfur and sulfurous acid.

thiote'pa. A white crystalline compound, $C_6H_{12}N_3PS$; an alkylating agent used as a palliative medication in malignant diseases.

thiou'racil. 2-Mercapto-4-hydroxypyrimidine; a compound that inhibits the formation of thyroid hormones.

thiou'rea. An antithyroid substance of the thiocarbamide group.

thirst. A desire to drink, often associated with an uncomfortable sensation of dryness in the mouth and pharynx.

  excessive t., polydipsia.

Thoma's counting chamber. Thoma-Zeiss hemocytometer; see under hemocytometer.

thorac-. Combining form denoting the chest.

thoracec'tomy. Resection of part of a rib.

thoracente'sis. The removal of fluid from the chest cavity by puncture; also called thoracocentesis.

thorac'ic. Relating to the thorax or chest.

thoracicoabdom'inal, thoracoabdom'inal. Relating to the thorax and the abdomen.

thoracicoacro'mial. See acromiothoracic.

thoracic outlet syndrome. Abnormal sensations of fingers (numbness, burning, etc.) formerly attributed to compression of the brachial plexus; now known to be due often to cervical disk or carpal tunnel syndromes.

thoracoabodom'inal. See thoracicoabdominal.

thoracocente'sis. See thoracentesis.

thoracolum'bar. Relating to the thoracic and lumbar regions of the spine.

thoracomyodyn'ia. Pain in the muscles of the chest.

thoracop'athy. Any disease of the chest.

thoracoplas'ty. Plastic surgery or repair of defects of the chest.

thoracopneumoplas'ty. Reparative surgery of the lung and chest.

thoracos'copy. Visual examination of the pleural cavity by means of an endoscope.

thoracos'tomy. The surgical creation of an open-

ing into the chest wall.

thoracot'omy. Surgical incision on the chest wall.

tho'rax. The chest; the upper part of the body between the neck and the diaphragm; it contains the chief organs of the circulatory and respiratory systems.

tho'rium. A radioactive metallic element; symbol Th, atomic number 90, atomic weight 232.038.

Thr. Symbol for threonine or its radical forms.

thread'worm. See pinworm.

thre'onine. An amino acid present in most proteins; essential to the diet of man and other mammals.

thre'ose. A monosaccharide containing four carbon atoms; $C_4H_8O_4$; one of the two aldoses, the other being erythrose.

thresh'old. The point where a stimulus just begins to produce a sensation; the intensity below which a mental or physical stimulus cannot be perceived.

  absolute t., stimulus t., the stimulus of least strength which will cause a response.

  auditory t., the intensity of the lowest perceptible sound.

  galvanic t., rheobase.

  radiologic t., the level of radiation dose below which there may not be permanent injury to the body.

  renal t., the level at which the kidney can no longer reabsorb all of a substance (sugar, ketones, etc.) presented, and some of it appears in the urine.

  stimulus t., see absolute threshold.

  t. of consciousness, the lowest gradient of sensation that can be perceived.

thrill. A tremor or vibration associated with a vascular or cardiac murmur and discerned by palpation.

throat. 1. The back part of the mouth extending to the beginning of the esophagus; generally the area from the nasopharynx to the larynx. **2.** The front of the neck.

  sore t., a throat condition characterized by discomfort, especially when swallowing, due to inflammation of the fauces, pharynx, tonsils, or larynx.

  strep t., streptococcal pharyngitis; see under pharyngitis.

throb. 1. To pulsate. **2.** A pulsation.

throe. A severe pang or seizure of pain, as experienced during childbirth.

thrombasthe'nia. Abnormality of the blood platelets in which they lack factors that are effective in blood coagulation; also called Glanzmann's disease.

thrombec'tomy. Surgical removal of a thrombus (blood clot).

thrombelas'tograph. Device for recording elastic variations of a thrombus during the process of

coagulation.

throm'bi. Plural of thrombus.

throm'bin. An enzyme in the blood derived from factor II (prothrombin) that converts fibrinogen into fibrin, thus producing a blood clot.

thrombin'ogen. Factor II (prothrombin).

thrombo-, throm-. Combining forms denoting a blood clot or thrombus.

thromboangii'tis. Inflammation of the wall of a blood vessel with clot formation.

  t. obliterans, disorder of the medium-sized arteries and veins, especially of the lower extremities; marked by inflammation of the wall of the vessel and surrounding connective tissue, resulting in tissue ischemia and gangrene; also called Buerger's disease.

throm'boblast. The giant cell precursor of the blood platelet (thrombocyte); more commonly called megakaryocyte.

thrombocytasthe'nia. A disorder of platelet function characterized by abnormal adhesion and/or aggregation; congenital varieties are known, and acquired forms are seen, especially in uremia.

throm'bocyte. A blood platelet.

thrombocythe'mia. A rare disorder of middle adult life, marked by abnormal proliferation of megakaryocytes with increase in circulating platelets; bleeding, thromboembolic diathesis, splenomegaly, and leukocytosis are frequently present.

thrombocytop'athy. General term denoting any disorder involving faulty function of blood platelets; also called thrombopathia.

thrombocytope'nia. Abnormally small number of platelets in the blood; also called thrombopenia.

thrombocyto'sis. Increase in the number of platelets in the blood.

thromboembolec'tomy. The removal of an embolism which obstructs the flow of blood through a vessel.

thromboem'bolism. Embolism (obstruction) in a blood vessel caused by a dislodged thrombus (clot).

thromboendarterec'tomy. The surgical removal of an obstructing blood clot together with the inner lining of the obstructed artery.

throm'bogen. Factor II (prothrombin).

thrombogen'ic. 1. Producing thrombosis or coagulation of the blood. **2.** Relating to factor II (prothrombin).

thrombol'ysis. The dissolving of a clot; also called thromboclasis.

thrombopath'ia. See thrombocytopathy.

thrombope'nia. See thrombocytopenia.

thrombophlebi'tis. Inflammation of the walls of a vein associated with formation of a thrombus

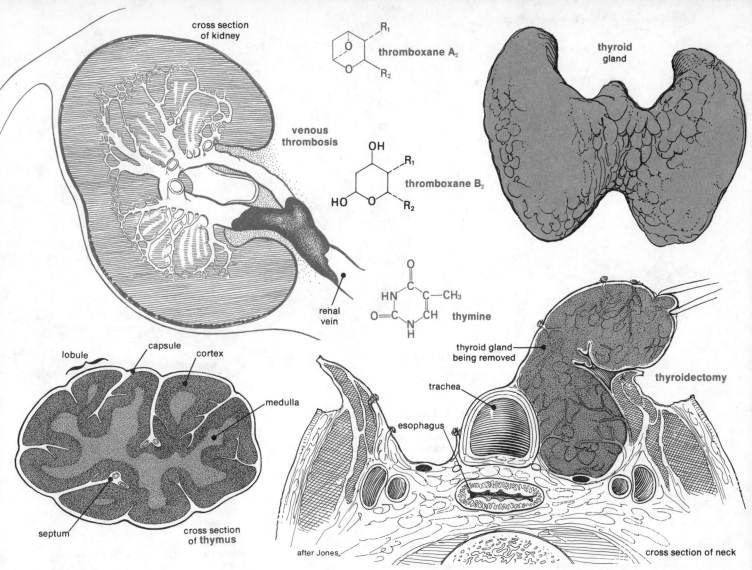

cross section
of kidney

thromboxane A₂

venous
thrombosis

thromboxane B₂

renal
vein

thymine

thyroid
gland

thyroid gland
being removed

thyroidectomy

trachea

esophagus

lobule   capsule   cortex

medulla

septum

cross section
of thymus

after Jones

cross section of neck

(blood clot).

puerperal t., thrombophlebitis of the great saphenous or femoral veins, causing a sudden painful swelling of the leg; it usually occurs in women with a low-grade infection of the birth canal after delivery; also called phlegmasia alba dolens and milk leg.

thromboplast′in. Factor III; a protein complex that initiates the clotting of blood.

plasma t., a complete thromboplastin capable of converting factor II (prothrombin) to thrombin directly.

tissue t., an incomplete thromboplastin requiring the presence of factor V, factor VII, and factor X in order to convert prothrombin to thrombin.

thrombopoie′sis. 1. The formation of a blood clot. **2.** The formation of blood platelets.

thrombo′sis. The formation or presence of a blood clot.

coronary t., the presence of a blood clot in an artery that supplies the heart muscle; a cause of heart attack.

venous t., arrest of circulation in a vein by a blood clot; also called phlebemphraxis.

thrombox′ane. A compound isolated from blood platelets (thrombocytes); it contains an oxane ring and is related to the prostaglandins; thromboxane exists in two forms; A₂ and B₂; the A₂ form appears to be much more potent than prostaglandin in some important biologic activities, such as smooth muscle contraction and platelet aggregation.

throm′bus. A blood clot, usually one located at the point of its formation, in a blood vessel or a chamber of the heart.

throw′back. An organism possessing characteristics which are absent in other contemporary members of the same species, but were present, or assumed to have been present, in members of remote generations.

thrush. Infection of the mouth with *Candida albicans*; marked by the appearance of white patches in the oral mucosa, which later become shallow ulcers; seen most commonly in infants or in patients receiving antibiotics or immunosuppressive drugs.

thu′lium. A metallic element of the lanthanide series, symbol Tm, atomic number 69, atomic weight 168.94.

thumb. The first digit on the radial side of the hand, apposable to each of the other four digits.

gamekeeper′s t., a subluxation of the metacarpophalangeal joint of the thumb.

tennis t., tendonitis accompanied by calcification in the tendon of the long flexor muscle of the thumb due to exercises in which the thumb is subject to great pressure and strain, as in tennis playing.

thymec′tomy. Surgical removal of the thymus gland.

-thymia. Combining form relating to the mind or emotions.

thy′mic. Relating to the thymus gland.

thy′midine. A condensation product of thymine with deoxyribose; a nucleoside in DNA.

thy′mine. One of the pyrimidine bases which is commonly found in deoxyribonucleic acid (DNA).

thymi′tis. Inflammation of the thymus gland.

thymo-. Combining form indicating a relationship to (a) the thymus gland; (b) the mind, soul, or emotions.

thy′mocyte. A lymphocyte that originates in the thymus gland.

thymogen′ic. 1. Originating in the thymus gland. **2.** Of hysterical origin.

thymokinet′ic. Stimulating the thymus gland.

thymo′ma. A tumor of the anterior mediastinum arising from the thymus gland; associated with a variety of diseases, including myasthenia gravis, agammaglobulinemia, and hematologic abnormalities; it may undergo malignant change.

thymop′athy. 1. Any disease of the thymus gland. **2.** Any mental disorder.

thy′mosin. An immunologically active thymic fraction of low molecular weight.

thy′mus. 1. A ductless glandlike lymphoid structure located just behind the top of the sternum; it appears to be the master organ in immunogenesis in the young and is believed by some to monitor the total lymphoid system throughout life; it consists of two lobes surrounded by a thin capsule of connective tissue; it grows quickly until the age of three years, after which it grows very slowly untill the age of about 13, at which time it begins to decrease in size; at old age, very little thymic tissue remains, having been replaced by fat and connective tissue; also called thymus gland. **2.** One of the organs of cattle called sweetbread.

thyro-, thyr-. Combining forms indicating a relationship to the thyroid gland.

thyroapla′sia. Congenital defects associated with faulty thyroid functioning.

thyroaryt′enoid. Relating to both the thyroid and arytenoid cartilages.

thyrocalcito′nin. See calcitonin.

thyrocricot′omy. Tracheostomy performed in extreme emergency conditions whereby the neck opening is made through the most superficial portion of the respiratory tract, the cricothyroid membrane. See also tracheostomy.

thyroglob′ulin. A protein produced and stored in the thyroid gland; a prohormone (precursor of hormone) which on hydrolysis yields iodinated tyrosines and thyroxin.

thyroglos′sal. Relating to the thyroid cartilage and the tongue.

thyrophy′oid. Relating to the thyroid cartilage and the hyoid bone.

thy′roid. 1. Pertaining to the thyroid gland; see under gland. **2.** Resembling a shield. **3.** A pharmaceutical preparation derived from the thyroid gland of certain domestic animals; used in the treatment of hypothyroid states.

thyroidec′tomy. Removal of the thyroid gland.

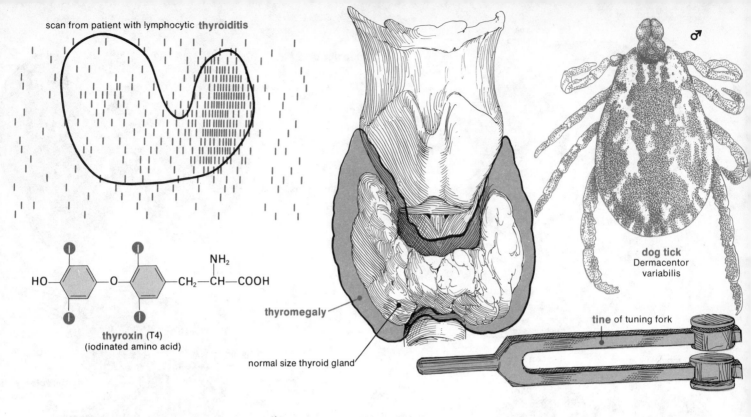

scan from patient with lymphocytic **thyroiditis**

thyroxin (T4)
(iodinated amino acid)

thyromegaly

normal size thyroid gland

dog tick
Dermacentor
variabilis

tine of tuning fork

---

thyroidi'tis. Inflammation of the thyroid gland.
  de Quervain's t., see subacute thyroiditis.
  granulomatous t., see subacute thyroiditis.
  Hashimoto's t., see lymphocytic thyroiditis.
  lymphocytic t., a form of chronic thyroiditis in which the thyroid gland is massively infiltrated with lymphoid and fibrous tissues causing destruction of the gland substance, goiter formation, and thyroid hormone insufficiency; thought to be an autoimmune disease; it occurs 20 times more frequently in women than in men, usually between the ages of 30 to 50; also called Hashimoto's thyroiditis and Hashimoto's struma.
  Riedel's t., a rare chronic condition in which the thyroid gland and adjacent structures are replaced by dense fibrotic tissue.
  subacute t., inflammation of the thyroid gland following viral infection, usually of the upper respiratory tract; also called de Quervain's or granulomatous thyroiditis.
thyromeg'aly. Abnormal enlargement of the thyroid gland.
thy'ronine. An amino acid present in proteins only as iodinated derivatives (iodothyronines).
thyroparathyroidec'tomy. Surgical removal of the thyroid and parathyroid glands.
thyrop'athy. Disease of the thyroid gland.
thyropri'val. Caused by removal of the thyroid gland or the arrest of its function.
thyropro'tein. 1. Thyroglobulin. **2.** Preparation made by iodinating protein (such as casein), having a physiologic action similar to that of thyroxin.
thyropto'sis. Downward displacement of the thyroid gland.
thyrot'omy. 1. Surgical division or cutting of the thyroid cartilage. **2.** Operative cutting of the thyroid gland.
thyrotoxico'sis. Toxic condition caused by an excess of thyroid hormone.
thyrotrop'ic, thyrotroph'ic. Stimulating the thyroid gland.
thyrot'ropin, thyrotroph'in. Thyrotropic hormone; see under hormone.
thyrox'in, thyrox'ine (T₄). An active iodine-containing hormone, existing normally in the thyroid gland, that aids in regulating metabolism; produced synthetically or extracted from the thyroid gland in crystalline form for treatment of thyroid disorders such as hypothyroidism, cretinism, and myxedema; also called tetraiodothyronine.
Ti. Chemical symbol of the element titanium.
tib'ia. The larger and medial of the two bones of the leg between the knee and the ankle; commonly called shinbone.
tibiofib'ular. Relating to both the tibia and fibula.

tic. An involuntary, brief, and recurrent twitching of a group of muscles, most commonly involving the face, neck, and shoulders.
  t. douloureux, spasmodic facial neuralgia, marked by piercing pain of short duration along the trigeminal nerve; also called trigeminal neuralgia.
tick. A mite of the families Ixodidae (hard shell ticks) and Argasidae (soft shell ticks), some of which are parasitic and the carriers of disease-causing microorganisms.
  dog t., Dermacentor variabilis, a hard shell tick that can transmit Rocky Mountain spotted fever; found on the East Coast of the United States; usually in mountainous, heavily wooded, or sagebrush areas; also called the American dog tick.
  Rocky Mountain wood t., Dermacentor andersoni, a hard shell, reddish-brown tick of the Western United States; most important vector of Rocky Mountain spotted fever; also conveys tularemia, Colorado tick fever, and Q fever, and is a cause of tick paralysis.
tick'le. 1. To feel a tingling or restless sensation. **2.** To excite the surface nerves by repeated light stimulation of the skin; also called titillate.
t.i.d. Abbreviation of Latin ter in die.
tide. An alternate rise and fall; a lapse of time.
  alkaline t., period following ingestion of food when the alkalinity of the urine is increased due to secretion of gastric juice; also called alkaline wave.
Tietze's syndrome. Pain and tenderness of the chest at the junction of ribs with cartilage; the pain may mimic that of coronary artery disease; also called costochondral junction syndrome and costal chondritis.
tim'bre. The characteristic quality of a sound whereby one may distinguish between two sounds of equal pitch and loudness.
  t. métallique, a high-pitched metallic second sound heard in dilatation of the aorta.
time. A degree or measure of duration.
  bleeding t., the duration of bleeding (normally from one to three minutes) from a small puncture made on the skin.
  circulation t., time required for blood to flow once through a given circuit of the circulatory system.
  clotting t., coagulation time.
  coagulation t., time required for blood to clot in a test tube.
  doubling t., in microbiology, the time needed for a population of cells to double in number; also called division or generation time.
  prothrombin t., time required for a clot to form when calcium and a preparation of thromboplastin (e.g., brain tissue) are added to plasma.

  reaction t., time elapsed between application of a stimulus and an observable response.
  recognition t., time elapsed between the application of a stimulus and the recognition of its nature.
  survival t., (1) interval between the completion or institution of a procedure and death; (2) the life span of cells.
tin. A malleable, silvery metallic element; symbol Sn (stannum), atomic number 50, atomic weight 118.69; a member of the subgroup containing carbon, silicon, germanium, and lead.
tinct. Abbreviation for Latin tinctura.
tinctor'ial. Relating to staining.
tinctu'ra (tinct, tr). Latin for tincture; used in prescription writing.
tinc'ture. An alcohol or hydroalcohol solution of nonvolatile animal or vegetable drugs or chemical substances, prepared usually by a percolation or maceration process; the strength is usually one to two parts by weight of the dry drug to ten parts by volume of the tincture, i.e., one to two grams per 10 milliliters.
  alcoholic t., one made with undiluted alcohol.
  belladonna t., an anticholinergic, antispasmodic, alcoholic preparation containing between 27 and 33 milligrams of alkaloids of belladonna leaf to 100 milliliters of tincture.
  hydroalcoholic t., one made with diluted alcohol in varied proportions of water.
  iodine t., a simple two per cent solution of iodine with two and a half per cent sodium iodide in water and 44 to 50 per cent alcohol; used as an anti-infective on the skin (iodine solution is generally preferred to the tincture as an antiseptic).
  opium t., a tincture containing 10 milligrams of morphine per milliliter; used for the symptomatic treatment of diarrhea.
  opium t., camphorated, see paregoric.
tine, pl. **tines. 1.** One of a set of slender prongs on a tuning fork. **2.** An instrument used for introducing an antigen, such as tuberculin, into the skin.
tin'ea. A superficial infectious condition of the skin caused by fungi belonging chiefly to the genera Trichophyton, Microsporum, and Epidermophyton; the fungi live on the dead horny layer of the skin and produce an enzyme that enables them to digest keratin, thus disintegrating hair, nails, and the keratinized cells of the skin; also called ringworm.
  t. barbae, tinea of the beard area; the lesions are dark red and dotted with perifollicular abscesses; it is prevalent in the United States, particularly in cattle-raising regions, where the usual causative organisms are Trichophyton mentagrophyes and Trichophyton verrucosum; also called barber's itch and tinea of the beard.

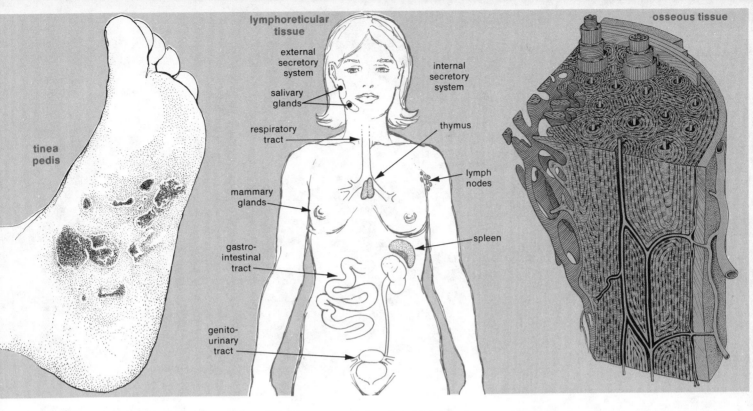

tinea pedis

lymphoreticular tissue

external secretory system

salivary glands

respiratory tract

mammary glands

gastro-intestinal tract

genito-urinary tract

internal secretory system

thymus

lymph nodes

spleen

osseous tissue

t. capitis, infection of the scalp and hair caused by species of *Microsporum* and *Trichophyton,* producing patches of round balding areas; likely sources of infection are hair clippers, theater seats, and domestic animals; also called tinea of the scalp and scalp ringworm.

t. corporis, a highly contagious form most commonly seen in children; caused by many species of *Microsporum* and *Trichophyton* and transmitted through contact with kittens, puppies, and other children; the typical lesion is round or oval, with a scaly center that usually tends to heal; the periphery of the lesion is an advancing circle of vesicles and papules; also called tinea of the smooth skin, ringworm of the smooth skin, and tinea circinata.

t. cruris, tinea involving the groin, perineum, and perianal region; most frequently caused by *Epidermophyton floccosum*; also called tinea of the groin, eczema marginatum, and epidermophytosis cruris.

t. pedis, a common infection of the feet; the acute form, caused by *Trichophyton mentagrophytes,* is characterized by blisters on the soles and sides of the foot and/or between the toes; the chronic form is caused by *Trichophyton rubrum* and the lesions are dry and scaly; also called athlete's foot, tinea of the feet, and ringworm of the feet.

t. sycosis, tinea barbae.

t. unguium, infection of the nails, especially the toenails, usually caused by *Trichophyton mentagrophytes, Trichophyton rubrum,* and *Epidermophyton floccosum*; also called tinea of the nails and onychomycosis trichophytina.

t. versicolor, a mild superficial infection of the skin, usually of the trunk, appearing as tan, irregularly shaped, scaly patches; caused by *Malassezia furfur.*

tin'foil. An extremely thin, pliable sheet of tin; a base metal foil used in dentistry as a separating material, as between a cast and denture-base material during flasking and curing procedures.

t. substitute, an alginate solution that serves as a separating medium.

tingle. To have a peculiar pricking or stinging sensation, as from an emotional shock or striking a nerve, such as the "funny bone" sensation.

tinkle. A metallic sound sometimes heard on auscultation over large pulmonary cavities, e.g., pneumothorax, or over a distended loop of bowel as in an ileus.

tinni'tus. Noises in the ear, such as ringing, buzzing, roaring, etc.

tintom'eter. An apparatus containing a standard color scale for determining by comparison the relative proportion of coloring matter in a fluid, such as blood.

tis'sue. A mass of similar cells and the substances that surround them.

adipose t., connective tissue composed of fat cells clumped together and surrounded by reticular fibers.

areolar t., a type of connective tissue composed of loosely woven collagenous bundles and elastic fibers with comparatively wide interspaces which are filled with a mucopolysaccharide ground substance.

bone t., see osseous tissue.

cancellous t., a honeycomb arrangement of bone cells as seen in the center of some bones such as the clavicle, vertebrae, the end of long bones, etc.

cartilaginous t., connective tissue with a solid, elastic matrix which may or may not have fibers embedded in it.

chondrogenic t., a connective tissue forming the inner layer of perichondrium, concerned with the formation of cartilagenous tissue.

connective t., a general term denoting any of the tissues that support and connect the various parts of the body except the nervous system; also called interstitial tissue.

elastic t., connective tissue composed chiefly of yellow elastic fibers; found in some ligaments and the walls of arteries and air passages.

epithelial t., see epithelium.

erectile t., tissue containing an abundance of vascular spaces which, when distended with blood, render the part firm.

fibrous t., connective tissue containing bundles of white fibers and a fluid ground substance; found in tendons, ligaments, aponeuroses, and such membranes as the dura mater.

hemopoietic t., tissue that is actively involved with the development of formed elements of the blood, as in the medulla of long bones.

interstitial t., see connective tissue.

lymphatic t., a network of fibers enclosing masses of lymphocytes.

lymphoreticular t., tissue that carries out the functions of immunity through a variety of cell types, each performing a specific function, either by direct cell action or through the elaboration of antibody.

mesenchymal t., see mesenchyme.

metanephrogenic t., portion of the intermediate mesoderm that eventually forms the excretory tubules of the kidney.

muscular t., tissue composed of threadlike fibers, either striated (skeletal) or nonstriated (smooth), which contract upon stimulation.

myeloid t., the red bone marrow which forms both red and white blood cells, consisting of the developmental and adult stages of erythrocytes, granulo-

cytes, and megakaryocytes in a stroma of reticular cells and fibers.

nervous t., tissue composed basically of nerve cells (neurons) supported by connective tissue (neuroglia).

osseous t., connective tissue with a tough, rigid, fibrous matrix containing deposits of mineral salts; also called bone tissue.

osteogenic t., a connective tissue forming the inner layer of periosteum, concerned with the formation of osseous tissue.

osteoid t., bone matrix prior to calcification; uncalcified osseous tissue.

reticular t., the most delicate type of connective tissue, composed of a network of fine fibrils; it surrounds individual cells, the acini of glands, and muscle fibers.

tita'nium. A low-density, amorphous metallic element of the carbon group, symbol Ti, atomic number 22, atomic weight 47.90.

t. dioxide, an exceptionally opaque white powder, TiO_2, used in creams and powders as a protectant against external irritations and solar rays; also called titanic acid.

ti'ter. 1. In chemistry, the standard strength of a volumetric test solution determined by titration; assay value of an unknown measure by volumetric means. **2.** The highest dilution of a material (serum or other body fluids) which produces a reaction in an immunologic test system.

ti'trate. To analyze the concentration of a solution by titration.

titra'tion. The process of estimating the quantity of a substance in solution by adding to it a measured amount of standard test solution until a reaction of known proportion is reached (shown by a color change in a suitable indicator, the development of turbidity, or the change in electrical state); from this the unknown concentration of the substance is calculated; also called titrimetry.

colorimetric t., one in which the end point is indicated by sudden change in color.

formol t., a process of titrating the amino group of amino acids by adding formaldehyde to the standard test solution (reagent).

potentiometer t., one in which the pH is constantly monitored, with a specific pH value serving as end point.

Tl. Chemical symbol of the element thallium.

TLC. Abbreviation for total lung capacity.

TLE. Abbreviation for thin-layer electrophoresis.

TLV. Abbreviation for threshold limit value.

TM. Abbreviation for (a) transcendental meditation; (b) tympanic membrane.

Tm. Symbol for (a) the element thulium; (b) tubular

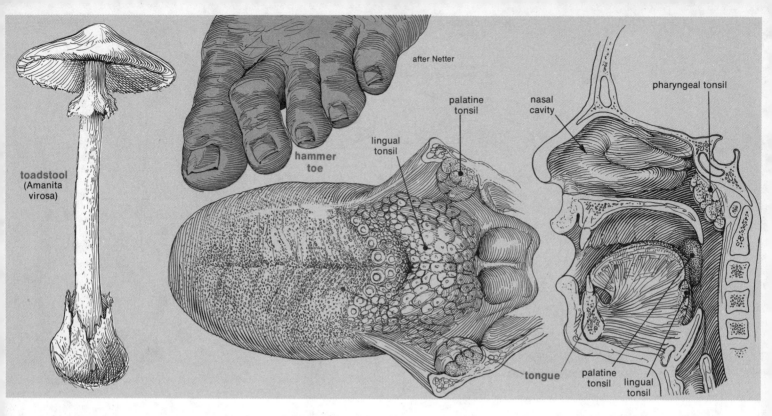

toadstool (Amanita virosa)

hammer toe

after Netter

palatine tonsil

lingual tonsil

nasal cavity

pharyngeal tonsil

tongue

palatine tonsil

lingual tonsil

maximum.

TMJ. Abbreviation for temporomandibular joint.

Tn. Abbreviation for intraocular tension.

toad′stool. Popular name for an inedible, umbrella-shaped mushroom; a poisonous mushroom.

tocodynamom′eter. An instrument for measuring the force of uterine contractions; also called tocometer and tokodynamometer.

tocoph′erol. See vitamin E.

α-tocopherol (α-T). A derivative of vitamin E; a light yellow, completely fat-soluble substance that occurs in the fatty portions of food; it is stored in the adipose tissue of man and functions in all tissues in the stabilization of the lipids of the cell's membranes; believed to play an important role in cellular metabolism.

toe. One of the digits of the feet.

clawing t.'s, an exaggerated dorsal contraction of the toes resulting from imbalance of the short intrinsic musculature and causing the toes to appear claw-like.

great t., hallux.

hammer t., deformity of a toe marked by dorsiflexion of the proximal phalanx with plantar flexion of the second phalanx; the second toe is most often affected.

mallet t., deformity of a toe marked by plantar flexion of the distal phalanx.

pigeon t., see pigeon-toe.

webbed t.'s, adjacent toes abnormally connected by a fold of tissue at their base; a form of syndactyly.

toe′nail. A horny plate on the dorsal surface of the tip of each toe. See also nail.

ingrown t., ingrowing t., a toenail, one edge of which is overgrown by the nail fold, producing a pyogenic granuloma; tight shoes, shrunken socks, and improper paring of the nail corners are common etiologic factors; trauma may also be a predisposing cause.

togavi′ruses. A large group of RNA viruses that multiply in the cytoplasm of cells; transmitted by arthropods, in which they also multiply; included are those causing yellow fever, hemorrhagic fever, and encephalitis.

toi′let. Local care and cleansing e.g., cleansing of a tracheostomy tube, of a wound and surrounding skin, of a patient after childbirth.

tola′zamide. An oral hypoglycemic drug that stimulates pancreatic secretion of insulin; Tolinase®.

tolazoline hydrochloride. A vasodilator with a direct relaxant effect on smooth muscle; used in treating frostbite sequelae, Raynaud's disease, and acrocyanosis; Priscoline Hydrochloride®.

tolbu′tamide. An orally active hypoglycemic drug (sulfonamide derivative), used in the management of certain cases of diabetes; it appears to act initially by stimulating the release of endogenous insulin from the pancreatic islet tissue; Orinase®.

tol′erance, tolera′tion. The capacity to assimilate a drug continuously or in large doses, or to withstand increased physiologic activities without experiencing unfavorable effects.

acoustic t., the maximum sound pressure level (SPL) that can be endured without harmful effects.

cross t., resistance to the effects of one drug resulting from an acquired tolerance to another, related drug.

g-t., tolerance to certain forces resulting from either acceleration or deceleration.

immunologic t., inability to react to the stimulation of a specific antigen.

individual t., unresponsiveness to a drug that the person has not received before.

species t., unresponsiveness to a drug existing as a characteristic of a particular species.

vibration t., the maximum vibratory movements that a person can endure without pain.

tol′erogen. An antigen that causes the immune mechanisms of an organism to be unresponsive to itself, resulting in a state known as tolerance; the opposite of immunogen.

tolnaf′tate. A topical antifungal agent effective against those species of *Epidermophyton, Microsporum,* and *Trichophyton* that cause dermatophytic infections (ringworms) in man; Tinactin®.

tol′uene. A colorless volatile liquid, $C_6H_5 \cdot CH_3$, used in organic synthesis and the manufacture of explosives and dyes; also called toluol and methyl benzene.

tolu′idine. A derivative of toluene.

tol′uol. See toluene.

-tome. Combining form indicating a cutting instrument.

tomo-. A combining form denoting (a) a section; (b) a cutting.

to′mogram. A roentgenogram made by tomography.

to′mograph. An x-ray machine designed to take sectional roentgenograms (tomograms) of the body.

computer-assisted t., a tomograph that utilizes a computer to reconstruct a section of the patient's body from scanned x-ray profiles; also called computerized axial tomograph.

tomog′raphy. The radiographing of a selected level of the body while blurring structures in front of and behind this level; the x-ray tube and film move in opposite directions during exposure so that the roentgenographic shadow of a selected bodily plane

remains stationary while the shadows of all other planes are in motion during exposure and therefore blurred; also called body section roentgenography.

computer-assisted t. (CAT), tomography utilizing a computer-assisted tomograph; also called computerized axial tomography.

tomoma′nia. 1. The tendency of certain surgeons to perform operations for minor ailments. **2.** A morbid desire to be operated upon.

-tomy. A combining form denoting the operation of cutting or incising.

tone. 1. The normal tension of a muscle or healthy state of an organ. **2.** The quality of sound or voice.

tongue. The extremely mobile mass of striated muscle covered by mucous membrane that arises from the floor of the mouth; it serves as the principal organ of taste and aids in mastication, deglutition, and the articulation of sound; also called lingua and glossus.

bifid t., a tongue that is split in its anterior portion by a longitudinal fissure; also called cleft tongue.

black t., hairy t., one with yellowish, brownish, or black furry patches on its dorsal aspect, made up of matted, overdeveloped papillae; the dark pigmentation is believed to be caused by microorganisms or by certain drugs; also called furry tongue.

cleft t., see bifid tongue.

coated t., one having a whitish appearance due to deposits of food particles, inflammatory exudates, sloughed epithelial cells, or fungus growths; occurring when secretion of saliva is insufficient, or when special diets eliminate chewing or certain vitamins.

fissured t., see furrowed tongue.

furrowed t., a tongue with several longitudinal grooves; also called fissured tongue.

geographic t., one with patches of papillary atrophy which fuse at their borders suggesting the appearance of a map.

hairy t., see black tongue.

magenta t., a tongue with a magenta coloration; occurring in riboflavin deficiency.

strawberry t., a tongue with a whitish coat and enlarged red papillae, occurring in scarlet fever.

tongue-tie. Condition in which tongue movements are restricted due to an abnormally short frenum.

ton′ic. 1. A state of sustained muscular contraction. **2.** A remedy that is supposed to restore vigor.

tonic′ity. 1. The normal condition of tension, as the slight continuous contraction of skeletal muscles; also called tonus. **2.** The effective osmotic pressure, usually compared to the osmotic pressure of plasma.

tonoclon′ic, tonicoclon′ic. Denoting muscular spasms that are both tonic and clonic.

tonofi′bril. One of the fine fibrils found in the cytoplasm of epithelial cells which gives a support-

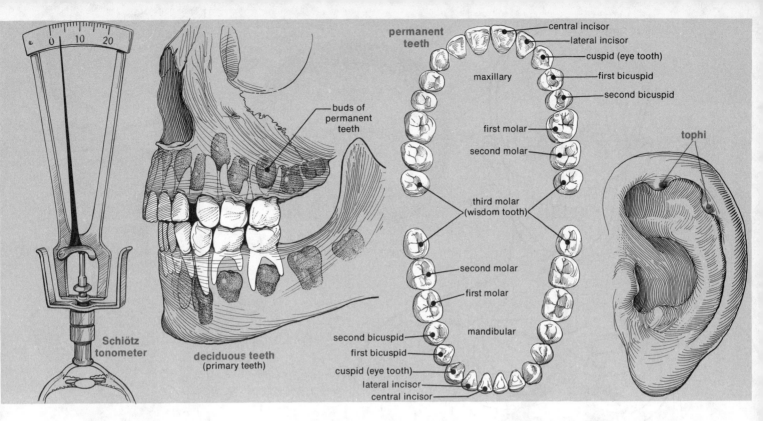

Schiötz tonometer

deciduous teeth (primary teeth)

buds of permanent teeth

permanent teeth

maxillary

central incisor
lateral incisor
cuspid (eye tooth)
first bicuspid
second bicuspid

first molar
second molar

third molar (wisdom tooth)

second molar
first molar

mandibular

second bicuspid
first bicuspid
cuspid (eye tooth)
lateral incisor
central incisor

tophi

ing framework to the cell.

tonofil′ament. A structural cytoplasmic protein, bundles of which form a tonofibril.

tonog′raphy. The continuous measuring and recording of changes in intraocular pressure with a tonometer.

tonom′eter. An instrument for measuring tension or pressure.

  Schiötz t., one which measures the intraocular pressure by determining the indentability of the cornea by a weighted plunger.

tonom′etry. The determination of tension of a part, as of pressure within the eyeball by means of an instrument (tonometer).

ton′sil. 1. A small mass of lymphoid tissue, especially the palatine tonsil. **2.** Any structure resembling a palatine tonsil.

  cerebellar t., a lobule on the undersurface of each cerebellar hemisphere.

  lingual t., an aggregation of lymphoid tissue on the posterior part of the tongue.

  Luschka's t., see pharyngeal tonsil.

  palatine t., one of two oval masses of lymphoid tissue, one on each side of the oral pharynx, between the pillars of the fauces.

  pharyngeal t., a collection of lymphoid tissue on the posterior wall of the nasopharynx; when enlarged it is known as adenoids; also called Luschka's tonsil.

  tubal t., a collection of lymphoid tissue near the pharyngeal orifice of the auditory (eustachian) tube; also called Gerlach's tonsil.

ton′sillar, ton′sillary. Relating to a tonsil, especially the palatine tonsil.

tonsillec′tomy. Surgical removal of the tonsils.

tonsilli′tis. Inflammation of a tonsil or tonsils.

tonsilloadenoidec′tomy (T & A). The surgical removal of both the palatine tonsils and the adenoids.

tonsil′lolith. A concretion or calculus in a tonsil.

ton′sillotome. An instrument, sometimes designed after a guillotine, for surgically removing a portion of a hypertrophied tonsil.

tonsillot′omy. The surgical removal of a portion of a hypertrophied tonsil.

to′nus. See tonicity (1).

tooth, *pl.* **teeth.** One of the bonelike structures embedded in sockets in the jaws, used for chewing.

  buck teeth, prominent projecting maxillary anterior teeth; upper front teeth in labioversion.

  canine t., see cuspid.

  dead t., nonvital tooth.

  deciduous teeth, the 20 teeth that generally erupt between the 6th and 24th months of life, and are later replaced by the permanent teeth; they

calcify partly before and partly after birth; also called primary, temporary, or milk teeth.

  eye t., see cuspid.

  Hutchinson's teeth, permanent incisors in which the edge is notched and narrow; considered a sign of congenital syphilis; also called notched teeth.

  impacted t., a tooth that, due to its position in the jaw, is unable to erupt or to attain its normal position after it has erupted.

  natal t., one that has erupted prior to birth.

  nonvital t., a tooth from which the pulp has been removed or one in which the pulp has died.

  notched teeth, see Hutchinson's teeth.

  permanent teeth, the 32 teeth that generally erupt from the sixth to the 21st years, belonging to the second or permanent dentition; they include four incisors, two cuspids, four bicuspids, and six molars in each jaw; sometimes called succedaneous teeth.

  primary teeth, deciduous teeth.

  snaggle t., a tooth out of proper line in relation to the others in the arch.

  spaced teeth, teeth which have shifted and lost proximal contact with adjacent teeth.

  succedaneous teeth, see permanent teeth.

  temporary teeth, deciduous teeth.

  unerupted t., a tooth prior to eruption through the gingiva.

  wisdom t., third permanent molar; erupts between the ages of 17 and 21 years.

tooth′ache. An aching pain in or about a tooth, usually due to caries, infection, or trauma; also called odontalgia.

tooth′pick. A wood sliver used to remove food particles from between the teeth.

  balsa wood t., a triangular wedge of balsa wood used to stimulate the interdental gingival tissues and to cleanse the interproximal surfaces of the teeth.

topagno′sis. Inability to identify the exact place where the body is touched.

topal′gia. Pain localized at one spot without any lesion or trauma to account for it; a symptom sometimes occurring in neuroses.

topec′tomy. Removal of a specific portion of the cerebral cortex in treating mental illness; a type of psychosurgery.

topesthe′sia. Ability to determine which part of the skin is touched.

topha′ceous. 1. Gritty. **2.** Having the features of a tophus.

to′phus, *pl.* **to′phi.** An accumulation of urate crystals usually deposited in the articular and periarticular tissues in gout; it has a firm gritty consistency; the areas most vulnerable are those of the elbows, feet, hands, and the helix of the ear; also

called chalk stone.

top′ical. Relating to a definite area.

topoanesthe′sia. Inability to determine the location of a cutaneous sensation.

topogno′sis. The ability to recognize the location of a sensation.

topogom′eter. A movable fixation target attached to the front of a keratometer for measuring the curvature of the cornea in its periphery.

topo′graphy. In anatomy, description of a limited area of the surface of the body.

toponarco′sis. Loss of sensation on a localized area of the skin.

tor′por. Sluggishness and slow response to stimuli.

torque. A rotary force capable of producing torsion and rotation about an axis, as one applied to a denture base; a twisting force.

tor′sion. The act of turning or twisting, or the condition of being turned or twisted, as the twisting of the spermatic cord.

  t. of a tooth, the rotation of a tooth on its long axis.

tor′so. The trunk.

torticol′lis. Spasmodic contraction of the muscles of one side of the neck, causing the head to be drawn and usually rotated to that side; commonly known as stiff neck and wryneck.

Tor′ula. Former name for *Cryptococcus.*

tor′ulus. A small projection; a papilla.

to′rus. 1. A protuberance or projection. **2.** A benign, localized exostosis.

  t. mandibularis, a torus located on the lingual surface of the mandible in the cuspid-bicuspid region.

  t. palatinus, an overgrowth of bone usually located in the midline of the hard palate.

  t. tubarius, a ridge posterior to the pharyngeal opening of the auditory (eustachian) tube; also called eustachian cushion.

totipo′tency. The ability to regenerate a whole organism from a part.

touch. 1. Special sense through which anything that comes in contact with the skin or mucous membrane is perceived; the tactile sense. **2.** To palpate or feel with the hands.

tour′niquet. Any device or constrictive wide band used for the temporary stoppage of arterial bleeding from an arm or leg.

tox-. Combining form denoting a poison; e.g., toxin.

toxe′mia. A condition caused by the presence in the blood of poisonous products of bacteria formed at a local site of infection.

  t. of pregnancy, a disorder of the last trimester of pregnancy characterized by hypertension, edema, and proteinuria; it may cause convulsions (eclamp-

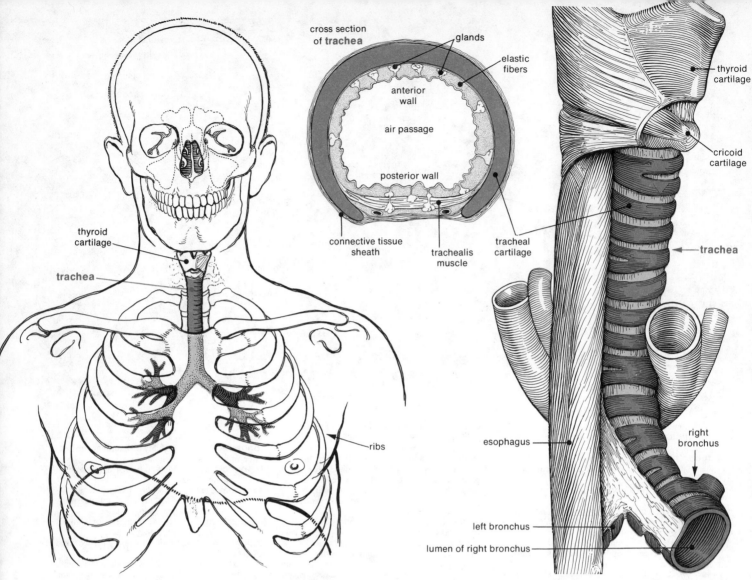

cross section
of **trachea**

glands

elastic
fibers

anterior
wall

air passage

posterior wall

thyroid
cartilage

cricoid
cartilage

connective tissue
sheath

trachealis
muscle

tracheal
cartilage

← trachea

thyroid
cartilage

trachea

esophagus

right
bronchus

ribs

left bronchus

lumen of right bronchus

sia) and is associated with an increased fetal and maternal mortality.

tox′ic. 1. Poisonous; harmful. **2.** Pertaining to a toxin. **3.** Caused by a poison.

t. blood level, see under level.

toxic-. See toxico-.

tox′icant. A poisonous or toxic agent; e.g., alcohol.

toxic′ity. The quality of being poisonous.

toxico-, toxic-. Combining forms indicating a relationship to a poison.

toxicoden′dron. Any of a variety of plants of the genus *Rhus* that cause skin lesions on contact, including poison ivy, poison oak, and poison sumac.

toxicoder′ma. Any skin disease produced by a poison.

tox′icodermati′tis. Skin inflammation produced by a poison.

toxicogen′ic. 1. Producing a poison. **2.** Produced by a poison.

tox′icoid. Producing effects like those of a poison.

toxicol′ogist. An expert on poisons and their antidotes.

toxicol′ogy. The study of the toxic or harmful effects of chemicals on the body; it deals with the symptoms and treatment of poisoning as well as the identification of the poison.

forensic t., diagnosis and treatment of intentional and accidental poisoning and the attendant legal implications.

toxicop′athy. Any disease caused by a poison.

toxif′erous. Poisonous.

tox′in. A poisonous substance produced by certain microorganisms.

extracellular t., exotoxin; toxin produced and released by bacterial cells as a normal physiologic process.

intracellular t., endotoxin; toxin produced and retained by bacterial cells and released only by destruction or death of the cells.

toxip′athy. Any disease caused by a poison.

Toxoca′ra. A genus of parasitic roundworms of the family Ascaridae.

toxocari′asis. Infection with roundworms of the genus *Toxocara.*

tox′oid. A toxin that has been rendered nonpoisonous by chemicals or other agents but is still capable of producing immunity.

tetanus t., the toxin from the tetanus bacillus, rendered nontoxic and used for immunization against the toxin produced by tetanus infection.

tox′ophore. The group of atoms in the toxin molecule that is responsible for its poisonous action.

Toxoplas′ma gon′dii. Intracellular protozoan parasite of the genus *Toxoplasma* causing toxoplasmosis in man.

toxoplasmo′sis. Disease caused by infection with *Toxoplasma gondii;* it may resemble a mild cold or infectious mononucleosis in adults; a disseminated form may lead to hepatitis, pneumonitis, myocarditis, or meningoencephalitis; involvement of the eyes occurs in another form; an infected pregnant woman can spread the disease to her unborn child, causing eye or brain damage or even death; eating raw meat from infected animals is the most common way in which the disease is acquired.

TPN. Abbreviation for triphosphopyridine nucleotide (former name for nicotinamide-adenine dinucleotide phosphate).

TPP. Abbreviation for thiamine pyrophosphate.

tr. Abbreviation for Latin *tinctura.*

trabec′ula, *pl.* **trabec′ulae.** A supporting, anchoring fiber of connective tissue; a dividing band.

septomarginal t., the moderator band that connects the septal band with the anterior papillary muscle and the parietal wall of the right ventricle.

trabeculae carneae, thick muscular bands on the inner walls of the ventricles of the heart.

trabec′ular. Relating to or marked by the presence of trabeculae.

trabecula′tion. The formation or the presence of trabeculae in a part.

tra′cer. 1. A substance which can be readily identified, such as a radioactive isotope, used to gain information. **2.** A device for recording the movements of the lower jaw.

tra′chea. A cartilaginous and membranous tube extending from, and continuous with, the lower part of the larynx to the bronchi; commonly known as windpipe.

tra′cheal. Relating to the trachea.

tracheal′gia. Pain in the trachea.

trachei′tis. Inflammation of the trachea.

tra′chelism, tra′chelis′mus. Spasmodic backward bending of the neck.

trachelo-, trachel-. Combining forms indicating the neck.

trachelor′rhaphy. Repair of the uterine cervix, as from lacerations.

tracheo-. Combining form denoting a relationship to the trachea.

tracheobron′chial. Relating to the trachea and a bronchus or the bronchi.

tracheobronchi′tis. Inflammation of the mucous membrane of the trachea and bronchi.

tracheobronchos′copy. Visual inspection of the interior of the trachea and bronchi.

tra′cheocele. Hernial protrusion of the mucous membrane through a defect in the wall of the trachea.

tracheoesoph′ageal. Relating to the trachea and the esophagus.

tracheolaryn′geal. Relating to both the trachea and the larynx.

tracheomala′cia. Softening and degeneration of the connective tissue of the trachea.

tracheoph′ony. The hollow sound heard on auscultation over the trachea.

tra′cheoplasty. Plastic surgery of the trachea.

tracheorrha′gia. Bleeding from the trachea.

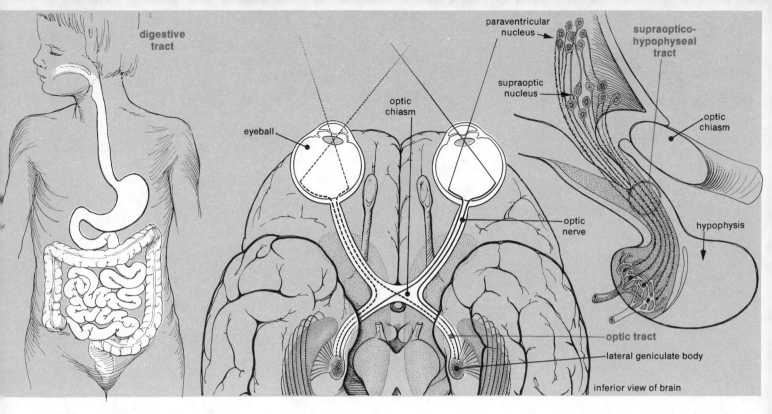

digestive tract

eyeball

optic chiasm

paraventricular nucleus

supraoptico-hypophyseal tract

supraoptic nucleus

optic chiasm

optic nerve

hypophysis

optic tract

lateral geniculate body

inferior view of brain

---

tracheos′chisis. Fissure of the trachea.

tracheos′copy. Visual examination of the interior of the trachea by means of a tracheoscope.

tracheosteno′sis. Constriction of the trachea.

tracheos′toma. An opening into the trachea through the neck.

tracheos′tomy. 1. A direct opening into the trachea through the neck to facilitate breathing or removal of secretions. **2.** The artificial opening or stoma so produced.

tra′cheotome. Tracheostomy knife.

tracheot′omy. Tracheostomy.

tracho′ma. A contagious viral infection of the conjunctiva and cornea caused by a large virus of the psittacossis-lymphogranuloma venereum group; at its onset the disease is characterized by inflammation followed by numerous follicles in the conjunctiva of the upper eyelid; after about six weeks these turn to large, red, hard papillae which last from several months to one or more years, ending with scar tissue formation which shortens and turns the eyelid inward and causes the conjunctiva and cornea to become dry; the disease is one of the chief causes of blindness in some parts of the world, especially the Middle East.

tracing. A line or a pattern of lines made by a pointed instrument on thin paper or plate representing movement (e.g., cardiovascular activity, mandibular movements) or pertinent landmarks of a cephalometric x-ray picture.

tracks. A slang expression for a series of tattoo-like needle scars from frequent narcotics injections.

tract. 1. A system of organs, arranged in series, that perform one common function; e.g., the respiratory tract. **2.** A collection of nerve fibers possessing the same origin, termination, and function.

   alimentary t., digestive tract.

   ascending t., any band of nerve fibers conveying impulses toward the brain.

   corticospinal t.'s, tracts composed of nerve fibers which originate from the cerebral cortex, pass through the medullary pyramid, and descend in the spinal cord.

   corticospinal t., anterior, the portion of the corticospinal tracts that descends through the cervical segments adjacent to the anterior median fissure of the spinal cord (the fibers decussate at their level of innervation); also called ventral corticospinal tract.

   corticospinal t., lateral, the portion of the corticospinal tracts that upon decussation (at the junction of the medulla and spinal cord) descends the length of the lateral part of the spinal cord; also called crossed pyramidal tract.

   descending t., any band of nerve fibers conveying impulses from the brain downward.

   descending V t., see spinal trigeminal tract.

   digestive t., the mucous membrane-lined passage from the mouth to the anus.

   geniculocalcarine t., nerve fibers that pass through the posterior limb of the internal capsule and terminate on the visual cortex of the occipital lobe; also called optic radiation.

   genitourinary t., the urinary passageway from the pelvis of the kidney to the urinary orifice through the ureters, bladder, and urethra; also called urogenital tract.

   iliotibial t., a strong, wide, thickened portion of the fascia lata of the thigh extending from the tubercle of the iliac crest to the lateral condyle of the tibia; it receives the greater part of the insertion of the gluteus maximus muscle.

   intestinal t., the part of the digestive tract between the pyloric end of the stomach and the anus.

   lemniscus t., lateral, lateral lemniscus.

   lemniscus t., medial, medial lemniscus.

   mammillotegmental t., nerve fibers which arise from the mammillary nucleus and descend into the reticular formation of the brain stem, terminating in the dorsal and ventral tegmental nuclei.

   mammillothalamic t., a bundle of nerve fibers which connects the mammillary body (medial mammillary nucleus) primarily to the anterior thalamic nuclear complex.

   olfactory t., a narrow band on the undersurface of the frontal lobe of the brain which connects the olfactory bulb to the cerebral hemispheres.

   optic t., a band of nerve fibers which extends from the optic chiasm to the lateral geniculate body, with some reflex fibers going to the spinal cord.

   pyramidal t., a term generally used to designate the corticospinal projections arising from the cerebral cortex and descending in the internal capsule, cerebral peduncle, and pons to the medulla oblongata; the term is restricted to mean nerve fibers that pass through the pyramid.

   respiratory t., the conducting airway consisting of the nose, mouth, pharynx, larynx, trachea, bronchi, bronchioles, and alveoli.

   rubrospinal t., a band of nerve fibers arising from the red nucleus (oval cell mass in the central part of the midbrain tegmentum); the fibers cross (decussate) and descend the length of the spinal cord.

   solitary t., a tract that begins in the upper medulla and extends to the cervical junction; it terminates along the course of the solitary nucleus; formed primarily by visceral afferent and taste fibers from the vagus, glossopharyngeal, and facial (intermediate) nerves; also called tractus solitarius.

   spinal trigeminal t., spinal V t., descending V t., afferent trigeminal root fibers that extend from the middle of the pons to the uppermost cervical spinal segments, where they terminate in the adjacent spinal trigeminal nucleus which forms a long cell column medial to the tract.

   spinocerebellar t., anterior, a band of nerve fibers that ascends along the lateral funiculus of the spinal cord to the cerebellum, via the superior cerebellar peduncle; also called ventral spinocerebellar tract.

   spinocerebellar t., posterior, a tract that lies in the lateral funiculus of the spinal cord and conveys nerve fibers from the thoracic nucleus to the cerebellum, via the inferior cerebellar peduncle; also called dorsal spinocerebellar tract.

   spinothalamic t., anterior, a band of nerve fibers in the anterolateral funiculus of the spinal cord that crosses over in the anterior white commissure before ascending to the ventral posterolateral (VPL) nucleus of the thalamus; also called ventral spinothalamic tract.

   spinothalamic t., lateral, a band of nerve fibers in the anterolateral funiculus of the spinal cord that ascends to the ventral posterolateral (VPL) nucleus of the thalamus, with some branches going to the reticular formation.

   supraopticohypophyseal t., a bundle of nerve fibers arising from the supraoptic and paraventricular nuclei of the hypothalamus and descending to the posterior lobe of the hypophysis (neurohypophysis), where these fibers branch profusely and form most of the bulk of the lobe.

   t. of Lissauer, poorly myelinated nerve fibers at the tip of the dorsal horn between the posteromarginal nucleus and the surface of the spinal cord, medial to the incoming dorsal roots; they are a continuation of the dorsal fibers that ascend and descend over two segments before terminating in the substantia gelatinosa; also called dorsolateral fasciculus.

   tuberohypophyseal t., a bundle of nerve fibers arising from small cells (arcuate nucleus) around the floor of the third ventricle and projecting to the infundibular stem of the hypophysis; also called tuberoinfundibular tract.

   urinary t., the urinary passageway from the pelvis of the kidney to the urinary orifice through the ureters, bladder, and urethra.

   urogenital t., see genitourinary tract.

   uveal t., see uvea.

trac′tion. Pulling or drawing; a method of treatment used in orthopedics to correct bone displacement by use of weights.

   skeletal t., heavy traction delivered to a broken bone by pulling directly on a metal pin or wire inserted into or through a bone; capable of deliv-

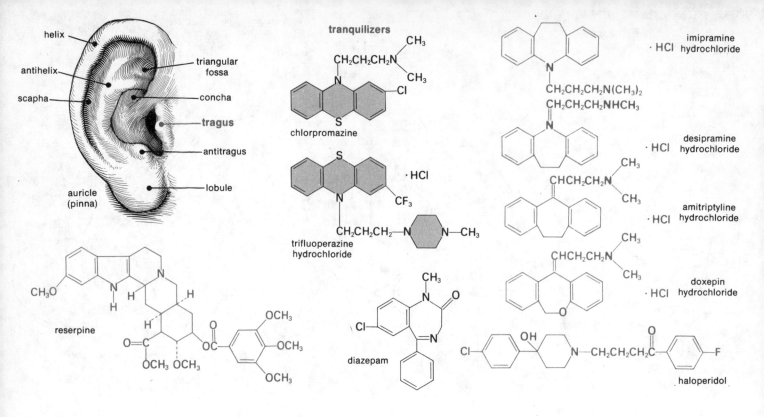

helix

antihelix

scapha

triangular
fossa

concha

tragus

antitragus

auricle
(pinna)

lobule

tranquilizers

chlorpromazine

trifluoperazine
hydrochloride

reserpine

diazepam

imipramine
· HCl hydrochloride

desipramine
· HCl hydrochloride

amitriptyline
· HCl hydrochloride

doxepin
· HCl hydrochloride

haloperidol

ering a traction force of approximately 40 pounds.

skin t., light traction delivered to a bone by pulling on adhesive strips attached to the skin of an extremity; capable of delivering a traction force of approximately 10 pounds; used frequently for the reduction of fractures in young children.

tractot'omy. Surgical severing of a nerve tract in the brain stem or spinal cord.

spinal t., cordotomy.

trigeminal t., severing of the descending root of the trigeminal nerve.

trac'tus. Latin for tract.

trag'acanth. The dried gummy exudation from the thorny shrubs of the genus *Astragalus,* especially *Astragalus gummifer;* used in pharmacy as a suspending agent; also called gum tragacanth.

tra'gus. The small projection of cartilage in front of the opening of the external ear.

trait. 1. In genetics, any inherited gene-determined characteristic; applied to any normal variation or to a disease, whether occurring in a recessive or a dominant condition. **2.** A particular pattern of behavior.

autosomal t., one determined by a gene which is present on any chromosome other than a sex chromosome.

dominant t., trait occurring when the responsible gene is present in a heterozygous state or single dose (i.e., having dissimilar alleles in corresponding loci of a pair of chromosomes).

recessive t., trait occurring when the responsible gene is present in a homozygous state or double dose (i.e., having identical alleles at corresponding loci of a pair of chromosomes).

sickle-cell t., term used in clinical medicine to denote a condition in which there is a tendency for the red blood cells to assume a sickle-like shape due to the presence of hemoglobin AS (the heterozygous state for hemoglobin S); individuals with the trait are usually asymptomatic but may manifest some of the complications of sickle cell disease.

trajec'tor. A device for following the path of a bullet in a wound.

trance. A state of detachment from one's physical surroundings, characterized by diminished activity and consciousness, resembling sleep; e.g., the state seen in hypnosis.

tranquiliz'er. A drug that allays anxiety and calms the patient.

trans-. Prefix denoting (a) across, through, beyond; (b) located on opposite sides of a molecule; (c) transfer of a chemical group from one compound to another.

transacetyla'tion. Metabolic reaction involving the transfer of an acetyl group.

transac'tion. The reciprocal interaction between two or more individuals involving simultaneous stimulation and response.

transam'inase. Any enzyme that catalyzes the transfer of amino groups (a reversible reaction); present in body tissues and blood serum; released into the serum in increased quantities upon tissue injury; also called aminopherase and aminotransferase.

glutamic oxaloacetic t. (GOT), enzyme that catalyzes the transfer of the amino group of aspartic acid to α-ketoglutaric acid, forming glutamic and oxaloacetic acids; present in all body tissues, especially in heart, liver, and skeletal muscle; serum levels may be elevated in acute myocardial infarction, active liver disease, or some disorders of muscle; also called aspartate aminotransferase and glutamate-aspartate transaminase.

glutamic pyruvic t. (GPT), enzyme that catalyzes the transfer of the amino group of alanine to α-ketoglutaric acid, forming glutamic and pyruvic acids; present primarily in the liver and to a lesser extent in kidney and skeletal muscle; serum levels are elevated in certain liver disorders; also called alanine aminotransferase and glutamate-alanine transaminase.

serum glutamic oxaloacetic t. (SGOT), glutamic oxaloacetic transaminase; present in blood serum; see glutamic oxaloacetic transaminase.

serum glutamic pyruvic t. (SGPT), glutamic pyruvic transaminase present in blood serum; see glutamic pyruvic transaminase.

transamina'tion. The reversible process of amino group transfer, catalyzed by enzymes that have been called transaminases, aminopherases, and aminotransferases.

transcrip'tion. 1. The process of transcribing, as in the transfer of the genetic code information from DNA to messenger RNA. **2.** See signature.

transdiaphragmat'ic. Across or through the diaphragm.

transdu'cer. A device that converts energy from one form to another.

Doppler ultrasonic t., a device that detects shift in sound (Doppler effect) from change in ultrasonic signal reflected from a bodily structure such as a blood vessel.

pressure t., a device that converts pressure differences into electric current which can then be readily amplified and recorded.

transduc'tion. 1. The change in the genetic makeup of a cell by transfer of DNA from a virus to the cell. **2.** The conversion of energy from one form to another.

transec'tion. 1. Cutting across. **2.** A cross section.

trans'ferase. An enzyme that catalyzes the transfer of a chemical grouping from one substance to another; also called transferring enzyme.

transfer'ence. 1. The shifting of symptoms from one part of the body to another. **2.** In psychiatry, the unconscious shifting of an individual's feelings from people important in his early life to those important to him at a later time, as seen in the patient-analyst relationship during psychoanalysis.

transfer'rin. Iron-binding β-globulin; it facilitates the transportation of iron to the bone marow and tissue storage areas; also called siderophilin.

trans'fer RNA. A type of RNA (ribonucleic acid) which binds and transports amino acids to the ribosome; see under ribonucleic acid.

trans'fix. 1. To pierce through with a pointed instrument. **2.** To immobilize as with terror. **3.** To impale.

transforma'tion. 1. In chemistry, a change of form or structural arrangement of atoms. **2.** In genetics, the genetic changes incurred by the incorporation into a cell of DNA purified from cells or viruses.

transfor'mer. A device used to transfer electric energy from one circuit to another, especially one that changes the voltage, current, or phase of an alternating current (AC).

transfu'sion. The introduction of a fluid, such as blood or plasma, into the blood stream.

direct t., the transfer of blood directly from one person (donor) to another (recipient) without exposing it to air; also called immediate transfusion.

exchange t., removal of blood containing a toxic substance (e.g., removal of blood containing high levels of bilirubin from a newborn with erythroblastosis fetalis) coupled with blood replacement using donor blood; also called substitution transfusion.

indirect t., transfer of blood from a donor to a suitable container and thence to the recipient; also called mediate transfusion.

reciprocal t., the transfer of blood from a person who has recovered from a contagious disease to a patient suffering with the same infection; an equal amount of blood is returned from the patient to the donor; used to confer passive immunity.

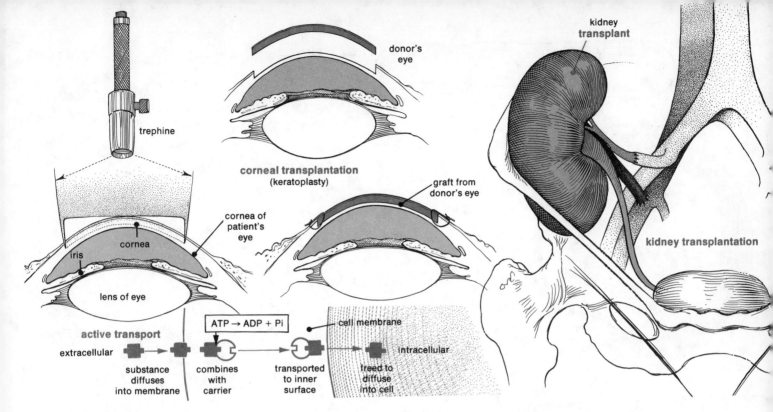

trephine

donor's
eye

corneal transplantation
(keratoplasty)

cornea of
patient's eye

graft from
donor's eye

cornea

iris

lens of eye

kidney
transplant

kidney transplantation

active transport

$$ATP \rightarrow ADP + Pi$$

extracellular

cell membrane

intracellular

substance
diffuses
into membrane

combines
with
carrier

transported
to inner
surface

freed to
diffuse
into cell

---

tran'sient. Short-lived; said of a heart sound.

transil'iac. Extending from one ilium to the other, as the transiliac diameter.

transillumina'tion. The examination of a body cavity by the passage of light through its walls.

transi'tion. A change from one state to another.

transla'tion. The process whereby the genetic data present in a messenger RNA (mRNA) molecule direct the order of the specific amino acids during protein synthesis.

transloca'tion. The transfer of part or all of one chromosome to another, nonhomologous chromosome.

translu'cent. Partially transparent; permitting light to pass through with sufficient diffusion to obliterate distinct images.

transmeth'ylase. See methyltransferase.

transmethyla'tion. The process in which methyl groups are transferred to the precursors of methylated compounds, e.g., creatine, choline, and adrenaline.

transmigra'tion. The normal passage of blood cells through the capillary walls.

transmis'sible. Capable of being passed from one person to another, as a disease.

transmis'sion. Conveyance; transfer, as of disease, from one person to another.

  duplex t., conveyance of impulses in both directions through one nerve.

  vertical t., prenatal transmission from mother to child.

transmu'ral. Through or across a wall, as the wall of a hollow organ or cyst.

transmuta'tion. A change of a chemical element into another, resulting from radioactive decay or nuclear bombardment.

transpep'tidase. Enzyme that promotes the transfer of an amino acid residue or a peptide residue from one amino compound to another.

transphenoi'dal. Through the sphenoid bone.

transphos'phoryla'tion. Chemical reaction in which a phosphate group is transferred from one organic phosphate to another.

transpira'tion. The passage of watery vapor or sweat through the skin or other tissue.

  pulmonary t., the passage of watery vapor from the circulating blood into the air of the lungs.

transpi're. To give off moisture through the skin or mucous membrane.

transplacen'tal. Denoting the movement of a substance through or across the placenta.

transplant'. 1. To transfer from one part to another, as in grafting. 2. The piece of tissue removed from the body for transplantation.

  Gallie t., narrow strip of fascia lata from the thigh, used as suture material.

transplan'tar. Extending across the sole of the foot; denoting muscular or ligamentous structures.

transplanta'tion. The transfer of tissue (graft) from one site to another.

  allogeneic t., transplantation of tissue between genetically dissimilar members of the same species.

  autoplastic t., one in which the graft is taken from another part of the same individual.

  corneal t., keratoplasty; replacement of the cornea or a portion of it (whole or partial thickness) with a graft usually taken from an eye of an individual who has recently died.

  heart t., replacement of a severely damaged heart with an entire organ from another person who has recently died.

  heterotopic t., transfer of tissue from one area of the body of the donor to another site in the recipient.

  homotopic t., orthotopic transplantation.

  kidney t., the transplantation of a kidney from one individual to another; the kidney transplant is usually obtained from a living relative with the same blood type or from a cadaver; also called renal transplantation.

  orthotopic t., transfer of tissue from an area of the body of the donor to an identical recipient site.

  renal t., see kidney transplantation.

  syngeneic t., transplantation of tissues between genetically identical or near-identical animals such as identical twins or highly inbred animals.

  syngenesioplastic t., the grafting of tissue to a recipient who is closely related to the donor, as from mother to her child.

  tendon t., the insertion of a slip from the tendon of a sound muscle into the tendon of a nonfunctioning (paralyzed) muscle.

  tooth t., the insertion of a tooth or tooth germ into a dental alveolus.

  xenogeneic t., transplantation of tissue between two different species, such as the transplantation of a chimpanzee kidney into a human.

trans'port. The conveyance of biochemical substances across cell membranes.

  active t., passage of a substance (ions or molecules) across a cell membrane by an energy-consuming process that permits diffusion to take place against an electrochemical gradient, e.g., toward the side of higher concentration (active uphill transport); coupling of an energy source to a downhill process may also occur, so that the net rate of movement of a substance is considerably greater than would occur from strictly passive transport (active downhill transport); active transport is carrier mediated.

transposi'tion. 1. The moving of tissues or structures from one place to another. 2. The presence of an organ on the wrong side of the body.

transsep'tal. Across a septum, as the transseptal fibers of the periodontal membrane, which go from the cementum of one tooth across the bony septum to the cementum of the adjacent tooth.

transsex'ual. 1. An individual with an overpowering desire to become the other sex. 2. An individual whose external sexual characteristics have been altered through surgery or hormonal intervention to resemble those of the other sex.

transsynap'tic. Denoting the transmission of a nerve impulse across a synapse.

transthorac'ic. Across the chest or performed through the chest wall.

transtra'cheal. Performed through the tracheal wall.

trans'udate. A fluid that passes through a membrane, such as a capillary wall, as a result of differences in hydrostatic pressure.

trans'uda'tion. The passage of a fluid through a membrane, as when parts of the plasma pass through the capillary walls into the tissue spaces; it differs from osmosis in that the fluid passes with most of the substances held in solution or suspension.

transure'thral. Via or through the urethra.

transvag'inal. Through the vagina.

transverse'. Cross-wise.

transver'sion. The eruption of a tooth in the wrong place or order.

transves'tism, transves'titism. 1. The practice of dressing in clothing of the opposite sex. 2. The overwhelming desire to be so dressed.

transves'tite. An individual who practices transvestism.

trape'zium. Name given to certain anatomic structures generally having a four-sided shape with no parallel sides.

trau'ma. Injury or damage.

  occlusal t., abnormal stresses and resulting pathologic changes on a tooth and surrounding tissues, caused by improper alignment of the teeth.

  psychic t., a painful emotional experience.

traumat'ic. Caused by or related to injury.

trau'matize. To injure or wound either physically or psychologically.

traumatogen'ic. Capable of causing injury or a wound.

traumatol'ogy. The branch of surgery concerned with injuries.

tray. A flat, shallow receptacle with raised edges

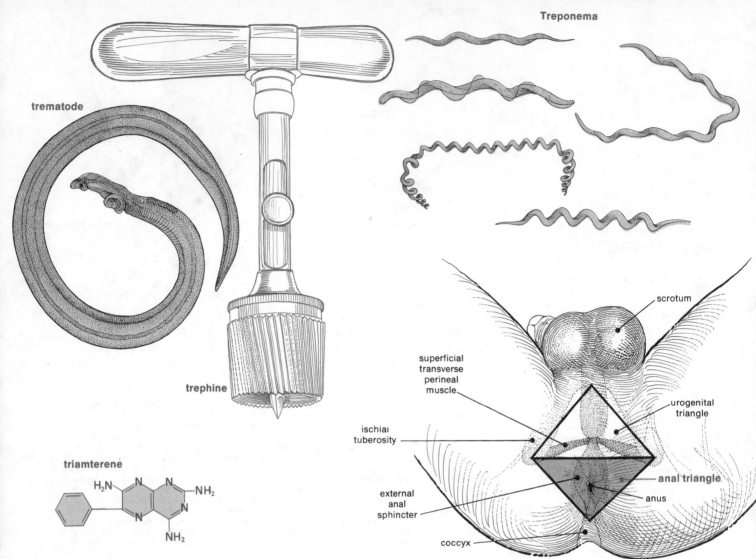

trematode

trephine

Treponema

triamterene

scrotum

superficial
transverse
perineal
muscle

ischial
tuberosity

urogenital
triangle

anal triangle

anus

external
anal
sphincter

coccyx

used for carrying or holding various items.

acrylic resin t., in dentistry, a custom-made impression tray of autopolymerizing acrylic resin for the individual patient.

impression t., in dentistry, a metallic or acrylic receptacle consisting of a flanged body and a handle for use in carrying impression material to the mouth and holding it in position against the teeth or oral tissues while the material sets.

surgical t., a tray for holding instruments in the operating room during a surgical operation.

tread′mill. A moving belt mechanism which permits individuals to walk or run in a stationary location under controlled conditions; used in studies of physiologic functions, particularly cardiac stress testing.

treat. To give medical aid to an individual by medicinal, surgical, dietary, or other measures.

treat′ment. The course of action adopted to care for a patient or to prevent disease.

conservative t., one in which any radical therapeutic or surgical measures are avoided.

drug t., treatment with medicines.

empirical t., one based on experience rather than scientific data.

expectant t., one aimed at the relief of symptoms until the nature of the illness is known; also called symptomatic treatment.

heroic t., the use of aggressive measures to preserve the life of the patient.

medical t., (1) one that employs medicines rather than surgical procedures; (2) treatment rendered by medical personnel.

megavitamin t., the use of huge doses (megadoses) of vitamins in treating disorders, such as the use of vitamin B₃ (nicotinic acid) for the treatment of schizophrenia; also called orthomolecular treatment.

palliative t., treatment aimed at mitigating symptoms rather than curing the disease.

preventive t., prophylactic t., treatment instituted to prevent a person from acquiring a disease to which he had been, or is expected to be, exposed.

root canal t., removal of the pulp of a tooth followed by obliteration of the root canal.

shock t., a type of psychiatric treatment in which a convulsive or comatose state is produced by the administration of an electric current, carbon dioxide, or insulin.

supportive t., supporting t., one aimed at maintaining the patient's strength.

surgical t., treatment by any cutting operation.

symptomatic t., see expectant treatment.

Tremato′da. A class of flatworms (including flukes) of the phylum Platyhelminthes; parasitic in man and animals.

trem′atode, trem′atoid. 1. A member of the class Trematoda; a fluke. **2.** Relating to a fluke.

trem′bling. An involuntary shaking, as from fever or fear; a shivering.

tre′mens. See delirium tremens.

trem′or. Trembling; rhythmic, involuntary, alternating contraction of opposing muscle groups, fairly uniform in frequency and amplitude.

trem′ulous, trem′ulant, trem′ulent. Quivering, trembling.

trench mouth. Necrotizing ulcerative gingivitis; see under gingivitis.

Trendelenburg's sign. See test, Trendelenburg's.

tre′panosome. Any protozoan of the genus *Trypanosoma*.

trephina′tion. Removal of a circular piece of skull with a trephine; also called trepanation.

trephine′. A cylindrical saw for cutting a circular piece of bone or other tissue, e.g., the cornea.

trephi′ning. The cutting of a circular portion of tissue with a trephine.

Trepone′ma. A genus (family Treponemataceae) of spiral bacteria, several species of which are pathogenic.

T. pallidum, the cause of syphilis in man.

T. pertenue, the cause of yaws.

trep′oneme. An organism of the genus *Treponema*.

treponemi′asis. Infection with bacteria of the genus *Treponema*.

TRF. Abbreviation for thyrotropin-releasing factor.

TRH. Abbreviation for thyrotropin-releasing hormone.

tri-. A combining form meaning three.

tri′ad. A group of three closely related signs or symptoms

Charcot's t., nystagmus, tremor, and scanning speech, seen in multiple sclerosis.

Hutchinson's t., parenchymatous keratitis, labyrinthine disease, and Hutchinson's teeth, seen in congenital syphilis.

Saint's t., hiatal hernia, diverticulosis, and gallstones occurring concomitantly.

triage′. The sorting of patients (as in a battlefield) to determine their priority for treatment.

triamcin′olone. A white crystalline powder, $C_{21}H_{27}FO_6$, used as an anti-inflammatory agent.

triam′terene. A drug that acts directly on renal tubules, producing sodium loss with potassium retention; when used in combination with thiazides, it enhances their hypotensive and diuretic effects; used to reduce edema associated with congestive heart failure, hepatic cirrhosis, and the nephrotic syndrome; Dyrenium®.

tri′angle. A figure or area formed by connecting three points with straight lines; a three-cornered area.

Alsberg's t., a triangular space formed by a line through the long axis of the femoral neck, a second through the center of the diaphysis, and a third transversely at the level of the base of the femoral head.

anal t., a triangular space with the angles placed

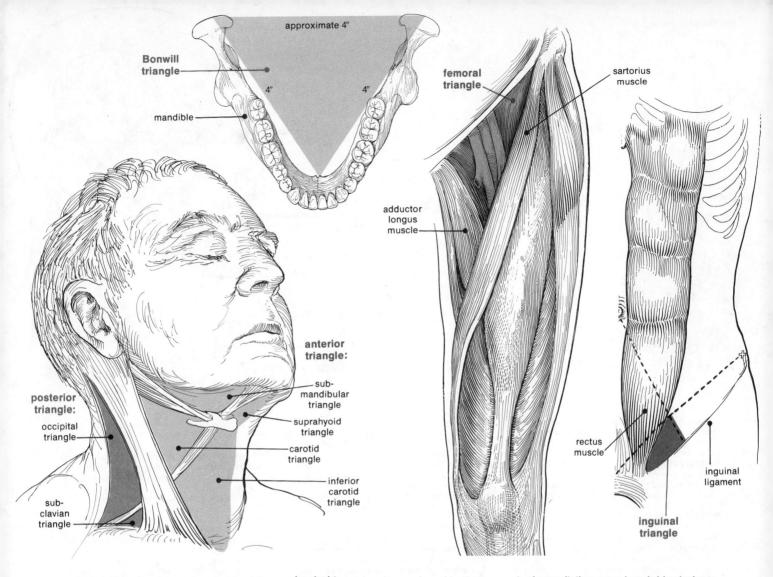

at both ischial tuberosities and at the tip of the coccyx.

anterior t., a triangular area in the neck, bounded by the mandible, the sternocleidomastoid muscle, and the midline of the neck.

axillary t., the triangular area formed by the inner aspects of the arm, the axilla, and the pectoral region.

Bonwill t., an equilateral triangle with the angles placed at the center of each mandibular condyle and at the mesial contact areas of the mandibular central incisors.

Bryant's t., a triangle whose base is from the anterior-superior iliac spine to the top of the greater trochanter; its sides are formed, respectively, by a horizontal line from the anterior-superior iliac spine and a vertical line from the top of the greater trochanter.

carotid t., the triangle of the neck, bounded above by the stylohyoid muscle and posterior belly of the digastric muscle, behind by the sternocleidomastoid muscle, and below by the omohyoid muscle.

crural t., the triangular area formed by the inner aspect of the thigh and the lower abdominal, inguinal, and genital regions, with the base traversing the umbilicus.

cystohepatic t., the triangular area formed by the liver, the cystic duct, and the hepatic duct; also called Calot's triangle.

Einthoven t., an imaginary equilateral triangle surrounding the heart, formed by lines representing the three standard limb leads of the electrocardiogram.

femoral t., a triangular space at the upper and inner part of the thigh, bounded by the sartorius and adductor longus muscles and the inguinal ligament; it is divided into two nearly equal parts by the femoral vessels; also called Scarpa's triangle.

Hesselbach's t., inguinal triangle.

inguinal t., a triangular area formed by the medial half of the inguinal ligament, the lateral edge of the abdominal rectus, and a line midway between the anterior-superior iliac spine and the pubic symphysis to the umbilicus; important area relating to inguinal hernia.

lumbar t., an area bounded by the edges of the latissimus dorsi and external oblique muscles and the crest of the ilium; also called lumbar triangle of Petit.

occipital t., the triangular area of the neck formed by the sternocleidomastoid, trapezius, and omohyoid muscles; the larger division of the posterior triangle.

olfactory t., a small triangular area just above the optic nerve near the chiasma, forming the posterior extremity of the olfactory tract where it diverges into the three roots; also called trigonum olfactorium.

omoclavicular t., subclavian triangle.

posterior t., a triangular area of the neck formed by the sternocleidomastoid muscle, the anterior margin of the trapezius muscle, and the middle third of the clavicle.

Scarpa's t., see femoral triangle.

subclavian t., the triangular area of the lower neck formed by the inferior belly of the omohyoid muscle, the clavicle, and by the posterior border of the sternocleidomastoid muscle; the smaller division of the posterior triangle.

submandibular t., the triangular area formed by the mandible, the stylohyoid muscle and posterior belly of the digastric muscle, and the anterior belly of the digastric muscle; it contains the submandibular gland.

suprahyoid t., submental t., region bounded laterally by the anterior belly of the digastric muscle, medially by the middle of the neck from the hyoid bone to the mental symphysis, and inferiorly by the body of the hyoid bone.

t. of auscultation, space bounded by the lower border of the trapezius muscle, the latissimus dorsi muscle, and the vertebral border of the scapula.

urogenital t., a triangular space with the angles placed at both ischial tuberosities and at the pubic symphysis.

vesical t., a triangular area in the bladder formed by the internal orifice of the urethra and the two orifices of the ureters; also called trigonum vesicae.

triatom′ic. 1. Denoting a molecule made up of three atoms. **2.** Possessing three replaceable atoms or radicals.

triba′sic. Denoting a molecule with three replaceable hydrogen atoms; denoting an acid with a basicity of three.

tribe. A taxonomic classification ranking just below a family or subfamily.

tri′ceps. Having three heads; denoting the muscle that extends the forearm.

trichatro′phy, trichatro′phia. Atrophy of the hair bulbs, characterized by brittleness, splitting, and shedding of the hair; a deterioration of the hair apparatus.

trichi′asis. Inversion of hairs about an orifice, as eyelashes that turn in and cause irritation of the cornea.

trichi′na. A larval worm of the genus *Trichinella*.

Trichinel′la. A genus of nematode parasites in the aphasmid group, i.e., those lacking postanal phasmids (chemoreceptors); the cause of trichinosis in man.

T. spiralis, an off-white, cylindroid worm about 1.5 mm in length; found coiled in a cyst in the striated muscle of various infected animals; a common cause of trichinosis in man; also called trichina or pork worm.

trichini′asis, trichinelli′asis. See trichinosis.

trichino′sis. A disease caused by the parasite *Trichinella spiralis*, usually ingested with raw meat, especially infested pork; the parasites become

triangle | **trichinosis**

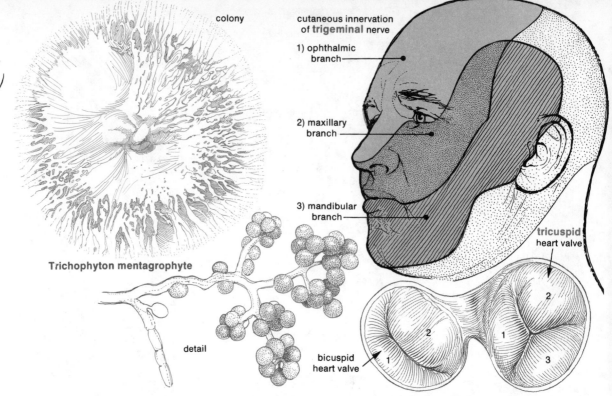

trichloroethylene

Trichomonas
vaginalis

colony

Trichophyton mentagrophyte

detail

cutaneous innervation
of **trigeminal** nerve

1) ophthalmic
branch

2) maxillary
branch

3) mandibular
branch

tricuspid
heart valve

bicuspid
heart valve

lodged in muscle, producing muscular stiffness and painful swelling, accompanied by nausea, diarrhea, fever, and sometimes prostration; also called trichiniasis and trichinelliasis.

trichloroeth′ylene. A sweet-smelling, nonflammable, volatile liquid with potent analgesic properties; used primarily as an analgesic in minor diagnostic surgical procedures and in obstetrics and dentistry; Trilene®.

trichlorometh′ane. Chloroform.

tricho-. Combining form meaning hair.

trichobe′zoar. A compact mass of hair in the intestinal tract, frequently occurring in cats.

tricholcla′sia, trichoc′lasis. Brittleness and eventual breakage of hair, as in monilethrix and trichorrhexis nodosa.

trichocrypto′sis. 1. Ingrown hairs. **2.** Any disease of the hair follicles.

tri′chocyst. One of the minute elongated cysts, arranged radially around the periphery of certain protozoans, capable of ejecting a bristle-like extension.

trichoepithelio′ma. A benign skin tumor originating in hair follicles; usually occurs on the face.

trichoesthe′sia. The sensation felt when one of the hairs of the skin is touched.

tri′chogen. Anything that stimulates hair growth.

trichoglos′sia. Black tongue; see under tongue.

tri′choid. Resembling hair.

tricholo′gia. Compulsive plucking of the hair.

trichol′ogy. The scientific study of hair—its anatomy, growth, and diseases.

Trichomo′nas. A genus of parasitic protozoan flagellates (class Mastigophora), species of which are characterized by three to five anterior flagella, a posterior flagellum, and an undulating membrane.

T. vaginalis, a species found in the vagina and in the urinary tract of men, sometime causing inflammation.

trichomoni′asis. Inflammation of the vagina and urethra caused by infection with *Trichomonas vaginalis*.

trichomyco′sis. Any infection of the hair with a fungus.

t. axillaris, infection of the axillary (and occasionally pubic) hair with *Corynebacterium tenuis*; it affects the cortex of the hair, but not the roots or surrounding skin, and occurs in persons past puberty; also called leptothrix.

trichonodo′sis. A hair condition characterized by knots or bulges; results when new hairs are not permitted to grow naturally from their follicles; also called beaded hair.

trichop′athy. Any abnormality of hair.

trichopho′bia. 1. A morbid revulsion at the

sight of loose hair on the clothing or elsewhere. **2.** An unwarranted fear of hair in excess of that considered normal for the area, especially on the face of women.

trichophytobe′zoar. A hard ball composed of hair and vegetable fibers sometimes found in the stomach of man and animals.

Trichoph′yton. A genus of pathogenic ringworm fungi (order Moniliales) possessing hyaline single-celled spores and being parasitic in the skin, nails, and hair follicles of man.

T. ceratophagus, *Trichophyton schonleini*.

T. interdigitalis, a variant of *Trichophyton mentagrophytes* that causes athlete's foot.

T. mentagrophytes, a superficial dermatophyte that causes ectothrix infections of scalp and beard hair (hyphae grow within and on the surface of hair shafts), and also of skin and nails; microconidia are numerous and occur in clusters at the ends of hyphae or singly alongside hyphae.

T. rubrum, a fungus with violet pigmentation of aerial mycelium; the cause of superficial infections in skin and nails.

T. schonleini, a fungus that causes favus, a severe form of chronic ringworm of the scalp, with destruction of hair follicles and permanent loss of hair in the infected area; in culture, the hyphae resemble reindeer horns and are sometimes referred to as favic chandeliers; also called *Trichophyton ceratophagus*.

T. tonsurans, a yellowish ringworm fungus that causes endothrix infections of hair (the hyphae grow only within the hair shafts).

T. violaceum, a fungus with purple mycelia; the cause of simple tinea capitis, black-dot ringworm, or favic lesions.

trichophyto′sis. A fungal infection caused by species of *Trichophyton*. See also tinea.

trichorrhe′a. Abnormal shedding of hair.

trichorrhex′is. Condition in which the hair breaks easily.

t. nodosa, nodular appearance of the hairs of the scalp, beard, and pubic area caused by transverse breakage of the shaft's cortex with subsequent longitudinal splitting into fine strands.

tricho′sis. Any disease of the hair.

Trichos′poron. A genus of fungi which may infect the hair; it characteristically sporulates on hair or hairlike structures.

T. beigelii, pathogenic species which is the cause of white piedra or trichosporosis.

trichosporo′sis. Any mycotic infection of the hair caused by a pathogenic *Trichosporon*.

trichostasis spinulosa. A common condition in which the hair follicle opening contains a dark

plug of from 10 to 50 short fine hairs in a horny mass; usually seen in persons with acne and seborrheic dermatitis.

Trichostron′gylus. A genus of worms (class Nematoda) which are intestinal parasites of herbivorous animals; they infest man only rarely and accidentally.

trichotilloma′nia. A compulsion to pull out or pluck one's own hair.

trichuri′asis. Infestation of the intestine with the whipworm *Trichuris trichiura*.

Trichu′ris. A genus of worms of the class Nematoda.

T. trichiura, an intestinal parasite of man; the anterior three-fifths of the worm is whiplike, the posterior two-fifths is thicker; eggs are brownish and lemon-shaped with pluglike translucent polar prominences; infection is acquired by direct finger-to-mouth contact or by ingestion of food, water, or soil containing larvae; also called whipworm.

tricus′pid. Having three cusps or points, as a valve in the heart or a tooth.

triethylene glycol. A compound $C_6H_{14}O_4$, used as an air disinfectant.

trieth′ylenemel′amine. A crystalline compound, $C_3N_3(NC_2H_4)_3$, used in the treatment of leukemia.

trifo′cal. Having three focal lengths.

trifo′liate. Having three leaflike parts.

trifurca′tion. Division into three branches or portions, as seen in the area of maxillary molars where the roots divide into three distinct portions.

trigas′tric. Denoting a muscle with three bellies.

trigem′inal. 1. Triple. **2.** Denoting the fifth cranial nerve.

t. pulse, see under pulse.

trigem′iny. A disturbance of the cardiac rhythm in which two premature beats follow each normal beat, or two normal beats are followed by a premature beat; also called trigeminal rhythm.

triglyc′eride. The most important of three groups of neutral fats; the basic unit consists of a molecule of glycerol in ester bond with three molecules of fatty acid; it serves as the major storage form of fatty acids and is practically the exclusive constituent of adipose tissue.

trig′onal. 1. Relating to a trigone. **2.** Triangular.

tri′gone. Triangle; a triangular space, eminence, or fossa.

collateral t., a somewhat triangular dilatation of the lateral ventricle of the brain between the posterior and descending horns.

fibrous t.'s, the two somewhat triangular masses of fibrous tissue that lie between the aortic arterial ring and the right and left atrioventricular rings.

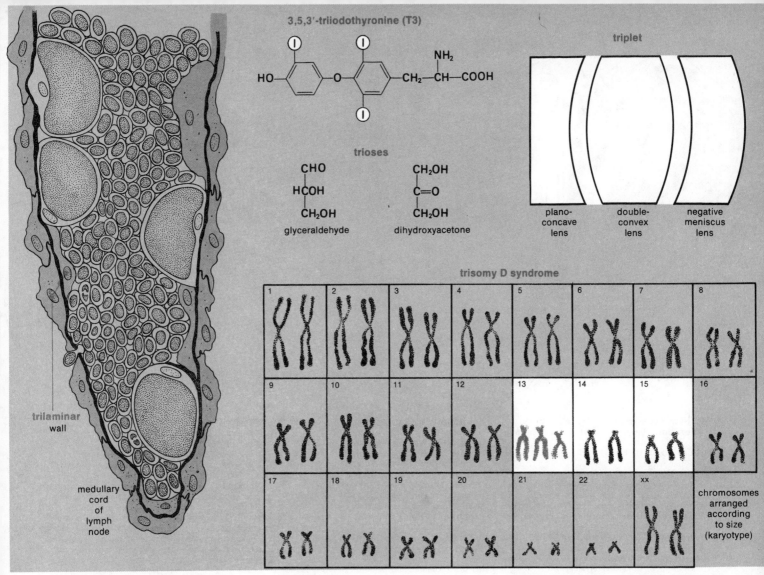

3,5,3'-triiodothyronine (T3)

trioses

glyceraldehyde

dihydroxyacetone

triplet

plano-concave lens

double-convex lens

negative meniscus lens

trilaminar wall

medullary cord of lymph node

trisomy D syndrome

chromosomes arranged according to size (karyotype)

habenular t., a depressed triangular area of the brain between the habenula and the thalamus, rostral to the superior colliculus on each side.

interpeduncular t., the fossa at the base of the brain between the two cerebral peduncles.

olfactory t., the small grayish triangular eminence at the posterior extremity of the olfactory tract where it diverges into the three roots; it lies above the optic nerve near the chiasm.

t. of the bladder, vesical trigone.

vesical t., a triangular, smooth area at the base of the bladder, whose apices are the openings of the ureters and the internal urethral orifice; in this area the mucosa is closely adherent to the muscular layer of the bladder wall; also called Lieutaud's triangle.

trigoni'tis. Inflammation of the urinary bladder, localized in the mucous membrane of the trigone; it usually follows an uncomplicated course and in most instances responds well to antibacterial agents.

trihy'drate. Compound with three molecules of water.

trihy'dric. Having three replaceable hydrogen atoms.

3,5,3'-triiodothy'ronine (T₃). A potent thyroid hormone containing three iodine atoms, normally present in the blood and thyroid gland; it usually represents about five per cent of the total thyroid hormone in blood; it is three times as active on a weight basis as thyroxin and because of differences in binding and metabolism it contributes to tissue metabolism equally with thyroxin.

trilam'inar. Composed of three layers.

trill. In speech, a sound produced by the vibration of a fluttering speech organ, most often the tongue; it causes a succession of closures and openings of the oral passage.

tril'ogy. A group of three related symptoms.

t. of Fallot, the combination of atrial septal defect, pulmonary stenosis, and ventricular hypertrophy.

trimes'ter. A period of three months; one-third of the length of a pregnancy.

first t., the period of pregnancy from the first day of the normal menstrual period to the 98th day; the first 14 weeks of gestation.

second t., the term of pregnancy from the 15th through the 28th week of gestation.

third t., the term of pregnancy from the 29th through the 42nd week of gestation.

trimeth'ylene. See cyclopropane.

trimor'phous. Occurring in three forms.

trinitroglyc'erin. See nitroglycerin.

trinitrophe'nol. See picric acid.

trinitrotol'uene (TNT). Explosive obtained by nitrating toluene.

trio'lein. A colorless oily substance occurring in many natural fats and oils; also called olein.

tri'ose. A three-carbon sugar; a monosaccharide, or sugar, possessing three carbon atoms in a molecule; e.g., glyceraldehyde and dihydroxyacetone; they represent the smallest carbohydrate molecules.

trip. Term used by drug abusers meaning (a) to take a narcotic or a hallucinogenic drug; (b) the effects produced by such drugs.

acid t., a hallucinatory experience following ingestion of LSD (acid).

ego t., anything done in order to boost one's self-esteem.

tripe. The muscular wall of the stomach of cattle, used as food.

triphosphopyridine nucleotide (TPN). Old term for nicotinamide-adenine dinucleotide phosphate (NADP).

trip'let. 1. One of three individuals born at one birth. 2. Three lenses cemented or mounted together as a single lens system to correct aberration.

triploblas'tic. Containing tissue derived from all three embryonic layers.

tri'ploid. A cell having three haploid sets of chromosomes in its nucleus.

triplo'pia. Visual defect in which one object is perceived as three instead of one.

trip'oli. A mild abrasive derived from certain porous rocks, suspended in a greaselike medium; used in dentistry for finishing dental restorations.

tris-. In chemistry, prefix denoting three of the substituents that follow.

Tris. Abbreviation for tris(hydroxymethyl)aminomethane.

trisac'charide. A carbohydrate with three monosaccharides in its molecule that upon hydrolysis yields three simple sugars; e.g., raffinose.

tris(hydroxymethyl)aminomethane (Tris). A buffer used in biologic preparations for in vitro studies, as with enzymes.

tris'mus. Difficulty in opening the mouth due to tonic spasm of the muscles of mastication; usually the first symptom of tetanus; also called lockjaw.

triso'mic. Denoting a cell or an individual having an extra chromosome.

tri'somy. The presence of an additional chromosome, homologous with one of the existing pairs, so that one particular chromosome is present in triplicate.

t. 21, Down's syndrome.

t. D syndrome. Cleft lip and palate, extra fingers or toes, abnormalities of the heart, abdominal organs, and genitalia, and defects of the central nervous system associated with mental retardation; caused by the presence of 47 chromosomes instead of the normal 46, the extra chromosome being of the group D; also called trisomy 13.

trit. Abbreviaton for Latin *trituratio*.

tritano'pia. Inability to perceive the color blue and reduced ability to perceive its combined forms (blue-greens and greens), except the violets; congenital tritanopia is rare; it occurs usually as a result of disease or detachment of the retina; also called blue blindness, blue-yellow blindness, and tritanopic vision.

trigone | tritanopia

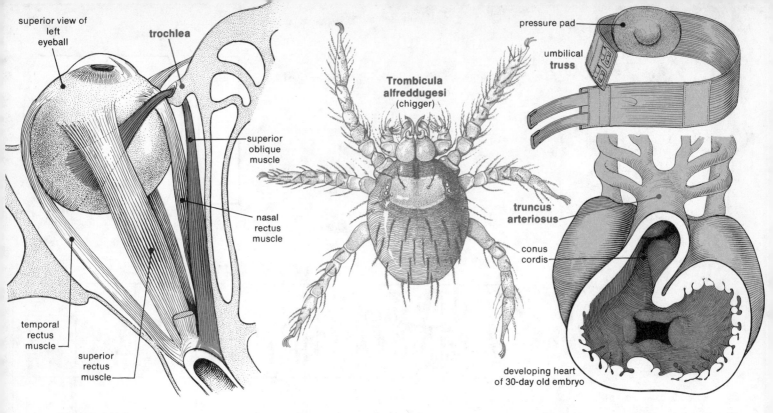

superior view of left eyeball

trochlea

superior oblique muscle

nasal rectus muscle

temporal rectus muscle

superior rectus muscle

Trombicula alfreddugesi (chigger)

pressure pad

umbilical **truss**

truncus arteriosus

conus cordis

developing heart of 30-day old embryo

trit′ium. See hydrogen-3.

trit′urable. Having the capability of being triturated.

tritura′tio (trit). Latin for triturate; used in prescription writing.

tritura′tion. 1. The process of reducing a solid to a fine powder by continuous rubbing, as the reduction of a drug to a fine powder (usually mixed thoroughly with milk sugar). **2.** In dentistry, the mixing of amalgam alloy either by itself or with mercury.

tritu′rium. A device used to separate immiscible liquids by virtue of their different densities.

triv′alent. Denoting an atom or radical with a valence of three; also called tervalent.

tRNA. Abbreviation for transfer ribonucleic acid.

tro′car. A sharp-pointed metal rod, used in a metal tube (cannula) for piercing the wall of a body cavity, after which it is withdrawn, leaving the cannula in place to permit evacuation of the fluid from the cavity; also written trochar.

trochan′ter. One of two prominences (major and minor) on the upper part of the femur.

tro′char. See trocar.

tro′che. Lozenge; a small medicated tablet.

troch′lea. Any pulley-like structure, especially the fibrous loop in the orbital cavity through which passes the tendon of the superior oblique muscle of the eyeball.

troch′lear. 1. Relating to a trochlea or pulley. **2.** The fourth cranial nerve; the trochlear nerve.

Trombic′ula. A genus of mites (family Trombiculidae) whose larvae have the ability to infest man.

T. akamushi, the kedani mite, a parasite of rodents; vector of rickettsial diseases.

T. alfreddugesi, a chigger; the larvae attack man, causing intensely irritating itching due to the injection of saliva into the skin.

trombiculi′asis. Infestation with mites of the genus Trombicula; also called trombiculosis.

Trombic′ulidae. A family of mites whose six-legged larvae (chiggers, red bugs, scrub mites, etc.) are parasitic on vertebrates, causing an irritating rash.

tro′phic. Relating to nutrition.

tropho-, troph-. Combining forms relating to nutrition; e.g., trophoblast.

tro′phoblast. The outer layer of flattened cells forming the wall of the blastocyst; it penetrates the uterine mucosa and develops into the placenta; it does not enter into the formation of the embryo itself.

trophoneuro′sis. Alteration of any tissue due to interruption of nerve supply to the part.

facial t., see hemiatrophy, facial.

trophopath′ia, trophop′athy. Any disorder of nutrition.

troph′otropism. Movement of living cells toward or away from nutritive material.

trophozo′ite. The young, ameboid, undivided stage of a sporozoan organism such as the malarial parasite, after it has been transmitted to man; the younger forms are ring-shaped; they eventually mature to form schizonts (the adult forms).

-trophy. Combining form indicating a relationship to nutrition.

-tropia. Combining form denoting abnormal deviation in the line of vision; e.g., esotropia, hypertropia.

tro′pia. Abnormal deviation of the eyes. See also strabismus.

-tropic. Combining form meaning (a) turning toward; (b) having an affinity for.

tro′pine. A poisonous alkaloid, 3α-tropanol; the major constituent of atropine and scopolamine, from which it is derived on hydrolysis; it possesses a tobacco odor and has medicinal value.

tro′pism. Tendency for parts of a living organism (e.g., leaves) to turn toward or away from a stimulus.

tropocol′lagen. The fundamental unit of collagen fibrils consisting of symmetric molecules with three helically arranged polypeptide chains.

tropom′eter. 1. A device for measuring the degree of rotation of the eyeball. **2.** A device for measuring the torsion of the shaft of a long bone.

tropomy′osin B. A fibrous protein concentrated in the Z line of muscle that can be extracted from dry powdered muscle; it has a different molecular weight from myosin.

tro′ponin. A protein in muscle that heightens the dependence of the ATP-induced contraction of actomyosin.

trough. A narrow shallow depression.

Trousseau's sign. Muscular spasm of the hand elicited by compression of the upper arm (as with a blood pressure cuff); a sign of latent tetany.

Trp. Symbol for tryptophan and its radicals; formerly abbreviated Try.

trun′cal. Relating to the trunk of the body or to any main branch.

trun′cate. Cut at right angles to the main axis.

trun′cus. Latin for trunk or stem.

t. arteriosus, the main arterial trunk of the fetal heart that gives rise to the aortic and pulmonary arteries.

trunk. 1. The human body excluding the head and the extremities; also called torso. **2.** The main part, usually short, of a nerve or vessel before its division. **3.** The main axis. **4.** A large collection of lymphatic vessels.

brachial plexus t.'s, the three trunks of the brachial plexus; see table of nerves.

brachiocephalic t., the large artery coming off the aortic arch that divides into the right subclavian and right common carotid arteries.

celiac t., the large artery arising from the abdominal aorta just below the diaphragm; it divides into the left gastric, hepatic, and splenic arteries.

intestinal lymphatic t., a short lymphatic vessel which drains lymph from the gastrointestinal tract and empties into the cisterna chyli.

lumbar lymphatic t.'s, two large collecting lymphatic vessels, right and left, that drain lymph upward from the lumbar lymph nodes to the cisterna chyli.

lumbosacral t., a large nerve formed by the union of the smaller part of the fourth and the entire fifth lumbar nerves; it enters into the formation of the sacral plexus.

pulmonary t., pulmonary artery; see table of arteries.

root t., the part of the multirooted posterior tooth situated between the cervical line and the points of bifurcation or trifurcation of roots.

sympathetic t.'s, two long chains of sympathetic ganglia on either side of the vertebral column extending from the base of the skull to the coccyx.

truss. A device consisting of a belt and a pressure pad, used to retain a hernia in place after reduction or to prevent the increase in size of an irreducible hernia.

Trypanoso′ma. A genus of parasitic protozoan flagellates (family Trypanosomidae), some of which are pathogenic.

T. cruzi, the species that causes Chagas' disease; endemic in Central and South America, especially in Brazil, Chile, Argentina, and Venezuela; found also in vectors in California, Arizona, and Texas.

T. gambiense, the species that causes West African or Mid-African sleeping sickness; transmitted by the tsetse fly; also called *Trypanosoma hominis*, *Trypanosoma ugandense*, and *Castellanella gambiense*.

T. rhodesiense, the species that causes Rhodesian trypanosomiasis (East African sleeping sickness); endemic in Rhodesia and Tanzania.

trypanosomi′asis. Any disease caused by infection with a protozoan parasite of the genus *Trypanosoma*; transmitted by the bite of the tsetse fly or by contamination of the bite wound of the kissing bug.

African t., disease of the central nervous system transmitted by several species of tsetse flies (genus *Glossinia*); the parasite (*Trypanosoma gambiense*)

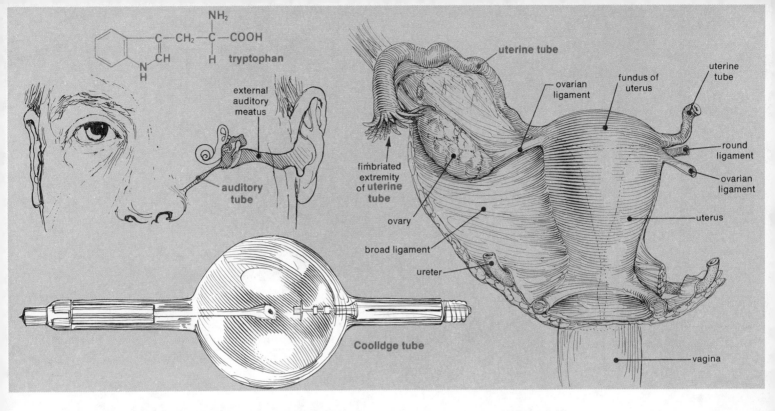

tryptophan

external auditory meatus

auditory tube

uterine tube

ovarian ligament

fundus of uterus

uterine tube

round ligament

ovarian ligament

uterus

fimbriated extremity of uterine tube

ovary

broad ligament

ureter

vagina

Coolidge tube

enters the circulation and becomes localized in the brain and lymph nodes; early manifestations include severe headache, fever, a feeling of oppression, and enlarged lymph nodes; wasting, mental deterioration, and drowsiness occur in the late stages and, if untreated, death occurs; also called African sleeping sickness.

American t., see Chagas' disease.

tryp′sin. One of the protein-splitting (proteolytic) enzymes in the pancreatic juice derived from trypsinogen.

trypsin′ogen, tryp′sogen. A substance secreted by the pancreas and converted, in the intestine, into trypsin by the enzyme enterokinase.

tryp′tic. Relating to the proteolytic enzyme trypsin.

tryp′tophan. An essential amino acid present in varying quantities in common proteins; deficiency may result in the development of pellagra.

tset′se. See *Glossina*.

TSH. Abbreviation for thyroid-stimulating hormone (thyrotropic hormone).

TSH-RF. Abbreviation for thyroid-stimulating hormone releasing factor.

tsp. Abbreviation for teaspoon.

tsutsugamushi disease. Infectious disease occurring in Southeast Asia; caused by *Rickettsia tsutsugamushi* and transmitted by mites; characterized by painful swelling of the lymphatic glands, fever, headache, eruption of dark red papules, and blackish scab on the genitals; also called mite-borne, scrub, or tropical typhus and island, tsutsugamushi, or Japanese river fever.

TTP. Abbreviation for (a) thrombotic thrombocytopenic purpura; (b) thymidine 5′-triphosphate.

tubal. Of or relating to a tube, especially a uterine tube.

tube. 1. A hollow cylinder. 2. A channel or canal.

auditory t., a channel connecting the cavity of the middle ear with the upper part of the throat (nasopharynx); it equalizes the pressure in the middle ear with the atmospheric pressure; also called eustachian tube.

Cantor t., a 10 foot long rubber tube with a mercury filled bag at the extreme end, used for intestinal intubation; it is usually introduced via the nose and directed into the stomach; with proper positioning of the patient the weight of the mercury bag helps to lead the tube through the duodenum and into the small intestine beyond.

Coolidge t., a hot-cathode x-ray tube that develops its electrons from a heated filament.

drainage t., one placed in a wound or cavity to allow the escape of fluids.

endotracheal t., a rubber tube inserted in the trachea as an airway in endotracheal intubation.

eustachian t., see auditory tube.

fallopian t., see uterine tube.

Geiger-Müller t., Geiger t., a gas-filled tube containing a cylindrical cathode and axial wire electrode, used to detect radioactivity; radioactive particles penetrate the tube's envelope and produce momentary current pulsations in the gas.

Levin t., a flexible tube introduced into the duodenum or stomach, usually through the nose, after an operation.

Miller-Abbott t., a double lumen 10 foot intestinal tube, used for diagnosing and treating obstructions of the small intestine.

photomultiplier t., apparatus used to amplify images of low intensity.

Rehfuss stomach t., one with a graduated syringe used for aspiration of stomach contents for analysis.

Sengstaken-Blakemore t., device consisting of three tubes, two with an inflatable balloon and the third one attached to a suction apparatus; used to stop bleeding from the esophagus.

Southey's t.'s, thin delicate tubes for draining fluid from subcutaneous tissues.

stomach t., a flexible 16-inch tube used for feeding or for washing out the stomach.

tracheotomy t., a metal or glass tube inserted into the trachea through a tracheotomy opening to facilitate breathing.

uterine t., one of two slender tubes, about four inches long, on either side leading from the uterus to the area of the ovary; it conveys the ovum from the ovary to the uterus and is usually where conception occurs; also called fallopian tube and oviduct.

vacuum t., glass tube from which air has been almost completely removed.

x-ray t., a vacuum tube used for the production of x rays; the enclosed electrodes accelerate electrons and direct them to an anode, where their impacts produce high energy photons.

tubec′tomy. See salpingectomy.

tu′ber, *pl.* **tu′bera.** A prominence.

t. cinereum, the small portion of the hypothalamus that protrudes into the floor of the third ventricle of the brain.

tu′bercle. 1. The specific lesion of tuberculosis. 2. A rounded elevation on a bone. 3. A nodule on the skin.

tuber′cular. Relating to or having tubercles; also called tuberculous; erroneously used instead of tuberculous to describe a person afflicted with tuberculosis.

tuber′culate, tuber′culated. Having nodules or tubercles.

tubercula′tion. The formation or presence of nodules.

tuber′culid. A skin lesion caused by the toxins of tuberculosis.

tuber′culin. A substance made from the toxins of the tubercle bacillus, used in the diagnosis and, to some extent, in the treatment of tuberculosis.

old t. (O. T.), a concentrated filtrate made from a six-week-old culture of tubercle bacilli in glycerol broth; it contains only the soluble substance produced by the bacilli during growth, not the microorganisms.

purified protein derivative of t. (P.P.D), an extract from tubercle bacilli prepared in the protein-free liquid medium.

tuber′culoid. 1. Resembling tuberculosis. 2. Resembling a tubercle.

tuberculo′ma. A tumor-like mass of tuberculous origin.

tuberculo′sis. A communicable disease caused by any of several species of *Mycobacterium* referred to as the tubercle bacillus; it manifests itself by the formation of tubercles or lesions in the tissues affected, most commonly the lungs; tuberculosis in man is caused by the human variety of *Mycobacteria* (*Mycobacterium tuberculosis*) and the bovine variety of *Mycobacterium bovis*) as well as some atypical bacteria.

acute miliary t., a form of tuberculosis in which the tubercle bacilli are carried in the blood stream throughout the body, thus affecting several organs simultaneously; also called disseminated tuberculosis.

cutaneous t., a rare group of skin diseases caused either by the presence of microorganisms in the skin or by allergic reactions to a previous bacterial infection.

disseminated t., acute miliary tuberculosis.

postprimary t., tuberculosis of the lung occurring as a reinfection or a reactivation of a dormant infection.

primary t., the phase of a tuberculous infection immediately following invasion of tissues by the tubercle bacilli.

pulmonary t., tuberculosis of the lungs, marked by ulceration and formation of cavities in the lungs, attended by fever and cough; formerly called phthisis and consumption.

tuber′culostat′ic. 1. Denoting an agent that inhibits the growth of the tubercle bacillus. 2. Arresting the growth of the tubercle bacillus.

tuber′culous. Afflicted with tuberculosis.

tuber′culum, *pl.* **tuber′cula.** 1. An elevation on a bone. 2. A nodule on the skin.

tuberos′ity. A rounded protuberance from the

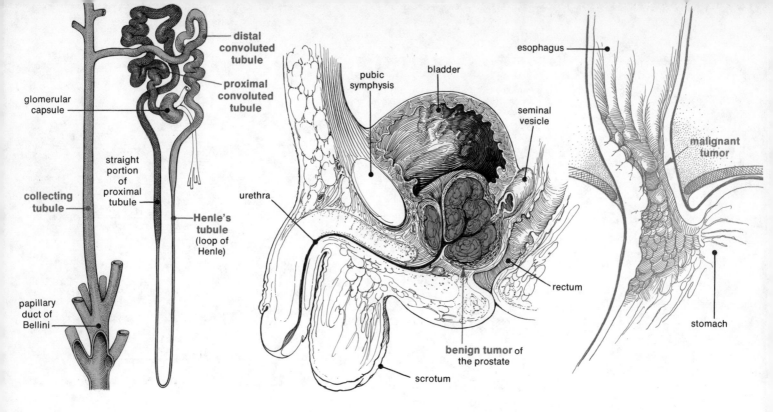

surface of a bone or cartilage.

tu′berous. Having many small rounded projections; lumpy; also called nodular.

tubocurarine chloride. An active alkaloid derived from *Chondodendron tomentosum* that produces skeletal muscle paralysis by occupying the receptors at the neuromuscular junction, thereby blocking the action of the neurotransmitter acetylcholine; used to produce muscular relaxation during surgical operations and to reduce the severity of muscle spasms in severe tetanus.

tubo-ova′rian. Relating to a uterine (fallopian) tube and ovary.

tu′bular. Relating to, shaped like, or consisting of a tube or tubes.

tu′bule. A small tube or canal; also called tubulus.

    collecting t., one of the straight tubules of the kidney (as opposed to the convoluted ones); it commences in the radiate part of the cortex, where it receives the distal convoluted tubule, and progresses to the renal pyramid in the medulla, where it empties into the papillary duct of Bellini; also called straight tubule and excretory duct.

    convoluted t., distal, the tortuous portion of the renal tubule leading from the terminal part of the ascending limb of Henle's (nephronic) loop to the collecting tubule.

    convoluted t., proximal, the tortuous portion of the renal tubule leading from the glomerular (Bowman's) capsule to the straight portion of the proximal tubule (pars recta) in the medullary ray; also called pars convoluta.

    dental t.'s, minute tubes or canals in the dentin of the tooth containing the dentinal fibers and extending radially from the pulp to the dentoenamel junction.

    Henle's t.'s, the straight descending and ascending limbs of a renal tubule which form Henle's (nephronic) loop.

    malpighian t.'s, slender tubular structures that emerge from the alimentary canal of some insects, usually between the midgut and hindgut.

    proximal t., the portion of the tubule leading from the glomerular capsule to the thin descending limb of the loop of Henle; it consists of a highly convoluted portion (pars convoluta) and a short straight segment (pars recta).

    renal t., the part of the nephron responsible for conveying the glomerular filtrate to the renal pelvis and transforming it into the final urine product; it consists of the glomerular (Bowman's) capsule, proximal tubule, Henle's (nephronic) loop, distal tubule, and the collecting tubule.

    seminiferous t.'s, long, threadlike, twisted tubules loosely packed in each lobule of the testis; the channels in which the spermatozoa develop and through which they are conveyed to the rete testis.

    transverse t.'s, invaginations of the sarcolemma.

tubuliza′tion. Protection of an injured or sutured nerve with an absorbable cylinder to promote healing.

tubulorrhex′is. Localized disintegration of epithelium and basement membrane of renal tubules; a characteristic lesion of acute tubular necrosis.

tuft. A cluster.

    malpighian t., see glomerulus (1).

tug, tug′ging. A pulling sensation.

tulare′mia. An infectious disease caused by the bacterium *Pasteurella tularensis*, transmitted to man by the bite of infected animals and marked by a prolonged or remitted fever and swelling of the lymph nodes; also called rabbit or deer-fly fever.

tumefa′cient. Causing a swelling.

tumefac′tion, tumes′cence. 1. A swollen condition. **2.** The process of swelling.

tu′mid. Swollen.

tu′mor. A neoplasm, an overgrowth of tissue.

    adenomatoid t., a benign, slow growing, graywhite nodules of uncertain origin, occurring in both male and female genital tracts.

    adipose t., see lipoma.

    benign t., one that does not form metastases or infiltrate and is unlikely to recur after its removal.

    blood t., one containing blood.

    carotid body t., chemodectoma.

    cellular t., one composed chiefly of cells of homogeneous stroma.

    desmoid t., see desmoid.

    Ewing's t., a malignant tumor occurring in the bones, especially the bones of the extremities, arising from medullary tissue; symptoms include fever, pain, and leukocytosis; also called Ewing's sarcoma and diffuse endothelioma of bone.

    fibrocellular t., see fibroma.

    giant cell t. of bone, a soft, reddish-brown, usually benign tumor of long bones, composed chiefly of multinucleated giant cells and ovoid or spindle-shaped cells; also called giant cell myeloma and osteoclastoma.

    glomus t., an extremely painful, small, bluish-red benign tumor in the skin, arising from cells of a glomus body; also called glomangioma.

    granular cell t., a benign, usually small tumor of uncertain origin, often involving peripheral nerves in skin, mucosa, or connective tissue; also called myoblastoma and granular cell myoblastoma.

    granulosal cell t., a rare, benign (potentially malignant) tumor of the ovary, occurring most frequently during the active reproductive age; it elaborates estrogen and is sometimes the cause of precocious puberty.

    heterologous t., a tumor composed of tissue different from the one in which it grows.

    homologous t., one made up of the same kind of tissue as the one from which it grows.

    Krukenberg t., a malignant, usually bilateral, tumor of the ovary, secondary to a mucous carcinoma of the stomach.

    malignant t., one which forms metastases, tends to recur after its removal, and eventually causes death; also called cancer.

    mixed t., one composed of more than one tissue or cell type.

    mixed t. of salivary gland, tumor believed to be derived from cells of salivary ducts or from embryonic cells of salivary glands; most frequently seen in the parotid gland; also called pleomorphic adenoma.

    mucoid t., see myxoma.

    osseous t., see osteoma.

    papillary t., see papilloma.

    phantom t., an abdominal swelling, simulating an ovarian tumor or pregnancy; a form of neurosis.

    pontine angle t., one located in the proximal portion of the acoustic nerve.

    Pott's puffy t., a circumscribed swelling of the scalp resulting from osteitis of the skull or from an extradural abscess.

    Schmincke t., tumor originating in the lingual and pharyngeal tonsils.

    Schwann's t., see neurofibroma.

    theca cell t., see thecoma.

    theca lutein cell t., see thecoma.

    transition t., a tumor originally appearing benign, recurring after removal, and then turning malignant.

    Warthin's t., papillary cystadenoma lymphatosum; see under cystadenoma.

    Wilm's t., a malignant tumor of the kidney, occurring mostly in young children; composed of embryonic elements.

    Zollinger-Ellison t., tumor of the pancreas causing the Zollinger-Ellison syndrome.

tumorigen′esis. The formation of a new growth.

tumorigen′ic. Causing tumors.

tu′morous. Resembling a tumor.

tung′sten. A chemical element with a very high melting point used as the target material of an x-ray tube as well as in electric light filaments; symbol W,

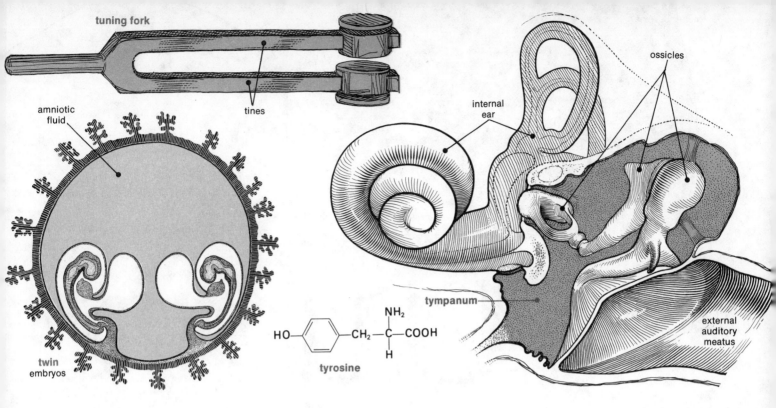

tuning fork

tines

amniotic fluid

twin embryos

tyrosine

$$HO-\text{⬡}-CH_2-\overset{\overset{\displaystyle NH_2}{|}}{\underset{\underset{\displaystyle H}{|}}{C}}-COOH$$

internal ear

ossicles

tympanum

external auditory meatus

atomic number 74, atomic weight 183.86.

tu′nica. A coat or enveloping layer of tissue.

t. adventitia, the fibrous outer layer of a blood vessel; also called tunica externa.

t. albuginea testis, the thick, fibrous, bluish-white membrane covering the testis.

t. dartos, the highly vascular layer of smooth muscle in the scrotum; its deeper fibers form a septum which divides the scrotum in two halves.

t. intima, the inner, serous layer of an artery.

t. media, the middle muscular layer of an artery.

t. vaginalis propria testis, a closed serous pouch investing the testis; it consists of a parietal and a visceral layer.

tuning fork. A forklike metal instrument with two prongs which, when struck, produce a sound of fixed pitch; used for testing hearing and vibratory sensation.

tur′bid. Cloudy.

turbidimet′ric. Relating to the measuring of turbidity.

turbidim′etry. Measurement of turbidity or cloudiness of a fluid.

turbid′ity. Cloudiness caused by the stirring up of sediment or suspended foreign particles, resulting in a loss of transparency.

tur′binate. 1. Shaped like an inverted cone or a scroll. **2.** A turbinate bone; see table of bones.

tur′bine. A rotary instrument activated by a stream of water.

turbinec′tomy. Surgical removal of a turbinate bone.

Turcot syndrome. The presence of polyps in the colon combined with brain tumors; transmitted as an autosomal recessive trait.

turges′cence. The process of swelling; the state of being swollen.

tur′gid. Congested; bloated.

tur′gor. Fullness.

turn. To move a fetus in the uterus from a malposition to one that will facilitate normal delivery.

Turner's syndrome. Condition due to a chromosomal anomaly (only one X chromosome); absence of ovaries or possession of only rudimentary structures, infantile female genitalia, short stature, and webbed neck are some of the symptoms.

tus′sis. A cough.

tus′sive. Relating to or caused by a cough.

twin. 1. One of two children born at one birth. **2.** Double; growing in pairs.

conjoined t.'s, twins having varying degrees of connection or fusion with each other; also called Siamese twins.

dizygotic t.'s., see fraternal twins.

fraternal t.'s, twins developed from two separate ova; they may or may not be of the same sex; also called dizygotic or heterozygous twins.

heterozygous t.'s, see fraternal twins.

identical t.'s, twins resulting from a single fertilized egg that splits at an early stage of development; they are always of the same sex, have the same genetic constitution, and have pronounced resemblance to one another; also called monozygotic or uniovular twins.

monozygotic t.'s, see identical twins.

Siamese t.'s, conjoined twins; originally applied to the publicized conjoined twins from Siam.

uniovular t.'s, see identical twins.

twinge. A sudden, short, sharp physical or mental pain.

twitch. 1. A brief involuntary or spasmodic contraction of a muscle fiber; usually phasic. **2.** To move sharply and suddenly; to jerk.

two-carbon fragment. The acetyl group CH_3CO-.

tylo′ma. Heavy callus formation.

t. conjunctivae, a localized cornification of the conjunctiva.

tylo′sis. 1. The formation of a callus. **2.** A callosity.

tympanec′tomy. Removal of the tympanic membrane.

tympan′ic. Relating to the chamber of the middle ear.

tympani′tes. Distention of the abdomen due to accumulation of gas in the intestines; also called meteorism.

tympanit′ic. 1. Relating to tympanites, as the sound produced by percussing over the distended abdomen. **2.** Tympanic or resonant.

tympanomastoidi′tis. Inflammation of the middle ear and the mastoid cells.

tympanomet′ry. The measurement of the flow of sound energy in the external auditory meatus; a means of detecting middle ear disease.

tympanoplas′ty. A general term denoting any of several operative procedures designed to restore hearing in patients with middle ear or conductive hearing loss.

type I t., see myringoplasty.

tympanosclero′sis. Scarring of the tympanic membrane (eardrum), causing hearing impairment; seen most commonly in children.

tympanosquamo′sal. Pertaining to the tympanic and squamous portions of the temporal bone.

tym′panum. The chamber of the middle ear, a cavity in the temporal bone housing the chain of ossicles.

tym′pany. A drumlike percussion sound.

type. A pattern of characteristics common to a number of individuals, chemical substances, diseases, etc., that serves to identify them as members of a particular group.

blood t., see blood group.

wild t., in genetics, the standard or the parent strain of an experimental microorganism; the most frequently observed form of an organism, or the one arbitrarily designated as normal.

typhe′mia. The occurrence of typhoid bacilli in the blood; also called typhoid bacillemia.

typhli′tis. Inflammation of the cecum; the term was formerly used for appendicitis.

typhlo-. Combining form meaning cecum.

ty′phoid. Resembling typhus.

ty′phous. Relating to typhus.

ty′phus. An acute infectious and contagious disease caused by a *Rickettsia* and marked by sustained high fever, severe headache, and a characteristic rash; also called typhus fever.

endemic t., see murine typhus.

epidemic t., one caused by *Rickettsia prowazekii* and transmitted by body lice.

flea-borne t., see murine typhus.

mite-borne t., see tsutsugamushi disease.

murine t., one caused by *Rickettsia mooseri* and transmitted by the rat flea; also called endemic or flea-borne typhus.

recrudescent t., see lymphoblastoma.

scrub t., see tsutsugamushi disease.

Tyr. Symbol for the amino acid tyrosine and its radicals.

ty′ramine. A colorless amine found in decayed animal tissue, certain cheeses, and ergot; produced by the decarboxylation of tyrosine; it has a weak sympathomimetic action but releases stored norepinephrine and has been used as a provocative agent in the diagnosis of pheochromocytoma.

tyrosinase′. A copper-containing oxidizing enzyme in bodily tissues which converts tyrosine into a red indole compound and thence to melanin; it catalyzes the oxidation of phenolic compounds; also called monophenol oxidase.

tyro′sine. A crystallizable amino acid, $C_9H_{11}NO_3$, that is sparingly soluble in water; present in most proteins; an essential constituent of any diet; a precursor of melanin and thyroxin.

tyrosino′sis. A hereditary disease of tyrosine metabolism; believed to be caused by lack of *p*-hydroxyphenylpyruvic acid oxidase, with resulting excessive excretion of *p*-hydroxyphenylpyruvic acid.

tunica | tyrosinosis

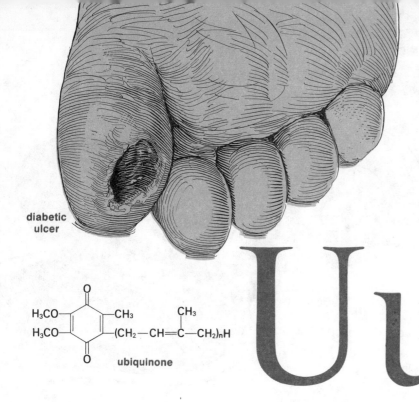

diabetic ulcer

ubiquinone

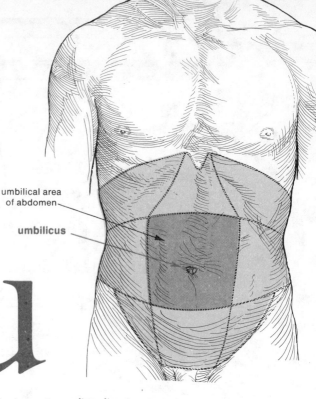

umbilical area of abdomen

umbilicus

Uu

U. Symbol for (a) kilurane, 1000 uranium units; (b) the element uranium.

u. Abbreviation for (a) unit; (b) upper.

ubiquin′one. 2,3-Dimethoxybenzoquinones, a hydrophobic compound that plays a role in electron transport in tissues; also called coenzyme Q (for quinone).

UCS. Abbreviation for unconditioned stimulus.

ud′der. The baglike mammary gland of animals such as cows, sheep, and goats.

UDP. Abbreviation for uridine diphosphate.

UDP-galactose. Abbreviation for uridine diphosphate galactose.

UDP-glucose. Abbreviation for uridine diphosphate glucose.

UDPG. Abbreviation for uridine diphosphoglucose (uridine diphosphate glucose).

UHF. Abbreviation for ultrahigh frequency.

ulal′gia. Pain in the gingiva (gums).

ul′cer. A depressed lesion on the skin or mucous membrane.

  Curling's u., one occurring in the duodenum as a result of severe bodily burns.

  decubitus u., ulcer of the skin, and sometimes muscles, occurring in pressure areas of bedridden patients allowed to lie in the same position for long periods of time; also called bedsore and pressure sore.

  diabetic u., one associated with diabetes, occurring most frequently in the lower extremities, especially the toes.

  duodenal u., ulceration of the mucous lining of the duodenum.

  esophageal u., one generally located at the lower end of the esophagus, frequently due to chronic regurgitation of gastric juice.

  gastric u., ulcer of the stomach usually on or near the lesser curvature.

  gummatous u., one occurring during the late stage of syphilis.

  indolent u., one that does not respond to treatment.

  peptic u., ulcer of the mucous membrane of the stomach or duodenum caused by the digestive action of acid-pepsin gastric juice.

  perforated u., one that has eroded through the wall of an organ, such as that of the stomach.

  rodent u., basal cell carcinoma of the skin.

  roentgen u., one caused by overexposure to x rays.

  stercoral u., ulcer of the colon caused by impacted feces.

  stomal u., ulcer in jejunal mucosa following (and occurring near) the surgical union of the jejunum and stomach.

  stress u., peptic ulcer associated with other conditions.

  transparent u., one occurring on the cornea and healing without opacity.

  trophic u., one due to impaired circulation to the part.

  varicose u., ulcer due to and overlying a varicose vein.

  venereal u., chancroid.

ul′cerate. To form an ulcer.

ulcera′tion. 1. The formation of an ulcer. **2.** An ulcer.

ul′cerative. 1. Causing the formation of ulcers. **2.** Marked by ulceration.

ulcerogen′ic. Causing the formation of ulcers.

ul′cerous. Characterized by the presence of ulcers.

ulerythe′ma. An inflammatory process that ultimately results in atrophy or scarring.

  u. ophryogenes, folliculitis of the eyebrows resulting in scarring and redness.

ul′na. The larger of the two bones of the forearm, extending from the elbow to the wrist on the side opposite to the thumb.

ul′nar. Relating to the ulna.

ulnora′dial. Relating to the ulna and radius (bones of the forearm).

ulot′omy. The cutting or sectioning of contracting scar tissue to relieve tension or deformity.

ultra-. A prefix denoting an extreme; a surpassing of a specified range; e.g., ultrastructure.

ultracen′trifuge. A convection-free high speed centrifuge (up to ±100,000 rpm); used in the separation of large molecules and for determinations of molecular weight.

ultrafil′ter. A semipermeable membrane (collodion, fish bladder, or filter paper impregnated with gels) used for performing ultrafiltration.

ultrafiltra′tion. 1. Filtration through a filter capable of removing all but the smallest particles, such as viruses. **2.** Filtration through a semipermeable membrane for the separation of colloids from their dispersion medium and dissolved crystalloids.

ultraliga′tion. Ligation or tying of a blood vessel beyond the point where a branch is given off.

ultramicrom′eter. A micrometer with an extremely accurate gauge, capable of measuring to one-millionth of a centimeter.

ultrami′croscope. A dark field microscope with high-intensity refracted illumination for viewing very minute objects or particles of colloidal size; the horizontal beam of light striking the particles is refracted and appears as bright spots against a black background.

ultramicroscop′ic. Too small to be visible under the ordinary microscope.

ultrami′crotome. An instrument for cutting tissue into very thin sections (0.1 μ thick, or less) for electron microscopy.

ultraso′nascope. An apparatus that sends sound impulses (at frequencies above the range audible to the human ear) toward an organ, which in turn bounces or echoes the sounds back; the patterns produced are graphically displayed on a fluorescent screen for interpretation.

ultrason′ic. Not perceptible to the human ear; relating to sound waves above 30,000 cycles per second.

ultrason′ogram. A record made by ultrasonography.

ultrasonog′raphy. The delineation of deep bodily structures by measuring the reflection of ultrasonic waves directed into the tissue.

ultrasonosur′gery. The use of ultrasound (high frequency sound waves) to disrupt tissues or tracts, especially in the central nervous system.

ultrasonot′omy. A psychosurgical procedure in which discrete brain lesions are produced, generally in the prefrontal lobes, by high frequency sound waves; used in the treatment of certain severe psychiatric disorders.

ul′trasound. Sound waves of frequency higher than the range audible to the human ear, or above 20,000 vibrations per second.

ul′trastructure. The ultimate structure or organization of protoplasm, as seen with the aid of the electron microscope; also called fine or submicroscopic structure.

ultravi′olet. Denoting a range of invisible radiation extending from the visible violet portion of the spectrum out to the low-frequency x-ray region of the electromagnetic spectrum.

ulula′tion. 1. The loud, inarticulate crying of emotionally disturbed persons, especially hysterical ones. **2.** Loud lamentation.

umbil′ical. Relating to or resembling the navel.

umbil′icated, umbil′icate. Dimpled; having a pit or depression that resembles the navel.

umbilica′tion. A depression or pit resembling the navel.

umbil′icus. The depressed area of the abdominal wall where the umbilical cord was attached to the fetus; also called navel.

um′bo, pl. **umbo′nes. 1.** A projection at the center of a rounded surface. **2.** The most depressed point on the outer surface of the tympanic membrane, formed by traction of the malleus on the inner surface of the membrane to which it is attached.

UMP. Abbreviation for uridine monophosphate (5′-phosphoribosyl uracil).

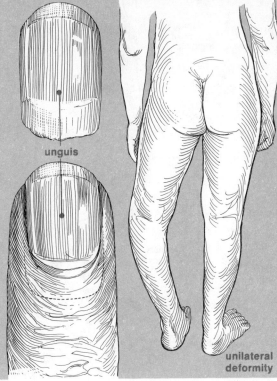

unguis

unilateral deformity

Units of Concentration	
molar (mol/liter)	M
parts per million	ppm
Units of Length	
meter	m
micrometer (micron)	μm (μ)
Angstrom (0.1 nm)	Å
Units of Volume	
milliliter	ml
microliter	μl
Units of Mass	
gram	g
microgram	μg
Units of Time	
hour	hr
minute	min
second	s, sec
Units of electricity	
ampere	amp
milliampere	mA
volt	V
ohm	Ω

Units of Energy and Work	
joule	J
calorie	cal
Units of Temperature	
degree centigrade	°
thermodynamic temperature (Kelvin)	K
Units of Radioactivity	
counts per minute	cpm
curie(s)	Ci
Miscellaneous **Units**	
revolutions per minute	rpm
cycles per second (hertz)	Hz
pascal (newton/meter$_2$)	Pa
lux	lx
candela	cd
lumen	lm

Prefixes to Names of **Units**

exa	10^{18}	E	milli	10^{-3}	m
peta	10^{15}	P	micro	10^{-6}	μ
tera	10^{12}	T	nano	10^{-9}	n
giga	10^{9}	G	pico	10^{-12}	p
mega	10^{6}	M	femto	10^{-15}	f
kilo	10^{3}	k	atto	10^{-18}	a
centi	10^{-2}	c			

un'ciform. Hook-shaped.

Uncina'ria. A genus of Nematoda characterized by a hooklike structure.

uncinari'asis. Ancylostomiasis; infection due to the presence of hookworms (species of Ancylostoma or Necator) in the intestine.

un'cinate. Hooked or shaped like a hook.

uncon'scious. 1. Inability to respond to sensory stimuli. **2.** In Freudian theory, the part of the mind containing feelings, urges, and experiences of which the individual is only briefly or never aware.

uncoup'ler. Any substance (such as dinitrophenol) that uncouples the usual linkage between oxidation and phosphorylation.

un'cus. The hooked anterior portion of the hippocampal gyrus.

undecylenic acid. An antifungal proprietary agent, $CH_2CH(CH_2)_8COOH$, used in treating dermatophytic infections.

underachiev'er. An individual, especially a student, who manifestly performs below his capacity as determined by tests of intelligence, aptitude, or ability.

un'dercut. 1. The portion of a prepared tooth cavity that mechanically locks the restorative filling, such as amalgam, into place. **2.** The portion of a tooth that lies between the gingiva and the crest of contour. **3.** The contour of a dental arch which prevents the proper insertion of a denture.

undernutri'tion. Any deviation below good nutrition; a condition resulting from a negative nutritive balance that occurs when metabolic utilization plus excretion of one or more essential nutrients exceeds the supply.

undescend'ed. Not descended to a normal position, as a testis that is retained in the abdomen.

undifferentia'ted. Not differentiated; usually applied to cells.

undo'. Psychoanalytically, to act out in reverse an unacceptable prior action (a defense mechanism).

un'dulate. 1. To fluctuate in wavelike patterns, as some fevers. **2.** Having an irregular, wavy border or appearance, as seen in the shape of a bacterial colony.

unerupt'ed. In dentistry, denoting a normal developing tooth or an impacted tooth that has not emerged or perforated the oral mucosa.

ung., ungt. Abbreviations for Latin *unguentum*.

un'gual. Relating to the nails; also called unguinal.

ung'uent. Ointment.

unguen'tum (ung., ungt.). Latin for ointment; used in prescription writing.

unguic'ulate. Having nails or claws.

un'guis, *pl.* **un'gues.** Latin for nail (either a fingernail or a toenail).

uni-. Prefix meaning one, single.

uniax'ial. 1. Possessing but one axis; e.g., a hinge joint. **2.** Developing chiefly in only one direction.

unicam'eral. Consisting of a single cavity; characterized by one compartment only.

unicel'lular. Consisting of one cell, as a protozoan.

unicus'pid. Denoting a tooth with one cusp.

u'niform. Consistent in appearance; without variation in form.

unigrav'ida. Primigravida; a woman pregnant for the first time.

unilam'inar. Possessing only one layer.

unilat'eral. Occurring only on one side.

uniloc'ular. Having only one compartment.

uninephrec'tomized. Having had one kidney surgically removed.

uninu'clear, uninu'cleate. Having only one nucleus.

unioc'ular. Relating to or having one eye.

union. The process of joining together of tissues; also called healing.

 delayed u., healing of a fractured bone which appears to be unduly slow.

 faulty u., a condition where tissues have united but not in their proper positions.

 primary u., healing which occurs without delay and without complicating infection; also called healing by first intention.

 syngamic nuclear u., the uniting of the nuclei of spermatozoon and ovum during fertilization.

 vicious u., a faulty union that produces a deformity.

unio'val, uniov'ular. Derived from one ovum.

unip'ara. A woman who has given birth to only one child.

unip'arous. 1. Giving birth to only one offspring at a time. **2.** Having given birth to only one offspring; also called primiparous.

unipen'nate. Resembling one half of a feather; said of certain muscles with a tendon on one side; also called unipenniform and demipenniform.

unipo'lar. Having, produced by, or located at one pole.

u'nit. An entity regarded as an elementary constituent of a larger whole.

 Angström u. (Å, AU, A), a unit of wavelength equal to one-tenth of a millimicron (nanometer).

 antigen u., the smallest amount of antigen that, in the presence of specific antiserum, will fix one unit of complement so as to prevent hemolysis.

 antitoxin u., the unit for expressing the amount of antitoxin that will neutralize 100 minimal lethal doses of toxin.

 Bodansky u., the amount of phosphatase in 100 milliliters of serum needed to liberate one milligram of phosphorus as inorganic phosphate from sodium β-glycerophosphate during the first hour of incubation at 37°C; a measure of alkaline phosphatase.

 British thermal u., (BTU), the amount of heat required to increase the temperature of one pound of water from 39° to 40°F.

 centimeter-gram-second u. (CGS u.), a metric unit denoting a rate of work.

 CGS u., abbreviation for centimeter-gram-second unit.

 coronary care u. (CCU), a facility designed to provide maximal surveillance and optimal therapy for patients suspected of having acute myocardial infarctions and other acute cardiac disorders requiring intensive and continuous monitoring.

 dental u., an operative unit in which are assembled items used in dental procedures, such as saliva ejector, compressed air, dental engine, operatory light, water supply, cuspidor, etc.

 electrostatic u. (esu), any fundamental electrical unit based upon the unit electrostatic charge which exerts a force of one dyne on a similar charge one centimeter away in a vacuum.

 gravitational u., a unit equal to one pound of force divided by one pound of mass.

 intensive care u. (ICU), a specially equipped facility in a hospital operated by trained personnel for the care of crtically ill individuals requiring immediate and continuous attention; also called medical intensive care unit (MICU); one designed to handle surgical problems is known as surgical intensive care unit (SICU).

 international insulin u., $^1/_{22}$ milligram of pure international standard zinc-insulin crystals.

 international system of u.'s, see under system.

 international u. (IU), a unit of biologic substance (e.g., vitamins) established by the World Health Organization (WHO).

 international u. of vitamin A, the biologic activity of 0.3 micrograms of vitamin A (alcohol form).

 international u. of vitamin D, the antirachitic activity of 0.025 micrograms of a standard preparation of crystalline vitamin D.

 King u., the amount of phosphatase which, acting upon disodium phenylphosphate at pH 9 for 30 minutes, liberates one milligram of phenol; a test of alkaline phosphatase activity; normal values in adult serum are five to 13 units.

 motor u., a motor nerve cell and the muscle fibers it innervates.

 photofluorographic u. (PF unit), an apparatus consisting of an x-ray tube and a generator coupled to a photographic camera to record miniature radiographs.

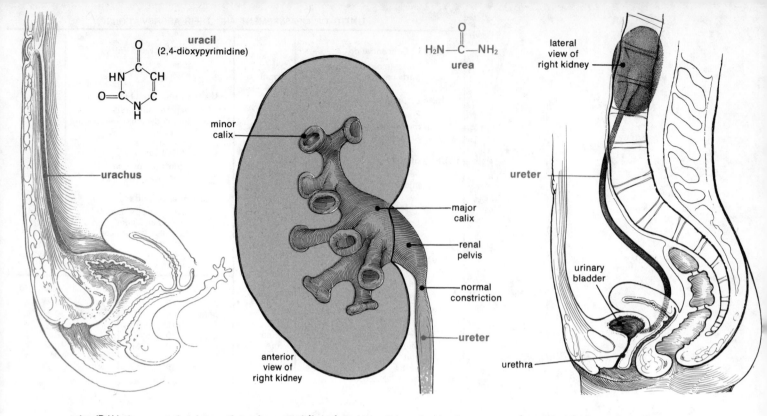

uracil
(2,4-dioxypyrimidine)

urachus

minor calix

major calix

renal pelvis

normal constriction

ureter

anterior view of right kidney

$$H_2N-\overset{\overset{\displaystyle O}{\|}}{C}-NH_2$$
urea

lateral view of right kidney

ureter

urinary bladder

urethra

rat u. (R.U.), the amount of a substance that under standardized conditions is just enough to produce a specified result in experimental rats.

Svedberg u., a unit of time and velocity measuring the sedimentation constant of a colloid solution, equal to 10^{-13} seconds.

u. of force, in the centimeter-gram-second (CGS) system, the dyne; the amount of force which accelerates a mass of one gram one centimeter per second.

u. of heat, in the centimeter-gram-second (CGS) system, the calorie; the amount of heat required to raise one milliliter of water from 14.5 to 15.5°C.

u. of oxytocin, the oxytocic activity of 0.5 milligram of the USP Posterior-pituitary Reference Standard; one milligram of synthetic oxytocin corresponds to 500 international units.

u. of penicillin, the penicillin activity of 0.6 microgram of the Food and Drug Administration master standard.

u. of vasopressin, the pressor activity of 0.5 milligram of the USP Posterior-pituitary Reference Standard.

USP u., a United States Pharmacopeia measure of the potency of any pharmacologic preparation.

United States Adopted Name Council (USAN). An enterprise that gives nonproprietary names to new drugs; it replaced the older AMA-USP Nomenclature Committee.

univa′lent. Having a valence of one; having the combining power of one hydrogen atom; also called monovalent.

unmy′elinated. Having no myelin sheath; a characteristic of some nerve fibers.

Unna's boot. A flexible and porous occlusive dressing, similar to a plaster cast but consisting of gauze bandage impregnated with a gelatinous substance and a paste; applied primarily to the foot and leg, especially in treating dermatitides and ulcerated conditions.

unsat′urated. 1. Not saturated; denoting a solution capable of dissolving more solute at a given temperature. **2.** Denoting an organic compound possessing double or triple bonds, as ethylene. **3.** Denoting a chemical compound in which all the affinities are not satisfied, thereby allowing other atoms or radicals to be added to it.

unsex′. To deprive of gonads or sexual attributes; to castrate.

unsta′ble. 1. Denoting emotional instability; psychologically maladjusted; not mentally fit to assume responsibility; unreliable. **2.** Tending strongly to undergo spontaneous change, said of a solution. **3.** Readily decomposing, as in radioactivity. **4.** Not steady or consistent in action or performance.

unstri′ated. Lacking striations; denoting the structure of the smooth muscle.

untoward′. Resistant to treatment.

up′per. Slang expression meaning an amphetamine pill.

up′take. The amount of a substance, especially a radionuclide, absorbed by any tissue; e.g., radioiodine (^{131}I) by the thyroid gland.

u′rachal. Of or relating to the urachus.

u′rachus. A canal present in the fetus between the umbilicus and the apex of the bladder; after birth it normally persists as a solid fibrous cord.

patent u., urachal fistula; a urachus which remains open after birth.

u′racil. 2,4-Dioxypyrimidine, a prevalent pyrimidine (base) found in nucleic acid.

ura′nium. A heavy silvery-white, radioactive metallic element, occurring in several minerals, especially pitchblende; it has a half-life of 4.5×10^9 years; symbol U, atomic number 92, atomic weight 238.07.

^{235}**U.**, a uranium isotope with a half-life of 713 million years; the first substance shown capable of supporting a self-sustaining chain reaction.

^{238}**U.**, the most common uranium isotope, with a half-life of 4.51 billion years.

uranostaph′yloplasty. A surgical procedure for repairing a defect (usually a cleft) of both the soft and the hard palate; also called uranostaphylorrhaphy.

uranostaphylos′chisis. Fissure or cleft of both soft and hard palate.

u′ranyl. The UO_2^{++} ion, as in such salts as uranyl nitrate, $UO_2(NO_3)_2$, and uranyl sulfate, UO_2SO_4.

u′rate. A salt of uric acid; occurs commonly in urinary deposits and calculi.

uratu′ria. An increase of urates in the urine.

Urd. Abbreviation for uridine.

ure-, urea-, ureo-. Combining forms indicating urea and urine.

ure′a. 1. $CO(NH_2)_2$; chief end product of mammalian protein metabolism, formed in the liver from amino acids and compounds of ammonia; the chief nitrogenous component of urine; an average person, in steady state and consuming average amounts of dietary protein, excretes about 30 grams of urea per day; also called carbamide. **2.** A preparation of hypertonic urea (30 per cent) used intravenously to temporarily reduce intracranial or cerebrospinal pressure in the control of cerebral edema; Ureaphil®.

urea clearance. See clearance, urea.

u′rease. An enzyme that promotes the breakdown of urea into ammonia and carbon dioxide; present in certain seeds and produced by certain microorganisms, especially *Proteus* bacteria.

urecch′ysis. Escape of urine into the tissues; e.g., in rupture of the bladder.

urede′ma. A swollen or edematous condition resulting from infiltration of extravasated urine into the tissues.

ure′do. 1. Urticaria. **2.** A burning or itching sensation in the skin.

urelco′sis. Ulceration of any part of the urinary passage.

ure′mia. A toxic condition caused by retention in the blood of waste substances normally excreted in the urine; the principal wastes which accumulate are products of protein metabolism; symptoms may include lethargy, loss of appetite, vomiting, anemia, blood clotting disorders, an abnormal mental state, pericarditis, and colitis.

ure′mic. Relating to uremia.

ureo-. See ure-.

ureol′ysis. The breaking down of urea into carbon dioxide and ammonia.

ure′sis. Urination.

u′reter. The long, slender, muscular tube that conveys urine from the pelvis of the kidney to the base of the bladder.

ure′teral. Relating to the ureter.

ure′terecta′sia. Distention of a ureter.

ure′terec′tomy. Surgical removal of a ureter or a segment of it.

ure′ter′ic. Of or relating to a ureter or ureters.

uretero-. Combining form denoting a relationship to a ureter.

ure′terocele. A cystlike dilatation at the lower end of a ureter, usually protruding into the bladder.

ureterocystos′tomy. See ureteroneocystostomy.

ure′teroenteros′tomy. The surgical procedure of forming an anastomosis between a ureter and the intestine.

ure′terogram. A roentgenogram of a ureter after injection of a radiopaque substance.

ureterog′raphy. The practice of x-raying the ureter after injection of a radiopaque substance.

ure′terolith. A stone in the ureter.

ure′terolithi′asis. The presence of a calculus in a ureter.

ure′terolithot′omy. Surgical removal of a stone from a ureter.

ure′terol′ysis. Rupture of a ureter.

ure′terone′ocystos′tomy. Transplantation of the distal part of the ureter to a site in the bladder other than the normal one; also called ureterocystostomy.

ure′teronephrec′tomy. Surgical removal of a kidney and its ureter.

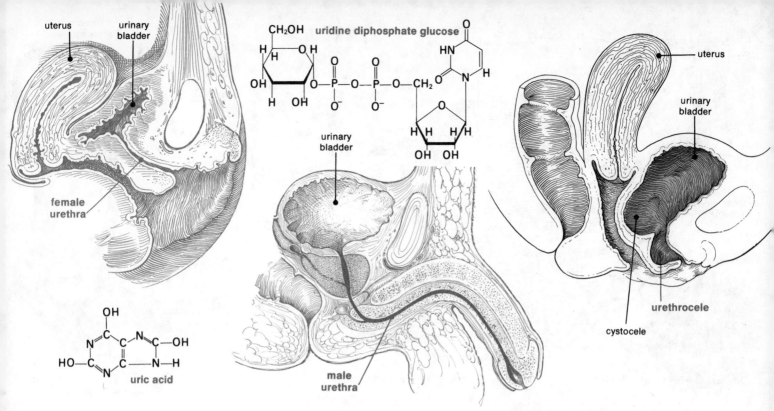

uterus | urinary bladder | female urethra

uridine diphosphate glucose | urinary bladder

uric acid

uterus | urinary bladder | urethrocele | cystocele | male urethra

---

ure´teropel´vic. Pertaining to a ureter and the adjoining renal pelvis.

ure´teropyeli´tis. Inflammation of a ureter extending up to and including the pelvis of the kidney.

ure´teropy´elogram. Pyelogram.

ure´teropy´eloneos´tomy. A surgical procedure for excising a portion of the ureter and inserting the remaining part through a new opening into the pelvis of the kidney.

ure´teropy´eloplas´ty. Reparative surgery of the ureter and pelvis of the kidney.

ure´teropyo´sis. Accumulation of pus in a ureter.

ure´terosig´moid. Pertaining to the ureter and the sigmoid colon.

ure´terosig´moidos´tomy. Surgical implantation of the ureters into the sigmoid colon.

ure´terosteno´sis. Abnormal stricture of a ureter.

ureterostomy, cutaneous. Attachment of the divided distal end of a ureter to the skin of the lower abdomen to create an external opening through which urine may be discharged when the bladder has been removed.

ure´terot´omy. Any surgical division of a ureter.

ure´terovag´inal. Relating to or communicating with a ureter and the vagina.

ure´teroves´ical. Relating to a ureter and the bladder, as the junction of the two structures.

ure´terovesicos´tomy. Surgical division of a ureter and its implantation to another site in the bladder.

u´rethane, u´rethan. Ethyl carbamate; a crystalline compound used in the treatment of leukemia.

urethr-. See urethro-.

ure´thra. The canal leading from the bladder and conveying urine to the exterior of the body.

  anterior u., the portion of the male urethra from the bulb to the tip of the glans penis; consisting of three parts, the bulbous, the pendulous, and the glandular parts.

  female u., a channel, about 1½ inches long, extending from the bladder to the urinary opening behind the clitoris.

  male u., a channel, about 8 or 9 inches long, extending from the bladder to the opening at the tip of the glans penis; it conveys spermatic fluid as well as urine.

  posterior u., the portion of the male urethra extending from the neck of the bladder to the bulb; it consists of two parts, the prostatic and the membranous parts.

ure´thral. Relating to the urethra.

urethral´gia. Pain in the urethra.

urethratre´sia. Occlusion or atresia of the urethra.

urethrec´tomy. Surgical removal of the urethra, or a segment of it.

ure´thremorrha´gia. Bleeding from the urethra; also called urethrorrhagia.

u´rethrism, urethris´mus. Irritability or chronic spasm of the urethra, usually associated with inflammation which may involve also the lower portion of the bladder.

urethri´tis. Inflammation of the urethra.

urethro-, urethr-. Combining form indicating a relationship to the urethra.

ure´throcele. 1. Prolapse of the female urethra. **2.** A sac or diverticulum of the wall of the female urethra.

ure´throcysti´tis. Inflammation of the urethra and bladder.

ure´throcys´topexy. Operation for the relief of stress incontinence in which the urethrovesical junction is sutured to the back of the pubic bone.

urethrog´raphy. The roentgenologic study of the urethra.

urethrom´eter. An instrument for measuring the caliber of the urethra.

urethrope´nile. Relating to the urethra and the penis.

urethroplas´ty. Surgical repair of a wound or a defect of the urethra.

ure´throprostat´ic. Relating to the urethra and the prostate gland.

urethrorec´tal. Relating to or communicating with the urethra and the rectum.

urethrorrhe´a. Abnormal discharge from the urethra.

ure´throscope. An instrument for inspecting the interior of the urethra.

urethros´copy. Visual examination of the urethra with a urethroscope.

ure´throspasm. Spasmodic contraction of the urethra.

ure´throsteno´sis. Narrowing or stricture of the urethra.

urethros´tomy. Surgical formation of an opening into the urethra for temporary or permanent diversion of urine.

ure´throtome. An instrument for dividing a urethral stricture.

ure´throt´omy. Division of the urethra for treatment of a stricture or removal of a foreign body.

ure´throvag´inal. Relating to the urethra and vagina.

ure´throves´ical. Relating to the urethra and the bladder.

uri-, uric-, urico-. Combining forms denoting a relationship in uric acid.

URI. Abbreviation for upper respiratory infection.

u´ric. Relating to urine.

u´ric acid. A white crystalline compound, $C_5H_4O_3$; a normal constituent of urine; also called lithic acid.

uricacide´mia. See uricemia.

urice´mia. An excess of uric acid and the urates in the blood; also called uricacidemia and lithemia.

urico-. See uri-.

uricol´ysis. The splitting up of uric acid molecules.

uricosu´ria. The passage of uric acid in the urine.

uricosu´ric. An agent that tends to increase the excretion of uric acid in the urine.

u´ridine. $C_9H_{12}N_2O_6$, a ribonucleoside containing uracil; important in carbohydrate metabolism; 1-β-D-ribofuranosyluracil.

  u. diphosphate (UDP), a nucleotide important in glycogen and galactose metabolism and in nucleic acid synthesis.

  u. diphosphate galactose (UDP-galactose), a nucleotide derivative of galactose, resulting from the reaction of uridine diphosphate glucose (UDP-glucose) and galactose-1-phosphate; also called diphosphogalactose.

  u. diphosphate glucose (UDP-glucose), a nucleotide derivative of glucose intermediary in glycogen synthesis; formed from the reaction of glucose-1-phosphate and uridine triphosphate (UTP); also called uridine diphosphoglucose (UDPG).

  u. triphosphate (UTP), a high-energy nucleotide which participates in glycogen metabolism.

uridro´sis. The presence of urea or uric acid in the perspiration, sometimes deposited on the skin as minute crystals; also written urhidrosis.

u´ridyltrans´ferase. See hexose-1-phosphate uridylyltransferase.

urin-, urino-. Combining forms indicating urine.

urinal´ysis. Analysis of urine.

  routine u., testing of the urine for the presence of abnormal amounts of protein or sugar, acidity, and specific gravity, and microscopic examination of the sediment from a centrifuged sample of urine.

u´rinary. Relating to urine.

u´rinate. To pass urine, to micturate.

urina´tion. The passing of urine; also called micturition.

u´rine. The fluid excreted by the kidneys, stored in the bladder, and discharged through the urethra; composed of approximately 96 per cent water and four per cent solid matter, chiefly urea and sodium chloride.

  residual u., the urine left over in the bladder after urination.

urinif´erous. Conveying urine, as the tubules in the kidney.

urino-. See urin-.

urinog´enous. Producing urine.

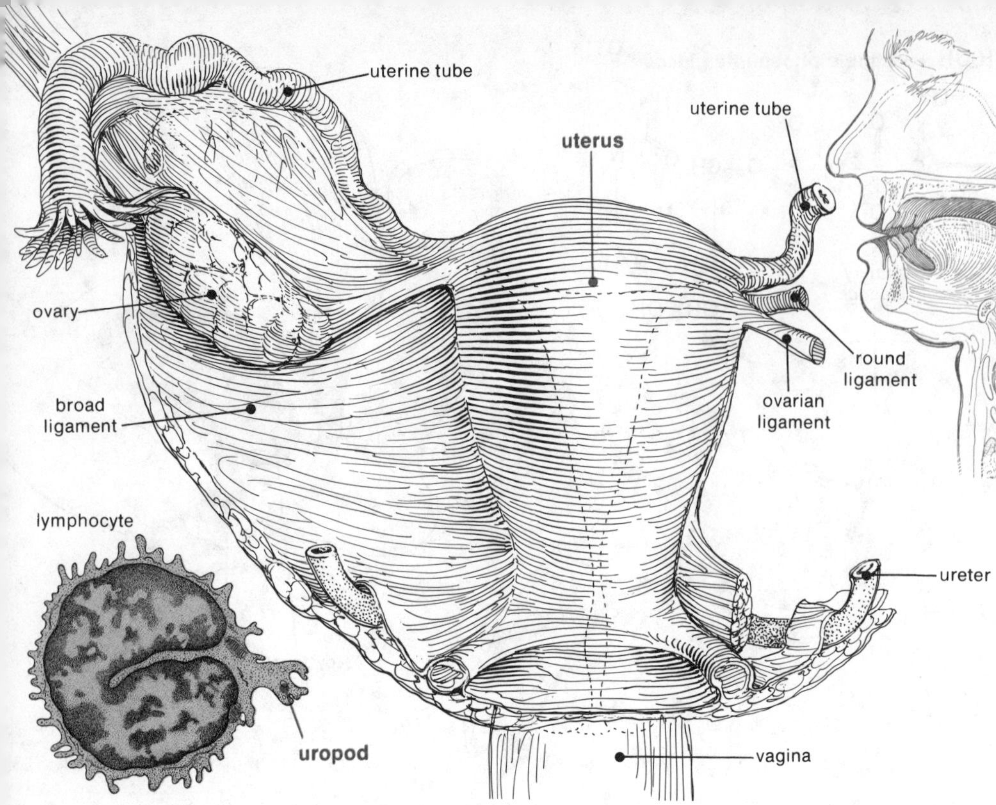
uterine tube
uterus
uterine tube
ovary
broad ligament
round ligament
ovarian ligament
ureter
vagina
lymphocyte
uropod

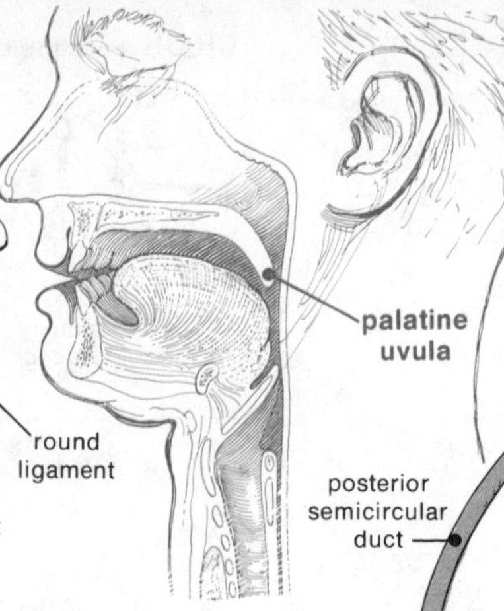
palatine uvula

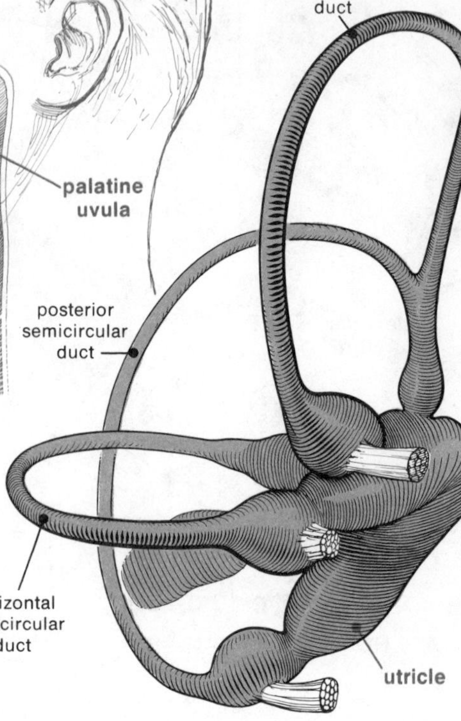
superior semicircular duct
posterior semicircular duct
horizontal semicircular duct
utricle

urinom'eter. A device used for determining the specific gravity of urine; also called urometer and urogravimeter.
uro-. Combining form relating to urine.
uroacidim'eter. An apparatus for estimating the degree of acidity of a sample of urine.
urobi'lin. A pigment normally found in small amounts in urine; formed by the oxidation of urobilinogen.
urobiline'mia. The presence of urobilin in the blood.
urobilin'ogen. A colorless compound present in large amounts in feces and in small amounts in urine; formed in the intestines by the reduction of bilirubin; upon oxidation it forms urobilin.
u'rocele. Distention of the scrotal sac with extravasated urine.
u'rochrome. A yellow or brownish substance believed to give urine its characteristic color.
urochro'mogen. A low oxidation product present in the urine of individuals in various pathologic states (e.g., pulmonary tuberculosis), which on further oxidation becomes urochrome.
urocys'tic. Of or relating to the urinary bladder.
urodyn'ia. Urination accompanied by pain or discomfort.
uroer'ythrin. A pigment sometimes present in urine; believed to be derived from melanin metabolism.
uroflo'meter. An instrument for measuring and graphically recording the rate of urine flow by weighing it during voiding; rate of urination indicator.
urogas'trone. A polypeptide extractable from normal urine in man and dog which, when injected into the body, inhibits gastric secretions.
urogen'ital. See genitourinary.
urog'raphy. Roentgenography of any part of the urinary tract.
excretory u., x-ray examination of the renal parenchyma, calices, pelves, ureters, and urinary bladder, following intravenous injection of a contrast medium which is rapidly excreted in the urine; also called intravenous pyelography.
retrograde u., urography after injection of a contrast medium into the bladder or ureters.
uroki'nase. A proteolytic enzyme in blood and urine that activates the fibrinolytic system by converting plasminogen to plasmin.
u'rolith, u'rolite. A calculus in the urinary tract.
urolithi'asis. The formation of urinary calculi and the resulting disease condition.
urolog'ic. Relating to urology.
urol'ogist. A specialist in urology.
urol'ogy. The branch of medicine concerned with the study, diagnosis, and treatment of diseases (especially by surgical techniques) of the urinary tract of both male and female, and of the genital organs of the male.
urop'athy. Any disease of the urinary tract.
uropla'nia. The escaping or extravasation of urine into the tissues.
ur'opod. An enlarged cytoplasmic extension from the surface of a cell; it is usually capable of developing microspikes and pinocytotic vesicles.
uropoie'sis. The formation of urine.
uropor'phyrin. A porphyrin, usually found in small amounts in the urine; excretion of an excessive amount may be seen in heavy metal poisoning or in cutaneous porphyria or congenital erythropoietic porphyria.
uros'chesis. Urinary retention or suppression.
urosep'sis. Sepsis resulting from the absorption and decomposition of extravasated urine in the tissues.
urti'ca. 1. The herb *Urtica dioica,* a weed that has stinging hairs. **2.** A wheal, pomphus, hive, or blister.
ur'ticant. 1. Any agent that causes itching or stinging. **2.** Producing an itching or stinging sensation.
urtica'ria. Eruption of transitory itchy wheals, often due to hypersensitivity to foods or drugs or to emotional factors; also called hives.
cold u., wheal formed upon exposure to cold.
papular u., a common and troublesome skin disease of childhood, characterized by the appearance of a wheal followed by a papule; although food allergy is widely accepted as a cause of the eruption, recent evidence favors a parasitic origin, such as bites from cat fleas and bedbugs.
u. pigmentosa, disorder characterized chiefly by yellow-brown macules and papules on the skin; may involve only the skin (juvenile type) or occur with other systemic symptoms (adult type); also called mastocytosis.
USAN. Acronym for United States Adopted Name Council.
USP. Abbreviation for United States Pharmacopeia.
USPHS. Abbreviation for United States Public Health Service.
ut dictum. Latin for as directed; used in prescription writing.
u'terine. Of or relating to the uterus.
u'terocystos'tomy. The surgical establishment of a communication between the cervix of the uterus and the bladder.
u'tero-ova'rian. Relating to the uterus and an ovary.
u'teroplasty. Reparative surgery of the uterus.
uterosa'cral. Relating to the uterus and the sacrum.
uteroton'ic. 1. Overcoming relaxation of the uterine muscle. **2.** An agent having such an effect.
uterotu'bal. Relating to the uterus and its tubes.
uterovagi'nal. Relating to the uterus and the vagina.
uteroves'ical. Relating to the uterus and the bladder.
u'terus. Womb; a hollow, muscular organ of the female mammal situated in the pelvis between the bladder and rectum; its function is the nourishment of the developing young prior to birth; the mature human uterus is pear-shaped, thick-walled, and about three inches long, reaching adult size by the 15th year and diminishing after the menopause; the upper portion of the uterus opens on either side into the uterine tubes and the lower portion opens into the vagina.
anomalous u., a malformed uterus.
gravid u., a pregnant uterus.
pubescent u., an underdeveloped uterus.
UTP. Abbreviation for uridine triphosphate.
u'tricle. The larger of the two sacs of the membranous labyrinth in the vestibule of the internal ear.
utric'ular. Relating to or resembling a utricle.
utriculosac'cular. Relating to the utricle and the saccule of the internal ear.
utric'ulus. Utricle.
UV. Abbreviation for ultraviolet.
u'vea. The middle, pigmented, vascular layer of the eye consisting of the choroid, the ciliary body, and the iris; also called uveal tract.
u'veal. Relating to the uvea.
uvei'tis. Inflammation of the uvea (choroid, ciliary body, and iris).
uveoparoti'tis. Vascular inflammation of the uvea (middle coat of eye) and the parotid gland; a manifestation of sarcoidosis; also called uveoparotid fever.
u'viform. Resembling grapes.
u'vula. From Latin, a small grape; any anatomic structure resembling a small grape; when used alone, the term designates the palatine uvula.
palatine u., the conical, fleshy mass of tissue suspended from the free edge of the soft palate above the back of the tongue.
vesical u., a mucosal ridge of the bladder just behind the internal urethral orifice, formed by the underlying median lobe of the prostate gland in the male.
uvulec'tomy. Surgical removal of the uvula.
uvuli'tis. Inflammation of the uvula.
uvulot'omy. Incision of the uvula or removal of a portion of it.

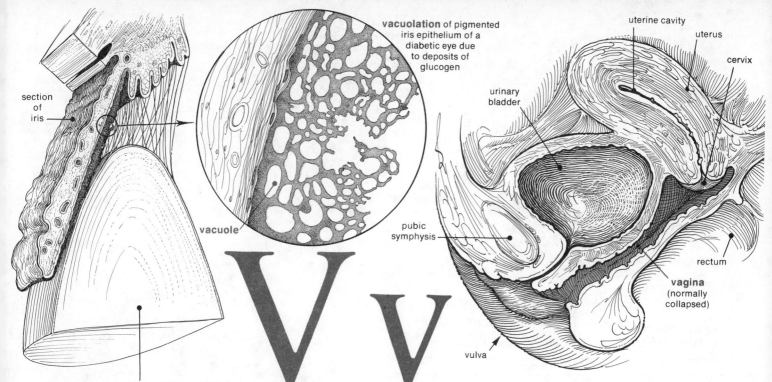

section of iris

vacuolation of pigmented iris epithelium of a diabetic eye due to deposits of glucogen

vacuole

section of lens of eye

pubic symphysis

uterine cavity

uterus

cervix

urinary bladder

rectum

vagina (normally collapsed)

vulva

V

V. 1. Abbreviation for (a) vision; (b) vitamin. **2.** Chemical symbol of the element vanadium.

V$_{max}$. Symbol for the maximum velocity in an enzymatic reaction.

v. 1. Abbreviation for (a) vein; (b) vicinal. **2.** Symbol for (a) velocity; (b) volt; (c) volume.

V$_1$, **V**$_2$, **V**$_3$, **V**$_4$, **V**$_5$, **V**$_6$. Precordial leads; see under lead.

V.A. Abbreviation for (a) Veterans' Administration; (b) visual acuity.

vac'cinate. To inoculate with a vaccine for the purpose of producing active immunity against a given infectious disease.

vaccina'tion. 1. Inoculation with the virus of cowpox, or vaccinia, as a means of producing immunity against smallpox. **2.** Injection or ingestion of an immunogenic antigen (vaccine) in order to produce active immunity against a given disease.

vac'cinator. 1. One who vaccinates. **2.** Instrument used in vaccination.

vac'cine. A preparation of dead, or live attenuated, viruses or bacteria used to prevent infectious diseases by inducing active immunity.

autogenous v., one made from organisms obtained from the individual to be inoculated.

bacillus Calmette-Guèrin v. (BCG vaccine), an attenuated, viable bovine tubercle bacillus vaccine which has proved to be highly effective in increasing the body's resistance against tuberculosis; possibly effective also in the treatment of certain neoplasms by a nonspecific stimulating effect on the body's immune system.

BCG v., abbreviation for bacillus Calmette-Guèrin vaccine.

Calmette-Guèrin v., bacillus Calmette-Guèrin vaccine.

cholera v., a sterile suspension of killed *Vibrio cholerae* organisms containing eight billion organisms per milliliter; given intramuscularly or subcutaneously in two doses one week to one month apart.

Cox v., see typhus vaccine.

diphtheria, pertussis, and tetanus v. (DPT), a triple vaccine for infants usually administered in three intramuscular injections one to three months apart, beginning at age six to eight weeks.

influenza virus v., a sterile, aqueous suspension of inactivated influenza virus grown in egg allantoic fluid and killed with formalin.

live v., one prepared from live organisms whose virulence has been reduced.

measles v., live, attenuated measles virus vaccine, given subcutaneously to children one year of age or older.

mixed v., one containing killed cultures of more than one species.

mumps v., a suspension of live attenuated mumps virus, given subcutaneously.

poliomyelitis v., vaccine against paralytic poliomyelitis; available in two forms: live, attenuated oral poliovirus vaccine (Sabin), and the formaldehyde-inactivated poliomyelitis vaccine (Salk) given by injection.

rabies v., a sterile suspension of killed, fixed rabies virus; usually given after exposure to the virus in a series of 14 to 21 daily doses injected in separate sites.

Sabin v. (OPV), live, oral poliovirus vaccine containing Types I, II, and III poliovirus strains; it produces a more rapid and longer lasting immunity than the Salk vaccine.

Salk v., a sterile suspension of formaldehyde-inactivated Types I, II, and III strains of poliovirus, now seldom used; immunization requires booster doses every two years.

typhoid v., a killed suspension of typhoid bacilli (*Salmonella typhosa*).

typhus v., a sterile suspension of the killed rickettsial organisms (*Rickettsia prowazekii*), which are cultivated in the yolk sac of eggs and treated with formalin; also called Cox vaccine.

yellow fever v., a live, attenuated strain of yellow fever virus grown in cell cultures and eggs.

vacci'nia. 1. A contagious disease of cattle caused by the vaccine virus; also called cowpox. **2.** A local reaction induced in man by the introduction of the virus for the purpose of immunization against smallpox; the reaction is usually limited to a single lesion at the site of inoculation.

generalized v., condition of secondary lesions of the skin following vaccination.

progressive v., widespread vaccinal lesions following vaccination; a severe, often fatal condition occurring in individuals who fail to produce antibodies; also called vaccinia gangrenosa.

v. gangrenosa, see progressive vaccinia.

vac'cinid. Allergic reaction to vaccination marked by localized eruption of vesicles or papules.

vaccin'iform, vac'cinoid. Resembling cowpox.

vaccin'ogen. A source of vaccine.

vac'uant. An agent that promotes emptying of the bowels.

vac'uolate, vac'uolated. Containing vacuoles.

vacuola'tion. The formation of vacuoles.

vac'uole. 1. A small space or cavity in the protoplasm of a cell. **2.** A small space in tissue.

vac'uum. A space devoid of gas or air; an empty space.

va'gal. Relating to the vagus nerve.

vagec'tomy. Removal of a portion of the vagus nerve.

vigilam'bulism. Condition, resembling sleepwalking but occurring in the wakeful state, in which the individual is unaware of his surroundings.

vagi'na. 1. The musculomembranous tubular structure extending from the vulva to the uterine cervix. **2.** Any sheathlike structure.

vag'inal. 1. Of or relating to the vagina. **2.** Relating to or resembling a sheath.

vaginalec'tomy. Surgical removal of a portion of the tunica vaginalis testis.

vaginali'tis. Inflammation of the tunica vaginalis testis.

vag'inate. 1. To form a sheath. **2.** Enclosed in a sheath.

vaginec'tomy. Partial or total excision of the vagina.

vaginis'mus. Painful spasmodic contraction of the vaginal walls on slightest touch.

vagini'tis. Inflammation of the vagina.

emphysematous v., a form characterized by the presence of numerous small gas-filled cysts in the upper vagina.

mycotic v., a form caused by a fungus; particularly common during pregnancy and in diabetes.

senile v., vaginitis occurring in elderly women, often causing adhesions which obliterate the canal.

vag'inocele. Colpocele; hernia protruding into the vagina.

vaginodyn'ia. Colpodynia; vaginal pain.

vaginofixa'tion. Colpopexy; suture of a prolapsed vagina to the abdominal wall.

vaginola'bial. Relating to the vagina and the labia; also called vulvovaginal.

vaginomyco'sis. Vaginal infection due to a fungus.

vaginop'athy. Any vaginal disorder.

vaginoperine'al. Relating to the vagina and perineum.

vaginoperineor'raphy. Colpoperineorrhaphy; repair of the vagina and perineum, as in cases of perineal tears.

vaginoperineot'omy. Enlarging the vaginal orifice by incising the vagina and perineum to facilitate childbirth.

vagi'nopexy. Colpopexy.

vaginoplas'ty. Colpoplasty; surgical repair of the vagina.

vagi'noscope. See colposcope.

vaginos'copy. Visual examination of the cervix and vagina, usually with the aid of a colposcope (vaginoscope).

vaginoves'ical. Relating to the vagina and the bladder.

vaginovul'var. Relating to the vagina and vulva;

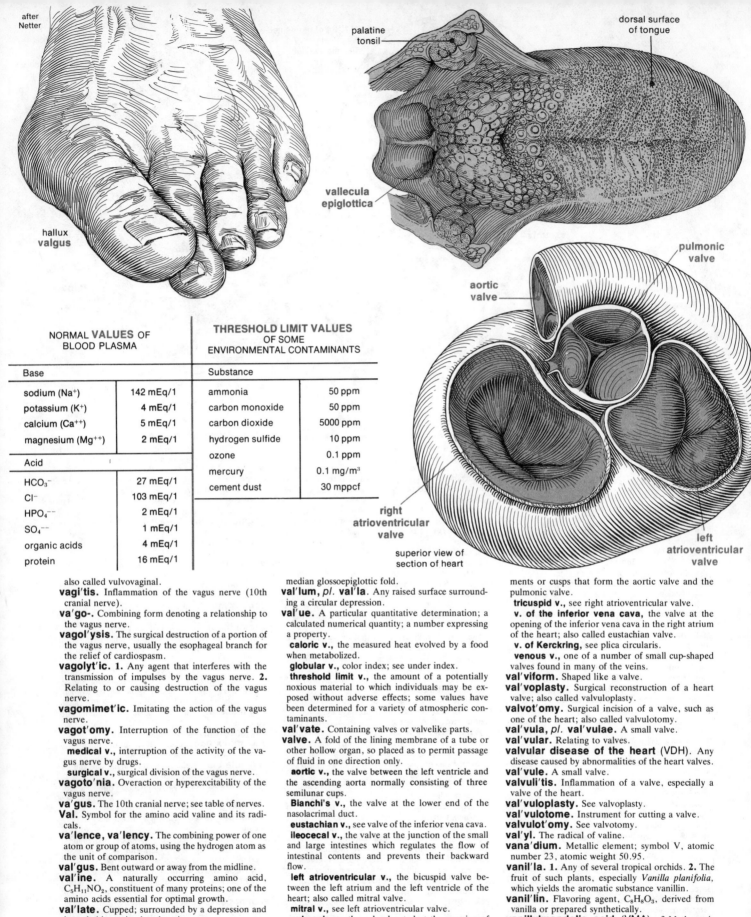

NORMAL VALUES OF BLOOD PLASMA

Base	
sodium (Na⁺)	142 mEq/1
potassium (K⁺)	4 mEq/1
calcium (Ca⁺⁺)	5 mEq/1
magnesium (Mg⁺⁺)	2 mEq/1
Acid	
HCO₃⁻	27 mEq/1
Cl⁻	103 mEq/1
HPO₄⁻⁻	2 mEq/1
SO₄⁻⁻	1 mEq/1
organic acids	4 mEq/1
protein	16 mEq/1

THRESHOLD LIMIT VALUES OF SOME ENVIRONMENTAL CONTAMINANTS

Substance	
ammonia	50 ppm
carbon monoxide	50 ppm
carbon dioxide	5000 ppm
hydrogen sulfide	10 ppm
ozone	0.1 ppm
mercury	0.1 mg/m³
cement dust	30 mppcf

also called vulvovaginal.

vagi′tis. Inflammation of the vagus nerve (10th cranial nerve).

va′go-. Combining form denoting a relationship to the vagus nerve.

vagol′ysis. The surgical destruction of a portion of the vagus nerve, usually the esophageal branch for the relief of cardiospasm.

vagolyt′ic. 1. Any agent that interferes with the transmission of impulses by the vagus nerve. **2.** Relating to or causing destruction of the vagus nerve.

vagomimet′ic. Imitating the action of the vagus nerve.

vagot′omy. Interruption of the function of the vagus nerve.

  medical v., interruption of the activity of the vagus nerve by drugs.

  surgical v., surgical division of the vagus nerve.

vagoto′nia. Overaction or hyperexcitability of the vagus nerve.

va′gus. The 10th cranial nerve; see table of nerves.

Val. Symbol for the amino acid valine and its radicals.

va′lence, va′lency. The combining power of one atom or group of atoms, using the hydrogen atom as the unit of comparison.

val′gus. Bent outward or away from the midline.

val′ine. A naturally occurring amino acid, C₅H₁₁NO₂, constituent of many proteins; one of the amino acids essential for optimal growth.

val′late. Cupped; surrounded by a depression and bounded by a circular elevation.

vallec′ula. In anatomy, a shallow groove, depression, or fossa.

  v. cerebelli, a deep hollow separating the inferior surface of the cerebellar hemispheres in which rests the medulla oblongata.

  v. epiglottica, the depression between the epiglottis and the root of the tongue, on either side of the median glossoepiglottic fold.

val′lum, *pl.* **val′la.** Any raised surface surrounding a circular depression.

val′ue. A particular quantitative determination; a calculated numerical quantity; a number expressing a property.

  caloric v., the measured heat evolved by a food when metabolized.

  globular v., color index; see under index.

  threshold limit v., the amount of a potentially noxious material to which individuals may be exposed without adverse effects; some values have been determined for a variety of atmospheric contaminants.

val′vate. Containing valves or valvelike parts.

valve. A fold of the lining membrane of a tube or other hollow organ, so placed as to permit passage of fluid in one direction only.

  aortic v., the valve between the left ventricle and the ascending aorta normally consisting of three semilunar cups.

  Bianchi's v., the valve at the lower end of the nasolacrimal duct.

  eustachian v., see valve of the inferior vena cava.

  ileocecal v., the valve at the junction of the small and large intestines which regulates the flow of intestinal contents and prevents their backward flow.

  left atrioventricular v., the bicuspid valve between the left atrium and the left ventricle of the heart; also called mitral valve.

  mitral v., see left atrioventricular valve.

  pulmonic v., the valve located at the opening of the pulmonary trunk.

  rectal v.'s, transverse folds of the rectum; see under fold.

  right atrioventricular v., the valve between the right atrium and the right ventricle of the heart; also called tricuspid valve.

  semilunar v., one of the crescent-shaped segments or cusps that form the aortic valve and the pulmonic valve.

  tricuspid v., see right atrioventricular valve.

  v. of the inferior vena cava, the valve at the opening of the inferior vena cava in the right atrium of the heart; also called eustachian valve.

  v. of Kerckring, see plica circularis.

  venous v., one of a number of small cup-shaped valves found in many of the veins.

val′viform. Shaped like a valve.

val′voplasty. Surgical reconstruction of a heart valve; also called valvuloplasty.

valvot′omy. Surgical incision of a valve, such as one of the heart; also called valvulotomy.

val′vula, *pl.* **val′vulae.** A small valve.

val′vular. Relating to valves.

valvular disease of the heart (VDH). Any disease caused by abnormalities of the heart valves.

val′vule. A small valve.

valvuli′tis. Inflammation of a valve, especially a valve of the heart.

val′vuloplasty. See valvoplasty.

val′vulotome. Instrument for cutting a valve.

valvulot′omy. See valvotomy.

val′yl. The radical of valine.

vana′dium. Metallic element; symbol V, atomic number 23, atomic weight 50.95.

vanil′la. 1. Any of several tropical orchids. **2.** The fruit of such plants, especially *Vanilla planifolia*, which yields the aromatic substance vanillin.

vanil′lin. Flavoring agent, C₈H₈O₃, derived from vanilla or prepared synthetically.

vanillylmandelic acid (VMA). 3-Methoxy-4-hydroxymandelic acid, the major urinary metabolite of adrenal and sympathetic catecholamines; the normal range for excretion is two to 10 milligrams per day; elevated levels of excretion suggest a pheochromocytoma.

va′por. The gaseous state of any substance that is liquid or solid at ordinary temperatures.

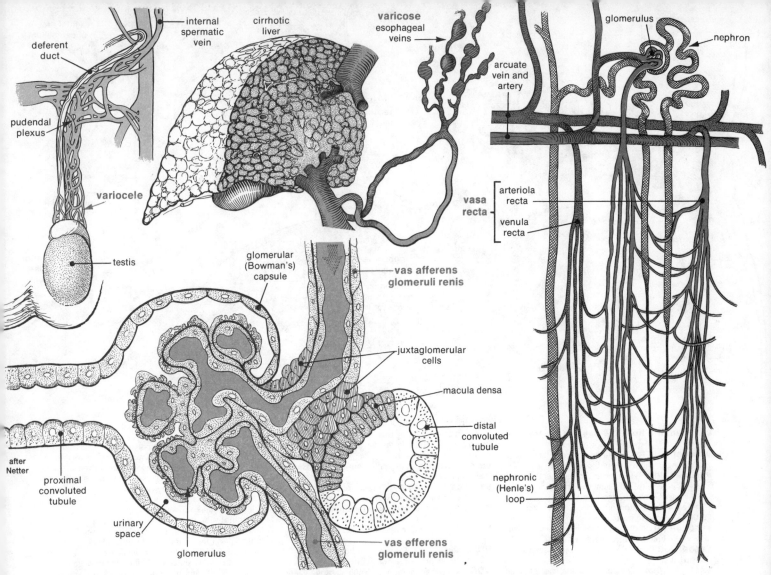

va'porize. To change into a vapor by heating.
va'porizer. An apparatus for reducing fluids to vapor for inhalation.
vapother'apy. The treatment of any disorder with vapor, steam, or spray.
var'iance. 1. A difference. 2. The act of varying.
  ball v., the changes occurring in the ball of a ball-valve prosthesis.
var'iant. Tending to deviate from a standard.
  L-phase v., a strain of bacteria with defective cell walls that has nutritive requirements similar to the strain from which it originated and is capable of reverting to its parental form; also called L-form.
varic-. See varico-.
varice'al. Relating to a varix.
varicel'la. See chickenpox.
varicel'liform. Resembling chickenpox.
var'ices. Plural of varix.
varico-, varic-. Combining forms denoting a varicosity or varix.
var'icocele. Dilatation of the veins of the spermatic cord in the scrotum.
varicocelec'tomy. Operation for removal of dilated veins of the spermatic cord (varicocele).
varicog'raphy. Roentgenologic visualization of varicose veins achieved by introducing a radiopaque substance.
varicophlebi'tis. Inflammation of varicose veins.
var'icose. Denoting abnormally dilated and tortuous vessels.
varicos'ity. 1. The state of being abnormally swollen. 2. A varicose vein.
varicot'omy. An operation for the removal of a varicose vein or varix.
varic'ula. A varicose condition of small veins, especially of the conjunctiva.
var'icule. A small varicose vein.
vario'la. See smallpox.
vari'olar. Relating to smallpox.
vari'oliform. In the shape or form of smallpox.

va'rioloid. A mild case of smallpox occurring in partially immune persons.
var'ix, pl. var'ices. A dilated and tortuous vessel, usually a vein.
  aneurysmal v., one resulting from the direct communication between a vein and an adjacent artery.
  esophageal varices, varicosities of the mucosal veins of the esophagus, usually the lower portion.
var'nish. A solution of a resin in a suitable solvent and an evaporating binder which when applied in a thin layer forms a hard, glossy, thin film.
  dental v., a solution of natural resins and gums in an organic solvent; it is applied over the walls and floor of the prepared tooth cavity; when the solvent evaporates, a thin film is left that protects the underlying tooth structure against the constituents of the restorative material and thermal shock.
var'us. Bent inward or toward the midline.
vas-. Combining form meaning vessel or fluid-conveying duct.
vas, pl. va'sa. A duct or canal through which a liquid, such as blood, lymph, chyle, or semen, is conveyed; a vessel.
  v. aberrans hepatis, any of the numerous, irregularly coursing, blind-ending bile ducts or associated blood vessels which are located in the coronary ligament, capsule, or fibrous appendix of the liver.
  v. afferens glomeruli renis, the afferent arteriole that conveys blood toward the glomerulus of the kidney.
  v. afferentia, a vessel entering a structure such as the lymph node.
  v. brevia, the small branches of the splenic artery supplying the greater curvature of the stomach.
  v. deferens, deferent duct; see under duct.
  v. efferens glomuli renis, the efferent arteriole that conveys blood away from the glomerulus of the kidney.
  v. efferentia, a vessel leaving a structure such as a

lymph node.
  v. lymphaticum, one that conveys lymph; there are two types: the afferent and efferent; also called lymphatic vessel.
  v. previa, an anomaly of the umbilical cord insertion in which the umbilical vessels traverse the lower uterine segment across the internal cervical os, and appear ahead of the fetal head at the opening of the uterus.
  vasa recta, the arterioles and venules that descend and ascend parallel to the nephronic (Henle's) loop in the pyramid of the kidney; the wider ascending limbs are often referred to as venulae rectae and the descending limbs are generally called arteriolae rectae.
  v. spirale ductus cochlearis, the largest blood vessel in the basilar membrane just beneath the tunnel of Corti in the ear.
  v. vasorum, one of many small blood vessels in the walls of larger arteries and their corresponding veins.
vas'cular. Pertaining to or containing vessels.
vascular'ity. The state of containing blood vessels.
vasculariza'tion. The formation of blood vessels.
vas'culature. The system of blood vessels of an organ.
vasculi'tis. Inflammation of a blood vessel or vessels.
vasculo-, vaso-. Combining forms denoting a relationship to blood vessels.
vasculogen'esis. Formation of the system of blood vessels.
vasec'tomy. Removal of the ductus (vas) deferens, or a segment of it; a means of male sterilization; also called deferenectomy.
vas'iform. Tubular.
vaso-. Combining form meaning blood vessel.
vasoac'tive. Having an effect on blood vessels.
vasocongest'ion. The state of being filled with

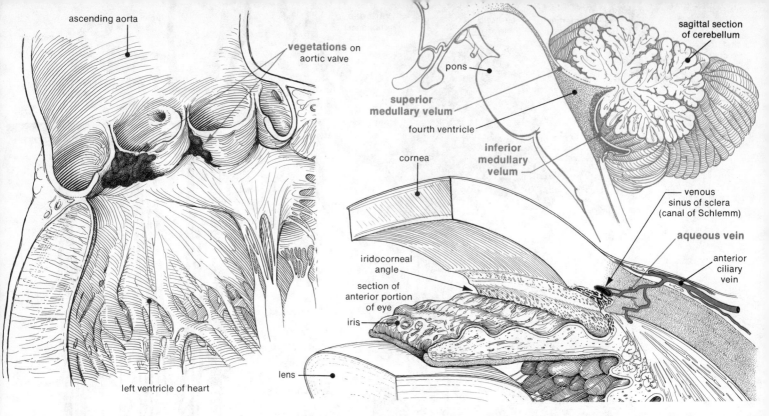

ascending aorta

vegetations on aortic valve

left ventricle of heart

sagittal section of cerebellum

pons

superior medullary velum

fourth ventricle

inferior medullary velum

cornea

iridocorneal angle

section of anterior portion of eye

iris

lens

venous sinus of sclera (canal of Schlemm)

aqueous vein

anterior ciliary vein

blood.

vasoconstric'tion. Narrowing of the lumen of blood vessels, expecially of arterioles.

vasoconstric'tor. A drug or nerve that causes narrowing of the lumen of blood vessels.

vasodila'tion. Widening of the lumen of the blood vessels, especially of the lumen of arterioles, leading to increased blood flow to a part.

  reflex v., dilatation of a blood vessel due to a reflex response to a stimulus.

vasodila'tor. A drug or nerve that causes a widening of the lumen of blood vessels.

vasodisten'tion. Vasodilation; opposite of vasoconstriction.

vasogan'glion. A glomus; a dense mass of blood vessels.

vasog'raphy. Roentgenography of blood vessels.

vasohyperton'ic. Causing increased tonicity in the smooth muscles of blood vessels; denoting increased arteriolar tension.

vasohypoton'ic. Causing reduced tonicity in the smooth muscles of blood vessels; denoting reduced arteriolar tension.

vasoinhib'itor. A drug that depresses the action of vasomotor nerves.

vasoinhib'itory. Restraining or reducing the action of the vasomotor nerves.

vasoliga'tion. Surgical ligation of the deferent duct (vas deferens).

vasomo'tion. Dilatation and constriction of blood vessels; also called angiokinesis.

vasomo'tor. Causing constriction or dilatation of blood vessels; denoting the nerves that have this action.

vasoneurop'athy. Any disease affecting the blood vessels and nerves.

vasoparal'ysis. Hypotonia of blood vessels; also called vasomotor paralysis.

vasopres'sin. Antidiuretic hormone; a hormone from the posterior lobe of the pituitary gland having a potent antidiuretic action and some vasoconstrictive action on the splanchnic circulation.

vasopres'sor. An agent that causes constriction of blood vessels and a rise in blood pressure.

vasosen'sory. Denoting sensory nerves going to the blood vessels.

vas'ospasm. Spasm or contraction of the muscular coats of blood vessels; also called angiospasm.

vasostim'ulant. 1. Stimulating nerves that cause dilatation or constriction of blood vessels. **2.** Any agent having such property.

vaso'tomy. Cutting into the vas deferens (deferent duct).

vasoton'ic. Relating to the tone of a blood vessel; an agent that increases tension of blood vessels.

vasotroph'ic. See angiotrophic.

vasotrop'ic. Tending to act on blood vessels.

vasova'gal. Relating to the action of the vagus nerve upon blood vessels.

vasovasot'omy. Surgical union of the ends of a severed deferent duct.

vasovesiculec'tomy. Surgical removal of a deferent duct and seminal vesicles.

vault. Any arched anatomic structure resembling a dome.

VC. Abbreviation for (a) color vision; (b) vital capacity.

VCG. Abbreviation for vectorcardiogram.

VD. Abbreviation for venereal disease.

VDG. Abbreviation for ventricular diastolic gallop (a third heart sound).

VDH. Abbreviation for valvular disease of the heart.

VDRL. Abbreviation for Venereal Disease Research Laboratories.

vec'tion. Transmission of causative agents of disease.

vec'tor. 1. An organism that transmits pathologic microorganisms from one host to another. **2.** Anything (electromotive force, velocity, etc.) that has a magnitude and a direction.

vectorcar'diogram. A graphic record of the magnitude and direction of the heart's action currents, displayed as a three-dimensional or spatial voltage loop.

vectorcardiog'raphy. The determination of the direction and magnitude of the heart's electric forces at any point in time; represented by vector loops.

  spatial v., three-dimensional voltage loop produced by the heart's action current and projected on the frontal, horizontal, and sagittal reference planes.

veg'an. One who does not eat food derived from animals (meat, milk, eggs, etc.).

veg'etarian. One who does not eat meat or animal products.

vegeta'tion. An abnormal plantlike outgrowth of tissue; specifically, growth composed of fibrin and fused blood platelets adherent to a diseased heart valve; circulating bacteria tend to plant at these sites.

veg'etative. Having a role in the processes of growth and nutrition.

ve'hicle. 1. In pharmacology, an inactive substance in which an active drug is dissolved or suspended; an excipient. **2.** Any inanimate carrier of an infectious agent from one host to another.

veil. Colloquial term for caul.

Veillonel'la. A genus of anaerobic, gram-negative bacteria normally found in the mouth and intestinal,

respiratory, and urogenital tracts of apparently healthy individuals.

vein. A vessel that carries blood toward the heart or one in the heart wall which returns blood to the right atrium. For specific veins, see table of veins.

  aqueous v.'s, minute vessels which transport aqueous humor from the venous sinus of the sclera (canal of Schlemm) out of the eyeball to the episcleral, conjunctival, and subconjunctival veins.

  cardinal v.'s, the major embryonic vessels which drain the cephalic part (anterior cardinal vein) and caudal part (posterior cardinal vein) and empty into the heart (via the common cardinal vein).

  emissary v.'s, veins which drain the intracranial venous sinuses and transport the blood to a vessel outside the skull; they serve as drainage channels in case of increased intracranial pressure.

  varicose v.'s, abnormally dilated, tortuous veins produced by prolonged, increased intraluminal pressure; most commonly seen in the superficial veins of the leg; varicose veins along with phlebothrombosis account for approximately 90 per cent of clinical venous disease.

  vitelline v.'s, veins which return blood from the yolk sac of an early embryo; they form an anastomotic network around the duodenum and in the liver and empty directly into the sinus venosus of the primitive heart.

velopharyn'geal. Relating to the soft palate and the pharynx.

vel'um. Any structure resembling a curtain.

  inferior medullary v., posterior medullary v., a thin sheet forming part of the roof of the cerebral fourth ventricle; composed of the cellular lining of the ventricle on the inside and pia mater on the outside.

  superior medullary v., anterior medullary v., a thin layer of white matter between the cerebellar peduncles, forming the anterior portion of the roof of the cerebral fourth ventricle.

  v. palatinum, soft palate.

ve'na. *pl.* **ve'nae.** Latin for vein.

  v. cava, see table of veins.

  venae comitantes, *sing.* **v. comitans,** veins (usually two) accompanying the corresponding artery.

vena'tion. The distribution of veins.

vene-. Combining form meaning poison.

venec'tomy. Phlebectomy.

veneer'. In dentistry, a porcelain or resin facing applied to a gold crown or pontic for esthetic purposes.

venena'tion. Poisoning.

venenif'erous. Bearing poison.

ven'enous. Poisonous; toxic; venomous.

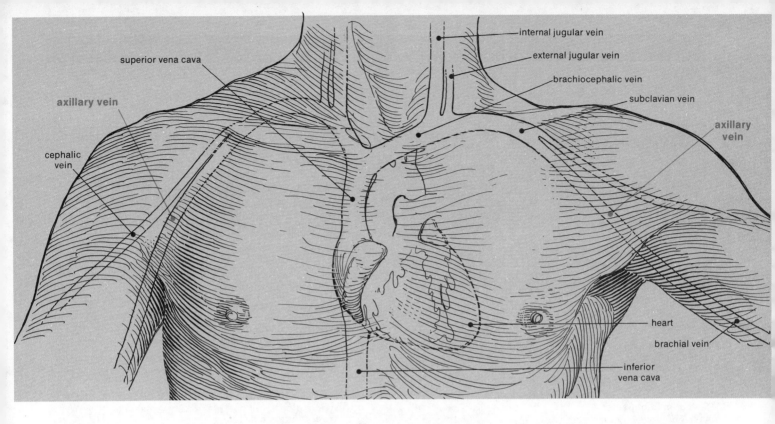

Labels on figure:
- superior vena cava
- axillary vein
- cephalic vein
- internal jugular vein
- external jugular vein
- brachiocephalic vein
- subclavian vein
- axillary vein
- heart
- brachial vein
- inferior vena cava

VEINS	LOCATION	DRAINS	EMPTIES INTO
alveolar v., inferior inferior dental v. *v. alveolaris inferior*	from mandibular canal it passes up the ramus of lower jaw	teeth of lower jaw	pyterygoid plexus
anastomotic v., inferior v. of Labbé *v. anastomotica inferior*	courses over temporal lobe of brain	superficial middle cerebral v.	transverse sinus
anastomotic v., superior v. of Trolard *v. anastomotica superior*	from lateral sulcus of brain aross parietal lobe	superficial middle cerebral v.	superior sagittal sinus
angular v. *v. angularis*	anterior angle of orbit and root of nose	formed by union of frontal and supraorbital veins; receives the infraorbital, superior and inferior palpebral and external nasal veins	anterior facial v. (behind facial artery)
antebrachial v., median	see median vein of forearm		
appendicular v. *v. appendicularis*	along the mesentery of the vermiform appendix	appendix	ileocolic v.
v. of aqueduct of vestibule *v. aquaeductus vestibuli*	through aqueduct of vestibule (accompanied by endolymphatic duct)	internal ear	superior petrosal sinus
arcuate v.'s of kidney *vv. arcuatae renis*	in corticomedullary zone of kidney	interlobular veins, *venulae rectae*	interlobar v.
auditory v.'s, internal	see labyrinthine veins		
auricular v.'s, anterior *vv. auriculares anterior*	front part of ear	external ear	superficial temporal v.
auricular v., posterior *v. auricularis posterior*	side of head in back of ear	plexus on side of head, tributaries from back of ear, stylomastoid v.	external jugular v.
axillary v. *v. axillaris*	upper limb from lower border of teres major muscle to outer border of first rib	junction of basilic and brachial veins; cephalic v., deep brachial comitans	subclavian v. (at outer border of first rib)
azygos v. *v. azygos*	from front of first lumbar vertebra it passes to right side of fourth thoracic vertebra where it arches over right lung	ascending lumbar, right subcostal, intercostal, hemiazygos, esophageal, mediastinal, pericardial, and right bronchial veins	superior vena cava
azygos v., left	see hemiazygos vein		

vein | vein

VEINS	LOCATION	DRAINS	EMPTIES INTO
basal v. *v. basalis*	from anterior perforated substance it passes posteriorly around the cerebral peduncle	anterior perforated substance; anterior cerebral v., deep middle cerebral v., inferior striate v.'s	internal cerebral v.
basilic v. *v. basilica*	from ulnar part of hand it passes up forearm and continues along the medial border of the biceps	dorsal venous network of hand; tributaries from ulnar side of forearm	joins brachial v. to form axillary v.
basivertebral v.'s *vv. basivertebrales*	tortuous channels in substance of vertebrae	vertebrae	anterior, external, and internal vertebral plexuses
brachial v.'s *vv. brachiales*	placed on either side of brachial artery	radial and ulnar veins, superior and inferior ulnar collateral veins, deep brachial v. (*v. profunda brachii*)	axillary v.
brachiocephalic v.'s innominate v.'s *vv. brachiocephalicae*	root of neck	right side: internal jugular, subclavian, internal thoracic, and inferior thyroid veins; left side: internal jugular, subclavian, and left highest intercostal veins	superior vena cava
bronchial v.'s *vv. bronchiales*	near bronchi	larger bronchi and roots of lungs	right side: azygos v.; left side: left highest intercostal or accessory hemiazygos veins
v. of bulb of penis *v. bulbi penis*	penis	expanded posterior part of the corpus spongiosum penis (bulb of penis)	internal pudendal v.
v. of bulb of vestibule *v. bulbi vestibuli*	vestibule	mass of erectile tissue on either side of vagina	internal pudendal v.
cardiac v.'s, anterior (three to four in number) *vv. cordis anterior*	ventral side of heart	ventral side of right ventricle	right atrium
cardiac v., great left coronary v. *v. cordis magna*	from apex of heart it ascends up to the back of heart	tributaries from left atrium and both ventricles; left marginal v.	left extremity of coronary sulcus
cardiac v., middle *v. cordis media*	ascends up back of heart from apex	tributaries from both ventricles	right extremity of coronary sulcus
cardiac v., small right coronary v. *v. cordis parva*	ascends up the heart from back of right atrium and ventricle	back of right atrium and ventricle; right marginal v.	right extremity of coronary sulcus or right atrium
cardiac v.'s, smallest (many minute veins) v.'s of Thebesius *vv. cordis minimae*	in muscular wall of heart	muscular wall of heart	mostly in atria, some in ventricles
cavernous v.'s of penis *vv. cavernosae penis*	penis	cavernous venous spaces in the erectile tissue of the penis (corpora cavernosa)	deep dorsal v. of penis, prostatic plexus
central v.'s of liver *vv. centrales hepatis*	middle of hepatic lobules	sinusoids in liver substance	sublobular v.
central v. of retina *v. centralis retinae*	from eyeball it passes out in the optic nerve	retinal veins	cavernous sinus, superior ophthalmic v.
cephalic v. *v. cephalica*	from radial part of hand it passes up forearm to groove along lateral border of biceps muscle of arm and more proximally between deltoid and pectoralis major muscles	radial side of dorsal venous plexus of hand; palmar and dorsal tributaries in forearm; thoracoacromial v.	axillary v. just caudal to clavicle
cephalic v., accessory *v. cephalica accessoria*	radial side of forearm	dorsal venous network of hand	cephalic v. at elbow
cerebellar v.'s, inferior *vv. cerebelli inferior*	bottom of cerebellum	inferior surface of cerebellum	transverse, superior petrosal, and occipital sinuses
cerebellar v.'s, superior *vv. cerebelli superior*	top of cerebellum (superior vermis)	upper surface of cerebellum	straight sinus and internal cerebral veins
cerebral v., anterior *v. cerebri anterior*	from upper surface of corpus callosum down through longitudinal fissure, above optic nerve to lateral cerebral sulcus	anterior perforated substance, lamina terminalis, rostrum of corpus callosum, septum pellucidum, striate v.	basal v.

vein | vein

502

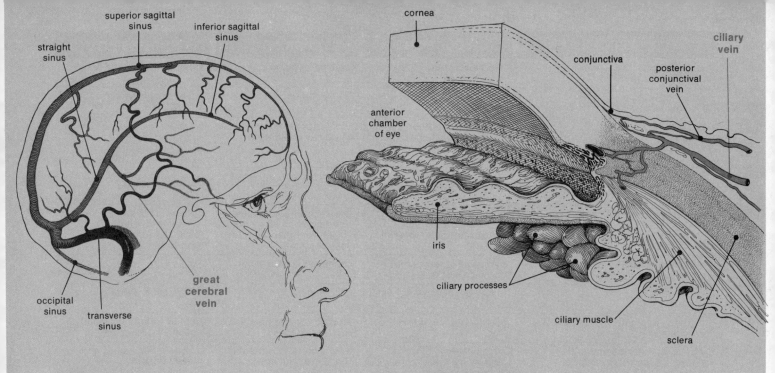

VEINS	LOCATION	DRAINS	EMPTIES INTO
cerebral v., deep middle deep Sylvian v. *v. cerebri media profunda*	lower part of lateral cerebral sulcus	tributaries from insula, neighboring gyri	basal v.
cerebral v., great great v. of Galen *v. cerebri magna*	around back part of corpus callosum of brain	internal cerebral veins	anterior extremity of straight sinus
cerebral v.'s, inferior *vv. cerebri inferior*	bottom of brain	inferior surface of cerebral hemispheres	frontal lobe portion: superior sagittal sinus; temporal lobe portion: cavernous, superior petrosal, and transverse sinuses; occipital lobe portion: straight sinus
cerebral v.'s, internal (two in number) v.'s of Galen deep cerebral v.'s *vv. cerebri internae*	from interventricular foramen they pass backward between the layers of the tela choroidea of the third ventricle	the deep parts of the cerebral hemispheres; thalamostriate, choroid, and basal veins	great cerebral v.
cerebral v., superficial middle superficial Sylvian v. *v. cerebri media superficialis*	lateral surface of brain	lateral surface of cerebral hemispheres	cavernous and sphenoparietal sinuses
cerebral v.'s, superior (8–12 in number) *vv. cerebri superior*	brain	superior, lateral, and medial surfaces of cerebral hemispheres	superior sagittal sinus
cervical v., deep posterior deep cervical v. posterior vertebral v. *v. cervicalis profunda*	from suboccipital region it follows deep cervical artery down neck	plexus in suboccipital triangle, occipital v., deep muscles of back of neck, plexuses around spinal processes of cervical vertebrae	inferior part of vertebral v.
cervical v.'s, transverse *vv. transversae colli*	parallel to transverse cervical artery	trapezius muscle and neighboring structures	subclavian v. or external jugular v.
choroid v. *v. choroidea*	lateral ventricle of brain	lateral ventricle, choroid plexus, corpus callosum	internal cerebral v.
ciliary v.'s (anterior and posterior) *vv. ciliares*	from outer surface of choroidal layer of eyeball they pass through the sclera	ciliary body, scleral venous sinus, conjunctiva	ophthalmic v.
cochlear v.'s *v. cochleares*	from lamina spiralis and basilar membrane to base of modiolus	cochlea	internal auditory v.
colic v., left *v. colica sinistra*	alongside the descending colon	descending colon and left colic (splenic) flexure	inferior mesenteric v.
colic v., middle *v. colica media*	transverse colon	transverse colon	superior mesenteric v.

VEINS	LOCATION	DRAINS	EMPTIES INTO
colic v., right *v. colica dextra*	ascending colon	ascending colon	superior mesenteric v.
conjunctival v.'s *vv. conjunctivales*	eye	bulba conjunctiva	superior ophthalmic v.
coronary v. gastric v. *v. coronaria*	from right to left along lesser curvature of stomach down peritoneum of lesser sac (omental bursa)	tributaries from both surfaces of stomach	portal v.
coronary v., left		see cardiac vein, great	
coronary v., right		see cardiac vein, small	
coronary sinus (wide venous channel about 2.25 cm in length) *sinus coronarius*	posterior part of coronary sulcus (covered by muscular fibers from left atrium)	great, small, and middle cardiac veins, posterior v. of left ventricle, oblique v. of left atrium	right atrium between opening of inferior vena cava and atrioventricular aperture
cubital v., median *v. mediana cubiti*	passes obliquely across bend of elbow	cephalic v. below elbow	basilic v.
cystic v. *v. cystica*	in liver accompanying cystic duct	gallbladder	right branch of portal v.
digital v.'s, plantar *vv. digitales plantares*	plantar surface of toes	plexuses on the plantar surface of toes	unite to form four plantar metatarsal veins
diploic v., anterior temporal *v. diploica temporalis anterior*	middle layer (diploë) of frontal bone and parts of parietal bones of cranium	frontal bone and anterior part of parital bones	sphenoparietal sinus and deep temporal v.
diploic v., frontal *v. diploica frontalis*	middle layer (diploë) of frontal bone of cranium	frontal bone	supraorbital v. and superior sagittal sinus
diploic v., occipital (largest of the four diploic veins) *v. diploica occipitalis*	middle layer (diploë) of occipital bone of cranium	parietal bone	occipital v. or transverse sinus
diploic v., posterior temporal *v. diploica temporalis posterior*	middle layer (diploë) of parietal bone of cranium	parietal bone	transverse sinus
dorsal v. of clitoris, deep (unpaired) dorsal v. of clitoris *v. dorsalis clitoridis profunda*	dorsal midline of clitoris	body and glans of clitoris	primarily into the vesical plexus
dorsal v.'s of clitoris, superficial *vv. dorsales clitoridis superficiales*	clitoris	subcutaneous layers of clitoris	external pudendal v.
dorsal v. of penis, deep (unpaired) dorsal v. of penis *v. dorsalis penis profunda*	dorsal midline of penis	penis	prostatic plexus
dorsal v.'s of penis, superficial *vv. dorsales penis superficiales*	dorsal midline of penis	skin and subcutaneous layers of penis	external pudendal v.
dorsal v.'s of tongue		see lingual veins, dorsal	
emissary v., condyloid *v. emissaria condylaris*	through condyloid canal of cranium	transverse sinus	deep veins of neck
emissary v.'s, foramen lacerum (two or three in number) *vv. emissariae foraminis lacerum*	through foramen lacerum of cranium	cavernous sinus	pterygoid plexus
emissary v., foramen of Vesalius *v. emissaria foraminis Vesalii*	through foramen of Vesalius (when present)	cavernous sinus	pterygoid plexus
emissary v., mastoid *v. emissaria mastoidea*	through mastoid foramen of cranium	transverse sinus	posterior auricular v. or occipital v.
emissary v., parietal *v. emissaria parietalis*	through parietal foramen of cranium	scalp	superior sagittal sinus
epigastric v., inferior deep epigastric v. *v. epigastrica inferior*	from area of umbilicus it descends to deep inguinal ring area	abdominal wall, ductus deferens in male, round ligament in female	external iliac v. about 1.25 cm proximal to inguinal ligament
epigastric v., superficial *v. epigastrica superficialis*	from umbilicus it runs downward and laterally toward inguinal ligament	lower and medial part of abdominal wall	great saphenous v.
epigastric v.'s, superior *vv. epigastricae superior*	from abdomen they ascend up toward diaphragm	skin and muscles of abdomen; xiphoid process, diaphragm	internal thoracic v.
episcleral v.'s *vv. episclerales*	in sclera close to corneal margin	angle of eye, sclera, conjunctiva	anterior ciliary veins
esophageal v.'s (several in number) *vv. esophageal*	along the esophagus	esophagus	azygos, hemiazygos and inferior thyroid veins

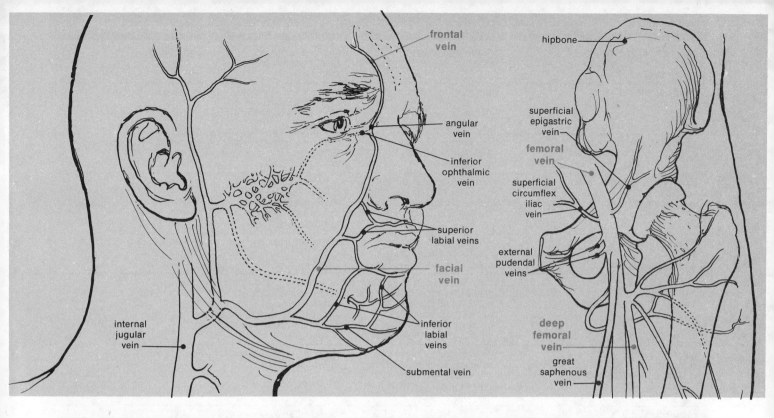

VEINS	LOCATION	DRAINS	EMPTIES INTO
ethmoidal v.'s *vv. ethmoidales*	ethmoidal sinuses	ethmoidal sinuses, frontal sinus, dura mater, walls and septum of nasal cavity	superior ophthalmic v.
facial v. anterior facial v. *v. facialis*	from medial angle of eye across face to neck	superficial structures of face; tributaries include: frontal, supraorbital, deep facial, superficial temporal, posterior auricular, occipital, and retromandibular veins	internal jugular v.
facial v., common	former term for the lower trunk of the facial vein (sometimes joined by retromandibular vein) which empties into the internal jugular vein		
facial v., deep *v. facialis profunda*	face	pterygoid plexus; small tributaries from buccinator, zygomatic, and masseter muscles	facial v.
facial v., transverse *v. facialis transversa*	from cheek it passes backward (just below zygomatic arch) to front of ear	muscles and related structures near the zygoma	superficial temporal v.
femoral v. *v. femoralis*	proximal two-thirds of thigh up to inguinal ligament	popliteal v., great saphenous v., profunda femoris v., muscular tributaries	external iliac v. at level of inguinal ligament
femoral v., deep profunda femoris v. *v. profunda femoris*	accompanies deep femoral artery	medial and lateral femoral circumflex veins; through muscular tributaries it anastomoses with the popliteal vein distally and the inferior gluteal vein proximally	femoral v.
femoral circumflex v.'s, lateral *vv. circumflexae femoris lateral*	winds around lateral side of upper femur	muscles of thigh, especially posterior muscles; lateral half of hip	femoral v.
femoral circumflex v.'s, medial *vv. circumflexae femoris medial*	winds around medial side of upper femur	muscles of upper thigh, especially posterior muscles; hip joint	femoral v.
fibular v.'s	see peroneal veins		
frontal v. *v. frontalis*	from forehead to root of nose	plexus of forehead and scalp	facial v.
gastric v.	see coronary vein		

vein | vein

VEINS	LOCATION	DRAINS	EMPTIES INTO
gastric v.'s, short (four or five in number) *vv. gastricae breves*	greater curvature of stomach	fundus and left part of greater curvature of stomach	splenic v.
gastroepiploic v., left *v. gastroepiploica sinistra*	from right to left along greater curvature of stomach	tributaries from ventral and dorsal surfaces of stomach and greater omentum	splenic v.
gastroepiploic v., right *v. gastroepiploica dextra*	from left to right along greater curvature of stomach	tributaries from greater omentum and parts of stomach	superior mesenteric v.
gluteal v.'s, inferior sciatic v.'s *vv. gluteae inferior*	from the proximal part of posterior thigh they enter the pelvis through the greater sciatic foramen	skin and muscles of buttock and back of thigh; medial femoral circumflex and first perforating veins	internal iliac v.
gluteal v.'s, superior gluteal v.'s *vv. gluteae superior*	from buttock through greater sciatic foramen to pelvis	tributaries from buttock	internal iliac v.
hemiazygos v. left azygous v. inferior minor azygos v. *v. hemiazygos*	in thorax, it ascends on left side of vertebral column to ninth thoracic vertebra before horizontally crossing over vertebral column to join the azygos v.	left ascending lumbar veins, caudal four or five intercostal veins, left subcostal v., esophageal and mediastinal veins	azygos v.
hemiazygos v., accessory superior minor azygos v. *v. hemiazygos accessoria*	descends on left side of vertebral column in thorax and usually crosses over vertebral column at eighth thoracic vertebra	fourth to seventh posterior intercostal veins	azygos v.
hemorrhoidal v.'s	see under rectal veins		
hepatic v.'s *vv. hepaticae*	liver	substance of liver; central, intralobular, and sublobular veins	upper group: three large veins drain into the inferior vena cava below the diaphragm; lower group: several small veins drain into the inferior vena cava lower down
hypogastric v.	see iliac vein, internal		
ileocolic v. *v. ileocolica*	ileocolic area	terminal ileum, appendix, cecum, lower part of ascending colon	superior mesenteric v.
iliac v., common *v. iliaca communis*	from sacroiliac articulation, ascends to fifth lumbar vertebra	internal and external iliac veins; iliolumbar and lateral sacral veins (in addition, the left common iliac v. receives the middle sacral v.)	unites with its member of opposite side to form inferior vena cava
iliac v., external *v. iliaca externa*	from under inguinal ligament, along brim of lesser pelvis, to sacroiliac articulation	lower limb and lower abdominal wall; inferior epigastric, deep circumflex and pubic veins	common iliac v.
iliac v., internal hypogastric v. *v. iliaca interna*	from greater sciatic foramen it passes upward to brim of pelvis	continuation of femoral v.; superior gluteal, inferior gluteal, internal pudendal, obturator, lateral sacral, middle sacral, dorsal veins of penis, vesical, uterine, vaginal	common iliac v.
iliac circumflex v., deep *v. circumflexa ilium profunda*	inner aspect of ilium	venae comitantes of deep iliac circumflex artery	external iliac v. about 2 cm above inguinal ligament
innominate v.'s	see brachiocephalic veins		
intercostal v.'s, anterior (12 pairs) *vv. intercostales anterior*	lower border of each rib	ribs and intercostal muscles	internal thoracic and musculophrenic veins
intercostal v., left highest left superior intercostal v. *v. intercostalis suprema sinistra*	posterior wall of thorax across arch of aorta	first two or three left intercostal spaces, left bronchial vein, and occasionally the left superior phrenic vein (it has a prominent anastomosis with the accessory hemiazygos v.)	brachiocephalic v.
intercostal v., left superior *v. intercostalis superior sinistra*	across arch of aorta	left second, third, and fourth intercostal veins	left brachiocephalic v. or accessory hemiazygos v.

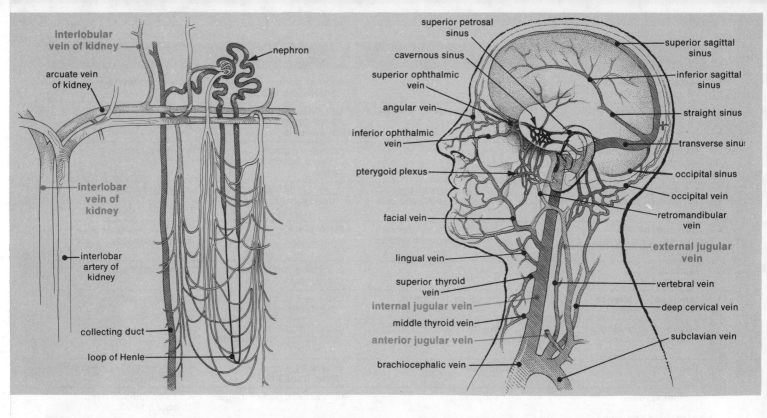

VEINS	LOCATION	DRAINS	EMPTIES INTO
intercostal v., right highest right superior intercostal v. *v. intercostalis suprema dextra*	posterior wall of upper thorax	upper two or three intercostal spaces	azygos v.
intercostal v.'s, posterior *vv. intercostales posterior*	one in each intercostal space	skin and muscles of the back and spinal tributary from vertebral plexuses	right side: azygos vein, right highest intercostal v.; left side: left brachiocephalic v., hemiazygos or accessory hemiazygos v.
intercostal v., right superior *v. intercostalis superior dextra*	posterior mediastinum	right second, third, and fourth intercostal spaces	azygos v.
interlobar v.'s of kidney *vv. interlobares renis*	between pyramids of kidney	arcuate veins	renal vein
interlobular v.'s of kidney *v. interlobulares renis*	cortex of kidney	cortex of kidney; stellate, capsular, and perforating veins	arcuate veins of kidney
interlobular v.'s of liver *vv. interlobulares hepatis*	in substance of liver between lobules	central or intralobular and sublobular veins	hepatic veins
intervertebral v.'s *vv. intervertebrales*	vertebral column	internal and external vertebral plexuses; veins from spinal cord	vertebral, intercostal, lumbar, and lateral sacral veins
intestinal v.'s (usually 10–15 in number) jejunal and ileal v.'s *vv. intestinales*	run parallel with superior mesenteric artery between layers of mesentery	walls of jejunum and ileum	superior mesenteric v.
jejunal and ileal v.'s	see intestinal veins		
jugular v., anterior (usually two in number) *v. jugularis anterior*	from near hyoid bone it passes down anterior part of neck	laryngeal and thyroid veins, neck muscles	external jugular or subclavian v.
jugular v., external *v. jugularis externa*	from substance of parotid gland it runs perpendicularly down neck	deep parts of face, exterior of cranium, retromandibular and posterior auricular veins	subclavian v., internal jugular v., or brachiocephalic v.
jugular v., internal *v. jugularis interna*	from jugular fossa it descends side of neck lateral to internal carotid artery, and then lateral to common carotid artery	brain, face, and neck; transverse sinus, inferior petrosal sinus, facial, lingual, pharyngeal, superior and middle thyroid and at times the occipital veins	brachiocephalic v.
jugular v., posterior external *v. jugularis externa posterior*	from occipital region down to middle third of external jugular	skin and superficial muscles of back of head and neck	external jugular v.

vein | vein

VEINS	LOCATION	DRAINS	EMPTIES INTO
labial v.'s, anterior *vv. labiales anterior*	vulva	anterior portion of labia majora; mons pubis	external pudendal v.
labial v.'s, inferior *vv. labiales inferior*	edge of lower lip to angle of mouth	labial glands, mucous membrane and muscles of lower lip	facial v.
labial v.'s, posterior *vv. labiales posterior*	vulva	posterior portion of labia majora; vestibule, labia minora	internal pudendal v.
labial v.'s, superior *vv. labiales superior*	edge of upper lip between mucous membrane and muscle	upper lip, tributaries from nose, nasal septum	facial v.
labyrinthine v.'s internal auditor v.'s *vv. labyrinthi*	from internal ear through internal acoustic meatus	internal ear	inferior petrosal sinus or transverse sinus
lacrimal v. *v. lacrimalis*	orbit	lacrimal glands, eyelids, conjunctiva	superior ophthalmic v.
laryngeal v., inferior *v. laryngea inferior*	dorsal part of larynx	muscles and mucous membrane of larynx	inferior thyroid v.
laryngeal v., superior *v. laryngea superior*	larynx	glands, mucous membrane, and muscles of larynx	superior thyroid v.
lingual v. *v. lingualis*	tongue	tongue by way of two or three tributaries	internal jugular or lower part of facial v.
lingual v., deep ranine v. *v. profunda linguae*	tongue	tip and deep part of tongue	vena comitans of deep lingual artery
lingual v.'s, dorsal *vv. dorsales linguae*	tongue	posterior part of tongue	lingual v.
lumbar v.'s (usually four in number on each side) *vv. lumbales*	lumbar walls	dorsal tributaries from skin and muscles of loin and by abdominal tributaries from abdominal wall; vertebral plexus	first and second drain into the ascending lumbar v.; third and fourth drain into the inferior vena cava
lumbar v., ascending *v. lumbalis ascendens*	ventral to transverse process of lumbar vertebrae	sacral and lumbar veins	right side: azygos v.; left side: hemiazygos v.
maxillary v. *v. maxillaris*	short trunk between the condyle of mandible and sphenomandibular ligament	pterygoid plexus	retromandibular v.
median v. of forearm median antebrachial v. *v. mediana antebrachii*	from base of thumb to middle of palmar forearm	venous plexus on palmar surface of hand	basilic v. and/or cephalic v., or median cubital v.
mediastinal v.'s anterior mediastinal v.'s *vv. mediastinales*	mediastinum	areolar tissue and lymph nodes of anterior mediastinum; pericardium	azygos v., brachiocephalic v., or superior vena cava
meningeal v.'s, anterior *vv. meningeae anterior*	over small wing of sphenoid bone	dura mater of anterior cranial fossa; cranium	ethmoidal and diploic veins, venous sinuses
meningeal v.'s, middle *vv. meningeae mediae*	from dura mater it leaves cranium via foramen spinosum of sphenoid bone	dura mater, internal surface of cranium, trigeminal ganglion	pterygoid plexus
mesenteric v., inferior *v. mesenterica inferior*	from rectum it ascends under cover of the peritoneum to the level of the pancreas	rectum; sigmoid and descending parts of colon	splenic v.
mesenteric v., superior *v. mesenterica superior*	from right iliac fossa it ascends between the two layers of the mesentery to the level of the pancreas	small intestine, cecum, appendix, and ascending and transverse parts of colon	portal v.
metacarpal v.'s, dorsal *vv. metacarpeae dorsales*	hand	dorsal metacarpal region	dorsal venous rete of hand
metacarpal v.'s, palmar *vv. metacarpeae palmares*	hand	palmar metacarpal region	deep palmar venous arch
metatarsal v.'s, dorsal dorsal interosseous v.'s of foot *vv. metatarseae dorsales*	run proximally in metatarsal spaces	dorsal digital veins at clefts of toes; metatarsal bones and neighboring muscles	greater saphenous vein
metatarsal v.'s, plantar *vv. metatarseae plantares*	between the metatarsal bones	plantar digital veins at clefts of toes; metatarsal bones and neighboring muscles	medial and lateral plantar veins

vein | vein

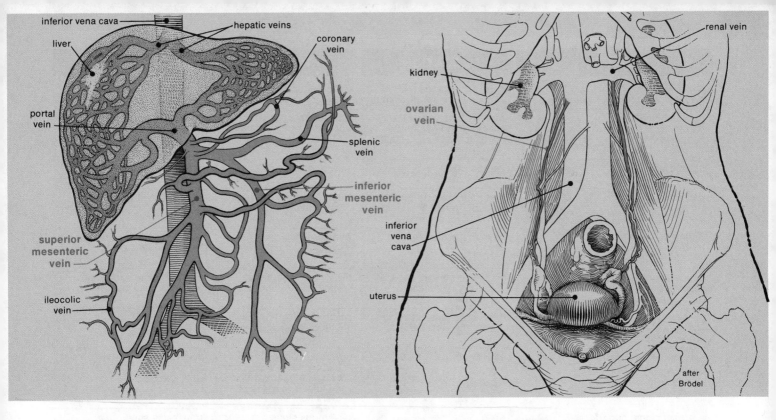

VEINS	LOCATION	DRAINS	EMPTIES INTO
musculophrenic v.'s *vv. musculophrenicae*	from diaphragm, along inner surface of costal cage at attachment of diaphragm, to sixth costal cartilage	diaphragm and lower intercostal spaces	internal thoracic v.
nasal v.'s, external (several in number) *vv. nasales externae*	from nose extending upward	external nose	angular and facial veins
nasofrontal v. *v. nasofrontalis*	anterior medial part of orbit	supraorbital and angular veins	superior ophthalmic v.
oblique v. of left atrium *v. obliqua atrii sinistri*	posterior wall of left atrium of hert	heart wall	coronary sinus
obturator v. *v. obturatoria*	from proximal portion of adductor region of thigh to pelvis through obturator foramen	hip joint and regional muscles	internal iliac v.
occipital v. *v. occipitalis*	from back part of scalp it passes into neck	plexus on posterior part of head; tributaries from posterior auricular and superficial temporal veins; parietal emissary, mastoid emissary, and occipital diploic veins	internal jugular or external jugular veins
ophthalmic v., inferior *v. ophthalmica inferior*	from floor of orbit it passes posteriorly to inferior back part of orbit	muscular and ciliary tributaries	cavernous sinus
ophthalmic v., superior *v. ophthalmica superior*	from inner angle of orbit, through orbit into cavernous sinus	eyeball, eye muscles, and eyelid	cavernous sinus
ovarian v.'s *vv. ovaricae*	in broad ligament near ovary and uterine tube	pampiniform plexus of broad ligament	right side: inferior vena cava; left side: left renal v.
palatine v., external *v. palatina externa*	palate region	tonsils and soft palate	pterygoid and tonsillar plexuses; facial v.
palpebral v.'s *vv. palpebrales*	eyelids	tributaries from eyelids	superior ophthalmic v.
palpebral v.'s, inferior *vv. palpebrales inferior*	lower eyelid	lower eyelid	facial v.
palpebral v.'s, superior *vv. palpebrales superior*	upper eyelid	upper eyelid	angular v. and superior ophthalmic v.
pancreatic v.'s *vv. pancreaticae*	at pancreas	tributaries from body and tail of pancreas	trunk of splenic v.

vein | vein

VEINS	LOCATION	DRAINS	EMPTIES INTO
pancreaticoduodenal v.'s *vv. pancreaticoduodenales*	head of pancreas and proximal part of duodenum	pancreas and duodenum	upper part of superior mesenteric v.
paraumbilical v.'s parumbilical v.'s Sappey's v.'s *vv. paraumbilicales*	from umbilical area they pass along ligamentum teres to liver	cutaneous veins about the umbilicus	accessory portal veins in liver
parotid v.'s *vv. parotideae*	parotid gland	part of parotid gland	retromandibular v. or superficial temporal v.
perforating v.'s *vv. perforantes*	perforate great adductor muscle to reach back of thigh	thigh muscles, especially hamstrings	deep femoral v.
pericardiac v.'s (several in number) *vv. pericardiaceae*	membranous capsule of heart	pericardium	brachiocephalic v. or superior vena cava
pericardiacophrenic v.'s superior phrenic v.'s *vv. pericardiacophrenicae*	parallel to phrenic nerve between pleura and pericardium	diaphragm; tributaries from pericardium	left brachiocephalic v. or superior vena cava
peroneal v.'s fibular v.'s *vv. peroneae*	from lateral side of heel up back of leg just below knee	calcaneus, leg muscles, tibiofibular syndesmosis	posterior tibial v.
petrosal sinus, inferior *sinus petrosus inferior*	inferior petrosal sulcus	cavernous sinus, internal auditory veins, veins from medulla oblongata, pons, and inferior surface of cerebellum	bulb of internal jugular v.
petrosal sinus, superior *sinus petrosus superior*	head	cavernous sinus	transverse sinus
pharyngeal v.'s (several in number) *vv. pharyngeae*	outer surface of pharynx	posterior meningeal veins and vein of the pterygoid canal; pharyngeal plexus	internal jugular v.
phrenic v.'s, inferior *vv. phrenicae inferior*	undersurface of diaphragm	substance of diaphragm	right side: inferior vena cava; left side: left suprarenal v. (often a second vein on the left side enters the inferior vena cava)
popliteal v. *v. poplitea*	from lower border of popliteal muscle, through popliteal fossa to adductor hiatus	anterior and posterior tibial veins	femoral v. at adductor hiatus
portal v. (about 8 cm in length) *v. portae*	in abdomen behind neck of pancreas	superior mesenteric, splenic, coronary, pyloric, cystic, and paraumbilical veins	divides into right and left before emptying into substance of liver
posterior v. of left ventricle *v. posterior ventriculi sinistri*	from apex of heart it travels parallel to longitudinal sulcus	diaphragmatic surface of left ventricle	great cardiac v.
prepyloric v. v. of Mayo *v. prepylorica*	end of stomach	pylorus	right gastric v.
profunda femoris v.		see femoral vein, deep	
profunda linguae v.		see lingual vein, deep	
v. of pterygoid canal Vidian v. *v. canalis pterygoidei*	from ear and throat through pterygoid canal to pterygopalatine fossa	middle ear, auditory tube, pharynx	pterygoid plexus
pterygoid plexus *plexus pterygoideus*	infratemporal fossa	tributaries from: inferior alveolar, middle meningeal, deep temporal, masseter, buccal, posterior superior alveolar, pharyngeal, descending palatine, infraorbital, pterygoid canal, and sphenopalatine veins	maxillary v.
pubic v. *v. pubis*	from dorsum of penis through obturator foramen to pelvis	pubic area	external iliac v.
pudendal v.'s, external external pudic v.'s *vv. pudendae externae*	from lower abdomen and genitalia to upper thigh	skin of lower part of abdomen; in male: anterior scrotal and	great saphenous v. or femoral v.

vein | vein

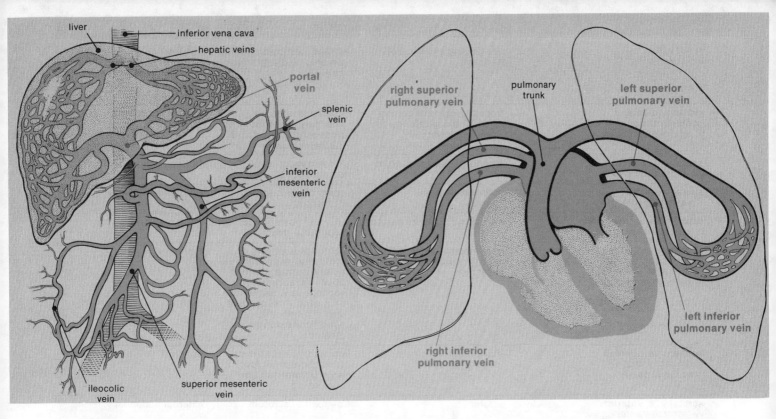

VEINS	LOCATION	DRAINS	EMPTIES INTO
		subcutaneous dorsal veins of penis; in female: anterior labial and subcutaneous dorsal veins of clitoris	
pudendal v.'s, internal internal pudic v.'s *vv. pudendae internae*	from perineum and genitalia to pelvis	perineum and genitalia	internal iliac v.
pulmonary v., left inferior *v. pulmonis inferior sinistra*	from left lung to heart	common basal segmental and lingual v.'s	left atrium of heart
pulmonary v., left superior *v. pulmonis superior sinistra*	from left lung to heart	superior division: apicoposterior and anterior and superior segmental v.'s; lingual division: superior and inferior segmental v.'s	left atrium of heart
pulmonary v., right inferior *v. pulmonis inferior dextra*	from right lung (inferior part of hilum) to heart	superior segmental, superior and inferior basal veins	left atrium of heart
pulmonary v., right superior *v. pulmonis superior dextra*	from left lung to heart	three tributaries from right superior lobe (posterior, apical, and anterior segmental v.'s) and one from the middle lobe of lung (midde lobe v.)	left atrium of heart
pyloric v. *v. pylorus*	along pyloric portion of lesser curvature of stomach	pylorus and lesser omentum	portal v.
radial v.'s *vv. radiales*	from hand, winds around lateral side of carpus up forearm to elbow	dorsal metacarpal veins	joined by ulnar veins to form brachial veins
ranine v.	see lingual vein, deep		
rectal v.'s, inferior inferior hemorrhoidal v.'s *vv. rectales inferior*	near anal canal and rectum	lower part of external rectal plexus	internal pudendal v.
rectal v., middle middle hemorrhoidal v. *v. rectalis media*	rectal area	rectal plexus; tributaries from bladder, prostate gland, and seminal vesicle	internal iliac v.
rectal v.'s, superior superior hemorrhoidal v.'s *vv. rectales superior*	from rectum to brim of pelvis	upper part of external rectal plexus	inferior mesenteric v.

vein | vein

VEINS	LOCATION	DRAINS	EMPTIES INTO
renal v.'s *vv. renales*	at right angle to hilus of kidneys	kidneys; testicular, inferior phrenic, and suprarenal veins	inferior vena cava (the right renal v. opens into the inferior vena cava at a slightly lower level than the left)
retromandibular v. posterior facial v. *v. retromandibularis*	from substance of parotid gland it passes alongside ramus of lower jaw	superficial temporal, maxillary, and tributaries from parotid gland and messeter muscle	external or internal jugular v.
sacral v.'s, lateral *vv. sacrales laterales*	anterior surface of sacrum	skin and muscles of dorsum of sacrum	internal iliac v.
sacral v., middle *v. sacralis media*	hollow of sacrum	region of posterior surface of rectum	left common iliac v.
saphenous v., accessory *v. saphena accessoria*	medial and posterior parts of thigh	inner and posterior parts of superficial thigh	great saphenous v.
saphenous v., great (longest vein in body) long saphenous v. *v. saphena magna*	from medial aspect of foot to 3 cm below inguinal ligament	tributaries from sole of foot; small saphenous v., anterior and posterior tibial v.'s, accessory saphenous v., superficial epigastric v., superficial iliac circumflex v., superficial external pudendal v.	femoral v.
saphenous v., small short saphenous v. *v. saphena parva*	from lateral ankle to middle of back of leg	lateral marginal v., deep v.'s of dorsum of foot, large tributaries from back of leg	popliteal v.
scrotal v.'s, anterior *vv. scrotales anterior*	scrotum	front part of scrotum	external pudendal v.
scrotal v.'s, posterior *vv. scrotales posterior*	scrotum	back part of scrotum	vesical venous plexus or internal pudendal veins
sigmoid v.'s (several in number) *vv. sigmoideae*	lower left side of colon	sigmoid colon and iliac colon	inferior mesenteric v.
spinal v.'s *vv. spinales*	in the pia mater of spinal cord where it forms a tortuous venous plexus	spinal cord and pia mater	internal vertebral venous plexus
spiral v. of modiolus *v. spiralis modioli*	modiolus of cochlea	cochlea	labyrinthine v.'s
splenic v. lienal v. *v. lienalis*	from hilus of spleen to vacinity of neck of pancreas	short gastric, left gastroepiploic, pancreatic, and inferior mesenteric v.'s	portal v.
stellate v.'s of kidney *vv. stellatae renis*	cortex of kidney near capsule	superficial part of cortex of kidney	interlobular veins of kidney
sternocleidomastoid v. sternomastoid v. *v. sternocleidomastoidea*	neck	sternocleidomastoid, omohyoid, sternohyoid, sternothyroid, and platysma muscles, skin of neck	internal jugular v.
striate v., inferior *v. striata inferior*	corpus striatum	anterior perforated substance of cerebrum	basal v.
stylomastoid v. *v. stylomastoidea*	descends vertically from stylomastoid foramen	mastoid cells, middle ear chamber, semicircular canals	retromandibular v. or posterior auricular v.
subclavian v. *v. subclavia*	from outer border of first rib to sternal end of clavicle	continues from axillary v.; external jugular v., anterior jugular v. (occasionally)	joined by internal jugular to form brachiocephalic v.
subcostal v. *v. subcostalis*	in abdominal wall along caudal border of 12th rib	lower abdominal wall	right side: azygos v.; left side: hemiazygos v.
subcutaneous v.'s of abdomen *vv. subcutaneae abdominis*	abdominal wall	superficial layers of abdominal wall	thoracoepigastric, superficial epigastric, or deep v.'s of abdominal wall
sublingual v. *v. sublingualis*	below the tongue	sublingual gland, mylohyoid and neighboring muscles, mucous membranes of mouth and gums, alveolar process of mandible	lingual v.
submental v. *v. submentalis*	below margin of mandible	submandibular gland; mylohyoid, digastric, and platysma muscles	facial v.

vein | vein

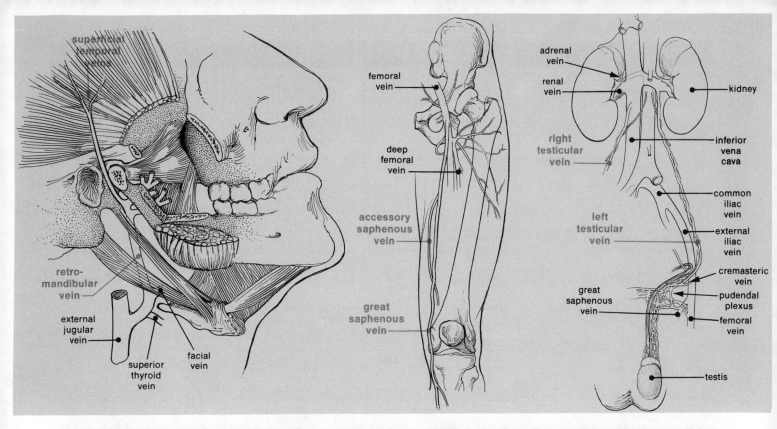

VEINS	LOCATION	DRAINS	EMPTIES INTO
supraorbital v. *v. supraorbitalis*	forehead	frontal muscle, frontal diploic v.	facial v.
suprarenal v., left *v. suprarenalis sinistra*	hilium of left adrenal gland	left adrenal gland	left renal v. or left inferior phrenic v.
suprarenal v., right *v. suprarenalis dextra*	hilium of right adrenal gland	right adrenal gland	inferior vena cava
suprascapular v. transverse scapular v. *v. suprascapularis*	from posterior surface of scapula it passes through scapular notch, runs parallel with clavicle and then crosses over brachial plexus and subclavian artery	shoulder joint, scapula, clavicle, and neighboring muscles and skin	external jugular v. or subclavian v.
supratrochlear v.'s (usually two in number) *vv. supratrochleares*	front and top of head	venous plexus of forehead	angular v.
temporal v.'s, deep *vv. temporales profundae*	side of head	deep areas of temporal muscle	pterygoid plexus
temporal v., middle *v. temporalis media*	from lateral angle of orbit, it passes to side of ear	temporal muscle; zygomaticoorbital v.	retromandibular v. or superficial and deep temporal v.'s
temporal v.'s, superficial *vv. temporales superficiales*	from scalp on side of head down to parotid gland	plexus on side of head; transverse facial, anterior auricular, and middle temporal v.'s	retromandibular v.
temporomandibular v.'s *vv. temporomandibulares*	temporomandibular joint (TMJ)	area surrounding temporomandibular joint; tympanic v.'s	retromandibular v. or maxillary v.
testicular v., left *v. testicularis sinistra*	from testis it ascends along spermatic cord through deep inguinal canal into abdomen	testis, epididymis	left renal v.
testicular v., right *v. testicularis dextra*	from testis it ascends along spermatic cord through deep inguinal canal into abdomen	testis, epididymis	inferior vena cava
thalamostriate v. *v. thalamostriata*	deep part of brain	corpus striatum, thalamus, and corpus callosum	internal cerebral v.
thoracic v., internal internal mammary v. *v. thoracica interna*	thorax	superior phrenic, superior epigastric, musculophrenic,	brachiocephalic v

VEINS	LOCATION	DRAINS	EMPTIES INTO
		perforating, anterior intercostal, sternal, thymic, mediastinal, and pericardiacophrenic veins	
thoracic v., lateral long thoracic v. *v. thoracica lateral*	lateral thoracic wall	lateral thoracic wall; costoaxillary v.'s	axillary v.
thoracoacromial v.'s acromiothoracic v.'s *vv. thoracoacromiales*	parallel with thoracoacromial artery	acromion, coracoid process, sternoclavicular joint, tributaries from deltoid, subclavius, pectoralis major and minor muscles	subclavian v.
thoracoepigastric v. *v. thoracoepigastrica*	anterior and lateral aspect of trunk (in subcutaneous tissue)	skin and subcutaneous tissue of anterolateral trunk	superiorly: lateral thoracic v.; inferiorly: superficial epigastric v.
thymic v.'s *vv. thymicae*	thymus gland	substance of thymus gland	left brachiocephalic and thyroid v.'s
thyroid v.'s, inferior (two to four in number) *vv. thyroideae inferior*	lower neck	venous plexus of thyroid gland; esophageal, tracheal, and inferior laryngeal v.'s	brachiocephalic v.'s
thyroid v.'s, middle *v. thyroidea mediae*	from thyroid gland it passes laterally over common carotid artery	lower part of thyroid gland; tributaries from trachea and larynx	lower part of internal jugular v.
thyroid v., superior *v. thyroidea superior*	from thyroid gland it passes up toward the head	superior part of thyroid gland; superior laryngeal and cricothyroid v.'s	upper part of internal jugular v.
tibial v.'s, anterior *vv. tibiales anterior*	from foot and ankle joint up front of leg between tibia and fibula	venae comitantes of dorsalis pedis artery; muscles and bones of anterior leg	popliteal v.
tibial v.'s, posterior (usually two in number) *vv. tibiales posterior*	from sole of foot to tibial side of leg where it ascends obliquely to back of leg just below bend of knee	muscles and bones of posterior leg	popliteal v.
tracheal v.'s (several in number) *vv. tracheales*	trachea	substance of trachea	thyroid venous plexus, brachiocephalic v., or superior vena cava
v. of tympanic cavity *v. cavum tympani*	middle ear	middle ear chamber (cavity), tympanic membrane, mastoid cells, auditory tube	pterygoid plexus and superior petrosal sinus
v.'s of tympanic membrane *vv. tympanicae membranae*	tympanic membrane (ear drum)	tympanic membrane	v.'s of tympanic cavity and external meatus
ulnar v.'s *vv. ulnares*	from hand it runs along border of wrist, up forearm to bend of elbow	deep palmar venous arches; superficial veins at wrist; palmar and dorsal interosseous v.'s	brachial v.'s
umbilical v. *v. umbilicalis*	traversing umbilical cord	placenta	fetus
uterine v.'s *vv. uterinae*	sides and superior angles of the uterus between the two layers of the broad ligament	uterine plexus	internal iliac v.
vaginal v.'s *vv. vaginales*	sides of vagina	vaginal plexus	internal iliac v.
vena cava, inferior (largest vein in body) *vena cava inferior*	from level of fifth lumbar vertebra it ascends along vertebral column to right side of heart	both common iliacs; lumbar, renal, testicular (male), ovarian (female), suprarenal, inferior phrenic, and hepatic veins	right atrium of heart
vena cava, superior (second largest vein in body) *vena cava superior*	from close behind sternum to upper portion of right side of heart	cranial half of body via brachiocephalic v.'s	cranial part of right atrium
vertebral v. *v. vertebralis*	from suboccipital triangle through transverse foramina of first six cervical vertebrae	suboccipital venous plexus, occipital v., internal and external vertebral venous plexuses, anterior cerebral v., deep cervical veins, first intercostal v. (occasionally)	brachiocephalic v.

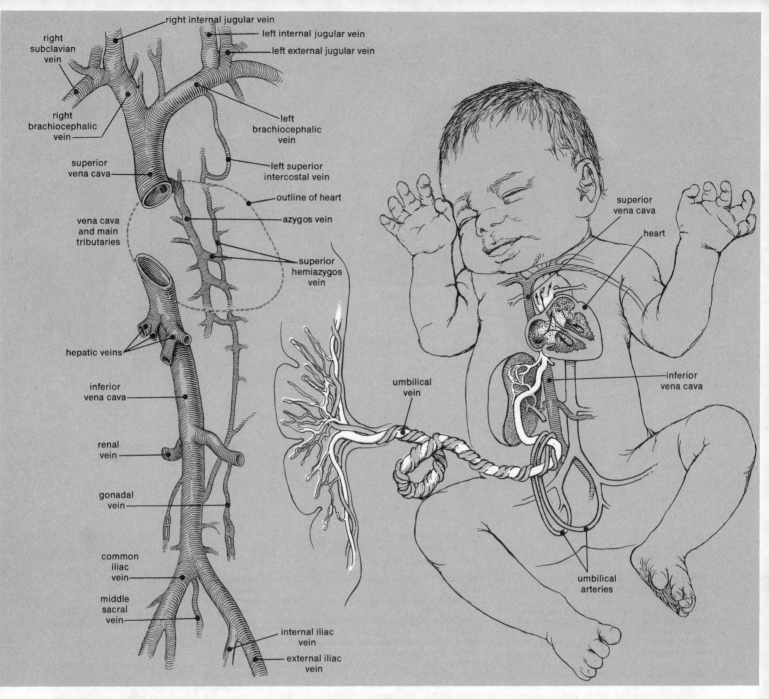

VEINS	LOCATION	DRAINS	EMPTIES INTO
vertebral v., accessory *v. vertebralis accessoria*	when present it accompanies vertebral vein and emerges through transverse foramen of seventh cervical vertebra	venous plexus of vertebral artery	brachiocephalic v.
vertebral v., anterior ascending cervical v. *v. vertebralis anterior*	from transverse processes of cervical vertebrae it descends between anterior scalene and longus capitis muscles (it accompanies ascending cervical artery)	plexus around transverse processes of cervical vertebrae	terminal part of vertebral v.
vesical v.'s *vv. vesicales*	back part of bladder and base of prostate gland	vesical plexus; anastomose with pudendal and prostatic plexuses	internal iliac v.
vestibular v.'s *vv. vestibulares*	internal ear	vestibule of internal ear	labyrinthine or internal pudendal v.
vorticose v.'s (usually four or five in number) vortex v.'s *vv. vorticosae*	eyeball, midway between cribosa and sclerocorneal junction	choroid layer of eyeball	superior or inferior ophthalmic v.'s

vein | vein

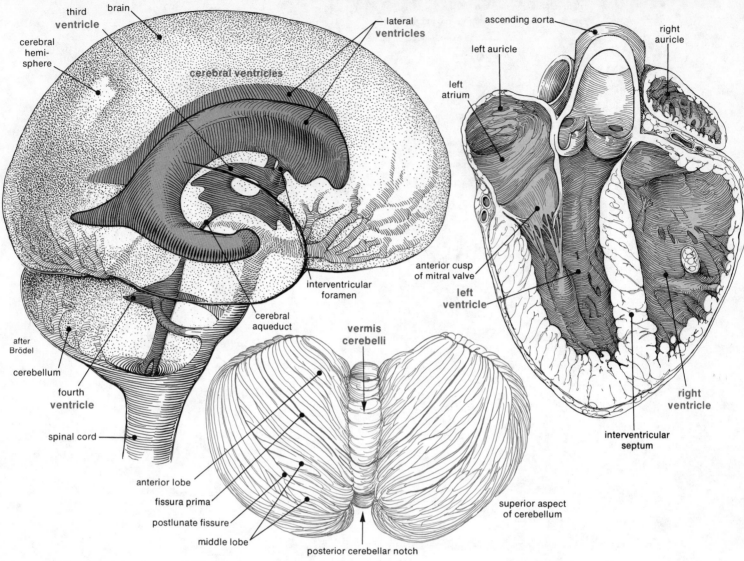

third **ventricle**
brain
lateral ventricles
cerebral hemisphere
ascending aorta
right auricle
left auricle
left atrium
cerebral ventricles
interventricular foramen
cerebral aqueduct
anterior cusp of mitral valve
left ventricle
after Brödel
cerebellum
fourth ventricle
spinal cord
vermis cerebelli
anterior lobe
fissura prima
postlunate fissure
middle lobe
posterior cerebellar notch
superior aspect of cerebellum
right ventricle
interventricular septum

vene′real. Relating to or resulting from sexual intercourse; the term is derived from the Latin *venereus*, love.

venereol′ogy. The study of venereal disease.

venesec′tion. Phlebotomy; withdrawing of blood through an incision of a vein.

veni-, veno-. Combining forms denoting veins.

venipunc′ture. The insertion of a needle into a vein.

venoc′lysis. The continuous injection into a vein of a medicinal or nutritive fluid; intravenous infusion of fluids by slow gravity flow or intravenous drip.

ve′nogram. A roentgenogram of a vein or veins after intravenous injection of a radiopaque substance.

venog′raphy. The making of a venogram; also called phlebography.

ven′om. A poisonous substance secreted by snakes or other animals.

venomo′tor. Causing changes in the internal diameter of veins.

venopres′sor. An agent which increases venous blood pressure by venoconstriction.

venosta′sis. See phlebostasis.

venot′omy. See phlebotomy.

ve′nous. Relating to a vein.

venovenos′tomy. Surgical connection of two veins.

ventila′tion. Physiologic process in which air in the lungs is exchanged with atmospheric air; a cyclic process of inspiration and expiration in which alternating fresh air enters the respiratory tract and an equal amount of pulmonary gas is exhaled.

   alveolar v., the amount of inspired gas which enters the alveoli each minute.

ventr-, ventro-. Combining forms denoting the abdomen.

ven′trad. Toward the ventral side.

ven′tral. 1. Relating to the abdomen. **2.** Anterior.

ven′tricle. A cavity, especially in the heart or the brain.

   cardiac v., one of the two lower and larger chambers of the heart.

   cerebral v.'s, the cavities within the brain (two lateral, the third, and the fourth).

   left v. (LV), the left lower chamber of the heart.

   right v. (RV), the right lower chamber of the heart.

ventricor′nu. The anterior column of gray matter of the spinal cord.

ventric′ular. Relating to any ventricle.

ventriculi′tis. Inflammation of the lining of the ventricles of the brain.

ventriculo-. Combining form indicating a relationship to a ventricle.

ventric′ulocisternos′tomy. Surgical establishment of communication between the ventricles of the brain and the subarachnoid space or cisterna cerebellomedullaris.

ventric′ulocordot′omy. Removal of a portion of each vocal cord of a dog to reduce the sound of its bark.

ventric′ulogram. A roentgenogram of the brain following the direct introduction of air or an opaque medium into the cerebral ventricles.

ventriculog′raphy. The making of x-ray films of the brain after replacing the cerebrospinal fluid of the ventricles with a gas.

ventriculopunc′ture. Introduction of a needle into a ventricle.

ventriculot′omy. Incision into a ventricle.

ventric′ulus, *pl.* **ventric′uli. 1.** Latin for ventricle. **2.** The stomach.

ventro-. See ventr-.

ventrofixa′tion of uterus. An operation for the correction of a retroplaced uterus by suturing the uterine fundus to the anterior abdominal wall; this procedure is no longer used but is of historical interest in the evolution of uterine suspension; also called hysteropexy and hysterorrhaphy.

ventros′copy. Laparoscopy.

ventrot′omy. Laparotomy.

ven′ula, *pl.* **ven′ulae.** Venule.

   venulae rectae, the numerous ascending venules that drain the medullary pyramids of the kidney and empty into arcuate veins.

   venulae stellate, the stellate venules in the renal cortex near the capsule.

ve′nule. A minute vein; usually one less than 100 μ in diameter.

   postcapillary v., unique venule marked by elongated endothelial cells, situated in the lymph node cortex where it allows lymphocytes to pass from the blood to the lymph.

verbigera′tion. Repetition of meaningless words or phrases; also called oral stereotypy.

verge. Margin.

   anal v., area between the perianal skin and the anal canal.

ver′gence. Movement of the eyes in opposite directions.

ver′micide. An agent that kills intestinal worms.

vermic′ular. Wormlike.

vermicula′tion. A wormlike motion.

ver′micule. 1. A small worm. **2.** Wormlike.

vermic′ulose, vermic′ulous. 1. Wormy. **2.** Wormlike.

ver′miform. Having the shape of a worm.

ver′mifuge. An agent that expels intestinal worms.

vermilionec′tomy. Excision of the vermilion border of the lip; the exposed area is generally resurfaced by advancing the undermined labial mucosa.

ver′min. Parasitic insects.

ver′minous. Infested with or caused by worms or any parasite.

ver′mis. Lating for worm.

   v. cerebelli, the narrow median part of the cerebellum which connects the two cerebellar hemispheres.

venereal | **vermis**

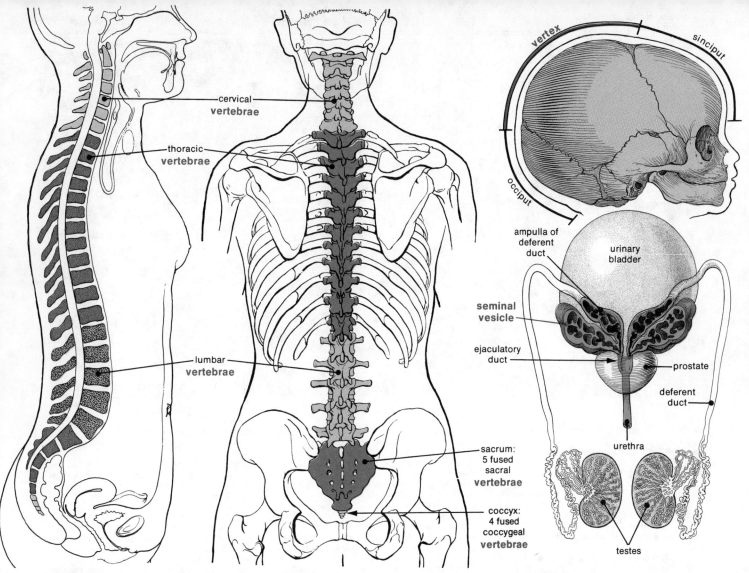

cervical **vertebrae**

thoracic **vertebrae**

lumbar **vertebrae**

sacrum: 5 fused sacral **vertebrae**

coccyx: 4 fused coccygeal **vertebrae**

vertex   sinciput

occiput

ampulla of deferent duct

urinary bladder

seminal vesicle

ejaculatory duct

prostate

deferent duct

urethra

testes

ver'mix. The vermiform appendix.
ver'nix. Latin for varnish.
  v. casesa, a fatty or cheesy substance on the skin of a newborn, consisting of stratum corneum, sebaceous secretions, and remnants of epithelium.
verru'ca. A wart.
verru'ciform. In the shape of warts or wartlike projections.
ver'rucose, ver'rucous. Resembling or covered with warts or wartlike roughness; denoting wartlike projections or elevations.
verruco'sis. A condition characterized by the presence of multiple warts or wartlike elevations.
verru'ga. Verruca.
verru'ga perua'na. The chronic form of bartonellosis; it usually, but not always, follows the anemic stage (Oroya fever); marked by a profuse skin eruption, chiefly on the face and limbs, which may persist from one month to two years. See also bartonellosis.
versic'olor. Marked by a variety of color; denoting turning or changing color.
ver'sion. 1. Turning of a fetus in the uterus to alter its position to a more favorable one for delivery. **2.** The state of an organ of being turned from its normal position. **3.** In ophthalmology, similar movement of the two eyes in the same direction.
  bimanual v., bipolar v., turning of the fetus with two hands; may be external or combined.
  Braxton Hicks v., seldom used procedure in which the forefinger and/or middle finger are introduced into the uterus to displace the presenting part of the fetus (often the shoulder) while the head is guided toward the birth canal by the operator's external hand.
  cephalic v., one performed in modern obstetrics only by external manipulations; each hand grabs one of the fetal ends and the head is gently pushed in the direction of the birth canal.
  combined v., one in which one hand is introduced

into the uterus and the other is placed on the abdominal wall.
  external v., manipulation by placing the hands on the abdomen and applying force gently and intermittently.
  Hicks v., Braxton Hicks version.
  internal v., direct turning of the fetus by introducing a hand into the uterus.
  podalic v., turning the fetus by seizing one or both feet and drawing them through the cervix.
  spontaneous v., one effected by contraction of the uterus alone.
ver'tebra, *pl.* **ver'tebrae.** One of the 33 bones that form the spinal column; they are divided into 7 cervical, 12 thoracic, 5 lumbar, 5 sacral, and 4 coccygeal vertebrae.
ver'tebral. Relating to a vertebra.
ver'tebrate. 1. Having a backbone or vertebral column. **2.** Any member of the subphylum Vertebrata, characterized by having a segmented vertebral column.
vertebrec'tomy. Surgical removal of a portion of a vertebra.
ver'tex. 1. The uppermost part of the head. **2.** In obstetrics, the crown of the fetal head.
ver'tical. Straight up and down; perpendicular, or at right angles, to the horizon.
ver'ticil. A whorl or circular arrangement; a collection of similar parts radiating about a point on an axis.
verticil'late. Characterized by or forming a whorl or whorls; circularly arranged.
ver'tigo. Illusion of revolving motion, either of oneself or of one's surroundings.
  auditory v., see Ménière's syndrome.
  aural v., vertigo caused by disease of the internal ear.
  ocular v., vertigo caused by errors in the refractive system of the eye or imbalance in the eye muscles.
  organic v., vertigo caused by brain damage.

verumontani'tis. Inflammation of the verumontanum (seminal colliculus).
verumonta'num. An elevation in the prostatic portion of the urethra, on either side of which open the prostatic and ejaculatory ducts; also called seminal colliculus.
vesic-, vesica-. Combining forms meaning (a) bladder; (b) blister.
vesi'ca. Latin for bladder and blister.
ves'ical. Of or relating to the bladder.
ves'icant. Any agent that produces blisters.
ves'icate. To blister.
vesica'tion. 1. The formation of a blister. **2.** A blister or blistered surface.
ves'icle. 1. A sac or hollow structure containing fluid or gas. **2.** A blister or circumscribed elevation on the skin containing serous fluid and ranging in size up to one centimeter, e.g., as in early chickenpox. Cf bulla.
  seminal v., one of the two sac-like glandular structures situated behind the bladder; its secretion is one of the components of semen.
  synaptic v.'s, a profusion of small spherical membrane-bound organelles in presynaptic nerve terminals that contain packages of protein-bound humoral transmitter substance; when released through the presynaptic membrane into the intercellular space, they cause changes in permeability and electric potential.
vesicobul'lous. Describing blister-like lesions containing serum.
ves'icocele. See cystocele.
vesicoc'lysis. Washing out of the bladder.
vesicoprostat'ic. Relating to the bladder and prostate gland.
vesicorec'tal. Relating to the urinary bladder and the rectum.
vesicot'omy. Cystotomy; surgical incision of the urinary bladder.
vesicoure'teral. Relating to the bladder and the

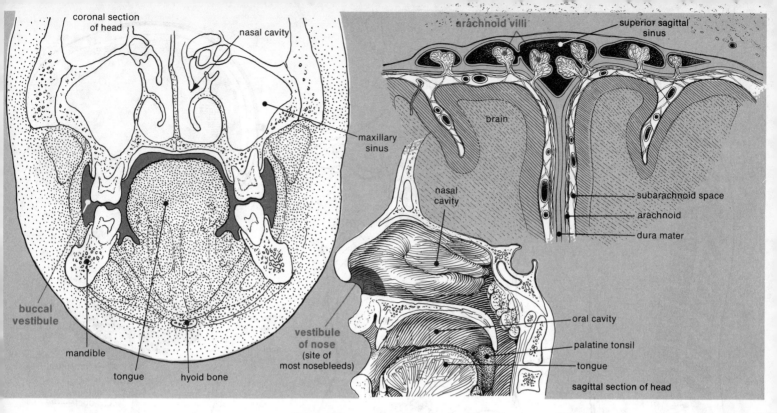

coronal section of head

nasal cavity

maxillary sinus

buccal vestibule

mandible

tongue

hyoid bone

arachnoid villi

superior sagittal sinus

brain

nasal cavity

subarachnoid space

arachnoid

dura mater

oral cavity

palatine tonsil

tongue

vestibule of nose
(site of most nosebleeds)

sagittal section of head

---

ureters.

vesicoure'thral. Relating to the bladder and the urethra.

vesicou'terine. Relating to the urinary bladder and the uterus.

vesicouterovag'inal. Relating to the bladder, uterus, and vagina.

vesicovag'inal. Relating to the bladder and vagina.

vesicovaginorec'tal. Relating to the bladder, vagina, and rectum.

vesic'ula, *pl.* **vesic'ulae.** A small bladder-like structure.

vesic'ular. 1. Of or relating to vesicles. 2. Containing vesicles.

vesicula'tion. The formation of vesicles or the condition of having numerous vesicles.

vesiculec'tomy. Removal of a seminal vesicle.

vesic'uliform. Having the shape of a vesicle.

vesiculi'tis. Inflammation of a seminal vesicle.

vesiculopap'ular. Relating to vesicles and papules.

vesiculoprostati'tis. Inflammation of the urinary bladder and the underlying prostate gland.

vesiculopus'tular. Relating to vesicles and pustules.

vesiculot'omy. Incision into a seminal vesicle.

ves'sel. Tubular structure that conveys fluids.

vestib'ular. Of or relating to a vestibule, especially the vestibule of the internal ear where balance functions are governed.

ves'tibule. A small chamber or space at the entrance to a canal.

  buccal v., the space between the teeth and gums and the cheek.

  labial v., the space between the teeth and gums and the lips.

  v. of aorta, a small space within the left ventricle just below the aortic opening; also called Sibson's aortic vestibule.

  v. of ear, the oval cavity in the middle of the bony labyrinth.

  v. of nose, the area just inside the nares.

vestibuloplas'ty. Operative procedure to deepen the labial sulcus (especially of the maxilla) and increase ridge height.

vestibulo'tomy. Surgical opening into the vestibule of the ear (labyrinth).

vestibuloure'thral. Relating to the vestibule of the vagina and the urethra.

vestib'ulum, *pl.* **vestib'ula.** A vestibule.

ves'tige. 1. A rudimentary structure; usually a remnant of an organ or part. 2. An imperfectly developed organ that has ceased to function.

vestig'ial. 1. Pertaining to a vestige. 2. A persist-

ing rudimentary structure.

vestig'ium, *pl.* **vestig'ia.** Remnant of a structure that was functional in the embryo.

veterina'rian. A person trained and licensed to diagnose and treat the diseases of animals, both domestic and wild.

vet'erinary. Relating to the diagnosis and treatment of diseases of animals.

vi'a, *pl.* **vi'ae.** Passage.

viabil'ity. The condition of being viable.

vi'able. Capable of living, as a fetus that has developed enough to be able to live outside of the uterus.

vi'al. A small glass container for holding liquid medicines.

vibra'tion. Oscillation; the act of moving back and forth rapidly; the rapid movement in alternately opposite directions of an elastic solid or a particle about an equilibrium position.

  sonic v., sound waves of ultrasonic frequencies used for disrupting cell structures in an aqueous medium.

vi'brator. A device that vibrates or causes vibrations.

Vib'rio. A genus of motile, gram-negative bacteria, occurring in salt and fresh water and in soil.

  V. cholera, a comma-shaped rod causing Asiatic cholera in man; also called cholera bacillus and *Vibrio comma.*

  V. comma, see *Vibrio cholera.*

vib'rio. Any bacterium of the genus *Vibrio.*

  El Tor v., bacterium isolated from six pilgrims who died of dysentery and gangrene of the colon at the El Tor Quarantine Station on the Sinai peninsula.

vibris'sa, *pl.* **vibris'sae.** One of the hairs within the nostrils.

vibrotherapeu'tics. Therapeutic use of vibrating devices.

vicar'ious. Acting as a substitute; occurring in a part of the body not normally associated with that specific function.

vic'inal (v.). Relating to or denoting the adjoining or neighboring position of radicals in an organic compound, as the 1, 2, 3 positions in the benzene ring.

vigilam'bulism. Condition, resembling sleepwalking but occurring in the wakeful state, in which the individual is unaware of his surroundings.

vig'ilance. Morbid wakefulness; insomnia; the state of being at vigil.

vil'li. Plural of villus.

villiki'nin. One of a group of gastrointestinal hormones believed to be responsible for the contraction of villi during digestion.

villo'ma. See papilloma.

villosi'tis. Inflammation of the villous aspect of the

placenta.

villos'ity. An aggregation of villi.

vil'lous. Covered with minute hairlike projections (villi).

vil'lus, *pl.* **vil'li.** A minute, vascular, hairlike projection from the surface of a membrane, such as the mucous membrane of the intestines.

  arachnoid villi, arachnoid granulations; see under granulation.

  chorionic villi, slender vascular projections of the chorion forming part of the placenta and through which all substances are exchanged between maternal and fetal circulations.

  intestinal villi, small projections on the surface of the mucosa of the small intestine; they are leaf-shaped in the duodenum and become finger-shaped, shorter, and sparser in the ileum; the sites of absorption of fluids and nutrients.

vinblastine sulfate. A salt of an antineoplastic alkaloid extracted from the periwinkle plant, *Vinca rosea*; Velban®.

Vinca rosea. See periwinkle.

Vincent's angina. Fusospirochetal pharyngitis; see under pharyngitis.

Vincent's disease, Vincent's infection, Vincent's stomatitis. Necrotizing ulcerative gingivitis; see under gingivitis.

vincristine sulfate. A salt of an antineoplastic alkaloid extracted from the periwinkle plant, *Vinca rosea*; used primarily in the treatment of acute leukemias, lymphomas, and solid tumors in children; Oncovin®.

vin'culum, *pl.* **vin'cula.** A frenum or restricting bandlike structure.

vin'egar. An impure, dilute (approximately six per cent) solution of acetic acid formed by the fermentation of alcoholic liquids (wine, cider, malt, etc.), or by the distillation of wood.

vinegaroon'. The nonvenomous whip-scorpion, *Mastigoproctus giganteus,* of southern United States and Mexico that emits a vinegary odor when disturbed.

vi'nic. Pertaining to or derived from wine.

viola'ceous. Denoting a violet or purple discoloration, usually of the skin.

vi'olet. A reddish-blue hue; the color evoked by radiant energy of wavelengths approximately 420 nanometers; seen in the most refracted end of the spectrum.

  ammonium oxalate crystal v., a stain composed of crystal (gentian) violet, ethyl alcohol, and ammonium oxalate mixed in distilled water; a type of Gram stain.

  crystal v., gentian violet.

  gentian v., a compound composed of one or sev-

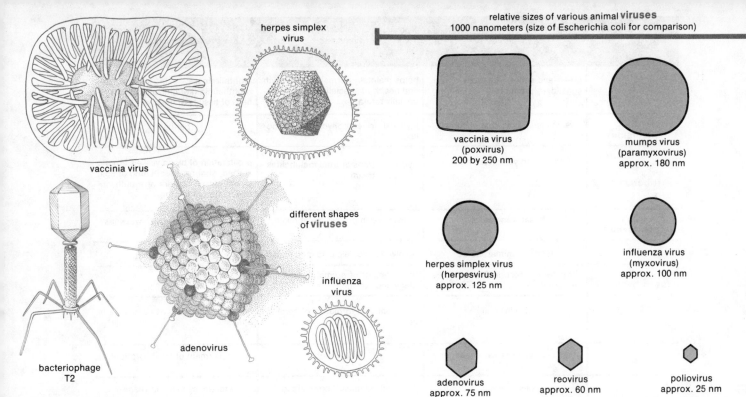

vaccinia virus

herpes simplex virus

bacteriophage T2

different shapes of **viruses**

adenovirus

influenza virus

vaccinia virus (poxvirus) 200 by 250 nm

mumps virus (paramyxovirus) approx. 180 nm

herpes simplex virus (herpesvirus) approx. 125 nm

influenza virus (myxovirus) approx. 100 nm

adenovirus approx. 75 nm

reovirus approx. 60 nm

poliovirus approx. 25 nm

eral methyl derivatives of pararosaniline; used as a biological stain, a bactericide in the treatment of minor lesions of the oral mucosa, and a fungicide in the treatment of moniliasis; also called crystal or methyl violet and methylrosanilin chloride.

Lauth's v., see thionine.

methyl v., gentian violet.

visual v., see iodopsin.

vios'terol. See vitamin D_2.

vi'per. A venomous snake of the family Viperidae and sometimes of the closely related Crotalidae.

European v., a common European viperine snake (*Vipera berus*), about two feet long with black markings patterned over a brownish-red to gray body; also called adder.

pit v., any of various venomous snakes of the family Crotalidae, characterized by a hollow, heat-sensitive pit between the eye and nostril; includes rattlesnakes, copperheads, and water moccasins.

Viper'idae. A family of snakes that includes many venomous species, characterized by movable, hollow, front fangs; included are the vipers and adders.

vi'ral. Relating to or caused by a virus.

vire'mia. The presence of virus in the blood.

vir'gin. A woman or man who has never had sexual intercourse.

virgin'ity. The state of not having experienced sexual intercourse.

vir'ile. 1. Relating to male sexual functions. **2.** Characteristic of masculine traits.

vir'ilism. The presence of male secondary sex characteristics in the female, caused usually be excessive amounts of androgenic hormones.

viril'ity. Masculine potency; manhood.

viriliza'tion. The appearance of secondary male characteristics, especially in the female.

vi'rion. A complete virus particle.

vi'roid. A folded, virus-like, single strand of low molecular replicating infectious RNA; the pathogen is smaller in size and simpler metabolically than a virus; it is thought to be linked to Creutzfeldt-Jakob disease.

virol'ogist. A specialist in virology.

virol'ogy. The study of viruses and diseases caused by them.

viromi'crosome. An incompletely formed virus released during the premature disruption of the host cell.

viropex'is. A process of phagocytosis in which cells engulf virus particles.

vir'ulence. Denoting the degree of pathogenicity of parasites within a species or the disease-producing capability of a microorganism; the state of being poisonous.

vi'rucide. Any agent destructive to viruses.

virulif'erous. Conveying viruses.

viru'ria. The presence of viruses in the urine.

vi'rus. An intracellular, infectious parasite, capable of living and reproducing only in living cells; virus particles usually range in size from 10 to 300 millimicrons, are visible under the electron microscope, and are spherical, polyhedral, or rod-shaped in form; each particle is composed of a protein shell which encloses a single nucleic acid, either ribonucleic acid (RNA) or deoxyribonucleic acid (DNA).

attenuated v., a virus so modified as to be incapable of producing a disease.

coxsackie v., see coxsackievirus.

dengue v., the causative agent of dengue, belonging to a group B arbovirus and transmitted through mosquitoes.

DNA v.'s, a class of viruses having an inner core of DNA and multiplying chiefly in the nuclei of cells; included are those causing herpes simplex, herpes zoster, chickenpox, smallpox, warts, and certain malignant tumors.

EB v. (EBV), a member of the herpesvirus group, first found in a lymphoma; the causative agent of infectious mononucleosis.

ECHO v., abbreviation for enteric cytopathogenic human orphan virus; see echovirus.

enteric v., enterovirus.

epidemic keratoconjunctivitis v., a type 8 adenovirus causing epidemic inflammation of the conjunctiva at the border of the cornea (shipyard eye); also associated with swimming pool conjunctivitis.

Epstein-Barr v., EB virus.

equine encephalomyelitis v., an insect-borne virus causing encephalomyelitis in horses and man; classified, according to the region where they occur, into eastern equine (EEE virus), Venezuelan (VEE virus), and western (WEE virus); transmitted by mosquitoes.

filtrable v., one small enough to pass through a porcelain filter or a filter of diatomaceous earths.

hepatitis A v., the causative agent of infectious hepatitis; it has a relatively short incubation period (two to six weeks) and is transmitted through ingestion of contaminated food or water.

hepatitis B v., the causative agent of serum hepatitis; it has a long incubation period (six weeks to six months) and is transmitted through contaminated blood or blood products as well as other routes, probably including saliva and possibly stool and urine.

herpes simplex v., see herpesvirus.

latent v., a virus that leaves its nucleic acid molecules (DNA) within a host cell; at a later date it may produce destructive viral proteins and destroy the cell.

lymphocytic choriomeningitis v. (LCM virus), the causative agent of congenital lymphocytic choriomeningitis in mice; believed to be associated with other inapparent and influenza-like infections.

measles v., see paramyxovirus.

mumps v., see paramyxovirus.

neurotropic v., one that thrives in nervous tissue.

oncogenic v., see tumor virus.

orphan v., one that has been isolated but not yet identified with any disease.

papilloma v., one causing warts; see papovaviruses.

poliomyelitis v., see picornaviruses.

rabies v., a relatively large, bullet-shaped, RNA virus that is the causative agent of rabies in man and other vertebrates; transmitted through the bite of an infected animal.

respiratory syncytial v. (RSV, RS virus), an RNA virus not yet classified but resembling a paramyxovirus; the cause of pneumonia and bronchiolitis in infants; derives its name from its capacity to fuse cells into a multinucleated mass (syncytium).

respiratory v., any virus that enters the body through and multiplies chiefly in the respiratory tract.

RNA v.'s, a large class of viruses having an inner core of RNA and multiplying chiefly in the cytoplasm of cells; included are those causing poliomyelitis, meningitis, yellow fever, encephalitis, mumps, measles, rabies, German measles, and the common cold; also called riboviruses.

Rous sarcoma v., see leukovirus.

RS v., abbreviation for respiratory syncytial virus.

rubella v., an RNA virus causing German measles (rubella); as yet unclassified but morphologically resembling a togavirus.

slow v., any virus causing a disease characterized by a long, unremitting course and gradual progression once the symptoms appear; slow viruses include etiologic agents of kuru, some cases of chronic hepatitis, and subacute inclusion body encephalitis.

tumor v., one capable of producing tumors, either benign or malignant, under natural or laboratory conditions; also called oncogenic virus.

varicella-zoster v., a member of the herpesvirus group causing chickenpox (varicella) and herpes zoster; see herpesvirus.

yellow fever v., see togavirus.

vis, *pl.* **vi'res.** Latin for force or energy.

vis'cance. A measure of the dissipation of energy in the flow of bodily fluids within cells and tissues or in tubes.

vis'cera. Plural of viscus.

vis'cerad. Toward or in the direction of the viscera.

VITAMIN	Sources	Functions	Deficiency
A	green and yellow vegetables, liver, eggs, dairy products	helps maintain normal body growth and health of specialized tissues especially retina	nightblindness, skin lesions, xerophthalmia (keratinization and dryness of tissues of the eye)
B_1 (thiamine)	yeast, meat, bran coat of cereals	involved in carbohydrate metabolism	beriberi
B_2 (riboflavin)	milk, egg yolk, fresh meat	hydrogen transfer from metabolites to blood stream	proliferation of blood vessels around cornea, abnormal reddening of lips, ulceration of corners of mouth, inflammation of tongue
B_6 (pyridoxine)	meat, vegetables	involved in protein metabolism	convulsions, muscular weakness, dermatitis of face
B_{12}	foods of animal source	involved in nucleic acid metabolism	pernicious anemia
C (ascorbic acid)	citrus fruits, green leafy vegetables, new potatoes	development of normal bones, cartilage and collagen	scurvy
D	fish liver oil	essential in formation of bone	rickets in children, osteomalacia in adults
E	green leafy vegetables, wheat germ, rice	antioxidant	impairment of fat absorption
K	fish, cereal	involved in clotting of blood	tendency to hemorrhage

vis'ceral. Pertaining to the internal organs.

visceral'gia. Pain in the viscera.

visceroinhib'itory. Restricting the function of the viscera.

visceromeg'aly. Abnormal enlargement of the viscera.

visceromo'tor. Causing functional activity of the viscera.

visceropari'etal. Relating to the abdominal organs and the abdominal wall.

visceropto'sia, visceropto'sis. Downward displacement of the abdominal organs.

viscerosen'sory. Relating to sensations in the viscera.

viscerotrop'ic. Affecting the organs.

vis'cid. Sticky.

viscid'ity. Stickiness.

viscosim'eter. Apparatus used to measure the viscosity of a fluid.

viscos'ity. The resistance to flow by a substance caused by molecular cohesion.

vis'cous. Sticky or glutinous; possessing a relatively high resistance to flow.

vis'cus, *pl.* **vis'cera.** Any large internal organ, especially in the abdomen.

vision. Sight.

binocular v., vision in which both eyes contribute to the formation of one fused image.

near v., ability to see objects clearly at normal reading distances (from 13 to 16 inches).

night v., ability to see clearly in reduced illumination.

peripheral v., ability to perceive objects outside of the direct line of vision.

scotopic v., lack of ability to distinguish colors and small details, without diminution of the ability to detect motion and low luminous intensities.

stereoscopic v., depth perception; see under perception.

tunnel v., one in which the visual field is severely contracted; also called tubular vision.

vis'ual. Relating to vision.

visual purple. See rhodopsin.

vis'ualize. 1. To make a mental image. **2.** To view.

visuau'ditory. Relating to both vision and hearing.

visuopsy'chic. Relating to the visual association areas of the occipital cortex of the brain, concerned with the interpretation or judgment of visual impressions.

visuosen'sory. Relating to perception of visual impressions.

vis'uscope. Instrument designed to identify the fixation characteristics of a partially blind (amblyopic) eye.

vi'ta. Latin for life.

vi'tal. Relating to life.

vital'ity. 1. Vigor, vital force, or energy. **2.** The capacity to live, grow, or develop.

vital'lium. A platinum-white, extremely hard cobalt-chromium alloy; used for orthopedic appliances and for cast dentures.

vitalom'eter. An electrical device used to determine the vital condition of a dental pulp; it could be either of high or low frequency; also called pulp tester.

vi'tals. 1. Viscera. **2.** Bodily parts and organs necessary for life.

vi'tamer. Substance performing a vitamin function.

vi'tamin. General term for any of several organic substances essential for normal metabolic processes and which, when absent in the diet, produce deficiency states.

v. A, a fat-soluble vitamin necessary for normal bone development and the health of certain specialized epithelial tissues, especially the retina for production of visual purple; present in green and yellow vegetables as a provitamin or precursor, which the body transforms into its active form; occurs in its preformed state in animal products (liver, eggs, and dairy products).

v. A_1, see retinol.

v. B, a member of the vitamin B complex.

v. B_1, see thiamine.

v. B_2, see riboflavin.

v. B_6, see pyridoxine.

v. B_{12}, a protein complex occurring in foods of animal source; lack of vitamin B_{12} causes pernicious anemia; also called cyanocobalamin, antipernicious anemia factor, and extrinsic factor.

v. C, see ascorbic acid.

v. D, a group of fat-soluble sterols that promote retention of calcium and phosphorus, thus aiding in bone formation; lack of vitamin D causes rickets in children and osteomalacia in adults; present primarily in fish liver oils; can be formed in the body upon exposure of the skin to sunlight; also called calciferol, the sun-ray vitamin, and antirachitic factor.

v. D_2, an irradiation product of ergosterol used as an antirachitic vitamin; also called ergocalciferol and calciferol.

v. D_3, a sterol of the vitamin D group formed by ultraviolet irradiation of the provitamin 7-dehydrocholesterol; also called cholecalciferol.

v. E, a group of naturally occurring fat-soluble substances which have antioxidant properties; in experimental animals, a lack of vitamin E may lead to sterility and muscular degeneration; also called tocopherol.

v. K, a group of fat-soluble compounds essential for clotting of blood; produced in the body by normal intestinal bacteria; also called antihemorrhagic factor.

v. Q, a vitamin essential for blood clotting; present in soybeans and probably in similar vegetables.

vitamin B complex. See complex, vitamin B.

vitel'lin. The main protein present in the yolk of eggs.

vitel'line. Relating to or resembling the yolk of an egg.

vitellogen'esis. Formation of yolk.

vitel'lus. The yolk of an egg.

vitilig'inous. Characterized by vitiligo.

vitili'go. Sharply demarcated, milky-white patches on the skin, usually on the face, neck, hands, lower abdomen, and thighs, caused by absence of melanin; also called acquired leukoderma.

vitrec'tomy. The surgical removal of the formed vitreous body from the eye.

radical anterior v., the surgical removal of the vitreous body within the eye's anterior half, usually performed during a full-thickness corneal graft procedure.

vit'reoretinop'athy. Disease of the eye involving the vitreous body and the retina.

vitr'eous. 1. Glassy. **2.** See body, vitreous.

vitrifica'tion. Conversion of dental porcelain into a glassy substance.

vitr'riol. 1. Any of various sulfates of heavy metals. **2.** Sulfuric acid.

blue, v., copper sulfate.

green v., ferrous sulfate.

oil of v., sulfuric acid.

salt of v., zinc sulfate.

white v., zinc sulfate.

viva'rium. Quarters in which animals are kept for observation or medical research; also called animal house.

vivi-. Combining form denoting alive or living.

vividial'ysis. Dialysis through a living membrane, as in lavage of the peritoneal cavity.

vividiffu'sion. The passage of blood through a membrane and its return to the living body without exposure to air; the principle used in the artificial kidney.

vivifica'tion. Assimilation and utilization of protein by the living cell.

vivip'ara. Denoting all forms of life whose eggs are developed within the body, thereby giving birth to living young.

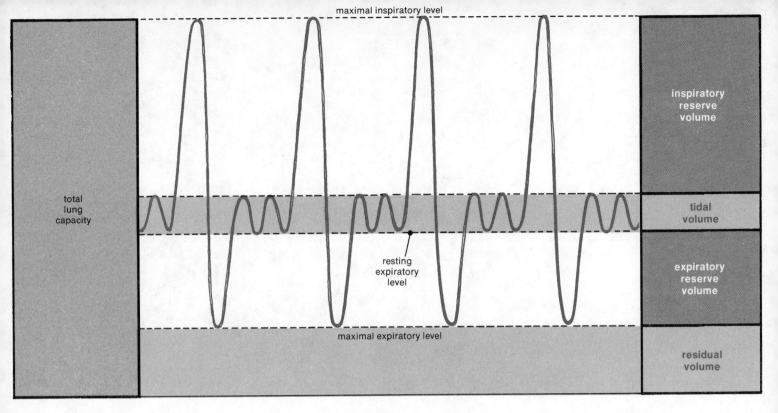

maximal inspiratory level

total lung capacity

inspiratory reserve volume

tidal volume

resting expiratory level

expiratory reserve volume

maximal expiratory level

residual volume

vivip'arous. Giving birth to living young developed within the mother's body; also called zoogonous.

vivipercep'tion. Study of vital processes in a living organism.

vivisec'tion. The performance of surgery on living animals for the purpose of experimentation.

VLDL. Abbreviations for very low-density lipoprotein.

VMA. Abbreviation for vanillylmandelic acid.

VNA. Abbreviation for Visiting Nurses' Association.

vo'cal. Relating to the voice.

voice. The sound produced by air passing through the larynx, upper respiratory tract, and oral structures of vertebrates, especially humans.

void. 1. To discharge a bodily waste, especially urine; to evacuate. **2.** Empty. **3.** Having no legal or binding effect or force; null.

vol. Abbreviation for volume.

vo'la. Lating for the palm of the hand or the sole of the foot.

vo'lar. Denoting the palmar surface of the hand or the plantar surface of the foot.

vol'atile. Having a tendency to evaporate rapidly at normal temperatures and pressures.

volatiliza'tion. Evaporation.

vol'atilize. To cause evaporation or to pass off in vapor.

vol'ley. A group of synchronous impulses.

volt. A unit of measure of electricity; a unit of electric potential necessary to cause one ampere of current to flow against one ohm of resistance on a conducting wire; named after the Italian physicist Alessandro Volta.

volt'age. Electromotive force expressed in volts.

voltam'meter. An apparatus for measuring the strength and quantity of current.

volt'ampere. A unit of electric power, equal to one volt times one ampere; one watt.

volt'meter. An electronic apparatus for measuring the potential differences in volts between two points.

vol'ume. The space occupied by matter in any state or form.

  blood v., the quantity of blood present in the vascular compartment of the body.

  expiratory reserve v. (ERV), the quantity of air that can be expelled from the lungs after a normal expiration; formerly called supplemental air.

  inspiratory reserve v. (IRV), the quantity of air that can be inspired after a normal inspiration; formerly called complemental air.

  minute v., (1) the volume of air expelled from the lungs per minute; (2) the volume of blood pumped by the left ventricle in one minute, normally four to five liters at rest.

  packed cell v., hematocrit (1); the volume of blood cells in a centrifuged blood sample, expressed as a percentage.

  residual v. (RV), the quantity of air remaining in the lungs after a maximal expiration; formerly called residual air and residual capacity.

  standard v., 22.414 liters, representing the volume of a perfect gas at standard temperature and pressure.

  stroke v., the quantity of blood expelled from each cardiac ventricle with each heartbeat.

  tidal v., the volume of air inspired and expired in a normal breath.

volumenom'eter. Instrument for measuring the volume of a body.

volumet'ric. Relating to measurement of or by volume.

vol'untary. Intentional; initiated by one's own free will; not obligatory.

volut'e. Rolled up.

volvulo'sis. See onchocerciasis.

vol'vulus. Twisting of a segment of intestine, causing obstruction.

vo'mer. See table of bones.

vom'ica. A pus-containing cavity, as in the lung.

vo'mit. 1. To expel the contents of the stomach forcibly through the mouth. **2.** The matter expelled from the stomach; also called vomitus.

vom'iting. The forceful expulsion of the stomach contents through the mouth.

  cyclic v., periodic or recurrent vomiting.

  pernicious v., persistent, uncontrollable vomiting.

  projectile v., expulsion of the stomach contents with great force, often not preceded by nausea.

  v. of pregnancy, vomiting occurring during pregnancy, especially in the early morning.

vom'itus. Vomited material.

von Gierke's disease. Type 1 glycogenosis; see under glycogenosis.

von Graefe's sign. See Graefe's sign.

von Hippel-Lindau disease. An inherited disorder of children marked by hemangiomas of the retina and hemangioblastoma of the cerebellum, medulla oblongata, and spinal cord; sometimes associated with cysts of several organs, especially the kidneys and pancreas; also called Hippel-Lindau or Lindau's disease and retinocerebral angiomatosis.

von Recklinghausen's disease. See neurofibromatosis.

von Willebrand's disease. Inherited disorder marked by deficiency of factor VIII and blood platelet abnormalities, resulting in prolonged bleeding time in the presence of normal platelet count and clot retraction; associated with bleeding from the gums, gastrointestinal tract, and uterus; also called Willebrand-Jurgeus syndrome, angiohemophilia, and constitutional thrombopathy.

vor'tex, *pl.* **vor'tices.** Latin for whirlpool; a general anatomic term designating a pattern involving rotation about an axis; a whorled design.

  v. cocygeus, the whorl of hairs sometimes present in the coccygeal region.

  v. cordis, the whorl of muscular fiber bundles at the apex of the heart.

  v. lentis, the whorl or star-shaped pattern of light lines visible on the surface of the lens of the eye.

  vortices pilorum, hairs arranged about an axis, as at the crown of the head; also called hair whorls.

vor'ticose. Having a whorled appearance, as the vorticose veins of the choroid layer of the eye.

vox. Latin for voice.

voyeur'. One who practices voyeurism; French for one who sees.

voyeur'ism. The practice of deriving sexual gratification from witnessing sexual acts of others or by observing the naked body.

VR. Abbreviation for vocal resonance.

VS. Abbreviation for volumetric solution.

VSD. Abbreviation for ventricular septal defect.

vul'canize. To combine rubber with sulfur or other additives under high temperature and pressure in order to improve its strength and resiliency.

vulga'ris. Ordinary; common; of the usual type; belonging to the multitude.

vul'va. The external female genitalia.

vul'var, vul'val. Of or relating to the vulva.

vulvec'tomy. Partial or complete removal of the vulva.

vulvi'tis. Inflammation of the vulva.

vulvocru'ral. Relating to the vulva and the crura of the clitoris.

vulvout'erine. Relating to the vulva and the uterus.

vulvovag'inal. Vaginovulvar; relating to the vulva and the vagina.

vulvovagini'tis. Inflammation of the vulva and vagina.

vv. Abbreviation for veins.

v/v. Abbreviation for a concentration expressed as volume (of solute) per volume (of solvent).

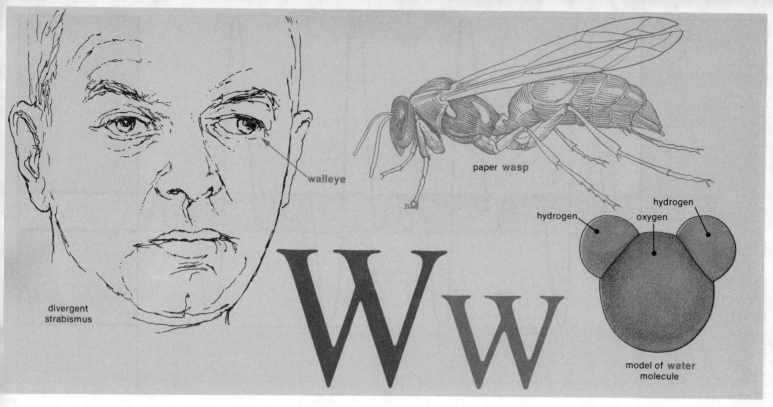

divergent strabismus

walleye

paper **wasp**

hydrogen hydrogen
oxygen

model of **water** molecule

W. 1. Abbreviation for wedge pressure. **2.** Symbol for (a) energy; (b) the element tungsten (wolfram). **w.** Abbreviation for watt.

Waardenburg's syndrome. A genetic defect characterized by anomalies of certain facioskeletal structures, congenital deafness, and pigmentary disorders; an estimated five per cent of individuals with congenital deafness have this genetic disease.

wad′ding. A soft layer of fibrous cotton or wool, used for surgical dressings.

wad′dle. To walk with short steps that cause the body to sway from side to side, as a duck; occurring in pseudohypertrophic muscular dystrophy and certain other nervous conditions.

waist. The part of the trunk between the bottom of the rib cage and the hips.

waist′ing. Shape of a bone in which the middle is narrower than the ends in transverse diameter.

Waldentrom's syndrome. Macroglobulinemia.

wale. Welt; a linear skin wheal.

walk. 1. To move on foot. **2.** The manner in which one moves when going on foot. See also gait.

wall. An investing structure that serves to enclose, divide, or protect an anatomic part; a part enclosing a cavity or space.

  cavity w., one of the enclosing surfaces bounding a prepared cavity in a tooth.

  enamel w., the part of the wall of a prepared cavity consisting of enamel.

wall′eye. 1. A dense, whitish opacity (leukoma) of the cornea. **2.** The eye that diverges in divergent strabismus.

wall′eyed. Having divergent strabismus.

ward. 1. A large room in a hospital usually with several beds for patients. **2.** A section of the hospital for special care and treatment of a particular group of patients.

  accident w., emergency room; see under room.

  isolation w., a ward in a hospital or institution where persons having or suspected of having a contagious disease are placed in quarantine.

  locked w., a ward in which mental patients are confined by locked doors.

  open w., a ward which is not locked.

  psychopathic w., a ward in a general hospital for the reception and treatment of mental patients.

war′farin. A colorless crystalline compound, 3-(α-acetonylbenzyl)-4-hydroxycoumarin, widely used as an anticlotting drug and rat poison; an acronym for Wisconsin Alumni Research Foundation + (Coum)arin.

warm-blooded. Homothermal; having a relatively high and constant body temperature independent of surrounding temperature.

warp. To distort out of shape.

wart. A small horny outgrowth on the skin, usually of viral origin; also called verruca.

  common w., a rough horny lesion varying in size from 1 mm to 2 cm in diameter; usually occurring on the hands; also called verruca vulgaris.

  filiform w., a long, horny, fingerlike projection, usually occurring in multiples; seen most commonly in adult males, in the bearded area of the face; also occurring on the eyelids and the neck.

  flat w., a smooth, small, skin-colored wart occurring in clusters of 30 or more; commonly seen on the face, neck, and dorsum of the hands.

  moist w., a soft, moist, pink to red mass, occurring as a single lesion or in clusters that resemble a cauliflower; usually seen around the genitalia and anus, less often between the toes and at the corners of the mouth; not usually of venereal origin; also called condyloma acuminatum and acuminate, venereal, or fig wart.

  plantar w., one occurring on the sole of the foot; also called verruca plantaris.

  venereal w., see moist wart.

wash. A lotion, often containing solid matter in suspension.

  eye w., see eyewash.

  mouth w., see mouthwash.

  red w., a lotion of zinc sulfate in compound tincture of lavender.

  yellow w., a suspension of mercuric oxide derived by precipitating a solution of mercuric chloride with calcium hydroxide.

wasp. An insect of the superfamilies Vespoidea and Sphecoidea, having a slender spindle-shaped body with elongated waist; it is second only to the bumblebee in frequency of reported fatalities from its sting.

waste. 1. To emaciate; to grow thin. **2.** Feces; the undigested residue of food voided from the bowels.

wasting. Emaciation.

water. A clear, colorless liquid, H_2O, present in all organic tissues and essential for life.

  alkaline w., water that contains appreciable amounts of the bicarbonates of calcium, lithium, potassium, or sodium.

  bound w., water in bodily tissues tenaciously held to colloids.

  distilled w., water purified by the heat-dependent process of distillation.

  free w., (1) water in the body that is not attached to colloids; it can be removed by ultrafiltration; (2) that amount of dilute urine formed per minute which can be considered free of solute assuming that the remainder of the urine is isotonic; C_{H_2O} (free water clearance) = V (urine flow in ml/min − C_{osm} (osmolar clearance).

  hard w., water containing ions, such as Mg^{++} and Ca^{++}, that form insoluble salts with fatty acids, especially water with more than 90 parts per million of calcium carbonate; it generally resists the action of soap to form a lather.

  heavy w. (D_2O), a compound analogous to water in which most of the hydrogen atoms are deuterium (heavy hydrogen); it differs from ordinary water in having higher boiling and freezing points; also called deuterium oxide.

  lime w., a solution of calcium hydroxide.

  metabolic w., see water of metabolism.

  mineral w., water that has appreciable amounts of mineral salts in solution.

  potable w., drinkable water free from contamination.

  saline w., water that contains neutral salts (chlorides, bromides, iodides, sulfates) in appreciable amounts.

  soft w., water than contains few or no ions that form insoluble salts with fatty acids, especially water with less than 80 parts per million of calcium carbonate; ordinary soap can lather in it easily.

  total body w., the total water content of the adult human body; equal to 50–70 per cent of the body weight.

  w. of combustion, see water of metabolism.

  w. of crystallization, water in chemical combination with a crystal, necessary for the maintenance of crystalline properties but capable of being separated by adequate heat.

  w. of hydration, water chemically united with a substance to form a hydrate, which can be removed, as by heating, without substantially changing the chemical composition of the substance.

  w. of injection, water purified by distillation for parenteral use.

  w. of metabolism, the water in the body derived from the oxidation of the hydrogen of a food element such as starch, glucose, or fat; the largest amount is produced in the metabolism of fat, approximately 117 grams per 100 grams of fat; also called metabolic water and water of combustion.

  w. on the brain, colloquial term for hydrocephalus.

water-borne. Conveyed by drinking water; describing certain diseases transmitted by contaminated water, such as cholera and typhoid fever.

water brash. The filling of the mouth with refluxed fluid from the esophagus, usually associated with heartburn.

Waterhouse-Friderichsen syndrome. A disorder of rapid onset marked by an extensive purpuric rash, bilateral adrenal hemorrhage, shock, and circulatory collapse; also called acute fulminat-

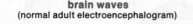

brain waves
(normal adult electroencephalogram)

frontal-central

central-occipital

frontal-temporal

temporal-occipital

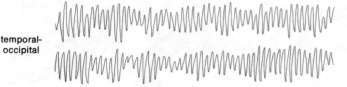

cannon wave

jugular venous tracing

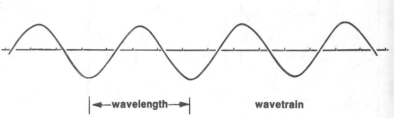

R wave

P wave

T wave

U wave

Q wave

S wave

normal electro-encephalogram

|←—wavelength—→| wavetrain

---

ing meningococcemia.

waters. Colloquial term for amniotic fluid, the fluid that surrounds the fetus.

bag of w., common name for amniotic sac; the closed sac of fetal membranes containing the amniotic fluid.

watt. The amount of electrical power produced by one volt with one ampere of current.

wat′tage. The amount of electric power, in watts, produced or consumed by an electrical device; amperage multiplied by voltage.

wave. A periodic increase and subsidence, as an oscillation propagated from point to point in a medium, characterized by alternate elevations and depressions.

alpha (α) w.'s, waves in the electroencephalogram with a frequency band from eight to 13 cycles per second; also called alpha rhythm.

arterial w., a wave in the jugular phlebogram due to the vibration produced by the carotid pulse.

beta (β) w.'s, waves in the electroencephalogram that have a frequency band from 18 to 30 cycles per second; also called beta rhythm.

brain w.'s, electrical potential waves of the brain.

cannon w., a large positive venous pulse wave produced by atrial contraction; it occurs when the right atrium contracts at the same time the tricuspid valve is closed by right ventricular systole, as in complete heart block and ventricular premature beats.

delta (δ) w.'s, (1) waves in the electroencephalogram that have a frequency band from 1/2 to 3 cycles per second; (2) the slow-rising, slurred, initial portion of the upstroke of the electrocardiographic R wave seen in the Wolff-Parkinson-White (W-P-W) syndrome, caused by preexcitation of a part of the ventricular myocardium.

dicrotic w., the second notch in the tracing of the normal arterial pulse.

f w.'s, small irregular waves or oscillations of the atria, characteristically seen in atrial fibrillation.

F w.'s, regular rapid undulating atrial waves seen in atrial flutter; thought to represent the manifestation of atrial depolarization and repolarization occurring in rapid succession from an ectopic focus.

fluid w., a sign of free fluid in the abdominal cavity; percussion on one side of the abdomen transmits a wave that is felt on the opposite side.

microelectric w., see microwave.

P w., the initial deflection of the electrocardiogram, representing depolarization of the atria; if retrograde or ectopic it is labeled P′.

pulse w., one originated by the impact of ejection of blood from the left ventricle into the full aorta and propagated to the periphery through the column of blood and the arterial walls.

Q w., the initial deflection of the QRS complex when such deflection is downward (negative).

R w., the first upward deflection of the QRS complex in the electrocardiogram (ECG).

radio w.'s, electromagnetic waves with wavelengths between one millimeter and 30 kilometers; also called Hertzian rays.

random w.'s, brain waves in the encephalogram produced by irregular changes of electric potential.

retrograde w., a distorted P wave pattern in the electrocardiogram, inverted in several leads where it should be upright, caused by an ectopic impulse from the ventricle spreading backward into the atria.

S w., a downward (negative) deflection of the QRS complex following an R wave.

sound w., system of longitudinal pressure waves passing through any medium; may or may not be audible.

T w., the deflection of the normal electrocardiogram which follows the QRS complex; it represents ventricular repolarization.

theta (θ) w., brain wave in the encephalogram having a frequency between four and seven cycles per second; also called theta rhythm.

Traube-Hering W.'s, Traube-Hering curves; see

under curve.

U w., a minor deflection of the normal electrocardiogram which occasionally occurs in early ventricular diastole following the T wave; especially prominent in persons with electrolyte imbalance.

wave′form. The mathematical graphic representation of a wave.

wave′length. One of three measurements of the vibration of a sound wave (others are amplitude and frequency); the longitudinal distance between the crests of two successive sound waves.

wave′train. A series of waves sent along the same axis by a vibrating body.

wax. A plastic, heat-sensitive substance secreted by insects, or obtained from plants or petroleum; consists essentially of high molecular weight hydrocarbons or esters of fatty acids; characteristically insoluble in water but soluble in most organic solvents.

baseplate w., a hard wax for making baseplates and occlusion rims.

bone w., one used for filling sterile bone cavities.

boxing w., a soft wax for boxing impressions for dental prostheses.

carnauba w., a hard wax with a high melting point used for the control of the melting range of various waxes; it is derived from the fine powder on the leaves of certain tropical palms.

casting w., a compound of various waxes with controlled properties of thermal expansion and contraction; used in making patterns which represent the exact reproduction of the missing tooth structure; it allows a mold to be made, into which the alloy is cast.

ear w., cerumen.

inlay w., wax used in making patterns for dental restoration from which an inlay is cast.

paraffin w., a white or colorless wax derived from the high-boiling fractions of petroleum; composed chiefly of a complex mixture of hydrocarbons of the methane series; also called paraffin.

sticky w., an adhesive wax used in dentistry for

523   **waters** | **wax**

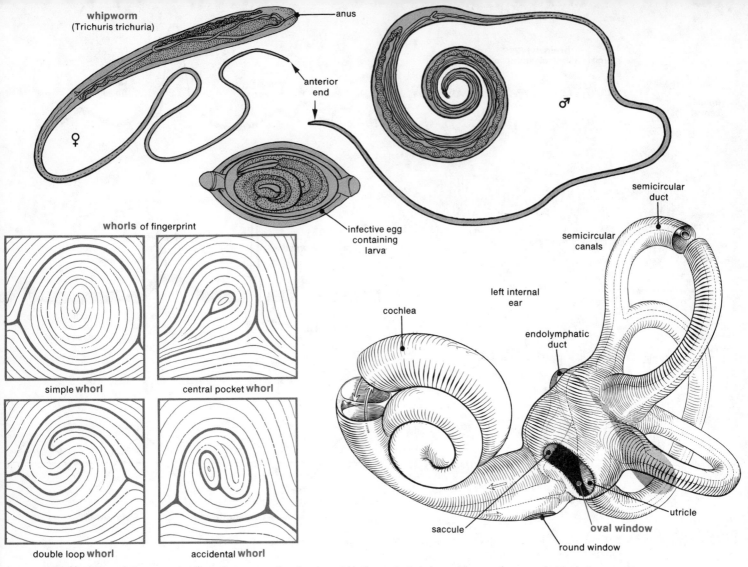

whipworm
(Trichuris trichuria)

anus

anterior
end

♂

♀

infective egg
containing
larva

whorls of fingerprint

simple **whorl**

central pocket **whorl**

double loop **whorl**

accidental **whorl**

semicircular
duct

semicircular
canals

left internal
ear

cochlea

endolymphatic
duct

saccule

utricle

oval window

round window

---

attaching a sprue pin to a wax restoration pattern.

wax′ing, wax′ing up. The shaping of a wax pattern or the wax base of a trial denture into the desired contours.

WBC. Abbreviation for white blood cell.

wean. To discontinue the breast feeding of an infant, with substitution of other nourishment.

web. A membrane or membranous fold.

  esophageal w., a condition marked by the presence of one or more membranous folds in the esophagus.

Weber-Christian disease. A disease of unknown cause marked by recurring fever and formation of subcutaneous nodules and plaques with atrophy of subcutaneous fat; the thighs and trunk are most frequently affected; also called relapsing febrile nodular nonsuppurative panniculitis.

weight. The measured heaviness of a specific object; the force with which a body is pulled toward the earth by gravity.

  atomic w. (at. wt.), the weight of an atom of any element compared with the weight of an atom of carbon-12 (^{12}C), which is taken as 12.00000; tables of atomic weights list a value of the element's isotopic weights.

  avoirdupois w., a system of weights and measures in which a pound equals 16 ounces, 7,000 grains, or 453.59 grams.

  combining w., gram equivalent; see under equivalent.

  equivalent w., see equivalent, gram.

  gram-molecular w., the numerical molecular weight of a substance expressed in grams; an amount of substance containing a weight in grams numerically equal to its molecular weight.

  molecular w. (mol. wt., MW), the sum of the atomic weights of all the atoms that make up a molecule.

weight′lessness. The state of experiencing no gravitational pull.

Weil's disease. Severe leptospirosis with jaun-

dice; disease caused by *Leptospira icterohemorrhagiae* transmitted to man by rats; characterized primarily by continued fever and hepatic disturbances, associated with jaundice, renal manifestations, and congestion of the conjunctiva; also called infectious spirochetal jaundice, icterohemorrhagic fever, and leptospirosis icterohemorrhagia.

Weiss' sign. See Chvostek's sign.

welt. A linear wheal, usually raised on the skin by a lash, blow, or flog; also called wale.

wen. Sebaceous cyst, especially of the scalp.

Wernicke-Korsakoff syndrome. Disorder of the central nervous system caused by abusive intake of alcohol and nutritional depletion, especially of thiamine; characterized primarily by sudden weakness and paralysis of eye muscles, double vision, and inability to stand or walk unaided; followed by derangement of mental functions, e.g., confusion, apathy, loss of retentive memory, and confabulation; it may terminate in death.

wet nurse. A woman who breast-feeds another woman's child.

wheal. A round or ridgelike transitory swelling on the skin; e.g., hives.

wheeze. 1. To breathe with difficulty, producing a whistling sound, usually due to bronchiolar constriction as in asthma. **2.** The sound thus produced.

whey. The watery part of milk that separates from the casein or coagulated part; also called serum lactis.

whip′lash. See injury, whiplash.

Whipple's disease. A rare systemic disorder characterized by anemia, increased skin pigmentation, arthritis, steatorrhea, and other signs of malabsorption; the intestinal wall and lymphatics are infiltrated by macrophages filled with glycoproteins; occurs predominantly among middle-aged men; also called lipophagic intestinal granulomatosis and intestinal lipodystrophy.

whipworm. *Trichuris trichiura*; a small whiplike roundworm, parasitic in the large intestine of man;

the cause of trichuriasis.

whis′key, whis′ky. An alcoholic liquid distilled from grain such as barley, maize, rye, and wheat, and containing 47 to 53 per cent ethyl alcohol by volume.

white′head. 1. A vernacular alternate for milium. **2.** Term colloquially used for a superficial skin lesion with a white purulent content.

whites. Colloquial term for leukorrhea; a thick whitish vaginal discharge.

whi′ting. A pure grade of chalk, $CaCO_3$; used in polishing metal and plastic structures, especially dental prosthetics.

WHO. Abbreviation for World Health Organization.

whoop. The shrill, noisy, paroxysmal gasp characteristic of whooping cough.

  systolic w., see honk, systolic.

whoop′ing cough. See under cough.

whorl. A spiral twist, such as any of the circular ridges of a fingerprint, the arrangement of muscular fibers at the apex of the heart, or the area of hair growing in a radial manner.

widow's peak. A V-shaped point formed by the hairline at the middle of the forehead; term derived from the superstition that it is a sign of early widowhood.

Wilms' tumor. See under tumor.

Wilson's disease. 1. (Samuel A. Kinnier Wilson) Hepatolenticular degeneration: see under degeneration. **2.** (Sir William J. E. Wilson) Exfoliative dermatitis; see under dermatitis.

wind′burn. Skin irritation due to excessive exposure to wind.

win′dow. An opening in a wall; also called fenestra.

  aortic w., a radiolucent area below the aortic arch formed by the bifurcation of the trachea and traversed by the left pulmonary artery, visible in the left anterior oblique roentgenogram.

  oval w., fenestra vestibuli; an oval opening in the

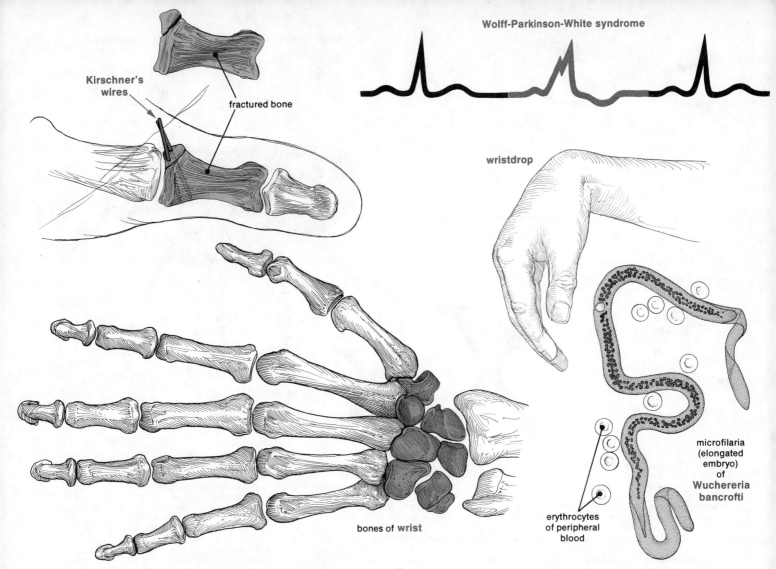

Kirschner's wires

fractured bone

wristdrop

microfilaria (elongated embryo) of **Wuchereria bancrofti**

erythrocytes of peripheral blood

bones of **wrist**

---

medial wall of the middle ear chamber, which leads into the vestibule of the internal ear; it houses the baseplate of the stapes.

round w., fenestra cochleae; a round opening in the lateral wall of the internal ear, which leads from the scala tympani of the cochlea to the middle ear chamber; it is closed by the secondary tympanic membrane.

wind′pipe. See trachea.

wing. Any anatomic structure resembling the wing of a bird.

wink′ing. The rapid closing and opening of the eyelids.

Winterbottom's sign. Swelling of the posterior cervical lymph nodes; indicative of early stages of African sleeping sickness.

win′tergreen. A low-growing evergreen plant of eastern North America, *Gaultheria procumbens*.

oil of w., see under oil.

wire. 1. A slender, pliable, metallic strand, used in surgery and dentistry. **2.** To bind structures with a wire or wires.

arch w., an orthodontic wire attached to molar bands positioned around the dental arch; used to provide tooth stabilization and/or maintain controlled pressure for tooth movement.

Kirschner's w., a heavy gauge steel wire used for applying traction in long bone fractures and for transfixation of fractured bones.

ligature w., a soft slender wire used to tie an arch wire to the band attachment around a tooth.

wiring. Fixation of the ends of broken bones by means of wire.

Wiskott-Aldrich syndrome. An X-linked recessive inherited syndrome of males, characterized by eczema, low platelet count, and increased susceptibility to infections due to a defect in cellular immunity; present primarily in infants and early childhood; bloody diarrhea is a common feature; also called Aldrich syndrome.

witch hazel. A liquid extract obtained from the dried bark and leaves of the plant *Hamamelis virginiana*; used as an astringent.

withdraw′al. A pathologic detachment or retreat from emotional involvement with people or the environment; seen in its extreme in schizophrenics.

withdrawal syndrome. Intense physiologic disturbances when abruptly discontinuing the administration of a drug that, by its prolonged use, induced physical dependence; also called abstinence syndrome.

Wolff-Parkinson-White syndrome. Anomalous atrioventricular excitation; congenital heart condition marked by irregular heart beat and distorted patterns of the electrocardiogram (shortened P-R interval and prolonged QRS complex); also called preexcitation syndrome.

womb. See uterus.

falling of the w., prolapse of the uterus.

wood alcohol. See alcohol, methyl.

wool fat. The fatlike substance obtained from sheep's wool, used in the preparation of ointments; also called anhydrous lanolin.

workahol′ic. A person who suffers from an abnormal, uncontrollable, habitual desire to work excessively.

working through. In psychoanalysis, all the processes in which a problem is actively explored by patient and therapist until a satisfactory solution has been found or until a symptom has been traced to its unconscious sources; it generally involves the recapture of infantile, repressed, unconscious material and its conversion into conscious thoughts and strivings.

World Health Organization (WHO). An agency of the United Nations concerned with health on an international level.

worm. Common name for any of various elongated invertebrates, as those of the phyla Annelida, Nematoda, or Platyhelminthes.

eye w., see *Loa loa*.

flat w., see flatworm.

guinea w., see *Dracunculus medinensis*.

heart w., see *Dirofilaria immitis*.

lung w., see lungworm.

Medina w., see *Dracunculus medinensis*.

pin w., see pinworm.

pork w., see *Trichinella spiralis*.

seat w., see pinworm.

serpent w., see *Dracunculus medinensis*.

trichina w., see *Trichinella spiralis*.

wound. Injury or trauma in any tissue.

contused w., injury to the tissues without a break in the skin.

incised w., a cut made with a knife or any sharp instrument.

lacerated w., a tear.

open w., one with an exposed opening.

penetrating w., one that enters a body cavity.

puncture w., a narrow wound made by a spiked instrument or weapon.

WPW. Abbreviation for Wolff-Parkinson-White syndrome.

wrin′kle. 1. A crease in the skin, especially one caused by habitual frowning or by atrophy of the corium, as in old age. **2.** A furrow or crevice on a normally smooth surface.

wrist. The carpal bones and adjoining structures between the hand and the forearm.

wrist′drop. Paralysis of the extensor muscles of the hand and digits.

wry′neck. See torticollis.

wt. Abbreviation for weight.

Wucherer′ia. A genus of parasitic nematode worms of the superfamily Filarioidea.

W. bancrofti, the Bancroftian filaria, formerly called *Filaria bancrofti* or *Filaria nocturna*; a parasite of the lymphatic vessels and the cause of elephantiasis.

wuchereri′asis. Infestation with worms of the genus *Wuchereria*.

w/v. Abbreviation for weight of solute per volume of solvent.

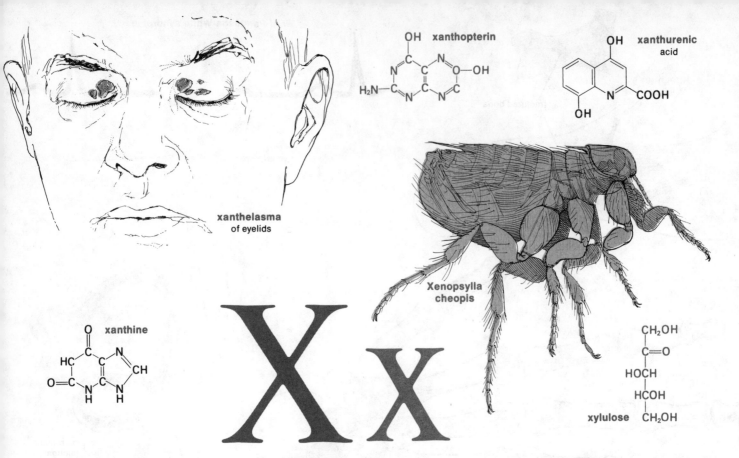

xanthopterin

xanthurenic
acid

xanthelasma
of eyelids

Xenopsylla
cheopis

xanthine

xyluloise

X. 1. Abbreviation for (a) exposure; (b) reactance; (c) sound particle displacement. **2.** Symbol for Kienbock's unit of x-ray dosage.

xanth-. See xantho-.

xanthelas'ma. A form of xanthoma; yellow, wrinkled, slightly raised patches on the skin, occurring on the eyelid, usually bilaterally near the inner angle of the eye; also called xanthelasma palpebrarum.

xanthe'mia. See carotenemia.

xan'thene. A crystalline compound which is the basic structure of many dyestuffs.

xan'thic. 1. Yellow. **2.** Of or relating to xanthine.

xan'thine. A white purine base present in most of the body tissues; sometimes found in urinary stones; converted by xanthine oxidase to uric acid.

xanthinu'ria. Passage of excessive amounts of xanthine in the urine.

xantho-, xanth-. Combining forms meaning yellow.

xanthochro'mia. A yellow discoloration of spinal fluid, usually an indication of a previous bleeding episode within the central nervous system.

xanthochrom'ic, xanthochromat'ic. Yellow colored.

xanthocyanop'sia. Abnormal color vision marked by inability to perceive red and green hues; vision is limited to yellow and blue.

xan'thodont. One who has yellowish teeth.

xanthogranulo'ma. Infiltration of tissue by lipid macrophahges.

xantho'ma. Slightly raised, yellow skin plaque, due to a disorder of fat metabolism.

  x. diabeticorum, diabetic x., the eruption of xanthomas in some cases of diabetes mellitus.

  x. tuberosum, x. tuberosum multiplex, the eruption of xanthomas in the form of yellow nodules of varying size chiefly of the knees, elbows, palms, and soles.

xanthomato'sis. The presence of multiple xanthomas; also called lipoid or lipid granulomatosis and xanthoma multiplex.

xantho'matous. Relating to a xanthoma.

xan'thophyll. A yellow carotenoid pigment in plants and egg yolk; also seen in human plasma as a result of ingesting food containing the pigment.

xanthop'sia. Condition in which everything appears yellow; also called yellow vision.

xanthop'terin. A yellow pigment present in many sources including butterfly wings and the integument of wasps and hornets; an inhibitor of xanthine oxidase.

xan'thosine. A nucleoside, xanthine-9-ribofuranoside, $C_{10}H_{12}O_6N_4$; formed by the deamination of guanosine.

xantho'sis. A yellow discoloration of the skin, sometimes seen in patients afflicted with cancer.

xanthurenic acid. 4,8-Dihydroquinaldic acid, large amounts of which are excreted during pregnancy and by pyridoxine-deficient individuals.

xan'thyl. The monovalent radical $C_{13}H_9O$ which occurs in xanthene.

X-chro'mosome. One of the sex chromosomes carried by the female in a double dose (two XX) and by the male in a single dose (one X and one Y).

Xe. Chemical symbol of the element xenon.

xeno-. Combining form meaning different; denoting a relationship to something foreign.

xenogene'ic. Relating to individuals of different species.

xenogen'ic. Originating outside the body or in a foreign substance within the body.

xen'ograft. A graft derived from a species different from that receiving it; also called xenogeneic graft, heterograft, and heterotransplant.

xenoimmune'. Denoting the condition of being immune to a xenogeneic antigen; also called heteroimmune.

xen'on. An odorless inert gaseous element found in minute proportions in the atmosphere; symbol Xe, atomic number 54, atomic weight 131.30.

xenon-133 (^{133}Xe). A γ-emitting radioactive inert gas with a physical half-life of 5.27 days; used to measure blood flow and regional pulmonary ventilation.

xenopho'bia. An undue fear of strangers.

xenophthal'mia. Inflammation of the conjunctiva due to injury or to the presence of a foreign body.

Xenopsyl'la. A genus of fleas.

  X. cheopis, the rat flea; vector of *Pasteurella pestis*, the causative bacillus of plague.

xeran'sis. Loss of moisture in the tissues.

xeran'tic. Causing dryness.

xero-, xer-, Combining forms denoting dryness; e.g., xeroderma.

xerochei'lia. Dryness of the lips.

xeroder'ma. A skin disease marked by roughness, dryness, and discoloration of the skin.

  x. pigmentosum, a congenital condition of the skin marked by extreme sensitivity to light which causes skin inflammation, freckles, superficial ulcer-

ations, glossy white spots due to thinning of the skin, and keratoses which become malignant; also called atrophoderma pigmentosum.

xerog'raphy. A dry photographic process in which an image formed by a resinous powder on an electrically charged photoconductive surface is transferred and developed on paper with carbon powder that adheres only to the electrically charged areas.

xeromammog'raphy. See mammography, zero.

xerome'nia. Occurrence of the usual general symptoms of menstruation without a blood flow.

xerophthal'mia. Xerosis of the conjunctiva; a degenerative condition, marked by extreme dryness and thickness of the conjunctiva with diminished secretions; also called ophthalmoxerosis.

xeroradiog'raphy. The making of nontransparent black and white prints of densities produced by x rays on a specially coated plate.

xero'sis. Abnormal dryness of the skin, conjunctiva, or mucous membranes.

xerosto'mia. Abnormal dryness of the mouth, caused by diminished or arrested secretion of saliva.

xerot'ic. Affected with abnormal dryness of the skin or conjunctiva.

xiphister'num. The xiphoid process or cartilage.

xiphocos'tal. Relating to the xiphoid cartilage and the ribs.

xiphodyn'ia. Pain in the area of the xyphoid cartilage.

xi'phoid. Sword-shaped.

X linkage. See under linkage.

X-linked. Determined by a gene located on the X chromosome; also called sex-linked.

x ray. See under ray.

XXY syndrome. See Klinefelter's syndrome.

xy'lene. A flammable hydrocarbon obtained from wood and coal tar, used as a solvent; also called xylol.

xy'lometazo'line. Compound used to reduce congestion of the nasal mucosa.

xy'lose. A pentose sugar (the molecule of which has five carbon atoms), $C_5H_{10}O_5$, found in beechwood, straw, etc.; the absorption of xylose from the intestine is used as a test in suspected cases of malabsorption syndrome; also called wood sugar.

xy'lulose. A pentose sugar found in two forms.

  D-x., an intermediate in pentose metabolism.

  L-x., an abnormal constituent of urine seen in essential pentosuria.

xy'lyl. The hydrocarbon radical, $C_6H_4(CH_3)CH_2$, consisting of xylene minus a hydrocarbon atom.

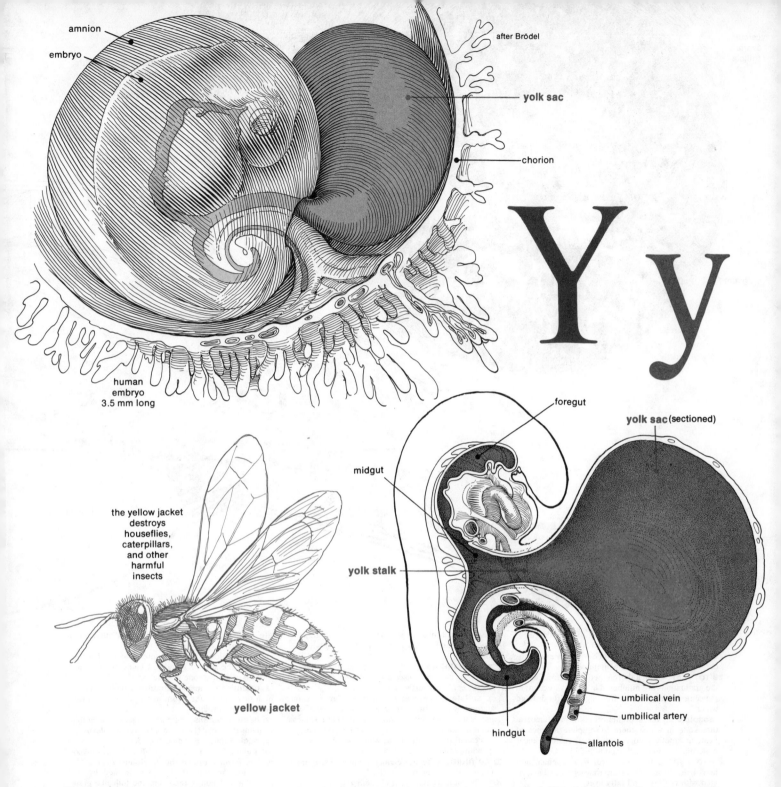

amnion

embryo

after Brödel

yolk sac

chorion

Y y

human
embryo
3.5 mm long

the yellow jacket
destroys
houseflies,
caterpillars,
and other
harmful
insects

foregut

yolk sac (sectioned)

midgut

yolk stalk

yellow jacket

umbilical vein

umbilical artery

hindgut

allantois

Y. Symbol for the element yttrium.

yaw. One of the lesions of the eruption of yaws.

yawn. A usually involuntary gaping of the mouth accompanied by a deep inspiration.

yaws. An infectious skin disease of tropical regions, marked by papular eruptions on the face, hands, and feet, and around the external genitals; caused by a spirochete, *Treponema pertenue*; also called frambesia, tropica, piǎn, and bouba.

Yb. Chemical symbol of the element ytterbium.

Y-chro′mosome. One of the sex chromosomes carried by the male in a single dose, i.e., one Y and one X.

yeast. 1. Any of several fungi of the genus *Saccharomyces* capable of fermenting carbohydrates. **2.** A commercial preparation, in either dry or moist form, used as a leavening agent or as a dietary supplement.

yel′low. 1. The hue of the spectrum between green and orange; evoked in the normal observer by radiant energy stimulation of wavelength approximately 580 nanometers. **2.** A dye or stain of this hue.

   brilliant y., an indicator dye that changes from yellow to orange or red at pH 6.4 to 8.0.

   visual y., all-*trans*-retinal; see retinal.

yellow jack. 1. A yellow flag on a ship or boat warning of disease on board. **2.** Yellow fever.

yellow jacket. Any of various small wasps of the family Vespidae, having yellow and black markings and usually constructing round, paper-like nests in the ground under logs or rocks; next to the honeybee, it is the most common stinging insect; also called yellow hornet.

-yl. In chemistry, a suffix used to designate a radical, especially a univalent hydrocarbon radical.

-ylene. In chemistry, a suffix used to designate a bivalent hydrocarbon radical.

yo′gurt, yo′ghurt. Curdled milk produced by the action of a ferment containing a lactic acid bacillus.

yolk. 1. The nutrient portion of an ovum, especially the yellow mass of the egg of a bird or a reptile. **2.** The fatty substance present in the unprocessed wool of sheep which, when purified, becomes lanolin.

yolk-sac. The highly vascular umbilical vesicle enveloping the nutritive yolk of an embryo; also called vitelline sac.

yolk-stalk. Omphalomesenteric duct; the narrowed passage between the intraembryonic gut and the yolk-sac.

ytter′bium. A bright silvery rare-earth element that has the ability to vary its valence in different environments; symbol Yb, atomic number 70, atomic weight 173.04.

yt′trium. A silvery metallic element; symbol Y, atomic number 39, atomic weight 88.90; always occurs with the rare earth minerals.

yt′trium-90 (⁹⁰Y). A radioactive isotope of yttrium (radioyttrium); has been used in the treatment of breast and prostatic cancer.

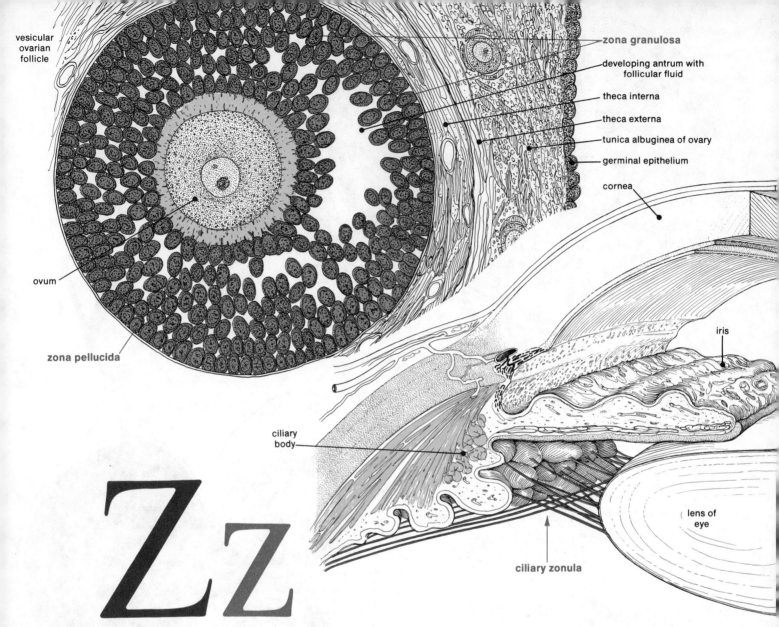

vesicular ovarian follicle

zona granulosa

developing antrum with follicular fluid

theca interna

theca externa

tunica albuginea of ovary

germinal epithelium

cornea

ovum

zona pellucida

iris

ciliary body

lens of eye

ciliary zonula

Zz

Z. Symbol for (a) atomic number; (b) impedance.

z. Abbreviation for (a) zero; (b) zone.

Zeitgeber. In biorhythmic behavior, an exact synchrony with any environmental cue.

ze′ro. The point on a thermometer scale from which the graduations are numbered in either direction; in the centigrade scale, the freezing point for distilled water.

absolute z., the hypothetical point in a temperature scale in which there is complete absence of heat; in kinetic theory, absence of relative linear molecular motion, reckoned as −273.2°C.

Zieve syndrome. Jaundice, hyperlipemia, and hemolytic anemia, occurring transiently and associated with cirrhosis and fatty liver.

zinc. A malleable and ductile metallic element; symbol Zn, atomic number 30, atomic weight 65.38.

z. chloride, a water-soluble caustic powder, $ZnCl_2$; used locally to destroy tissues.

z. gelatin, see under gelatin.

z. oxide, a white powder, ZnO, insoluble in water; a mild astringent and antiseptic incorporated in ointments, lotions, and dusting powders; used to prevent sunburn and to treat skin disorders (eczema, ringworm, psoriasis, varicose ulcers, and ivy poisoning); the main ingredient of calamine lotion.

z. oxide and eugenol (ZOE), compound used widely as a base material beneath tooth restorations, a temporary filling, an impression paste, and root canal filling; also used as a hardening agent for demineralized dentin.

z. permanganate, dark brown, water-soluble crystals, used in solution as a germicide.

z. peroxide (ZPO), a yellowish powder, ZnO_2, insoluble in water; used as a wash for oral infections

(suspended in four parts of water) and to disinfect, deodorize, and promote healing of wound infections.

z. stearate, white, greasy granules, insoluble in water; an antiseptic used as a dusting powder to protect epithelial surfaces and wounds.

z. sulfate, white, water-soluble powder, used in solution as an eyewash to treat mild eye irritations and as a lotion (white lotion) to treat skin diseases and infections (acne, impetigo, and ivy poisoning); also called salt of vitriol and white vitriol.

z. white, zinc oxide.

zirco′nium. A metallic element, symbol Zr, atomic number 40, atomic weight 91.22.

Zn. Chemical symbol of the element zinc.

zo-. See z-.

ZOE. Abbreviation for zinc oxide and eugenol; see under zinc.

zoet′ic. Relating to life.

Zollinger-Ellison syndrome (Z-E syndrome). Syndrome caused by a gastrin-secreting tumor of the pancreas, producing a high concentration of hydrochloric acid in the stomach; ulcers are formed in the esophagus and upper intestinal tract; symptoms include malabsorption, diarrhea, pain, and nausea; often associated with other endocrine abnormalities, especially hyperparathyroidism.

zo′na. 1. A zone, especially an encircling region distinguished from adjacent parts by some distinctive feature. **2.** Herpes zoster.

z. adherens, see zonula adherens.

z. fasciculata, the intermediate layer of radially arranged cell cords in the cortex of the adrenal gland, between the zona glomerulosa and zona reticularis; together with the zona reticularis, it is the

site of formation of adrenal steroids other than aldosterone.

z. glomerulosa, the thin outermost layer of the cortex of the adrenal gland just below the capsule; the site of aldosterone production.

z. granulosa, a mass of stratified cuboidal epithelium surrounding the ovum within a vesicular ovarian (graafian) follicle.

z. hemorrhoidalis, the part of the anal canal that contains the rectal (hemorrhoidal) venous plexus.

z. occludens, see zonula occludens.

z. pellucida, a refractile, gel-like neutral glycoprotein formed around the developing ovum; it is about four microns thick and is formed by the mutual interaction of the ovum and follicular granulosa cells; it degenerates and disappears just prior to implantation to the endometrium.

z. reticularis, the inner layer of the cortex of the adrenal gland where the cell cords form an irregular network; together with the zona fasciculata, the site of production of adrenal steroids other than aldosterone.

z. spongiosa, (1) horizontal strata; see under stratum; (2) older term for the most posterior layer of the dorsal horn of the spinal cord, now known as Rexed's lamina I.

z. vasculosa of Waldeyer, the highly vascular stroma in the center of the ovary; also called medullary substance.

zonesthe′sia. A constricting sensation, as by a girdle.

zon′ula. A small zone, usually a circular one.

ciliary z., z. of Zinn, the suspensory apparatus of the crystalline lens consisting of numerous delicate fibers that originate in the ciliary body and attach to

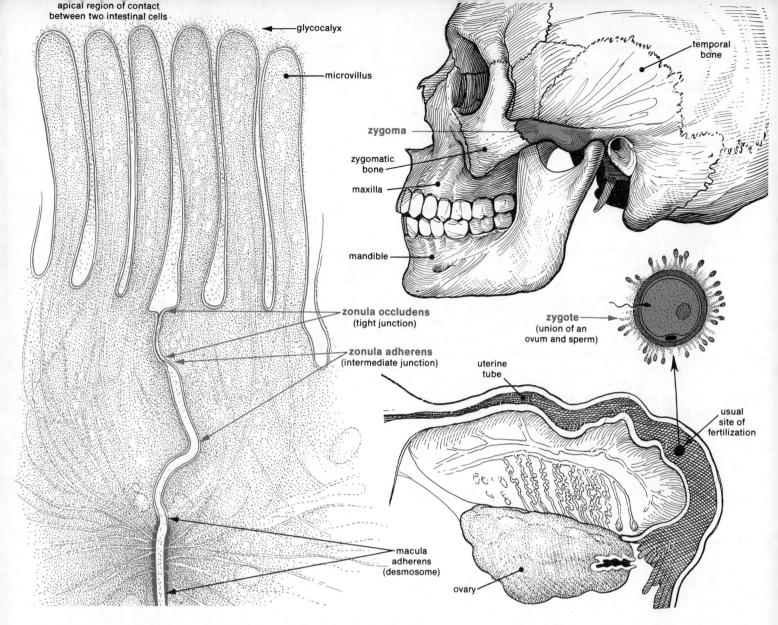

apical region of contact between two intestinal cells

glycocalyx

microvillus

zonula occludens (tight junction)

zonula adherens (intermediate junction)

macula adherens (desmosome)

temporal bone

zygoma

zygomatic bone

maxilla

mandible

zygote (union of an ovum and sperm)

uterine tube

usual site of fertilization

ovary

---

the anterior and posterior surface of the capsule of the crystalline lens; as the ciliary muscle contracts, the tension of the fibers vary, thus determining the degree of convexity of the lens.

z. adherens, that part of the junctional complex of epithelial cells where the adjacent cells have a narrow (~200 Å) space between apposing membranes; also called zona adherens.

z. occludens, that part of the junctional complex of epithelial cells where adjacent cell membranes are fused, with obliteration of the intercellular space; also called zona occludens.

z. of Zinn, see ciliary z.

zo′nular. Relating to a zonula.

zonuloly′sis. Dissolving of the ciliary zonule by an enzyme, such as chymotrypsin, to facilitate removal of the lens in some cases of cataract extraction.

zoo-, zo-. Combining forms denoting a relationship to an animal or animal life.

zooanthropono′sis. A disease of vertebrates that can be naturally acquired from humans when they are the maintenance host; e.g., human tuberculosis. Cf anthropozoonosis and amphixenosis.

zoochem′istry. The chemistry of animal tissues.

zoogen′ic, zoogenet′ic. Caused by animals.

zoog′onous. Viviparous; giving birth to living animals which derive nutrition directly from the maternal organism.

zo′oid. 1. An animal cell capable of independent movement within a living organism; e.g., spermatozoon and ovum. **2.** Resembling an animal.

zool′ogist. One who specializes in zoology.

zool′ogy. The branch of biology concerned with the study of animals.

zoono′sis. Any disease acquired from animals or

shared by man and other vertebrates.

zoopar′asite. An animal parasite.

zo′ophilic. Denoting a preference for animals.

zoopho′bia. Abnormal fear of animals.

zo′ospore. A motile, flagellated, asexual spore, as of certain fungi; also called swarm spore.

zootox′in. A substance found in snake venom and the secretions of certain insects.

zos′ter. An encircling belt or pattern; a girdle.

herpes z., see under herpes.

zos′teroid. Resembling herpes zoster.

ZPG. Abbreviation for zero population growth.

Z-plas′ty. A technique for repairing contracted scar tissue.

Zr. Chemical symbol of the element zirconium.

zwit′terion. Dipolar ion; an ion that possesses both negative and positive charges.

zygo-, zyg-. Combining forms denoting a yoke, especially joining together in the manner of a yoke.

zygodac′tyly. Fusion of the skin and connective tissue between fingers or toes without fusion of bones.

zygo′ma. 1. The zygomatic process of the temporal bone. **2.** The zygomatic arch. **3.** Term sometimes applied to the zygomatic bone (cheekbone).

zygomat′ic. Relating to the zygoma.

Zygomyce′tes. A class of fungi that reproduce by the union of gametes of equal size.

zygo′sis. Fusion of two unicellular organisms, including exchange of nuclear material.

zygos′ity. The condition of being developed from one or more eggs; said of multiple births.

zy′gote. The single fertilized cell formed by the union of two gametes.

zy′gotene. In meiosis, the second stage of pro-

phase in which the homologous chromosomes approach each other and begin to pair.

-zygous. Combining form denoting a zygotic constitution; e.g., heterozygous.

zy′mase. Obsolete term for enzyme.

-zyme. Combining form denoting an enzyme; e.g., lysozyme.

zymo-, zym-. Combining forms denoting a relationship to fermentation or to enzymes; e.g., zymolysis and zymophore.

zy′mogen. See proenzyme.

zymogen′esis. The formation of an active enzyme from a proenzyme (inactive precursor).

zymogen′ic, zymogen′ous. 1. Pertaining to a proenzyme or to zymogenesis. **2.** Producing a fermentation.

zy′moid. Resembling an enzyme.

zymol′ogy. Enzymology.

zymol′ysis. Chemical process or fermentation brought about by means of an enzyme.

zymolyt′ic. Fermentative.

zy′mophore. The active portion of an enzyme molecule.

zymoplas′tic. Participating in the formation of enzymes.

zy′mosan. An insoluble anticomplementary factor derived from the walls of yeast cells and used in the assay of the protein properdin; composed of lipids, polysaccharides, proteins, and ash of variable concentrations.

zy′mose. Invertase.

zymo′sis. 1. Fermentation. **2.** The development of infectious diseases.

zymot′ic. 1. Relating to or caused by fermentation. **2.** Denoting any infectious disease.

zonula | **zymotic**

ILLUSTRATION CREDITS

The authors acknowledge the following publications as sources from which the listed original illustrations for this dictionary were derived by permission.

American Family Physician, American Academy of Family Physicians, Kansas City, Mo.
Adrenal glands, ampulla, anesthesia, antibody, bone cement, table of bones (lunate), constrictor muscles of pharynx, descensus testes, dialysis, diverticulum, dog tick, ductus arteriosus, fetal membranes, flexion, glaucoma, hookworms, hymenopterans, Jackson-Pratt drain (interstitial and ventricular), omphalo-mesenteric cyst, ovary, pancreas, pleura, proglottid, prostatic massage, pyemotic ventricosus, rheumatoid arthritis, spur, strain, and tooth designation.

Bellanti, J. A.: *Immunology* (II), ed. 2, W.B. Saunders Co., Philadelphia, 1978.
Afferent, hilus, and lymph node.

Dorland's Illustrated Medical Dictionary, ed. 25, W.B. Saunders Co., Philadelphia. 1974.
Auricle.

Grollman, S.: *The Human Body: Its Structure and Physiology*, ed. 3, MacMillan Publishing Co., Inc., New York, 1974.

Nerve (vestibular and cochlear), osseous labyrinth, pathway, and retina.

Kruger, G. O.: *Textbook of Oral Surgery*, ed. 4, The C. V. Mosby Co., St. Louis. 1974.
Alveolectomy and impaction.

Langley, L., Telford, I., Christian, J.: *Dynamic Anatomy and Physiology*, ed. 4, McGraw-Hill Book Co., New York, 1974.
Acromion, aperature of sinus (sphenoid and maxillary), table of bones (femur and sphenoid), calvaria, chamber, ciliary body, ethmoidal infundibulum, navicular bone, optic axis, sacrum, vertebral arch, and vertebral body.

Melloni, B. J., Stone, P. Y., Hurd, J. A.: *Anatomy and Physiology* (I and III), McGraw-Hill Book Co., New York, 1971.
Air cells, basion, table of bones (ethmoid), canaliculus, cephalic index, cochlear duct, concha, conjunctiva, crista ampullaris, lacrimal gland, lacrimal sac, mastoid, nasal septum, opisthion, orbit, ossicles, scala, spinal ganglia of cochlea, and visual pathways.

Smith, D. R.: *General Urology*, ed. 9, Lange Medical Publishers, Los Altos (in press).
Benign.

NOTES

NOTES

NOTES

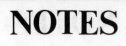

NOTES

NOTES

NOTES